History of the
Royal College of Physicians
of Edinburgh

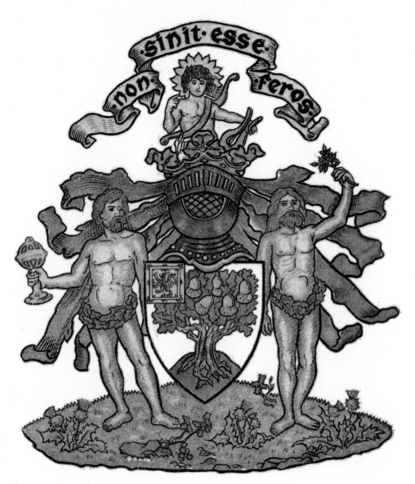

Coat of Arms of the Royal College of Physicians of Edinburgh

History of the
Royal College of Physicians
of Edinburgh

W. S. Craig
BSC MD FRSE FRCP(ED)

BLACKWELL SCIENTIFIC PUBLICATIONS
OXFORD LONDON EDINBURGH MELBOURNE

© 1976 Blackwell Scientific Publications
Osney Mead, Oxford OX2 0EL
8 John Street, London WC1N 2ES
9 Forrest Road, Edinburgh EH1 2QH
P.O. Box 9, North Balwyn, Victoria 3104, Australia

British Library Cataloguing in Publication data
Craig, William Stuart
   History of the Royal College of Physicians
     of Edinburgh.
   Bibl.—Index.
   ISBN 0-632-00088-0
   1. Title
   610'.6'24134 R35
   Royal College of Physicians of Edinburgh—
     History

Distributed in the United States of America by
J. B. Lippincott Company, Philadelphia
and in Canada by
J. B. Lippincott, Company Ltd., Toronto

Printed in Great Britain by
T. & A. Constable Ltd.

CONTENTS

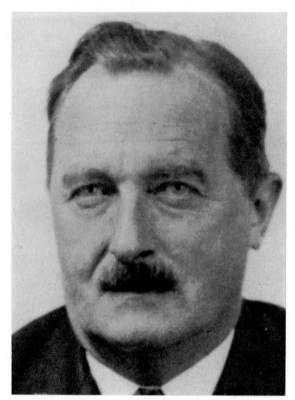

Professor W. S. Craig (1903–1975)

FOREWORD

This foreword had already been written in draft and the proofs of the History had begun to come off the press when we were deeply shocked by the sudden death of Professor Stuart Craig just when his formidable undertaking was all but complete. It was some years ago that the approach of the Tercentenary of the College stimulated the then President, Dr Christopher Clayson, and his Council to commission a History of the College, fuller and more comprehensive than the previous brief and now out-of-date work. Professor Craig undertook his challenging task with great energy, untiring industry and remarkable speed, so that it has been completed well ahead of our Tercentenary date but will be published to coincide with another major Edinburgh celebration in which the College is clearly concerned, the 250th Anniversary of the foundation of the Faculty of Medicine of Edinburgh University. The book will be a splendid memorial to a fine physician and a devoted Fellow of the College.

The College is most grateful to Sir Derrick Dunlop, who has taken a close interest in the book throughout, for agreeing, after Professor Craig's death, to see it through the Press.

The older medical Royal Colleges of Great Britain and Ireland were originally unique to these islands. Their example later stimulated the formation in the United Kingdom of other Royal Colleges concerned with newer disciplines. Abroad, several English-speaking countries founded Colleges similar to our own, but such institutions do not exist elsewhere in Europe.

Taking its original inspiration in medical education and standards from the University of Leyden in the Netherlands, the Royal College of Physicians of Edinburgh, after several attempts over a number of years, was finally founded in 1681. In its earlier period it was chiefly concerned with the establishment of standards of practice and later with undergraduate education, but later still, it became, like its sister Colleges, increasingly occupied with postgraduate education and the standards and quality of medical care. The examination for the Membership of the College became a hallmark of quality for those undergoing training for specialist practice in Medicine. The high reputation of that examination, and of postgraduate training in Edinburgh, attracted candidates from all over the world. At the time of writing, we have some 2000 Fellows and 2400 Members in 60 different countries, beside 4100 holders of the M.R.C.P.(U.K.) who since 1969 are jointly Members of this College, of the Royal College of Physicians and Surgeons of Glasgow and of the Royal College of Physicians of London.

An important feature of the Royal Colleges is their independence from Government control. Their concern with quality and standards, and the fact that most of the leading members of the medical profession are Fellows of one or another, give the Colleges a unique prestige. This prestige leads to their advice being sought by Governments and allows them to proffer unsought advice in the knowledge that it will receive close attention.

The evolution of the College, and the development of its high standing in the national and international community, is fascinatingly outlined in Professor Craig's pages. He sought to put the College, at all periods, into its historical context, clarifying both the influence of contemporary society on the College and of the College on society. As in all institutions there were great men, good men and some, in spite of Lord Acton, who were both great and good. Also, of course, there were many very ordinary men, sometimes doing their best, sometimes squabbling, but always being fascinatingly and delightfully human. In this book Professor Craig has captured the good, the bad and the indifferent for the arbitrament of posterity.

If a civilized society is one which has the collective moral imagination to feel a sense of responsibility for its afflicted members, this College has a proud record of concern. Through its efforts and those of its Fellows, it has played a leading part in the foundation of hospitals, Trusts and many other organizations for the service of the sick. One should mention in particular the Royal Infirmary of Edinburgh in 1736 and the Royal Edinburgh Asylum in 1807. Academically, besides its own activities, it was one of the initiating bodies in the foundation of the Faculty of Medicine of the University of Edinburgh, a Faculty which, as already mentioned, celebrates its 250th Anniversary in the year this History is published. The College was also closely concerned in the foundation and evolution of the National Health Service and has been constantly active in its improvement.

Throughout its existence the College has often worked closely with other bodies for common ends. It is worth recalling, in these days when it is the fashion for problems of pollution to receive very proper attention, that in its early days the College co-operated with the City administration in dealing with pollution in the Nor' Loch; both bodies were later concerned with the appointment of the first Medical Officer of Health in Scotland. Although in the past our College was from time to time at odds with its fellow Colleges, recent years have shown closer and closer co-operation in their work for the public weal. The intangible sense of community and friendship which has characterized our own College has been increasingly extended to Fellows and Members of our sister institutions at home and overseas.

Ancient and well-established institutions are notoriously prone to malignant infiltration by the cancer of complacency. This is why we must welcome criticism and controversy. Only the cut and thrust of argument will keep us alert and creative. Nevertheless, after some 300 years, we are, I think, entitled to look back with well-founded pride on the achievements of three centuries. We can be equally proud of the wit and scholarship with which Professor Craig has chronicled them.

Finally we must thank Mr Per Saugman of Blackwell Scientific Publications for the enthusiasm and generosity with which he agreed to publish this book on a non-profit-making basis and the Carnegie Trust for helpful financial support.

JOHN CROFTON
President

PREFACE

*There is nothing that more divides civilised from semi-savage men than to be conscious of
our forefathers as they really were.*

G. M. Trevelyan

The Royal College of Physicians is an integral part of the life of Scotland and of
Edinburgh medicine. Its history cannot be considered in isolation. Throughout an
existence of almost three centuries the College has been subject to the influences of
national and civic trends to which it has itself often contributed. This is exemplified
by a study of the social, economic, political and legal histories of the country.

At its inception the College encountered obstruction from the surgeons, the
Universities and the Church. Timely aid was forthcoming from King James VI and
later King Charles II. For a long period, mutual hostility characterized relationships
between physicians and surgeons. Relative status was at stake. The apothecaries, to
some extent, were not unwilling pawns in the pursuit of worldly precedence: one
outcome, aided in no small measure by the College, was the evolution of the
nineteenth-century general practitioner. Concerted efforts at reform in that century eventually brought about rational order in place of professional chaos, and
encouraged better understanding between rival Licensing Authorities north and
south of Tweed. Later the probings of the University Commissioners gave rise to
acute but happily temporary conflict between the medical Corporations and the
Universities.

The College was directly involved in these medical and medico-political events,
and often with good reason sought to protect Scottish interests from dominance
by policies emanating from a remote Whitehall. At times patriotic fervour betrayed excessive national sensitivity and, when Scottish inter-city disagreements
intervened, parochial patriotism was liable to assume an aggressive form. These
reactions were typical of the political climate in which our forebears lived. The same
is true of the vindictive and often scurrilous pamphlets indulged in by professional
men—the more extraordinary in that they contrasted markedly with the formal and
obsequious courtesy of contemporary memorials and reports.

Basically, to quote Trevelyan, 'politics are the outcome rather than the causes of
social change'. This is very evident in the history of the College. Nor is it surprising

when account is taken of the sweeping social changes which have happened in Scotland since 1681. These have been related to the recurrent periods of devastating destitution and attendant epidemics; the procrastination in introducing the economic benefits of the Treaty of Union; industrialization coupled with the arrival of Irish immigrants in large numbers; the introduction of compulsory education; and within recent times, the creation of a vast framework of social legislation culminating in the growth of a Welfare State of which the National Health Service and the conception of Community Medicine are now entrenched components.

In 1681, the newly incorporated College had as one of its main objects the establishment in Scotland of professional standards comparable with those obtaining in Holland and Paris. Today the College remains dedicated to further advancement of medical science and is concerned to promote the interests of patients, the responsibility of the National Health Service. Continuous adjustment and adaptation have proved necessary over the years, due in large measure to social changes and also, within recent decades, to the increasingly scientific content of medicine.

Economics enter largely into political, social and medical history. Inevitably they have had a profound influence on the activities of the College. In an age when administrators and those nebulously referred to as 'planners' exert disproportionate influence in the execution of political policies, the College is confident of the strength it derives from preservation of financial and political independence. The gratifying response to the Public Appeal in 1972 was evidence of the extent to which this confidence is shared by others.

At a recent informal gathering outside the College, the altogether surprising view was expressed that in the past Edinburgh medicine had lacked initiative. As already stated, the College is an integral part of Edinburgh medicine and there can be no denying that its accomplishments give the direct lie to such an irresponsible generalization. The origin of the College was itself solely attributable to visionary initiative. Many of its Fellows have since been recognized internationally as pioneers in clinical medicine. There are, however, aspects of medicine other than the purely clinical. The College was in the vanguard among those making provision for the poor and necessitous; advocating hospitals for the care of the physically and mentally ailing; urging, contrary to the tenets of the redoubtable Divine, the Reverend Dr Chalmers, humanization of measures for relief under the Poor Law; condemning the notoriously insanitary conditions prevailing in Edinburgh, and focussing attention on the plight of those in the Highlands and Islands. More than a hundred years ago one of our most eminent Presidents was expressing concern at the atmospheric pollution resulting from industrial processes, and towards the end of last century the

College, in a corporate capacity, successfully memorialized Parliament with a view to the appointment of a Royal Commission on Venereal Diseases. While the First World War was at its height the College was engrossed in measures for the rehabilitation of disabled ex-servicemen and, much more recently, has conducted research into the problems of the aged and made constructive recommendations in connection with their needs.

Invaluable research and extensive routine services were features in times of peace and war of the work of the College Laboratory during the sixty-three years of its existence. Restricted by the terms of its original Charter in the sphere of medical education, the College was not deterred from giving weighty support to the School of Medicine of the Royal Colleges of Edinburgh (1895–1948); and has taken an active and notably effective part in the deliberations of the Edinburgh Post-Graduate Board for Medicine. Nor is it out of place to go further back in history and recall the generally acknowledged important part played by the College in fostering the creation of a Faculty of Medicine in the University of Edinburgh in 1726. In these and other ways the College can justly claim to have made worthy contributions to the education of undergraduate and postgraduate students of medicine. Moreover, at different times, this influence has extended in varying degrees to the continents of America, Asia, Australasia and Africa.

In a unique way the Library bears testimony to the initiative and continuity typifying College progress throughout the centuries. The beginnings consisted of a gift of books from Sir Robert Sibbald in 1682. Today it constitutes a most precious heritage, is surpassingly rich in both ancient and modern literature and is accepted as being one of the finest medical libraries in the country.

This History aims at presenting these and other accomplishments in perspective. References to Members and Fellows are numerous but deliberately they are in no sense biographical. It is hoped that readers will be conscious of the true, vital spirit of Fellowship underlying corporate Collegiate activities. Fellows, it is felt, would wish to be remembered less as individuals than as active contributors to that Fellowship. No corporate gathering can expect to escape periods of dissension. Our College has been no exception. No attempt has been made to conceal the parts played by those inclined to be 'contumacious' but they occupy only a small portion of the canvas depicting 'our forefathers as they really were'.

Mindful of the many Members and Fellows overseas who knew the late Sir James Cameron and of his concern for their interests, it is not inappropriate to give the following excerpt concerning him from the College Minutes of 6th May 1969:

'Only two days before he died he was discussing what the College should do about
its tercentenary in twelve years' time—an event he well knew he would not see.
His idea was that the College should mark the event by re-writing or at least
bringing up-to-date the History of the College.'

To have been entrusted with the task has been a very great privilege and a source
of humble pride for one who has for long harboured a deep and enduring affection
for the College.

W. S. CRAIG

Mellendean,
Gifford, 1975.

ACKNOWLEDGMENTS

So many Members and Fellows have responded to verbal and written requests for information that anything approaching adequate acknowldgement is out of the question. It is hoped that they will understand and feel none the less, that their generous co-operation has been used to good purpose and with discretion. Suffice it to say that of over 150 of our Diplomates in over seventeen countries, who were written to, only one failed to respond.

The same is true for Fellows of sister Colleges: the late Mr Norman Dott, Mr A. B. Wallace and Sir John Bruce; Sir Donald Douglas, Mr Tom Hamilton, Sir Charles Illingworth, Mr J. A. Ross, and Sir Michael Woodruff of the Royal College of Surgeons of Edinburgh; Dr E. C. Fahmy (a Fellow of our College) and Dr John Sturrock of the Royal College of Obstetricians and Gynaecologists; the late Sir Charles Harris, and Lord Amulree, Professor Elaine Field, Dr Neville M. Goodman, C.B., and Dr C. E. Van Rooyen of the Royal College of Physicians of London. Of these a number were friends of long standing. The same applies to Professors J. H. de Haas and H. A. Snellen of the Netherlands; and to Dr Thos. E. Cone, jun. of Boston, Massachusetts who spared no effort in dealing with many enquiries.

Great assistance was obtained from members of professions other than medicine including the Very Reverend A. C. Craig, M.C., D.D., the Reverend A. I. Dunlop, B.D. and the Reverend R. Murray, B.D. Facts concerning 'resurrectionists' in Crail were provided by the Reverend A. J. Moncrieff, B.D. Other help was obtained from Professor I. M. Campbell of Edinburgh University and Emeritus Professor Gillies of Leeds University. Together Professor John Craig, F.R.C.P. and Mr A. A. Cormack, D.Litt. of Aberdeen made it possible to trace a great grandson (F. A. G. Poole, Esq.) of Richard Poole (F.R.C.P. 1825); and chance observation of a paragraph in the Press led to an approach to Lady Patricia Fisher, M.P., a great grand-daughter of Samuel Smiles, M.D. Mr Poole and Lady Fisher were most helpful in giving information about their distinguished ancestors. Similar help was forthcoming about two past Presidents from near neighbours—Mrs M. E. Stevens, a third generation descendant of Sir Robert Christison (1838 and 1846), and M. E. Beilby, Esq. a great grandson of William Beilby (1844). Miss M. Maclagan very kindly volunteered information concerning the photograph of her forebears (illustration between pp. 960 and 961).

Valuable assistance was obtained in acquiring information and photographs from the relatives of certain other Fellows: from the late Lady Cameron; Dr Robin (F.R.C.Path.) and Miss Barbara Harvey about Colonel W. F. Harvey and Mrs Lennox Hunter, Mrs Joyce Matthew and Colonel Hamish Mackay, D.S.O. about Colonel A. G. McKendrick. Further information concerning Fellows in the Indian Medical Service was supplied by a number of individuals, including Sir George McRobert, C.I.E., Lt. General Sir Neil Cantlie, K.C.B., K.B.E., M.C., Maj. Generals A. MacLennan, O.B.E. and A. Sachs, C.B., C.B.E.; Brigadier R. M. Vanreenen, Q.H.S. and Colonels H. W. Mulligan, C.M.G. and P. H. Addison. Points raised about personnel in the Royal Navy were kindly dealt with by Vice Admiral Sir R. D. Caldwell, K.B.E., C.B. and Rear Admiral Buckley, C.B., D.S.O. and Dr Hugh Maingay. Information about Sir Robert Philip was given by the late Dr Harley Williams, about Chalmers Hospital by the late Dr W. N. Boog Watson, and about Edinburgh Academy by Mr Magnus Magnusson, M.A.

Help in other fields was given by the Secretary of the Royal Society of Edinburgh (Mr W. H. Rutherford, F.C.I.S., F.R.S.E.); the Hon. Secretary of the Scottish Society of the History of Medicine (Dr H. P. Tait); the Clerk to the Heriot Trust (Mr D. Morris, B.L.); the Secretaries of the Dean Orphanage Trust (Mr K. M. Croft, LL.B., W.S.), the Longmore Hospital (Mr R. L. Dickson, B.L., F.H.A.); the Edinburgh Medical Missionary Society (Dr J. L. Tester, O.B.E.) and the Royal Scottish Corporation (Mr H. McLeod); the Archivist of the Edinburgh Royal Infirmary (Mrs P. M. Eaves-Walton, M.A.); Mr T. W. Hurst, J.P., F.H.A., F.C.I.S., formerly Secretary and Treasurer to the Royal Infirmary and now of 'ASH'; and Mr John A. Myers, B.Pharm., F.P.S., LL.B., D.P.A., A.C.I.S., Regional Pharmacist of the former S.E. Region Hospital Board.

Without exception Librarians responded generously to requests for help. They included those associated with the Royal College of Surgeons of Edinburgh (Miss D. U. Wardle, A.L.A.), the Royal College of Physicians of London (Mr L. M. Payne, M.B.E., F.L.A.), the College of Physicians of Philadelphia (Miss L. M. Holloway, Associate Curator, Historic Materials), the University of McGill (Miss M. Fransiszyn, Osler Library), the University of St Andrews (Mr R. N. Smart, M.A.), the University of Leyden, the National Library of Scotland, the Central Public Library, Edinburgh, and the Royal Medical Society. Mr Leonard J. Jolley, M.A., F.L.A., now in Australia, and Professor G. R. Pendrill, M.A., Dip.Lib., F.L.A., now in Canada, both former Librarians of the College, gave valuable help. Further assistance was obtained from the Scottish Record Office and the Office of the Lord Lyon King of Arms.

Throughout, unstinted help was received from successive Presidents, Members of

Council and other Officers of the College not forgetting the Clerk (Mr Alexander Macfie, W.S.). The Treasurer (Dr William Macleod) belied his official designation by his consistently generous understanding, and the Honorary Librarian (Dr Chalmers Davidson) gave freely of his bibliographical knowledge. A special debt of gratitude is owed to my officially appointed mentors: Sir Derrick Dunlop, Dr Ronald F. Robertson and Dr Alex. J. Keay. The two last-named will not begrudge it being said that Sir Derrick in particular was a fount of sage advice, graciously dispelling doubts and curbing excessive exuberance!

Happily, shameless importuning fostered no overt enmities: certainly new friendships have been made and many old ones revived.

As to the staff of the College Library—they could not have constituted a more enthusiastic team. The Librarian, Miss Joan Ferguson, M.A., A.L.A., never flinched whether dealing with a barrage of disconnected questions, searching for long-forgotten manuscripts in dust-laden basements and windswept attics, or reading proofs in the 'wee sma' 'oors'. Her assistants, Miss E. J. Eaglesham, M.A., A.L.A. and Mrs S. G. Le Touze, B.A., Dip.Lib., were proficiency personified as they relentlessly pin-pointed inaccuracies and wayward references. Miss D. McKay's industry vied with that of her colleagues. Her skill in deciphering atrocious scripts coupled with her ability to induce metal fatigue in a modern typewriter were beyond praise. Nor can the contributions of Miss M. C. Oliver and Miss C. M. Lownie of the Administrative Staff go unacknowledged. Despite thinly disguised apprehension they never failed to produce loose 'Minutes-awaiting-binding' with a hint of patronage in a way reminiscent of Whitehall administrators when dealing with their professional counterparts!

A special debt of gratitude is owed to the publishers in the persons of Mr Per Saugman (Managing Director) and Mr Nigel Palmer (Edinburgh domiciled Director) who were unremitting in their enthusiastic support of the project, and ever ready with advice on technical aspects.

No acknowledgments would be complete without loving tribute being paid to my wife for her toleration, encouragement and practical assistance sustained over the years from first word to last.

Errors of omission and commission will inevitably reveal themselves. Responsibility rests solely with the author.

Illustrations
Captions to illustrations indicate the sources of material. Grateful thanks are extended to the various individuals, publishers and institutions (at home and abroad) who so

readily agreed to use of the material; Mr Scott for photographs and photographic reproductions of highest standards; and Her Majesty's Stationery Office for permission to extract sections of official Reports. The Rev. Alec. Shillinglaw, B.D., himself an international cricketer of no mean prowess, was instrumental in obtaining the photograph of W. G. Grace.

LIST OF ILLUSTRATIONS

Chapter I

THE BACKGROUND:
HISTORICAL AND SOCIAL

. . . Superficial it must be, but I do not disown the charge. Better a superficial book, which brings well and strikingly together the known and acknowledged facts, than a dull boring narrative, pausing to see further into a mill-stone at every moment than the nature of the mill-stone admits. Nothing is so tiresome as walking through some beautiful scene with a minute philosopher, a botanist or pebble-gatherer, who is eternally calling your attention from the grand features of the natural scenery to look at grasses and chucky-stones. Yet, in their way, they give useful information; and so does the minute historian . . .

. . . Gad, I think that will look well in the preface. My bile is quite gone. I really believe it arose from mere anxiety. What a wonderful connection between the mind and body . . .

Sir Walter Scott (1771–1832) (entered in his *Journal* before commencing to write the *Life of Napoleon*)

The Royal College of Physicians of Edinburgh was granted its Charter in 1681, the 'great seal' being appended on St Andrew's Day of that year. It is not sufficiently realized that the idea of such a College had been conceived more than sixty years before. For this all credit is due to a small group of physicians with knowledge of the practice and teaching of medicine on the Continent. Unlike their surgical counterparts they had no status in the form of a town tradesman's or craftsman's guild. Their proposals met with obdurate opposition from the surgeons, the Church and the Universities. The influence of these and other interests did not cease with the successful erection of the College. Indeed throughout its development and to the present day the activities of the College have been inseparable from the changing outlook and changing emphases in national and civic affairs. An inevitable consequence is that the History of our College cannot be considered in isolation. To do so would be to ignore Scott's 'grand features of the natural scenery' of which the College has been an integral part for some three hundred years.

B

In this context it is appropriate to mention that it has been said of Sir Robert Sibbald, the arch-protagonist of our College, that 'Sibbald, like the Gregories, the lawyers Stair and Mackenzie and the architect Bruce who lived in the same period, was one of the fathers of the Scottish enlightenment of the post-Union age'. In the self-same passage the statement is made that the Royal College of Physicians 'was the first small germ of Scotland's later reputation for great medical education'.[1]

THE NATION AS A WHOLE

No nation in Europe can look with a more just pride on their past than the Scots, and no young Scotsman ought to grow up ignorant of what that past has been.

James Anthony Froude

You come of a race of men the very wind of whose name has swept to the ultimate seas.

Sir J. M. Barrie (Rectorial Address, University of St Andrews)

Every Scottishman has a pedigree. It is a national prerogative as unalienable as his pride and his poverty.

Sir Walter Scott

Religious and political strife were characteristic of the national life in Scotland throughout the sixteenth and seventeenth centuries. The period covered the reigns of Mary Stuart, James VI (I of England), Charles I and Charles II; the duration of the Protectorate; and the years of kingship of James VII (II of England) followed by the revolution leading to acceptance of the Crown by William of Orange.

During Mary Stuart's reign a struggle persisted between the nobility and the Crown and although civil war broke out on occasions, it was not widespread and interference with the life of the community at large was limited. In subsequent reigns, as the power of the nobility in relation to the Crown declined, an increasing influence on national affairs was exerted by merchants in the towns and small land-owners in the country. Fear of domination by France, coinciding with a growth of opinion favouring Protestantism under the dominating influence of John Knox contributed ultimately to the Religious Reformation. Thus there was established the nation's adherence to Protestant principles based upon the simplicity of the original gospel. This was no sudden achievement, and the reign of James VI was associated with a protracted struggle between the conception of Presbytery on the one hand, and Episcopacy with its implied creation of bishops on the other.

It is interesting to note that James VI took with him to England his Scottish physician, John Craig, a graduate of Basel. Craig's admission as a Fellow of the London College of Physicians did not take place without doubts being expressed about his foreign origin: and was probably furthered by deference to the wishes of the King who intimated that ' "Wee purpose" to naturalize Craig "out of hand"; but "things are now between the two nations in such termes, as no man of judgment can accompt them two, but one" '.(2)

Some ten years after James VI took up residence in the south, members of the enlarging Scottish community in London formed a society named 'The Scots Box' intended to assist the less successful among their number. This society was the forerunner of the Royal Scottish Corporation of today which was granted its first Charter in 1665. Among its activities were succouring victims of the Plague and burying those who died 'with as much decency as the publick calamity would permit'; and making special provisions at the time of the Great Fire. At the present time pensioners and disabled ex-service men rank high among those benefiting at the hands of the Corporation.(3)

The religious struggle continued after James VI of Scotland succeeded to the English throne in 1603 and was inherited as a legacy by Charles I. Nevertheless a new stimulus was experienced by trade in Scotland and a fillip given to education with the foundation by James VI in 1583 of the College of Edinburgh—or King James' College as it was sometimes called. At the same time as granting a Charter for the erection of a College, the King made available the lands and collegiate church of St Mary in the Fields (The Kirk o' Field).(4) The College was a Town College: the Town Council being vested with all the authority of patrons and governors, and with powers to elect and depose professorial staff. Sixteen years later (1599) the Crown granted a Charter establishing the Faculty of Physicians and Surgeons of Glasgow. Charged with the duty of drafting a Constitution for a new church, Protestant ministers delivered their historic *Book of Discipline* in 1561. In this book there were included proposals for providing for the necessitous poor and the establishment of a school in every parish. Effect was not given at the time to the latter proposal, and in 1616 an Act, which was not immediately effective, was passed requiring that provision of schools be made.

Perhaps Scotland has never been ruled by a sovereign so out of touch with his people as Charles I. This was demonstrated by his obduracy in seeking to impose by divine right, measures completely antagonistic to the convictions of those who had willed the Reformation. The Covenant produced in Greyfriars Kirkyard in 1638, and the Solemn League and Covenant pronounced by the General Assembly in 1643 were direct results of the King's attitude. None the less the execution of a Scottish prince royal, in the person of Charles I, at the hands of the English was not generally acceptable. Under the Protectorate which followed, justice was more effectively and impartially administered, and peace and order more successfully maintained. Attempts by Cromwell to secure union between Scotland and England were however unsuccessful, largely because of lack of unanimity among religious sects. The restoration of the monarchy in 1660 with the crowning of Charles II was followed by a renewal of lay patronage in the appointment of ministers of religion, a procedure which had been abolished at the instance of the Covenanters immediately after the revolution of 1649.

TEST ACT

In July 1681 James, Duke of York, acting as Royal Commissioner, opened Parliament in Edinburgh and used the occasion to impose on Scotland a Test Act based on a similar English enactment of 1673. The Act applied to State officials, clergymen, judges and magistrates and any dangerous or suspected persons: and required acknowledgment of the King's supremacy in ecclesiastical and civil matters and a declaration that covenants and armed rebellion were unlawful.

Tradition has it that while in Edinburgh the Duke frequently played golf on Leith Links and he is credited with arranging the first match between Scotland and England.[5]

James, Duke of York, who had imposed the Test Act, became King (James VII of Scotland and II of England) in 1685. He was an avowed Roman Catholic and attempts to overthrow him were not long delayed. Indications were not lacking that his inclinations were for the re-introduction of his religion to Scotland, and his persecution of the Covenanters was intensified. The birth in 1688 of a Prince of Wales was a signal for alarm on the part of Scottish presbyterians and English episcopalians lest a catholic succession to the throne be established. Events moved rapidly. Known to be abroad, James VII was deposed. The Crown was offered to William of Orange and his reign saw the re-establishment of presbyterianism in Scotland but was marred by two events which fostered distrust in the Union of Parliament (1707) achieved in the time of his successor Queen Anne. The first of these was the treacherous massacre of Glencoe; and the second, the failure of the Darien Scheme, a failure contributed to by the attitude of English politicians and traders. Many were convinced that Union had involved surrender of Scottish nationality. Protests were many and varied, and disillusionment increased with the arrival of zealous tax officials from south of the border. Taxation gave an impetus to smuggling which was, in part, the root cause of the Porteous riot and other disturbances.

There were two ill-fated attempts—in 1715 and 1745—to restore the House of Stewart. Sir John Pringle, a Fellow of the College, successor to Sir Isaac Newton as President of the Royal Society and Physician General to His Majesty's Forces under Cumberland, devoted a chapter in his *Observations on the Diseases of the Army* to the campaigns of 1745 and 1746 which included the battle of Culloden.[6] It was not until some years after the collapse of the '45 Jacobite rising that the country began to enjoy increasing prosperity in so far as central Scotland and the Lowlands were concerned. Not so the Highlands. There a process of depopulation began which has continued to the present time. By way of contrast a great increase of population took place in the area between the Forth and Clyde where the metal industries expanded as the Industrial Revolution gained momentum. In the course of time the area came to be known as the 'industrial belt'. Nevertheless as Pryde points out, for many years after the Union 'to the Londoner, the Scot was not only poor, backward and rude: he was also a Jacobite, open or concealed. To the Scotsman, the "auld enemy" was rich and arrogant, cruel and heartless.'[7] On the same subject Cameron has written 'in spite of the surrender of independent political sovereignty, there still remained the acceptance of the idea that Highland or Lowland, Saxon or Gael, were and remained *Scotsmen*, subjects of an ancient kingdom whose unity . . . still commanded a deep seated if not always unbroken loyalty'.[8]

PERIODS OF DEARTH

As to the previous economy of the country as a whole, there is no gainsaying that Scotland was poor if not actually impoverished. Strangely, however, there was occasional conflict of opinions. Thus a continental physician of the name of Perlin, visiting Scotland in the middle of the sixteenth century, concluded that 'the country is but poor in gold and silver, but plentiful in provisions'.[9] Writing of the seventeenth century Pryde maintained that the dilemma facing Scottish economy 'became acute . . . though it is easy to overlook it amid the drama of religious conflict and civil strife'.[10] Allowing that commercial development at home, and trade with Ireland, Holland and more especially France underwent a measure of development in the reign of James VI, the fact remains that in Scotland there was much poverty. Of this there could be no more conclusive evidence than that contained in a report made in 1699 by Sir Robert Sibbald of our College. He wrote:

'God Almighty . . . requireth of us, a due Care for the Relief of the Poor; This is one of the Tributes we owe to Him, and he hath Dispersed the Poor amongst us, as his Substitutes and Receivers, to whom it is to be payed . . . This Charity to the Poor . . . is an Act of the greatest Policy and civil Prudence: For Poverty and Want Emasculate the Mindes of many, and make those who are of dull Natures, Stupid and Indisciplinable, and unfit for the Service of their Countrey: these that are of a firy and active Temperament, it maketh them unquiet, Rapacious, Frantick or Desperate. Thus, where there are many Poor, the Rich cannot be secure in the Possession of what they have . . . And such Considerations ought now to be la'id to Heart, when the Bad Seasons these several Years past, hath made so much Scarcity and so great a Dearth, that for Want, some Die by the Way-side, some drop down in the Streets, the poor sucking Babs are starving for want of Milk, which the empty Breasts of their Mothers cannot furnish them: Every one may see Death in the Face of the Poor, that abound everywhere; the Thinness of their Visage, their Ghostly Looks, their Febbleness, their Agues and their Fluxes threaten them with sudden Death, if Care be not taken of them. And it is not only common wandering Beggars, that are in the case; But many House-keepers, who lived well by their Labour and their Industrie, are now by Want, forced to abandon their Dwellings, and they and their little Ones must Beg; and in this their Necessity they take what they can get: Spoiled Victual; yea some eat these Beasts which have died of some Disease, which may occasion Plague amongst them.'[11]

The basic situation was aggravated by the periodic occurrence of epidemics and famine resulting from the failure of crops. Periods of dearth have been described as occurring 'with monotonous regularity' in the seventeenth and eighteenth centuries. The causes were varied. A major famine in 1698–9 followed seven lean years of harvest with many dependent on nettles for spring greens and upon wild herbs and mustard seed for sustenance. A particularly severe winter in 1739–40 with ice and snow in unprecedented amounts brought mills to a stop and so contributed to a scarcity of meal. In 1848 a situation of the utmost gravity followed failure of the potato crop which at the time was relied upon to provide the primary source of food.[12] These are but major instances of a social problem varying in seriousness and extent but constantly recurring, and inseparable from vagrancy and large scale destitution. It is significant that a new Act was passed in 1579 having as dual objective the 'punishment of the strong and idle beggars' and the 'relief of the poore and impotent'.

Another and contrasting social situation within the community was the plight of workers in the salt and coal mines of the lowlands. Their life was one of unmitigated serfdom. By law, miners were compelled to remain for life with the same employer, or should the employer leave, with his successor. Not until 1775 was a law passed which abolished the bondage which would otherwise have been automatically imposed on those who after that year 'shall begin to work as colliers and salters'. Twenty-four years passed before unconditional freedom was given to all by Law. It is a measure of the degradation of human relationships that prior to 1775 miners desperate to discharge debts would pledge the future freedom of their children to the coalmaster, these children in turn being condemned to future life-servitude.[13]

Many years elapsed before the needs of the mentally deranged in the community received any attention—provided always that they were harmless. This is well illustrated by an entry in the records of one West of Scotland parish in the year 1816. An unfortunate individual was described as 'deranged and at large—sleeping in stairs and closes through the town from choice; is sometimes a bishop, and at other times a duke, as the mania operates: quite harmless.[14]

HOUSING

Over the centuries, housing was a no less serious and even more persistently chronic problem. While standards differed as between the dwellings of the laird and the artisan, few homes could be described as large and attractive, much less extravagant. Inevitably provisions in rural districts contrasted with those in the towns, but all were subject to changes as the distribution and occupation of people altered. The houses of rural workers and those on the fringe of towns were built of stones without mortar, the gaps between stones being filled with heather or bracken, and a hole in the roof serving as chimney. Furnishings were minimal and overcrowding unavoidable. As homes, the buildings scarcely merited the picturesque description of 'but and ben'. In the towns tenements were the standard form of housing for the poor and more fortunate alike. Here again overcrowding was acute—overcrowding in an environment deprived of sunlight and lacking the most elemental services fundamental to sanitation and hygiene. The poor and the nobility occupied different floors in the same tenement and to quote Cameron again, 'enforced physical proximity in the Old Town of Edinburgh brought intimacy and recognition of a community of life'.[15] Lockhart gave expression to rather similar views when he wrote 'People visit each other in Edinburgh with all the appearance of cordial familiarity who, if they lived in London, would imagine their difference in rank to form an unpassable barrier against such intercourse'.[16] And the attitudes in town extended to the golf course! To quote the Statistical Account of Scotland 'the greatest and the wisest of the land were to be seen on the Links of Leith mingling freely with the humblest mechanics... all distinctions of rank were levelled by the joyous spirit of the game'.[17] Following in the wake of early industrialization there were massive movements of population seeking proximity to areas of growing industry or to those places where developing railways were making inordinate demands for casual labour. With redeployment of population there was transfer of overcrowding, and overcrowding in circumstances which had little if any regard for religious persuasions or ethnic origins.

As recently as 1952 it was written 'It was Bannockburn and John Knox that carried Scotland through, and she is not quite through yet, on housing'.[18]

DESTITUTION

Nothing in the world delights a truly religious people so much as consigning them to eternal damnation.

James Hogg

For centuries there was no form of poor relief other than charity forthcoming from religious institutions and private philanthropists. The churches had poor-boxes into which parishioners deposited their contributions when attending divine service. According to Robertson, throughout the seventeenth century the church collections and the issue of begging badges together were 'the general if not the sole system of relief'. In 1700 poor rates were levied in only three parishes throughout the length and breadth of Scotland.[19] With time, relief of destitution became a rather more formal, established function of the Kirk. The trend was consolidated when, before the Union of the Crowns, Parliament laid down the principle that each parish should, with its Kirk Session as agent, be responsible for the sustenance of the native poor. This remained the basis of Scottish poor law for more than two and a half centuries. Although an unrelenting advocate of social reform, even the famous divine Thomas Chalmers was violently opposed to anything in the nature of what today would be termed a 'means test' in providing for the poor. To him Poor Relief as administered in England created the evil it set out to treat, corrupted character, and caused class hatred.[20] In the words of Burleigh, Chalmers was a Tory who looked to the vanished past of pre-industrial Scotland with its effective parochial system.[21] It has been said that Chalmers is to be regarded as a disciple of Malthus.[22] The Church was reluctant to relinquish its functions in connection with the necessitous poor, even in the face of inadequate resources. This was particularly evident when proposals were advanced for a system of compulsory relief; and an already difficult situation was aggravated when after the Disruption of 1843 churches drew on their limited relief resources for members of their own denominational persuasions only. Conditions deteriorated to such an extent in the nineteenth century that a Commission on Poor Relief was appointed. To quote Grant, the systems of poor relief of England and Scotland '. . . erred in opposite directions, that of England in too easy largesses, that of Scotland in a too griping economy'.[23] By an Act of 1845 a Central Board of Supervision was established in Edinburgh, and Parochial Boards and Inspectors of the Poor were created. In 1616 the minister of the Kirk in every parish was required by law to keep a register of marriages, baptisms and deaths.

A contribution of altogether immense importance to the subject was made by a one-time President of the College—Dr William Pulteney Alison. His *Observations on the Management of the Poor in Scotland*[24] is today an insufficiently appreciated classic, although at the time it 'won the public ear, and the result was the Act of 1845, and the appointment of the Board of Supervision'.[23] It constituted an irrefutable indictment of Society, and while maintaining an exemplary moral tone eschewed dramatization and emotionalism. While critical, the theme of the book was essentially constructive and based upon long experience of hospital and dispensary practice and upon an intensive study of conditions as they obtained in Glasgow, Dublin and continental countries. Such comparisons as are drawn were far from favourable to Edinburgh or Scotland in general. Allied to astute clinical observation and epidemiological interpretation there were throughout the *Observations* humanism and compassion totally devoid of mawkish sentiment. Dr Alexander Wood, another distinguished President, was a protégé of Alison: and wrote 'having been indoctrinated in sanitary science by Dr Alison, I became a zealous sanitary reformer'.[25] None other than Thomas Carlyle wrote of 'the brave and humane Doctor Alison, who speaks what he knows'.[26]

Alison described the destitution and suffering of the poorer classes and while not declaring destitution to be a prime cause of contagious fever he considered it to be a major factor in spread. While allowing that 'deficient nourishment, want of employment, and privations of all kinds, and the consequent mental depression' were variously assessed as causes of spread, he stated categorically that their influence is much greater than 'any cause external to the human body itself'.[27] He deplored how unfavourably the Scottish poor compared with the English in the matter of 'habitual cleanliness', and describing the lot of female field labourers concluded that 'the fact is, they live in a condition to which that of most domestic animals is a luxury'.[28] Such observations were substantiated by facts. Discussing measures for the relief of the poor he was highly critical of the prevalent attitude of discouraging relief of mere poverty because it ignored the overriding importance of means for the prevention of disease. Quite obviously Alison regarded the popular public view that relief of poverty was injurious by discouraging the poor to depend on their own resources as a shibboleth; nor could he countenance the opinion of many of his countrymen that voluntary measures for relief were more effective than their statutory counterparts in England. He viewed with gravest concern the prevailing policy of 'repressing the claims on charity of indigence, independently of disease'.[29] About the time the book was written the public were being made aware of 'combinations among skilled workmen to raise the amount of wages'.[30] To Alison this was understandable in the context of his medical thesis. In making recommendations, he frankly admitted to being faced with one particular difficulty—the continual importation of the Irish poor. His recommendations included the establishment of a central authority for administering relief; increase and greater uniformity of relief rates applicable to indigence from lack of employment, independently of disease; and the provision of work-houses with associated fever wards.

In his introduction Alison allowed that he might have exposed himself to criticism for entering a discussion which was outside his province. In reality, in 1840, he courageously established for all time the importance of the contribution to be made by the far-sighted physician to the prevention of disease, whether in terms of public health, social medicine, community medicine or any other modern connotation. Alison's views were shared by his brother Archibald Alison, Sheriff of Lanarkshire, whose publication *The Principles of Population* appeared in 1840.[32] Not without justification Guthrie referred to Pulteney Alison as 'the "Chadwick" of Edinburgh'.[31]

In a number of respects views not dissimilar from those of Alison had been expressed more than fifty years previously by William Buchan, another Fellow of the College, who at different times practised in Edinburgh, Yorkshire and London. While in Yorkshire he was the mainstay in establishing one of the first Foundling Hospitals and proved to be an outstanding pioneer in the reform of paediatric care. His outlook however extended far beyond the age of childhood as evidenced in his book *Domestic Medicine* and embraced preventive and social medicine. Unique at the time of publication (1769) the book soon won an international reputation for the author and is considered by many today to be a classic. A native of Roxburghshire, Buchan was buried in Westminster Abbey in 1805.

EPIDEMICS

Just as periods of dearth occurred with monotonous regularity so also did epidemics. The association needs no elaboration. Nor does the connection between frequent rampant epidemics on the one hand and intolerable conditions of housing and over-crowding on the other. To this was added almost total disregard of the needs of hygiene in the matter of providing water supplies and the disposal of sewage. Intolerable as housing conditions were, they were not comparable with those pre-vailing in common lodging houses. In the case of some epidemics and contagious diseases, there is little doubt as to their nature; in the case of others there is some confusion more especially where the records admit uncertainty in the free indetermin-ate use of the term 'fever'.

Fever—'hectic fever' to be precise—was a term commonly applied to tuberculous infection in the older literature. What better description of scrofula could there be than Shakespeare's in his *Macbeth*—'Strangely-visited people, All swol'n and ulcerous, pitiful to the eye, The mere despair of surgery . . .'? Wasting was almost synonymous for phthisis, and Keats, himself a victim, recognized the vulnerability of youth when he wrote 'Youth grows pale, and spectre thin, and dies'. Reliable mortality records were not available until the nineteenth century was well advanced, but there is no escaping the fact that Scotland's history in this connection was a depressing one.

Records for the period 1870–90 show that the mortality rate due to tuberculosis in Scotland far exceeded that in England and even Ireland. Furthermore it was not until the end of the century that the extent to which bovine infection in Scotland con-tributed to morbidity was fully appreciated. Dr (later Sir) Sims Woodhead while Superintendent of the College Research Laboratory was the first to focus atten-tion on the risk of human infection from milk containing tubercle bacilli.[32a] Ultimate practical realization of the danger was the result of the pioneer work of (Sir) Robert Philip and (Sir) John Fraser. Sir Robert's subsequent achievements in the field of prevention within the community are dealt with elsewhere (Chap. XVIII). Why did tuberculosis in Scotland assume all the characteristics of a national social scourge? A multiplicity of factors rather than any one is to be incriminated. Thus in the earliest days of industrialization everything was in favour of infection and the spread of infection—destitution, malnutrition and unbelievable overcrowding in circumstances devoid of effective sanitation and ventilation. The incorporation of cow byres in dwelling-houses undoubtedly accounted for a great deal of the bovine tuberculosis in both town and country. Together virtual total ignorance of the rudiments of hygiene and the uncontrolled mass movements of population added to the hazards.

Reasonably reliable facts are known, however, about the existence of syphilis in Scotland. It was first noted in Aberdeen about 1497 and as pointed out by J. Y. Simpson, a connection with the 'syne of venerie' was suspected from the first.[33] Introduction of the disease has been attributed to foreign adventurers accompanying Perkin Warbeck. It is known too that leprosy was endemic in the Shetland Islands for many years where it persisted until late in the seventeenth century. The last native leper in Great Britain came from the Shetlands and died in 1798.[34] Plague struck Shetland early in the fourteenth century and recurred throughout Scotland at frequent intervals until the mid-seventeenth century, earning the name 'foul death of the English' because on one occasion it was brought back by Scottish raiders returning north from across the Border. By the greatest of good fortune the 'Great Plague' of 1665–6 of London and other English centres did not reach Scotland. There is in the College Library an unpublished manuscript entitled *A History of the Plague in Scotland* by Dr John Ritchie. The tragedy is the author died before his outstanding work could be published.[35] Scrofula was common in the seventeenth century, dysentery and smallpox in the eighteenth, and cholera in the nineteenth century.[36]

Dunblane was one of the many townships severely affected by cholera. There, deaths were so numerous that tolling of the church bell for funerals was dispensed with; and because one side was principally involved fires of tar were lit in the High Street to prevent spread to the other side. It is said that when the doctor 'was called to a case of cholera his first act was to take measurements of the patient for his coffin'.[37]

In the early 1800's smallpox, measles and whooping-cough in that order were the most fatal diseases among children. As early as 1755 Dr Francis Home gave trial to measles vaccine during an Edinburgh epidemic.[38] Dr Alison of the College was one of the first physicians to report in 1817 on the beneficial effects of vaccination against smallpox.[39] In 1765, Francis Home gave the first clinical description of what more than half a century later was named diphtheria. Describing the 'white, soft, thick preternatural coat or membrane' lining the upper respiratory tract in fatal cases he remarked upon the ineffectiveness of 'any internal or external medicine . . . to effectuate a solution of the membrane after it is once . . . consolidated'; and went on to argue 'We have, then, no method remaining to save the patient's life, but that of extraction. That cannot be done through the glottis. When the case is desperate may we not try bronchotomy?'[40] He found the condition prevalent in Ayrshire, Galloway and Fife although rare in Edinburgh. Typhus became prevalent in the nineteenth century at the time when overcrowding was exacerbated by population movements, and the importation of Irish labour. A President of our College in comparatively recent times had memories of losing his general practitioner father at an early age as a result of typhus. The infection was contracted in Caithness from the crew of a ship engaged in the Baltic Trade.[41] Relatively common in the seventeenth and eighteenth centuries in rural areas, ague or malaria disappeared by 1840 or thereabouts, probably as a result of the drainage and cultivation of marshy areas.[42] Christison, speaking to the Social Science Association in 1863, said that ague had completely disappeared.[43]

CARE OF THE SICK AND AILING

Today medical care is interpreted in terms of that provided by the physician, the surgeon, the obstetrician, the general practitioner and those concerned primarily with community medicine. Confusion attached to the historical evolution of the spheres of influence of these different disciplines, and not all accounts are agreed as to the exact course of events. On one aspect there is agreement. Almost all forms of medical care can be traced back to the compassionate services provided by monks, whether itinerant or attached to the *hospitia* of monasteries in different parts of the country.

For many centuries many varieties of disease were treated by clerics, but a papal edict was issued debarring operations involving contact with blood. The cleric met the situation by employing as deputy his barber colleague who with shaving already combined the art of phlebotomy. From this embryonic craft new developments arose. According to inclination or ability the individuals concerned concentrated on operative activities, continued to undertake operations and to shave, or limited their activities to those of barber. They nevertheless combined to form trades guilds to preserve their common interests, and in Edinburgh the Guild of Surgeons and Barbers together with other guilds was incorporated in 1505 under the Seal of Cause from the Town Council. The Seal was ratified by the King in the following year.

In so far as medicine was concerned, this became the special interest of the monks prohibited from practising surgery; but the separation of medicine and surgery prompted the creation of yet another specialty—that of the apothecary interested in the composition of drugs and the study of materia medica. Two apothecaries—James Borthwick and Thomas Kincaid—were admitted into the company of the surgeons in 1645. Subsequently some surgeons in Scotland, in contrast to England, combined the functions of apothecary with their craft, but a considerable number preferred to limit their activities to those of a pharmacist. These last came to be known as 'simple pharmacists'. Appreciation of the origins of such terms as barber–surgeon and surgeon–apothecary is essential to understanding of some of the problems faced by physicians prior and subsequent to their obtaining a charter of incorporation.

What were the circumstances which led the apothecaries and surgeons to develop a working alliance, albeit of limited duration? Two tolerably reliable accounts are available, although both are to some extent charged with emotion. Of these the first is by Dr William Eccles, a one-time President of our College and not one disposed to view surgeons kindly! To him the Corporation of Surgeons was 'the Masterful Deaconery' which acquired such superiority that the surgeons 'soon did overtop' their fellow Deaconeries. According to Eccles 'the Trade as well as Word Chirurgion Apothecary were unheard of . . . untill . . . 1657, two Chirurgions that had been bred in the Army, did upon their return think Washing and Barbarizing too mean, and Pharmacy both more honourable and profitable'. One outcome was that the Town Council were prevailed upon to conjoin by an Act (25.ii.1657) the apothecaries with the surgeons and by doing so to create 'a new heterogenious Imployment'. Not all apothecaries and surgeons took advantage, if advantage it were, of the new edict— 'severals of both Trades keeping themselves by their distinct Imployments'.[44]

In the course of time the simple apothecaries, resentful of the autocratic control imposed upon them by the Surgical Deaconery, became erected into a Fraternity. When in 1680 the Fraternity took steps to sever connection with the Barber–Surgeons, the apothecaries recalled the background history in a *Representation for the Apothecaries against the pretended Chirurgeon-Apothecaries*. The representation maintained that creation of a Deaconry notwithstanding the surgeons had evidenced 'neither skill in, nor pretence to Pharmacy'; and then went on to explain how 'when the Scots Army went to England, some of the Apothecaries prentices went along as Mates to the Chirurgeons'. The wars over, the two named James Borthwick and Thomas Kincaid returned to Edinburgh and on reassuming 'the employment of Apothecary to which they were bred . . . found so much favour with the Chirurgeon–Barbers as to be received into their number . . .'.[45]

As will be appreciated later, these events although apparently domestic as between apothecaries, surgeons and the various intermediate grades proved to be of considerable if unforeseeable importance in the days immediately preceding the granting of a Charter to the Royal College of Physicians (Chap. III).

Those who sought to become physicians eventually found the intimate, direct association of medicine with clerics inappropriate, but continued to attach value to broad academic training. An incidental result of the different approach to training was that socially the physician was recognized as a gentleman, the surgeon accepted as a handicraftsman.[46] At the end of the sixteenth century the Scottish general practitioner of the period was the barber–surgeon, with training limited to that of having been a barber–surgeon apprentice. Not a few apothecaries practising as pharmacists visited patients, prescribed for them and even performed certain minor surgical operations provided always that there was no opposition on the part of local surgeons. In the more remote parishes the kirk minister and farmer were frequently looked to for such help as they could give and in a number of areas undertook inoculation against smallpox. To meet the situation the physicians in Edinburgh agreed to take part in a plan whereby students of Divinity at the University would be taught the technique of inoculation.[47] Physicians in the strict sense of the term were few and far between, there being one or at most two in the few larger towns all having had academic training in Holland, Italy or France. There were in addition many with valueless claims to knowledge or experience who professed to be practising physicians, surgeon–barbers and barbers but who deserved the label of quack or mountebank, even in the light of prevailing conditions.

In 1858 the General Superintendent of the Poor remarked upon the want of confidence in medical men among the rural population. Ten years previously the Board of Supervision had issued a circular, stating that to be qualified to undertake medical relief a medical practitioner must possess a degree or diploma of physician or surgeon of a University or other body in Great Britain or Ireland legally entitled to confer or grant such a degree or diploma.

EDINBURGH

> *Now, God in Heaven bless Reekie's town*
> *With plenty, joy and peace!*
> *And may her wealth and fair renown*
> *To latest times increase! Amen.*
>   Robert Burns (in a letter to his friend Dr Fyffe)

Although national events had their repercussions on Edinburgh, their effect varied in degree; and events in Edinburgh itself did not by any means always influence the position elsewhere in the country. By 1603 Edinburgh had consolidated and actually added to its dominant position among Scottish burghs. In 1633 Charles I created a fourteenth bishopric and, with St Giles as its cathedral church, Edinburgh assumed the status of 'city' and acquired formal recognition as the 'capital'. The approximate population in 1603 was 25,000 and remained more or less stationary until after the failure of the '45 Rising. Thereafter it rose progressively to 50,000 in 1750, 100,000 in 1800 and 200,000 in 1850.[48] Subsequent figures were 319,247 and 471,897 for 1911 and 1939 respectively.[49, 50]

HOUSING

Despite the increasing congestion, policy determined that such limited new construction as did take place should be in the neighbourhood of the Royal Mile, Cowgate and Grassmarket and should not extend beyond the surrounding Flodden Wall. As a result building took place upwards; tenements rose to as many as eight, ten or even more storeys but in 1698 the number above the causeway was limited to five by Act of Parliament.[51] Construction involved considerable fire-risk, the high-pitched roofs were thatched, the gable ends and frontages faced with wood, and the stairs tortuous, narrow and steep. To add to the risk the custom prevailed of stacking heather, broom, whin and other fuels in the closes and wynds. By law this practice was stopped and the use of slates, lead or thackstone instead of thatch or deal boards made compulsory.[52] Not all legislation was so far seeing. A window tax was levied in 1696 being based at first on each inhabited house, and later on each and every window thus penalising tenements in particular. This tax was not revoked until 1806.

Numerous taverns and coffee houses dispersed throughout the Old Town served as places to which to escape from squalid homes, and as places for business, professional and social contacts and relaxation.

WATER SUPPLY

Water was at a premium. For centuries any supply had been dependent upon private and public pump wells, until in 1672 water was led from Comiston and the Pentland Hills to a tank on Castlehill and thence distributed by taps throughout the town. With the piping of water, the age-long service provided by 'water caddies' ceased. Many houses of the poor had no direct service until an Act in 1862 compelled proprietors to install water. No matter the improvement, it is open to question whether, as was claimed, 'no city of its bulk in modern Europe is better furnished with . . . supplies of feuel and water'.[53, 54]

SEWAGE AND REFUSE DISPOSAL

Certainly no comparable claim could be made in the matter of sewage and refuse disposal. In actual fact, Edinburgh was notoriously dilatory in this respect, and it was not until the nineteenth century that sewers and drains were accepted as essential, integral parts of the city's sanitary provisions. Part reason for the lack of enthusiasm was reluctance by some to forfeit the material benefits of carting and using sewage for agricultural enrichment. Irrigation of the Meadows in this way created an utterly intolerable nuisance by present day standards.

As early as the sixteenth century and for many years after, the custom in Edinburgh was on the sounding of the St Giles bell at ten of an evening, for sewage and refuse of every kind accumulated during the previous 24 hours, to be discharged from the windows of every house into the street below. The consequent state of loathsome, filthy agglomeration beggars description and is best left to the imagination. Effective cleansing of streets, alleys, closes and wynds was impossible if even seriously attempted, although it is recorded that, when Lord Provost, Sir James Dick removed fulzie from the streets on the backs of horses to his estate at Prestonfield.[55] That was in 1686. In the same century, following a visit to Edinburgh, King James complained to the city magistrates about the 'shameful filthiness', and later an Act in the reign of William III required the removal of dung and fulzie, the cleansing of common stairs and the prohibition of keeping swine in dwelling-houses.

John Wesley gives his impression and reactions after a visit to Edinburgh in his Journal:

> 'Monday May 11, 1761. I took my leave . . . The situation of the city . . . is inexpressibly fine; and the main street so broad and finely paved, with the lofty houses on either hand . . . is far beyond any in Great Britain. But how can it be suffered, that all manner of filth should still be thrown . . . into this street continually? Where are the magistracy, the gentry, the nobility of the land? Have they no concern for the honour of their nation? How long shall the capital city of Scotland, yea, and the chief street of it, stink worse than a common sewer?'[56]

Wesley visited Edinburgh again in 1772. On this occasion he became indisposed and his medical attendant Dr James Hamilton called in, in consultation, Dr James Gregory and Dr Alexander Monro *secundus*.[57]

The foundation-stone of the first house of the New Town was laid in 1767 and accomplishment of the first phase of the scheme including Princes Street and George Street was achieved with completion of Charlotte Square about 1800. Later extensions took place North beyond Heriot Row, East towards Calton Hill and North-

West to the feu of the Earl of Moray.[58] Previously the well-to-do and the poor had lived in the same wynds and closes, differentiation being as it has been described aptly 'vertical rather than horizontal'.[59] Proximity encouraged an element of mutual understanding and preparedness to help regardless of class and income; a rich feature of human relationships still prevalent in those parts of the Lowlands and Highlands of Scotland removed from the materializing influence of industry and city life.

As the New Town took shape the materially more fortunate or gentry as they were then called, removed to it from the Old Town. No relief was afforded the latter into which vast numbers of new arrivals came to fill the vacancies, with the result that congestion became worse than it had ever been. Living by any decent standard was impossible.[60] Of the single-roomed houses in the city in 1861, 1530 had 6–15 persons living in each 'house', and 121 of the rooms had no windows and many were cellars. Elsewhere one common stair served 59 rooms none of which had water, water closet or sink and which accommodated a total of 248 people.

It was in the year 1861 that a house in Chalmers Close collapsed with the loss of over 35 lives—'the building ran together with a hideous uproar and tumbled story upon story to the ground'.[61, 62] Indirectly this tragic incident was a factor in the appointment of the city's first medical officer of health in the person of (Sir) Henry Littlejohn. Dr Alexander Wood of our College was in the forefront of those further-ing the appointment.[63] In fairness it should be made clear that Edinburgh was not alone in the matter of disgraceful housing standards. There is ample evidence of this in the Poor Law Commissioners' Report in 1842 on the *Sanitary Condition of the Labouring Population*.[64]

Gas lighting was introduced into Edinburgh in 1820 but many years elapsed before it was available for other than the rich and the illumination of the principal thorough-fares.

FAMINE, DESTITUTION AND PESTILENCE

'Tis infamous, I grant it, to be poor.
Hark ye, Clinker, you are a most notorious offender. You stand convicted of sickness,
hunger, wretchedness and want.

Tobias Smollett

Water shortage was a frequent occurrence and was probably worst at the time of the great drought in 1652,[65] and throughout the century scurvy and scrofula were common. Of the Castle garrison of 300 men who capitulated in 1640, it is said that

160 died of scurvy.[66] Although the Union ultimately proved beneficial, the immediate effects on the Scottish capital were disturbing and depressing. Commercial activities tended to stagnate and the East Coast trade was virtually destroyed: and an element of inertia overcame the city as illustrated by a reluctance to restore houses involved in the many fires of the period.[67] Famine was prevalent in 1740 but assumed even severer form during the period of 1782–8 as a result of the failure of the crops, and prompted the City Council to import grain for public consumption.[68] Towards the end of the eighteenth century starvation was still rife, working committees were organized, public kitchens established and over ten per cent of the population were dependent for sustenance on charity. Writing of the year 1816 Cockburn remarked upon the great distress among the poor, which he described as less severe but greater in extent than in 1797.[69] According to the same authority employment was provided by having the Bruntsfield Links cleared of whins and old quarries, and paths built on Calton Hill and at the base of Salisbury Crags.

Plague is known to have reached Edinburgh in 1431 and to have recurred at intervals over a period of two centuries. Especially serious outbreaks took place in 1503 and 1588; despite regulations imposed by the Town Council and the voluntary evacuation of many citizens, deaths in 1588 exceeded 1400 in number. Vagrants and beggars abounded and recognition of their liability to spread disease was the reason for special regulations (1575) being drawn up to control their movements and activities. Despite these measures vagrancy reached a fresh peak in 1578.[70] Other regulations provided for the appointment by the City Council of surgeons to visit the sick poor and, where plague was suspected, the occupants of a house were removed to hastily erected wooden huts on the Burgh Muir. It is known that in one year about 2500 people died of the plague. By 1584 the Town Council had established a small hospital for lepers which seven years later was replaced by a converted former monastic building at Greenside. Five patients were admitted in 1591 and were subject to rigid control; and as a reminder of the possible penalty for disobedience a gallows was erected at the gavel of the hospital.[71] The last patient with leprosy in Scotland was diagnosed after admission to the Edinburgh Royal Infirmary in 1798.[72]

Early references to typhus fever are limited but Ferguson mentions that it was present in Edinburgh in 1735.[73] A particularly severe outbreak took place in 1817, with recurrences in 1826–9, 1837, 1842–3 and 1846–8. These outbreaks imposed a well-nigh impossible burden on the Royal Infirmary in the absence of any special 'fever' hospital. Ordinarily the Infirmary reserved at least two wards for infectious diseases but, to cope with the demands of the 1817 epidemic permission was obtained to use the unoccupied Queensberry House Barracks. Closed in 1818 at the end of the outbreak, the improvised overflow hospital had to be reopened on the occurrence of a further epidemic in 1826, and no fewer than 150 beds were in constant occupation additional to those in the Infirmary. When a third epidemic developed in 1837 the Queensberry House Barracks were not available. The Infirmary having more accommodation of its own, earmarked nine wards representing a total of 140 beds for 'fever', and secured the temporary use from the City of a house which had previously functioned as the Lock Hospital for venereal disease. Over a fifteen months' period 2771 patients were treated. Two even more extensive epidemics occurred in 1842–3 and 1846–8. Additional to improvised arrangements in the past, tents were pitched in the vicinity of the Infirmary and use made of the chapel. During the period 1841–8, 17,542 patients with infectious fevers were treated. Patients in the last two epidemics included an outstandingly large proportion of 'wandering Irish' among whom it was thought the disease first appeared.[74]

In 1828 an 'epidemic fever' with new features gave rise to uncertainty and a certain amount of diagnostic confusion among practitioners in Edinburgh. The most striking characteristic was its distribution. It occurred among the well-to-do and 'instead of occupying the Cowgate, the Grassmarket and the High-street, the usual haunts of typhus, this fever had its head-quarters in Heriot-row and Great King-street; and . . . extended . . . in the direction of the Water of Leith . . . and . . . along the shore to Musselburgh'.[75] The epidemic came to be referred to in both East and West Scotland as the *'Edinburgh New Town Epidemic'*.[76]

Christison had experience of the epidemic fever both in Queensberry House and the Infirmary and stated that seventeen attacks had been personally experienced by twelve senior medical staff over a period of two years in the Infirmary.[77] His thesis for the Doctorate of Medicine at Edinburgh University was based on this experience and he described epidemic fever as presenting in one of three forms—one in keeping with the synocha of Cullen nosology, another consisting of a mild variety of typhus (the typhus mitior of Cullen) and the third, a form intermediate between the two others. Remarking on the tendency of the third form to be ignored Christison wrote with enviable sagacity—but not in his thesis—'There certainly it was, in spite of the scepticism of "Young English Physic", who is prone to believe only in what he himself has seen, and will not grant the like privilege to his predecessors'.[78]

Another outbreak occurred fifteen years later and a detailed account of 220 patients was given by Dr Halliday Douglas, a Fellow of the College, under the title *Statistical Report on the Edinburgh Epidemic Fever of 1843–44*.[79, 80]

Although smallpox outbreaks occurred at intervals throughout the seventeenth and eighteenth centuries it did not appear to be so geographically extensive in Scotland as in England. Moreover Edinburgh did not suffer to the extent of other towns such as Aberdeen, but it did share with other places the tendency for mortality to be high among children. Edinburgh experienced a particularly severe outbreak during the period 1740–2, when 2700 victims died of whom more than half were under 5 years of age. Between 1744 and 1763 about one in every ten of all deaths was attributable to smallpox.[81] In his *History of England*, written in 1848, Macaulay described how 'smallpox was always present, filling the church yards with corpses, tormenting with constant fears all whom it had not yet stricken, leaving on those whose lives it spared the hideous traces of its power'.[82]

Cholera, present elsewhere in Scotland, extended to Edinburgh in 1832, via Port Seton having been brought originally by ships trading with Riga and other Baltic seafaring towns.[82a] In the following year the Cholera Acts were placed on the Statute Book. During a period of $11\frac{1}{2}$ months there were 1886 victims of whom 1065 died. According to the *Scotsman* of the period rioting took place as a form of protest against admission to hospital where doctors were thought to be experimenting on their patients.[83] Another outbreak in 1848–9 appeared to originate in Edinburgh and of 810 known cases 478 died. To deal with the situation a special hospital for cholera victims was opened, and this had to be re-opened for the second of two subsequent outbreaks in 1853 and 1854. The Hall used for the purpose and known as Drummond Street Cholera Hospital was in actual fact the old Surgeons Hall only recently vacated by, but still the property of the Surgeons.[84] The Janitor of Edinburgh Academy succumbed in the epidemic of 1854. Fortunately his death occurred during the school holidays which allowed books to be fumigated, woodwork to be oil-painted and drains to be overhauled before the start of term.[84a] Henry Littlejohn had ample justification for his statement that 'Edinburgh is notorious for its epidemics of fevers'.[85]

Arnot referred to 'the contagious plague, called the grandgore' recognized between 1490 and 1500 and explained by him as due 'to intercourse with the natives of America'.[86] The management of those afflicted consisted of removal, until health had been restored, to the Island of Inchkeith, an adequate supply of food being given. Rules were rigid and the penalty for infringement 'burning of the cheek'. 'Grandgore' was one of the names by which syphilis was then known. Little does Edinburgh realize its past indebtedness to the many islands of the Forth for the incarceration of fugitive prisoners, and dread disease.

Nor did Edinburgh escape the ravages of tuberculosis. The disease did not respect any social class. There were no fewer than 171 byres, some located under dwelling houses, within the City of Edinburgh in 1853.[87] In 1865 the mortality due to phthisis in Morningside was astoundingly high, and twice as high in terms of percentage of deaths as in the Grassmarket. In the opinion of the Medical Officer of Health this was explained by 'the number of invalids who flock' to Morningside 'during winter and spring'.[88]

COMMUNITY LIFE AND ORDER: SOME ASPECTS

Acts of civil disobedience and rioting are interspersed throughout the history of Edinburgh. The city in 1570 has been described as 'the centre of endless disorders and feuds';[89] in the seventeenth century as the scene of 'great Disorders committed in the streets';[90] and in the early eighteenth century as still having an 'unenviable notoriety for its street riots'.[91] Few incidents lacked rational explanation when account is taken of the contrasting political and religious convictions held by many in the community. Inevitably strife arose between adherents of Knox and those of the Pope; Jacobite and Royalist; pro-unionist and anti-unionist. Scarcity and the high price of food, unemployment and ill-paid employment under harsh conditions, intolerable home conditions and destitution were understandable causes of ventilated resentment.

Civil disorder took the form typical of any age even to the extent of having student participants. On two occasions (1580 and 1595) pupils at the High School were detained in the Tolbooth prison on account of rioting and 'holding the school'. In 1580 there were no serious consequences but in 1595, a pupil shot dead the baillie who was leading town officials on their way to force the school doors.[92] University students in 1680 rivalled those of modern times in their excesses, burning down and destroying the contents of the Roman Catholic Lord Provost's house. The Lord Provost's private secretary and accountant was George Watson who later endowed the Edinburgh school which bears his name to this day.[93] In due course the house, Prestonfield, was restored and in the middle of the following century a President of the College (Sir Alexander Cunningham Dick) acted as host to Johnson and his biographer Boswell;[94] and to Benjamin Franklin and John Morgan of Pennsylvania. Morgan was the first American Licentiate and Fellow of the College. Dick was described by Johnson as 'the only Scotsman liberal enough not to be angry that I could not find trees, where trees were not'.[95] In a letter to Boswell dated 11th February 1784 Johnson was instructed to 'ask your physicians about my case; and desire Sir Alexander Dick to write me his opinion':[96] and in a second letter (2nd March 1784) he was told to 'return Sir Alexander Dick my sincere thanks for his kind letter; and bring with you the rhuburb which he so tenderly offers me'. Boswell added that the rhuburb was from Dick's garden at Prestonfield from a crop awarded 'a gold medal by the Society of London for the Encouragement of Arts, Manufactures, and Commerce'. Others from whom Boswell sought advice concerning his employer were Doctors Cullen, Hope, Monro and Gillespie.[97] Some years previously (1777) Dick had occasion to write thanking Johnson for the gift of *Journey to the Western Islands of Scotland*.[98]

One historian explained the occurrences of student unrest as evidence that after the Restoration 'Students . . . appear to have been pretty much tainted with the fanatick principles of the covenanters'—[99] processions, burning of effigies, apprehensions and custody. A sequel to rioting on this occasion was that Doctor Alexander Monro together with other Senators was among those summoned to stand trial before 'Visitors' sent at the instance of Parliament.

While sundry efforts were made to promote some degree of order in the city the first officially sponsored organization was the creation of a Town Guard in 1641[100] whose recruits in the main were ex-Highland soldiers still possessed of musket or Lochaber axe. In 1805 unarmed police were appointed to take over the functions of the original Town Guard.

Penalties to which those breaking the law were liable were many, varied and drastic. There is ample evidence of this in the records of the Old Tolbooth. A suspected murderer could be submitted to the ordeal of 'touching the corpse', guilt being established should blood issue from the orifices or the wound of the body. Special medical interest attaches to the hanging of a person who was 'both man and woman, a thing not ordinar in this kingdome'. The crime was irregular conduct and the irregular conduct that 'his custome was always to goe in a woman's habite'. 'When opened by certain doctors', Margaret Rannie as the person had been known in life, 'was found to be two every way, having two hearts, two livers, two every inward thing'.[101, 102] In 1659 a woman was 'whipt throw the heighe street from the castle hill to the netherbow' for stealing.[103] For bearing false witness 'Sundry persons . . . had their ears nailed to the Trone . . . and one . . . had his tongue pierced with a hot iron'.[104] A man of 75 years was burnt at the Gallo-lay for incest: his sister aged 60 was hanged, having confessed to incest and witchcraft.[105]

Witchcraft was a crime with an aura all its own. In a land almost fanatically dedicated to Protestantism, even idolatry was dealt by the law with greater compassion. Death was decreed as penalty for witchcraft by an Act of 1563 and was not removed from the Statute Book until 1736. While in operation it was applied 'with the terrible literalism' of the text 'Thou shalt not suffer a witch to live' and the most fervid applicants were 'the ministers, Presbyterian and Episcopalian alike'.[106] The Record of Judiciary for 13th September 1678 contains the following:— 'Ten women were accused of witchcraft . . . They were all convicted on their own confessions, condemned to be strangled at a stake and burned'. Of those incriminated the vast majority were women. No less an authority than Brown considered it was impossible to assess the total number of victims in Scotland and that 'it is by thousands and not by hundreds that they must be reckoned'.[106] The last 'witch' in Scotland was condemned to death by law in 1727. She was strangled.[107] Strangling consisted of being 'bund to ane staik and wirreit' as distinct from the sentence reserved for the 'more atrocious' cases, 'brunt in assis, quick (alive) to the death'.[108]

Apparently much less zeal was shewn in the discharge of the other pastoral duties related to the keeping of a Register. It was written in 1779 'of the register of births and burials in Edinburgh . . . they have been kept in such manner as to render them . . . the infallible sources of error. The register of burials is kept by people whose faculties are impaired by drinking, who forget to-day what was done yesterday . . . they enter not into the list of burials any who have died without receiving baptism: nor those whose relations are so poor, as not to be able to pay for the use of a mort-cloth . . . As for the register of births it does not deserve the name.'[109]

Edinburgh differed from most of Scotland in that it was better documented. Dr James Stark, the Registrar of Mortality, took advantage of this to attempt a simple statistical analysis. His conclusion was that reversal of the trend of falling death rate between 1780 and 1820 was attributable to a combination of recurrent epidemics, physical and moral degradation and Irish immigration precipitated by a great commercial 'slump' in 1829.[110] In England, medical statistics associated with the name of John Graunt had first appeared in the mid-seventeenth century.

Despite Stark's appraisal, Edinburgh had no justification for complacency. A Committee appointed in 1867 by the Lord Provost to enquire into prevailing misery and destitution published a Report on *The Condition of the Poorer Classes*. Basing their conclusions on the findings of a Subcommittee with Dr Alexander Wood of our College as Chairman, those responsible estimated that 1344 preventable deaths took place each year. Dr Wood was well equipped for his task and he was soon actively engaged in the foundation of the *Association for Improving the Condition of the Poor*.[111]

PHYSICIANS, SURGEONS AND APOTHECARIES

I do remember an apothecary—
And hereabouts he dwells,—which late I noted
In tatter'd weeds, with overwhelming brows,
Culling of simples; meagre were his looks,
Sharp misery had worn him to the bones:
And in his needy shop a tortoise hung,
An alligator stuff'd, and other skins
Of ill-shaped fishes; and about his shelves
A beggarly account of empty boxes,
Green earthen pots, bladders and musty seeds,
Remnants of packthread and old cakes of roses,
Were thinly scatter'd to make up a show.

William Shakespeare (*Romeo & Juliet*)

Following their incorporation as a Guild, the surgeons and barbers progressively extended their sphere of influence. Additional to what may be described as their essentially clinical activities there is evidence in the Town Council records that they appeared as expert witnesses, and submitted reports in medicolegal cases. In 1589 a surgeon–barber who had been deeply involved in a professional capacity with plague victims was retained 'to treat the poor of the town'. Apothecaries and pharmacists competed with the surgeons and barbers in that they both prescribed and dispensed medicines. A decree issued by the Provost and Baillies in 1575 forbidding apothecaries and others who were not members of the Surgeons' Guild from practising in this way, was only partially effective. Of physicians there were only a limited number in the latter half of the sixteenth century, the majority if not all of whom were possessed of degrees from or had trained at universities abroad.[112] A former President of our Sister Edinburgh College advanced the view that 'Scottish physicians were in little repute among us for more than a century after James IV'. In support of this he refers to the undeniable fact that at the time in question, those with the influence and means showed a predilection for consulting foreign physicians. He instanced the employment of a French physician by Mary Queen of Scots (1552), and of French and Italian physicians by the affluent Archbishop Hamilton of St Andrews (1547).[113]

In point of fact, there being no other form of training than that of apprenticeship to a barber–surgeon, resort had to be made to foreign universities for a medical education. Leyden University in particular attracted many Scots and the teaching there of Boerhaave was to exert an immense influence in future years on the Medical School in Edinburgh. There was no effective University medical faculty until 1726 and virtually no teaching of medicine in Scotland until the last quarter of the seventeenth century.[114] Meanwhile in Italy, the absence of university faculties in some cities had been a factor in creating medical corporations intended to counterbalance pre-existing powerful guilds of surgeons.[115]

Physicians, surgeons, barbers and apothecaries were alike in that, even as they knew competition among themselves, they had in common the need to contend with the impostor. Flagrant quackery was practised in Edinburgh no less than in Scotland as a whole throughout the sixteenth, seventeenth and to a lesser extent the eighteenth century. Anderson pills, first concocted in the early seventeenth century, were available and in demand for over two centuries. In 1687 a case relating to these pills was recommended by the Lords of Session 'to the College of Physicians to consider the petition'. The task can have been no easy one when account is taken of Fountainhall's reservation that 'if the physicians should require the receipt to see if the composition be wholesome, this would divulge the secret and prejudge the parties of their intended benefit'![116] Whereas the poor depended upon traditional folklore and the nostrums of the mountebank, the rich in the towns sought advice from the apothecary, the barber–surgeon and the physician. As from 1657 apothecaries were by an Act of the Town Council required before practising to be examined by members of the Guild of Surgeons and Barbers. The activities of quacks acquired a deserved notoriety among the laity no less than among those concerned to enhance the status of the medical profession. They made full use of handbills and erected public stages to publicize themselves and disseminate extravagant claims for their 'infallible cures'. John Ponthus was a quack about whom there are reliable known facts. He visited Scotland in 1633, 1643 and 1662. From Fife as a base of operations he made visits to Perth, Stirling, Glasgow and Edinburgh. Lamont recorded of him 'Every tyme he had his publicke stage erected, and sold thereon his droggs to the peopell . . . Each tyme he had his peopell that played on the scaffold, ane ay playing the foole, and ane other by leaping and dancing on the rope. The two last tymes he was hire, both his printed peapers, and his droggs were one and that same.'[117] One occasion on which this same Ponthus was in Edinburgh is mentioned in the Records of Edinburgh for 5th June 1663 in the following terms:

> 'Grants libertie to John Ponteyus, professour of Physick to build a stage doun about Blackfreir wynd head, for publict view, they acting no obscene thing to give offence . . .'[118]

On this same subject the following quotation from Arnot is of interest in that it refers to the erection of our College:

'In this period the Royal College of Physicians was erected by patent. Before that the city was over-run with quacks and mountebanks. There is a lively instance of the deplorable state of the science of medicine in the records of the privy council. One JOANNES Michael Philo physician, sets forth to the privy council, that his Majesty had allowed him to practise his proffesion in England, and for that purpose to erect public stages: and he entreats the same liberty in this kingdom. The council, accordingly, allow him to erect a stage in the City of Edinburgh; but they also appoint the petition to be intimated to, and answered by, the Master of Revells, against the next meeting of the council; and, in the meantime, discharge the physician to practice rope-dancing.'[119]

Writing facetiously on this subject to Dr William Cullen, President of the Edinburgh College of Physicians, Adam Smith said:

'Stage-doctors, I must observe, do not much excite the indignation of the faculty: more respectable quacks do. The former are too contemptible to be considered as rivals: they only poison the poor people; and the copper pence which are thrown up to them in handkerchiefs could never find their way to the pocket of a regular physician. It is otherwise with the latter: they sometimes intercept a part of what perhaps would have been better bestowed in another place. Do not all the old women in the country practice physic without exciting murmur or complaint? And if here and there a graduated doctor should be as ignorant as an old woman, where can be the great harm?'[120, 121]

Mention must be made of one other, however, who although he was born (1745) and studied medicine in Edinburgh must be regarded as a psychopath rather than a purely mercenary character. By name James Graham, few could vie with his Bohemian conceptions and wild dramatizations. Having practised in England, he returned there after a period in America, and established a 'Temple of Health' in Pall Mall. In it therapeutic reliance was placed on art, statuary, music and 'the powers of electricity and magnetism'. In 1783 he returned to Edinburgh where he gave lectures assisted by a young lady of some beauty who later was to become Lady Hamilton. There was no dearth of patients. Among them was (Sir) Walter Scott who at the age of 14 years having been stricken with poliomyelitis, was referred for 'electrical' treatment by his maternal grandfather, a Fellow of the Edinburgh College. Eventually Graham was placed under restraint on account of insanity.[122, 123]

Persistence of the quack problem prompted *Punch* in 1845 to prescribe 'A dose for the Quacks'. The quack was described as 'a personage too essential to the comfort of a large class of society, to be deprived of his vocation. He is, in fact, the Physician of the Fools.' *Punch* went on to propose 'that every Quack should not only be suffered to call himself what he is not, but should be compelled to call himself what he is!'

PROGRESS IN MEDICINE AND OTHER ARTS

Despite the handicap imposed by political and religious strife, the seventeenth century saw progress in the arts of peace and this acquired increasing momentum and purpose in the two succeeding centuries. In the field of medicine the Royal College of Physicians was incorporated by Charter in 1681 and a Royal Charter was granted to the Sister College of Surgeons in 1778; and the embryonic (Royal) Infirmary was opened in 1729, to be followed in 11 years by the first institutional Work-house for the poor (1740) and in 47 years by the first Dispensary—The Old Town Dispensary (1776) in Edinburgh. In 1726 the University of Edinburgh established a Faculty of Medicine and in 1732 the Medical Society was formed. This Society was succeeded by the Philosophical Society, which was temporarily disbanded at the time of the '45 rebellion but revived in 1752.

The eighteenth century was the century of the Hunters—William (1718–83) and John (1728–93)—David Hume (1711–76), Adam Smith (1723–90) and Robert Burns (1759–96). The lives of such other national figures as James Watt (1736–1819), Sir Henry Raeburn (1756–1823) and Sir Walter Scott (1771–1832) extended from the eighteenth into the nineteenth century, in which last Robert Louis Stevenson was born and died. A deeply disturbing event was the Disruption (1843) arising from renewed and acute discontent over the patronage attached to the appointment of incumbents. The origins were to be found in the restoration of Church patronage a few years after the Treaty of Union (q.v.). Happily the ultimate outcome was one of gradual reunion and not permanent secession. The Patronage Act of 1712 was eventually repealed in 1874. Another statutory advance was the Education Act of 1872 which by implication gave effect to recommendations, dating back to the original *Book of Discipline* but not implemented, for schools for every parish. None the less it is salutary to remember that reporting on pauperism in Edinburgh as late as 1865 Henry Littlejohn, Edinburgh's first Medical Officer of Health, felt compelled to write:

> 'The pittances that are given to paupers through the proverbial economy of boards, representing the rate-payers of our city, are only intended to allow of life being maintained at a legal flicker and by no means at a steady flame.'[124]

Discussing the eighteenth century of Scottish medicine the Bulloughs were impressed by the benefit to Edinburgh in particular of effective alliance of population growth, urbanization, prosperity and opportunities for schooling.[125]

The general trend was to a fuller life for all, and a richer life for the more fortunate.

There were the ennobling advances of architectural planning attributable to the Adams, Playfair and Craig; the growing interest in and cultivation of music with the eventual creation of a concert hall; and readier access to the printed word whether in the form of journals such as the *Edinburgh Gazette*, the *Edinburgh Review* and *Blackwoods Magazine* (founded in 1699, 1802 and 1817 respectively) or in the form of daily newsprint (the *Scotsman* was first published in 1817).

To compare the days of early organization in the field of medicine with those of industry in more modern times is illuminating. In many but not all ways, the evolution of incorporations of Surgeons and Physicians has been mirrored in the growth of the trade union movement. Common to growing professional and industrial status and influence, there has developed an increasing concern over differentials in terms of spheres of influence, and over ability to exercise power in determining policy. Historical perspective compels recognition of the fact that the motives underlying past altercations between surgeons and physicians differed little, if at all, from those giving rise to twentieth century 'chalk-line' demarcation disputes between boilermakers and shipwrights.

Today in a rapidly changing society there are within the community those who harbour unfriendly sentiments to the point of envy and prejudice towards the medical profession. There are cells of discontent even within the ranks of the profession, which find difficulty in understanding or accepting the rôle of administrative bodies. How right Robert Louis Stevenson was when he wrote:

> 'Age may have one side, but assuredly Youth has the other. There is nothing more certain than that both are right, except perhaps that both are wrong.'

How, it may be wondered, would Stevenson have reacted to the attitude of Dr Andrew Duncan, a one-time President of our College. Annually Duncan used to publish *Medical Commentaries* and in 1791 enlisted the aid of his son. Having done so, Duncan, sen. was constrained to write of his newly acquired assistant in the Preface:

> 'Notwithstanding his youth, and want of experience in literary composition, I yet trust, that he has not failed in retaining the sense of the Authors whose writings he has analyzed:—And, if the language which he employs should sometimes appear deficient in accuracy or perspicacity, the Indulgent Reader will I hope, permit me to offer for him, the apology which the illustrious Haller made for his son, "Condonandum aliquid juveni octodecim annorum".'[126]

In due course Andrew Duncan Junior held three University chairs at different times, and was one of the first in Scotland to give serious trial to Laennec's stethoscope.

Whether it be Youth or Age musing on the past or setting sights for the future it behoves us all as individuals, corporate bodies or academic institutions to ponder over the following extract which relates to a legal case in which the College was involved and which is culled from Lord Fountainhall's *Decisions* (2nd February, 1686).

> 'It was represented against the Physicians, that power was inebriating, and therefore thir Gentlemen, tho' very worthy persons, are ready to abuse it, not being accustomed to it; and it may degenerate the sooner into oppression and tyranny, that they are concerned; therefore their power was limited.'[127]

If medical practice was in a state of chaos in the seventeenth century, extreme confusion persisted perhaps in slowly lessening degree in the eighteenth and nineteenth centuries. By the early nineteenth century physicians were engaged in attending to the more economically fortunate in the community and in philanthropic activities; together, surgeons and apothecaries dealt with the bulk of what may be described as general practice; and large numbers of nondescript quacks, some claiming to apprenticeships but none with qualifications, continued to practise at will. Samuel Smiles—in turn doctor, business executive, philanthropist and author of *Self Help*—has left a description of his experience after being bound in 1826 as an apprentice for five years to two doctors in Haddington. 'I had' he recalled 'to learn the nature and the qualities of drugs, and how to make up prescriptions, pills, mixtures, potions, ointments, blisters, infusions, tinctures and such like . . . I learnt the arts of bleeding and bandaging. I had to assist in attending the poorer class of patients.'[128] According to Comrie, Thomas Keith is reputed to have been the last medical apprentice in Edinburgh. That was in the year 1845.[129]

Restiveness among the profession and the community assumed sizeable proportions. Different schemes to deal with the situation were suggested in 1805 by Dr Latham in London and Dr Harrison (an Edinburgh graduate) in Lincoln. Neither scheme won favour. At this stage the apothecaries in London came into the picture and during the course of negotiations Dr Fothergill suggested the term 'general practitioners' to describe the work of the apothecaries—possibly the first time that the term had been used. In 1815 a new Law—the Apothecaries Act 1815—was placed on the Statute Book. In accordance with the provisions of the Act the Society of Apothecaries became the administrative and licensing authority, established a Court of Examiners, insisted upon a five years' apprenticeship and conferred a diploma of licentiateship on successful candidates (L.S.A.). In a way which seems at variance with customary British justice the Society was empowered to act on information provided by an informer who frequently proved to be a fellow practitioner prompted by motives of jealousy. It has been said that the Apothecaries Act 'for over forty years was the official charter for general practitioners'.[130] The statement applied to England. None the less the Edinburgh College was involved in so far as implementation of the Act as interpreted by the Society of Apothecaries bore hardly on Licentiates of the College practising in the south. This was one of many circumstances which kept alive discontent and stimulated demands for further and more effective medical reform.

Between 1840 and 1858 no fewer than eighteen Bills were brought before Parliament in an endeavour to reform the general state of medical practice. The frustration and obstruction experienced almost vied with that known to those promoting legislation to curb child labour. The eighteenth and successful Bill was given the Royal Assent on 2nd August 1858 and thus there came into existence the Medical Act of 1858. Under the Act the General Council of Medical Education and Registration composed of qualified medical practitioners and with a Subsidiary Council for Scotland (and Ireland) was created. The Council was charged with the responsibility of maintaining an annual Medical Register; disciplining those guilty of infamous conduct in a professional respect, and supervising and co-ordinating the examinations of the many licensing bodies. It was under obligation to compile and publish the British Pharmacopoeia and in all matters was responsible to the Privy Council.

Sir John Simon, one of the most eminent civil servants of all time, was Medical Officer to the newly constituted General Medical Council and was strongly in favour of devising an administrative framework whereby entry to the medical profession would be by one portal and subject to candidates passing an examination by a national board. Simon's immaculate administrative mind must have been aghast at prospects of having dealings with some seventeen licensing bodies of which one was none other than the Archbishop of Canterbury himself! It is not difficult to understand why Simon in his search for administrative tidiness contemplated relegation of the qualifications granted by the Universities and the medical and surgical Corporations to an entirely subsidiary role. Had his policy been adopted these qualifications would not have carried entitlement to registration. It would have rested with the individual to decide whether to obtain a University Degree or Corporation Licence before or after passing the examination of a national board, or indeed whether to consider taking them at all.

Tacit support for Simon's projected policy was forthcoming from a Royal Commission on the Medical Act in 1881. The Commission included in its number the doughtiest of able administrators in the person of (Sir) William Turner: professor of Anatomy, later Principal of the University of Edinburgh, and the 'bonniest of fechters'. In a minority report he forcibly enunciated the reasons why the universities and medical corporations should continue to grant qualifications; but, at the same time, argued convincingly that a licensing body not granting a complete qualification embracing medicine, surgery and midwifery should combine with another appropriate body in order that qualifications granted should be complete. Turner's recommendations were embodied in the Medical Act of 1886. Individual licensing bodies continued to grant their own qualifications but the General Medical Council possessed power to appoint examiners to those bodies which did not, of their own, provide complete qualifications. In 1859 the Royal College of Physicians of Edinburgh, the Royal College of Surgeons of Edinburgh and the Faculty of Physicians and Surgeons of Glasgow joined forces to establish a Conjoint Examining Board for Scotland.

The latter half of the nineteenth century saw amendments to the Medical Reform Act, initial acceptance of the place of women in the medical profession, the beginnings of statutory public health and school medical services, and recommendations of a Royal Commission on the Scottish Universities. Meanwhile with advances in medical science and training, pathology and physiology were acquiring increasing importance. Bacteriology followed suit. Soon after the turn of the century biochemistry and virology were firmly established as of major significance. The physical state of army recruits at the time of the Boer War spotlighted the basic bearing on national health of nutrition and environment. Among important administrative developments influencing the outlook of the Medical Corporations were the National Insurance Act of 1911, and the creation of the Department of Health for Scotland in 1929. The Department of Health became responsible for public health measures formerly undertaken by the Local Government Board for Scotland established in 1897. Special provision for the Highlands and Islands was made by Acts passed in 1913 and 1917. A maternity and child welfare service was launched while World War I was in progress. Under the Local Government Act for Scotland of 1929 responsibility for statutory public health services and for the administration of hospitals formerly run by boards of guardians, was vested in the councils of the large towns and counties.

The entire structure of hospital administration and staffing was fundamentally changed with the coming into force of the National Health Service as an essential, integrated part of the Welfare State in 1948. While the place of the consultant and specialist seemed assured, the ultimate precise rôle of the general practitioner was not clearly outlined. Inevitably these many and various administrative developments over the last eight or nine decades had an impact on the work of the College with its

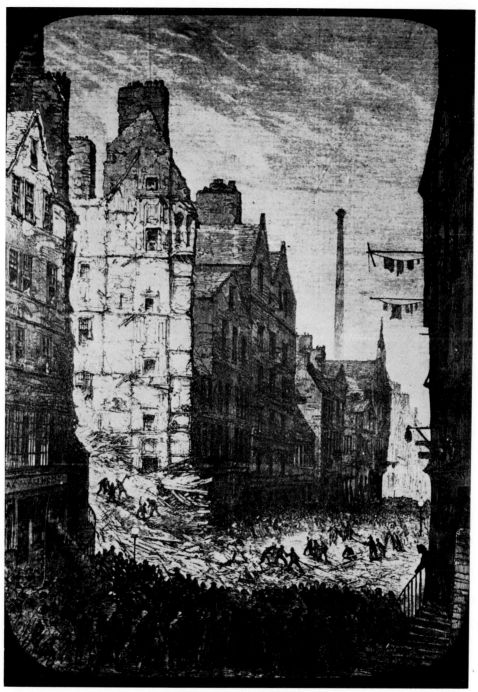

PLATE I 'Heave awa' land
By courtesy of Edinburgh Public Libraries; photograph by A. G. Ingram Ltd.

centuries-old record of active interest in virtually all aspects of medical practice and medical education. Necessarily the College has made successive adjustments to deal with the changing national and local situation. Of adjustments one of the most important in recent times has been dealing with the problems given rise to by the recommendations of the Royal Commission on Medical Education contained in the Goodenough Report (1944).[131]

The Chapters which follow give an account of the work entailed over the centuries in the College's endeavours to keep abreast of the times and prepare for the future.

REFERENCES

(1) SMOUT, T. C. (1972) *A History of the Scottish People, 1560–1830*, Rev. Edition, pp. 174–5. London: Collins/Fontana.

THE NATION AS A WHOLE

(2) CLARK, Sir G. (1964) *A History of the Royal College of Physicians of London*, vol. 1, p. 193. Oxford: Clarendon Press.

(3) McLEOD, N. (1974) Personal communication.

(4) DICKINSON, W. C. (1965) *Scotland from the Earliest Times to 1603*, 2nd Edition (rev.), p. 376. (New history of Scotland ser.—vol. 1.) London: Nelson.

(5) POTTINGER, G. (1972) *Muirfield and the Honourable Company*, p. 4. Edinburgh: Scottish Academic Press.

(6) PRINGLE, Sir J. (1755) *Observations on the Diseases of the Army*, 7th Edition, p. 39. London: W. Strahan.

(7) PRYDE, G. S. (1962) *Scotland from 1603 to the Present Day*, p. 116. (New history of Scotland ser.—vol. 2.) London: Nelson.

(8) CAMERON, J., *Lord Cameron* (1967) Scott and the Community of Intellect. In *Edinburgh in the Age of Reason*, p. 49. Edinburgh: University Press.

(9) BROWN, P. H., ed. (1891) *Early Travellers in Scotland*, p. 73. Edinburgh: David Douglas.

(10) PRYDE, G. S. Op. cit., p. 24.

(11) SIBBALD, Sir R. (1699) *Provision for the Poor in Time of Dearth and Scarcity*, pp. 2–3. Edinburgh: James Watson the Younger.

(12) FERGUSON, T. (1948) *The Dawn of Scottish Social Welfare*, p. 29. London: Nelson.

(13) COCKBURN, H. (1910) *Memorials of his time*, New Edition, pp. 70–2. Edinburgh: Foulis.

(14) GORDON, S. & COCKS, T. G. B. (1952) *A People's Conscience*, p. 103. London: Constable.

(15) CAMERON, J., *Lord Cameron* Op. cit., p. 51.

C

(16) LOCKHART, J. G. (1820) *Peter's Letters to his Kinsfolk*, 1st American, from the 2nd Edinburgh Edition, p. 121. New York: Printed by C. S. Van Winkle for A. T. Goodrich and Co. *et al.*

(17) POTTINGER, G. Op. cit., p. 5.

(18) ROSS, Sir J. S. (1952) *The National Health Service in Great Britain*, p. 62. London: Oxford University Press.

(19) ROBERTSON, D. (1953) *The Princes Street Proprietors and other Chapters in the History of the Royal Burgh of Edinburgh*, p. 255. Edinburgh: Oliver & Boyd.

(20) BROTHERSTON, J. H. F. (1952) *Observations on the Early Public Health Movement in Scotland*, p. 70. London: H. K. Lewis.

(21) BURLEIGH, J. H. S. (1960) *A Church History of Scotland*, p. 316. London: Oxford University Press.

(22) MECHIE, S. (1960) *The Church and Scottish Social Development, 1780–1870*, p. 48. London: Oxford University Press.

(23) GRANT, Sir A. (1884) *The Story of the University of Edinburgh*, vol. II, p. 408. London: Longmans, Green & Co.

(24) ALISON, W. P. (1840) *Observations on the Management of the Poor in Scotland and its Effects on the Health of the Great Towns*. Edinburgh: Blackwood.

(25) BROWN, T. (1886) *Alexander Wood, M.D., F.R.C.P.E.: A sketch of his life and work*, p. 134. Edinburgh: Macniven & Wallace.

(26) CARLYLE, T. [1843] *Past and Present*, p. 5. London: Chapman & Hall.

(27) ALISON, W. P. Op. cit., p. 21.

(28) Ibid., p. 32.

(29) Ibid., p. 43.

(30) Ibid., p. 187.

(31) GUTHRIE, D. J. (1954) *The Medical School of Edinburgh*, p. 21. Edinburgh: The University.

(32) ALISON, Sir A. (1840) *The Principles of Population and their Connection with Human Happiness*, 2 vols. Edinburgh: Blackwood.

(32a) WOODHEAD, G. S. (1889) Tabes mesenterica and pulmonary tuberculosis. In *Reports from the Laboratory of the Royal College of Physicians, Edinburgh*, ed. by J. Batty Tuke and G. S. Woodhead, vol. 1, pp. 179–212. Edinburgh: Young J. Pentland.

(33) SIMPSON, J. Y. (1872) *Archaeological Essays*, vol. 2, p. 326. Edinburgh: Edmonston & Douglas.

(34) COMRIE, J. D. (1932) *History of Scottish Medicine*, 2nd Edition, vol. I, p. 199. London: Baillière, Tindall & Cox.

(35) RITCHIE, J. (c. 1955) *A History of the Plague in Scotland*. (Ms.)

(36) CREIGHTON, C. (1891–4) *A History of the Epidemics in Britain*, 2 vols. Cambridge: University Press.

(37) BARTY, A. B. [1944] *The History of Dunblane*, p. 233. Stirling: Eneas Mackay.

(38) COMRIE, J. D. Op. cit., vol. I, p. 319.

(39) Ibid., vol. II, p. 430.

(40) HOME, F. (1765) *An Enquiry into the Nature, Cause and Cure of the Croup*, p. 59. Edinburgh: Kincaid & Bell.

(41) ALEXANDER, W. A. (1974) Personal communication.

(42) COMRIE, J. D. Op. cit., vol. II, p. 431.

(43) CHRISTISON, Sir R. (1885) *Life of Sir Robert Christison, Bart*, vol. I, p. 376. Edinburgh: Blackwood.

(44) [ECCLES, W.] (1707) *An Historical Account of the Rights and Priviledges of the Royal College of Physicians and of the Incorporation of Chirurgions in Edinburgh*, p. 14. Edinburgh: Privately printed.

(45) POOLE, R. (1838) *Preparatory Notes for a History of the College*, p. 37. (Ms.)

(46) DUNCAN, A. (1896) *Memorials of the Faculty of Physicians and Surgeons of Glasgow, 1599–1850*, p. 5. Glasgow: Maclehose.

(47) SINCLAIR, Sir J. (1792) *The Statistical Account of Scotland*, vol. II, p. 126. Edinburgh: W. Creech.

EDINBURGH

(48) FERGUSON, T. Op. cit., p. 70.

(49) REGISTRAR-GENERAL FOR SCOTLAND (1914) *Fifty-seventh Annual Report . . . 1911*. Glasgow: H.M.S.O.

(50) REGISTRAR-GENERAL FOR SCOTLAND (1944) *Eighty-fifth Annual Report . . . 1939*. Edinburgh: H.M.S.O

(51) MAITLAND, W. (1753) *History of Edinburgh*, p. 112. Edinburgh: Hamilton, Balfour & Neill.

(52) Ibid., p. 62.

(53) ARNOT, H. (1779) *The History of Edinburgh*, p. 340. Edinburgh: W. Creech.

(54) FERGUSON, T. Op. cit., pp. 152–4.

(55) BAIRD, W. (1911) George Drummond: an eighteenth century Lord Provost. In *The Book of the Old Edinburgh Club*, vol. 4, p. 12. Edinburgh: Constable.

(56) CAMPBELL, R. H. & DOW, J. B. A. (1968) *Source Book of Scottish and Economic History*, pp. 230–1. Oxford: Blackwell.

(57) WRIGHT-ST. CLAIR, R. E. (1964) *Doctors Monro; a medical saga*, pp. 79–80. London: Wellcome Historical Medical Library.

(58) SMOUT, T. C. Op. cit., pp. 458–9.

(59) PRYDE, G. S. Op. cit., p. 84.

(60) FERGUSON, T. Op. cit., p. 9.

(61) Ibid., p. 52.

(62) EDINBURGH. City corporation (1929) *Edinburgh, 1329–1929* [Sexcentenary], p. 16. Edinburgh: Oliver & Boyd.

(63) BROWN, T. Op. cit., pp. 145–7.

(64) *Report on the Sanitary Conditions of the Labouring Population of Great Britain* (1842) Local reports on Scotland. Presented to Parliament, July, 1842. pp. 23f.

(65) LAMONT, J. of Newton (1830) *The Diary of Mr. John Lamont of Newton. 1649–1671*, ed. by G. R. Kinloch. (Maitland club, no. 7), p. 45. Edinburgh: James Clarke & Co.

(66) FERGUSON, T. Op. cit., p. 26.

(67) BAIRD, W. Op. cit., p. 5.

(68) FERGUSON, T. Op. cit., p. 21.

(69) COCKBURN, H. Op. cit., p. 294.

(70) FAIRLEY, J. A. (1911) The old tolbooth: with extracts from the original records. In *The Book of the Old Edinburgh Club*, vol. 4, pp. 93–4. Edinburgh: Constable.

(71) ARNOT, H. Op. cit., pp. 257–8.

(72) COMRIE, J. D. Op. cit., vol. I, p. 199.

(73) FERGUSON, T. Op. cit., p. 118.

(74) TURNER, A. L. (1937) *Story of a Great Hospital; the Royal Infirmary of Edinburgh, 1729–1929*, pp. 157–60. Edinburgh: Oliver & Boyd.

(75) Notices, statistical and historical, respecting the prevalence of dysentery in Scotland. (1831) *Glasgow Medical Journal*, **IV**, 13, 7–8.

(76) HUME, J. (1831) Case of the Edinburgh New Town epidemic. *Glasgow Medical Journal*, **IV**, 15, 229.

(77) CHRISTISON, Sir R., Op. cit., p. 145.

(78) Ibid., p. 144.

(79) DOUGLAS, A. H. (1844) Statistical report on the Edinburgh epidemic fever of 1843–44. *Northern Journal of Medicine*, **2**, 7, 8–22.

(80) DOUGLAS, A. H. (1845) Statistical report on the Edinburgh epidemic fever of 1843–44. *Northern Journal of Medicine*, **2**, 10, 209–20; **2**, 11, 269–78.

(81) FERGUSON, T. Op. cit., pp. 111–2.

(82) MACAULAY, T. B. (1914) *The History of England from the Accession of James the Second*, vol. V, p. 2468. London: Macmillan.

(82a) PASSMORE, R. & ROBSON, J. S., eds. (1974) *A Companion to Medical Studies*, vol. 3, p. 12.48. Oxford: Blackwell Scientific Publications.

(83) TAIT, H. P. (1957) The cholera board of health, Edinburgh, 1831–34. *Medical Officer*, **98**, 235–7.

(84) TURNER, A. L. Op. cit., p. 160.

(84a) MAGNUSSON, M. (1974) *The Clacken and the Slate; the story of the Edinburgh Academy, 1824–1974*, p. 178. London: Collins.

(85) LITTLEJOHN, Sir H. D. (1865) *Report on the Sanitary Condition of the City of Edinburgh*, p. 7. Edinburgh: Colston & Son.

(86) ARNOT, H. Op. cit., pp. 259–60.

(87) PRYDE, G. S. Op. cit., p. 253.

(88) LITTLEJOHN, Sir H. D. Op. cit., p. 22.

(89) FAIRLEY, J. A. Op. cit., p. 93.

(90) MAITLAND, W. Op. cit., p. 57.

(91) BAIRD, W. Op. cit., p. 22.

(92) FAIRLEY, J. A. Op. cit., p. 100.

(93) WAUGH, H. L. (1970) *George Watson's College; history and record, 1724–1970*, p. 4. Edinburgh: George Watson's College.

(94) THIN, R. (1927) *College portraits*, p. 57. Edinburgh: Oliver & Boyd.

(95) BOSWELL, J. (1958) *The Life of Johnson*, vol. II, p. 95. London: Dent (Everyman's Library).

(96) BOSWELL, J. Op. cit., p. 498.

(97) Ibid., pp. 499–500.

(98) Ibid., p. 73.

(99) ARNOT, H. Op. cit., p. 392.

(100) Ibid., p. 504.

(101) LAMONT, J. Op. cit., p. 53.

(102) FAIRLEY, J. A. Op. cit., p. 111.

(103) Ibid., p. 131.

(104) LAMONT, J. Op. cit., p. 13.

(105) Ibid., p. 218.

(106) BROWN, P. H. (1911) *History of Scotland to the Present Time*, vol. II, p. 354. London: Cambridge University Press.

(107) SMOUT, T. C. Op. cit., pp. 190 and 192.

(108) FAIRLEY, J. A. Op. cit., p. 91.

(109) ARNOT, H. Op. cit., pp. 322–3.

(110) STARK, J. (1847) *Inquiry into Some Points of the Sanatory State of Edinburgh*. Edinburgh: A. & C. Black.

(111) BROWN, T. Op. cit., pp. 148–52.

(112) COMRIE, J. D. Op. cit., vol. I, pp. 167–79.

(113) GAIRDNER, J. (1864) *Sketch of the Early History of the Medical Profession in Edinburgh*, p. 17. Edinburgh: Oliver & Boyd.

(114) DUNCAN, A. Op. cit., p. 5.

(115) POLLAK, K. (1968) *The Healers; the Doctor, then and now*. In collaboration with E. Ashworth Underwood, p. 109. London: Nelson.

(116) POOLE, R. Op. cit., p. 115.

(117) LAMONT, J. Op. cit., p. 158.

(118) EDINBURGH. City council. Archives (1940) *Extracts from the Records of the Burgh of Edinburgh, 1655 to 1665*, ed. by M. Wood, p. 322. Edinburgh: Oliver & Boyd.

(119) ARNOT, H. Op. cit., p. 168.

(120) RAE, J. (1895) *Life of Adam Smith*, p. 276. London: Macmillan.

(121) THOMSON, J. (1859) *An Account of the Life, Lectures and Writings of William Cullen, M.D.*, vol. I, p. 476. Edinburgh: Blackwood.

(122) COMRIE, J. D. Op. cit., vol. I, pp. 336–8.

(123) KAY, J. (1842) *A Series of Original Portraits and Caricature Etchings . . . with Biographical sketches and Anecdotes*, Vol. I, p. 30. Edinburgh: Paton.

(124) LITTLEJOHN, H. D. Op. cit., p. 42.

(125) BULLOUGH, V. & BULLOUGH, B. (1971) The causes of the Scottish medical Renaissance of the eighteenth century. *Bulletin of the History of Medicine*, **45**, 1, 20.

(126) Medical Commentaries for the year 1791 . . . Collected and published by Andrew Duncan. (1792), vol. VI. Edinburgh: Peter Hill.

(126a) CRAIG, J. (1972) A general dispensary practice 150 years ago. *Aberdeen University Review*, **XLIV**, 4, 362–3.

(127) LAUDER, Sir J., *Lord Fountainhall* (1759) *The decisions of the Lords of Council and Session from June 6th, 1678, to July 30th, 1712*. (2.ii.1686), vol. I, p. 399. Edinburgh: Hamilton & Balfour.

(128) SMILES, S. (1905) *The Autobiography*, ed. by T. Mackay, pp. 28–9. London: John Murray.

(129) COMRIE, J. D. Op. cit., vol. II, p. 606.

(130) POLLAK, K. Op. cit., p. 158.

(131) SCOTLAND. Dept. of Health (1944) *Report of the Inter-departmental Committee on Medical Schools* (The Goodenough Report). London: H.M.S.O.

Chapter II

SEEKING A CHARTER OF INCORPORATION: THREE ABORTIVE EFFORTS

There is not a fiercer hell than the failure in a great object.

John Keats

Success in obtaining the Charter of the College was the culmination of strenuous efforts exerted over a period of more than sixty years by physicians resident in the City of Edinburgh. On no fewer than three occasions, organized attempts towards this end failed when within reasonable distance of achievement. All attempts had as primary objective the remedying of the generally recognized far from satisfactory standards of medical practice in the City and bordering areas. Implied in the objective was the desire to improve the status of physicians in the community, and in relation to others practising the art of healing in a multitude of ways.

1617–21
(In the reign of James VI—I of England)

The first attempt was made in the year 1617 on the occasion of a visit to Edinburgh by the then reigning monarch, James VI of Scotland (I of England). An approach was made to the King to whom the views of the physicians as to the desirability of establishing a Society or Corporation were presented. There can be little doubt that the King issued orders dated 3rd July 1621 to Parliament directing that a College of Physicians be established in Edinburgh, in the following terms:

'Order by King James VI. to the Parliament, for a Colledge of Physitians there.
JAMES R.
Commissionaris and Estates of Parliament, we greit you heartilie well.
For sa meikle as we are certainlie informet of the gryte abuse done and practised

be ane number of ignorant and unskilfull persons, quha without knowledge of the science and facultye of medicine, being nather learned not graduat therin, presumes at thair awen hand to profess and practice physik and medicine, to the gryt and evident hazarde and danger of the lyffes and healthes of many of our subjects, quhilk evill is becume so ryff and frequent, that the samyne is lyklie to produce gryte harme and detriment except the samyn be tymouslie prevented; and seeing it perteines to us, out of our princelie and royall cair, to sie to the guid of that our realme, and to appoint and establish tharin sik convenient and cumlie order, as is observet in this our kingdome of Ingland, and other foreigne nationes, in the like caices: Therefor, it is our will and pleasure, that thair be ane Colledge and incorporation of the Professors of Medicine erected within that our kingdome, consisting of the number of seven persones, of quhom ane sall be elected and chosen yeirlie President and Deane of Facultie; quhilk seven persones and their successores to be chosen and elected in the places and roomes of the deceissand, sall have the liberties, priviledges, and immunities dew to ane Colledge and Incorporation, and sall be capable of all gifts, donationes, legacies, and other commodities to be gifted, disponed, or left to them, be whatsumever persone or persons; and sall have power to persue and defend in judgment, as ane body and incorporatione, and sall have and injoy the liberty of meitings and conventiones, all sik tymes as they pleise, for considering and adviseing upon all things necessar and expedient for the good of the said Faculty and Professors thereof; and to that effect sall have ane common seill, quhilk sall be callet the seill of the Facultie: And because we are not particularlie informet anent the persones who are fitt to make up the first Incorporatione; Therefor, it is our will, that ye informe yourselves theirof, and name and appoint seven persons, being Doctors and Professors of Physik and Medicine, of the best skill and estimation among yow, whom ye sall take sworne; and because the grytest hurt and skaithe done be the saide ignorant persones who presumes but (*without*) warrande to practise physik, is done and committeit within our burgh of Edinburgh, and countrie thereabout: Thairfor, it is our will that ye declaire and ordaine, that it sall not be lawfull to any persone or persons to presume to exerce and practise the said arte and science of physick and medicine within oure saide towne of Edin^r· or . . . miles about the samyn, except he be tryed be the saide Colledge and Incorporatione, and approven be their testimonial under thair subscription and common seill of the said Facultie: And siclyk, that ye give warrand to the said Colledge and Incorporation to make choise yeirlie of three of their number, who sall have the cair and charge, to searche and try the freschness and sufficiencie of all drogges, wares, and medicaments, being within all and whatsumever Apothecaries choppes within our said burgh of Edinburgh, and gif they be found corrupt and insufficient, to destroy the samyne, and that ye sett down penalties against the refusers or contraveners of the said statute: And also that ye resolve and conclude upon sik uther order and remedies quhilk sall be thought fitt or necessar by you for eschewing of the foresaids inconveniencies within the rest of the parts of our said Kingdome.

Given at our Manor of Otelandes, the third day of Julie 1621.

This conteynes your Majesties warrant to the Commissioners and Estates of Parliament for erecting of a College of Physitianes, and prohibiting wemen and ignorent persons to practice that arte in Scotland.

2nd August 1621.   GEORGE HAY.
The Lordis remittis the consideratione of this Article and Articles given in heirwith, to the consideration of the Lords of Secret Counsill, and whatsoever the saids Lords sall determine and ordain therintill, sall have the force of ane Act of Parliament, and stand in strength quhil it be alterit be sum public act againe.'[1]

DR GEORGE SIBBALD (OF GIBBLISTON)

Almost simultaneously with the issue of this order certain Articles were delivered to Parliament 'for the Facultie of Medicine, to be considered be the Estates'. Dr George Sibbald, uncle of (Sir) Robert Sibbald was one of the prime movers in the endeavours of the Edinburgh physicians. Among papers which, in the course of time, came into the hands of his nephew was one outlining the Articles. The historical value of this particular document, 'the first draught', cannot be over-estimated. It read as follows:

'Articles for the Facultie of Medicine to be considered be the Estates of Parliament.

First, it is humblie cravit that the saids Estates nominate and designe sevin persones of the profession of Medicine, to make up the number of the Incorporatione prescrivit be the statute signit be his Majestie.

Item, it is humblie cravit, that the saids estatis of parliament declaire and ordaine, that it sall not be lawfull to any person to take upon them the Arte of Apothecarie, except he be tryed and approvin be the said facultie, with the concourse of the bretherein of Apothecaries.

Item, that it sall not be lawfull to no person to practise Chyrurgerie, except he be tryed and approvin be the said facultie, with the concourse of the Bretheren of the Chirurgians.

Item, that it be defendit and forbiddin, that na person not being ane Apothecar, presume to sell medicinal drogues by smalls to his Majesties Lieges, but allenarly that they sell the samen be greattes to the Apothecaries, who hes skill and knowledge to try and consider of the freshness and goodness of the saids druggs, and who, by the statute, are ordeaned to be answerable for the samyne.

Item, It is humbly cravit that penalties be sett down be the said estatis, to be exacted from the contraueners of the said statute, and that order be appoynted for exacting of the samyne.

.   .   .   .   .

Item, that the said estaits give power and commission to the Lords of his Majestie's Secreit Counsell, to hear and considder of the saids overtures, and to conclude and determine thereupon, and upon all uther guid and expedient meanes whilk may furder and promote the said Facultie of Medicine within the kingdome, as the samen sall be proponed to their Lordships, be the brethren of the facultie in all tyme cumming.'[2]

SUPPORT LACKED FINALITY

Despite the apparent incisiveness of the order of July 1621, finality had not been reached as evidenced by a cautionary passage contained in the Articles sent for the consideration of the Estates. This particular passage observed:

> 'anent the ordour to be observed in the uther pairtes of the countrie, because the samin cannot be resolved without long deliberation, theirfor, it is humbly desyred that the said estaits give command and direction to the said Facultie to consult, advise, and resolue upon fittest and most expedient means for establishing of good order in the haill parts of the countrie, concerning the Professors and Practisers of Medicine, and to exhibit the samine to the Lords of his Majesties Secret Counsell.'[3]

STRENGTH AND SOURCE OF OPPOSITION

The proposals for the establishment of a College came to naught as a result of opposition, in the main by the Bishops of the Church, but in part by the chirurgeons of the time. Dealing with the power of the Bishops in the Secret Council and referring to the events of 1621 a physician wrote some forty years later:

> 'His Majesty (James VI) referring to the consideration thereof to his Council, whereof in these times the Bishops were come to make up a great part, and were become in that Consistory so powerful that they did indeed sway all,—they finding the petitioners most of them inconform to the innovations in worship they were then about establishing, did in this withdraw their favour so from them, that though they were ashamed to be found professed owners of such horrid impiety, to stop or deny openly and absolutely notions and desires so liquidly just, yet became obdured to own so much of it as to work the equivalent, by even proroguing from day to day the honest intenders, till they got them at last wearied out.'[4]

This comment must be evaluated in the light of the prevailing position whereby the Archbishops and Bishops were the Chancellors of the three older Universities which possessed exclusive rights for the conferment of degrees. While the Bishops may have had genuine doubts about the known or alleged religious non-conformity of those submitting a case for a College, they were also apprehensive lest their prescriptive privileges should be restricted. Likewise the Corporation of Surgeons in Edinburgh were fearful that serious curtailment of their rights and activities might eventuate.

1630–4
(In the reign of Charles I)

Efforts by the physicians of Edinburgh were renewed in 1630. Charles I was on the throne by this time and he referred the entire subject to his Privy Council. Subsequently a decreet of the Lords instructed the physicians of Edinburgh, specified by name 'to give in some heads and articles' for the erection of a College of Physicians. The physicians gave effect to the instructions by submitting seventeen Articles ostensibly by 'the Graduate Doctors in that facultie, Inhabitants of the Towne of Edinburghe, and in the name of all uther Graduate Doctors in the said Facultie within the Kingdome'.[5]

PROPOSALS SAVOURED OF AUTHORITARIANISM

The following were among features of the Articles:

(1) an implication that the Graduate Doctors to constitute the College would be 'of the reformed religion, received, and publikly professed, within this Kingdome'.

(2) authority to have 'a Counsell-house within the towne of Edinburgh, Canongait, or Suburbs, or within a mile theirof'.

(3) possession of a Common Seal, to be called 'The Seale of the Facultie of Medicine'.

(4) choice of the President and Councillors should always be 'out of the number of the Graduate Doctors of the Societie . . . of Edinburgh'.

(5) prohibition of the sale of 'any drogues of dangerous quality . . . to any whatsomever, except allenarly either to the Apothiquhers, or to the Physitians of the foresaid Incorporation, or Licentiats from the said Colledge, or to such others as has their warrand and ordinance for the same'.

(6) no Chirurgeon or Apothecary to practise their arts without previous trial and examination by the College, the examination to be made 'with concurrence of the "masters and freemen in Chirurgerie within Edinburgh",' and that of the Apothecaries in particular to be 'in presence of the Masters, Apothiquhers, and freemen of the said towne for the tyme'.

(7) '. . . the tryall and examination of the Licentiats or (persons) to be promoted to the degree of Doctorate, be made in the whole Societie and Fellowshipe of Edinburgh, with liberty to whatsoever other Graduate Doctors of the whole incorporation through the Kingdome, to concurr with them in the said tryall and examinatione, if they please; but the Promoters to the degree of Doctorate to be only the Graduate Doctors of the fellowship of Edinburgh, and these *per vices*, the eldest Physitian of Edinburgh beginning, and so consequently by order.'

(8) prohibition against the practise of medicine, except by the Doctors of the College, and those authorised and licensed by letters-testimonial.

(9) within Edinburgh 'and 24 miles round about' practice to be the sole preserve of the physicians of the 'said Societie and fellowship of . . . Edin[r].'—but, without 'prejudice always, to whatsoeuer Graduate Doctors within the Kingdome, of the incorporatione, to be called and admitted at the desyre of the patients to consultations withe the Physitians of the said fellowship, within the said towne . . .'

(10) measures for dealing with 'manie abusers and ignorant persons, never trained up, nather in medicine nor good literature' who take to themselves the style of Doctors of Medicine. All existing Graduate Doctors and all new Graduated Doctors were to appear in Edinburgh with their credentials and matriculate with the 'Colledge and Incorporation, as Members thereof'. Exception was provided for those entitled to the style of Doctor acquired at 'some famous University abroad' or from the College and Incorporation.

(11) no Chirurgeon within Edinburgh should 'take blood of any person, or undertake the cure of any aposteme, ulcer, fracture, or wounde, or any other thing requiring chirurgicall operatione, which may be deadlie or dangerous for the life of the deseased or a wounded person (such as are the woundes of the head, stomach, diaphragme, bellie, bladder, lightes, and liuer or great vessels,) without the advise and counsell of one of the . . . Physitianes of Edin[r]., except in case of present necessitys, and that no deposition be given up, to any Judge whatsoever be chirurgians anent any wounded person, or the quality of the wounde or woundes, but at the sighting, and under the hand and subscriptione and forme of the Doctors of the said Societie, together with the Masters in Chirurgie of the said Towne . . .'

(12) the institution of measures for the warning and summoning of delinquents, to enlist the co-operation of magistrates, and to ensure that 'all keepers of wardes and prissons . . . accept and receaue . . . all and every such persone or persones so offending, as sall be committed to them from the . . . Colledge'.[6]

Among the papers inherited by (Sir) Robert Sibbald from his uncle Dr George Sibbald was a draft copy of the above Articles. With them was a scroll of a petition in Dr George Sibbald's hand to Parliament, 'the substance wheirof is as followeth:

The graduate doctors humbly sute and crave, that their persons, their callings, their dwelling houses, may obtane and injoy these immunities, liberties and priviledges, which, with much tyme, travell and charges, is obtained over seas from divers Schooles and Universities, and haue been granted for many ages by the most of Princes and Republiks in Christendome to presbiters, mediciners and lawers, that their persons be not pressed to any military service, that their callings be not vilified with the name or condition of any trade or traffick, and that their lodgings and dwelling-houses be not troubled nor molested with any sojors or quarterings whatsumever, for that they use no merchant trade, nor traffick with money, and doe not agree for fies or rewardes with any man, nor craue the same after they haue deserved them, and their persons ought to be (as they are ever readie) quatenus fert valetudo, aetas, &s. to visite and attend their ordinarie and customable patients, according to their urgent simptomes and necessities, quod in bello fieri nequit: that their persons be not oblidged to watch or waird any towne, castell or fortresse, nor yett stented, taxed, or compelled to pay any soume of money for any of the said military duties for maintenance of their Guards or Garrisones, or maintenance of any souldier, "Presbiteri, Medici, Juris periti, Doctores, Professores, etc. debent esse immunes ab omnibus belli muniis, oneribus, sumptibus, hospitationibus, etc."

Item, that every Graduate Physitiane of the Colledge ought and may exerce and practise any parte of Physike, and namely, of Surgery, according to the licences and priviledges of their Doctorate: that some of the Physitians be made censores of all other parts and offices of physike, to haue the inspection and censure thereof, and namely, in the matter of admitting prentises to be masters in Surgery, and in the censuring of faultes admitted by these prentises, or by the Surgeons themselves in the work of their calling, to judge thereupon, togither with the Masters of the said calling; and that because of the manifold abuses that arise dayly upon the admission of ignorant prentises, and euen because of the unskilfulness of the extortion of the Lieges for their fees, or other fautes in diligence, dyet etc. admitted too oftine be many common Surgions.'[7]

DISILLUSIONMENT

There is little in the way of precise information to account for the lack of any developments after submission of the above Articles by the physicians. Basically the reason may well have been the unsettled state of public affairs in general.

The position in which the King found himself was by no means easy. This is apparent in the following recommendation submitted by him to 'his Privie Counsel':

'Right trustie and weelbeloved Cousin and Counsellor . . . and trustie and weelbeloved Counsellors wee greete you weell. Whereas we understand that our late royall Father did wrythe to his privie Counsell signifying that though he gave warrant for ane act to pass in parliament in favore of the physitians for restraining the practice of ignorant and unskilfull, yett it was not his meaning that they should prejudge the Chyrurgians in their auncient and lawfull priviledges. To whitche purpose a complaint hath beene made to us in behalfe of the Chyrurgians that they may not be wronged as they informe us is intendit by the physitians. Wee being willing to take the lyke course that our late father did and that none of them do trench upon others by making use of the misteries and skill peculiar to their severall arts. Our pleasure is that you call the cheife of both within Edr. and Canongaitt befor you and so compose and order the differences among theme as they may not wrong ane another, upon such penalties as you and all thinke fitt to prescribe. And whereas the Chirurgians have petitioned that wee wold be pleased to recommend to you to cause setle and ratifie some overtures amongst themselfes and their apprentices for the better discharging of their trade and goode of our subjects according to the enclosed note of their demands. Our further pleasure is that you consider theirof recommending for you to caus such of theme to be settled and ordered as you upon hearing of theme sall condescend upon. Which recommending to your care wee bid you fairwell. From our Court at Whythall the 28 of October 1634.'[8]

Nevertheless there is interest in the following extract from a manuscript of 1657, a copy of which is in the possession of the College:

> 'They were, as said is, from time to time, from Parliament to Parliament, always delayed till the year 1633, that King Charles came to Scotland to be crowned. Then the business having been strongly recommended by the Lords of the Articles chosen for that Parliament,—nothing using by them to be so recommended but what was really concluded by them to be of unquestionable utility for the public, and necessary should be enacted,—to the Parliament: they being not to sit any time, were pleased to enact its reference to the Privy Council for despatching it,— which act may be seen inrolled among the unprinted Acts of that Parliament, 1633, where it resteth to this hour. The well-meaning petitioners, being become by that time many of them aged, but all of them wearied out with toil, did of necessity desist thereafter from any further prosecution of it, but left it with them, and till the last year it was never publickly spoken of.'[9]

Doubt exists as to the authorship of the manuscript. It has been attributed to Sir Robert Sibbald but this is not generally accepted.[10] Almost certainly the writer was an older man. One possibility is that it was Dr George Sibbald who was as active in furthering the petition of 1630 as he had been that of 1617; another possibility is that the writer was Dr George Purves who was particularly involved in the third later effort to obtain a Charter. Writing of his uncle's terminal efforts Robert Sibbald said 'This is all I finde done in my uncle his tyme, he heth this reflectione upon it, that the maitter was delayed and abstructed by those men, as sould and ought most to haue furthered the same for their own private ends and interests'.[11]

1656–60
(In the time of Oliver Cromwell, Lord Protector)

Not what they want but what is good for them.

Oliver Cromwell

Following the death of Dr George Sibbald new proposals were drawn up for the creation of a College of Physicians. Minutes of meetings arranged for this purpose were signed by the following eighteen Doctors[11]:

A. Ramsay	D. Balfour	D. Oughterlony
Al. Meirting	Wm. Macgill	T. Gordon
Ja. Leslie	J. Saintserf	Silvester Rattray
Thomas Gleg	Ro. Strachane	D. Moire
Tho. Forbesse	Alexr. Yeoman	George Purvass
Ro. Burnett	D. Bethune	D. Patone

PRELIMINARIES

According to Robert Sibbald, the 'project for the Colledge was mainly managed by Doctor George Purvass, a man of great parts, and of much boldness and vivacity of spirit, and who was of a pragmatick temper, and did not spare charges nor paines for to accomplish the designe'.[12]

On one occasion in 1657, bearing a letter signed by five of his colleagues Purves (or Purvass) visited the Royal College of Physicians of London where acting on instructions the registrar gave him every assistance in looking through the statutes. It would seem that tact and diplomacy were on occasion among Purves' 'great parts' because the letter which he took with him praised the London College for 'its discoveries of the hidden secrets of nature, admired by the whole world'.[13] Those signing the letter included Robert Burnett, George Rayns, Henry Henryson, Robert Cunningham and James Calhoun. By some misunderstanding, the history of the London College referring to Dr Purves' visit in 1657 describes him 'as a representative of a newly founded college of physicians' in Edinburgh, and later makes the comment 'The Edinburgh college seems to have been shortlived'.[13]

In passing it should be mentioned that Comrie suggested that Alexander Ramsay, rather than Purves 'was the first, and presumably therefore the most outstanding' among those urging the application for a Charter.[14] This is debatable. Ramsay graduated M.D. in Basel (1610): became a Fellow of the Royal College of Physicians of London (1618): and was a physician to Charles I in 1635.

'PUBLIK ABUSES'

Two documents relevant to this third attempt to establish a College of Physicians in Edinburgh are of importance. Of them the first is one 'giving' in the words of Robert

Sibbald 'account of the publik abuses in maitters of medicine'. These abuses were recorded by those of Purvass' time as:

(1) The frequent murders committed universallie in all parts . . . by quacks, women, gardiners and others grossly ignorant . . .

(2) The unlimited and unaccountable practises of Chirurgeons, Apothecaries and Empericks pretending to medicines . . . all these undertaking the cure of all diseases without advice or assistance of Physitanes.

(3) The unwarrantable vending of drugs, simple and compound, by Drugists and Apothicaries, not only in common sale, but in the dispensing Physitianes receipts . . . without security taken from the buyer, or any other restraint, as is found by the great difference in medicines in their operatione here from what is found abroad.

(4) The exorbitant prices of drugs . . .

(5) The great abuse lately established in Edinburgh and other cities, by ingrossing promiscuously these two Trades into one Incorporatione, whence many not bred in these airts sett up to the greate prejudice of the patient and discredite of the Physitians.

(6) The great charges and difficulties Students of Medicine are putt to in travelling abroad for educatione and degrees in the science of Medicine . . .

(7) The great losse Physitians are at, in not improving their learning by Professors.

(8) The advantages would accrue to all the nation, if, as other well governed Countries, they had such settlements of privileidges for Physitians here, and Literature would to the nations honour advance.[15]

INVESTIGATIONS AT CROMWELL'S BEHEST

The document concerning 'publik abuses' together with articled proposals for a Societie and Colledge of Physitians were submitted to Cromwell, then Lord Protector. In June 1656, the Lords of Council in the course of reviewing measures for the improvement of medical practice appointed a Commission or Board of Physicians to obtain information and offer advice. The Commission numbered five and included two Englishmen, Doctors Wright and Bate, both of whom were physicians to Cromwell.[16] Wright is reputed to have been in particular favour with his political master. Unanimous agreement was reached by the Commission as to the expediency of establishing a College, and their recommendations to the Lords of Council to that effect incorporated particular proposals concerning the constitution. The Council conveyed their conclusions to the Protector in the form of a letter signed by one of their number (the Lord President of Cromwell's Council in Scotland). Referring to the complaints concerning charlatan practice and the abuse of drugs, the signatory

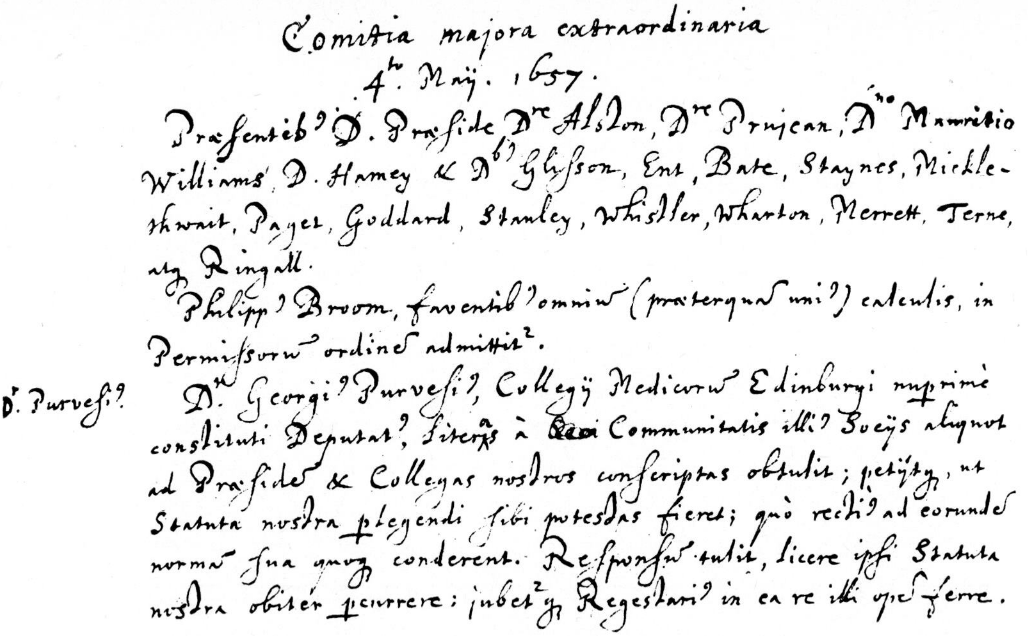
Comitia majora extraordinaria
4to Maij. 1657.

Praesentibus D. Praeside Dre Alston, Dre Prujean, Dno Mauritio Williams, D. Hamey & Dris Glisson, Ent, Bate, Staynes, Micklethwait, Paget, Goddard, Stanley, Whistler, Wharton, Merrett, Terne, atque Ringall.

Philippus Broom, faventibus omnium (praeterquam unius) calculis, in Permissorum ordinem admittitur.

D. Purvesius Dr Georgius Purvesius, Collegij Medicorum Edinburgi nuperrime constituti Deputatus, literasque à Communitatis illius Socijs aliquot ad Praesidem & Collegas nostros conscriptas obtulit; petijtque, ut Statuta nostra perlegendi sibi potestas fieret; quo rectius ad eorundem normam sua quoque conderent. Responsum tulit, licere ipsi Statuta nostra obiter percurrere; jubeturque Registrarius in ea re illi operam ferre.

PLATE 2a Extract from Minutes of Royal College of Physicians of London. (*See* Appendix B)

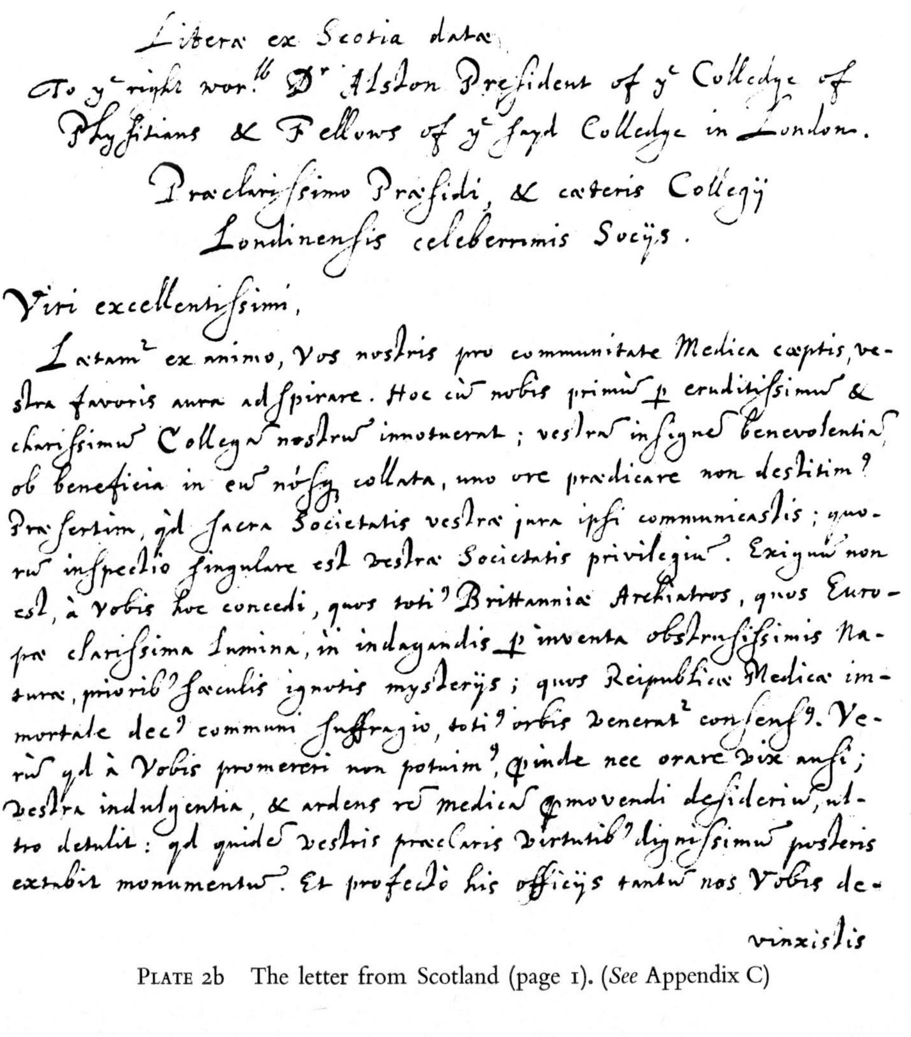
Litera ex Scotia data

To ye right wor.ll Dr Alston President of ye Colledge of Physitians & Fellows of ye sayd Colledge in London.

Praeclarissimo Praesidi, & caeteris Collegij Londinensis celeberrimis Socijs.

Viri excellentissimi,

Laetamur ex animo, Vos nostris pro communitate Medica coeptis, vestrae favoris auram adspirare. Hoc cum nobis primum per eruditissimum & charissimum Collegam nostrum innotuerat; vestram insignem benevolentiam, ob beneficia in eum nostrûmque collata, uno ore praedicare non destitimus. Praesertim, quod sacra Societatis vestrae jura ipsi communicastis; quorum inspectio singulare est vestrae Societatis privilegium. Exiguum non est, à vobis hoc concedi, quos totius Brittanniae Archiatros, quos Europae clarissima lumina, in indagandis per inventa obstrusissimis Naturae, prioribus saeculis ignotis mysterijs; quos Reipublicae Medicae immortale decus communi suffragio, totius orbis veneratur consensus. Verum quod à Vobis promereri non potuimus, quod inde nec orare vix ausi; vestra indulgentia, & ardens rem medicam promovendi desiderium, ultro detulit: quod quidem vestris praeclaris virtutibus dignissimum posteris extabit monumentum. Et profecto his officijs tantum nos Vobis de-

vinxistis

PLATE 2b The letter from Scotland (page 1). (*See* Appendix C)

dinxistis, ut quibꝰ verbis gratias agamꝰ, vehementer hae-
sitem? Sunt enim in Vobis omnia augustiora, quã quo cona-
tus nostri infirmitas ꝓvenire queat. Supersunt tamen vota; &
si non beneficijs vestris parē, nostro tamen in Vos studio,
quantã cogitando consequi possumꝰ, meritas debitãꝗ gratias
referimꝰ. Et ꝓ officia, quæ præstitistis, ꝓ medicinæ honorē,
ꝓ vestra dignitate, ꝓ generis humani in hoc regno sanita-
tē, obnixè rogamꝰ obtestamúrꝗ, ut Medicinã inter nos
oberrantis commiseceamini; cui vim inferunt Empirici,
agyrtæ, chirurgi, pharmacopæi, & omnes ψευδίατροι.
Submissè etiã petimꝰ, ut consuetã humanitate Parvesiũ
nostrũ complectamini, omnibúsꝗ consilijs, commune rei
Medicæ bonũ spectantibꝰ opitulemini, & ulteriori ve-
strorũ Actorũ inspectione dignemini. Sic Vos nostræ
reipublicæ medicæ eritis promotores; sic Vestri nominis
splendor Scotiæ τò σκότος irradiabit; neꝗ ulla rerũ
humanarũ vicissitudine, aut excedentis ævi viribꝰ dele-
bit², sed æternitati consecrabit². Valete.

V. V. Excell.   Ro. Burnett? Geo. Rayus
observantissimi.   Henr. Henrysonꝰ. Ro. Cunningamiꝰ
                                        Ja. Cathonni?.

PLATE 2c   The letter from Scotland (page 2)

Litera responsoria

Excellentissimis ornatissimisq̃ Viris D.D.
Præsidi & Socijs Collegij Medicoru᷎
Edinburgi nuper constituti. —

Clarissimi ornatissimiq̃ Viri,

Sæviente apud Nos nupâ belli civilis procellâ, met᷎ erat
ne infami plurimis naufragijs ƥopulo illideren᷎ ᷍& ludibrio
essem᷎ ijsdẽ ventis. Nempe inter Varia Reipublicæ turbamen-
ta, nostra quoq̃ Ars auctoritate suâ non paru᷎ mulctata fuit?
du᷎, semoto legu᷎ metu (quaru᷎ neglectu fomenta subdunt᷎ atq̃
alebria improbitati) tenebriones, agyrtæ, seplasiarij, tonsores,
an᷎ fatidicæ, aliaq̃ id gen᷎ vitulamina, sperabilis indemnitatis
aurâ affulgente, sacra nostra involabant. Nimiru᷎ acre in-
citamentu᷎ audendi quæslibet, lucru᷎ est: præsertim illis, qui ad
esuritionis incitas redacti, Libitinæ vota sua exsolvere per-

timescunt.

PLATE 2d   The reply (page 1). (*See* Appendix D)

timescunt. Sed nos servavit Apollo: debita scil. tam
praeclara Arti reverentia, & concessa jus olim à summis Po-
testatib? irrefragabilis auctoritas, extegis illis medendi licen-
tias plurimũ retulit; restituétq; brevi (uti speram?) in in-
tegrũ tã nobili tibiq; necessaria Professioni suũ decus. Qua-
propter & Vobis etiã gratulamur plurimũ, Viri doctissimi, qd
ad eandes normã Collegiũ extruere, & è face plebis Vos exi-
mere statuistis, amplisq; privilegijs auctoritate vestrã commu-
nivistis. Quippe ijs legib? effrenatã impitorũ Medicastrorũ
audaciã coercebitis, qui temerarijs ausis morborũ sibi incogni-
torũ medelas aggrediuntur: artisq; dignitas foedè commaculata,
resarcietur in posterũ. Accedit & aliud commodũ: quòd so-
ciatis hoc pacto operis, animisq;, Medicinã pomoeria feliciùs
promovebitis, Viriq; ad ornamentũ seculi; artisq; Apollineæ
gloriã nati, quib? honesto prudentiãq; cordi pect? est, ala-
crius scientiã nostrã fines proferent, ejusdéq; dignitate praeclaris suis virtutib? constabilient. Convénit nos, Vir huma-
nitatis atq; eruditionis singularis, D. Purvesi? literásq; vestras
gratissimas obtulit: eidéq; Statuta nostra, ac regiminis for-
mã plustrandi copiã fecim?: & si qua alia in re opã nostrã
Vobis uti commodũ videbit; scitote, nos desiderijs vestris
nequaquã defuturos: simúlq; salutes interminã, ac prospera
omnia ex animo apprecamur. Valete.

Datũ Londini 7°
Maij. An° supra mille-
simũ & sexcentesimũ
quinquagesimo septimo.

Geor. Enti? M. D. Coll.
Lond. Soci? & Regestrar?

wrote piquantly 'Your Highness' Council were more clearly convinced of the evil than of what might be an effectual and adequate remedy.' Continuing he explained that the Council 'found, that, as the want of a College of Physicians in Scotland occasioned the ill, so the erection of a College . . . might cure it,—at least in a high and good degree lessen and prevent it'.[17]

The writer of the letter, being indisposed, delegated responsibility for delivering the letter to Dr Purves, explaining to the Protector at the same time that 'being necessitated for some time to repair to the country to follow more undisturbedly a little course of physic, I have presumed humbly by letter to impart this unto your Highness: lest the bearer hereof, Dr Purves, might wait too long . . . Dr Wright, and several others in this city are informed of the thing itself, and convinced of the necessity and advantages of it, who, together with Dr Purves, may give your Highness satisfaction in many doubts which may arise . . .'[18]

Cromwell with little delay commended the various documents and their contents to the Council, which in turn appointed a Committee of three of their members to give the proposals for a College in Edinburgh urgent and serious consideration. This committee obtained reports from physicians of the College of London, and the legal opinions of the Attorney- and Solicitor-Generals; and examined 'an agreement upon the explication and restriction of every one of the articles between, and mutually signed by, the Provost [of Edinburgh], then the City's Commissioner at London, and him of our number [most probably Dr Purves] who was by us commissioned for prosecution of obtainment of the patent'.[19]

CHARTER CONDONES IRRATIONAL CLAIMS

A Charter was duly sealed and sent to Scotland, requiring the erection within the city of Edinburgh of a 'Societie and Colledge of Physitians . . . which should consist of a President and Fellowes under the name of a President and Colledge of Physitians of Scotland . . . who should have power and authoritie to oversie, rule, and order what may concerne the right administratione of Physike to the people of Scotland, in all pairts . . . with power to them to censure and punish all persones who shall presume to practise, exercise or profess Physick or give Medicines, or ordaine Physicall praescriptiones in any pairts or place in Scotland, being not Members of the said Colledge, or not being approved and licensed by the said President and Colledge under the common seall.' On the pretext that 'the science of Physick doth comprehend, include and containe in it the knowledge of Chirurgery, being a speciall part of the same and member thereof' the President and College were to be em-powered to practise the Art of Chirurgery 'save only within the cities of Edinburgh and Glasgow'. Under the Charter the examination and licensing of Apothecaries and the inspection of their shops were to become the responsibility of the College. Apothecaries approved by the College were to be answerable to Censors appointed by the College in the matter of the 'Sufficiencie of their Simples and Compoundes, imployable for the use of the people'. A final provision was to the effect that the College was entitled to accept from the magistrates of cities and burghs and the Sheriffs of counties 'such dead bodies of malefactors executed, as they shall desyre, for making of dissection and anatomie . . .'[20]

By the terms of the Charter, the Colledge

> 'for the time was to be made up of Alexr. Dowglass, William Macgill, George Rae, John Balfour, William Patoun, James Beatoun, George Purvess, Robert Cuninghame, Andrew Moire, Alexr. Martine, Alexr. Yeoman, Robert Burnett, Thomas Gleg, George Hepburne, Silvester Ratra, Henry Henrysone, James Leslie, William Moire, John Sinserfe and James Colhoune.'[21]

VARIED AND VIOLENT PROTESTS

The terms of the Patent produced severe, indeed violent reactions in many quarters. In Edinburgh and elsewhere burgh councils took umbrage at what they regarded as threatened infringement of their liberties. The City of Glasgow allied itself to the opposition, being influenced by the existence of the Charter possessed by the City Faculty which with physicians, embraced chirurgeons and apothecaries. Surgeons in Edinburgh were in the forefront of those protesting and, in virtue of their associa-tion as members of a trade guild with the Town Council, were in a position to enlist civic support for their resistance. With reason, the surgeons saw in the terms of the Charter belittlement of their experience and ability, and restriction of their activities. While of only limited significance, the provisions made for supplies of dead bodies to the physicians contrasted with the one malefactor's body per year which had been the prerogative of the barber–surgeons over decades.

At the time in question the surgeons were conscious of invasion of their territory by two types of practitioner—the 'unincorporated physicians and incorporated apothecaries' and their reaction was intensified by the conviction that since the early sixteenth century surgeons had been 'the sole teachers and almost the sole practitioners' in Edinburgh.[22] Moreover, exception was taken to the fact that, for the most part, medical degrees held by those pressing for a College of Physicians had been awarded by foreign universities. At the time, few degrees had been awarded by Scottish Universities and none by the University of Edinburgh, and there were fears that the proposed College would model itself on continental customs which encouraged a medical aristocracy with surgeons as their subservient underlings. One form of immediate protective action taken by the Corporation of Surgeons was to transmit a petition asking that ambiguities in the Patent should be cleared up, and that before the Charter acquired final acquiescence in law the Council of State should be enabled to give full consideration 'to every one's just rights and privileges'. Inevitably consideration of the petition led to delay.[23]

Wrath was not confined to the surgeons in Edinburgh. Those in Glasgow were quick to notice that Cromwell's Charter contemplated the establishment in Edinburgh of a College of Physicians for Scotland. As members of the Glasgow Faculty they speedily enlisted support and at a meeting of the Faculty in June 1657 they 'did all in one voice Commissionat and Impower Johne Hall and Mr. Arch. Grahame to goe to Edg^r to advocat and oppose the sam, before the Counsall of Stait'. It has been suggested on good evidence that a clandestine approach to the Glasgow Faculty was at one time made with a view to obtaining support for the Edinburgh project. This could explain why the deacon of chirurgeons was summoned as officer of a city guild to appear before the City Council and given implicit instructions. Leaving the Council he reported to the Faculty and 'did demand of them whither they would adher to ther old gift or joyne w^t the prīt calling of Physitianes. They did all in on voyce adher to ther old gift.'[24]

The universities added their weight to the growing resistance. In particular this applied to the University of Aberdeen which maintained that there had been 'an actual profession of Medicine many years erected, established, and stipended, with a learned Doctor of Medicine in the place, for some years ago, exercing and orderly teaching and professing Medicine in all its parts'. Because by its Charter this University could 'licence every of their graduates to teach and exerce their respective professions, into which they are graduated, as wide as any who take their degrees at Paris or Bononia (Bologna) i.e. *hic et ubique terrarum*', it considered that the powers contemplated for the College of Physicians in respect of granting licences and imposing examinations would of necessity 'exceedingly injure . . . the just rights and powers' of their University.[25]

A MEETING OF PHYSICIANS AT DUNDEE

The Aberdeen views were given at a meeting in July 1657 at Dundee attended by physicians from Edinburgh and Aberdeen, and called for the express purpose of considering the policy and some of the possible repercussions arising from the proposed College of Physicians. Following discussion the Physicians from Edinburgh conceded that there should be no encroachment or lessening of the existing privileges of the Universities where graduating students or bona fide qualified persons were concerned. Among those present from Edinburgh were Alex^r Yeoman, Sylvester Rattray, Alex^r Martin, John Saintserf, David Balfour, D. Bethunn, D. Ochterlony, John Paton and George Purves. An account of the conference written by the last named and transcribed by Dr John Boswell eventually came into the possession of Mr Alexander Boswell, one time Clerk to the College. At the conclusion of the conference the Physicians of Edinburgh were empowered to draw up an explanatory account of the 'true state of the business on hand'. The probability is that Purves' account was the official one in this sense.[26]

No surgeons were present at the meeting. None the less discussion of surgical and pharmaceutical considerations was not precluded. Whatever the conflict on matters academic, there was an impressive if not altogether surprising unanimity of views concerning the desirable limits to apply to the activities of surgeons. In many respects the limitations considered desirable corresponded to those set out in the Articles submitted to Charles I by the physicians of Edinburgh. Two elaborations deserve mention. Liberty was granted to surgeons 'to cure the Lues Venerea—as full liberty as they have hitherto been in custom of': and those of 'the inferior grade' were to be permitted to undertake vivisection. Inferior grade presumably referred to the apothecaries or maybe the barbers. Small wonder that in later years a senior surgeon delivering a historical lecture saw fit to declare that 'The self-conceit of the physicians of those days took a dangerous direction, for they thought themselves the proper persons to govern the untitled members of the profession': and that surgeons saw in the proposals of 1657 'nothing short of annihilation as a body, and subjection, as individuals, to the caprices of a pragmatic and irresponsible depotism'.[27] In the words of a physician of the time 'The Chirurgeons . . . made . . . a buzzling and a stour, and wanted not their prop likeways, as now they have from the Town of Edinburgh.'[28] Such was the persistent deep-seated embitterment of the surgeons that even although by their delaying tactics, they had successfully contributed to rejection of the Charter of 1656–7, they continued to regard it as having been a calculated, malicious 'plot'. Determined to forestall a recurrence their Edinburgh Guild approved and passed a motion in 1672 'for erecting the Colledge of Edinburgh into ane Universitie' as 'a caveat against all hazards by a Colledge of Phisitians'.[29]

With the death of Cromwell proposals for the establishment of a College of Physicians lapsed into abeyance; and with some justification it can be said, those who aimed at fulfilling them 'by grasping at too much, lost all'. As to the prime mover of the venture in 1656, John Lamont in his diary, records:

> 'Doctor Puruis [sic] phesitian, depairted out of this life att Edenboroughe, and was interred ther, Decr. 1661. Some say that he was loath to die, and said, "What! can nether God nor money save a life?" And afterward—"Bot now I sie that all men are mortall." '[30]

Review of the three abortive attempts to erect a College of Physicians reveals how with the passage of time the aspirations of the physicians underwent elaboration and extension. The orders (1621) of James I to his Parliament contemplated the College having Edinburgh as its sphere of influence and authority: but the Charter of the Lord Protector (1633) proposed legislation for the erection in Edinburgh of a College of Physicians of Scotland with national responsibilities. Whereas by the terms of the Charter of 1621 the College was to consist of not more than seven persons, the number was increased to nine in 1633. Moreover, whereas initially vacancies were to be filled by choice and election, the second Charter accepted that those granted the right to practise were automatically held eligible as successors on the occurrence of vacancies in the College, although in the ultimate, inclusion in the College was determined by election. In the Charter of 1633 there was reference for the first time to the award by the College of a degree of Doctorate. In contrast with their Articles of 1621 which made no more than a plea for trial and approval of those contemplating surgery, the physicians in 1633 recommended proposals which can be described unequivocally as almost wholly obnoxious. At the same time and with greater reasons, the Articles of 1633 proposed the tightening of existing regulations relating to the activities of Apothecaries.

Criticism of the early efforts of the Edinburgh physicians is easy on the score of acquisitiveness, aggressiveness and impetuosity. Robert Sibbald's views in this connection are of special interest. He gave them in a letter presumed to have been sent by him to Lord Perth. The letter opened with reference to communications concerning her health from 'my Lady Murray' and 'Doctor Needham her ordinary who is a physician of very great reputation'. The letter then continued 'My Lord there is an affaire now in agitation wherein I am deeplie concerned . . . and . . . beg your favour and assistance. It is this—the Physicians in and about this place have been long waiting the opportunitie of seeking to be created into a Colledge or Society. . . .' Having summarized steps taken towards this end in previous years the writer continued—'Thereafter some of the Physicians in this place, particularlie Doctor Purvas endeavoured in the tyme of the late rebellion to obtain a patent from Oliver but in regard it contained many exorbitancies and encroachments upon the Universities, it met with so much opposition as made it ineffectual; but by none was it more withstood than by the Surgeons.'[31]

When all is said and done the facts about the sixteenth and seventeenth centuries are sparse. The fault of the physicians then, if faults they were, are to be found to this day in our present-day society. What should not be forgotten in any consideration of the abortive efforts to found a College of Physicians in Edinburgh are the prodigious pioneer efforts of such men as Dr George Sibbald and Dr George Purves. They lived in tempestuous times. Religious and political strife were always near at hand. To travel long distances was no mean task—nor always safe. (Robert Sibbald in his autobiography tells of meeting highwaymen on one occasion, and of being pursued by a dragoon 'with a drawen Bagonet' on another.[32]) As pioneers the early physicians were suspect by those with whom they had to negotiate, and had to contend with the eternal wariness of central authority. Overshadowing all was the deplorable state of medicine whether as an art or science. Standards could not bear comparison with those on the Continent or for that matter with contemporary England. No matter their stature, they faced these difficulties with pertinacity and conviction, and in doing so unwittingly paved the way to ultimate success. It is not without significance that Sir Robert Sibbald referred so fully in his memoirs to his uncle Dr George Sibbald, and to George Sibbald's successor Dr George Purves.

Nor is it irrelevant to quote here Sibbald's tribute to his uncle on another matter. 'By the advice of my uncle by the Father side, Doctor George Sibbald, Physician in Edinburgh, I sucked till I was two yeers and two moneths old, and could run up and down the street, and speake, because my other brothers and sisters had dyed hectick: which long sucking proved, by the blessing of God, mean to preserve me alive.'[33] The wet-nurse became for many years a devoted retainer in the Sibbald household. Dr George Sibbald's paediatric prowess has been given less publicity than his persistent pioneering.

REFERENCES

1617–21

(1) SIBBALD, Sir R. (1837) *Memoirs of the Royal College of Physicians at Edinburgh*, pp. 3–5. Edinburgh: Thomas Stevenson.

(2) Ibid., pp. 5–6.

(3) Ibid., p. 6.

(4) [PURVES, G.] [1657] Account of the rights of the professors of medicine. In *Mss. collections . . . in relation to the rights of a physician in general, and of the Royal College of Physicians of Edinburgh in particular*, p. 72.

1630–4

(5) SIBBALD, Sir R. Op. cit., p. 7.

(6) Ibid., pp. 7–13.

(7) Ibid., pp. 14–15.

(8) POOLE, R. (1838) *Preparatory Notes for a History of the College*, p. 1. (Ms.)

(9) [PURVES, G.]. Op. cit., pp. 72–3.

(10) R.C.P.E. (1833) *Report on Examination of Medical Practitioners*, p. 8. Edinburgh: Neill.

(11) SIBBALD, Sir R. Op. cit., p. 15.

1656–60

(12) Ibid., p. 18.

(13) CLARK, Sir G. (1964) *A History of the Royal College of Physicians of London*, vol. 1, p. 284. Oxford: Clarendon.

(14) COMRIE, J. D. (1932) *History of Scottish Medicine*, 2nd Edition, vol. I, p. 267. London: Baillière, Tindall & Cox.

(15) SIBBALD, Sir R. Op. cit., pp. 15–16.

(16) MUNK, W. (1878) *The Roll of the Royal College of Physicians of London*, 2nd Edition, rev. and enl., vol. 1, 1518 to 1700. London: Royal College of Physicians.

(17) R.C.P.E. Op. cit., p. 11.

(18) Ibid., pp. 11–12.

(19) Ibid., pp. 12–13.

(20) SIBBALD, Sir R. Op. cit., pp. 16–18.

(21) Ibid., pp. 16–17.

(22) GAIRDNER, J. (1860) *Historical Sketch of the Royal College of Surgeons of Edinburgh*, p. 8. Edinburgh: Sutherland & Knox.

(23) R.C.P.E. Op. cit., p. 13.

(24) DUNCAN, A. (1896) *Memorials of the Faculty of Physicians and Surgeons of Glasgow, 1599–1850*, pp. 69–70. Glasgow: Maclehose.

(25) R.C.P.E. Op. cit., p. 15.

(26) Ibid., p. 16.

(27) GAIRDNER, J. (1864) *Sketch of the Early History of the Medical Profession in Edinburgh*, pp. 19–20. Edinburgh: Oliver & Boyd.

(28) R.C.P.E. Op. cit., p. 7.

(29) GAIRDNER, J. (1860) *Historical Sketch of the Royal College of Surgeons of Edinburgh*, p. 9. Edinburgh: Sutherland & Knox.

(30) LAMONT, J. of Newton (1830) *The Diary . . . 1649–1671*, p. 142. Edinburgh: James Clarke.

(31) POOLE, R. Op. cit., pp. 17–18.

(32) SIBBALD, Sir R. (1833) *The Autobiography of Sir Robert Sibbald*, KNT., M.D., p. 38. Edinburgh: Thomas Stevenson.

(33) Ibid., p. 12.

Chapter III

A CHARTER OF ERECTION GRANTED: 1681

Despite the imperfections of your betters we leave you a great inheritance, for which others will one day call you to account.

Sir J. M. Barrie

Efforts to establish a College of Physicians were eventually rewarded in 1681 in which year Charles II granted a Charter. It has long been recognized that a major and dominating rôle was exercised by (Sir) Robert Sibbald in promoting and directing the successful negotiations. To this extent Robert Sibbald's contribution to the Edinburgh College can be likened to that of Linacre's to the Sister College in London.

DIFFICULTIES PERSIST

Sibbald has left an account in his *Autobiography* of events which preceded the King's decision to grant a Charter.[1] From this account it is evident that as in the days of his uncle and Purves, difficulties were raised by the old time contestants—the Surgeons, the Town Council and the University.[1] That Sibbald did not exaggerate is borne out by the fact that when the Surgeons heard that promotion of a Charter for a College of Physicians was in progress, their Corporation appointed a Committee of sixteen members to deal with the situation. The purpose of the Committee was to organize resistance with all available resources because the Surgeons were fearful that the Charter 'might mightily encroach upon their privileges and tend to other prejudices'. Consideration was even given by their Corporation to seeking a new Charter with the object of consolidating their position in anticipation of eventualities, but the plan did not materialize.[2] Opposition to the Surgeons' plan was not confined to Edinburgh. Petitions against it were sent in 1682 to the Duke of York, the High

Commissioner, by four Dundee doctors ('Tho. Forbes M.D., Alexander Arbuthnott M.D., A. Lamb M.D. and Jo. Campbell M.D.') and two in Montrose ('Ja. Dixon D.M. and Jo Gordon D.M.'). None of the physicians named was associated with the Edinburgh College of Physicians.[3]

Some idea of the problems confronting Sibbald and his colleagues can be gleaned from 'Answers to the objections given in to the Lords of His Majesties Privie Counsel against the Signature given in by the Physicians in and about Edin.' The document was discovered by Poole. Appearing after the above title were the words 'wrote before 1681', and the text was 'written in different hands but pertaining to the like subject'. The 'answers' constituted a refutation of accusations advanced in the main by the Surgeons. To the imputation that they sought to establish a monopoly, the Physicians replied that 'a tryall' was necessary to exclude 'the illiterate and unskilful' but that anyone proving 'sufficientlie qualified' would be licensed by the College. Suggestions of parsimony met with an indignant retort to the effect that 'it never will be doubted that Physicians have enlarged hearts and the bowels of compassion towards the poor' and the Surgeons were challenged to give 'an instance of any Physician living in this place that ever refused to give advice to the poor . . .'.

While these answers were factual there was another of a more intriguing character. It was maintained by the Surgeons that the patent desired by the Physicians would invest them with 'jurisdiction within themselves' involving reference to the Burgh magistracy only as to 'their concurrence' in executing the physicians' laws 'against contraveeners'. By way of reply the Physicians did not accept that the Surgeons were competent to object on that score and referred to the powers already given 'to the societie of Physicians in London'. The attitude of the Physicians was further elaborated in a way to which today the most bigoted surgeon could not take exception. Explaining their purpose to 'restrain the arbitrary and licentious practice of illiterate and unqualified persons', the Physicians 'humblie' conceived 'that it will hardlie be possible to make the designe effectual' without judiciary rights; 'besides it seems to be inconsistent with reason that the Physicians who are a superiore order to Surgeons and Apothecaries should be brought before them in a Towne Counsel whereof they (Surgeons etc.) are members. The person, contraventious whereof, possibilie themselves may be guiltie.' Then there was quietly inserted a suggestion that the Lords of His Majesty's Privy Council might think fit 'to adde any of their owne number or of the Senators of the College of Justice or of the Magistrats of the burgh and that it shall be sufficient if any one of these three concurre with us in giving sentence against any that are not members or licentiats of the Colledge, we shall humblie acquiesce'. But the draughtsman seems to have known apprehension over his boldness, because he apparently attempted to score out reference to the College of Justice and burgh Magistracy. Poole writing in 1838 threw out the suggestion that herein may have been engendered first ideas about 'the election of such Honorary Fellows as were Members of the Court of Session'.[4]

Eventual, if grudging acceptance by the Surgeons was facilitated by the absence of any clause in the new Charter contemplating control by the Physicians of the practice of Surgery. The Charter of 1681 ordained in no dubious terms that 'the Edinburgh Surgeon Apothecaries are to have the power of treating every kind of wounds, contusions, practises, dislocations, tumours, ulcers, and other evils of that kind which fall under surgical operations and the accidents thence arising'. However a measure of protection was provided for the physician by decreeing that the Surgeons 'shall by no means have the care of diseases originally internal, solely to be undertaken under the prescription and direction of the physicians of the said College'.[5] Another point calculated to reduce surgical antagonism was the omission of any claim by the Physicians to bodies for dissection, thereby implying relinquishment of intentions to teach anatomy. Surgeons and Physicians alike of the Faculty of Physicians and Surgeons of Glasgow understandably saw reason for reassurance in the College being defined as of Edinburgh and not of Scotland, and indeed this withdrawal of the territorial claims of 1656 dispelled the Faculty's opposition to the Charter of 1681. By the terms of their own Charter the Faculty had for a number of years been linked with clearly defined parts of the West of Scotland.

There is reason to believe that the proposal to erect an Edinburgh College of Physicians had the positive support of the Apothecaries. The evidence consists of a document or scroll described by Poole. Dated 1681 the document appears to be a copy, lacking signatures but having on the reverse side thirteen names 'all in the same handwriting'. It purported to be 'The Apothecaries' Approbation of the erection of the College of Physicians'. 'Wee', it stated, 'the Apothecaries living in the City of Edinburgh, being informed that the Doctors of Medicine resideing in the said City and the places adjacent are endeavouring to obtain the erection of a College of Physicians for the regulating of the practice of Physick and restraining of Quacks Gardeners women and other ignorant and unskilfull persons after due and serious consideration doe judge it our interest more especially above any of the Leidges to declare our consent and approbation thereof . . . and wee declare wee are ready if need be to supplicate for the samin.'[6] Two experiences which may have influenced the attitude of the apothecaries were prosecution of some of their number by the surgeons, and participation of the physicians in the Court of Session case between apothecaries and surgeons (q.v.).

CONCESSIONS AND CONCILIATION

In the words of Sibbald 'it took a long tyme of dispute befor the counsell, in answering the objections of the Chirurgeons and of the Town of Edinburgh' against the creation of a College of Physicians.[7] In this connection account must be taken of the close links between the Town and the Surgeons. The Surgeons were members of a town guild with a Deacon recognized by the Town Council, and close identity of interests between town and guild was inevitable. Moreover as patrons of the Town's College the Town was again in a favourable position to influence the attitude of the future University. Nor were the interests and attitudes of the other universities wholly separable from that of the Church, the Chancellors of St Andrews, Glasgow and Aberdeen Universities being Bishops (or Archbishops) of the Church. None the less, the Physicians secured agreement with the Church and Town's College first. This was undoubtedly favoured by concessions to the effect that the College of Physicians would not be empowered to erect a medical school or confer degrees; and that any patent granted the College of Physicians would be without prejudice to the rights and privileges of 'The University or College' of St Andrews, Glasgow, Aberdeen and Edinburgh. A third concession was that graduates of the Scottish Universities could practise Medicine in the other University towns, and that although subject to the Bye-laws of the College of Physicians if they resided in Edinburgh, all University Graduates could claim to be made licentiates of the College of Physicians without examination or fee.[8]

Sibbald set course for the creation of a College of Physicians well aware of the errors in tactics, lack of diplomacy and excess of emotional propaganda which had made for the failure of those who had tried in earlier years. His first approach was to his fellow-physicians in Edinburgh and was made in circumstances which in retrospect seem to have been almost fortuitous.

In 1680 a dispute arose between the surgeons and apothecaries of the town arising from the alleged usurpation of the functions of surgeons by an apothecary. The ensuing legal case came before the Judges of the Court of Session, the crucial point at issue being the apothecaries' claim that pharmacy and surgery should be recognized as separate crafts or professions. A suggestion that the advice of 'disinterested, learned and skilful' physicians be sought was agreed to by the judges who thereupon required the opinion of Dr Stevensone, elder, Dr Hay and Dr Balfour.[9] Subsequently Dr Burnet was called upon in addition. The four physicians were looked to for an opinion 'about the Chirurgion Apothecaries, whither ther were any such conjunction of these employments in other countryes, and whither or not it was expedient for the Leidges, they should be joined in one person here'.[10] Thinking 'it possible that the physicians bore them no good will' for having opposed all attempts to erect a College of Physicians in Edinburgh and, that their advice to the judges would be prejudiced, the surgeons objected to the membership and constitution of the committee without avail.[9] As events turned out final judgment was in favour of the apothecaries. Before submitting their conclusions to the Judges of the Court of Session the four members of committee saw fit to get the views of other physicians in the Town. For this purpose they all adjourned to Dr Hay's place of abode on a day in July 1681.

D-DAY

Discussion of the report in course of preparation completed, Sibbald recorded in his *Autobiography*:

> 'I took the occasion to represent to them, that this being the first tyme we had all mett, I thought it was our interest to improve the meeting to some furder use, and I downright proposed we might take into consideration, the establishment of a Colledge to secure our priviledges belonged to us as doctors, and defend us against the incroachments of the Chirurgion Apothecaries, which were insupportable. This gave the first ryse to our meetings thereabout, . . .'.[7]

In this way Sibbald won the co-operation of his physician colleagues and brought about concerted action. Almost certainly he was helped in this by his previous close professional acquaintanceship with, among others, Dr Burnett, Dr Stevensone, Dr Balfour and Dr Pitcairne who used to meet at Sibbald's lodgings 'once a fourthnight or so, wher we had conferences'[11] (Chap. IV). Of those attending the meetings Balfour was probably best known to Sibbald. They had previously met in France while pursuing their independent foreign travels and, because of a common interest in, among other studies, natural history, an increasingly close understanding grew up between them when later, they were both practising in Edinburgh.

A visit to Edinburgh of the King's High Commissioner, in the person of the Duke of York, offered a possible opportunity to bring aspirations for the establishment of a College to the notice of the King. To this end Sibbald consulted Sir Charles Scarborough, the King's First Physician who had arrived in Edinburgh only a short time after the High Commissioner. The fact that Sibbald in his own words found Scarborough 'our very great friend and very ready to give us his best assistance' with the High Commissioner and the King, speaks for itself.[7] Likewise approach to the Earl of Perth served to dispel much of the opposition prevailing among the nobility. There was ample justification for this approach in the mutual friendship already developing between the two men. Writing in his *Autobiography* about events towards the end of 1678, Sibbald recorded how 'About this time the Earle of Perth began to employ me as his Physitian to his family, and introduced me with his friends'.[12] Assessment of the extent of the Earl's influence is a matter of conjecture. It is fashionable to belittle the old nobility but there can be little doubt that, at a time when the aristocracy and barons were conscious of waning power, the Earl of Perth's efforts were a major factor in winning their support for the cause of the Edinburgh College. Nor is it without significance that, on the occasion of his Knighthood in 1682, Sibbald afterwards wrote 'The Earle of Perth and Sir Charles Scarborough had concerted the matter, wee indeed knew nothing of the designe'.[13] The Knighthood was conferred at Holyrood Palace in 1682.

ROYAL FAVOUR

Still pursuing his objective Sibbald seized the opportunity of being received in the Royal presence to give to the King, Charles II, the Warrant of James VI dated 3rd July 1621 and issued to Parliament concerning the establishment of a College of Physicians in Edinburgh. According to Sibbald '. . . his Royall Highness, who, so soon as he saw it superscribed by King James, said with much satisfaction, he knew his grandfather's hand, and he would see our byseness done, and from that moment acted vigourously for us, so that it was resolved there should be ane colledge of Physitians . . .'.[7]

Scarborough at the time of his Edinburgh visit was one of the Council of the College of Physicians of London[14]: had been a pupil of Harvey and has been described as his friend and his protégé[15]; and had previously met Balfour when the latter was in London[16] and who like himself had studied under Harvey. There was yet another devotee of Harvey among the Edinburgh contingent in the person of Archibald Pitcairne, noted for his ardent advocacy of Harveian teachings. This association of interests among those concerned with the creation of an Edinburgh College has been interpreted as evidence that Harvey 'though dead . . . had an influence over these earnest and intelligent men in favouring the conception of the scheme and the preparation of its design'.[17] Significance too may attach to the fact that one of those in the list of petitioners for a Charter was (Sir) Thomas Burnet who was physician to the King, an appointment held also by Scarborough.[18]

SIBBALD'S ESPECIAL CONTRIBUTION

Of one thing there can be little doubt. Scarborough on the one hand, and Sibbald and his Edinburgh colleagues on the other had in common a zealous, almost passionate concern for the advancement of medicine as a science and as a reputable service to the community. It is in this context that debate concerning the creation of an Edinburgh College of Physicians is to be seen. Deliberations were not concerned with national and local politics. There can be nothing but admiration for the judicious deployment of his resources as, phase by phase Sibbald unfolded and applied his plan of campaign. Throughout he paid heed to errors of the past, gave consideration to contemporary advice, and at the outset won the esteem and confidence of Edinburgh colleagues for the future. Legitimately he sought and earned support in circles outwith his own strictly professional sphere. He succeeded where others had failed by conciliation and concession without sacrifice of principle or professional dignity.

Some might argue that the requirements regarding surgical practice in the Charter of 1681 constituted something approaching a complete *volte-face* on the part of the physicians. In reality the disputations between physicians and surgeons, whether about surgical practice or pharmaceutical alliance differ little in bases from the 'chalk-line demarcation disputes' and inter-union rivalry of our century. But what of the attitude of Sibbald and his confrères as conciliators? The terms of the Charter implied acknowledgment of past misjudgments and the withdrawal of past exorbitant demands. Requiring emphasis are the honest intent and purpose underlying this adjustment in policy—an adjustment brought about without resort to any self-deceptive 'face-saving' formulae so indispensable to settlement of disputes in the present age.

THE FACTOR OF RELIGION

A man's religious convictions are the concern of his own private conscience. Vacillation on the part of Sibbald certainly lost him friends and made him enemies. His conversion to, and later recantation of the Roman faith both bear the hallmark of sincerity to judge by his *Autobiography*.[19] The fact that he did not undertake teaching after being appointed Professor of Medicine in the Town College has been ascribed to his religious leanings at the time but this is open to question. These were heart-searching times and Poole after detailed study of all available papers obviously found the greatest difficulty in assessing the attitude of the College. He did not evade the inference that the favour in which it found itself at Court had been contributed to by expedient submissiveness. At the same time Poole stoutly maintained that not all Fellows were 'equally loyal and submissive'. In support of this latter view he cites the examination of Dr Matthew Brisbane at an inquisition at the time of Drumclog and Bothwell Bridge. That was about 1679. In 1684, according to the same source 'Some of the College . . . out of pique to some of their Members, as Doctors Burnet, Hardy and Stevenson, obtained from the Privy Council an order that all who practised medicine within Edinburgh should take the test, else they might be debarred'. Apparently these members were by the terms of the relevant Act of Parliament omitted *per expressum*, and subsequently the 'test was . . . offered *ex super abundanti* for their Preses and Censors of the Faculty, and now they would stretch to them all'. Poole was careful to point out however that opposition to the Test did not necessarily arise from political or religious persuasions. Several episcopalians and presbyterians took exception to the Test, and others for unspecified reasons were exempted from its obligations. None the less it is on record that Fountainhall referred to Sibbald as 'The Apostate Doctor Sibbald'.[20]

THE ORIGINAL FELLOWS

While all credit must be given to him for his sagacious leadership, administrative adroitness, temperamental equilibrium, and balanced persuasive personality Sibbald would almost certainly have wished that credit be apportioned to the group of physicians as a whole. To read Sibbald's writing is to have constantly borne in on one his sincere, unaffected humility. This applies particularly to those of his writings which outline events preceding the eventual award of a Charter to the Royal College of Physicians. As he acknowledged help received from this or that source, and mentioned obstruction encountered in this or that quarter one is apt to forget how deeply involved he was, and the intensity of the unrelieved strain to which he must undoubtedly have been submitted. He wrote of his contributions as a co-operative participant and not as the constructive leader which in reality he was.

And what of the physicians who united to further the prospects of the original patent? They numbered 21, of whom 11 were graduates or students of the University of Leyden; and 6 had been to other continental universities. Knowledge of these men

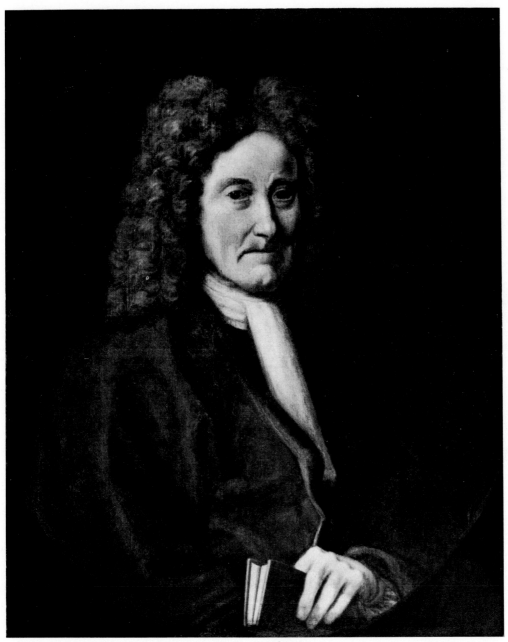

PLATE 3   Sir Robert Sibbald (1641–1722)
Reproduced from portrait in the College by John Alexander; photograph by Tom Scott

is negligible in the case of some, limited in the case of others, and not inconsiderable in the case of a few. They are all included in the list of Fellows in the original patent, and the following are a few details concerning them, in the order they appear in the patent:

(Sir) David Hay (?–1699)
    Physician-in-ordinary to the King—1684.
(Sir) Thomas Burnet (1638–1704): M.D., Montpellier—1659
    P.R.C.P.Edin.—1696. Physician to four reigning monarchs.
Matthew Brisbaine (?–1699): M.D., Utrecht—1661
    Honorary F.R.C.P.Edin. Later F.F. of P. & S. Glasgow: became town physician
    to Glasgow—1682: Rector of Glasgow University—1677.
(Sir) Archibald Stevensone (1629?–1710): M.D., Leyden—1661
    First P.R.C.P.Edin.: 1681–4.
(Sir) Andrew Balfoure (1630–94): M.D., Caen—1661: Student at Blois and Paris
    P.R.C.P.Edin.—1685.
(Sir) Robert Sibbald (1641–1722): Student at Leyden—1660
    Secretary R.C.P.Edin.—1682. Second P.R.C.P.Edin.—1684. F.R.C.P.Lond.—
    1686. Physician to the King in Scotland: Geographer for the Kingdom of
    Scotland to the King—1678. Voluminous writer on medical, archaeological
    and historical subjects. Deeply concerned with preparation of College
    Pharmacopoeia.
James Livingstone (?–1682)
    Councillor and Censor at time of erection of the College.
Robert Crawfurd (1644–c. 1699): Student at Leyden—1668
    Member of College Pharmacopoeia Committee: actively interested in Dis-
    pensary.
Robert Trotter (1648–1727): M.D., Leyden—1672
    Treasurer and Censor R.C.P.Edin.—1684. P.R.C.P.Edin.—1694 and 1700.
    Member of College Pharmacopoeia Committee.
Matthew Sinclare (St. Clair) (1654?–1728): Student at Leyden—1674
    P.R.C.P.Edin.—1698 and 1708. Last survivor of the 21 original Fellows.
James Stewart (1652–84): Student at Leyden—1674
    Interested in Pharmacopoeia.
William Stevensone (?)
    Second Treasurer R.C.P.Edin.—1682. First Librarian R.C.P.Edin.—1683.
    Name disappears from minutes after 1684. In sympathy with Covenanters.
Alexander Cranstone (?–c. 1699)
    Treasurer R.C.P.Edin.—1683. First Vice-President and Censor R.C.P.Edin.—
    1694. Active in Dispensary.
John Hutton (?): ? M.D., Padua
    First Treasurer R.C.P.Edin.—1681. Resigned 1682 on leaving Scotland: may be
    doctor of same name who joined R.C.P.Lond. in 1690.
John M'Gill (?)
    Member of Pharmacopoeia Committee. Name disappears from minutes after
    1684.

D

William Lauder (1652–?): Student at Leyden—1674

John Lermonth (1656–?): Student at Leyden—1675
    Censor R.C.P.Edin.—1684.

James Halket (1655–?): Student at Leyden—1675
    P.R.C.P.Edin.—1704. Took part in examination of first candidate to receive the
      degree of M.D. from the Town's College—1705.

William Wright (?)
    Took part in preparation of College Pharmacopoeia.

Patrick Halyburton (?)
    Took part in preparation of College Pharmacopoeia.

Archibald Pitcairne (1652–1713): M.A., Edin.—1671: M.D., Rheims—1680:
    Studied in Edinburgh and Paris. M.D., Aberdeen—1699
    Youngest of original Fellows of College. Second Secretary R.C.P.Edin.—1684.
    Professor of Medicine, University of Leyden: 1692–3. Sought association with
    R.C. Surgeons Edin. and made F.R.C.S.Edin—1701. Fervid Jacobite and
    contentious episcopalian.

REALIZATION

Reviewing events in retrospect in his *Autobiography*, Sibbald wrote concerning difficulties with the Surgeons and the Town of Edinburgh that: 'We soon did agree with the universities and Bishops, and there were some conditiones insert in the patent in their favours, and they became strong solicitours for us, so that after long debates, the matter was concerted, and the draught of the patent agreed to by the Counsell, was sent up, and very soon thereafter, by his Royall Highness his procurement, returned signed by the King; the very next day I turned it into Latin, and the day thereafter gave it in to the Chancery chamber, and waited upon it till it was written in parchment, and ready for the great seall, which was appended to it upon the 29th of November, 1681, being St. Andrew's day . . . The patent is very honourable for our Society, and contains a jurisdiction within ourselves, which the publick judicatures are obliged to see executed.'[21]

Johnson's Boswell claimed to have the 'Life of Sir Robert Sibbald, the celebrated Scottish antiquary, and founder of the Royal College of Physicians at Edinburgh, in the original manuscript in his own handwriting'. He believed it to be 'the most natural and candid account of himself that ever was given by any man'. When Boswell referred to Sibbald's return to the Protestant fold after temporarily embracing Roman Catholicism, it brought forth from Johnson the comment '. . . a man loves to review his own mind. That is the use of a diary, or journal.'[22]

THE CHARTER SUMMARIZED

The Charter commenced by emphasizing the necessity for the examination of those proposing to practise a profession, and the dire results accruing from the lack of regulations appertaining to Medicine. It envisaged correction by the College of prevailing abuses. Importance was attached to Edinburgh's pre-eminence as the Metropolis and seat of Supreme Judicial Courts. The College was to consist of certain named individuals and of others who might be chosen by them as Colleagues and Fellows of their Society within the city of Edinburgh, its Suburbs and Liberties: so that they and their successors should be united and conjoined into one Body, Community, and College in all time coming. Those 'named' corresponded with those already given (q.v.) as appearing in the patent.

Provision was made for the election of a Council, President, and other Office-Bearers: and the College was empowered to enact for its government and welfare and for promoting the Science and regulating the practice of Medicine within the City of Edinburgh and Leith, their Suburbs and Liberties.

The Charter prevented, under certain penalties, any one from practising Medicine within the jurisdiction of the College who had not obtained its Licence or Diploma. Under certain regulations the College was enabled to call before it and fine unlicensed practitioners; and to punish Physicians, Doctors of Medicine, Licentiates and Fellows practising within their jurisdiction, who might violate any of the Laws of the College. It was obligatory on the College to confer, without examination or fee, a licence to practise on any applicant in possession of a degree of any Scottish University.

Under the terms of the Charter, the College could together with a magistrate and chemist examine the medicines in Apothecaries' shops and destroy those found to be unsatisfactory in quality: and magistrates were unable to allow any one to open an Apothecary's shop until the applicant had satisfied the President and Censors of the College that he had a competent knowledge of drugs.

The Charter provided that no Fellow of the College should be called upon to act as juror at any assize in town or country or called out to watch or ward, or on any pretext whatever be withdrawn from his patients.

The *Charta Erectionis Regii Medicorum Collegii apud Edinburgum* dated 29th November 1681 is reproduced in translated form in Appendix E. This Charter was followed by a Charter of Ratification in 1685 (Appendix F).

Preservation of perspective justifies mention of two other events of 1681—one of metropolitan interest: the other of fundamental far-reaching national significance.

Of these the first was the granting of a Charter to the Merchant Company of Edinburgh, the second was the publication by Lord Stair of his *Institutions of the Law of Scotland*. According to Poole, Dr Thomas Dalrymple admitted a Socius in July 1694 was the fourth son of the author.[23] To quote Lord Cameron the '*Institutions* . . . laid the foundation of a system flexible and harmonious and readily capable of development and adaptation to the needs of a developing and changing society'.[24]

In 1682 the Advocates' Library, now the National Library of Scotland, was founded by Sir George Mackenzie of Rosehaugh. That same year our College was in receipt of books from Sir Robert Sibbald which were the beginnings of its Library (Chap. VI).[25]

Events were to prove that the Royal College of Physicians of Edinburgh had its own special contribution to make to this developing and changing society.

REFERENCES

(1) SIBBALD, Sir R. (1833) *The Autobiography of Sir Robert Sibbald, Knt., M.D.*, pp. 29–31. Edinburgh: Thomas Stevenson.

(2) CRESWELL, C. H. (1926) *The Royal College of Surgeons of Edinburgh. Historical Notes from 1505–1905*, p. 119. Edinburgh: Oliver & Boyd.

(3) POOLE, R. (1838) *Preparatory Notes for a History of the College*, pp. 25–6. (Ms.)

(4) Ibid., pp. 8–13.

(5) R.C.P.E. (1925) *Historical Sketch and Laws of the Royal College of Physicians of Edinburgh*, p. 251. Edinburgh: Royal College of Physicians.

(6) POOLE, R. Op. cit., pp. 15–16.

(7) SIBBALD, Sir R. Op. cit., p. 30.

(8) GRANT, Sir A. (1884) *The Story of the University of Edinburgh*, vol. I, p. 223. London: Longmans, Green & Co.

(9) CRESWELL, C. H. Op. cit., p. 116.

(10) SIBBALD, Sir R. Op. cit., p. 29.

(11) Ibid., p. 28.

(12) Ibid., p. 26.

(13) Ibid., p. 32.

(14) RITCHIE, R. P. (1899) *The Early Days of the Royall Colledge of Phisitians, Edinburgh*, p. 58. Edinburgh: G. P. Johnston.

(15) Ibid., p. 60.

(16) Ibid., p. 57.

(17) Ibid., p. 54.

(18) COMRIE, J. D. (1932) *History of Scottish Medicine*, 2nd Edition, vol. I, p. 277. London: Baillière, Tindall & Cox.

(19) SIBBALD, Sir R. Op. cit., pp. 37–41.

(20) POOLE, R. Op. cit., pp. 77–8.

(21) SIBBALD, Sir R. Op. cit., pp. 30–1.

(22) BOSWELL, J. (1958) *Life of Johnson*, vol. II, pp. 165–6. London: Dent (Everyman's Library).

(23) POOLE, R. Op. cit. (Matters in reference to persons and history of College.)

(24) CAMERON, J., *Lord Cameron* (1967) Scott and the Community of Intellect. In *Edinburgh in the Age of Reason*, p. 53. Edinburgh: University Press.

(25) MEIKLE, H. W., ed. (1947) *Scotland: a description of Scotland and Scottish life*, p. 225. Edinburgh: Nelson.

Chapter IV

PHYSICIANS' 'HALLS'

It is a reverend thing to see an ancient castle or building not in decay.

Francis Bacon

Public buildings being the ornament of a country, it establishes a nation, draws people and commerce, makes the people love their native country.

Sir Christopher Wren

One of the first problems facing those who had succeeded in their petition for the erection of a College of Physicians was to find a suitable place for their regular meetings. A number of years were to pass before the College possessed anything meriting the designation of 'hall'. Of necessity use had to be made of make-shift provisions during this time.

Sibbald tells in his *Autobiography* of meetings at about fortnightly intervals in his lodgings attended during 1680 by Doctors Burnett, Stevensone, Balfour and Pit-cairne.[1] He goes on to describe how the subjects discussed were 'letters from these abroad, giving account of what was most remarkable a doing by the learned, some rare cases had happened in our practice, and ane account of Bookes, that tended to the improvement of medicine or naturall history, or any other curious learning'. The programme bears a strong resemblance to that of present-day medical departments. Continuing Sibbald said that the meetings continued 'till the erection of the Colledge of Physicians' and that they were 'forborne then upon the introducing of such conferences once a moneth in the Colledge'.[1] Available evidence does not warrant the assumption that the monthly College conferences took place in Sibbald's lodgings or for that matter in Dr Hay's house where the first historic meeting already mentioned (Chap. III) was held. Two factors making for uncertainty are that Minutes for the period 1685 to 1692 are missing and those Minutes which are available do not record the place of meeting. The first reference in this connection is on 1st February 1694 to the effect that the Treasurer reported that 'he hath payed the rent for the

Colledge meeting-house'.[2] That is all. There follows on 14th September 1695 a Minute tersely headed 'mett at the President's lodgeings being denyed the keys of the Colledge by Dr. Steivenston'.[3] The President was Dr Trotter and the incident occurred at a time when serious misunderstandings were brewing among the Fellows (Chap. XIX). A justifiable inference is that use was being made of Dr Stevensone's rooms for College proceedings, but a Minute dated 29th September 1696 gives rise to doubts on this point.[4] It records that 'it was carried nemine contradicente yt* Dr. Stevensone should be ordained to pay ye money due to him to ye colledge for yt pt of ye house ye colledge formerly mett in and possessed by him'. In November of the same year there followed in place of a deleted minute a recorded instruction to two Fellows 'to demand Dr. Stevensones discharges he pretends to have of yt money due him to ye colledge'.[5] And then references to the subject ceased. What was the true situation—was the College a tenant of Dr Stevensone, or Dr Stevensone a tenant of the College? Academic although this question now is, Ritchie deduced from the fact that because Stevensone continued to live in the same quarters for at least four years after he refused entry to his fellow *Socii*, the College had in all probability been occupying a chamber in his lodging.[6] Uncertainty apparently still prevailed, as the next record stated that the Treasurer had been ordered on 24th May 1697 to pay 'to Mr. William Livingstoune ffourty two punds Scotts for a years rent of the meeting room of the colledge'.[7] The rent was to be supplemented with 'a dollar' for the maid.

On 27th April 1698 the momentous decision was taken to buy a house.[8] Two Socii were deputed to make enquiries, and in a week's time reported 'They see none fitter for the College than the house presentlie possessed by Mr. William Livingstone'. An offer was made for the house but, being unsuccessful the tenancy arrangements continued.[9, 10] Shortly afterwards Mr Livingstone must have died because in 1700 a minute recorded paying what was due to the deceased including 'a crown for coals'.[11]

Some years later (13th July 1704) a proposal was considered to apply 'ffor a Right to the housse and ground possesst by Mistress Lidderdale'.[12] It was decided that the President should wait upon the Lord Provost with a view to ascertaining his reaction. As there is no further mention of the proposal, it was presumably unacceptable.

FOUNTAIN CLOSE (1704)

Within a month (15th August 1704) a Committee of six doctors was appointed to consider another possibility. The Committee was required 'to meet and agrie with

---

* Spelling of quoted extracts has been taken from the original transcription.

Mr. James McKenzie for his Land yairds lyand at the foot of the ffountoun Closse for the use and behove of the Colledge . . .'.[13] At the next meeting of the Council (24th October 1704) the Committee together with the President was instructed 'to end and agrie with the said Sir' (no longer Mr) 'James Mackenzie yranent, and to get ane Dispositione yrof in ffavors of the Colledge and if need beis to take the advyse of Lawzers in the matter'.[14] Payment 'of thrie thousand fyve hundreth marks' was agreed on 1st December 1704 representing 'the pryce of the hous and yairds'.[15] In a little over six months (29th June 1705) it was recorded 'that there are severall reparationes necessary to be made in the hous lately purchast for the Colledge yr place of meeting'.[16] This is the first specific mention of possession of a meeting place by the College in its own right. Repairs apart, improvements in the form of a new stair and gate 'for secureing the entry to the Colledge and Gardens' were decided upon as necessary. After repairs there followed extensions.[17, 18] In 1711 the College acquired from a city merchant of the name of William Jeffrey 'the houss, ground and pertinents Lyand att the foot of the under yaird of the Colledge be east the wall'.[19] The ground in question lay between that originally purchased and the then fashionable Cowgate, and the attractions of the garden now possessed by the College prompted the aristocracy of the neighbourhood to ask that access be given to them by way of a favour. Agreement was readily forthcoming.

After almost four years, consideration was given to the building of a new pavilion or hall but the unsatisfactory state of College finances prevented implementation of the plan. In the meantime the College had embarked on another scheme, difficult to understand fully in the light of modern times. An 'old ruinous houss in the Cowgate att the foot of the Lower yaird' together with other buildings in a similar state of advanced disrepair were converted into a Cold Bath[20] which as described elsewhere (Chap. V) was made available to the public at a charge. This was to prove a costly venture. The possibility of reviving the proposal for a pavilion was raised in 1715 only to be again rejected on the score of lack of funds[21]—but some years later money was borrowed from a city merchant and a new hall was erected in 1722.[22] As had been the practice in the old building, space was made available in the new hall for the attendance of the ailing poor. The new 'housse' was equipped 'with a pavilion-rooffe' to which successive Minutes appeared to attach considerable importance, and was of at least two floors. As now, so then 'there seems some things to be over Charged' and there had to be further borrowings.[23]

Again reminiscent of modern trends, the Fountain Close Hall was found before long to have inadequate provision for unanticipated expansion and development. There would seem to have been minor irritations also, because in 1751 the College appointed a Committee to consider how best to deal with the abuse of 'washing and drying of Cloaths, skins etc.' in the garden to which all and sundry evidently had access.[24] In 1760 the decision was arrived at to build yet another new Hall within the curtilage of the then existing College property.[25] In the words of Dr Beilby, 'Notwithstanding all the sums that had been expended in the erection of a *new* building, and in the repair of the *old*, the former seems to have been slight and insufficient, and the latter was in so dilapidated a condition . . . it was resolved to build a new Hall . . . and a plan was obtained and approved, the execution of which was to cost £800 . . .'. Before proceeding further the College sought the expert opinion of Mr Robert Adam who declared the plan to be unsuitable and 'quite unworthy of the Body for whom it was intended'. Without cost to the College Adam produced a plan of his own conception. The attractions of the plan were immense but wisely the College exercised restraint and resisted temptation in the face of an estimated cost of between £5000 and £6000.[26] In passing it is interesting to note that one elaborate set of plans submitted when prospects of a new Hall were first mooted, came from as far afield as Rome.[27]

TEMPORARY ASYLUM

Resigned to carry on without the new Hall, the College was eventually compelled by events and the local climate to take drastic action. Books in the Library which were already a legitimate source of historic and professional pride were deteriorating seriously and rapidly. Their removal from Fountain Close became a matter of the utmost urgency. An appeal was made for accommodation, or as an earlier history terms it 'Temporary Asylum', to the Managers of the Royal Infirmary which was then situated near the Old College of the University. They responded generously and when the old buildings in Fountain Close were sold in 1770, put a spare apartment at the disposal of the College Library and 'most chearfully granted liberty to the College to meet about their affairs' in the Managers' Board Room.[28] Advantage was taken of these privileges for fifteen years. There could be no better illustration of the happy relation existing between the College and Infirmary than the action of the Managers of the latter at this time 'directing the Treasurer "to make their most Respectfull Compliments to the College, and assure them its with a very sensible pleasure they embrace this opportunity of showing the sence they have of the Colledge merit with this Charitable Corporation in having had the honour in a great measure to be the projectors of it." '[29]

As might be expected, neighbours were aware of the dilapidated state of the College. In 1763 a memorial was received by the College from one 'presently possessed' of property 'lying immediately to the North of that ruinous old House which the Learned Faculty formerly used as Their Liberary and Gardeners Dwelling'.[30] No matter whether reference to the 'Liberary' was correct or incorrect, there can be no question about the fact of dilapidation! The premises in Fountain Close were sold for £800.[31] Used in succession by an episcopal church and 'several dissenting bodies', the site was ultimately acquired by the Roman Catholic Church of St Patrick's.[32-34]

These troubles of the physicians became acute at a time when construction of Edinburgh's New Town was in an embryonic stage and the College would have been failing in its declared dedication to progress had it not given serious thought to establishing headquarters in the New Town. Following a petition to the Edinburgh Town Council for a site, negotiations were entered into for the land on which the Register House now stands. The negotiations were just on the point of final agreement when acting on behalf of the Government, the architect Mr Robert Adam successfully pressed the overriding claims of his design for the Register House. By way of consolation the College were offered as an alternative the site now occupied by the Scott Monument. This they rejected and were then given the choice of a site in George Square or another in George Street. They chose the latter.

GEORGE STREET HALL (1781)

The man who builds and wants wherewith to pay
Provides a home from which to run away.

E. Young

Building on the George Street site began in 1775. Although first occupied on 7th August 1781 during the Presidency of Alexander Monro *secundus*, the Hall was not completed in the literal sense of the word until about 1830.[35]

Arnot in his *History of Edinburgh* explained that the College of Physicians 'did not chuse to build' on their previous site and that 'they, therefore, disposed of the ground to the gentlemen of the episcopal communion in Edinburgh who have there erected the English chapel'. He then described the new Hall in considerable detail.

'The College of Physicians feued from the town of Edinburgh a large area, in the centre of the divisions of George's-street, in the extended royalty, on which they have erected a magnificent hall, the design of Mr. Craig, who planned the New Town. The foundation-stone was laid by Dr. Cullen, assisted by all the medical professors on 27th November 1775.* This building extends upward of eighty feet in front. It is adorned with a portico, the pediment of which is supported by four superb Corinthian columns, which stand at the distance of six feet from the wall. The platform on which they are erected, is about seven feet above the level of the street, and the ascent to it by a flight of steps thirty feet wide.

'The under floor contains lodging for a librarian and porter, and some other apartments. The second floor, to which the entry is by the stair leading to the portico, consists of four apartments, a lobby, which is a cube of thirty-five feet, lighted by five windows, two on a level with the door, and three above. On the right hand is a room of twenty-four by eighteen, and fourteen high; and on the left, another of the same dimensions. One of these apartments is intended for the ordinary meetings of the college; the other for a waiting room to accommodate those who may have business with the college at their meetings: But the principal apartment is destined for the reception of the library, and the different curious productions belonging to this society. This room is upwards of fifty feet long, by thirty broad, and twenty high. It is lighted by two rows of windows, five in each row, and on three sides is surrounded with a gallery. Besides these, there are some smaller apartments where the members of the college may read or write, when they borrow books from the library which they do not chuse to carry home with them.'[37]

The architecture did not please everyone. Youngson from studies of prints and elevations, accepted the Hall as having been reasonably well proportioned but referred to Farington's criticism on the score that 'the capitals are a third too large for the pillars'.[38] Nevertheless Youngson accepted the building as a 'chaste and elegant imitation of ancient Grecian architecture'. Craig—nephew of the poet-author of *The Seasons*[36]—both designed and built the Hall and as events turned out it was 'the only important building by Craig in Edinburgh'.[38] The magistrates of the City conferred on him with the Freedom of Edinburgh a gold medal in a silver box as a reward for having designed the best plan of the new town. Evidence exists to suggest that Craig's original plan had been first submitted to a Mr Stuart, author of the *Antiquities of Athens*.[36]

Building of the George Street Hall plunged the College into debt. The contract with Craig to cover design and construction had originally been for £2725, but payments had amounted to £3850 by November 1779.[38] Ultimately the expenditure involved was of the order of £4800. Nor, it would appear, was the architect

---

* The date had been deliberately advanced to take place before the end of the presidency of Dr Cullen who had been largely responsible for advancing the project.[36]

without difficulties because, in a letter to the College dated 11th November 1779, he wrote 'If the Committee does not pay me the account of Extraordinary work I presented to Dr. Grant the 2nd curt. amounting to £105 beside the rise of wages which I was obliged to pay the masons and wrights etc, owing to their Combination, I shall repent the day I ever laid a stone of their building—The Royal College are all Gentlemen as individuals, how far they will behave genteely as a Society time must soon determine.'[39] As in the twentieth, so also in the eighteenth century fixed-price contracts had their pitfalls!

Intensive efforts to procure subscriptions were ineffective: and the Hall was immediately mortgaged to cover a deficit of almost £100. The College was strangely unorthodox in its ways of business. After deciding to disallow certain not inconsiderable claims made by Craig, it straightway agreed 'to make him a present of £60 sterling . . . upon his granting the College a proper Discharge of every claim . . .'.[40] One year later the College were still harrying Craig because he 'has never yet moved the stones belonging to him', much less repaired certain structural damage.[40]

Such was the despondency which prevailed among the ranks of the Fellows that, even before occupation of the new building a proposal to sell the Hall was submitted. To this end, negotiations were entered into with interested parties to convert the building into Assembly Rooms. The aim of the parties was to appease those fashionable young ladies who were becoming disillusioned by the unattractiveness of their social apartments in Bell's Wynd on the south side of the town. Negotiations had reached the stage of agreement about price and the College had virtually approved their Committee's action, when those seeking to purchase changed their mind and withdrew their offer of £3750. All references to the transactions were erased from the Minutes but it is known that the ladies' 'second thought' served to strengthen a resolution previously drawn up by some objecting Fellows seeking to get the transaction rescinded by an appeal to the law. Beilby for his part considered that the trend of events saved the College 'from the indelible disgrace into which it was plunging',[42] but he does not make clear whether the disgrace he feared was one of total bankruptcy, or of a 'Swinging Edinburgh' in the 80s—the 1780s. Nor did he mention that previously in 1758, when plans for a new College Hall were at a preliminary stage the 'Gentlemen of the musical society' had 'expressed their desire to have their musical hall or Concert room in the same building'. A second approach was not made at that time.[43, 44]

Be that as it may, the College put an end to further delay and on 7th August 1781 assembled in the New Hall for the first time despite an as yet unfinished interior stage. Still handicapped by precarious finances the College had no option but to proceed cautiously with outstanding work which was considerable. In actual fact, final completion of the original design did not take place until about 1830. Having in mind Arnot's glowing account (q.v.) it comes as something of a surprise to read that from the outset internal arrangements had proved inconvenient.[45] Beilby went so far as to say that all the Fellows had felt, and many had complained of the unsuitableness and discomfort of these arrangements: and that a 'wish was very commonly expressed by those especially who made most use of it, that we could obtain a more commodius edifice, though it were of less imposing exterior'.[46] A purely personal impression is that these arguments represented no more than a part of the truth and that in reality the College was rightly unable to rid itself of apprehensions concerning poverty and indebtedness.

Uncertainty gained momentum. The College had no funded capital. Entrance fees paid by Fellows were the only source of income. On the face of it the College had lived courageously. The stage was set for retrenchment at the first favourable opportunity. That opportunity came in 1843 when an offer of £19,500 was made for the New Hall, George Street by the Commercial Bank of Scotland.[47]

The sum desired by the College was £19,950. 'Haggling' rather than bargaining ensued and notes exchanged between the College's lawyer and the Bank's spokesman betrayed increasing irritation. On 5th June (1843) the latter wrote:

> '£365 is as you say *all* the difference . . . It is a mistake to think because an offer has been made for a Bank, that a further concession of hundreds will be made . . .'[48]

Eventually a price of £19,700 was agreed, the Bank paying the expenses of conveyance and obtaining entry within 14 to 28 days.[49] It was considered that the sum accepted would prove adequate to build another Hall of greater capacity and convenience, while being less impressive. While that was the realistic appraisal of the situation there was genuine heart-burning among many Fellows acutely conscious of the sacrifice entailed in the loss of an imposing building.

There was a curious delayed sequel. In May 1868, by which time the College had been long since comfortably settled in its Queen Street Hall, the President stated that a 'Dr. Craig of Ratho had mentioned . . . that a large stone having a floral wreath with an Aesculapian Lyre in the centre cut thereon and believed to have stood over the pillars . . . of the Old Hall of the College in George Street, had, on the removal of the Old Hall, come into the possession of the late Mr. Paul, Manager of the Commercial Bank, that Mr. Paul had been frequently requested to hand it over to the College, but had always expressed his unwillingness to part with it, that during his last illness he had requested it to be given to Dr. Craig . . . .'.

With discretion in keeping with his Collegiate Office, the President made no mention of Dr Craig's relationship to Mr Paul—whether bank client, professional attendant, or both! What Dr Craig had made clear, having had the stone refaced, was that the College could have the stone 'at a price'.[50] The stone was purchased and removed to the College.

When a decision was made to establish a Public Dispensary, later known as the Royal Public Dispensary, the College placed apartments in the George Street Hall at its disposal until the managers were able to obtain a building of their own.[51]

IN 'LODGINGS' AGAIN (1843)

The George Street Hall sold, the College was homeless. Perforce a house had to be rented. That selected was 119 George Street, now part of the site occupied by the Church of Scotland offices, and it functioned as meeting place for the College of Physicians from 1843 to 1846.[52]

QUEEN STREET HALL (1846)

The foundation-stone of a new Hall in Queen Street was laid on 8th August 1844 by the President in office, Dr Robert Renton. In the course of extensive structural alterations, the foundation-stone of the old Hall in George Street was unexpectedly unearthed. It was found to have on it an appropriate inscription, and to have enclosed in it a bottle which in turn contained a Parchment Roll with written on it the names of the Fellows of the College at the time. Also in the bottle were some British coins bearing the date 1771, and two silver medals. One of the medals bore the College coat of arms on one side, with the names of the President and architect ('Jac. Craig') on the obverse side. The other medal had a facsimile of the George Street Hall with, under it, the Aesculapian serpent and rod; and on the obverse side Craig's name was inscribed together with the designation 'Architecto Propter Optimam Edinburgi Novi Ichnographiam'.

Returning to the Queen Street foundation-stone ceremony in 1844, this took place in the presence of the Fellows of the College, Civic and University representatives and others: and on this occasion the symbolic bottle encased in the ceremonial stone contained a copy of the last edition of the *Edinburgh Pharmacopoeia* with a list of the Fellows of the College, an old printed account of past private affairs of the College, an *Edinburgh Almanac* for 1844, several British coins of the period and a piece of silver plate bearing an appropriate Latin inscription.[53]

The new Queen Street Hall was designed by Thomas Hamilton, a distinguished Edinburgh architect whose masterpiece was the Royal High School. In some respects the design of the College resembles that of the High School. Referring to the exterior Youngson describes it as

> 'somewhat square and severe in its proportions, but is relieved by a portico which frames the central window of the upper floor; mounted on each side of the lower portico is a large classical figure, and a third figure, equally large, is poised on top of the pediment of the upper portico. The effect is extraordinary but not unpleasing, although it might be better if the building were somewhat wider. The interior is in a similar style. The entrance hall and stairway are severe and yet grand, while the main hall is a magnificent apartment in the construction of which expense has clearly not been spared. Slightly longer than it is broad, and high in proportion to its size, it is surrounded by eighteen free-standing marble columns, above each of which, along the frieze, stands a life-size classical figure. The effect is spectacular, although it is perhaps not unfair to say that it is more Victorian than Roman.'[54]

To this should be added that the main hall has an impressively effective enriched ornamental ceiling: and that the main hall today is larger than the original, extensions having been completed in 1868. A series of plaques adorn the frieze. These consist of profiles—to the West, of Harvey, Monro (primus), Cullen, Jenner and Baillie; to the South, of Galen, Hippocrates and Avicenna; to the East, of Gregory, Hunter, Smellie, Boerhaave and Sydenham; and to the North, of Abercrombie and Thomson.

The exterior sculptures are of Hygieia, Aesculapius and Hippocrates, the sculptor being Alexander Ritchie, a pupil of Thorwaldsen. Another feature is the plaque inserted in the north wall of the New Library. A tablet below records that it was removed 'From the Old College Hall/George St./1776' (q.v.).

A wholly unexpected and to this day unexplained finding was a coat of arms carved in the stonework of the underpassage of the College building. The Lord Lyon considered that the arms are those of the Nairns of St Fort or Sandford in Fife, but another authority was equally convinced they are the arms of the Nairns of Strathord or Strathaird and in particular of William Nairne, Lord Nairne, husband of Carolina, Baroness Nairne the poetess.[55]

Expense of the entire project was high. In the first place the College paid £2750 for the two houses (Numbers 9 and 10 Queen Street) which had to be demolished to free the site. The contract price for the building, signed in 1844, was £4838 but increasing expenses led to this being revised before long to £5415. When rendered, the contractor's account was £5898. Additional work together with furnishings brought the final bill to £7194—£9944 when allowance is made for initial clearance of the site. A salutary figure for progressives to ponder over when translated into terms of current values.

Not unnaturally the Hall was a source of interest outside strictly medical spheres. It was visited in 1886 by the Architectural Association[56], but strangely in 1911 the Council was 'not prepared to agree' to the Edinburgh Merchant Company entering the Hall 'to take measurements'.[57]

In 1902 electric lighting was installed.[58] Previously illumination had been by gas and a Minute recorded that the lamps in front of the College had to be 'regularly lighted'. Whether for the benefit of the public or for the safe descent of the steps by Fellows was not stated![59] The provision of hand pumps, metal pails and hoses were recommended by the City Firemaster and written across the recording Minute in bold lettering is the word 'Fire!'.[60] During the Second World War a Fire-watcher was appointed, an Air Raid Shelter provided in accordance with the requirements of the Civil Defence Act 1939, and arrangements made for the protection of pictures and books.[61, 62] The College was fortunate in suffering no structural damage, as experienced by the Sister College in London.[63] In 1956 the premises were entered by burglars, but the small amount of silver plate stolen was recovered. The same did not apply to the delectable contents of a number of bottles.[64, 65]

A First Extension: 8 Queen Street (1864)

Within no less than nineteen years the need for yet further accommodation became apparent. This was attributable to two factors—the great increase in the number of Fellows since reduction of the entry fee, and the rapidity with which additions had been made to the Library. An opportunity arose to purchase property immediately adjoining the Hall on the east. Past experience pointed to the need for weighty consideration but 'after long . . . and much delicate negotiation No. 8 Queen Street was acquired for £6000'.[66] The house had been designed by Robert Adam and had an interesting history. Built in 1770 it was the first house to be erected in Queen Street, the feuar being Lord Chief Baron Ord. There are three main storeys, on each of which are suites of intercommunicating rooms, well lit and of large, lofty dimensions. In several rooms there are mantelpieces of white statuary marble, and door-

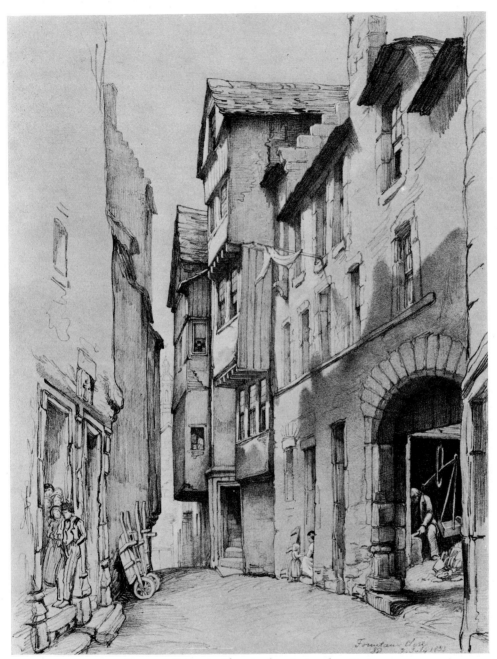

PLATE 4 Fountain Close in the nineteenth century
Reproduced from *Old Edinburgh* (Edinburgh, 1879) by James Drummond; photograph by Tom Scott

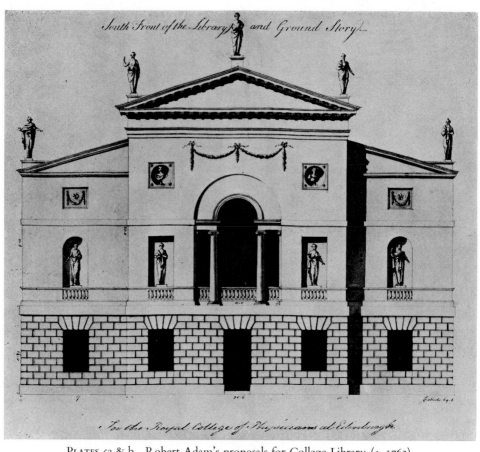

South Front of the Library and Ground Story

For the Royal College of Physicians at Edinburgh

PLATES 5a & b   Robert Adam's proposals for College Library (*c.* 1762)
By courtesy of the Trustees of Sir John Soane's Museum

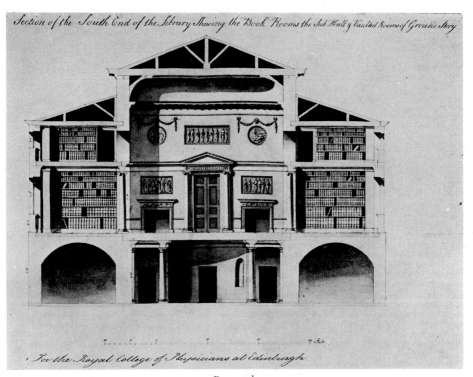

Section of the South End of the Library Shewing the Book Rooms the Sub Hall & Vaulted Rooms of Ground Story

For the Royal College of Physicians at Edinburgh

PLATE 5b

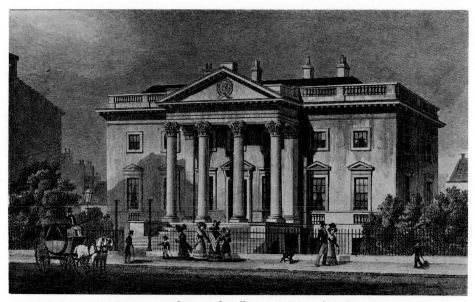

PLATE 6 Physicians' Hall, George Street (1825)
Reproduced from a Thomas Shepherd engraving

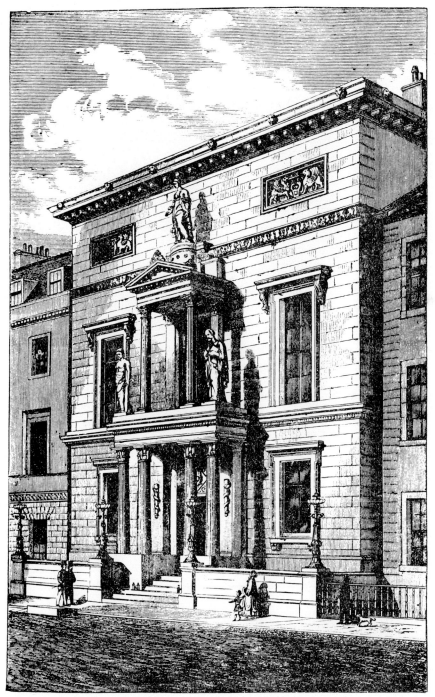

PLATE 7   Physicians' Hall, Queen Street (1846)

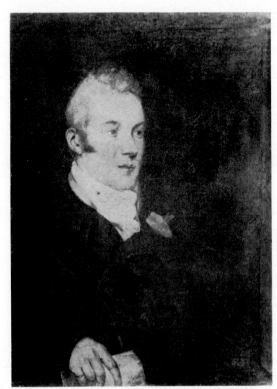

PLATE 8   Dr William Beilby (1783–1849)
By courtesy of M. E. Beilby, Esq.

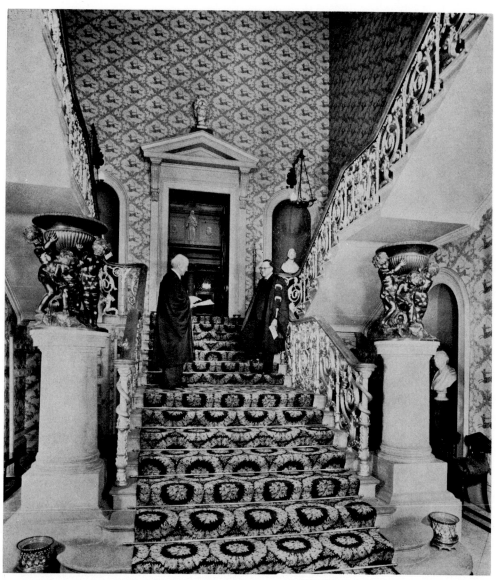

PLATE 9   Queen Street: Grand Staircase
Photograph by Tom Scott

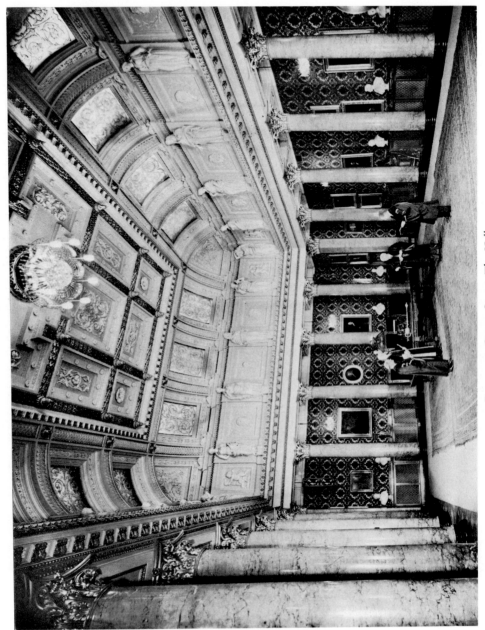

PLATE 10 Queen Street: The Hall
Photograph by Tom Scott

heads supported by scrolled consoles and enriched with fluting.[67] The property was purchased in 1864 from the trustees of the Headmaster (Dr Alexander Reid) of the Edinburgh Institution (forerunner of Melville College) which continued to use the premises for several years in accordance with the terms of the lease. In 1868, when the Main Hall at 9 Queen Street was enlarged, a spacious hall—the New Library—was erected at the back of No. 8, the basement being leased to the Institution for a term of years. At a later date this new accommodation was adapted for further Library purposes.

When the Edinburgh Institution finally moved to Melville Street in 1920, No. 8 Queen Street was re-let to a Government Department until about 1951. The College then occupied the first floor of the house to provide a Fellows' Room, a Members' Room and supplementary Library accommodation. Rooms used for these purposes together constitute what has been described as 'the finest Adam Suite in Edinburgh'. Especially noteworthy are the fine enriched ceilings, and the oil paintings enclosed in some of the mouldings on the ceilings. In 1955 restoration, redecoration and furnishing were carried out in a way appropriate to the period when the house was built.[68] Rooms on the ground floor were adapted for use as office accommodation and cloakrooms.

The house is officially listed as a Historical Monument.

An interesting remnant of the past is the continuation of one of the front cellars below Queen Street to emerge in the Queen Street Gardens. The original intended purpose was to provide safe access to drying greens. Comparatively recently, in the 1960s, the need arose to summon the fire brigade when the basement of No. 8 was filled with swirling smoke. The source of the trouble?—gatherings of fallen leaves being burnt inadvertently at the garden end of the subterranean passage: a quixotic situation when account is taken of the sale by the College in 1917 of the subway to Edinburgh Corporation on condition that the College was freed 'from all responsibility in connection with the subway, and also that the City will undertake to build up the south entrance to the subway if and when required by the College . . .'[69]

On different occasions the Queen Street Hall or other parts of the accommodation have on request been made available to, among other scientific bodies, the Harveian Society and the Psychological Society of England.[70, 71] In 1957 on the occasion of their Bicentenary Dinner the Royal Medical Society had arranged for use of the Hall but because of the number of applications the venue had to be changed.[72] Early in the previous century when this same Society had decided to build new premises Dr Bennet, a Fellow of the College, delivered two lectures in the Queen Street Hall, 'in aid of the Building Fund of the Royal Medical Society'.[73]

A Second Extension: 11 Queen Street (1970)

In 1970 the property adjoining the Main Hall (No. 9 Queen Street) on the west was purchased. This house, No. 11, remains an integral part of the original Georgian Queen Street but no information is available about the architect or builders. Owned at one time by the *Edinburgh Gazette* it was thereafter, until purchased by the College of Physicians, occupied by a succession of commercial concerns. The new addition will be integrated pending improvements to and expansion of facilities in the College.

Flowers that Bloom in the Spring Tra-la

A Council Minute in 1911 states to the Treasurer having been authorized 'to arrange for the permanent maintenance of window boxes with flowers in the College'.[74] Successive Treasurers seem to have been oblivious of their responsibility in this connection—but too many of them have been involved for any one to claim historical notoriety in the manner of supposedly contumacious Dr Oliphant of old.

REFERENCES

(1) SIBBALD, Sir R. (1833) *The Autobiography*, p. 28, Edinburgh: Thomas Stevenson.
(2) College Minutes, 1.ii.1694.
(3) Ibid., 14.ix.1695.
(4) Ibid., 29.ix.1696.
(5) Ibid., 13.xi.1696.
(6) RITCHIE, R. P. (1899) *The Early Days of the Royall Colledge of Phisitians, Edinburgh*, p. 152. Edinburgh: G. P. Johnston.
(7) College Minutes, 24.v.1697.
(8) Ibid., 27.iv.1698.
(9) Ibid., 29.iv.1698.
10) R.C.P.E. (1925) *Historical Sketch and Laws*, p. 39. Edinburgh: Royal College of Physicians.
(11) College Minutes, 8.vii.1700.
(12) Ibid., 13.vii.1704.

FOUNTAIN CLOSE (1704)

(13) Ibid., 15.viii.1704.
(14) Ibid., 24.x.1704.

(15) Ibid., 1.xii.1704.

(16) Ibid., 29.vi.1705.

(17) Ibid., 6.iii.1706.

(18) Ibid., 5.viii.1706.

(19) Ibid., 7.viii.1711.

(20) Ibid., 4.iii.1712.

(21) Ibid., 3.v.1715.

(22) Ibid., 2.viii.1720.

(23) Ibid., 1.v.1722.

(24) Ibid., 5.xi.1751.

(25) R.C.P.E. Op. cit., p. 41.

(26) BEILBY, W. (1847) *Address Delivered at the Opening of the New Hall of the Royal College of Physicians, November 27, 1846*, pp. 29–30. Edinburgh: Constable.

(27) PENDRILL, G. R. (1959) *The Halls of the Royal College of Physicians of Edinburgh.* [Typescript.]

TEMPORARY ASYLUM

(28) College Minutes, 4.xi.1766.

(29) EDINBURGH ROYAL INFIRMARY (1909) *Notes and Excerpts from the Minutes, &c. as to the relationship of the University and the Royal Colleges of Physicians and of Surgeons to the Institution. 1728–1908*, p. 4. [Edinburgh: R.I.E.]

(30) R.C.P.E. (1763) *Miscellaneous Papers*, no. 187: 1.xi.1763.

(31) R.C.P.E. (1925) *Historical Sketch and Laws*, p. 42. Edinburgh: Royal College of Physicians.

(32) DRUMMOND, J. (1879) *Old Edinburgh.* Edinburgh: G. Waterston, Sons & Stewart.

(33) *Edinburgh: Scotland's Capital* (1967) with . . . photographs, by Alan Daiches [and others], p. 52. Edinburgh: Oliver & Boyd.

(34) R.C.P.E. (1925) *Historical Sketch and Laws*, p. 48. Edinburgh: Royal College of Physicians.

GEORGE STREET HALL (1781)

(35) WRIGHT-ST. CLAIR, R. E. (1964) *Doctors Monro: a medical saga*, p. 80. London: Wellcome Historical Medical Library.

(36) THOMSON, J. (1859) *An account of the Life, Lectures and Writings of William Cullen, M.D.*, vol.II, p. 85. Edinburgh: Blackwood.

(37) ARNOT, H. (1779) *The History of Edinburgh*, pp. 322–3. Edinburgh: W. Creech.

(38) YOUNGSON, A. J. (1966) *The Making of Classical Edinburgh, 1750–1840*, p. 95. Edinburgh: Edinburgh University Press.

(39) R.C.P.E. (1779) *General Correspondence*, 10.xi.1779.

(40) College Minutes, 1.viii.1780.

(41) Ibid., 12.ix.1781.

(42) BEILBY, W. Op. cit., p. 32.

(43) College Minutes, 7.ii.1758.

(44) Ibid., 2.v.1758.
(45) PENDRILL, G. R. Op. cit.
(46) BEILBY, W. Op. cit., p. 33.
(47) College Minutes, 11.v.1843.
(48) Ibid., 8.vi.1843.
(49) Ibid., 23.vi.1843.
(50) Ibid., 5.v.1868.
(51) R.C.P.E. (c. 1850) *Abstracts of the Minutes, AD 1682–1731.* By George Paterson. p. 103. (Ms.)

IN 'LODGINGS' AGAIN (1843)

(52) College Minutes, 1.viii.1843.

QUEEN STREET HALL (1846)

(53) R.C.P.E. *Historical Sketch and Laws*, pp. 43–6. Edinburgh: Royal College of Physicians.
(54) YOUNGSON, A. J. Op. cit., p. 280.
(55) Council Minutes, 29.x.1929.
(56) Ibid., 12.xi.1886.
(57) Ibid., 14.vii.1911.
(58) Ibid., 28.x.1902.
(59) Ibid., 10.xii.1877.
(60) Ibid., 24.x.1883.
(61) Ibid., 25.iv.1939.
(62) Ibid., 28.i.1941.
(63) COOKE, A. M. (1972) *A History of the Royal College of Physicians of London*, vol. 3, p. 1074. Oxford: Clarendon.
(64) Council Minutes, 4.xii.1956.
(65) Council Minutes, 11.xii.1956.
(66) R.C.P.E. (1925) *Historical Sketch and Laws*, p. 46. Edinburgh: Royal College of Physicians.
(67) ROYAL COMMISSION ON THE ANCIENT MONUMENTS OF SCOTLAND (1951) *An Inventory of the Ancient and Historical Monuments of the City of Edinburgh*, p. 197. Edinburgh: H.M.S.O.
(68) PENDRILL, G. R. Op. cit.
(69) College Minutes, 6.ii.1917.
(70) Ibid., 18.iii.1884.
(71) Ibid., 6.ii.1866.
(72) GRAY, J. (1952) *History of the Royal Medical Society, 1737–1937*, p. 311. Edinburgh: Edinburgh University Press.
(73) Ibid., p. 202.
(74) Council Minutes, 31.x.1911.

Chapter V

CERTAIN EARLY PROJECTS AND THEIR EVENTUAL OUTCOME

Sibbald . . . was one of the fathers of the Scottish enlightenment of the post-Union age.
                                                                              T. C. Smout

Once in possession of its Charter the College lost no time setting in motion various projects in keeping with the declared aims of those who had signed the petition. All these projects proved their value. In the course of time, some were in danger of outliving their usefulness and were quietly terminated.

THE PHYSICK GARDEN: [1667]–1761

Strictly speaking, this was not in any sense a product or preserve of the College. None the less, it owed its origin to two leading Edinburgh physicians, both of whom were to become Presidents of the College—(Sir) Andrew Balfour and (Sir) Robert Sibbald. These two men had in common an intense interest in natural history. Moreover, as doctors they recognized the dictum of the period that knowledge of botany and anatomy was fundamental to the study of medicine. Already the surgeons had made provision for the study of anatomy and it remained for the physicians to do likewise for botany. Having previously met on the Continent, the friendship between Sibbald and Balfour soon ripened when, in 1667, Balfour came from St Andrews to settle in Edinburgh. They decided to join forces in creating a physic garden. What transpired is best described in Sibbald's own words:

> 'I had become acquaint with Patrick Morray, Laird of Levingstone . . . ; and I frequently went to Leviston, wher he had collected of plants . . . neer to a thousand. I made Dr. Balfour his acquaintence with Levistone, which, . . . gave the rise to the designe of establishing the medicine garden at Edinburgh. Doctor Balfour and I

first resolved upon it, and obtained of John Brown, gardner of the North Yardes in the Abby, ane inclosure of some 400 foot of measure every way . . . By what we procured from Leviston and other gardens . . . we made a collection of eight or nyne hundred plants ther.'[1]

The co-operation of a number of physicians was obtained. At first 'dreading that it might usher in a Coledge of Physitians', the chirurgeon–apothecaries were obstructive but eventually capitulated in face of Balfour's persuasiveness to the extent of assisting in obtaining from the Town Council a lease of the garden belonging to Trinity Hospital. This in effect was a second garden additional to that at Holyrood Abbey, and both were supervised by James Sutherland who later held the titular office of Professor of Botany in the Town's College.[2] Balfour and Sibbald were appointed Visitors of the garden by the Town Council. Early resentment by the surgeons may well have arisen from the fact that they themselves had previously established a Physick Garden in 1656.[3]

Sutherland was succeeded in the chair of botany by Dr Charles Preston, a Fellow of the College, and he in turn in 1712 by his brother George Preston—a Druggist and Apothecary. The last named successfully sought a recommendation in his favour from the College. Preston was followed in 1729 by Dr Charles Alston, who in his day had matriculated at Leyden and graduated at the University there. Doubtless his association with Leyden explained his inclusion in a list of subscribers for what proved to be a classic botanical book, published by Boerhaave on behalf of his deceased Parisian friend Vaillant.[4]

In 1689 the North Loch was drained as a defence measure during the siege of the castle, with the result that uncontrolled water drained for several days over the grounds at Trinity Hospital and almost destroyed the garden. To compensate, the garden at Holyrood was extended. Many years later (1761) the two gardens were disbanded and a new one developed on the west of Leith Walk only to be replaced in sixty years' time (1822–4) by the present Botanic Garden in Inverleith Row.[5] Without hint of either approval or disapproval Cockburn wrote of the Physic Garden being a 'favourite open-day haunt of the literature and polite flirtation of Edinburgh'.[6]

Realization of Sibbald's garden project took place during the very years he was intent on marshalling resources for the furtherance of the establishment of a College of Physicians. There may well be significance in his almost simultaneous appointment by Charles II as His Majesty's 'Geographer for the Kingdome of Scotland' and His Majesty's 'Physitian ordinary' for the Kingdom of Scotland.[7] Sibbald gave an indication of his approach when he wrote 'I had from my Settlement here [Edinburgh] a designe to informe myself of the naturall history this country could affoord, for I had learned at Paris that the simplest method of Physick was the best, and these that the country affoorded came nearest to our temper, and agreed best with us, so I resolved to make it a part of my studie to know what animalls, vegetables, mineralls, metalls and substances cast up by the sea, were found in this country, that might be of use in medicine, or other artes usefull to human lyfe . . .'.[8]

Words no doubt sounding strangely in a modern world of internationally pill-dominated pharmacy, but which, none the less, possessed a core of persisting perspective.

Day after day, day after day the same—
A weary waste of water.

Robert Southey

Mention has been made of the property in the College grounds of Fountain Close (Chap. IV). In February 1712 because 'the hauss . . . was turning ruinous and Inhabit-able' a Committee including the President was appointed 'to goe with a knoweing Tradesman to visit the said houss, and to Consider if they should be repaired, or what uther us can be made yrof that they be more beneficiall to the Colledge'.[9] The Committee reported within less than a week and their recommendation that the 'old Tenement . . . should be Imployed for erecting of a Cold-bath by way of Pavilion Conforme' was approved.[10] On 24th July 1713 it was reported that 'the Cold-bath Lately built . . . was now finished' and the College thanked a member of the Com-mittee 'for the Care and payne . . . taken in bringing the . . . Bath to such perfec-tion'.[11]

No particulars as to clientèle appear in the Minutes but, it is recorded that for each attendance a charge of 12 Shillings Scots was made with over and above 'tuo pence to the servant for every tyme': but, anyone willing to pay a guinea yearly was entitled to use of the bath 'as frequently as they please'.[11] At first a Committee of physicians appears to have attended 'to receive the fees and superintend the ablutions'.[12] The situation as seen in the light of present-day customs, must have been extraordinary to the point of being bizarre: and the mind 'boggles' at the thought of successful phys-icians themselves critical of the commercial activities of surgeons and pharmacists, acting as bath superintendents. They were in effect, purveyors of water with no therapeutic value other than that of cleanliness and hygiene. Professionally they were doing no more than offsetting the disadvantages of Edinburgh's notorious domestic water supply. It is small wonder that the physicians relinquished their duties as attendants for those of Period Visitors. As Visitors they were required to report to the College at regular intervals about the structure, equipment and general functioning of the bath-house.

In October 1714 the Cold Bath had 'turned insufficient and not serviceable at present'. Thereafter followed a sad and sorry tale extending over some thirty years. Advice was obtained from 'Massones or other Tradesmen'.[13] What transpired is not noted but within five days a Minute recorded that discussions had taken place with a merchant and Writer to the Signet about letting the Cold Bath.[14] Agreement was reached in two days, the rental being fixed at twenty guineas per annum and the College undertaking to make the Bath 'sufficient and serviceable' forthwith. Not surprisingly difficulties arose in due course and in February 1716 one of the joint tenants applied for an abatement of the rent on the score of 'The Rigor of the Seasone and the present calamity by the warr and the Losse of tyme for the Space of sex weeks that the . . . Cold-bath was a repairing'.[15] An abatement of two guineas was allowed by the College in respect of 'the Sex weeks tyme that the . . . bath was a repairing'.[16] Rent arrears were the next development[17] but representations, initially at least, put matters right.[18] There followed the need for more repairs and a contract was entered into with 'the Massone' who undertook then, to 'maintain [the "Cold Bath"] water-tight . . . for payment of Ten Shillings starling yearly'.[19] Late in 1719 the College terminated the lease of the Bath, no precise reason being given in the Minutes.[20] Relations between the contracting parties did not benefit. Bearing in mind that negotiations eventually involved personal contact, the physicians deputed to further the aims of the College were not to be envied! Recourse was made to threat of legal proceedings.[21, 22] Happily settlement of the issue was reached, whereby although deprived of his tenancy, the Writer to the Signet was allowed by the College 'his bathing in the said Cold-Bath for himself only and that Gratis Dureing their pleasure'.[23]

At this stage consideration was given to disposing of the Bath. As it turned out a new tenant was found in the person of 'an appothecary and Druggist'. His annual rent was £25, this being an increase on that agreed by the former tenants[24, 25]: within three years he too defaulted.[26] Protestations were less effective on this occasion, producing no more than assurances by the tenant. In February the tenancy arrangements came to an end and a Committee was instructed once again to 'consider the State of the Cold Bath and to sett it by Tack or any other way they think fitt'.[27]

Another tenancy was the outcome—this time granted to two 'Chirurgeons in Edinr. . . . for five years at Eighteen pound Sterling yearly'.[28] Because of losses incurred by the surgeons the College agreed to reduction of the rent by 'Two pounds six shillings and six pence sterg.' for one year only.[29] Troubles with maintenance and the inadequacy of those undertaking repairs recurred.[30] Another agreement with yet another tradesman was arrived at 'anent the keeping the Cold Bath in Sufficient Repair yearly',[31] but in the matter of months the College, obviously disturbed, arrived at a decision to call in Mr McGill or Mr Norman Adam for their advice as architects.[32] The advice given, which involved major structural renovations and the use of new materials, was accepted but with insistence by the College upon rigid terms of contract to cover unsatisfactory workmanship. Execution of the work involved the College in borrowing yet again.[33]

In August 1734 frustration gave way to exasperation as evidenced by a Minute to the effect 'That notwithstanding all that John Wyllie has done to ye Cold Bath ye same is still unsufficient and does not answer the proposed designe for Bathing'.[34] The repairs seemed to be giving satisfaction three months later as doing 'at present . . . very well'[35] but when approached again two years later Wyllie expressed inability to proceed 'about repairing ye Cold Bath But the season being so far advanced the same must be delayed till harvest'.[36] When he did effect repairs, the result did not satisfy the College who reminded him of the penalty clause in the contract.[37]

Over all the years to date there was no mention of a specific fault or defect but on 5th August 1740 the President stated to having been informed that the 'Cold Bath . . . was in so bad Condition That it did Run out about ane Inch deep in the Space of ane hour.[38] Nothing significant appears to have been done until the next year when an estimate of 'Nynteen pound five Shillings and Six pence Sterl.' was obtained for 'the expence of Lyning the Cold Bath with Lead'.[39] On completion of the work the College was informed 'That the Preses [President] advanced him ten pound Sterl. of ye money before the work was Begun'; and that 'Mr. Campbell's accot. for finishing ye Cold Bath . . . exceeds the estimate formerly given in in upwards of Seven pound Sterl.'[40] What eventuated when Mr Campbell was 'conferred with' does not seem to have been recorded.

Otherwise the Minutes contain only a few more references to the Cold Bath—one to the effect that 'The Colledge allow the use of the Cold Bath Gratis to any in the Infirmary who shall have ane order for that purpose from the Physician attending, The other persons attending the Cold Bath being always first served'.[41] Another is really the only Minute in the entire series conveying a vestige of satisfaction. It explained that 'application had been made to the good town of Edinr. Setting forth That the well which Supplys the Cold Bath being of Publick use to the town, the good town ought to Repair and keep it up which was readyly Granted by the town Councill'. But, as though the administration were twentieth and not eighteenth century, the Minute concluded with 'But as yet nothing has been done in that affair.'[42]

The last Minutes on the subject refer to the renting of the Bath to a surgeon who was with peculiar appropriateness 'agent to the Navy in North Brittain'.[43] The navy's agent was evidently very much on the alert because he secured a refund from the College of moneys received by the 'Gardiner . . . from persons attending the Bath'.[44] Discreetly, the Minutes do not detail the exact circumstances!

That was in 1757 and the Minute books contain only one more reference to the Cold Bath (7th November 1758). Perhaps the troublous times were the death knell of the ruinous houses. Whatever the reason and no matter the circumstances in which it occurred, the end of the Bath-house came none too soon. Cryptic although the recorded Minutes are, there is no concealing the persistent indecisiveness of the College almost deserving today's popular political connotation of 'stop-and-go'. Equally evident is the difficulty experienced by the physicians in dealing with recalcitrant tenants and awkward workmen against a background of financial expertise which would not stand actuarial scrutiny. Some consolation may be derived from the fact that the College of Surgeons was equally unsuccessful in a similar venture. The Infirmary was no more fortunate despite lavish expenditure on paving and tiling with white marble imported from Holland.[45]

THE DISPENSARY: CARE OF THE NECESSITOUS: 1682–1749

It is greatly to the credit of the College that on the occasion of their first recorded Quarterly Meeting on 6th February 1682 they resolved 'that att the next meeting of the Colledge some persouns be appoynted by the Colledge to be physitians for the poore'.[46] Considerable time must have been devoted to the subject at the next meeting because, additional to it being 'ordered that Doctors Burnett and Crawfurd shall untill the next electione of the College serve the poore of the Cittie and suburbs', it was recommended 'to the President and Censors to acquant the Provost of the Colledges Resolutione, and to desyre the Provost to acquant the Councill . . .'. The hope was also expressed that the Council would 'nominat some persone to be apothecary': and that the 'Ministers of severall Kirk Sessions' should be informed with the intention that they would 'give certificates that the poore that are sick are in there bounds'. To ensure a reliable service 'Doctors nominat are authorized to Deput any of the Colledge In caise of there necessary absence for some space'. With an approach which would have done credit to the Civil Service they 'resolved that for the good of the Society and keeping of good order therein a promisory paper be drawn up by the Councill and offered to the next meeting of the Colledge to be agried to, and as the samen shall be agried to by the Colledge to be signed by all the Members'.[47]

There is no evidence that any promissory paper evolved, or that the Town Council nominated anyone as apothecary. But the physicians developed and maintained the service undeterred, contributing to the cost of medicines if not directly from their own pockets, from such sources as fines for absence from or late attendance at Quarterly Meetings of the College, and for failure to attend at the prescribed times to 'the sick poore'.[48] At a later date fixed contributions to the Dispensary were required of each Fellow on election.[49] Paradoxically, funds for medicines for the poor were raised at Assembly Hall sessions which did not find favour with some at the time when the sale of the College's George Street Hall was being contemplated.[50]

From the Minutes it appears physicians for the poor were appointed for a period of twelve months, two at a time.[51, 52] In 1705 the College 'unanimouslie agried . . . That tue of their number shall attend at their place of meeting [Fountain Close] every Munday Wedensday, and ffryday betwixt thrie and four in the afternoone for giveing advyce to the sicke and poore Gratis'[53]: and two years later the College agreed to the use of the College Hall for a Repository for Medicines when required.[54]

An apothecary was appointed to the Dispensary after an interval of almost seven years[55] and on his decease an agreement was reached with a Doctor Murray 'anent the keeping and Dispenseing of the Druggs and Medicaments belonging to the Colledge'.[56] In June 1707 the College was one of the beneficiaries when the estate of 'Mary Erskine relict of James Hair Druggist Burges of Edgr' was distributed. The legacy to the College amounted to 'the soume of Twelve hundred and ffiftie merks Scots money which is to be Laid out upon security and the rent thereof to be yearly imployed for buying and furnishing of Druggs and medicaments to the sick poore who have theire advyce gratis from the said Royall Colledge'.[57] Not altogether surprisingly the gift stimulated great interest, and at least seven meetings took place in less than twelve months to consider how best to use the legacy while at the same time adhering strictly to the terms laid down. Eventually it was decided that the sum of money involved be made available for lending out 'to such of the members of the Colledge who have subscrybed for setting up a Repository for furnishing of Medicines to the sick poore at the Intrinsick value'.[58] The Repository was established in 1708, and the College allowed 'the College Hall for what meetings the subscrybers for the said Repository shall appoynt'.[59] The custom prevailed in a number of nineteenth and twentieth century hospitals of calling their out-patient departments 'dispensaries' although no medicines were dispensed: and dated back to the establishment by the Edinburgh and London Colleges of dispensaries in which diagnostic and dispensing services were combined.

Another of Mary Erskine's major benefactions was to the Merchant Maiden Hospital—now the Mary Erskine School.

In 1712 there was another significant development. The College 'appoynt that for the future the Licentiats shall give their advyce and attendance on the said poore alswell as the ordinary members'. Of special interest is that the decision was preceded by the comment 'Considering the Charity in gieving punctuall attendance on the sick poore'.[60] It suggests that demands on the dispensary had increased but that humanitarian considerations were not forgotten as they sometimes are in hardpressed modern hospital out-patient services. Individually, however, members and licentiates cannot all have been perfectionists because, at a later date, the College found it necessary to instruct 'their officer to give a billet to every member (whose turn it is to attend the sick poore) weekly or oftener as their attendance is to be made; and the Exacting of the fynes for being absent therefrom or from the quarterly meetings be Delayed till next meeting of the Colledge and no Longer'.[61]

Inevitably the establishment of the Infirmary in 1729 posed problems for the Dispensary, more especially as physicians on the staff of the former were drawn from among Fellows of the College. A Minute on the subject dated 5th May 1730 reads:

> 'The Oppinion of the Council in Relation to ye attendance on ye Infirmary and Sick poor being Reported to the Colledge the same was approven of And the Colledge did yrupon order That in Place of two phisicians who ordinarily attended the hall formerly, only one shall wait on And when the present Course is over, The Eldest phisician shall begin, And So in Course go on as formerly . . . And that all the fellows and Licentiats shall be obleidged to attend both at the Hall and Infirmary in yr turns Or Send oyrs of ye Colledge Number for them And who does not observe these Rules shall be subject to the Censure of ye Colledge.'[62]

Such bureaucratic utterances might almost have emanated from a Government or regional office. Fortunately a realistic solution eventuated. The Infirmary, with medical staff consisting solely of Fellows of the College, took the initiative and the

College, probably well alive to the advantages, readily co-operated. A College Minute of 2nd May 1749 sums up the sequence of events.

> 'It haveing been proposed by the Managers of the Royal Infirmary That in place of the Colledge their giveing attendance upon poor patients at their own hall twice a week They will be pleased in time Coming in their turn to attend the poor out patients at the Infirmary upon Monday and friday weekly at three afternoon The managers haveing Resolved that the out patients Shall get medicines gratis from the Infirmary Shop The above desire of the Infirmary was agreed to by the Colledge.'[63]

None the less, the College took umbrage at the way in which the Infirmary implemented the agreement. The trouble arose from 'the Statut of the Royal Infirmary Relateing to their attendance on the out Patients . . . Which had been printed without any previous Concurrance of the Colledge.' However the College 'afterwards agreed to on ane apology haveing been made' to give trial to the Infirmary proposals. The upshot was that 'finding it upon tryal very Inconvenient for the Same Physician to attend the Infirmary in the forenoon And the out patients in the afternoon Doe therefore Resolve and agree That in time Comeing the attendance on the Infirmary and out patients shall be by two different Physicians . . . And the Colledge appoint this Resolution to be Intimat to the managers of the Royal Infirmary . . . by Such of the members of the Colledge as are managers of the Infirmary'.[64]

The managers of the Infirmary 'agreed to and approved of' the Resolution[65] and so with transfer from the College of the work of 'physitians for the poore' the Infirmary benefited from the long accumulated experience of the College, and together the College and Infirmary agreed staffing arrangements in 1749 for 'in time coming' which have continued to this day.

THE PHARMACOPOEIA: 1699–1864

> *What rhubarb, senna, or what purgative drug,*
> *Would scour these English hence?*
> William Shakespeare (*Macbeth*)

> *I firmly believe that if the whole materia medica could be sunk to the bottom of the sea, it would be all the better for mankind,—and all the worse for the fishes.*
> Oliver Wendell Holmes

The very first item in the first Minute of the College relates to the *Pharmacopoeia*. It reads 'Remitted to the former Committee named for forming a pharmacopea to meet and prepair the samen as was apoynted'.[66] From this it is evident that some form of professional gathering or Committee had already been at work on the subject in advance of official meetings of the newly created College. The names of those on the Committee are not known but on 8th March (1682) five doctors were appointed 'as a Comittee to Consider of the draught of a Pharmacopea as the samen is already drawn by the Comittee formerly named for that effect . . . and conjunctly or seperatly to revise the samen, and to also mark on a paper apart what is there opinion to add or diminish . . .'.[67] From this it can be reasonably surmised that preparation of a draft was already considerably advanced, and it would seem that the new Committee was intended either to replace or formally reconstitute the old. Certainly no time was lost and the question arises why was the subject given something akin to 'top priority'?

Without exception all petitions for a Charter had enlarged upon the literally chaotic situation prevailing in the selection, preparation, issue and costs of drugs and medicaments (Chap. II). These conditions were still prevalent in Scotland at the time of the erection of the College. In England the situation was less perturbing due in some measure to a pharmacopoeia having been drawn up by the College of Physicians of London in 1618. At least six editions of this pharmacopoeia had been published but its jurisdiction did not extend further north than Berwick-on-Tweed and its formulae were not binding on the apothecaries of Scotland. Although the Edinburgh College had legal power to visit the shops and inspect the drugs of apothecaries a need remained for the guidance if not actual control of those dispensing medicaments.

Despite the underlying purpose and despite the apparent urgency of the need, the *Edinburgh Pharmacopoeia* was an inordinately long time in being published. Conflicting personalities in the College were almost certainly at the root of this, together with a desire on the part of one or more Socii not to give offence to the apothecaries. By his own confession Sir Archibald Stevensone was consistently opposed to the idea of the *Pharmacopoeia* (q.v.).

In March 1682 a special Committee of five was appointed to 'revise the severall parts of the Pharmacopea as they are now mended'.[68] Instructed 'to bring in his part of the Pharmacopea' at the meeting seven days previously,[69] Dr Balfour on 20th August 1683 'gave account that he had agried with David Lindsay for printing the pharmacopea who had undertaken to give the Colledge Copies of each of the Impressions for the use of the Colledge whereto the Colledge agries and appoynts each Member to revise their oun part, and the Preses Doctors Balfour Sibbald and Pitcairne to be revisers of the haill, and that the Preses Doctors Balfour and Sibbald or any tue of them enter into a Contract with the printer'.[70]

Despite the encouraging progress reflected in these Minutes there is no further mention of the *Pharmacopoeia* until December 1684, three days after Sibbald's election as President. At the first sederunt over which he presided in that capacity he and seven Fellows were 'appoynted to be a Quorum for Considering the Pharmacopea and Improvement of Medicine'.[71] Stevensone in his 'Information' allowed to having been highly critical of 'this so much magnified Dispensatory' but he categorically attributed suppression of it to the 'Learned Doctor Balfour of Worthy Memory'. According to Stevensone, the Dispensatory was 'altogether useless to the Apothecaries, nor was it ever agreed to by the Society [College] but was only the Work of Doctors Sibbald, Trotter, and two or three more to whom that Affair was committed'. The doctors concerned were those appointed as a special Committee by the College in December 1684. Defending himself against Trotter's probably legitimate insinuations, Stevensone claimed to have concurred with Sibbald's close friend Balfour 'to suppress this ill shaped Bratt they seem so fond of, which could never have endured the Light'.[72] Stevensone's account was tinged too much by hurt pride and emotion to be accepted as accurate.

It is at this stage in the College's history that there is an extensive absence of Minutes, and when they are resumed in 1693 the records show evidence of a number of Minutes having been deleted. One such deletion follows a recording that seven Socii, including the President and Sibbald had been named in February 1696 'to revise the pharmacopea and make ther report to the colledge and to appoynt ther owne meetings'.[73] This after an interval of twelve years, and thirteen years since contact with a printer had been authorized!

In about a year's time—thirteen months to be precise—another revisory Committee was appointed to review 'the severall papers relateing to the dispensatory . . . given in by the severall Comities with ther remarks upon them'.[74] Not without reason an element of urgency crept into affairs and within two weeks 'the colledge appoynts the Comitie appoynted for the dispensatory to meet every Munday at eleven acloak ay and whill the affair be at ane end'.[75] Sibbald about this time resigned from the Committee which continued from time to time to report to the College desirable amendments, deletions and additions. The College took one further hesitant step forward in September 1698 when it 'heard all the objectiones made against the pharmacopea unto the oyles and have approven it soe farr'.[76] And finally with what would appear to be an understandable admixture of shame and new faith, in March 1699 it was recorded that 'the colledge takeing into ther consideratne yt the dispensatory which hath been aggried upon haveing been severall tymes comitted by the colledge to severalls of the members thereof to be revised and ther reports made, In pnce of the colledge The colledge being now satisfied with the draught yrof ordaines the samen to be printed and appoynts the president and dr Eizat or in any of yr absence dr Mitchell to agrie with the printer revise the sheits and correct the press'.[77]

The apologia, if such it was, cannot have satisfied Sibbald. From first to last he had regarded production of a pharmacopoeia as of supreme importance and had put his every endeavour into furthering and hastening the project. His reactions to persistent frustrations have been told by himself in his *Autobiography*:

> 'In the tyme I was president . . . The Pharmacopaea Edinburgensis was composed, and licensed to be printed by the Chancellor, and the Printer agreed to print it gratis, and give the College a competent number of copies, and take his hazard of vending the rest; bot by the malice of some, it was laid aside for ten yeers ther- after.[78]

Elsewhere, referring to agreement given by the College, he concluded 'and yett a faction obstructed them'.[79] Words of a disappointed man, yes—but dignified words when account is taken of the polemics and vituperation indulged in by those of his period and subsequently.

Paterson gave a less restrained version. 'Another fierce contention' he quoted 'arose from the question of publishing a Dispensatory which had been prepared under the sanction of the College. Stevensone's party opposed its publication on the ground of its being "barely a transcript of the London one, ill-copied and worse explained". Dr Pitcairne was attacked in a virulent pamphlet which charged him with the inconsistency of having written a commendatory preface to a book which he afterwards represented as worthless.' The pamphlet was entitled 'Information for Dr Arch^d Pitcairn against the abdicate Professor . . . or a Mathematical demonstration that liars should have good memories . . . Whereby the College of Physicians is vindicated from the Calumnies contained in Dr. Stevenson's last information relating to the Dispensary'.[80]

Paterson considered that the first edition of the *Edinburgh Pharmacopoeia* was published in 1683 and not in 1699 as stated by Beilby. In point of fact the edition of 1699 was the delayed production of the *Pharmacopoeia* first contemplated in 1682.

Did the *Edinburgh Pharmacopoeia* attain its objectives? The answer is an unquali- fied yes. First appearing in 1699, twelve subsequent editions were brought out—in 1722, 1735, 1744, 1756, 1774, 1783, 1792, 1803, 1805, 1817, 1839 and 1841. There were in addition reprint editions in 1807, 1808, 1809 and 1813.[80a] Before the second new edition was sent for printing, the draft was revised and agreed 'as to the Metho- dus Componendii' with representatives of the Surgeons.[81, 82] A letter was received

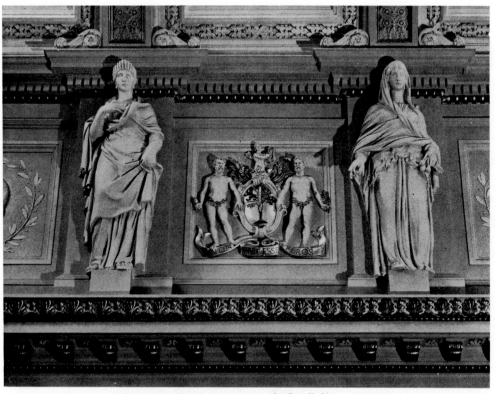

PLATE 11 Queen Street: Detail of Hall decoration.
Reproduced by permission from *Scottish Field*; photograph by George B. Alden

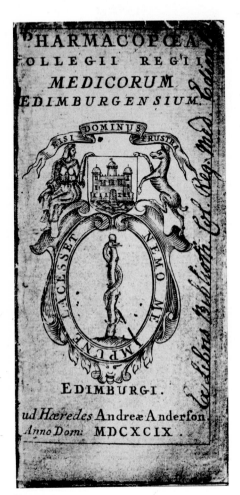

PLATE 12

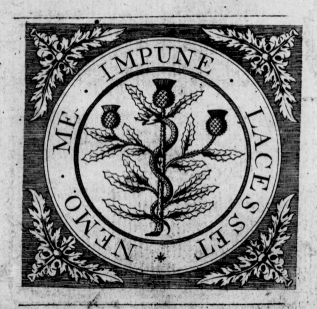

PLATE 13

PLATE 12 *Edinburgh Pharmacopoea*: Title page, 1699
PLATE 13 *Edinburgh Pharmacopoeia*: Title page, 1735
Photographs by Tom Scott

from Dr Gray at London 'in verie civill terms thanking the Colledge for sending him a copie'.[83] As with the second, agreement with the Surgeons was arrived at before publication of the third edition, the first meeting for the purpose being 'on ye first Tewsday of December next [1732] at Johns Coffee house at three afternoon'.[84] A factor which accelerated publication of the third edition was the unauthorized production in London of a 'pirated' copy.[84a] Commenting on the fourth edition in a letter to William Cullen who had superintended the revision, Sir John Pringle remarked 'I should judge that in point of simplicity and elegance of composition, where composition is required, the new Edinburgh Pharmacopoeia has got as far before the last London Pharmacopoeia (1746) as that work excelled all others preceding it'. There followed a forecast applicable to reviewers of all generations: '... we shall have fault found with several things, by some for having so far cast off the old farrago, and by others for not having availed ourselves of all the new lights'.[85]

Cullen was assisted in his revisionary work by Dr John Clerk whom he described as 'the person who chiefly introduced into Scotland judgment, accuracy and elegance in private prescriptions'.[86] In 1821 on the motion of the President (Dr Buchan) a special vote of thanks was accorded Dr Hope for his effective refutation of criticisms in the *Annals of Philosophy* and his defence of 'the Chemical processes recommended by the College'.[87]

The successive editions were in general use throughout Scotland until the appearance of the *British Pharmacopoeia* in 1864. There is some indication of the appeal of the *Edinburgh Pharmacopoeia* in the fact that over 2000 copies of the 6th edition[87a] and the entire 9th edition were sold within about a year of being first issued[87b] and: that less than two years elapsed between issue of the first and second editions in English (q.v.). Issued by the General Medical Council under the terms of the Medical Act, 1858, use of the *British Pharmacopoeia* became obligatory throughout the United Kingdom.

A pharmacist's appraisal is not out of place. It ran as follows:

'Edinburgh has been a prolific source of official and unofficial pharmaceutical literature, some of it of classical rank. Pride of place is taken by the Edinburgh Pharmacopoeia ... As was inevitable, the earlier editions retained many medieval survivals, and fearsome witches' cauldron brews, but even apparently irrational examples of *modus operandi*, have later turned out to have a scientific *raison d'être*. Thus, in the second edition (1722) under "Bufo Praeparatus", the apothecary is directed to place living toads in an earthen pot, dessicate them at a moderate temperature, and reduce the residue to powder. This looks suspiciously like a hocus-pocus business, but it is now known that the skin of the toad contains a glycoside akin in action to digitalis.'[88]

E

As was to be expected the *Edinburgh Pharmacopoeia*, or *Pharmacopoea Collegii Regii Medicorum Edinburgensium* to give it its first and more ornate title, was subject to drastic and extensive changes in the course of its existence. Although perpetuating such ancient lore as *Album Graecum* (dog's dung) and *Cranium hominis violenta morte extincta* (the skull of a murdered man) the first edition has been described as more selective than the London Pharmacopoeia at that time.[89] In the sixth edition of 1774 the term 'Simples' was replaced by that of 'Materia Medica' and in the picturesque phraseology of Cowen 'Homo and his parts were completely removed'.[89a] Digitalis was first introduced into the Pharmacopoeia in 1699, retained in the second, third and fourth editions and then discarded only to be reinstated in the seventh edition of 1783. Selection of preparations for inclusion was subject to profound discrimination, despite which and as a result of rapid and vast increase in knowledge 'of the 1,009 drugs and forms of medicament in the Ph. Ed., 1741 [*Edinburgh Pharmacopoeia*] less than 100 survive' to the extent of being included in the *British Pharmacopoeia* of 1932.[89] Innovations of nomenclature in the last edition (1841) earned general approval but perhaps one of the most far-seeing and practical features was the inclusion of directions in English for the compounding of preparations. Sheer force of necessity may partly explain the tardy employment of English when it is remembered that among the approved pharmaceutical compounds included in the first edition there were 'some which contained from forty to seventy articles in each' ![90] (Sir) Robert Christison provided a commentary on the *Pharmacopoeia* in his *Dispensatory* (1842). In it he dealt with the physical and chemical properties of drugs and with their influence on the human body.

In its day the *Edinburgh Pharmacopoeia* acquired international fame. It was translated into Dutch and German additional to being produced in Latin by publishers in, among other continental centres, Bremen, Göttingen, Leipzig, Rotterdam, Venice, Milan and Geneva. Furthermore Cowen of New Brunswick has stressed the significance of 'the direct role of the Edinburgh Pharmacopoeia as the progenitor of American Pharmacopoeias'. His remarks applied particularly to the Pharmacopoeia of the *Massachusetts Medical Society* (1808), the greater part of which was subsequently included in the first *United States Pharmacopoeia* (1820).[91] Cowen's historical study of *The Edinburgh Pharmacopoeia* is admirably comprehensive and should be consulted by anyone interested in the subject.

Robert Christison acted as Chairman of the General Medical Council Committee entrusted with the task of compiling the first 'Pharmacopoeia of Great Britain and Ireland'.[92] Edinburgh and Dublin applauded the result—but not so London. In Christison's own words 'the critical clamour in London is nothing more than the progeny of a similar outcry which arose there on the publication of the last London Pharmacopoeia, of the last Edinburgh one, and of my Dispensatory. By-and-by all these works outlived defamation, and were rapidly sold off. I prophesy that the same will be the fate of the British Pharmacopoeia.'[93] His prophesy was speedily vindicated.

Poole revealed an interesting sidelight. Some days after his examination by the Parliamentary Committee (July 1834) he had a private conversation with Mr Warburton who apparently considered that the *Edinburgh Pharmacopoeia* compared more than favourably with that of London, and that in the matter of chemists London did not have an equal 'to our Christison'.[94]

In 1862 the College took the initiative in pressing for adoption of the decimal system in the new *Pharmacopoeia*.[95]

TWO 'MUSEUMS'

At different times the initiative and enthusiasm of Fellows were responsible for the creation of two museums representing contrasting interests and redounding greatly to the credit of the College. Both eventually ceased to function as College entities under the relentless pressure of competitive interests and the problem of costs, as rival interests multiplied. The process is a continuing one and Fellows of today like their predecessors of the past are faced with the challenging decision of what, and how much of the proven past to jettison in order to make way for a partially unproven present and a wholly uncertain future.

Natural History Museum: 1706–70

Attention has already been drawn to Sibbald's wide vision of natural history in its relation to medicine and allied sciences: and to his interest in 'animalls, vegetables, minerals, metalls and substances . . . that might be of use in medicine'. His *Letters*[96] to a variety of people were strewn with evidence of his constant search for more knowledge and tangible confirmation of his impressions. He enlisted the aid of the local minister 'to gett me the best account of . . . two whales came in at Culross shortly'. To another minister he wrote of skate and 'poirpoises', 'of fossils', of a 'substance lyke Corall . . . brought from Cantyre and other parts' and again 'of the figures stones, and of the mineralls and metalls found in the Shire (of Ranfrow)'.

Correspondence and the giving of interesting specimens were not all one way. A letter to Sibbald told of 'a spoon of a mixed metall which was found with the Roman coin of Faustina . . . about a mile from Saltcoats'; 'a bibula of silver . . . gote within a mile of Port Glasgow . . . and with it . . . Saxon coins'; of an inscribed cornelian stone, a snail stone, a 'Gothish' ring 'found somewhere beneith Stirling'. In all Sibbald's writings there was a constant quest for books and manuscripts. Such then were some of his innumerable interests and they serve to explain in part how in 1706 he was in a position to offer specimens to the College. His offer which was accepted is recorded in a Minute of 12th March 1706 as follows:

> 'The said day Sir Robert Sibbald offered to give a Large Parcell of Curiosities to the Colledge Provyded he have the power of keeping and ordering them, ffor which offer he had the thanks of the Colledge, and the Thessrer was desyred to Provyde a Convenient Presse in the Colledge for them.'[97]

No details are given concerning the curiosities themselves, nor is there any further reference in the Minute books to Sibbald's gift or its ultimate disposal. It is interesting that nine years previously (1697) Sibbald gave a collection of specimens to the Town College and with them a catalogue dedicated to the Town Council and entitled *Auctorium Musaei Balfouriani e Musaeo Sibbaldiano*.[98] The catalogue classified objects in the collection according as they were minerals; the more rare substances taken from plants; the more rare productions from the Animal Kingdom; Works of Art, manuscripts and rare books. Although his gift to the Town's College was made first, the articles given by Sibbald to the College of Physicians were possibly, indeed probably similar in character. Another interesting fact is that Sibbald concentrated in the main on collecting indigenous curiosities of particular value in relation to the Natural History of Scotland: and he considered his collection to be supplementary to that of his close friend Balfour whose specimens had been gathered over many more years from a great variety of countries the world over. In this connection there is a Minute (24th September 1696) to the effect that 'the colledge considering that Dr. Balfour's curiosities are in the colledge of Edgr. and amongst them the oars of the boat and the shirt of the Barbarous man yt was in the boat belonging to the colledge of physitians and that the same boat is lykelie to be lost they haveing noe convenient place to keep it in doe give the said boat to the colledge of Edgr. ther to be preserved and that it be insert ther yt its gifted by the Royall Colledge'.[99]

From this it would seem that Balfour's contribution to any Royal College museum of Natural History was on a much more moderate scale than that of Sibbald, who had probably originally intended that his curiosities should be the equivalent of visual aids for lectures and colloquia. What happened to Sibbald's curiosities in the College of Physicians is not known. What is certain is that his gifts to the Town's College were added to those of Balfour. To quote Grant '. . . interest in the Natural History collections . . . was not maintained; the objects fell into disorder, deteriorated, or were abstracted. By 1770 . . . the Sibbald Museum had disappeared.'[100]

Thus the College of Physicians, the Town College and its successor the University each in their several ways failed to discharge their obligations in the matter of preserving Sibbald's collections which he himself so valued, that he desired in his lifetime to 'have the power of keeping and ordering them'.

Sporadically, a rare specimen or 'curiosity' was given to the College as for instance 'a Gravell-stone of a prodigous bigness which was past by a woman in Zetland above 60 years of age and yet alyve' by Sir Edward Eizatt[101]; and some 'anatomicall preparationes' gifted by 'John Monro Chirurgeon'.[102] There is no mention in the Minutes of how or where these were stored.

Materia Medica Museum: 1835–96

A Committee appointed to consider the sale or improvement of the College Hall in George Street indicated in its report (4th August 1835) that 'it had occurred to the Committee that it might be desirable to commence a Museum of Materia Medica, for the reception of which the Hall, or other part of the building, might gradually, and as required be fitted up'.[103] Dr Christison pointed out the great benefit that would arise from the formation of such a Museum, and a Subcommittee with him as convener and Dr Gregory as one of the five other members was appointed to further the proposal. Minutes of this Committee exist from 1837 to 1885. Bound in heavy leather they are interspersed with detailed monumental lists of the many items accumulated over the years. Two things in particular about the Minutes are impressive. Firstly the meticulous care taken in what Sibbald would have termed 'keeping and ordering them' which obviously involved repeated review and radical amendment of the catalogued items: and secondly the old-world gracious phraseology of the Minutes themselves, perhaps employed to placate the Council when moderate financial encouragement was being periodically sought.

Early steps were taken to secure the co-operation of the profession and of officials in the Colonies, and to obtain exhibition cases suited to the preservation of specimens. A particular difficulty proved to be the provision of effective lighting. If for a period, the Council was hesitant on the score of even modest expenditure, this was due to uncertainty about possible repercussions on College funds should the Medical Amendment Bill being considered in 1878, pass through Parliament. This hesitancy is not to be construed as evidence of disinterest on the part of the College because, previously when the Queen Street Hall was opened in 1846, the then President was at pains to pay high tribute to Professor Christison in this connection. He attributed to Professor Christison's zeal and industry 'the commencement and the progress already made, in the formation of a museum of Materia Medica; for the indefinite enlargement and effective display of which we now possess ample and suitable accommodation'.[104]

Cold analysis of the contents of the museum would savour of a miniature encyclopaedic inventory. Fortunately there is no need for this because, lying loosely between the leaves of the Minute book, there were notes on scraps of paper written by an unknown but undoubtedly authoritative hand. The character and trend of the notes suggest they were intended for reference on some open occasion when summary of the museum's progress over the years was intended. The following extracts from the notes convey better than anything else the enthusiasm of those responsible for the museum, and the success attending their efforts.

'Museum

On Aug. 4th 1835 Dr. Spens proposed the commencement of a Museum of . . . On that occasion Dr. Christison pointed out the great benefit which would arise from it . . .

On Nov. 3rd of same year 1835 the first donation was presented by Dr. Davidson and consisted of 3 essential oils viz. Cajeput oil, oil of Cloves and Indian oil of grass (andropogom) . . .

On 2nd Feb. 1836 the first Curator or *Keeper* of the Museum as he is called was appointed in the person of Dr. Spittal.

In 14 months afterwards by April 29th 1837 no fewer than 48 additional specimens had been contributed by Drs. Christison, McLagan, Traill, Clark Aberdeen, the Pharmacopoeia Committee and Mr. Duncan Druggist.

On 6th August 1839 Dr. Stark succeeded to the Curatorship and on Nov. 22nd 1839 we find Dr. Christison again . . . contributing to the Collection other 15 Specimens and in addition we find Dr. Craigie, Dr. Shortt; Mr. Duncan also contributed no fewer than 26 Substances. The Pharmacopoeia Committee also gave some. 57 new specimens were thus added to the museum which now contained 108 substances. We also find the Committee authorizing Dr. Stark the Curator to expend the sum of £25 Sterling granted by the College for that purpose—and on Feb. 4th 1840 we find a considerable addition from this source 41 specimens having been purchased and two donations having been received from Mr. McFarland Druggist and our pr. Dr. Christison—By this time the infection seems to have spread and 4 days later viz Feb. 8th ["18th" was probably intended] Messrs

Peter Lawson & Son presented a very fine collection of cereals and other substances to the extent of 37 articles

.   .   .   .   .

On July 1st 1840 the indefatigable Curator Mr. Stark showed that he had been judiciously expending more of the pecuniary grant of Nov. 22nd 1839 for 55 interesting specimens had been added making in all 258 specimens.

.   .   .   .   .

A great accession was made on Janu. 15th 1841 by the Royal Botanical Soc. of Ed. having presented . . . "A Collection of British Medical Plants" constituting a hortus siccus of 338 specimens . . .

On Feb. 14th 1841 Dr. Graham set a good example by cutting a spray in fruit of the Laurus Cassia and presenting it to the Museum.

Fresh purchases were also being effected for on March 22nd 1841 52 specimens of remedies entirely from the Mineral Kingdom were added; while on Nov. 9th 1841 the vegetable world seems with the exception of Petroleum to have been solely called upon to yield its treasures thence we have volatile and fixed oils, and Resinous exudations and balsams.

On Nov. 4th 1843 the obstructed channel was again opened by the fruit of castor oil and Capsules of Quassia amara being presented by Dr. Douglas McLagan and Fruit of Adamsonia digitata (Monkey Bread) by Dr. Christison.

Till Oct. 1846 another lull occurred but on that occasion Dr. J. H. Davidson presented a very fine large crystal of alum while in the following month (Nov. 19th 1846) a most interesting contribution was made by Prof. J. Y. Simpson being no less than the Brass Pestle and Mortar with wh. the famous Cullen and no less celebrated Wm. Hunter compounded galenicals . . .

Such were the gradual additions amounting in all to 366 when a magnificent collection of cinchona barks was contributed by John Eliot Howard Esq. of Tottenham near London which was augmented from time to time by additional grants of cinchonas and their alkaloids and of the lichens growing connected on the barks till on 4th Nov. 1856 he crowned his munificient gift of additional cinchonas by presenting to the library a volume containing his valuable papers on these trees. The specimens sent . . . furnishing such a complete and varied collection as is not, I suppose equalled by any Museum in the United Kingdom . . . and I trust we shall never forget our obligations to the generous donor whose contribution in 1856 was the last we were destined to receive from any source for at least 21 years, but I do trust a new era in the history of the museum may this year be inaugurated and that such a peculiarly valuable collection will receive large accessions by contributions from Fellows and others.

.   .   .   .   .

On Nov. 9th 1848 Quillaia and Copalcki Barks were also presented by Mr. Howard while Dr. Christison still exhibited his interest . . . by a contribution of Native Nitrate of Potash and Orkney Kelp—on Aug. 5 1851 by Messrs. T. & H. Smith whose fame as successful experimentalists is so well known sent us a beautiful specimen of Crystallized Gallic Acid . . . About this time apparently a large accession of the objects of materia medica was made by the purchase fr. Dr. Theodore Martius of Erlangen of a vast number of specimens in excellent condition amounting apparently in all to about 160 animal preparations 1395 vegetable do ... and 309 chemical substances giving a total of 1864 specimens ...

On June 15th 1854 the Curator himself (Dr. Stark) presented the now famous cocoa leaves and also Paraguay Tea and I am glad to be able to add that even America lent us a helping hand for a specimen of the Slippery Elm was presented to this College by Dr. Storer of Boston U.S. I trust that from friends in all parts of the world we may receive liberal contributions and that central africa so recently revealed to us may enrich our Museum by many illustrations of her Medicinal Flora.

. . . . .

The first valuable gift of 57 specimens was presented by Col. Michael from the Indian Department of the Forestry Exhibition which was held in Edr. in 1884.

In 1886 the North British Branch of the Pharmaceutical Society of Great Britain very kindly presented us with 29 very interesting specimens.

In Nov. (1887) a very fine collection of new and rare Drugs amounting to 93 specimens was most generously sent to our Museum by Messrs. Thomas Christy & Company London, so well known for their ability zeal and success in their publications ...

In July 1888 our museum was further enriched by 16 specimens being . . . valuable Medicinal plants from Brisbane, Queensland along with 2 . . . of much interest viz Akazza and ordeal Bark and Follicles of Strophanthus hispidus.

Messrs. Burroughs Wellcome & Co. London kindly sent us a follicle of Strophanthus hispidus.'

The last record in the Museum Minute book was dated 1885: and the last event in the above draft notes was in 1888. In 1896 the College accepted the recommendation of a specially appointed Committee to discontinue the Museum and use the room thus vacated as additional Library accommodation. Earlier in 1862 there had been indefinite proposals that the College Museum should be transferred as a gift to the newly opened Museum of Science and Art, but these never materialized. The decision of 1896 was however final and the College Materia Medica Museum was transferred to the Pharmaceutical Society of Great Britain.

At the same time as accepting the transfer the Pharmaceutical Society agreed to preserve the collection separate and intact, with a distinctive mark or inscription: and that Fellows of the College should have free access to the Collection, while Licentiates of the College and Students of Medicine would have access on producing 'an order' by any Fellow of the College.[105]

Library demands, considered as paramount, accounted for the demise of the College Materia Medica Museum. Today within their own walls libraries are being driven to expediency measures in endeavours to preserve intact their historically rich possessions competing for space with an avalanche of current literature of vastly varying standards. But irreplaceable treasures are to be found elsewhere than in libraries. A need of the late twentieth century is to guard against precipitate under-estimation of the value of past acquisitions, and of too highly emotional appraisal of all that is new.

THE LABORATORY: 1887–1950

The work of the Laboratory started in 1887[106] and ceased in 1950.[107] It could be argued that inclusion of the Laboratory among 'early projects' is not justified. On the other hand the Laboratory had in common with the Physick Garden, the Dispensary and the Pharmacopoeia that during its existence it made an altogether outstanding major contribution to the advance of medical science and the fame of the College of Physicians. Moreover there is justification in continuity. The Laboratory came into being as College Museum activities ceased.

Birth Pangs

In 1885 a Committee was appointed to consider means for furthering research as part of the activities of the College. The original motion to this end was moved by Dr (later Sir) Batty Tuke, and reflected the College's awareness of the wide-ranging extent and almost breathless speed of advances being made in scientific medicine and in the destruction of entrenched dogma. Creation of a laboratory was recommended by the Committee and won the support of the College when proposed formally. As, however, the majority of those in favour was less than the three-quarters necessary for the application of College property 'to other than the ordinary purposes of the College', the motion was not carried. Brought forward once more some nine months later, the proposal met a similar fate in similar circumstances. Undaunted, four months later, influential sponsors of the scheme submitted a Petition to the Council drawing attention to the lack of laboratory facilities. A new and third Committee was appointed, and its Report in terms similar to those previously submitted was accepted unanimously by the College at each of three successive readings. Except in so far as no subtle personalities or disguised delaying tactics were involved, the events were mildly reminiscent of those concerned with Sibbald and the Pharmacopoeia. Dr Clouston, whom none could accuse of reactionarism, uttered a warning of as great significance today as when first given. He declared 'A College of Physicians going to work to encourage Research and omitting any encouragement to the Study of Clinical Medicine and Therapeutics except through a Laboratory, is surely outdoing the play of Hamlet without the Prince of Denmark.'[108] Final approval of the Report took place on 15th February 1887[109]—and the outcome?—the creation of the first laboratory for medical research in Britain.

From the outset it was intended that the Laboratory should be harnessed to 'the prosecution of Original Research' and that it 'should be open, without Fee to Fellows of the College, to Members, to any Licentiate who shall obtain the sanction of the Curator and Committee to use the Laboratory for purposes of Scientific Research, [and] to any Medical Man or Investigator who shall obtain the sanction of the Council . . . to use the Laboratory for purposes of Scientific Research'.[110] It redounds to the credit of the College that the resources of the Laboratory were made so freely available. One criticism voiced in the earliest days of debate had been 'it would be unjust in the highest degree so to limit our Scheme of Research encouragement that only Edinburgh men could take advantage of it'.[111] In the course of time workers were drawn from places as far apart as Lithuania and Hong Kong; specimens were received from Scotland, many parts of England and sources as different as Kansas and Cairo, Lagos and Teheran and in collaboration in epidemiological research with workers in India.[112]

Accommodation

The first building to be occupied by the Laboratory was near to, and leased from, the Royal Infirmary at 7 Lauriston Place. Opened towards the end of 1887 provision was made in it for Chemistry, Histology, Bacteriology and photographic Micropathology.

Dr (later Sir G. Sims) Woodhead, the first Superintendent gave a detailed description profusely illustrated with line drawings, in the opening article of the first volume of the Laboratory Reports, of all that was involved in adapting the building.[113] In the last article of the same volume Woodhead illustrated his subject of *Tabes Mesenterica* and *Pulmonary Tuberculosis* with whole lung sections, some in colour.[114] His equipment included what was then a novelty—a large microtome. Initially most use of the facilities was made by those who were primarily clinicians anxious to offset the disadvantage of divorce from academic and teaching pursuits.

Dr Woodhead left to take charge of a laboratory then being started by the College of Physicians of London. One of his major accomplishments was to found the *Journal of Pathology and Bacteriology* of which he was the first editor.

By 1892 the premises were proving inadequate and steps were taken to purchase 42–44 Lauriston Place, but did not materialize because the Superior of the property was a rigidly confirmed opponent of experiments on animals. At this stage the Infirmary assisted the College by extending the lease of 7 Lauriston Place until more suitable accommodation was found. Eventually in 1895 property was purchased in Forrest Road which had served as the Headquarters of the Rifle Volunteer Brigade and which appeared in the title deeds as 'The Charity Work house called by the name of Bedlam'. All had not been sunshine in Lauriston Place: indeed the reverse at times held good. The Report of the Laboratory for 1895 began 'The work . . . was much interfered with during January, February and March, first through the freezing of all the water pipes, and second, through the epidemic of influenza. It was only in May that the various workers commenced their usual regular attendance.' Worse was to follow. A serious fire in 7 Lauriston Place compelled accelerated transfer to Forrest Road which was to be the home of the Laboratory throughout the remainder of its existence.[115] Dr Noel Paton was Superintendent of the Laboratory at this time. Any one who knew him in his later years can readily picture his elegant figure, impeccably dressed and with immaculately creased trousers, moving around in unperturbed fashion 'come frozen pipes, come consuming fire'.

Accommodation was loaned to the Asylums Board for one of their pathologists for over three years.

In passing it should be mentioned that in 1893 the Royal College of Surgeons of Edinburgh were thinking of developing a laboratory of their own. The possibility of joint action by the Colleges of Physicians and Surgeons was discussed but the former were unable to accept a suggestion that the College of Physicians should maintain the Library which was to be made available for a fee to Fellows of the College of Surgeons, while the Surgical College were to maintain their museum, already open to the public. Negotiations along these lines soon lost their urgency, but in 1899 the College of Surgeons offered to contribute £200 annually for three years towards the cost of maintaining the Laboratory. Not unnaturally the offer was accepted and the Surgeons were invited to nominate one of their Fellows to serve on the Laboratory Committee. Co-operation along these lines continued until closure of the Laboratory.

Research

Although often interwoven and overlapping, the work of the Laboratory can best be considered in terms of research and routine investigations. Inevitably persistence of the ever-expanding influences which first prompted conception of the Laboratory was reflected in the changing emphases in research conducted throughout the 63 years of its existence.

During the last decade of the nineteenth century much time and effort was spent on producing a diphtheria antitoxin of greater effectiveness than those then procurable elsewhere in Britain. Technical difficulties similar to those encountered in English centres were successfully overcome. Production was eventually stopped because of the economic limitations of small-scale production, the improved reliability of commercially produced sera, and interference with the other activities of the Laboratory. About this time an investigation into the physiological changes associated with migration in the life history of salmon was carried out at the behest of the Fishery Board of Scotland. This was the first work undertaken by the Laboratory for a Government Department. Another study was the condition of the air in coal mines. There followed in 1900 an investigation into the diet of labouring classes in Edinburgh, the Town Council making a contribution to help defray the expenses incurred.

Research in the early years of the present century concentrated on nutrition, comparative anatomy, experimental physiology with special reference to ductless glands, and to an increasing extent, bacteriology. Of published papers two dealt with *Observations on the movements of the Pollution of the River Tyne during the summer of 1891.* This was by no means the only study by the Laboratory which anticipated the late twentieth century's global concern about pollution. Thirty-three years later (1924) a report was requested by, and sent to the Board of Health on the nature of deposits of black mud on the shores of the Clyde estuary. During World War I research on trench frostbite, the 'late' bacteriology of wounds, and on means for combating poison gas was undertaken: and vaccines were prepared for use by the Belgian Army against typhoid, *staphylococci* and *streptococci*.

After the war little was carried out in the way of anatomical and physiological research, but pathology and bacteriology more than retained their interest, while chemistry and to a rather lesser extent statistical surveys came in for study. The development, commencing in 1928, of a cabinet gallery of tumours for morphological studies of cancer deserves special mention. Internationally known, and associated particularly with the name of Colonel William Harvey, it incorporated specimens contributed from centres all over the world. Prior to World War II chemical research was becoming increasingly interested in organic studies and less so with metabolic and dietetic problems; and was attracted by the colloidal factors of immunity and by the synthetic preparation of antibiotics. Study by individuals of the accidental or incidental finding was being replaced by organized long-term investigations by teams. World War II brought research to a summary end although in 1947 a bacteriological examination of 2000 specimens of milk per annum from Midlothian and West Lothian was undertaken at the instance of the Department of Health for Scotland. An unusual request was met when Scottish Command in the person of the Sanitary Officer asked for facilities to undertake research for the Army. Accommodation was reserved for the Army Officers involved from 1903 to 1919.

A complete account of the research activities of the Laboratory is beyond the compass of this history but from review of the papers published in the Laboratory Reports other interests of those associated with the Laboratory included the physiology and pathology of pregnancy and parturition; neuropathology; antenatal pathology and pharmacology. In his Convocation Oration to the American College of Physicians in 1964 Dr W. W. Spink recalled with satisfaction how some months previously he had given the Freeland Barbour Fellowship Lecture before the Royal College of Physicians of Edinburgh. His subject was *The Dilemma of Bacterial Shock*.[116]

Although never professing to be a Teaching Department, the Laboratory made a valuable contribution to the understanding of applied science by organising fortnightly 'colloquia'. These dealt with research and experimental medicine, and were attended by University staff but had to be discontinued in 1939 after being held for seventeen years.

Routine Services

As in the case of research, routine services were subject to changing pressures and changing emphases. Reports on morbid specimens rose from 50 in 1890, to over a thousand in 1898: and for many years bacteriological reports represented about 70 per cent of the total. In 1900 the Town Council was approached and a tariff agreed for the examination of specimens of sputum, urine and milk. Comparable arrangements were made later in connection with samples for bacteriological diagnosis of diphtheria and typhoid. Previously the Town Council had insisted on a proviso that the arrangements should apply 'only for cases where the parties themselves are in poor circumstances and quite unable to pay the fees which would be asked for such examination'. With extension of the service they were providing, the College stipulated firmly that 'no limitation be made regarding the facilities for such examination to certain classes of citizens'.[117] In 1905 the Local Government Board arranged that their Medical Officers should send all specimens for bacteriological examination to the Laboratory of the College. Previously the same Board, on the occasion of the appearance of plague in Glasgow in 1900, had asked the Laboratory to have arrangements made for the bacterial diagnosis of any suspected cases which might arise in Scotland. As events turned out only two specimens were received for examination. An ever-increasing problem known to most laboratories to this day was abuse by clientèle—the sending of specimens which should have been within the competence of the medical practitioner; for investigations unlikely to be of any practical use; and without any accompanying information of value. Another abuse, still prevalent in some centres, was the sending of routine specimens to the Laboratory by hospitals themselves equipped with all necessary facilities.

After the outbreak of war in 1914 a much depleted staff accepted responsibility for the pathology requirements of the Royal Navy base at Granton, and of Scottish Command which had no R.A.M.C. Medical Officer available. Very considerable demands were made on the Laboratory, reaching their maximum at times of outbreaks of cerebro-spinal fever. Another wartime commitment was the manufacture of stock vaccines to meet increasing demands for distribution by Messrs. Duncan, Flockhart & Co. Tuberculin was manufactured to make good the loss of supplies from Germany. Public Health (V.D.) Regulations 1916 prompted a steadily increasing number of blood specimens for Wassermann examination. In 1918 it was agreed with the Town Council that specimens sent by the Medical Officer of Health or city Medical Practitioners would be dealt with by the Laboratory, and that the Laboratory would provide facilities for information to be given to medical practitioners about methods employed in the investigations.

To cater for increase and elaboration of general services a bacteriologist was appointed to the staff in 1909; and in 1920 a specialist in biochemistry (Dr Kermack) as whole-time Superintendent. The latter was an expert statistician, and a statistical department was soon established by him. In 1946 a Special Haematological Department was developed to deal with the increasing number of blood samples sent for examination in a widening variety of clinical circumstances.

Envoi

As can so easily happen success bred demand, and demand in turn, financial strain. Never blessed with large financial resources for research, the Laboratory was constantly in the dilemma of balancing the needs of research with the demands for greatly appreciated routine reporting services. Income derived from routine services was at best only moderate. Furthermore complications arose from the vacillations in policy of local authorities and indeed, on at least one occasion, of the University. Thus in 1902, entirely contrary to the expressed wish of the Public Health Committee and medical profession, the Edinburgh Town Council accepted an offer of the Trustees of the Lister Institute to undertake all bacteriological examinations on behalf of the Medical Officer of Health, the City Fever Hospital and the medical practitioners of Edinburgh.[118] In 1939, as part of a policy of retrenchment, the University withdrew financial support, the origins of which dated back to 1913. Then came the wartime regional laboratories of World War II, harbingers of the framework of laboratory services in the National Health Service. From the beginning these laboratories encroached on areas which for many years had been a source of income to the College Laboratory. Still further large-scale loss of income was foreseen as an inevitable result of laboratory schemes proposed and pending under the National Health Service. In the new world dominated by administrators and planners there was no viable place for the College of Physicians Laboratory. It is not to be wondered at, therefore, that the Laboratory's staunchest philanthropic supporter, the Carnegie Trust, should feel obliged firstly to reduce and then to withdraw financial support.

Deliberately, previous mention has not been made of the indebtedness of the Laboratory to the Carnegie Trustees. It is not possible to overestimate the generosity and encouragement shewn by the Trustees from the time they were originally approached by the College in 1903. The financial position of the Laboratory was then extremely precarious, with services continuing to expand and research gravely handicapped by lack of income. A five years' agreement was reached between what can only be described as benefactors on the one side and suppliants on the other. The Carnegie Trustees for the Universities of Scotland purchased the Laboratory for £10,000 and assumed responsibility for the entire cost of maintaining it. For their part the College undertook to pay to the Trustees £750 per annum and to transfer to them any sums received from the Royal College of Surgeons of Edinburgh. Four years later the Trustees made a grant of £600 for equipment and apparatus, and in 1908 the original agreement was renewed for a further five years. After the death of

Lord Lister in 1912 plans were set on foot for a suitable Memorial. The Royal Colleges of Edinburgh, the University and the Carnegie Trustees were involved; and under the scheme jointly proposed, it was contemplated that the Laboratory would without losing identity or name be merged into a proposed Lister Memorial Institute.

By the terms of the 1903 agreement between the Carnegie Trustees and the College the former were under obligation, if the agreement was not renewed, to reconvey the Laboratory to the College, who for their part were required to repay the purchase amount of £10,000. With the object of enabling the College to make 'a commensurate contribution' to the Lister Memorial project, the obligation on the part of the College to repay £10,000 was annulled and the Trustees became owners of the Forrest Road Laboratory buildings. Progress on the Lister Memorial Scheme was brought almost to a halt by the hostilities of 1914–19 and the Laboratory continued to function under the old arrangements.

Having survived a second world war, and despite having made a significant contribution to its prosecution, it became manifest that the College of Physicians Laboratory would not long survive the establishment of the National Health Service. No possibility existed of reviving the Laboratory as a Research Unit, and research ceased in 1949. In the following year professional and technical staff were absorbed by other services, and the Forrest Road buildings were handed over to the University by the Carnegie Trustees. The only way to grasp how much the Laboratory accomplished in its relatively short lifetime is to read conscientiously the annual reports. They reveal industry and imagination on a scale which even those who paid frequent visits could not appreciate. During the sixty years of its existence the results of original research carried out in the Laboratory provided material for over 600 published papers, a number of which were accorded international recognition.

Although incomplete the above facts afford ample evidence of the debt of gratitude owed to the Carnegie Trustees by the College. That the activities of the Laboratory came to an end was in no way due to lack of magnanimous philanthropic support, or to lack of faith and zeal on the part of those who worked in the Laboratory. Rather it was the result of submergence by the popular tidal wave of planning on a national scale. Those who remember the College Laboratory and the quiet unceasing industry of its staff, cannot but subscribe to the regrets of a one time Superintendent:

'That in the brave new world . . . no place could be found for an institution so long established, so widely known and with so high a reputation may seem strange to us, and to future generations perhaps inexplicable.'[119]

REFERENCES

THE PHYSICK GARDEN: [1667]–1761

(1) SIBBALD, Sir R. (1833) *The Autobiography*, p. 21. Edinburgh: Thomas Stevenson.
(2) College Minutes, 5.viii.1712.
(3) GUTHRIE D. J. (1964) *The Medical School of Edinburgh*, p. 7. Edinburgh: Edinburgh University Press.
(4) LINDEBOOM, G. A. (1968) *Herman Boerhaave; the man and his work*, p. 147. London: Methuen.
(5) COMRIE, J. D. (1932) *History of Scottish Medicine*, 2nd Edition, vol. I, p. 266. London: Baillière, Tindall & Cox.
(6) COCKBURN, H. (1910) *Memorials of his Time*, p. 407. Edinburgh: Foulis.
(7) SIBBALD, Sir R. Op. cit., p. 41.
(8) Ibid., p. 21.

THE COLD BATH-HOUSE: 1712–58

(9) College Minutes, 26.ii.1712.
(10) Ibid., 4.iii.1712.
(11) Ibid., 24.vii.1713.
(12) R.C.P.E. (1925) *Historical sketch and laws*, p. 40. Edinburgh: Royal College of Physicians.
(13) College Minutes, 26.x.1714.
(14) Ibid., 2.xi.1714.
(15) Ibid., 7.ii.1716.
(16) Ibid., 14.iii.1716.
(17) Ibid., 5.xi.1717.
(18) Ibid., 6.v.1718.
(19) Ibid., 4.xi.1718.
(20) Ibid., 29.ix.1719.
(21) Ibid., 3.xi.1719.
(22) Ibid., 10.xi.1719.
(23) Ibid., 2.ii.1720.
(24) Ibid., 3.v.1720.
(25) Ibid., 17.v.1720.
(26) Ibid., 5.iii.1723.
(27) Ibid., 1.ii.1726.
(28) Ibid., 3.v.1726.
(29) Ibid., 7.ii.1727.
(30) Ibid., 5.viii.1729.
(31) Ibid., 3.xi.1730.
(32) Ibid., 3.viii.1731.
(33) Ibid., 2.xi.1731.

(34) Ibid., 6.viii.1734.
(35) Ibid., 5.xi.1734.
(36) Ibid., 4.v.1736.
(37) Ibid., 7.xii.1736.
(38) Ibid., 5.viii.1740.
(39) Ibid., 2.ii.1742.
(40) Ibid., 3.viii.1742.
(41) Ibid., 2.ii.1742.
(42) Ibid., 5.xi.1745.
(43) Ibid., 3.ii.1756.
(44) Ibid., 1.ii.1757.
(45) TURNER, A. L. (1937) *Story of a Great Hospital; the Royal Infirmary of Edinburgh, 1729–1929*, p. 105. Edinburgh: Oliver & Boyd.

THE DISPENSARY: CARE OF THE NECESSITOUS: 1682–1749

(46) College Minutes, 6.ii.1682.
(47) Ibid., 10.ii.1682.
(48) Ibid., 6.v.1707.
(49) BEILBY, W. (1847) *Address Delivered at the Opening of the New Hall of the Royal College of Physicians, November 27, 1846*, p. 20. Edinburgh: Constable.
(50) DRUMMOND, C. G. (1953) *Pharmacy and Medicine in Old Edinburgh*, p. 26. London: Pharmaceutical Press.
(51) College Minutes, 15.xi.1694.
(52) Ibid., 5.xii.1695.
(53) Ibid., 25.x.1705.
(54) Ibid., 4.xi.1707.
(55) Ibid., 1.vi.1714.
(56) Ibid., 10.xi.1719.
(57) Ibid., 27.vi.1707.
(58) Ibid., 3.ii.1708.
(59) Ibid., 4.xi.1707.
(60) Ibid., 4.xi.1712.
(61) Ibid., 3.v.1715.
(62) Ibid., 5.v.1730.
(63) Ibid., 2.v.1749.
(64) Ibid., 1.viii.1749.
(65) Ibid., 7.xi.1749.

THE PHARMACOPOEIA: 1699–1864

(66) Ibid., 18.i.1682.
(67) Ibid., 8.iii.1682.

(68) Ibid., 21.iii.1682.

(69) Ibid., 13.viii.1683.

(70) Ibid., 20.viii.1683.

(71) Ibid., 7.xii.1684.

(72) R.C.P.E. (1696) *Miscellaneous Papers*, no. 98.

(73) College Minutes, 6.ii.1696.

(74) Ibid., 9.iii.1697.

(75) Ibid., 22.iii.1697.

(76) Ibid., 12.ix.1698.

(77) Ibid., 24.iii.1699.

(78) SIBBALD, Sir R. Op. cit., p. 34.

(79) Ibid., p. 42.

(80) R.C.P.E. (c. 1850) *Abstracts of the Minutes, AD 1682–1731*. By George Paterson. (Ms.)

(80a) COWEN, D. L. (1957) The Edinburgh Pharmacopoeia. *Medical History*, **1**, 2, 342.

(81) College Minutes, 5.ix.1721.

(82) Ibid., 7.xi.1721.

(83) Ibid., 7.viii.1722.

(84) Ibid., 7.xi.1732.

(84a) Ibid., 30.vi.1732.

(85) THOMSON, J. (1859) *An Account of the Life, Lectures and Writings of William Cullen, M.D.*, vol. II, p. 84. Edinburgh: Blackwood.

(86) THIN, R. (1927) *College Portraits*, p. 39. Edinburgh: Oliver & Boyd.

(87) College Minutes, 1.v.1821.

(87a) Ibid., 14.ix.1775.

(87b) Ibid., 6.xi.1804.

(88) GILMOUR, J. P. (1938) Phases of pharmacy in Edinburgh: an historical sketch. *Quarterly Journal of Pharmacy and Pharmacology*, **XI**, 361.

(89) PENDRILL, G. R. (1961) The Royal College of Physicians of Edinburgh, its origins and functions. *Scottish Medical Journal*, **6**, 527.

(89a) COWEN, D. L. Op. cit., pp. 124–5.

(90) BEILBY, W. Op. cit., p. 35.

(91) COWEN, D. L. Op. cit., p. 134.

(92) CHRISTISON, Sir R. (1886) *Life of Sir Robert Christison, Bart.*, vol. II, p. 173. Edinburgh: Blackwood.

(93) Ibid., p. 232.

(94) POOLE, R. (1834) *Notes etc. regarding . . . evidence before the [Parliamentary] Committee on medical education*, pp. 37–9. (Ms.)

(95) College Minutes, 25.x.1862.

NATURAL HISTORY MUSEUM: 1706–70

(96) SIBBALD, Sir R. (1837) *Letters of Sir Robert Sibbald*. Edinburgh: Thomas Stevenson.

(97) College Minutes, 12.iii.1706.

(98) GRANT, Sir A. (1884) *The Story of the University of Edinburgh*, vol. I, p. 374. London: Longmans, Green & Co.
(99) College Minutes, 24.ix.1696.
(100) GRANT, Sir A. Op. cit., p. 375.
(101) College Minutes, 22.viii.1717.
(102) Ibid., 6.v.1718.

MATERIA MEDICA MUSEUM: 1835–96

(103) College Minutes, 4.viii.1835.
(104) BEILBY, W. Op. cit., p. 37.
(105) College Minutes, 23.vi.1896.

THE LABORATORY: 1887–1950

(106) RITCHIE, J. (1953) *History of the Laboratory of the Royal College of Physicians of Edinburgh*, p. 11. Edinburgh: Royal College of Physicians.
(107) Ibid., p. 106.
(108) College Minutes, 25.v.1886.
(109) R.C.P.E. (1925) *Historical Sketch and Laws*, pp. 93–4. Edinburgh: Royal College of Physicians.
(110) Ibid., pp. 95–6.
(111) RITCHIE, J. Op. cit., p. 6.
(112) Ibid., p. 7.
(113) TUKE, J. B. & WOODHEAD, G. S., eds. *Reports from the Laboratory of the Royal College of Physicians, Edinburgh*, vol. I, p. 3. Edinburgh: Young J. Pentland.
(114) Ibid., p. 179.
(115) College Minutes, 4.ii.1896.
(116) SPINK, W. W. (1964) The tradition of the College. (Convocation address, Forty-fifth annual session of the American College of Physicians.) *Annals of Internal Medicine*, **61**, 150.
(117) RITCHIE, J. Op. cit., p. 28.
(118) Edinburgh. Bacteriological examinations for the city (1902) *British Medical Journal*, **1**, 805.
(119) RITCHIE, J. Op. cit., p. 107.

Chapter VI

THE LIBRARY

These are the tombs of such as cannot die.
George Crabbe (*The Library*)

How pure the joy when first my hands unfold
The small, rare volume, black with tarnished gold.
J. Ferriar, M.D. (*Bibliomania*)

Medical literature . . . is the currency or medium of exchange by which a man contributes to
or borrows from the common stock of knowledge and experience, and the volume of this
currency and the character of its metal are of the greatest importance to us all.
Sir Robert Hutchison

Whatever the outcome of other early projects one is pre-eminent in virtue of being
the earliest, of uninterrupted progress, and of unimpaired vitality as the tercentenary
of the College approaches. It is the founding, expansion and maintenance of a Medical
Library. To refer even in retrospect to the Library as a 'project' is as unseemly as it is
mundane. Today the Library of the Royal College of Physicians of Edinburgh is the
largest medical library in Scotland, and the third largest in the United Kingdom.
Size of itself is no criterion of worth. Above all it is the richness of the literature
accumulated on the shelves which makes for the greatness of the Library: a richness
derived from ancient medical classics of priceless value, from native and foreign
medical writings published in the life-time of the College, and from a comprehensive
collection of periodicals publicising modern advances awaiting proof or disproof of
their contribution to progress. The Library is financed entirely from College funds.
In so far as contributions by Fellows of the College and alumni of the University ot
Edinburgh are concerned, the Library provides a readily accessible mine of information. Acquisition of this has followed judicious purchasing on some occasions, but
to an equally great extent has been fostered by generous gifts and legacies from Fellows of the College, and others.

Among the latter, two deserve special mention. The first is Mr David Laing, Librarian to the Society of Writers to the Signet. In 1820 he recognized that a purchase made by him had come by devious paths from the College of Physicians and forthwith arranged for its return. The book in question was a copy of the printed catalogue of a deceased President's (Dr John Drummond) library[1] which had been presented to the College in 1741; and which contained legal documents of conveyance and acceptance of the original bequest. Loss of the copy probably took place during removal of the College Library from the Cowgate to the Infirmary in 1766. The unexpected recovery of property not known to have been lost stimulated Dr Andrew Duncan, sen. to inscribe on the title page:

'Ex Libris Collegii Regii Medicorum Edinburgensium. Quesitum ipsis kal. Decembris, 1820 et quisquis sustulerit ultimus suorum moriartur. Script A. Duncan, Sen. Pr. Emer. et Collegii Pater'[2]

The other special benefactor was a surgeon—Mr William Brown, F.R.C.S.E. He too was concerned in the recovery of a catalogue. The particular catalogue, dated 1767,[3] was the first to be printed of the Library. No copy was preserved in the Library and apparently no one was aware of its existence by the middle of the nineteenth century. Mr Brown, finding it bound with a number of pamphlets in his personal library, generously presented it to the College—the title *Catalogus bibliothecae collegii regii medicorum, 1767.*[4]

PROBLEMS—PREDICTABLE AND UNPREDICTABLE

Inevitably the Library has shared in the vicissitudes of the College but from study of the history it is abundantly clear that from the time of its foundation the Library had a prior claim on the sympathies and resources of the Fellows. No less interesting is the fact that this attitude to the development of the Library does not appear to have abated even at times of prolonged internal dissension or of such absorbing external pressures as those involved in medical and university reform. To say this is not to imply that the Library has lacked domestic problems. Financial difficulties have never been far removed. Some easement of the situation followed the sale in 1756 to booksellers of the copyright of the *Pharmacopoeia* as return for a considerable number of books.[5] Previously the policy had been established of selling books which were duplicates or unsuited to retention, new medical books being purchased with the proceeds.[6] Fellows were given first option on books listed for auction.[7] A century later, because of 'the low state of the Finances' it was decided in 1830 to institute an annual levy of 'Two Guineas, as an additional fund for the purchase of Books'[8] but there is no evidence that action along these lines was ever taken. Accommodation crises, formerly recurrent, later assumed the characteristics of chronicity. An aspect of library administration apt to be forgotten is that of maintaining a tolerably adequate catalogue. This can be harassingly time consuming, and the problem has been gravely aggravated by the indiscriminate, it might almost be said irresponsible, spate of medical printed works in modern times. The onus on library committees to exercise their powers of selection wisely, is immense. The technical difficulties in the way of facilitating intelligent and at the same time prompt availability of resources make a reliable up-to-date cataloguing procedure indispensable. This involves reliance upon experienced staff, subject to the inescapable hazards of indisposition and decease, as the history of the Library bears witness. Small wonder then, that crises can and do occur. One such event synchronized with transfer of the Library in 1846 to the present Queen Street Hall from the temporary premises at 119 George Street. It had been arranged that on transfer a new alphabetical catalogue would be prepared. Hardly had the work been commenced when the individual mainly involved took ill, and before long died. Effective continuity was precluded by the subsequent illness of the Librarian 'who was for a considerable time rendered incapable of superintending the work'. To their lasting credit certain members of the Library Committee took up the task of comparing the manuscript catalogue left by the deceased member of staff with the books themselves, and in the words of a grateful Librarian 'by great exertions, brought the work, in 1849, to a successful termination'. The number of volumes in the Library at this time was about nine thousand.[9] Sheer necessity compelled the abandonment of the printed-book catalogue and the last printed catalogue was published in 1898. Since that date a card sheaf catalogue has been maintained.[10]

SIBBALD'S INITIATIVE

The spontaneous and enthusiastic response to the 1849 crisis by the Library Committee would have warmed the heart of Robert Sibbald to whom the Library largely owed its origin. Moreover, Sibbald was one who favoured 'keeping and ordering'. How did Sibbald contribute to the beginnings of the College Library? When writing in his *Autobiography* of 'our conferences in the Colledge frequently' he said 'I gave about this tyme [1682] a presse with three shelfs full of books, to the Colledge of Physitians, amongst which were Galen's works, 5 volumes Greek, and five Latine, Hippocrates in Greek, of Aldus' edition, Gesner his history of animals, 3 volumes, Paris bind, and some other valuable books'.[11] Available evidence points to Sibbald's gift being the first to the College Library, it being recorded as the first entry in the earliest record of donations in the following terms: 'Dominus Robertus Sibbald, Eques Auratus, Medicus Regis Ordinarius et Collegii Regii Medicorum apud Edinburgum Censor et Registrarius Bibliothecae pro dicto Collegio fundamenta posuit'.[12]

From time to time in subsequent years the records refer to gifts of books being made by Socii and in 1696 'it was agried to nemine contradicente that every intrant be requryed to give a book one or moe as they please to the colledge library'.[13] This edict did no more than confirm an established tendency. Writing in 1779, Arnot says of the College Library, it 'contains many valuable books, chiefly in natural history, the greatest part of which belonged to Dr. Wright of Kersie; and, upon his death, a donation was made of them by his heir to the College in consequence of an inclination to that effect, expressed by the deceased'.[14] Dr Wright was a former Fellow and the College did benefit in the way stated. In other respects Arnot's account does scant justice to the progress and expansion achieved by the Library, and is more of a socially contemporaneous impression than an assessment based on intimate knowledge. In point of fact, as Jolley pointed out, Sibbald's original gift was speedily followed by others from eminent individuals in Scotland, in England and on the Continent. Benefactors included Bishop Burnet, Sir Hans Sloane, Sir Isaac Newton and George, Earl of Cromartie.[15]

'LIBERARIUS APPOYNTED'

Sibbald was Censor during the years 1682 and 1683 during which time (Sir) Archibald Stevensone was President.[16, 17] Appointment of the first Librarian of the College is recorded in the Minutes for 7th May 1683 as follows:

> 'It being moved that their should be a Liberarius Chosen for the Colledge and
> voted there should be one, and Dr. Stevensone yor appoynted to be the persone and
> Doctor Pittcairne to be Deput Liberarius.'[18]

Two Stevensones were present at the sederunt—the President, Archibald Stevensone and Dr Stevensone yo[r]. The latter was William Stevensone, one of the Fellows in the Original Patent, who was the second Treasurer in the history of the College[19] which office he resigned after being appointed Librarian. His resignation was accepted 'Upon a motion made in behalf of Doctor Stevensone yor Thesaurer to the College That in regaird of his Indispositne of body, some fitt persone might be named Thesaurer in his place and his accompts taken off his hand, Doe grant his Desyre . . .'.[20] Importance attaches to the designation '*yo*ʳ' as this was used in the Minutes to differentiate William Stevensone from his senior Archibald Stevensone. It was not customary to enter Christian names in Minutes. As Ritchie rightly pointed out previous historians of the College failed to recognize the differentiation with the result that Archibald Stevensone instead of William Stevensone Yoʳ has sometimes been credited with being Treasurer.[21] When elected President Archibald Stevensone was referred to as 'Doctor Stevensone *older*'[22] and occupied the Presidential chair at the sederunt which appointed William Stevensone Yoʳ as Librarian. Lest William Stevensone's retiral from the Treasurership to take up the post of Librarian be interpreted as pointing to the latter being a sinecure, aspiring Librarians should ponder over the fact that according to Fountainhall the 'physicians . . . out of pique to . . . Stevenson Younger, obtained . . . an order that all who practised medicine within Edinburgh should take the test . . .'. [23] (The 'test' referred to was the 'Act anent Religion and the Test' Acts of the Parliaments of Scotland, 31st August 1681.)

COMMITTEES

Some years elapsed after the creation of the Office of Librarian before a Library Committee was formed. In 1705, Sibbald together with the President, Censors, Library Keeper and three other Fellows were 'appoynted Curators and oversiers of the Colledge Librarie ffour with the Librarie Keeper to be a Quorum'.[24] From time to time modifications of committee approach were adopted in an endeavour to promote efficiency. Thus in 1801 a special Committee was appointed 'to look into the present state of the Library' at the time of a change of Librarian, and 'to take the charge of his [the retiring officer's] hand in order to be delivered over to his Successor'.[25] Underlying this move was disquiet over missing books. A salaried Assistant Librarian was first appointed in 1823[26]—the facetious might argue that his appointment provided a scapegoat for vanished volumes. Some years later the Library Committee was authorized, subject to safeguards, to make temporary regulations relating to the Library with the object of dispensing with the inconvenience and delay involved in making formal application to the College in every situation, no matter how trivial.[27]

Even library administration was not wholly devoid of personalities. There was one occasion when the Librarian 'laid hands upon the Officer and forcibly ejected him from the Library'. Efforts to mollify the Librarian were quite ineffectual. After giving an assurance that in similar circumstances he would 'act in the same manner', he wrote 'as to accepting [!] my resignation, that the Council cannot help, for I have refused to withold or to withdraw it'.[28, 29]

ORIGINAL SIN

Missing and unreturned books—the College Librarians in common with their brethren elsewhere can be forgiven if they ascribe these in one way or another to Man's Original Sin. Strewn throughout the Minutes of the College are not so much plaintive as despairing appeals for help for restoration of property borrowed many years before an age of polluting non-returnables. The situation in 1823 is admirably summed up with due decorum and without libel in the *Historical Sketch* of the College—'Up to this time, and indeed throughout the whole history of the Library, much difficulty seems to have been experienced in preventing the books from being taken away in an irregular manner, and in getting the whole of the borrowed books returned'.[26] Surprisingly, trial of compulsory annual recall of all borrowed books was not made until 1800,[30] but the results were far from encouraging. Little benefit accrued from fines of one shilling per day per book.[31] Many years later it was determined that Fellows resident more than ten miles from Edinburgh had to obtain the special permission of Council before borrowing books.[32] Even the equivalent of black lists included in the Minutes proved unavailing. Superficially there would appear to be some relationship between academic eminence and exalted amnesia! In a desperate attempt to discipline one well-known miscreant, who had shewn no sign of response to five successive appeals to return what he had borrowed, an edict was issued requiring that replacements be ordered at his expense and that the customary fines be exacted in full.[33] Discretion rules out analysis of the sinners drawn from the ranks of more ordinary mortal Fellows.

ATTEMPTS TO POOL RESOURCES

First attempts at co-operation between the College and the University in so far as library services were concerned were sincere although unsuccessful. In 1763 several proposals were considered. The first, through the agency of Alexander Monro *primus* was submitted by the Principal of the University 'for uniteing' the medical libraries of the College and University. Separate and joint meetings of College and University Committees followed, but the College felt constrained to withdraw from the proposed 'coalition' as the inconvenience and expense entailed would more than offset any advantages. There was no question of hurt feelings on the part of anyone and the College gave 'their hearty thanks to Doctor Robertson Principal of the University for this mark of his attention'.[34]

That the conception of co-operation between the two Libraries had an appeal for a number of Fellows is certain. About this same time different proposals to this end were submitted by three Fellows, including Dr Robert Whytt, but none found favour with a Committee appointed to consider them. Among the reasons for the Committee's decision were undesirability of separating the Library from the Hall, the increased risk of loss, and the problems of alienation of property.[35]

Later efforts to achieve a pooling of library resources met with chilling receptions. At a Quarterly Meeting in 1793 a written proposal was received and approved en-titling every University Professor to have the same facilities as Fellows for borrowing books from the College Library, 'upon condition that every Fellow of the College . . . shall be entitled to borrow Books from the University Library on the same footing as Professors, or as Members of the College of Surgeons'.[36] Mention of the Surgeons referred to an agreement entered into by their College with the University, whereby the former having made over their Library to the University undertook to pay the University £5 per annum. Fellows of the College of Surgeons obtained privileges equal to a Professor in respect of consulting and borrowing books.[37] The proposal was considered in turn by the Senatus Academicus who agreed it should continue in force for one year 'but thereafter to Cease if it shall be found to have been attended with any inconvenience'.[38] Cease it apparently did but owing to what inconvenience is nowhere stated.

COLLEGE V. TOWN AND GOWN

A desire for access to the University Library persisted among Fellows, and a Com-mittee was appointed to further their objective. In the course of time the Committee memorialized the Patrons of the University (The Town Council). The Memorial was dated 1st June 1829. It was, it must be frankly admitted, a communication begging assistance in the form of access to the University Library on three counts: viz. the expense of necessary medical books; the inadequacy of funds available to the College; the fact that the University Library, established for public benefit, had the advantage of superior pecuniary contributions and of the receipt without cost of copies of all new works published in Great Britain.[39] Wrapped up in sentimentalities the supplications do not make elevating reading, and did not succeed in their objective. The civic authorities informed the College in the briefest and bluntest terms 'that it was inexpedient to grant the request' in a letter dated August 13th 1829.[40] In fairness it should be mentioned that in replying to our College, the University patrons may have been indirectly influenced by acute differences prevailing at the time between the University and the Edinburgh College of Surgeons in the matter of library facilities.[41]

Nothing daunted the College Committee then memorialized 'the Commissioners for visiting the Universities and Colleges of Scotland'. Dated 16th October 1829, this Memorial was no more skilfully drafted than that to the Patrons of the University. In a mildly bombastic way it recapitulated the part played by the College in establishing the Infirmary, in founding the Museum of the University, in examining Candidates for Degrees in Medicine and in the fostering of a University Medical Faculty. The impression given is one of injured dignity rather than one of frustrated enthusiasm. Once again the College experienced a rebuff in a letter which, though less cryptic than the previous one, was none the less emphatic, the Commissioners seeing 'no reason to differ from the opinion expressed by the Town Council on the subject'.[40]

But the matter was not entirely ended. On 30th October (1829), presumably after receipt of the Commissioners' reply dated 20th October, the College again memorialized the Town Council as University Patrons. In effect this second communication regretted the failure of their previous one 'to detail the particular obligations of the University to the College' and endeavoured to make good the omission. Reference was made to the fact that the decision to reject Principal Robertson's advances in 1763 (q.v.) had not influenced 'the donation of the College at an after period for the present buildings of the University . . .'. The sole result of this Memorial was a letter from the City Clerk asking for details of Professor Robertson's proposals. These the College provided, only to be informed that the magistrates and Council had approved a report of a Committee of the Senatus Academicus urging that 'the prayer of the [College] Memorial should be again refused'.[40]

The whole is a sad reflection on the persisting antagonism among professional interests dating back to the previous century while the Town Council continued to exercise its authority—in some ways an operatic presentation of Town and Gown—with the University Commissioners already within the City Walls!

As to arrangements with our sister Royal College of Surgeons of Edinburgh, a motion at an ordinary meeting in 1903 was moved to make the Library of the College of Physicians accessible to Fellows of the College of Surgeons. The motion was ruled out as being incompetent on the score of applying part of the property of the College to a purpose other than 'ordinary'.[42, 43] With cavalierish gallantry the Royal College of Surgeons resolved to grant the use of their Library to Fellows of the Royal College of Physicians. That was in 1906.[44] In 1923 the College of Physicians accorded full Library privileges to Fellows of the College of Surgeons working in the Laboratory, subject to nomination by the Council of the Surgeons' College.[45] Greater magnanimity was shewn in 1953 when the College approved regulations drawn up by Council to favour increased co-operation with the Library of the Royal College of Surgeons. The new arrangements provided for inter-library lending; co-operative selection of periodicals and books; and permission for Fellows of each College to read in either Library. Conditional arrangements for reading in the Library were extended also to certain specified categories of research workers.[46]

GIFTS AND BEQUESTS

The first Catalogue of the Library printed in 1767 and rediscovered by Mr Brown contained a list of 2346 works.[47] By the middle of the nineteenth century the number of volumes was in the neighbourhood of 9000,[48] and an estimate of the contents of the Library at the end of that century was 39,800 volumes.[49] During the inclusive period 1767–1896 at least 12 catalogues or appendices to catalogues were prepared. By 1925 the number of volumes had risen to approximately 100,000,[50] and to 200,000 in 1970.[51]

It is not possible to mention more than a few selected examples of books at present in the Library, and any impression conveyed must necessarily be superficial. One of the earliest purchases was the library of the Laird of Livingstone (Chap. V) in 1705[52] and a few years later in 1741 the library of Dr John Drummond (q.v.) came into the possession of the College. Included in this collection was an important non-medical manuscript—a fifteenth-century copy of the *Cursor mundi*. Another such manuscript in the Library is the original of Dr John Brown's *Rab and his friends* written in 1859 in an ordinary exercise book the worse for wear. According to Thin this particular manuscript was presented in 1906 by several Fellows who were instigated by Sir William Osler to purchase it.[53] In the words of an American Professor of Medical History 'as a piece of prose the medical profession may well be proud of it'.[54]

Brown was not, as stated, at any time President of our College. On one occasion William Hunter was an intending contender at a forthcoming sale but a letter written by William Cullen is extant in which Hunter is warned that the College were determined to secure all the important works.[55] At the time of the removal of the College to the New Hall in George Street Sir John Pringle gave to the College a series of volumes of manuscript annotations. He made it a condition that they should never be published and never be allowed out of the College building.[56] This condition has been respected faithfully: only comparatively recently the College Council had occasion on "moral or ethical" grounds regretfully not to accede to a Continental University's request for photostatic reproductions.[57]

In his day Pringle had had a distinguished career in the Army (Chap. XXVII) and in civil life. His wife was a daughter of Dr William Oliver whose name is associated with the Bath Oliver biscuits. Boswell was a friend of Pringle but failed to establish a friendly relation between him and Johnson. 'Sir John was not sufficiently flexible . . . the repulsion was equally strong on the part of Johnson; who, I know not from what cause, unless his being a Scotchman, had formed a very erroneous opinion of Sir John.'[58]

There then followed the purchase of books at the sale of Dr William Cullen's library and after an interval the bequest by Dr Andrew Duncan, sen. of a large collection of manuscript notes and lectures of the founders of the Edinburgh School of Medicine. Shortly before his death another ex-President, Dr James Home, gifted over two hundred volumes which included the lectures in manuscript of such past outstanding men as St. Clair, Alston, Cullen, Rutherford, Black, Francis Home, and Gregory. Other personal notebooks in the Library include those of Sir Robert Sibbald, Sir Archibald Pitcairne, Sir Robert Christison's immaculately scribed records of Gregory's lectures, and William Cullen's copies of his own consultation letters.

Donations were received also on their death from Dr Abercrombie who became President and a consultant after many years in general practice; the Begbies, father and son; and among distinguished academics, Hughes Bennett and J. Y. Simpson. Gifts of their own works were made by Sir Alexander Morison and Dr Paine of New York. A series of original drawings by Pieter Camper for Smellie's Midwifery was received from Dr Burt, and a copy of the original Bills of Mortality of the City of London for the year of the great plague from Dr Maclagan. Additional manuscripts of Dr William Cullen were gifted by Drs Thomson and Craigie and in 1862 the Library Committee bought the library of a former Fellow and Librarian of the College—Dr John Clerk. Many of the volumes of the latter bear his doctor-father's book-stamp with a crest surrounded by his name 'Ihone Clerk'. Further considerable additions to the Library were made between 1860 and 1880. They included parts of the libraries of outstanding physicians in Germany and of Professor Russel, Dr Robert Ferguson and Professor Goodsir. A bequest from Dr Craigie contained purchases made by him in life from the libraries of well-known physicians at home and abroad, including Professor Traube of Berlin.[59]

More recent additions to the Library have included a collection of medical works belonging to Sir James Young Simpson; a portion of the primarily neurological library of Dr Ninian Bruce; the diaries and case books of Dr Alexander Hamilton; and autograph letters of, among others, Florence Nightingale, Robert Christison and Edward Jenner.[60] Other interesting additions were Sir Walter Scott's Law Thesis for admission to the Faculty of Advocates formerly in the possession of the paediatrician Dr John Thomson; and Pitcairne's *Dissertationes Medicae* gifted by Dr Douglas Guthrie on the occasion of the tercentenary of Pitcairne's birth.[61]

The Simpson Collection gifted to the College by Sir Alexander Russell Simpson in 1913 contained many books and manuscripts from the library of Sir James Y. Simpson. In all there were 1575 volumes including the first edition (1628) of William Harvey's *De Motu Cordis*. Although recorded in the original J. Y. Simpson catalogue the existence in the collection of the historic Harveian copy was not generally known until 1961 when it was discovered by the College Librarian, Mr G. R. Pendrill.

It is gratifying to note that gifts were given as well as received. In Duncan's Memorials of the Glasgow Faculty, the 'College of Physicians, Edinburgh' appears as the last entry in a list of 'The names of such worthie persons as have gifted books to the chierurgions Librarie in Glasgow'.[62]

LIBRARY POLICY

Fundamentally, while making effective provision for adjustment, the policy of the College has not changed through the centuries. From the time of its inception to the present day the Library has been 'one of the foremost of their [the College's] activities and the chief burden on their income'.[63] Money has always been spent lavishly in relation to available sources of revenue, a policy which has benefited from donations by individual Fellows over the years. Purchases and gifts have not been confined to major works of the past but have included 'transitory pamphlets of the present'.[64] A direct result is that there are in the Library virtually complete sets of the unrestrainedly vicious and scurrilous pamphlets which etiquette did not prevent being published by warring factions in the days of Pitcairne and Gregory. To read these pamphlets is revealing—revealing in a professionally salutary sense. It is at least to the credit of the College that, if such dubious literature had to be collected, strict impartiality was preserved, and the explosive vilifications and at times verging blasphemous declarations of the contestants of both sides were religiously retained. The Library has gained. Bibliographically it has been, if not elevated, at least enriched historically.

A former Librarian has in recent times admirably reviewed the place of the College Library. Discussing the more modern section of the Library he commented on the importance attached to periodicals, of which there is an excellent collection of British, Continental and American examples extending back in most instances to the first issue.[63] Today periodicals present an especial problem on account of rising costs. Their number has increased out of all recognition as subspecialization has grown apace. Of necessity increasing circumspection has had to be exercised in deciding which new periodicals should be purchased and which old ones disposed of or discontinued. A comparable problem with regard to books as distinct from periodicals arose as early as 1704.

'The Library of the Royal College of Physicians', wrote Jolley, 'combines a well-maintained modern library with a rich historical collection. But the special interest of this historical collection is that it is merely the residue of the modern library of the past. Of the 16 medical incunabula on the shelves, only the very fine *editio princeps* of Celsus's *De re medicina* was purchased as a historical rarity. The rare books are on the shelves because they were the working books of the past and this is true not only of the seventeenth- and eighteenth-century books but even of the very numerous sixteenth-century works. The special attraction of the library is that for nearly 300 years it has carried out the same function for the same class of reader.'[63]

Events leading up to purchase might almost be described as fatalistic. On 1st March 1894 an entry was made in the Library suggestion book to the effect that 'the Library Committee purchase the first edition (1478) of Celsus' *De re medicina*'. Beneath the entry the Honorary Librarian (Dr G. W. Balfour) added the laconic comment 'Declined'. Some six weeks later it is recorded in the Library Committee Minutes that on instructions from Council it had been agreed to purchase that which had been previously 'declined'.[65]

The cost to the College was 15 guineas. Today the first edition Celsus is one of the College's priceless irreplaceable possessions.

In 1953 part-use was made of a bequest (Sydney Watson Smith) to provide

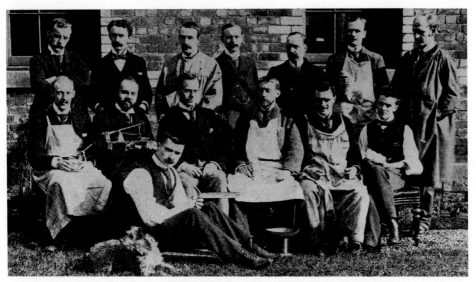

PLATE 14   Royal College of Physicians Laboratory Group (1894)
Reproduced from a photograph in the College by Tom Scott

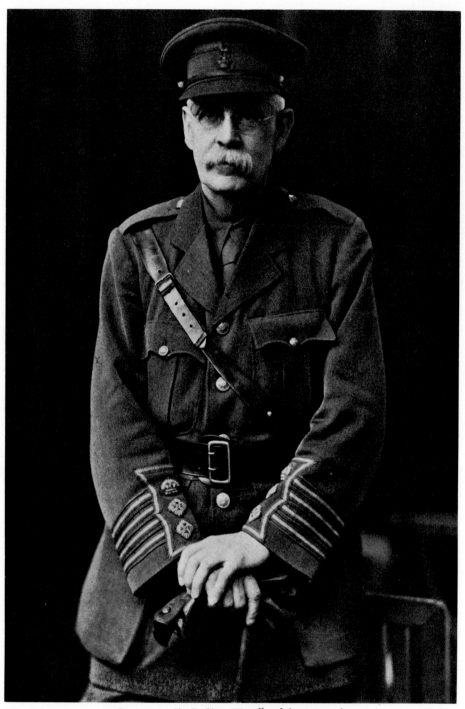

PLATE 15   Sir G. Sims Woodhead (1855–1921)
Reproduced from a photograph in the College by Tom Scott

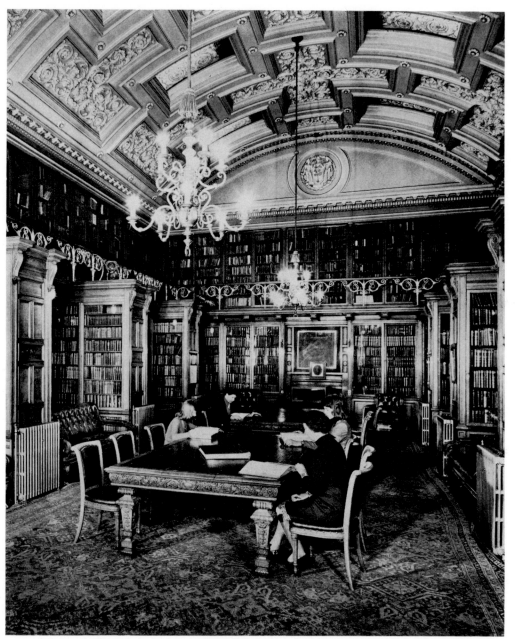

PLATE 16   The New Library, Queen Street
Photograph by Tom Scott

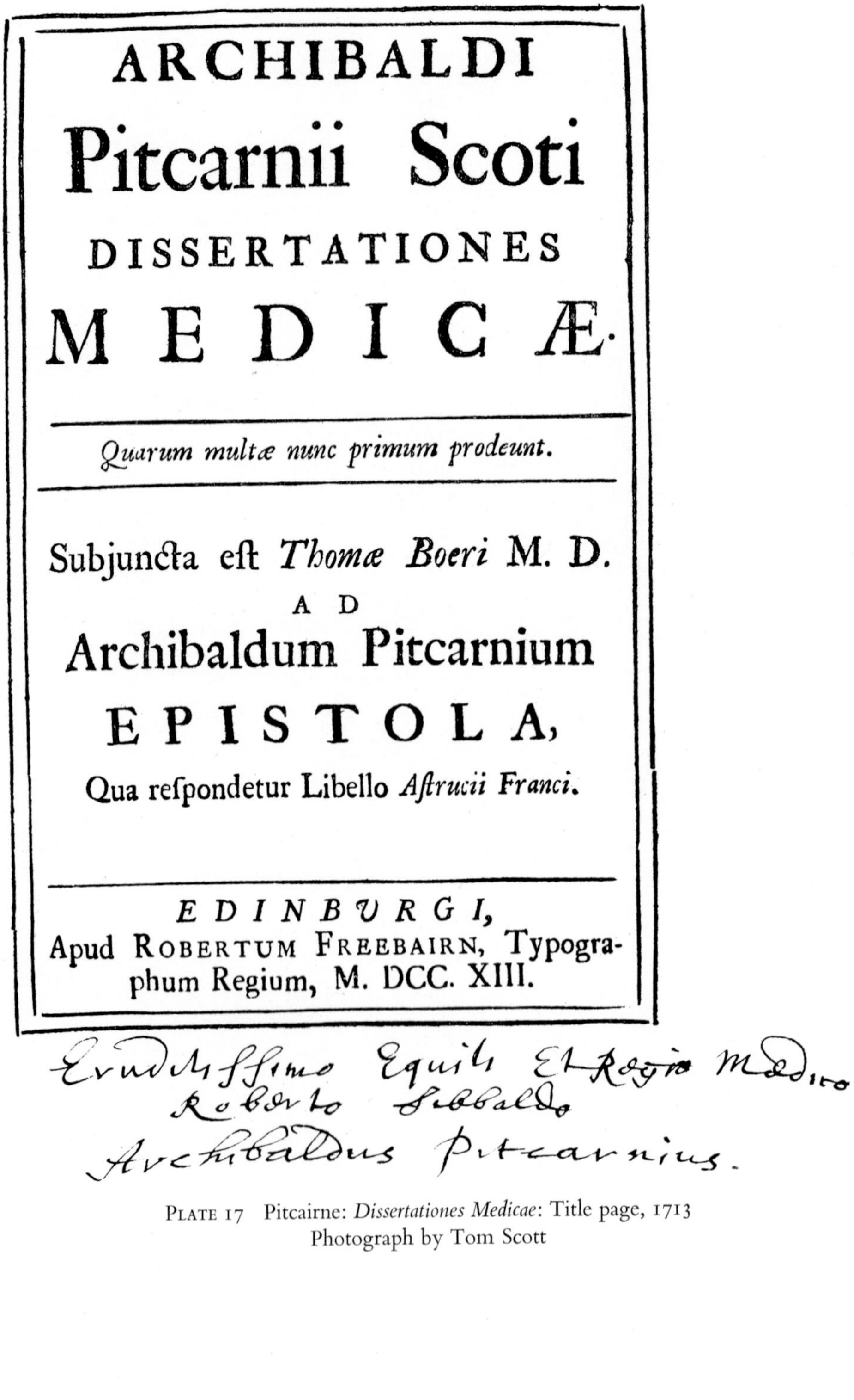

ARCHIBALDI

Pitcarnii Scoti

DISSERTATIONES
MEDICÆ.

Quarum multæ nunc primum prodeunt.

Subjuncta est *Thomæ Boeri* M. D.

A D

Archibaldum Pitcarnium

EPISTOLA,

Qua respondetur Libello *Astrucii Franci.*

EDINBURGI,
Apud ROBERTUM FREEBAIRN, Typogra-
phum Regium, M. DCC. XIII.

Eruditissimo Equiti Et Regio Medico
Roberto Sibbaldo
Archibaldus Pitcarnius.

PLATE 17   Pitcairne: *Dissertationes Medicae*: Title page, 1713
Photograph by Tom Scott

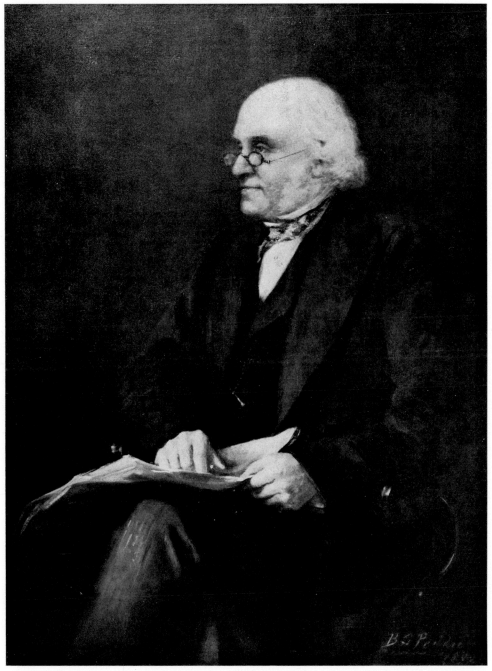

PLATE 18 Dr John Brown (1810–1882)
Reproduced from portrait in the College by Barbara Peddie; by permission from *Scottish Field*;
photograph by George B. Alden

equipment for photocopying and to establish arrangements for the translation of articles needed by medical research workers.[66, 67]

As is to be expected, the repair and maintenance of items in the Library is a constant problem and the College was indebted in 1958 to the Wellcome Trust for a substantial contribution towards the rebinding of early medical books.[68]

A comparatively recent bequest with sentimental associations was left to the College by Mr John Matheson Shaw, M.A., who had been Librarian for seventeen years (1886–1903). The bequest was intended to provide for lectures 'to bring before General Practitioners and Students at the hands of a Specialist the most recent advances and developments in the Science of Medicine and the allied Sciences'.[69]

POSSIBLE FUTURE DEVELOPMENTS

In May 1966 the President reported that informal discussions had taken place with representatives of the Royal College of Surgeons, the University and the National Library of Scotland to consider the desirability and practicability of a centralized medical library.[70] Thereupon the College appointed a Special Committee to review Library policy. At a subsequent working dinner, the impression was gained that while the University and our College viewed prospects of collaboration favourably the attitude of the Royal College of Surgeons was less encouraging.[71] A Report presented by the Special Committee was considered by the College some 18 months later. Apparently the attitude of the Surgeons had not changed but the University could be expected to welcome participation by the College in their efforts to provide additional Library Buildings at the University. Our College approved the Committee's recommendation that while priority must be accorded College interests a justifiable case existed for limited affiliation. Dr W. A. Alexander and Sir James Cameron were appointed as a negotiating team with power to co-opt an additional Fellow.[72] In November of the same year the College was informed that it had been decided to support in principle the concept of a single library of current medical literature in a new building adjacent to the new University Library. There was frank admission that formidable difficulties would have to be overcome and fruition might not take place for ten years.[73]

Another Report was submitted by the Special Committee in 1969 and embodied detailed proposals which had had the support of Sir James Cameron before his untimely death. A large number of problems remained unsolved, including doubts whether the facilities available to Fellows and Members in the Central Library would

F

be equivalent to those enjoyed in the College Library. There appeared to be some uncertainty also as to whether the Central Library would function as a Borrowing or a Reference Library. Acting on a suggestion put forward by the President (Dr Christopher Clayson) the College agreed by 27 votes to 5 to approve in principle the negotiating party's proposals, subject to details being given later and to eventual assurance on doubtful issues including those relating to finance.[74]

At the time of writing (1972) negotiations are continuing for the erection of a unified Medical Library for current medical publications. Prospects have improved with a decision by the University to devote a recent large Australian legacy towards a new Medical Library, but this will not of course absolve the College from making their financial contribution. In the course of time the College will require to give monetary support to a project under way since 1971 for the creation of a unified catalogue of early medical books in Edinburgh libraries. The project aims at ultimately including all books published before 1850 and is being undertaken by a Librarian appointed by the Royal Medical Society who has been granted free access to the College Library.

MEMORIES AND PORTRAITS

On the occasion of his address as President on the opening of the College Hall in Queen Street, Dr Beilby referred to 'the formation of a good medical library, select rather than extensive' as a cherished object of the College. With disarming persuasiveness he went on to suggest to 'fellow-members' that in their private libraries there might well be many volumes the historical value of which would be enhanced were they to be transferred from their present 'isolated state' to the shelves of the College Library. In furtherance of his argument he drew attention to the improved arrangement and accessibility of the Library possessions consequent upon the opening of the new Hall.[75] Dr Beilby was not to know then that within twenty years additional library accommodation would have to be constructed in proximity to the Main Hall[76]: and that of even greater significance, continuing pressure on shelf accommodation would compel coversion of a large section of the basement of No. 8 Queen Street into a Storage Library. Twenty five thousand volumes were stored in the new acquisition.[77]

On the walls of the Hall in which Dr Beilby delivered his address there hang the portraits of many distinguished past office bearers of the College, serving as reminders of their contributions over the years to the eminence of the College and the advancement of medicine. The portraits are among the College's proud historical possessions, and Dr Robert Thin in his book *College Portraits* has left to posterity a series of informative biographical sketches of a number of those personages whose portraits are in the Hall of the College.[78]

Artists responsible for original portraits include David Alison (Sir Byrom Bramwell), Andrew Gamley (Alexander Keiller), Sir John Watson Gordon (Alexander Wood; William Seller), Robert Home (David Berry Hart), Cornelius Janssen (King James VI; Queen Anne of Denmark); John Lorimer (Sir Robert Christison), Sir Henry Raeburn (Andrew Duncan), Sir George Reid (Sir John Sibbald), Fiddes Watt (Sir Thomas Clouston), and Philip Westcott (Sir Alexander Morison). There are in addition copies of Raeburn's original portraits of James Gregory and Daniel Rutherford, and of Belluci's (jun.) original of Robert Whytt: and several medallion portraits including three by Tassie of William Cullen, John Hunter and James Hutton and one of Andrew Duncan by Henning. The College possesses also an impressive series of busts and a valuable collection of engravings. Dr Thomas Spens presented four engraved prints of medical practitioners in 1833 with the express object of encouraging the beginning of the collection.[79]

REFERENCES

(1) DRUMMOND, J. (1701) *Catalogus librorum Joannis Drummond, M.D.* Edinburgh: Privately printed.

(2) R.C.P.E. (1925) *Historical Sketch and Laws*, p. 80. Edinburgh: Royal College of Physicians.

(3) R.C.P.E. (1767) *Catalogus bibliothecae collegii regii medicorum Edinburgensium.* [Edinburgh]: Royal College of Physicians.

(4) R.C.P.E. (1925) *Historical Sketch and Laws*, p. 82. Edinburgh: Royal College of Physicians.

(5) Ibid., p. 81.

(6) College Minutes, 5.v.1713.

(7) Ibid., 3.xi.1713.

(8) Ibid., 2.xi.1830.

(9) R.C.P.E. (1898) *Catalogue of the Library*. Preface, p. xxi. Edinburgh: Royal College of Physicians.

(10) FERGUSON, J. P. S. (1973) Personal communication.

(11) SIBBALD, Sir R. (1833) *The Autobiography*, p. 33. Edinburgh: Thomas Stevenson.

(12) R.C.P.E. (1725) *Catalogue of Donations to the Library, 1681–1725*. (Ms.)

(13) College Minutes, 29.ix.1696.

(14) ARNOT, H. (1799) *The History of Edinburgh*, p. 324. Edinburgh: W. Creech.

(15) JOLLEY, L. (1952) Medical libraries of Great Britain. II. Medical libraries of Scotland. *British Medical Bulletin*, **8**, 2–3, 256.

(16) College Minutes, 30.xi.1682.

(17) Ibid., 6.xii.1683.

(18) Ibid., 7.v.1683.

(19) Ibid., 1.v.1682.

(20) Ibid., 20.viii.1683.

(21) RITCHIE, R. P. (1899) *The Early Days of the Royal College of Physicians, Edinburgh*, p. 103. Edinburgh: G. P. Johnston.

(22) College Minutes, 30.xi.1682.

(23) LAUDER, Sir J., *Lord Fountainhall* (1759) *The Decisions of the Lords of Council and Session, from June 6th, 1678, to July 30th, 1712.* [20.ix.1684.] Vol. I, p. 304. Edinburgh: Hamilton & Balfour.

(24) College Minutes, 13.xii.1705.

(25) Ibid., 3.xi.1801.

(26) R.C.P.E. (1925) *Historical Sketch and Laws*, p. 83. Edinburgh: Royal College of Physicians.

(27) College Minutes, 7.v.1844.

(28) Council Minutes, 2.v.1862.

(29) Ibid., 9.v.1862.

(30) College Minutes, 5.viii.1800.

(31) Ibid., 7.xi.1826.

(32) Ibid., 2.v.1876.

(33) Council Minutes, 7.xii.1909.

(34) College Minutes, 29.iii.1763.

(35) Ibid., 21.iv.1763.

(36) Ibid., 5.xi.1793.

(37) GRANT, Sir A. (1884) *The Story of the University of Edinburgh*, vol. II, p. 177. London: Longmans, Green & Co.

(38) College Minutes, 3.ii.1794.

(39) Ibid., 22.vi.1829.

(40) Ibid., 3.xi.1830.

(41) CRESWELL, C. H. (1926) *The Royal College of Surgeons of Edinburgh*, pp. 86 f. Edinburgh: Oliver & Boyd.

(42) College Minutes, 3.ii.1903.

(43) R.C.P.E. (1925) *Historical Sketch and Laws*, p. 158. Edinburgh: Royal College of Physicians.

(44) College Minutes, 19.vi.1906.

(45) College Minutes, 17.vii.1923.

(46) Ibid., 5.v.1953.

(47) R.C.P.E. (1898) *Catalogue of the Library*. Preface, p. xviii. Edinburgh: Royal College of Physicians.

(48) Ibid., p. xxi.

(49) Ibid., p. xxiv.

(50) R.C.P.E. (1925) *Historical Sketch and Laws*, p. 87. Edinburgh: Royal College of Physicians.

(51) FERGUSON, J. P. S. (1973) Personal communication.

(52) R.C.P.E. (1925) *Historical Sketch and Laws*, p. 78. Edinburgh: Royal College of Physicians.

(53) THIN, R. (1927) *College portraits*, p. 30. Edinburgh: Oliver & Boyd.

(54) CLENDENING, L., comp. (1942) *Source Book of Medical History*, p. 346. New York: Hoeber.

(55) CULLEN, W. (1769) Letter to Dr Hunter, from Edinburgh, 11th February 1769. In *An Account*

of the Life, Lectures, and Writings of William Cullen, M.D. Thomson, J. (1859) Vol. I, p. 555. Edinburgh: Blackwood.

(56) R.C.P.E. (1925) *Historical Sketch and Laws*, p. 82. Edinburgh: Royal College of Physicians.

(57) Council Minutes, 24.x.1961.

(58) BOSWELL, J. (1958) *Life of Johnson*, vol. II, p. 46. London: Dent (Everyman's Library).

(59) R.C.P.E. (1898) *Catalogue of the Library*. Preface, pp. xviii f. Edinburgh: Royal College of Physicians.

(60) R.C.P.E. (1925) *Historical Sketch and Laws*, p. 86. Edinburgh: Royal College of Physicians.

(61) College Minutes, 3.ii.1953.

(62) DUNCAN, A. (1896) *Memorials of the Faculty of Physicians and Surgeons of Glasgow, 1599–1850*, p. 216. Glasgow: Maclehose.

(63) JOLLEY, L. Op. cit., p. 257.

(64) Ibid., p. 256.

(65) Library Committee Minutes, 12.iv.1894.

(66) R.C.P.E. (1955) *Report by the President* [Sir Stanley Davidson] . . . *1953–54*. Edinburgh: Royal College of Physicians.

(67) College Minutes, 5.v.1953.

(68) Ibid., 4.ii.1958.

(69) Ibid., 6.xi.1951.

(70) Ibid., 3.v.1966.

(71) Ibid., 1.xi.1966.

(72) Ibid., 7.v.1968.

(73) Ibid., 5.xi.1968.

(74) Ibid., 22.vii.1969.

(75) BEILBY, W. (1847) *Address on the Opening of the New Hall of the Royal College of Physicians, November 27, 1846*, p. 37. Edinburgh: Constable.

(76) R.C.P.E. (1925) *Historical Sketch and Laws*, p. 47. Edinburgh: Royal College of Physicians.

(77) Ibid., p. 88.

(78) THIN, R. Op. cit.

(79) R.C.P.E. (1925) *Historical Sketch and Laws*, p. 84. Edinburgh: Royal College of Physicians.

Chapter VII

LICENTIATES: PRIOR TO 1858

The moment of vocation had come
. . . the world was made new to him.

George Eliot

It is as much of the business of a physician to alleviate pain, and to smooth the avenues of
death, when unavoidable, as to cure diseases.

John Gregory (1725-73)

In fact he did not find M.D.'s Worth one D—M.

Thomas Hood

While today there can be no doubts as to the significance of such designations as
Licentiate, Member, Collegiate Member and Fellow, care is necessary in interpreting
their implied meaning when referring to Minutes and historical documents of the
earlier days of the College. For many years 'Socius' and 'Fellow' were employed somewhat indiscriminately and the compelling spirit of fellowship which has long been
an especial feature of our College is largely attributable to the reluctance of those first
in office to conceive of any difference between Socius and Fellow. The Membership
was a creation of the late nineteenth century but in the preceding two hundred years
frequent use had been made of the term 'Member' when referring to those attending
Sederunts.[1] In 1822 it was specifically enacted that the term 'Member' should be
debarred in references to Licentiates. Confusion is liable to arise also from the
inconsistent use over many years of the qualification 'honorary' whether in relation
to Fellows or Members. By way of contrast, even allowing that the Licence was
discontinued for a period, the terms 'Licentiate' and 'Licentiateship' have never lost
their original basic significance in relation to the right to practise medicine.

LICENTIATESHIP

The avowed object of all petitioners associated with each attempt, unsuccessful and successful, to obtain a Charter was a general raising of the standards of medical care. Likewise all Articles submitted in favour of successive pleas for a Charter had in common the need for some form of control of medical practice, whether of 'mountebank' or seemingly more orthodox form. Authority to license, granted by the Charter of 1681, gave to the College the opportunity to give trial at least to the efficacy of control.

What powers of control did the College actually possess? In the first place practice in Edinburgh and its precincts without a licence from the College was prohibited; and being a Scottish graduate was not a sufficient reason for being excused the penalty of a fine if convicted of practising without a licence within the area of the College's jurisdiction. By August 1682 the need for tightening regulations became evident and it was 'resolved and agried . . . that hereafter no persone shall be Licensed to practise Medicine in the Citty of Edgr or Suburbs yrof Except he be first ane graduat Doctor of Physick'. Again subject to the overriding condition that he must already be in possession of a Doctorate of Medicine, 'any persone in the Countrey' could petition for a licence; and provided that the 'Examinatne and tryall of the qualificatne' proved satisfactory, the College was prepared to 'grant a Licence or Certificat to him as a fitt persone sufficiently qualified for practiseing of Medicine in the Countrey'. There then follows a caveat in the Minute of no little significance— 'But if such a persone shall happen to Come in to Edgr. he shall not have allowance to practise yr, without a new Examinatne and Licence and be first a graduat Doctor'.[2]

In drawing up these regulations the College took account of the effect of the College patent on the individual practitioner. It was provided that 'any Physitian graduat befor the patent, upon applicatione to the Colledge for a Licence to practise in Edgr. he shall without any examinatne upon payment to the Thesaurer of ffyve pounds Star: have a licence to practise in Edgr. he keeping his ordinary residence in the Countrey, and giving bond to pay uther ffyve pounds Star: if he shall happen to come in to inside and practise in Edgr.' According to Paterson 'if any persons were licensed for the Country . . . no trace of the fact is to be discovered in the Minutes'.[3]

But what of the individual seeking a licence to practise in Edinburgh who became a graduate doctor at a date after receipt by the College of its patent? He, it was

ordained 'shall be obleidged imediatly to Consigne in the Thesaurers hands befor
he abyde Examinatne ffyve pounds Star: and if he be not after Examinatne found
Sufficient he shall Losse ffytie Shillings starling thereof'.[2] In the event of his being
found sufficient, the total disbursements involved in getting a licence were the same
as a colleague possessed of a doctorate of medicine before the College patent. Payment by bonds was a procedure employed when necessary, and one which proved
over the years to be a source of trouble to the Treasurer and Council. A clause of
fundamental importance in the Charter was one which enabled a medical graduate of
any of the Scottish Universities to claim exemption from examination, and the
award of the College licence to practise on payment of recognised dues.

Summarized—to practise in Edinburgh and neighbourhood required the College
licence obtainable by examination from which Scottish University graduates were
exempt: and the licence, although not obligatory, was available also to those practising in the country outwith the area of the College's jurisdiction, subject to their
satisfying examiners and to payment of appropriate dues.

INEXPERIENCED HASTE

With such a complicated background it is not surprising that procedure for licensing
was characterized by a number of curious anomalies and occurrences in the earlier
years. To some extent this was contributed to by the fact that 'Our predecessors were
manifestly too hasty'.[4] Initially the College implemented the business of admission
and election with what now appears altogether unseemly haste. Thus a large number
of instances are on record of an applicant for a licence succeeding in his plea, being
advanced to the intermediate step of Candidate so styled, and chosen a Fellow at one
and the same sederunt. According to circumstances this rapid procedure was applied
irrespective of whether or not the petition for Licence indicated preparedness to be
examined. To add both to inconsistency and unpredictability the College concluded
their decisions on 12th August 1682 by adding that 'when the Colledge shall find it
necessar to Call any Candidat to be of their number That the oldest Candidat shall be
the persone requyred to enter'.[5] This last clause has been quoted as evidence that,
'in a certain sense, the College made Fellowship, or the step towards it, compulsory
on licentiates; and the fact is indubitable,—a condition being for some time attached
to the petition for a licence—namely, that the individual "obliged himself to enter
Candidate, and thereafter a Fellow of the College".'[6, 7]

FIRST LICENTIATE BY EXAMINATION

On 4th December 1682 it was reported that a Dr Kello had 'addressed a Bill to the Colledge to be received as one of the Society and offering himself to abyde a tryall conforme to the rules of the Colledge . . .'. This was the first application, appeal or prayer as it was variously called to be received by the College. Despite what today the public relations officer would naively excuse as 'a failure in communications' (q.v.) Dr Kello was successful, 'the Colledge being well satisfied . . . admitts him to be a Licentiat and appoynts him to have a warrand therefor under the Subsnes and seale of the Colledge Conforme to the former acts made yranent'.[8]

INJURED DIGNITY

There was one at least who about this time took affront at such powers as the College were able to exercise—a Dr Christopher Irving. In part his attitude may have been explained by his Irish origins. He was very conscious of his position as official historiographer for Scotland and Physician to James VII: and understandably resented ejection from his Irish patrimony and the Town College of Edinburgh by the demands of the Covenant. To him the erection of the Royal College of Physicians was a source of intense irritation. Basing his arguments on a presentation of his education, degrees, army commissions and services he applied to the Privy Council that he should not be suffered 'to be stated under the partial humours or affronts of the new College composed of men altogether his juniors (save Dr Hay) in the studies of philosophie and practice of physick'. The Privy Council in their wisdom found justification in Irving's remonstrances, and absolved him from submitting himself to the adjudication of the Royal College. Their decision was confirmed by an Act of the Scottish Parliament in 1685.[9, 10] Ironically John Monro, father of Monro *primus*, was 'booked apprentice' in 1688 to Irving who had been a Freeman Surgeon as well as practising physician for thirty years. The apprenticeship has been interpreted as a subterfuge to circumvent the Regulations of the Surgical Incorporation.[11] In the course of time the position was regularized, Monro's apprenticeship to Borthwick being confirmed.

Another interesting sidelight concerning Irving is that about 1658, at a time when attempts to found our College were unavailing, he dedicated a drama in Latin to Dr George Sibbald.[10]

Although it is known that prayers were received and elections made during the period for which no recorded Minutes exist, there is no information concerning procedures followed. On the resumption of records the first candidate to be examined was a Dr Oliphant, who having satisfied the examiners was licensed to practise and the College 'by another vote In respect of his good qualificationes admitt him Candidat'.[12] He was 'Admitted . . . to be a Socius and Member of the Colledge and received him to sitt and vote with them' six months later.[13]

Within a short period of time and for a considerable number of years, the College developed the practice already mentioned of granting a licence and advancing to Fellowship at one sitting. Not every applicant was dealt with in this way, but the Minutes contain references to many benefiting from this phenomenal acceleration 'on any particular reason being assigned'. An amazing variety of reasons were forthcoming. Cause for favour by the College was seen in the past appointment of one petitioner as physician in the Imperial Court of Czarist Russia,[14] and of another as physician to the Emperor and Empress of Germany.[15] A reason advanced by more than one Candidate was that elevation would ensure the appearance of their names in new editions of the Pharmacopoeia due for early publication. The predilection for aspiring medicals to appear in print has a long history!

Not surprisingly in view of its largely lost function the intermediate status or ranking of Candidate was discarded about 1710.[4] A partial attempt to control the situation was made a number of years later by stipulating that at least one year should elapse between being granted a licence to practise and admission as a Fellow.[16] Practice however did not by any means always accord with legal theory—as evidenced by Minutes so recent as those in the early nineteenth century.

EARLY OFFENDERS

None the less the impression must not be gained that in discharging its responsibilities under the Charter, the College disregarded the crucial significance of constant care in the granting of licences and unremitting watchfulness in the matter of unlicensed practice within their area of jurisdiction. Indeed pursuit of these two objectives was a frequent source of anxiety and of expenditure which could be ill afforded. Thus in January 1699 legal advice had to be sought in dealing with a Doctor Ford who refused to pay a fine imposed on him by the College for unlicensed practice, he having failed or been unwilling to produce evidence of a Scottish University degree.[17] Six months later he is recorded as 'compearing before the colledge and declaring yt he was sensible of his being in the wrong in standing out'. He was subsequently admitted a Licentiate after producing his patent from the University of Aberdeen. In the same month a 'Dr. Preston', who had failed to explain practising without a licence, appeared before the College 'and acknowledged that it is about two years since he came to this towne and that he has severall times practised physick since within the towne of Edgr. . .'.[18] Within three days 'Mr. Charles Prestone indweller in Edger, and pretended practitioner of physick ther, was decerned at the instance of . . . pror ffiscall to pay to [the] treasurer of the colledge ffyve pounds Sterling. . .'.[19]

Another who was reported for 'unlicensed practiseing' was Dr Walker.[20] He asked that 'the Colledge would Indulge him in a little more time to determine himself whether he Shall fix upon the practise of Physick or Surgery'.[21] Five years later a Dr Innes applied for a licence without examination but was unsuccessful as he failed to produce evidence of the diploma he claimed to possess. Dr Innes applied a second time within a few weeks producing his diploma but 'he Refuseing to Conform himself yrto Or to Signe the obligation . . . The President . . . haveing asked the opinion of the College They unanimously Resolve not to Grant Dr. Innes a Licence . . . untill he agree to Submitt to the Rules of the Society . . .'.[22] Occasionally failure of a petitioner to produce his diploma of medical doctorate was overcome by Socii at a sederunt testifying to their personal knowledge of the petitioner's qualifications and diplomas. One such crisis was resolved in this way when a Candidate claimed to have left his diploma in Paris.[23]

A REACTIONARY REFORMED

A second case involving considerable costs in securing legal opinion concerned Mr Martin Eccles who combined pharmacy with the practice of medicine and who, although a Doctor of Medicine of St Andrews University, possessed no licence to practise in Edinburgh. The gravamen of Mr Eccles' attitude was that he was not 'satisfied that there is any thing inconsistent or incompatible in the exercise . . . by the same person' of medical and pharmaceutical practices. Unfortunately perhaps the College, on legal advice, did not respond to a conciliatory letter from Mr Eccles. The case went to Court, the verdict going against Mr Eccles who, before accepting defeat, unsuccessfully referred the matter to a Court of Appeal.[24-29] In May 1756 it was recorded that the College were 'disposed to treat him with all the Gentleness and Lenity Especially as he had Come to wait on the Colledge'. None the less on their implicit instructions 'The President Rebuked him', and at the same time told Dr

Eccles 'that it was hoped he would behave so for the future as may make the Colledge take no furder nottice of this affair'.[30] The whole suggests a Gilbertian version of the General Medical Council of a later century, the more Gilbertian in that 'Mr.' Eccles now 'Dr.', joined the College as a Licentiate in 1771 and became a Fellow in the same year.[31]

In direct contrast in 1833, Dr Allison tendered his resignation as 'having made an arrangement to succeed Mr Scott, Apothecary and Druggist . . . I am under the painful necessity, according to the Laws, of resigning my place as a Fellow'. It is pleasing to note that 'while the College received his resignation, he had the best wishes of the College for his welfare and prosperity'.[32]

FEES

Fees were another source of trouble, and there is no concealing the fact that the state of the College's finances conditioned policy in the matter of the scale of fees levied. Adjustment took its extreme form when it was decreed that 'such physitians as shall apply to the Colledge to be made Licentiats without submitting themselves to Examinatione shall pay ane thousand merks Scots to the Colledge for their Licence'.[33] The enactment was probably intended to counter the privilege of exemption from examination granted to graduates of Scottish Universities under the College Charter. If so the reduction in the number of applicants was in accordance with national caution and common sense, and the fee was reviewed ere long!

EXTORTION BREEDS RESENTMENT

Nevertheless the College's attitude had some basis because there were at least two instances of men indicted for practising without being licensed hurriedly remedying the situation by obtaining a degree from the University of Aberdeen. Dr Drummond was one such. Spoken to '. . . anent his practising without being Licentiat . . . doctor Drummond did requyre some further tyme befor he should give a determinate answer'.[34] On 7th January 1704 he produced the necessary patent from Aberdeen, was licensed to practise, accepted as candidate and admitted as Socius before the day was out.[35]

Such are the bald facts to be obtained from the College Minutes which have been modified by deletion and erasure. Poole had access to earlier versions of the Minutes in which the original alterations had been only partially effective. In his words, 'The deleted Minutes and a certain printed paper tell another tale'.[36] Certainly in 1702 it is recorded that 'the Colledge allows the president to consult more Advocates in the actione against Dr. Drummond'—reference to which was deleted in the original Minutes.[37] As to the 'paper' mentioned by Poole—this was printed and consisted of a Statement entitled 'Information for Doctor Drummond and the University of Aberdeen, As also for the other three Universities within the Kingdome for their Interest; against the Colledge of Physicians of Edinburgh'.[38]

The 'information' was verbose in the extreme, poor in logic, and might well have carried more weight had drafting been in more competent hands. In brief, Drummond did not accept the jurisdiction of the College in so far as they sought to prevent a University Doctor of Medicine practising medicine. He should he maintained 'if the College understood either power, or their interest' have been offered his licence *gratis*. Without doubt he was incensed that the process taken out against him was 'altogether new and the first that has been heard of, of this nature before your Lordships'. Then followed the stinging topicality incapable of convincing refutation . . . 'who are the Colledge, in as much as the Company of the Physicians concerned, are notourly divided, each of the two parties acclaiming the power of the Colledge and having now a process depending betwixt themselves before the Lord Rankeilor: So that until the process be determined, the Defender doth not know who are the Colledge and to whom to apply'.[39] The case came before Lord Fountainhall who apparently recorded no opinion and Poole came to the conclusion that the case was 'probably settled in a private way, favourably towards the College'.[40] It may have been that together with being the first victim, the scale of fees proved irksome, because while the case was proceeding another Aberdeen graduate (Dr John Hay) was granted his licence after it had been ordained that he must first 'satisfie the Treasurer . . . befor extract of his licence'.[41]

Drummond's experience was in marked contrast with that of John Thatcher who was licensed in 1815 and failed to be elected by ballot for election as Fellow in both 1816 and 1817. Eventually he became a Fellow in 1828. Study of the Minutes points to his recurrent experience being unique. What was the reason?—wild oats, youth or prejudice? College papers do not provide the answer, but a letter in the files signed 'John Thatcher' and dated '2 o'clock P.M. May 7 1816' stated to 'having accidentally & most unexpectedly, learnt that somewhat of an unfavourable impression has been made respecting me'. Asserting his conduct had been appropriate to that of a Gentleman, the letter concluded by saying that he would be found 'unimpeachable' by any fair and candid enquiry.[42] No matter—once won, his spurs were used to good purpose in Council and on Committees for a number of years, and he proved to be the first of four successive generations practising medicine in Edinburgh, his great grandson Dr Lewis Thatcher being a Fellow until his decease in 1970.

In so far as blood-relationship is concerned, it is interesting that in 1797 Dr Alexander Monro *secundus'* successful petition for a licence was 'signed by Dr. Alexander Monro Senior for his Son'.[43] Previously in 1744 an Edinburgh physician presented a petition 'on behalf of . . . his Brother Physician at Kingstoun in Jamaica'.[44] The dues having been paid, the College granted both a Licence and Fellowship, noting at the time that the successful petitioner 'may be serviceable to the Colledge by keeping up a Correspondence with them, and Sending what Curiositys the places may affoord where he shall Reside . . .'. This partiality for curiosities on the part of the College was not infrequently cited as a particular reason for assignment when granting of a licence or elevation to the Fellowship was involved. Acceptance of the validity of a particular reason being assigned was not uncommonly qualified by such words as 'without allowing what has been done in this particular case to be drawn in precedent in time coming'.[44]

Petitioners were not always readily forthcoming with payment. In 1725 a request for special consideration prompted the reply that the petitioner 'can have no Dimunutione or ease of the money that he is due to the College Conforme'.[45] Not to be rebuffed a few months later the doctor in question gave in a petition, 'Craving that some part or the haill of the money payed by him for being Licentiat . . . might be Restored again to him In regaird he aplyed to the Colledge for being Licentiat out of a particular view of being Chandaj Professor of Medicine at St. Andrews but, being Disapoynted thereof . . .'.[46] The Minutes go on to record that 'the Desyre yrof was Refused as being both unprecedented and of bad Consequence'. Perhaps less unprecedented was a proposal made by another individual to pay overdue fees in accordance with conditions which he himself specified but which were rejected as inadmissible by the College.[47] Defaulters were a source of anxiety to most Treasurers and it is not uncommon to read in the Minutes such words as 'and if the Dor. refuse . . . the Colledge appoynts the Thessrer to pursew him for the same'.[48]

SECOND THOUGHTS

Occasionally persistence rather than pursuit was manifested in the other direction. In 1764 a Dr Abernethy wrote asking that his name be omitted from any lists of Licentiates, a request with which the College felt unable to comply.[49] Nine years later the College received a letter from a Dr 'Abernethy Drummond' stating that 'the practice of physick . . . has long since ceased to be the object of my pursuit [and] that seeing the privileges of a Licentiate are to me of no manner of significancy I hereby resign them into your hands'.[50] The resignation, or as the College preferred to regard it, the renunciation was accepted. Although there is no conclusive evidence, the probability is that the two 'Abernethys' were one and the same individual. A sequence of events with a happier ending occurred in connection with Dr Andrew Halliday. In 1820 he asked in writing that his name 'be expunged from the Records of the College as a Licentiate'.[51] It was not considered possible to accede to the request, but it was agreed to delete his name from future lists. In a letter dated 13th April 1827 from Hampton Court, Dr—now Sir Andrew Halliday, wrote in the following terms to the President:

> 'As President of the Royal College of Physicians, I beg you will express to that learned body . . . my sincere regret at having written a Letter some years ago desiring my name to be withdrawn from the List of Licentiates, and at the same time say that I shall feel honoured in being restored to that List, and that I hope I may yet be found worthy to be raised to the rank of a Fellow.'[52]

His hope was fulfilled in August 1827.[53]

EARLY OVERSEAS LINKS

Selection of individual names for mention is invidious but for historical purposes there is justification for noting that two pioneers of medicine on the American continent, John Morgan and William Shippen, obtained the College licence in 1765 anf 1767 respectively.[54, 55] A medical graduate of Edinburgh University, Morgan 'had furder Improved himself at London Paris and Several places in Italy and proposed Soon to Settle at Pensylvania in America and tho he never Intended to practise at Edin yet he was very desirous to be admitted a Licentiat'. This being so, there is an element of inverted magnanimity in the rest of the Minute '. . . the College They admitt the Said Doctor John Morgan a Licentiat . . . with power to practise medicine within the City of Edinr. and Libertys thereof.'! Shippen's successful petition was couched in very similar terms but was submitted after he had begun 'practiseing as a physician at Philadelphia'. Both he and Morgan were made Fellows with little delay.

On 1st November 1763 the Licentiateship was made a necessary stepping stone to the Fellowship and it was decreed that 'no person resideing in Edinburgh . . . Shall be admitted a Fellow . . . Sooner than one full year after the day he has obtained his Licence.'[56] An unforeseen result of this was that Fellows were subjected to a double tax by the Government. To meet the situation the Regulation was rescinded in 1829, Fellows thereafter being elected without passage through a preliminary phase of Licentiateship.[57] In consequence the order of Licentiate, dating back to the admission of Dr Kello in 1682, fell into disuse.[58] It was resuscitated in an entirely new form in 1859.[59]

TOWN AND COUNTRY

But what was the exact value of the licence of the Edinburgh College to the practitioner? In Edinburgh and suburbs it was a legal obligation: in the rest of Scotland it was, without being obligatory, an added professional status symbol, except in those areas which by law came under the jurisdiction of the Faculty of Physicians and Surgeons of Glasgow. The areas in question were the counties of Lanark, Renfrew, Ayr and Dunbarton and the Royal Burgh of Ayr. In them the Licence of the Faculty was the only one with legal backing, the position resembling that in the three Lothians, and the Counties of Fife, Roxburgh, Berwick, Selkirk and Peebles additional to the City of Edinburgh where the licence of the Edinburgh surgeon–apothecaries alone carried the weight of authority to practise surgery or pharmacy.

LIONS RAMPANT AND COUCHANT

The position with regard to England was very different. By an Act of Parliament in the time of Henry VIII it was decreed

> 'that noo person from hensforth be suffered to exercyse or practyse in Physyke through England until such time that he be examined in London by the said President and three of the said Electys (of the College of Physicians); and to have from the said President or Electys Letters Testimonialae of their approving and examination.'[60]

As Munk explained, this statute aimed at disposing of ambiguities in the Letters Patent of 23rd September 1518 constituting the London College. The decree determining the conditions to be satisfied before anyone might practise concluded with the incontestable caveat 'except he be a Graduate of Oxford or Cambridge, which hath accomplished all things for his form without any grace'.[61] Degrees from these two Universities carried with them authority to practise 'per universum Anglicae regnum' which in practice was interpreted to include Scotland. It is not without significance that in 1827 the belligerent editor of the *Lancet* saw occasion to remark upon 'the odious self-complacency and malicious arrogance of the graduates of Oxford and Cambridge, often decrying, as they are known to be, and always oppressing, the physicians of other Universities'.[62]

Some fifty years previously the philosopher Adam Smith had expressed himself on the subject in a letter to Dr Cullen. He wrote:

> 'Had the Universities of Oxford and Cambridge been able to maintain themselves in the exclusive privilege of graduating all the doctors who could practise in England the price of feeling a pulse might by this time have risen from two and three guineas . . . to double or triple that sum; and English physicians might and probably would, have been at the same time the most ignorant and quackish in the world . . . Had the hopeful project of the rich and great universities succeeded, there would have been no occasion for sense or science . . . Our regular physicians in Scotland have little quackery, and no quack accordingly has ever made his fortune among us.'[63]

Adam Smith was not blindly biased because he expressed agreement, giving his reasons, with the rejection by the London College of certain Edinburgh graduates because 'they were ignorant of their profession'.[64]

These diverse forms of authority were in no sense part of a reciprocal arrangement. However graduates from Scotland practising south of Tweed were not impeded in any way by the English Universities. In marked contrast it was the College of Physicians of London which by prosecution and fine sought to impede and hamper immigrant doctors holding degrees of Scottish Universities or licences of one of the Scottish medical corporations. Writing in 1870 of the London College, Chapman stated '. . . While all the efforts of the College to prevent ignorant persons from practising, and to shield the public from their destructive nostrums, notoriously failed, it used its authority to restrain surgeons, apothecaries and Scotch physicians, from competing with its own fellows and licentiates.'[65] Power to restrain the ambitious, immigrant Scot was vested also in the Apothecaries Society under the Apothecaries Act of 1815. Given powers to ensure that only those possessed of the Company's diploma should practise the art of the apothecary, the Company conducted what had all the appearance of being a campaign as selective as it was vindictive and persistent, against those among practitioners coming from Scotland.

As evidence of the situation in which a Licentiate of the Edinburgh College might find himself if practising in England, the following extract from a letter submitted to a Committee in 1834 is informative:

'I studied the medical profession in Edinburgh, and during the seven years I was at the University I attended the following classes: Practical Medicine (Professor Gregory); Institutes of Medicine (Professor Duncan); Anatomy, Surgery and Dissection (Professor Barclay); Surgery and Pathology (Professor Munro); Chemistry (Professor Fife); Materia Medica, Dietetics and Pharmacy (Professor A. Duncan); Midwifery and Diseases of Women and Children (Professor Thatcher, to whom I was assistant); Surgery (Professor Allen); Royal Infirmary, where I was a dresser and assistant (Mr. Macdonald); Clinical Lectures at the Royal Infirmary (Professor Russell). I was matriculated four years in the University of Edinburgh. I returned to England in 1824, and have been practising here ever since I was induced to take up my residence at a town—. The second year, I was unanimously elected medical attendant for the poor to the parish, and surgeon to the Yeomanry Cavalry. About a year ago, information to the Apothecaries' Society was given of my practising; and I received a notice, through their solicitor . . . that proceedings were to be instituted against me immediately for practising as an apothecary without a licence. Considering that I had a right to dispense medicines to my own patients, I defended the action for recovery of penalty of £20, which defence cost me £400. After this action, to enable me to dispense with impunity, I took a partner, who was a licentiate of the Society, and also a fellow (? Member) of the London College of Surgeons; and I have now received another notice, that another information has been laid against me, and that proceedings are again to be commenced forthwith.'[66]

Then as now, in trade or profession, informers were not far to seek among rival 'colleagues'. In attempting to bring order out of chaos, the Medical Act of 1858 aimed at eradicating the animosities and jealousies arising from the multiplicity of vested interests with historical and legal origins, and with obsessions of power and materialism originating from age-long parochial and national antagonisms.

AN EXAMINATION FOR LICENTIATESHIP

Examination of the first candidate, Dr Kello (q.v.), took place in December 1682 and consisted of three parts. Of these the first was conducted by Doctors Balfour and Cranstoune on the 4th of the month and the examination was 'upon Severall materiall questions viz. De purgatione et venisectione'. The second part was held four days later when Doctor Balfour in company this time with Dr Sibbald 'severally examined him (Dr Kello) upon tuo aphorismes . . . formerly intimat to him'. Doctors Crawfurd and

Pitcairne were the examiners 'appoynted to examine him for the Last tyme . . . upon tuo severall caises of Medicine' on 11th December. After being told 'the caise he was to Insist upon' he was 'publickly examined' before the assembled Socii of the College. Passage from one part of the examination to another was preceded by an expression of satisfaction on the part, not of the active examiners but of all the assembled Fellows of the College. Whether failure in any one part would have resulted in failure in the whole examination is an open question. Certainly there were no opportunities for 'compensation' as practised in recent times. The reference in the Minutes 'to examine him for the Last tyme' has about it an intense nostalgically echoing air which has survived the centuries in the individual case, whether for good or ill.

The only flaw in the arrangements was that Doctor Crawfurd failed to appear in his capacity as appointed co-examiner 'without Intimating to Dr. Kello or the President the caise he designed the Doctor should be examined upon'. Faced with a nonplussing situation 'The Colledge ffinds it not just that his admissione should be delayed upon Dr. Crawfurd's Neglect, and Thairfor haveing now reconsidered the severall Examinatnes, and Doctor Kellos anssrs Have admitted and admitts him to be a Licentiate . . .'.[67-69]

The form of the first examination provided the basis of subsequent 'tryalls'; and the third part was to prove the forerunner of the essentially clinical assessment of candidates to which to this day so much importance is attached by the College and the University of Edinburgh. From the fact that the Minutes repeatedly refer to the 'caice' and not 'the disease' which the candidate 'was to judge upon' it has been surmised that clinical material was provided for examination purposes.[70] A point possibly favouring this view is that in 1724 a successful candidate 'payed Twenty shilling starling to the Thessrer for the use of the Dispensary belonging to the Colledge'.[71] If the supposition be correct the probability is that the College depended upon their Dispensary to provide any clinical material required.

In the course of time the term 'Institutions of Medicine' came to be applied to the first part of the examination. When precisely is doubtful but it was certainly in use by 1695 in which year it appeared in the Minutes of 25th September[72]; and it was employed also by Sibbald who wrote of studying 'the institutions and practice, under Sylvius'.[73] Implied in the new designation was the basic importance of anatomy and physiology, the latter as propounded by Harvey.

A major modification was decided on in 1694 when the College considered 'what furder Tryall should be imposed on Intrants after their examinatne'. In their determinations they 'thought fitt that the Intrant shall have a Subject of a Discourse prescribed him by the Colledge upon which he is to Treat when appoynted either to be Delivered viva voce or by papers'.[74] The first Intrant subject to this new demand was not ready with his discourse on the appointed day. His omission was excused once, but not a second time. One month later it is recorded how the College 'amerceit' him 'in ane Rex Dollar . . . for being absent from this meeting and not sending his Discourse in wryte'.[75] Inexorably the mode of examination tended to expand and in 1723 written 'explanations' crept into the picture, when the College ordained 'that for hereafter all the Candidates and Licentiats . . . shall give in just Copies of the severall Explanatnes of their aphorismes and of their severall opinions of the practicall caices to be given them at any tyme hereafter to the Secretarius . . .'.[76, 77]

Quite apart from the format of the examination, consideration was given to other aspects. Thus as early as December 1684[78] Doctor Sibbald was 'desyred to revise the severall acts anent the electing and admitting of Intrants', and three weeks later, having been elected President, he moved that 'the Colledge take to their Consideratione the minimum quid sic of the time that a Licentiat should study before he be Licensed'. There is no evidence of what transpired as Minutes lost include all those of Sibbald's tenure of the Presidency.

A subject which at one time gave rise to controversy within the College was the appointment of examiners or examinators as they were then called. Originally the practice had been followed of appointing special examiners either at the Sederunt before which the Intrant appeared or at the preceding Sederunt. At some time during the period for which records were lost, procedure must have been modified. The changes assumed more or less precise form in 1693[79] when it was recorded that the College 'Doe think fitt that there be ffyve Examinators appoynted to Continew till the next electione of the President etc. and that there be nominat by the President and Colledge from year to year . . . and there shall be no examinatne unless thrie of these Examinators be present, and the President or propreses and as many of the Colledge as with the Examinators present shall make up a full Quorum, and It is ordained that for the greater Solemnity the whole members be warned to be present at the Examination of Intrants and the Colledge doth appoint the next meeting to be this day eight days . . . which tyme the Examinators are to be appoynted and nominated'.[80]

The new régime was still in operation at the end of 1694,[81] but in September of the next year it was 'put to the vote whither the old law anent the examination of intrants as it was at the first errection or the new law appoynting examinators for a whole year together should be observed in tyme comeing'.[82] Eventually following three sittings on the subject it was carried that 'the old law should be revived and the new abrogat nemine contradicente'.[83]

REFERENCES

(1) College Minutes, 5.xi.1822.

LICENTIATESHIP

(2) Ibid., 7.viii.1682.

(3) R.C.P.E. (c. 1850). *Abstract of the Minutes, AD 1682–1731*. By George Paterson. [Fellowship and License.] (Ms.)

(4) R.C.P.E. (1833) *Report on Examination of Medical Practitioners*, p. 53. Edinburgh: Neill.

(5) College Minutes, 7.viii.1682.

(6) R.C.P.E. (1833) *Report on Examination of Medical Practitioners*, p. 56. Edinburgh: Neill.

(7) College Minutes, 4.xii.1682.

(8) Ibid., 7.xii.1682.

(9) GAIRDNER, J. (1860) *Historical Sketch of the Royal College of Surgeons of Edinburgh*, p. 22. Edinburgh: Sutherland & Knox.

(10) COMRIE, J. D. (1932) *History of Scottish Medicine*, 2nd Edition, vol. I, p. 245. London: Baillière, Tindall & Cox.

(11) WRIGHT-ST CLAIR, R. E. (1964) *Doctors Monro; a medical saga*, pp. 7–8. London: The Wellcome Historical Medical Library.

(12) College Minutes, 15.v.1693.

(13) Ibid., 9.xi.1693.

(14) Ibid., 19.viii.1762.

(15) Ibid., 4.xi.1755.

(16) Ibid., 1.xi.1763.

(17) Ibid., 21.vi.1699.

(18) Ibid., 27.vi. 1699.

(19) Ibid., 30.vi.1699.

(20) Ibid., 30.vi.1699.

(21) Ibid., 3.xi.1761.

(22) Ibid., 8.xii.1761.

(23) Ibid., 5.xi.1771.

(24) Ibid., 11.ii.1755.

(25) Ibid., 6.v.1755.

(26) Ibid., 20.v.1755.

(27) Ibid., 17.vii.1755.

(28) Ibid., 4.xi.1755.

(29) Ibid., 3.ii.1756.

(30) Ibid., 4.v.1756.

(31) Ibid., 5.xi.1771.

(32) Ibid., 7.v.1833.

(33) Ibid., 25.x.1705.
(34) Ibid., 25.viii.1701.
(35) Ibid., 7.i.1704.
(36) POOLE, R. (1838) *Preparatory Notes for a History of the College*, p. 245. (Ms.)
(37) College Minutes, 31.xii.1702.
(38) POOLE, R. Op. cit., p. 246.
(39) Ibid., pp. 246–7.
(40) Ibid., p. 249.
(41) College Minutes, 16.xi.1702.
(42) R.C.P.E. (1816) *General Correspondence*, 7.v.1816.
(43) College Minutes, 7.xi.1797.
(44) Ibid., 15.v.1744.
(45) Ibid., 16.ii.1725.
(46) Ibid., 3.viii.1725.
(47) Ibid., 6.viii.1782.
(48) Ibid., 22.viii.1717.
(49) Ibid., 7.ii.1764.
(50) Ibid., 2.ii.1773.
(51) Ibid., 1.viii.1820.
(52) Ibid., 1.v.1827.
(53) Ibid., 7.viii.1827.
(54) Ibid., 5.iii.1765.
(55) Ibid., 3.xi.1767.
(56) Ibid., 1.xi.1763.
(57) R.C.P.E. (1925) *Historical Sketch and Laws*, p. 56. Edinburgh: Royal College of Physicians.
(58) College Minutes, 5.iv.1859.
(59) R.C.P.E. (1925) *Historical Sketch and Laws*, p. 57. Edinburgh: Royal College of Physicians.
(60) 14 and 15 Henry VIII, c. 5 (1523).
(61) MUNK, W. (1878) *The Roll of the Royal College of Physicians of London*, 2nd Edition, vol. I, p. 10. London: Royal College of Physicians.
(62) Editorial (1827) *Lancet*, **XII,** 665.
(63) RAE, J. (1895) *Life of Adam Smith*, p. 278. London: Macmillan.
(64) Ibid., p. 276.
(65) CHAPMAN, J. (1870) *The Medical Institutions of the United Kingdom: a history exemplifying the evils of overlegislation*, p. 41. London: John Churchill.
(66) Ibid., p. 42.

AN EXAMINATION FOR LICENTIATESHIP

(67) College Minutes, 4.xii.1682.
(68) Ibid., 8.xii.1682.
(69) Ibid., 11.xii.1682.

(70) RITCHIE, R. P. (1899) *The Early Days of the Royall Colledge of Phisitians, Edinburgh*, p. 100. Edinburgh: G. P. Johnston.
(71) College Minutes, 4.ii.1724.
(72) Ibid., 25.ix.1695.
(73) SIBBALD, Sir R. (1833) *The Autobiography*, p. 16. Edinburgh: Thomas Stevenson.
(74) College Minutes, 4.i.1694.
(75) Ibid., 1.ii.1694.
(76) Ibid., 5.iii.1723.
(77) RITCHIE, R. P. Op. cit., p. 115.
(78) College Minutes, 1.xii.1684.
(79) Ibid., 19.xii.1684.
(80) Ibid., 14.xii.1693.
(81) Ibid., 6.xii.1694.
(82) Ibid., 14.ix.1695.
(83) Ibid., 21.ix.1695.

Chapter VIII

OF THE FELLOWSHIP: 1682–1858—
RELATING MAINLY TO DOMESTIC ISSUES

You are a subtle nation, you physicians.

Ben Jonson

. . . give place to the physician for the Lord hath created him; let him not go from thee, for thou hast need of him. There is a time when in their hands there is good success.

Ecclesiasticus, xxxviii, 12, 13

The heading has been deliberately chosen. If there is one feature which pervades the spirit of the College today it is the atmosphere of Fellowship—impossible of definition but none the less constantly present. Fellows who have spent their professional lives in Edinburgh may not be fully alive to this, taking the apparently inevitable for granted. Those who, in exile, regularly return to the College, cannot but be acutely conscious of it. Participating in this Fellowship is the outstanding privilege of being a Fellow. The privilege is the greater when account is taken of its evolution over the centuries—an evolution admittedly punctuated from time to time by fierce disagreement and violent controversy, but none the worse for that.

The first Fellows of the Royal College of Physicians were those whose names appear in the original patent (Chap. III). They numbered twenty-one. As already mentioned (Chap. VII) the first to be admitted under the terms of the Charter as a Colleague and Fellow was Dr Kello on 5th February 1683.[1] A second Fellow (Dr Abernethy) was admitted in December of the following year. Records including Minutes are missing for the inclusive period 22nd December 1684 to 21st March 1693 but details concerning subsequent sederunts indicate that five additional Fellows were admitted during those years. An early Law determined that a Socius and ordinary member was one 'who is duly graduate examined and approved off by ye colledge is a residenter in Edgr and payd ye whole deus'[2] and, 'ys is ye law for ane ordinary socius to dinstinguish him from ane extraordinary or honorary socius'.[3]

QUORUM

The first sederunt of the College was held on 18th January 1682 being attended by twelve of the twenty-one Fellows of that time. For a number of years, views as to what constituted a practicable rather than a desirable quorum varied. In 1693 the quorum was reduced from a previous ten to six but at the same time it was stipulated that 'the whole members are to be dewly advertised to attend each meeting appoynted if they be in Toun, and this restricted Quorum to make no Law till what is proposed for a new Law be heard in thrie severall meetings'. The need for restriction was attributed to 'the death of some and absence of severalls of the members . . . liveing at a Distance . . .'.[4] Two and a half years later the College reverted to the old Law 'ordaining ye sederunt to consist of ten members and ye president . . .'[5] only to decide within another three months that 'eight and the president are a sufficient quor- to doe everything competent . . .'.[6] Still not satisfied, yet another decision was arrived at in the same year to the effect that 'considering that many of the members are frequently absent wherby the meetings are often frustrat . . . sex and the president be a sufficient Quorum . . .'.[7] Vacillations continued—the number was reduced to five in 1701 'considering that the full quor cannot be gote to meet . . .': and raised to nine again in 1704 as 'the former Quorum . . . was made up of too ffew . . .'.[8, 9]

Results were not as desired. Not for the first time there was no quorum in May 1717 and it is recorded that the President (Dr William Stewart) is to 'get the Colledge to have there meetings more full and Expecially the quarterly meetings Compleat at Least to a full Quorum. Otherwayes those that shall be absent (without a Lawll. Excuse . . .) to be unLawed in a greater Mulct than contained in the former acts . . .'[10] There was need for a further appeal some ten years later when, there having been no quorum at a Quarterly Meeting, the President commented that 'notwithstanding of the former Acts made annent the due attendance of the quarterly meetings and the sick poor Yet severall of the members . . . were Negligent in attending . . .'. Continuing, he moved that 'ane former act . . . made anent fyning of absent members might be putt in Execution for the future . . .'. At this point in the Minutes there is the delightfully rich marginal annotation—'Fynes paid for absence for bygones and to be exacted in time coming' indicative of both retrospective and prospective action. As an indication of the ruthlessness of the Act once adopted, the President was fined for absence despite having been in the country for health reasons and despite having ensured the attendance as deputy of 'the pro-preses' ![11]

FINES

As a disciplinary weapon, fines acquired increasing favour if not popularity. A relatively early Intrant who had been deemed worthy of a licence was 'amerceit . . . in ane Rex Dollar . . . for being absent from this meeting and not sending his Discourse in wryte . . .'.[12] Whereas that default related to an individual, corporate failings were not lacking. Thus it is recorded in 1706 'The Colledge taking into consideratione how much it is for the honor reputatione and advantage of the Societie, That the members attend the meetings either for the sick poor or other business Does Recommend to all a Due attendance . . . and Sieing ther are four quarterly meetings appoynted . . . more particularly designed for the managdement of the affairs of the Society Thairfor the College Doth enact . . . that each member Doe attend the quarterly meetings and the sick poore under the penalty of ffourty Shillings Scots toties quoties . . .'. Provision was made for a 'relevant excuse' but a fine of seven shillings Scots toties quoties was the fate of any member arriving late by more than half an hour.[13] Socii over 60 years of age were exempt from fines for non-attendance at Quarterly Meetings.[14]

For a time those failing to abide by the regulations relating to 'Discourses or Speeches' were liable to even greater penalties. 'The Colledge taking into their Consideratne the decencie and usefulness of the members of their punctuall observeing the dayes appoynted . . . Do Statut . . . That such members as shall be appoynted . . . to have such Discourses or Speeches shall punctually observe the tyme . . . under the penalty of thrie punds Scots for every such omissione . . .'. Provision was made for a discourse to be read by any of the Socii were the author necessarily absent.[15] Surprisingly there was something of a *volte face* in 1714. In that year it was adjudged that 'the restricting of the said fynes would be a better means for the Due attendance . . . than if continued . . .', but at the same time it was recommended that the record book be 'Inspected and read every Quarterly Meeting'.[16] Subsequently it was determined that only indisposition was an acceptable reason for absence from Quarterly Meetings[17] to which some fifty years later was added 'being furth of Scotland'.[18] All was not ruthlessness, however, because there is a note recording the College's readiness to accede to a petition of a Fellow that regular attendance be not insisted upon because of his 'Valetudinary state of health'.[19] In due course and in truly democratic spirit, a member of Council proposed that the policy of fines should be extended to those of the Council who were guilty of absence or tardy appearance at Ordinary and Extraordinary Meetings of the Conncil.[20]

Late arrivals continued to be a persistent source of irritation, and explained a decision that 'every member who shall hereafter Come a quarter of ane hour after three o'Clock to be Regulat by the watch of the President for the time Shall forfeit a fine of Sixpence, and whoever shall Come in half ane hour after three o'clock Shall forfeit one shilling . . .'.[21] Premature departure from meetings was regarded with almost equal disfavour. In the absence of leave from the chair the fine was one shilling[22, 23] which went the supposed way of all fines to the Tavern Fund. The expense of Tavern bills was a recurrent subject of comment on the score of delayed and inadequate payment. To meet the situation and defray the expense of Suppers an annual levy was proposed.[24] A victim of the situation was the Treasurer (Dr John Boswell) who was sadly out of pocket until matters were righted by enforcing an allowance for entertainments from money paid by new Fellows.[25] With the passage of years the sophistication which accompanies progress required that the more elegant term 'Entertainment Fund' be used in preference to 'Tavern Bills'!

As today, hours of meeting have a bearing on attendance. These were changed from 4 p.m. to 5 p.m. in 1778[26] and from 5 p.m. to 3 p.m. 'exactly' 13 years later.[27] In 1848 there appeared a surprising Minute of great precision—Meetings of the College should be held by Greenwich time'.[28]

Were all fines paid? A Committee appointed to examine a late Treasurer's accounts observed 'two members only have paid fines during the course of last year . . . although there were certainly more fines incurred . . .', and begged leave 'to propose, that the List of fines shall be called over at the beginning of every meeting and the money immediately paid to the President who shall also call for the fines from all those that are sero, as soon as they enter the Room . . . .'.[29] That was in 1795—rather recent for invidious comparison with 1981!

Not until 1896 did Council agree 'to accept a general statement of such . . . infirmity from age . . . as a sufficient reason for remitting fines which may be incurred through absence from College Meetings'.[30]

CONCESSIONS

Contrasting with their policy of fines was the preparedness of the College to grant concessions in special circumstances. Examples are the giving of a monetary gift to the widow of a past President[31]; and an annuity to the grand-daughter of another past President.[32] The widow of another Fellow asked that her deceased husband's 'bond of ffour hundred merks' be returned to her . . . 'in regaird her circumstances were such that she could not pay it . . .'.[33] Again unanimously, the College 'aggried to that dureing her lyftime she shall not be troubled either for prinle or interest of the said bond . . .', agreement being granted on Christmas Day.[34] Again unanimously, a monetary gift was given to a Fellow of forty-two years' standing who in his day was a notably active participant in College affairs. The gift was given 'to free him from his present embarrasments'.[35] Very occasionally a disturbing situation arose when unexpected death prevented a Fellow whose fees had been paid, from taking his seat. Policy in these circumstances was somewhat at variance. After discussion in sederunt, the money involved was returned to the deceased's family in one case but not in another.[36, 37] On another occasion a grant was given to the destitute widow of a late 'officer' (servitor).[38]

An appeal of an exceptional kind was received by the Treasurer (Dr James Hay) in February 1775. It was submitted by Mary Mead, a niece of Dr Richard Mead of London, on behalf of herself and her two children.[39] The College authorized the Treasurer to pay a sum of five pounds.[40] Dr Mead had been an Honorary Fellow of our College in his lifetime and, according to Boswell, his success as a London physician prompted Johnson to remark that 'Dr. Mead lived more in the broad sunshine of life than almost any man'.[41]

DOMESTIC FINANCE

It is natural to pass from fines to finance. To say that is not to suggest that the College was primarily concerned with mercenary matters. On the contrary the history of the College is one of constant pursuit of the socio-medical objectives declared in the petitions for incorporation, and of generosity in terms of professional skill and monetary beneficence against a background of hazardously limited resources. Mention of major hazards is made elsewhere in various chapters. Over and above these there were relatively minor problems of finance reflecting the growing pains of a newly born administratively inexperienced corporation.

The state of the general finances was subject to great variation. Thus early in the life of the College quarterly collections were made for defraying expenses[42]; and in the College Regulations of 1789 there appeared—'The expence of the supper usually given to the College by a Resident Fellow on his admission shall be limited to £5, 5s.

If the expence exceed this the additional charge shall be defrayed from the same fund as other suppers of the College.'[43] Early in the next century (1804), because expenditure had very considerably exceeded income over a number of years a Committee was appointed to investigate.[44] Retrenchment must have produced results because in a little over a decade the Treasurer described 'the present situation of the Funds . . . to be in a flourishing state'.[45] Within a few years it was recorded that 'the Council had taken into consideration in what manner the sense of the College could best be expressed . . . of its marked appreciation of his [the Treasurer's] conduct in various situations, but particularly in the zealous discharge . . . as treasurer for the last twenty five years'. The upshot was his acceptance of a sum of money, large even by present day standards 'for a piece of Plate, or to be disposed of by him in any other manner he should think proper'.[46]

Euphoria was not to last long. Within ten years the 'low state of the finances' prompted an unsuccessful proposal that each member should pay two guineas annually to make possible the purchase of more books.[47] Then metaphorically and literally came a tightening of belts. In 1835 it was decreed that there should be 'no College Dinner in May next nor Breakfast previous to the Election Meeting in December next, with the view of leaving an additional Sum, for the purchase of Books . . .'.[48] Furthermore the College steeled itself to renew the interdict the following year.[49] A Minute for November 1838 suggests that restrictions were relaxed because 'it was agreed that the College should give a Breakfast biennially on the Saturday after the Election day to which the President of the College of Surgeons and his Council should be invited'.[50]

Then, however, came a warning from the Finance Committee of the imminence of a possible crisis situation. Expenditure over a number of years had greatly exceeded income and there had been encroachment on capital. Basically the situation had arisen as a result of reduced income consequent upon a decline in the number of entrants. Recommendations submitted included the sale of Bank Stock, the discontinuation of Newspapers, withdrawal of contributions to public charities and appreciable limitation of Library expenses. There was general approval of the recommendations but not of a desire expressed by the Finance Committee 'that the Fellows will for this year at least be prepared to forego the pleasure attendant on the annual dinner and to allow the amount received for contributions and fines . . . to go towards the current expences of the College'. Stoicism would appear to have waned since 1835.[51]

The eighteenth century brought a new nightmare, but as later generations have come to learn, only the beginnings of one. In May 1799 in anticipation that 'some requisition would probably be made by Government', the President and Treasurer were appointed as a 'Committee to attend to the Interest of the College in that matter'.[52] Apprehensions were more than justified. Six years later to the day, the College was informed by the Treasurer that 'a considerable demand had . . . been made upon the College for Property and Income Tax which he considered as considerably overcharged'.[53] Reporting in 1808, he referred to a heavy demand for Property Tax and to his efforts to get 'the proper deduction . . . in regard to the Income of the College'. Then as now, 'various communings had taken place' and in this instance a tolerable compromise was reached.[54] Forty years later the outcome was different. Reporting success in his claim for exemption from Assessed and Local Taxes,[55] the Treasurer had to announce within five months that an appeal by the local taxation authority had resulted in the Justices of the Peace making an award against the College.[56] Events had a ring familiar to twentieth-century descendants! Over 100 years were to elapse before the College was granted Charitable Status by the Inland Revenue Authorities. This followed an application made by the College after a ruling in the House of Lords in the Bland-Sutton Will dispute that the Royal College of Surgeons of England was a Charity.[57]

Previously, at the turn of the century, the College had reason to learn how wide the Department of Inland Revenue casts its net. An application to obtain duty free spirits for 'chemical analysis research and the preparation of microscopic specimens' was subjected to close scrutiny. Eventually authority was obtained 'to receive Duty-free spirits to an extent not exceeding 20 bulk gallons annually'.[58]

To add to his worries the Treasurer had to cope with the problem of overdue bills and dishonoured bonds. Elsewhere (Chap. V) mention has been made of difficulties experienced in collecting rent due for tenancy of the cold bath-house. On occasion Fellows were unco-operative in response to demands for overdue subscriptions,[59] but in pleasing contrast the Treasurer was able on one occasion to report that he 'had Received from the Lord President of the Session ffour hundred Merks for his Brother . . . Deceased who had not paid any dues to the Colledge as a fellow of it . . .'.[60] It was customary for a proportion of Members to deposit bonds when unable immediately to pay their entry fees and these bonds 'often occasioned trouble and were sometimes unproductive or relinquished'.[61] One example will suffice. It concerned an account of a bond 'granted . . . of ffour hundreth merks . . . the debt being ill to resolve and almost Desperat . . . has trans-acted the samen for tuo hundreth merks'.[62] The extent to which the College was prepared to assert itself is illustrated by the case of a Fellow 'suspended from siting and voting in the colledge ay and while he satisfie ye colledge for his contumacious refusing to pay ye money due by him to ye colledge . . .'.[63]

Of defaulters the most celebrated were probably two whose names appear in the List of Fellows in the Original Patent. Sibbald in his *Autobiography* referred to them specifically by name when describing events in connection with the affixation of the seal to the Charter of 1681. He wrote 'it cost a great deal of money to defray the charges of the plea, and for getting it signed at court, and sealed here. Wee payed considerably each of us, except Dr. Hay, who would not contribute one farthing, though his name be the first insert in the patent. Dr. Brisban payed nothing either, and so they were declared by the Colledge to be onlie honorarie members.'[64] According to the Minutes they were to remain 'honorary' until they 'apply and pay ye dews' which they never appear to have done.[65]

'Honorary' maybe, but in the most strict, literal and deservedly critical sense.

Difficulties with Stamp Duties in connection with Licentiates and Fellows have been mentioned (Chap. VII). In 1812 enquiries were made as to the extent to which such Duty applied to Honorary Fellows only to be informed that there could be no exemption for Honorary Fellows whether *ex officio* or not.[66] The matter was taken up again, this time with the Chancellor of the Exchequer, the point being made that the attitude of the Stamp Office prevented the College from conferring the Honorary Fellowship.[67] The answer received would have done for any subsequent decade or century—a promise in the meantime to look into the matter, 'altho' he [the writer] is of course unable to express any opinion . . . at present'.[68]

Impartiality requires admission that events of the utmost rarity would seem to cast doubt upon the technical efficiency or maybe even absolute integrity of one Treasurer at least. Uncertainty on the part of the College constrained them on one occasion to order that 'The Clerk and Officer get a List of the Tennents names . . . with ane accompt of their yearly payable rents . . . as also they ordain the Clerk to draw ane List out of the Book of any Dors that has been entered Licentiate or made Socius Dureing the tyme that Dr. . . . was Thessrer yrto in order to make a Charge against him either for what money he had received belonging to the Colledge or bonds or precepts granted for the samen . . .'.[69] At this time in history it is the principle, not the names of those concerned, which is of significance. The same subject is touched on in the *Report on Examination of Medical Practitioners* when, referring indirectly to the collegiate dispute associated with the name of Stevensone and others (Chap. XIX), it circumspectly recorded 'Very probably, a dispute which long agitated the College, was connected with something having the aspect of irregularity or remissness on the part of the Treasurer at this time'.[61]

A curious sequence of events occurred in 1731. At a time when Bonds were due for payment, £100 was borrowed from a Fellow who was made Treasurer at the next election.[70]

PROCEDURES

Throughout the life of the College, Committees responsible to Council have formed an essential part of the procedural framework. To enumerate them would be as pointless as it would be impossible. Nevertheless what can only be described as a whirlwind onset by one President (Dr Andrew Duncan, sen.) deserves recording. Elected in accordance with custom around St Andrew's Day, within two months he 'represented that he was desirous to have proper Committees appointed for consideration of various subjects of a public nature . . .': and there and then appointed four Committees for the Lunatic Asylums; Inoculation; Vapour-Baths; and Cold Bathing—and these additional to standing and other special Committees.[71]

With the number of new enactments passed at successive Quarterly Meetings, revision of the Laws and Regulations was necessary at fairly frequent intervals. Revision was an occasion for the confrontation of opposed views and could tax the Chairman's tact to the limits. The following motion of Council bears this out. 'The College taking into consideration the concern which the President has had in the late revisal of the Laws, and the great trouble and attention he has bestowed on this, are of opinion, however different the sentiments of the different members may be upon that subject, that he has acted from the purest motives, and in the most honourable manner . . .'.[72]

In 1771 it was decided that admission of a Fellow should be 'by Ballot in place of voteing as formerly'. At the same time it was decreed that 'no member shall Engage himself to the Candidate before the time of Balloting nor thereafter Reveal to any person in what manner he had Balloted, under the penalty of being held as one who has Broke his honour and faith to the College'.[73] Previously it had been decided that proposals for admission of a Fellow should lie on the table until the next Quarterly Meeting,[74] and that no person residing and licensed to practise medicine in Edinburgh could be admitted a Fellow 'Sooner than one full year after the day he has obtained his Licence . . .'.[75] The probationary period was extended from one to three years in 1896.[76] In the 1805 edition of 'Charter and Regulations' the word 'Members' was amended for the first time to 'Fellows'[77]: and indiscriminate use of the term Member gave rise to a resolution, unanimously accepted, that 'the term . . . be applied to Fellows exclusively'.[78] There is in the College Library a copy of the

Regulations for 1789, and in it the Promissory Engagement has deleted from it in heavy red crayon the last words 'and a good Christian'. The deletion has remained in all subsequent editions, the Promissory Engagement finishing 'as I desire to be holden and reputed an honest man'.[79]

The College did not differ from other Societies in showing obeisance to precedence. In 1758 it was laid down that members were to be called in the Roll according to the dates of their admission as Fellows,[80] and in 1789 that the senior Licentiate in the event of two or more Licentiates being moved for admission 'shall be always first balloted'.[81]

HONORARY FELLOWSHIP

Honorary Fellowship was first conferred in 1696. Except in so far as there are no recorded facts during the period of lost Minutes, it is known that between 1696 and 1809 there were 52 recipients of whom 17 were laymen and 35 doctors. Of the doctors at least 16 possessed continental degrees, many being of foreign nationality. Edward Jenner was made an Honorary Fellow in 1806 and on being informed wrote to the President on 31st July as follows:

> 'Gentlemen
> I beg leave to return my sincerest acknowledgements for the high honor you have conferred upon me by presenting me with your Diploma.
> The benefits which the Vaccine Inoculation has diffused among mankind, have induced many public Societies to grant me marks of distinction, all which I value most highly; not only because they are grateful to my own feelings, but because they materially contribute, by the sanction attached to them, to extend more widely the practice I had the happiness to announce to the world.
> Highly as I prize every honor which I receive, yet I will acknowledge that yours was more than ordinarily gratifying, both on account of its rarity and of the high reputation which your College enjoys of never acting from sentiments of favor and unmerited partiality.
> I have the honor to be, Gentlemen, with profound respect your ever obliged and very faithful humble Servant.
> (Signed) Edwd. Jenner'[82]

In a recent article *Three Scots in the Service of the Czars* Dr J. B. Wilson, F.R.C.P. described the accomplishments of two Honorary Fellows—Dr James Mounsey and Dr John Rogerson.[83] Although not a Fellow of the College the third doctor mentioned, Sir James Wylie, arranged at the age of 83 years for the College to be

G

informed of the thirteen decorations awarded him by various Royal Households during his active lifetime. Wylie, retired in St Petersburg, thought that the College would be interested.[84]

One or two letters were received from persons abroad applying to become Honorary Members, which by way of reply were told that the College 'never yet assumed any Honourary member upon Petition But of their own proper motion.' There was even more convincing evidence of the College's concern that the privileges of honorary association should be jealously guarded in a Minute of 1773. At the same time as determining that the number of Honorary Fellows should not exceed ten, it added 'three of whom only to be admitted on accot. of their rank and fortune &c. and seven on account of literary merit'.

Another needlessly perplexing situation arose from the fact that by the terms of the College Charter, University Professors of Medicine were entitled to demand admission as Honorary Fellows 'upon a proper application'. Accepting the legally irrevocable position, the College determined that 'in any lists or rolls . . . the persons so to be admitted shall be distinguished by some proper mark . . .'. The mark adopted was an asterisk, but to distinguish from whom? In a way capable of more than one interpretation the act explained—'from the honorary members admitted by voluntary act of the College' ![87]

After 1809 no more Honorary Fellowships were conferred until 1919, in which year H.R.H. The Prince of Wales was admitted as an Honorary Fellow under regulations previously determined by an enactment dated 1904.

BIZARRE ENQUIRIES

Considered in the context of major administrative policy these may seem rather trivial aspects of the College's work. Nevertheless, account must be taken of difficulties in the past related to existing forms of communication and transport and of distances involved. Distractions were many, and on occasion irrelevant. There were the diplomatic challenge successfully met of dealing with a Surgeon-neighbour's request to take down a wall of old College property[88]; the necessity, in the light of past experience, for the proper recording of Minutes and keeping of all College papers[89]; and the summoning of Fellows to serve on a jury 'albeit by the College Charter . . . members of the College are Expressly Exeemd from attending any juries . . .'.[90] Many years later, a Fellow appointed by the College to be one of the managers of the Charity Work House announced that he had been served with a

Summons at the instance of the Royal Bank of Scotland. The Summonses were against the Treasurer and Managers, and were served on the managers jointly and severally as individuals. 'Quite preposterous' was the unfortunate Fellow's masterly understatement.[91]

A number of approaches, some of which seem bizarre in the circumstances of today, were made to the College for an opinion. In 1708 a minister of the Gospel sought encouragement 'for his endeavors in finding out severall new mechanicall Inventiones as pleases' and members were recommended to give 'incouradgement in what manner they thought proper . . .'.[92] Two gentlemen sought 'the Approbation of the Colledge about the new method of their Cureing Ruptures . . .'[93] and after an interval of five months the President did 'Signe And Recomendation In favours' of the applicants. The Recommendation was based on personal observations made by Fellows of the College and on information derived from other sources.[94] In 1744 it was minuted that a notorious John Taylor 'who designs himself Doctor of Physick and oculist to his majesty, has Inserted in the news papers . . . advertisements Stuffed with gross injurious falsehoods . . .'. The College countered with a Declaration in the newspapers which concluded with the words that 'as he is to Leave this place very Soon, Wee have no other view in publishing this declaration Than to prevent unwary people in oyr places . . . from being Imposed on . . .'.[95] That was in July. Four months later there arrived 'a Treatise on the diseases of the eye by Dr. Taylor oculist dedicat to the Colledge, and which was Sent by him . . . as a present to the Colledge'.[96] There is no mention of acknowledgement by the Colledge! The College of Surgeons was no less agitated by Taylor's presence in the City and protested volubly but ineffectively at the presentation to him of a Burgess Ticket by the Town Council. Whether the sister college was gifted by Taylor with a copy of his publication is not known![97]

Then there was an occurrence with an almost Pandoric aura. It was decided to open three boxes 'which have long been in the possession of the College'.[98] Findings were no more gruesome than specimens of Lead Ore, Marbles, Fossils, Shells, Corals and the like.[99] Something akin to bio-engineering in elementary form came to the fore in 1807 with the receipt by the College of 'a Deliniation and description of a Machine for conveying sick or wounded persons . . .'. After inspection of the machine a Committee of the College approved of it 'as an easy ingenious and inexpensive conveyance' for its intended purpose.[100] Later in the century a practitioner offered to lay before the College 'certain views on the nature of the Inflammation . . .'. His suggestion that a series of evening meetings might be arranged met with difficulties, and a Committee was appointed to consider alternatives.[101] There is no mention of the outcome, possibly because at the time the College was deeply involved searching for a new hall. As a last instance of the diverse situations requiring to be dealt with there was the case of a self-styled Lecturer on Political Economy who laid claim in an advertisement to being a Fellow of the College. Enquiries confirmed that in fact he was a non-resident Fellow. The College accepted the advice of Council to let the matter drop 'believing that any notice taken . . . would only injuriously force it upon public attention'. Before tendering their advice, however, Council did put to the sederunt 'That if the associating the name of the College with the proposed Lectures be very offensive to Members' it might be a question whether the College should encourage his voluntarily surrendering his right to designate himself, Fellow.[102, 103]

PUBLICATIONS

Early in the history of the College consideration was given to control of publications linked with its name. The question was first raised in 1694 when it was decided publications should be subject to approval by the College at several fully attended meetings and subject to two-thirds of those present not dissenting.[104, 105] A number of years later a Committee was appointed to meet a Fellow 'to inspect a Specimen of the work he Intends to publish . . .'. Somewhat astonishingly entitled 'A full view of the publict transactions in the Reigne of Queen Elizabeth &c', it earned the Committee's unqualified approval as 'one of ye most Curious and usefull performances', and as 'equally instructing and Entertaining'.[106] Appreciation was confirmed by the College who 'did unanimously agree that so Great Application Accuracy and Skill in Compileing So Noble and Valuable a work, deserve all Suitable and Generous Encouragement'.[107]

An allied subject brought to the notice of the College was the possibility of publishing a volume of medical essays and observations. The project was first proposed in a letter from Mr William Monro, an Edinburgh bookseller who expressed the hope that Fellows would 'patronize the work and each . . . Contribute to the promoteing of it'. One who expressed his 'decided disapprobation' was a past President, Dr James Hamilton Junior. In a letter dated 10th January 1826 he stated in trenchant terms that previously men of eminence had not considered the publication of transactions expedient; the number of Periodical Journals was already more than sufficient; and the London College had 'by no means added to' its respectability by publishing transactions. Some of Hamilton's views may have been reactionary at the time, but could be applied with reason now.[108] This did not dissuade the College who

'Resolved to Contribute all they Can to the promoteing So good a designe and undertakeing'.[(109)]

Behind Mr Monro's initiative was a recently formed Society of medical practitioners (the *Edinburgh Society for the Improvement of Medical Knowledge*—founded in 1731) anxious to encourage the publication of medical and surgical papers. Active participants included the University professors Monro *primus*, Charles Alston, James Crauford, James Innes, Andrew Plummer, John Rutherford, William Porterfield and Andrew St Clair; and the following additional Fellows of the Royal College— Drs John Drummond, sen., Francis Pringle, John Clerk, Robert Louis, William Cochran, John Learmont and James Dundas. The surgeon Mr John Macgill was also a member of the Society of which Monro was the first Secretary.[(110)] The first volume of the Society was published in 1733 and entitled *Medical Essays and Observations, revised and published by a Society in Edinburgh*.[(111)] Further volumes consisted of one each in 1734, 1735 and 1737. Volume V is in two parts; part one being dated 1742 and part two 1744. The various volumes went through several editions including French, German and Dutch versions.[(112)] Contributors were from all parts of Scotland, from England north and south and even from Ireland and the Continent.

Monro *primus* made several contributions of which one in particular was of importance. This was 'An Essay on the Nutrition of the Foetus' which was published in three parts. Nor according to Wright-St Clair was this Monro's first excursion into the perinatal field to be explored by another Fellow of the College, J. W. Ballantyne, more than a century and a half later. There is in the Library of the University of Otago a student notebook of Monro in which the first entry made in 1717 is a full translation of Bellinger's *Tractatus de Foetus nutritu*. The translation was made while Monro was studying in London.[(113)]

Duncan in his *Memorials* of the Glasgow Faculty commenting on the first appearance of the *Glasgow Medical Journal* in 1828 says appreciatively that 'the medical periodical press of Edinburgh, and occasionally of London—the *Medical and Philosophical Commentaries*, *Medical Essays and Observations*, *The Edinburgh Medical and Surgical Journal* and the *Lancet*—afforded outlets to the intellectual activities of a few Glasgow men, such as John Paisley, James Calder, Robert Watt, John Burns, and others'.[(114)]

Amidst a galaxy of authors, Fellows of the Royal College figure in all the volumes, but their contributions have been criticized as failing to give all credit due to previous pioneer efforts of the College. To subscribe to this view is to ignore the catholicity shewn in the acceptance of papers. Taking full account of the conditions prevailing at the time of publication the *Medical Essays* are intriguing; and in particular, the reviews of Recent Progress under 'Observations' are entrancing. There can be no question that the five volumes of *Medical Essays and Observations* contributed to the international reputation of Edinburgh Medicine. Linnaeus described them as 'for physicians the most excellent proceedings of all the Learned Societies'. The first volume was dedicated to the President of the Royal Society, Sir Hans Sloane, and the Essays as a whole have been described as 'the first *periodical* publications dedicated to a defined and restricted branch of natural knowledge'.[115]

Eventually about 1737 the Society underwent a fundamental change and became the Society for improving Arts and Science, and particularly Natural Knowledge. The subsequent history of this new Society, which later assumed the name of the Philosophical Society, is dealt with in Chapter XXXIV.

In 1825 a meeting was called by the President (Dr Alexander Monro) to consider 'the propriety of the College publishing Transactions in the same manner as the Colleges of London, Dublin and Paris'.[116] The proposal obviously provoked considerable discussion at each of three Extraordinary Meetings and it was only at the following Quarterly Meeting a majority vote decided 'That it is expedient that the Royal College should publish a Volume of Transactions as soon as a sufficient number of papers which may appear of such importance as to deserve publication shall have been collected'.[117] Later, regulations were approved. Papers submitted were to be read at a monthly meeting arranged for the purpose, and decisions as to suitability for publication were to rest with the result of a ballot by one of several Committees. There were four Committees, one for each of the following—Practical Medicine and Pathology; Chemistry and Pharmacy; Materia Medica and Botany; and Midwifery.[118]

A very different problem presented in 1829 with the appearance in the *Caledonian Mercury* of an advertisement 'intituled "Royal College of Physicians" . . . inserted most improperly without the knowledge or Sanction of the College'.[119] The Minutes did not give any precise indication of the contents of the advertisement but did have 'engrossed' in them unanimously approved 'Resolutions by the Royal College of Physicians'. Copies of the Resolutions were sent to the *Courant* and *Mercury* Papers for insertion: and to the Secretary of State for the Home Department, the Lord Advocate for Scotland, and the late Chairman of the Committee of the House of Commons on Anatomical Instruction. Simultaneously the Editor of the *Caledonian Mercury* was directed to insert a paragraph clearly indicating that the College disclaimed responsibility for the insertion of the advertisement. The Resolutions deplored the recent disclosure of crimes; declared belief in the necessity for anatomical instruction while allowing that evils did exist in connection with the teaching of anatomy: and urged, at the same time as expressing readiness to co-operate, the need for new legislation. Whatever the exact terms of the original advertisement, the contents and date (7th January 1829) of the Resolutions point to some relationship, however indirect, to circumstances surrounding the Burke and Hare trial in December 1828.[120]

The advertisement appeared on 5th January and the College first heard of it at an Extra-Ordinary Meeting called in response to a requisition addressed to the President (Sir Alexander Morison) by several members and dated 2nd January 1829. The requisition asked for consideration of 'any measures . . . with a view to tranquillize the public mind on the subject of the late atrocities committed by Burke and his Associates, to prevent their repetition, and to relieve the Medical profession generally from the odium justly excited by them'.[121]

Decision to initiate the *College Publication Series* was not arrived at until 1954.[122]

CLINICAL FIELD STUDIES

Initiative, investigation and publication were not, it must be made clear, confined to 'Resident Fellows' on the Roll of the College. To read Samuel Smiles on this subject is salutary. Writing of his apprenticeship with a Fellow, Dr Lewins of Haddington, he said 'I once witnessed the doctor in the throes of literary composition. It was a tremendous business. We went into a back bedroom in the furthest corner of the house, so as not to be disturbed by the noises in the kitchen. The doctor dressed himself in his long, hanging shawl-gown; strode about the floor, and dictated. The product was an article on Infantile Remittent Fever . . . It was full of rather long words such as "intromittent" "exacerbations"; and so on.'[123]

That was in the early 1800s. Trials and tribulations in these circumstances have not altered greatly with the years! However, the article referred to by Smiles eventually appeared in the *Edinburgh Medical and Surgical Journal*.[124]

DISCOURSES AND ASSEMBLIES

Historically the subject of discourses and publications extends back to pre-Charter days when Sibbald met with colleagues in his lodgings. Having outlined 'the matters we discoursed upon' Sibbald went on to say 'Severall of the discourses are inserted in a book I call Acta Medica Edinburgensia. They were forborne then upon the introducing of such conferences once a moneth in the Colledge.'[125] The first of the discourses delivered under the aegis of the newly erected College was on 7th January 1684 and was undertaken by Sir Archibald Stevensone. Ten more took place between then and the time for which no Minutes now exist.[126-135] There is doubt about a twelfth which on 3rd November 1684 a Dr Halyburtoune was appointed to give. Although he chose the subject of his discourse there is no record of his having delivered it, or for that matter of his having attended at another sederunt.

When available Minutes resume: first mention of discourses occurred on 9th November 1693 when regulations were drawn up for 'The ffirst Thursday of every moneth . . . in place of the first Munday formerly appoynted for their meeting, and that . . . one of the Members according to there seniority have ane discourse either upon ane aphorisme of Hippocrates or any other point of Medicine of his own Choise . . .'.[136, 137] Results must have been rewarding because within two months it was decided that 'furder tryall should be Imposed on Intrants' in the form of a discourse![138] In July of 1694 it was decided to discontinue discourses 'the tyme of the vaciance'[139] but as events turned out they were not resumed until 5th February 1697 when one was given by Sibbald.[140] He gave another eight years later and the tragedy is that it is not available for the purposes of this History, having had as subject 'ane historicall account of such Doctors of Medicine as were Scotsmen and particl. of those that practised in Scotland and what they had written in Physick, or philosophie.'[141]

In later years the question of meetings for Fellows cropped up sporadically in sederunts; in some respects the various proposals considered were confusing and it is not altogether clear that they all had furtherance of the same object in mind. What is significant is the irrepressible if not vociferous desire for meetings of some kind. Thus in 1705 a proposal for weekly Monday afternoon meetings 'To conferr about Medicine and other parts of Learning' was 'relished . . . very well'.[142] Then followed the institution of fines for malattendance at discourses. An abrupt Minute in 1708 referred to orders that every Wednesday afternoon be reserved 'for Conferrences'.[143] In passing it should be mentioned that alone among original Fellows, Archibald Pitcairne persistently failed to give effect to repeated instructions to deliver a discourse. On each occasion he incurred the penalty of fine but whether with equanimity on the part of that petulantly turbulent man the Minutes do not disclose. Discourses ceased to be held at some time between 1710 and 1712. As Ritchie pointed out, weekly and other conferences were distinct from the discourses at sederunts and, not being recorded in the Minutes, it is not known how long they continued.[144]

Many years later a Fellow of undisguised zeal moved that one evening each month should be reserved for an assembly of members to converse and communicate 'information on all matters relative to Medicine and General Science'. Attendance was to be optional. Tavern traditions being discarded 'the refreshment of Tea' was to be introduced.[145] Apparently the proposal received somewhat timorous support at first. Within the ranks of the College however there was one possessed of caution worthy of a Treasury Official. He urged that a list of those interested should be made, and unless they did not amount to a simple majority of the Fellows the expense involved was not warranted: and that 'at least one officer or functionary' should attend for the purpose of making records.[146] Things appear to have lain dormant until, with possible tactical subtlety the mover of the original motion proposed that 'the Hall of the College is not maintained for general accommodation; and that without the regular sanction of the College no other meetings whatever be held therein'. He failed to get a seconder.[147] Undaunted he returned to his initial proposal a year later but the College took the line that until a majority favoured evening meetings 'no part of the funds of the College should be applied to that purpose'.[148] That was in 1835. In 1838 this admirably irrepressible Fellow was again to the fore, making 'some observations as to having evening meetings' with as sole result 'the College . . . again directed the wishes of the Fellows to be ascertained by circulating a paper . . . for the signature of those . . . in favor . . .'.[149] And there the account ended. Perhaps as can happen, inconvenient questionnaires went astray. No matter, the pertinacity of the member in question epitomizes a spirit the College should always welcome in its midst.

But there was not a total lack of progress in this sphere. Within a few years it was suggested that evening meetings with tea should give way to Lectures followed by 'Tea and Coffee'. The proposals emanated from the Council and the Lecturers were to be given by individuals 'qualified to undertake the duty' at monthly intervals at '8 o'clock evening'. Invitations were extended to 'the Fellows of the Royal College of Surgeons and a few distinguished Strangers'.[150]

UNLICENSED PRACTICE AND OTHER IRREGULARITIES

On a number of occasions it is recorded that the 'College recommends to the President to speak to such Physitians as are in Toun who have not entered to the College that they come in and enter yrto'.[151] The defector if he can be termed such, proved a problem for many years although in the course of time the number 'pursued by the College' lessened notably, in part due to greater awareness of the Charter rights of the College. The College strove the while to uncover illicit 'general practice' and to exercise care in the admission of members. A case in point, early in the history of the College was lodgement of a protest against a proposed admission as Socius on the grounds that the Intrant had not undergone the requisite three years study of medicine.[152]

Within a few months of being granted a Charter the College dealt with an indidividual peddling 'poysonous tabblets . . . as a Vomitur tablett . . .'[153] and a few months later with 'a pretended chirurgeon . . . hath taken upon him to administrat Physick and use Chirurgery upon some persones . . . To the hazard of their lives . . .'.[154] On one day in May 1683 it was ordered that 'three be persewed for unwarrantable practiseing'[155] and in June of the same year 'John Saar Montebank . . . apprehended together with a Remitt from the Lords of Sessione' was ordered 'to make payment of thriescore punds Scots money for ilk month more than thrie months yt he had practised Medicine without . . . Licence'.[156] Partial acquittal was granted in some instances as in the case of an individual who claimed ignorance of the College jurisdiction and who was allowed 'to continue his practise as formerly . . . haveing payed . . . fourty rex Dollars and promeist to pay his quarter dues as the rest of the Colledge does'.[157]

Events in connection with a Doctor of Divinity who confessed to having practised medicine in Edinburgh 'for a long tyme' had an eventual even more gratifying outcome. When 'enquyered at by the president if he intended still to doe soe without any license from the colledge, He answered he was not weell resolved and could give no positive answer . . .'. He was given one week 'to resolve in'.[158] There is no clear statement of what transpired within seven days. However the College did not miss the opportunity to give practical expression to the virtues of Faith, Hope and Charity. In less than two years it granted a licence to practise to the Divine who in the interval had acquired a Doctorate of Medicine at Harderwick.[159, 160]

Two notable and as it turned out legally costly cases concerned Surgeons—James Nisbet and Martin Eccles (Chap. VII). Nisbet was fined 'Fyve punds Sterling . . . for his haveing undewly and illegally practised medicine . . .'. He having made 'ane submissive acknowledgement Declaratione and promeise . . . to be more Cautious and not to comitt the Lyke in tymecoming' asked for and was granted a remission of his fine and discharge.[161] Another instance of the College's vigilance was illustrated by enquiries conducted into the activities of a Fellow practising in Putney, who had been publicly accused of selling drugs and thereby infringing the Bye-Laws of the College. The Fellow's explanation more than satisfied the College which agreed with his expressed disapproval of the 'General practice system as it commonly prevails in England'; and took the 'opportunity of formally expressing their regret that the state of practice in any part of the Country should still be such as to compel any class of Physicians to keep their own drugs . . .'.[162]

A curious case was dealt with in 1847 involving the 'head of a hydropathic Establishment at Wharfdale' and Fellow of the College. 'Certain certificates in . . . favour had been extensively circulated' and one of them contained 'a notice regarding his admission to the College inconsistent with the Truth'. The doctor in question disavowed being accessory to the publication of the document but this did not prevent the College from roundly condemning him and requiring that he 'give to his disavowal as extensive a circulation as that of the original misstatements . . .'.[163] What eventuated is not recorded; nor is there any exact indication of his misrepresentations. Furthermore his name has been retained in all lists of past Fellows.

In the latter half of the eighteenth century much confusion arose from indeterminacy of policy in the matter of Fellows practising Midwifery and Surgery. The circumstances involved are dealt with in Chapter XIX. New regulations for the examination of foreign graduates were passed defining the conditions permitting dispensation of examination, and outlining a desirable format for examinations.[164, 165]

Homeopathy was a source of much discussion. In 1842 a practitioner known to be an adherent of Homeopathy was not admitted, some members at the sederunt thinking that admission would seem to suggest College 'sanction to the system'.[166] The case concerned a potential Intrant. A different situation arose nine years later when a Fellow of the College openly professed to being a practising homeopathist and through a colleague asked that this be made known to his Edinburgh friends. An immediate outcome was submission to the College by Council of four Resolutions indicating its unqualified unpreparedness to admit a homeopathist to membership; expressing regret at the defection of some members, emphasizing the impossibility of Fellows meeting homeopathists in consultation; and stating to the College reserving the right to disclaim as it may wish or decide defectors amongst its Fellowship. As to the self-confessed, honest miscreant if he can be called such, no arbitrary action was taken against him except in so far as he had sent to him a copy of the Resolutions and a clear indication that he and his like should withdraw from the College.[167] If College action, as distinct from resolve, was chary this could well be explained by awareness of current moves in the matter of medical reform which might bring their own solution to the ethical problem.

Events prompted Dr Alexander Wood to publish a treatise entitled *Homeopathy Unmasked*, which earned for him strongly worded criticism from homeopathists. He responded with a second treatise which was commended by physicians in different parts of the country.[168]

Whatever the muted feelings of the College as a whole, another eminent Fellow (Sir Robert Christison) did not refrain from referring to a particular homeopathist as one 'who treated . . . with drops of nothingness, powder of nonentity, and *extractum nihili*'.[169]

REFERENCES

(1) College Minutes, 5.ii.1683.
(2) Ibid., 1.xi.1695.
(3) Ibid., 4.xi.1695.

QUORUM

(4) Ibid., 15.v.1693.
(5) Ibid., 1.xi.1695.
(6) Ibid., 12.ii.1696.
(7) Ibid., 29.xi.1696.
(8) Ibid., 16.v.1701.
(9) Ibid., 12.i.1704.
(10) Ibid., 7.v.1717.
(11) Ibid., 1.xi.1726.

FINES

(12) Ibid., 4.i.1694.
(13) Ibid., 5.viii.1706.
(14) R.C.P.E. (c. 1850) *Abstracts of the Minutes, AD 1682–1731*. By George Paterson. [Fines.] (Ms.)
(15) College Minutes, 6.v.1707.
(16) Ibid., 28.xi.1714.
(17) Ibid., 7.xi.1727.
(18) Ibid., 2.ii.1768.
(19) Ibid., 6.v.1794.
(20) Ibid., 5.xi.1833.
(21) Ibid., 3.ii.1761.
(22) Ibid., 3.xi.1830.
(23) Ibid., 1.v.1849.
(24) Ibid., 3.v.1785.
(25) Ibid., 7.viii.1798.

(26) Ibid., 4.viii.1778.
(27) Ibid., 1.xi.1791.
(28) Ibid., 1.ii.1848.
(29) Ibid., 4.viii.1795.
(30) R.C.P.E. (1898) *Letter book*, 24.vi.1898.

CONCESSIONS

(31) College Minutes, 7.xi.1727.
(32) Ibid., 4.ii.1777.
(33) Ibid., 25.xii.1696.
(34) Ibid., 5.ii.1697.
(35) Ibid., 18.v.1841.
(36) Ibid., 6.vi.1828.
(37) Ibid., 19.v.1838.
(38) Ibid., 2.viii.1853.
(39) R.C.P.E. (1775) *General Correspondence*, 28.ii.1775.
(40) College Minutes, 20.iii.1775.
(41) BOSWELL, J. (1958) *Life of Johnson*, vol. II, p. 253. London: Dent (Everyman's Library).

DOMESTIC FINANCE

(42) College Minutes, 1.ii.1709.
(43) R.C.P.E. (1789) *Charter and Regulations of the Royal College of Physicians of Edinburgh*, p. 53. Edinburgh: Murray & Cochrane.
(44) College Minutes, 1.v.1804.
(45) Ibid., 6.ii.1816.
(46) Ibid., 2.v.1820.
(47) Ibid., 2.xi.1830.
(48) Ibid., 3.ii.1835.
(49) Ibid., 2.ii.1836.
(50) Ibid., 6.xi.1838.
(51) Ibid., 1.xi.1842.
(52) Ibid., 7.v.1799.
(53) Ibid., 7.v.1805.
(54) Ibid., 3.v.1808.
(55) Ibid., 6.ii.1844.
(56) Ibid., 7.v.1844.
(57) Ibid., 22.vii.1952.
(58) R.C.P.E. (1903) *Letter Book*, 28.i.1903.
(59) College Minutes, 6.viii.1782.
(60) Ibid., 1.xi.1726.

(61) R.C.P.E. (1833) *Report on Examination of Medical Practitioners*, Appendix (B), p. 57. Edinburgh: Neill.
(62) College Minutes, 19.i.1705.
(63) Ibid., 7.viii.1696.
(64) SIBBALD, Sir R. (1833) *The Autobiography*, p. 31. Edinburgh: Thomas Stevenson.
(65) College Minutes, 7.xi.1695.
(66) Ibid., 4.v.1813.
(67) Ibid., 2.viii.1825.
(68) Ibid., 1.xi.1825.
(69) Ibid., 7.ii.1716.
(70) R.C.P.E. (c. 1850) *Abstracts of the Minutes, AD 1682–1731*. By George Paterson. [Financial transactions.] (Ms.)

PROCEDURES

(71) College Minutes, 1.ii.1791.
(72) Ibid., 5.ii.1805.
(73) Ibid., 5.ii.1771.
(74) Ibid., 7.viii.1759.
(75) Ibid., 1.xi.1763.
(76) Ibid., 23.vi.1896.
(77) R.C.P.E. (1805) *Charter and Regulations*, p. 3. [Edinburgh: Royal College of Physicians.]
(78) College Minutes, 5.xi.1822.
(79) R.C.P.E. (1789) *Regulations of the Royal College of Physicians of Edinburgh*, p. 53. Edinburgh: Murray & Cochrane.
(80) College Minutes, 1.viii.1758.
(81) Ibid., 3.ii.1789.

HONORARY FELLOWSHIP

(82) Ibid., 5.viii.1806.
(83) WILSON, J. B. (1973) Three Scots in the service of the Czars. *Practitioner*, **210**, 569–74, 704–8.
(84) R.C.P.E. [1851] *General Correspondence*.
(85) College Minutes, 6.v.1760.
(86) Ibid., 3.xi.1773.
(87) Ibid., 24.ii.1774.

BIZARRE ENQUIRIES

(88) Ibid., 1.xi.1763.
(89) Ibid., 6.v.1707.

(90) Ibid., 6.viii.1765.

(91) Ibid., 6.v.1834.

(92) Ibid., 3.ii.1708.

(93) Ibid., 2.xi.1725.

(94) Ibid., 3.v.1726.

(95) Ibid., 11.vii.1744.

(96) Ibid., 6.xi.1744.

(97) CRESWELL, C. H. (1926) *The Royal College of Surgeons of Edinburgh. Historical notes from 1505 to 1905*, p. 110. Edinburgh: Oliver & Boyd.

(98) College Minutes, 1.viii.1786.

(99) Ibid., 7.xi.1786.

(100) Ibid., 3.xi.1807.

(101) Ibid., 2.v.1843.

(102) Ibid., 18.v.1841.

(103) Ibid., 28.v.1841.

PUBLICATIONS

(104) Ibid., 16.x.1694.

(105) Ibid., 23.x.1694.

(106) Ibid., 4.ii.1735.

(107) Ibid., 6.v.1735.

(108) R.C.P.E. (1826) *General Correspondence*, 10.i.1826.

(109) College Minutes, 4.v.1731.

(110) GRAY, J. (1952) *History of the Royal Medical Society, 1737–1937*, p. 2. Edinburgh: University Press.

(111) RITCHIE, R. P. Op. cit., p. 132.

(112) INGLIS, J. A. (1911) *The Monros of Auchenbowie*, p. 66. Edinburgh: Constable.

(113) WRIGHT-ST. CLAIR, R. E. (1964) *Doctors Monro; a medical saga*, p. 50. London: Wellcome Historical Medical Library.

(114) DUNCAN, A. (1896) *Memorials of the Faculty of Physicians and Surgeons of Glasgow, 1599–1850*, p. 208. Glasgow: Maclehose.

(115) SHAPIN, S. A. (1971) *The Royal Society of Edinburgh: a study of the social context of Hanoverian science*, p. 85. (Thesis.)

(116) College Minutes, 14.xii.1825.

(117) Ibid., 7.ii.1826.

(118) Ibid., 14.iii.1826.

(119) Ibid., 6.i.1829.

(120) Ibid., 7.i.1829.

(121) Ibid., 6.i.1829.

(122) Ibid., 4.v.1954.

CLINICAL FIELD STUDIES

(123) SMILES, S. (1905) *The Autobiography*, ed. by T. Mackay, p. 132. London: John Murray.
(124) LEWINS, R. (1832) Pathological and practical observations on infantile remittent fever. *Edinburgh Medical and Surgical Journal*, **37**, 110, 115–23.

DISCOURSES AND ASSEMBLIES

(125) SIBBALD, Sir R. (1833) *The Autobiography*, p. 28. Edinburgh: Thomas Stevenson.
(126) College Minutes, 4.ii.1684.
(127) Ibid., 3.iii.1684.
(128) Ibid., 7.iv.1684.
(129) Ibid., 6.v.1684.
(130) Ibid., 2.vi.1684.
(131) Ibid., 7.vii.1684.
(132) Ibid., 8.ix.1684.
(133) Ibid., 20.x.1684.
(134) Ibid., 3.xi.1684.
(135) Ibid., 1.xii.1684.
(136) Ibid., 9.xi.1693.
(137) Ibid., 15.xi.1693.
(138) Ibid., 4.i.1694.
(139) Ibid., 30.vii.1694.
(140) Ibid., 5.ii.1697.
(141) Ibid., 12.i.1705.
(142) Ibid., 30.viii.1705.
(143) Ibid., 9.xii.1708.
(144) RITCHIE, R. P. Op. cit., p. 130.
(145) College Minutes, 5.viii.1834.
(146) Ibid., 12.viii.1834.
(147) Ibid., 4.xi.1834.
(148) Ibid., 3.xi.1835.
(149) Ibid., 1.v.1838.
(150) Ibid., 24.xii.1850.

UNLICENSED PRACTICE AND OTHER IRREGULARITIES

(151) Ibid., 5.ii.1712.
(152) Ibid., 18.xi.1695.
(153) Ibid., 28.iv.1682.
(154) Ibid., 6.xi.1682.
(155) Ibid., 7.v.1683.

(156) Ibid., 15.vi.1683.

(157) Ibid., 22.ii.1684.

(158) Ibid., 7.vii.1696.

(159) Ibid., 13.iv.1698.

(160) Ibid., 27.iv.1698.

(161) Ibid., 19.ii.1708.

(162) Ibid., 1.ii.1848.

(163) Ibid., 3.viii.1847.

(164) Ibid., 2.xi.1841.

(165) Ibid., 7.xi.1843.

(166) Ibid., 1.ii.1842.

(167) Ibid., 9.v.1851.

(168) BROWN, T. (1886) *Alexander Wood, M.D., F.R.C.P.E. A sketch of his life and work*, p. 55. Edinburgh: Macniven & Wallace.

(169) CHRISTISON, Sir R. (1885) *Life of Sir Robert Christison, Bart.*, vol. I, p. 382. Edinburgh: Blackwood.

Chapter IX

OF THE FELLOWSHIP: 1682–1858— RELATING TO EXTERNAL POLICY

With us ther was a Doctour of Phisik;

.   .   .   .   .

He knew the cause of everich maladye,
Were it of hoot, or collde, or moyste, or drye,
And where they engendred, and of what humour.
He was a verray, parfit praktisour.

Geoffrey Chaucer

You doctors have a serious responsibility. You call a man from the gates of death, you give
health and strength once more to use or abuse. But for your kindness and skill, this would
have been my last book, and now I am in hopes that it will be neither my last nor my best.
R. L. Stevenson (inscription in a volume gifted to his physician)

With the passage of years the College acquired increased status in the eyes of the civic authorities, those responsible for the national health and the medical profession in general. Matters of external policy assumed increasing importance in the deliberations of the College and domestic problems were accorded rather less priority where claims on the time of Fellows were involved.

EPIDEMIC DISEASE

APPROACH BY TOWN COUNCIL

Inevitably, as College activities extended and expanded, contacts with the Town Council became more frequent and were related to a constantly widening range of common interests. One of the earliest approaches to the College by the Town

Council was in the year 1721. It took the form of a Memorial 'Desyreing the Colledge their opinion and advyce to Guard against any Pestilentious Infection'. The opinion of the College was sought as to the necessity of certain projects before difficult and expensive measures were embarked on; and as to the desirability of 'a prescription or recept for a Perfume proper to be used . . . in their houses as a fence against Infectious air . . .'. Questions were also raised about the provision of drugs, liquids which might be of value and 'ffoods which ought to be avoyded'. Finally the Memorial gave a hint that the Magistrates contemplated securing the agreement of physicians, surgeon–apothecaries and 'Reverend Ministers of the Citty . . . Not to abandon the Citty when it has most need of their assistance . . .'.[1]

Recommendations made by a College Committee appointed for the purpose were transmitted by the President (Dr James Forrest). They were lengthy and detailed and among other recommendations, advised the draining of the Nor'-Loch 'with all Imaginable Expedition . . . leaving a Canall in its middle . . . with a Constant Current of running water from the ffountains'; removal of the slaughter houses 'to some Convenient Distance from the Toun'; Carrion to 'be burried and not exposed as usuall to rot above ground': removal of 'dunghills': frequent cleaning of the streets preferably with water: provision of 'housss of office . . . att Convenient distances': and waggons to call for 'what is gathered in privat ffamilies . . . and non to be allowed . . . to throw out any kynd of nastiness over windows or in the Staires or closses'. In addition the need for prisons, hospitals and public work houses being kept clean, gardeners to bury useless Plants, and vagrants to be removed, was stressed.[2]

Some sixty years later, the Town Council again asked for the College's opinion as to the desirability of removing the 'Slaughtering houses . . . in the centre between the old and new Toun'. As was to be expected the College were emphatic that, as then situated, the 'slaughtering houses' could prove prejudicial to the health of the inhabitants.[3] This time more effective action may have been taken because in 1785, acting on a predecessor's suggestion the President (Dr John Hope) sent 'a letter of thanks . . . to the Lord Provost and Magistrates of Edinburgh for the vigorous and public spirited measures which they are now carrying forward for the extention and improvement of this City'.[4]

Some years later at a time when scarcity of meal and destitution had assumed serious proportions, the College received 'a Card' from the Lord Provost seeking their support in the form of subscriptions to meet the expense incurred in supplying the poor.[5] In 1817 a new Police Bill was being proposed and a Committee of the College was appointed to consider the Draft. This was the first occasion on which such a Bill had been laid before the College for consideration. The Committee's report, which won the approval of the College, stated that 'by far too little time has been allowed for the attentive consideration'; power of imprisoning for 90 days vested in any one Judge might expose the personal liberty to hazard which would not be sanctioned by Law; and that the proposed increased expenditure was objectionable as imposing or entailing new burdens. Other subjects dealt with concerned the maintenance of engines for extinguishing fire. The boldness of the physicians has to be admired! They did however write with unquestionable authority when they concluded with the opinion 'that the Superintendent of Police should be entitled to compel all whom it concerns without exception, to keep the pavement at all times in proper order to which at present there seems in some districts a blameable inattention'.[6]

When the Committee reported on the second draft they reiterated their view that the Superintendent of Police 'should be imperatively directed to enforce the removal and the prevention of the formation in future of the enormous dung-hills which present themselves at every avenue to the Town'. In further support of their contentions they indicated that 'it is the decided opinion of all well informed Medical men that the exhalations from putrid and putrescent matter have given rise to the most malignant fevers . . .'.[7]

A sequel was the receipt by the President (Dr Thomas Hope) of a letter dated 19th October 1817 from the Lord Provost with 'a Request, that you will have the goodness to ascertain . . . the present State of Fever in this city, and what proportions such may be at the present season compared to that of any former period . . .'. Members of the College gave deliberate consideration to the enquiry. The reply sent indicated that 'this Fever is more frequent in Edinburgh than it usually is at this season', but at the same time gave a cogent explanation of why comparison with experience at other times would be unreliable. Not content with answering that which had been asked, the letter wound up with a peroration on the benefits to be expected from 'inculcating among the ranks of the lower classes due attention to . . . ventilation, cleanliness, separation of the sick from the healthy, purification of apartments, bedding and Clothes etc.'.[8]

THE NEED FOR A FEVER HOSPITAL

Twenty-six years later it remained for a Fellow of the College to declare at a Quarterly Meeting 'that the present state of Fever in Edinburgh called loudly for the support of the public in establishing a Fever Hospital that liberal subscriptions were required to accommodate the patients in Surgeon Square, which was not supplied with Furniture, and whose patients altho' the Infirmary was crowded, could not at present consequently be admitted'.[9] A formal motion, involving a donation by the College, was submitted but had to be withdrawn on technical grounds. In lieu another motion was adopted, requiring a Committee to represent to the Dean of the Faculty of Advocates the opinion of the College 'that there should be no farther delay' in applying a recent bequest left by the late Mr Chalmers 'for the erection of an Hospital . . . for the benefit of the sick and hurt'.

SMALLPOX

In 1771 yet another letter was received from the Lord Provost.[10] On this occasion the College was urged to consider 'the most effectual means to prevent the plague at present raging in other countries from taking place' in Edinburgh. A College Committee advised the President who was asked to reply, but in what terms is not recorded.[11] About this time plans for an Inoculation Hospital were discussed with the 'Society of Surgeons'[12] and the desirability 'of a general inoculation for the small pox at certain fixed periods' as successfully carried out in other parts of Great Britain was later considered.[13] Eventually on the advice of a special Committee the College offered free inoculation to 'the Children of the lower ranks' during the months of September and October annually, and suggested that the Infirmary and Public Dispensary should do likewise.[14] An advertisement was inserted in the newspapers publicizing the College decision, and the College and the Surgeons jointly approached the clergy to secure their help in recommending use of the proffered service.[15] Use was also made of a pamphlet[16] and the success which followed the first newspaper advertisement encouraged the College to repeat the insertion,[17] with, as events proved, even better results.[18]

In 1806 a letter was received from the Royal College of Physicians of London, asking the Edinburgh College to provide information in order that a report on the state of vaccination required of them by the House of Commons might be complete 'for every Part of the United Kingdom'. It must be admitted the Edinburgh reply was both surprising and revealing—and on the surface at least not very helpful. Opening with the admission that the Edinburgh College 'have but little opportunity themselves of making observations on Vaccination, as that practice is entirely conducted by Surgeon apothecaries and other Medical Practitioners not of their College, and . . . the aid of a Physician is never required'. The negligence or ignorance of parents, mistaken notions concerning impropriety, and difficulty in country districts of procuring vaccine were given as reasons why adoption of vaccination had not been general.[19]

CHOLERA

Turning to cholera, the College had advance warning of possible European involvement when in 1821 it received from the East India Company a printed report on the Epidemic Cholera Morbus which had ravaged the territories of Bengal.[20] Ten years later, by which time cholera had secured a hold on a number of countries in Europe, a Fellow expressed surprise that no communication on the subject had been received from the Government and he urged that the College should show initiative by offering advice on measures needed to prevent spread to this country.[21] Within a few months a communication was received from the Royal College of Surgeons suggesting a joint Conference with the same object in mind, the College of Physicians having already written to the Secretary of the Board of Health in London.[22] A small Committee of the College of Physicians, previously appointed to advise the Lord Provost and magistrates, recommended the Lord Provost to convene a meeting of representative citizens at which a Board was established. On the Board there was weighty representation of the College and of practitioners who had acquired knowledge of cholera in the Far East.[23] Considering that cholera reached Edinburgh and its environ in mid-January 1832 and that the epidemic persisted throughout the year, there are inexplicably few references to the subject in the College Minutes. The same applies to the period 1833–4 when there was a more brief but equally severe outbreak. That is not to say that the College exerted no influence. It undoubtedly did so in the persons of such Fellows as Drs Abercrombie, Alison and Christison, all of whom were on the Board. At the request of the Board, Dr Abercrombie, using information obtained from colleagues in Haddington, Newcastle and Sunderland, brought out a pamphlet for the clinical guidance of practitioners.[24] Christison wrote with a vehement conviction characteristic of his authoritative contributions to College debates: and Alison directed the attention of the College to their neglect of the daily reports of cholera received from the City Board of Health and to the need for the documents being preserved if only because of their future historical value.[25]

With the near approach of cholera once more, the Town Council sought a conference with the College in 1848, the result of which was a decision to 'renew intercommunication' but not to be precipitate in taking any immediate steps.[26] In

October of the same year a full meeting was held at the instigation of the Presidents of the two Edinburgh Colleges and attended by representatives from the local Parochial Boards. At the meeting mention was made of difficulties encountered following the centralization of responsibility in the General Board required by the new Act for the Prevention of Epidemic Diseases. Additional to formal appeal to London the College President (Robert Christison) was in the fortunate position of having the personal acquaintanceship of the redoubtable and powerful Mr Chadwick on the General Board—an acquaintanceship which appears to have been used to good purpose. The General Board forthwith established a Local Board. That anxiety was acute, is evident from the following excerpts from a letter written on 5th October 1848 to Chadwick by the College President:

> '. . . in at least two separate localities here, a disease indistinguishable from malignant cholera has broken out . . .'
>
> 'If this be the advent of the Epidemic we are taken quite unprepared . . .'
>
> 'It is more than a month since . . . I was empowered by the College to put myself in communication with the City authorities on the Subject of making preparations for the disease . . . but its slow progress on the Continent led us here, as it seems to have also led you all in London, to be slow to believe that any great preparation would be necessary.'

Having delivered to central authority a subtle homily with courage beyond that of modern local government the President gives it as his opinion that 'preparation must be begun instantly and with energy', and goes on to deplore the delay stemming from the rigidity of central control.[27]

A full account of his actions was given by the President to the College which in return expressed its entire approval. Asked concerning the 'utility or necessity of Hospitals in the treatment of malignant Cholera' the College gave a somewhat equivocal reply. They considered that other things being practicable in the matter of treatment, patients should not be removed from home, but that as a large proportion of cases occur 'among the lowest population . . . it is . . . unsafe for the healthy to remain in attendance'. Having said which, the College decided 'it is most undesirable that the healthy be exposed in treating the sick, provided the removal of the sick be practicable'. Whereupon the College was then asked if its members favoured the use of gentle laxatives to correct a tendency to constipation as a measure for the prevention of cholera. On this occasion there was unanimity, and the College saw no reason why mild laxatives should be discouraged basing their opinion in part on the unfortunate results of directions to the contrary issued by a Board of Health in the epidemic of 1833.

Eventually a copy of the College Resolutions was sent to the General Board of Health. These recommendations contemplated among other developments, small hospitals for the removal of the lowest poor; dispensaries for the supply of medicines at all hours; a list of men prepared to act as cholera physicians; and Houses of Refuge or Quarantine for the Healthy.[27] Two replies were received—the first platitudinous, the second interim but more realistic and embodying a deserved tribute to the College President as an eminent contributor 'to the progress of Sanitary Improvements'. Paradoxically the President on the same day as referring to this correspondence had to announce that because the General Board of Health had no power to delegate, the Local Board of Health had had to be dissolved. How often in administrative spheres does an impasse of this kind occur at a time of crisis! It fell to the College of Physicians Committee of Investigation in co-operation with a Committee of the Royal College of Surgeons to continue to operate in the absence of a Local Board.[28]

In 1852 Council reported to the College concerning correspondence with the General Board of Health about the Returns of Cholera Cases. The report referred to the frustrations of 1848; indicated approval of the appointment by the General Board of a Medical Council, albeit in London; and stated to the two Royal Colleges in Edinburgh having prepared directions, regulations and schedules on behalf of the Board for use in Scotland which had proved eminently successful. In the course of the early part of the negotiations, the Colleges expressed to the Board their extreme apprehension that the returns issued by the Board 'will from their number and complexity, entail an amount of labour on medical men, which few amid the labour and anxiety of Cholera Cases would be found willing to undertake'. The continuing ability of administrative departments to issue inopportune questionnaires has, it would seem, a dynastic origin!

Approached by the Board for assistance in applying measures for the control of cholera the President of the College in his letter of reply included a comment 'that the appointment of a Medical Council to aid the General Board of Health, cannot but be acceptable to the College being in conformity with opinions which have been repeatedly expressed to successive governments. It may be doubtful, however, how far a Medical Council composed exclusively of English Practitioners can advise beneficially for Scotland, when the laws, customs and habits of the people are in many respects, so very different.' The same letter drew attention to difficulties arising from the Poor Law Board having been invested with 'the whole power—to the exclusion of all Medical Authority'.

Another aspect brought to the Board's attention was that (in 1854) the cases of cholera were 'not by any means . . . confined to the pauper classes, but have shewn themselves extensively in a class who can choose their own medical attendants'. This the College pointed out meant that whereas returns would be required from Workhouse doctors, 'they must be asked as a favour from other Medical men'. The Secretary may well have permitted himself a wry smile because almost simultaneously he was advising the Board that the cholera, having fortunately disappeared, the time for using the returns was probably past. Circulation of the forms raised problems. Asked to circulate them the College drew attention to the strain on their finances in the absence of repayment, and recommended that distribution should be the responsibility of the Parochial Boards. Eventually, officially franked envelopes were promised the College.[29]

CONTAGIOUS FEVER

Yet another epidemic condition which brought the College and Town Council into mutual consultation was contagious fever, which in all probability was synonymous with typhus fever although possible confusion between typhus and typhoid fever cannot be ruled out. In May 1817 a Committee was appointed by the College to investigate reports of 'a contagious fever existing in Edinburgh' and to draw up any regulations that might seem desirable.[30] They found that a continued fever was more prevalent than usual, but being of a mild character did not call for any special measures on the part of the College. In the interval an enquiry had been received from the Lord Advocate asking in particular if 'the masses of putrescent matter which have been collected for Sale in the Vicinity by the Commissioners of Police or their Lessee' were in any way to blame.[31] The reply sent to the Advocate, perhaps sensitive to possible legal interpretations, did not incriminate the specified 'putrescent matters' but instead enlarged upon the detrimental effects of 'offensive vapors and effluvia' in general. As to the fever itself—it was referred to as one 'of the Typhoid character' and ascribed to contagion, lack of ventilation, offensive exhalations, fatigue, intemperance and bad or too little food—many of these commonly operating at one and the same time.[32]

Prompted by reports emanating from the Society for relief of the Destitute Sick about this time, the Lord Provost enquired from the College as to 'the present State of Fever in this City' and was sent a reassuring reply couched in terms similar to those of the letter sent to the Lord Advocate. Once again the opportunity was taken to focus attention on the fundamental importance of deplorable social conditions as a cause of epidemic disease and its dissemination.[33] Still on the subject of contagious fever a letter, together with a Minute of the Committee for preventing contagious fever, was received from a minister of religion with the object of procuring the support of the College. No other details are minuted, and all that can be deduced is that apprehension was probably still extensive and that the importance of the College as a professional body was fully recognized.[34]

BILLS OF MORTALITY

. . . there is a definite task before us—to determine from observation, the sources of Health, and the direct causes of death in the two sexes at different ages and under the different conditions. The exact determination of evils is the first step towards their remedies.

William Farr

Over a number of years the College had been worried about the inadequacy of returns necessary for the reliability of Bills of Mortality, and to secure improvement submitted a plan to the City Magistrates.[35] Included in the plans were proposals that those responsible for 'the superintendance' of the Bills as General Inspectors should be the Lord Provost, the Senior Clergymen of the City and the Presidents of the two Edinburgh Colleges.[36] Although approved of by the magistrates, circumstances prevented effect being given to the plan. In 1806 the College again took the matter up and appointed a Committee to determine how greater accuracy of returns could be secured.[37] Four years later the College received a Report 'relative to the number of Funerals and the Epidemic diseases' which had prevailed in the city during the previous two quarters[38]; and after the reading of a similar Report the next year it was decided that the presentation of such Reports should become a regular feature of Quarterly Meetings of the College.[39]

REGISTER OF BIRTHS, DEATHS AND MARRIAGES

DEARTH OF RELIABLE INFORMATION

In 1840 recommendations drawn up by the Statistical Section of the British Association dealing with the need for an improved system of Registration of Births and Deaths and Marriages in Scotland was considered by the College. A resolution was then passed by the College to the effect that it fully recognized 'the essential advantages to be derived to Medical Science from an accurate Registration of Births and Deaths, together with the causes of death'. This was followed by the appointment of a Committee to consider ways and means of furthering this objective.[40] Following discussion with a Committee of the Royal College of Surgeons a communication was sent to the Lord Advocate. This communication referred to previous failure to procure a legislative enactment for Registration in Scotland comparable to that already applicable to England, largely as a result of the opposition of Session Clerks throughout the country; pointed out that a system of Registration has been in operation for a number of years in the City of Glasgow under the auspices of the Municipal Authorities; and advocated the establishment by law of a system of Registration for 'the whole Country or at least as extensively as may be practicable'. The Lord Advocate's reply was guardedly encouraging and while recognizing such considerations as personal interests, popular prejudices and pecuniary difficulties, invited suggestions without pledging himself to their adoption or even to the fulfilment of his 'own desire in regard to this important matter'.[41]

About the same time a Memorial was forwarded by the College to the Secretary of State for the Home Department which declared that Registration not being general, many births and marriages were not being recorded; and such records as were kept of burials had no value as indications of causes of deaths, or of the incidence of deaths in different classes of society and in different parts of the country. It was argued further that regular and accurate records were essential for answers to 'all those questions in vital statistics which may enable the Physician to understand the causes of diseases epidemic, endemic and sporadic, and to adopt the means most likely to prevent diseases susceptible of prevention, to diminish mortality, to improve health, and to extend if practicable, the average duration of human life'. Finally, and despite previous rebuffs in Parliament, the strongest of pleas was submitted for legislation in Scotland 'similar to that which has been for several years in operation in England'. Copies of the Memorial were sent to the Lord Advocate and the Lord Provost.[41]

When a Bill was brought into Parliament the proposed clauses were considered in detail by the College. Criticism was voiced by some concerning certain details, more especially about the form of schedule. It was felt that by shortening it and by simplification of disease nomenclature, it would more accurately reflect the needs of Scotland without sacrificing scientific precision and value, or making comparison with English records impossible.[42] A Committee appointed at the time, later had what was described as a very satisfactory interview with the Lord Advocate and came away heartened by amendments of the pending Bill in keeping with the desires of the College.[43]

ENGLISH NOSOLOGY SUSPECT

On 2nd May 1854 the College was given notice that 'a Bill, for the better Registration of Births, Deaths and Marriages in Scotland, had reached Edinburgh'. Thereupon another Committee was appointed and reported back within a week,[44] the Report including a most excellent summary of the Bill. The College accepted the Report unanimously and resolved to petition Parliament in favour of the Bill—customarily referred to as Lord Elcho's Bill. A formal petition was submitted to the Commons, and sent to Lord Elcho together with a covering letter. The letter drew attention to the College's objections to the possible use of the English System of Registration of the causes of death. Earlier in debate the College had had their attention drawn to the absence in the Bill of any instructions to Registrars about the form enquiries as to causes of death were to take.[45] Replying, Lord Elcho made clear his intention to submit points made by the College to 'a Select Committee of the Scotch members', whereupon the College straightway sent a circular on their own to each of the 'Scotch members' together with copies of the College Resolutions. These members were, it would appear, assumed to be of high intellect and particularly receptive because, in the letter sent them, the College's opposition to the wholesale importation of English practice was elaborated, and elaborated with clarity. 'The College finds in the nosology (systematic classification of diseases) adopted by the Registrar General of England, and made the basis of his system, a very complete and elaborate view of Pathological Science admitting of considerable criticism—The College are therefore of opinion that the use of this Nosology tends to introduce into Medical Science both errors and questionable propositions, and they are desirous of having an opportunity of suggesting a simpler, and more practical nomenclature . . . for . . . consideration . . .'.[46]

BUREAUCRACY

But this was not to be the end of the matter of Registration. A new clause was added to the Bill savouring not a little of State dictatorship and selective nationalism. The clause aimed at imposing a penalty on medical men for not reporting deaths that occurred in their practice. Moreover as the College were quick to point out to the Lord Advocate 'English medical men are not so treated, and the clergy have obtained an exemption from the penalty'. Protests called for tact and diplomacy lest they might be misconstrued as signifying opposition to the entire Bill. Unwittingly Lord Elcho's response to protests might have been a prototype for mid-twentieth century!—'I regret . . . the clause . . . should be deemed objectionable . . . But the intention is, that Medical men should be furnished with printed forms . . . which they will have to fill up, and I hope this will not be found inconvenient in practice.' A local Member of Parliament endeavoured to use his influence with Lord Elcho, after hearing from the College. Additional to formal approach to selected individuals the Secretary of the College, on instructions, wrote an official letter to the Edinburgh newspapers outlining the purpose of the new Bill and the part played in the preliminaries by the College, and recommending that a medical man should be 'conjoined with the Registrar'.

There then appears a note in the Minutes which requires reproduction in full to allow of interpretation being unbiased!

> 'Understanding that the execution of the Bill would devolve upon Mr. Pitt Dundas, the Deputy Registrar General, and that he would have to appoint a Secretary, Dr. Alison has, through a mutual friend, put himself in communication with Mr. Dundas, pointing out the advisability of naming a medical man to the office, and has been assured by that friend, that the feeling of the College should be duly laid before Mr. Dundas.'[47]

Wheels within wheels—then as now!

CARE UNDER THE POOR LAW

The idea of poor law relief is to to do as little as possible, as late as possible, and for as short a time as possible.
> Sir Arthur Newsholme (concerning the position prior to the Royal Commission of 1905)

ENQUIRIES INVITED

A resolution was passed at a Quarterly Meeting on 4th February 1840 to send a petition to H.M. The Queen 'praying that the Enquiry of the Poor Law

Commissioners may be extended to Scotland'.[48] The petition consisted of a communication addressed to the Secretary of State for the Home Department. Referring to the enquiries being made by the Commissioners into 'the Sanatory condition of the labouring Classes both in England and Wales' it asserted that that of the Labouring Classes in Scotland 'equally demands investigation'. In support of this contention the petition declared that in Edinburgh and Glasgow conditions were 'worse in several respects and particularly as regards the liability to contagious Fever than that of the labouring Classes in most if not all of the great Towns in England'. The Home Secretary replied on 19th February 1840 to the effect that the Poor Law Commissioners had 'undertaken to extend their labours to Scotland'.[49] Developments were not long in taking place. Application for an enquiry into the present state of the Poor Law in Scotland and for information relative to Epidemic Disease in Edinburgh was made by the Secretary to the Commissioners; and the College made it abundantly clear that they considered such an enquiry to be highly necessary and that they 'would as a Body and as individuals afford every facility to the investigations'.[50]

SCOTTISH PRACTITIONERS AT A DISADVANTAGE

A fundamental flaw in understanding between College and the Commissioners however declared itself unexpectedly. It concerned the qualifications of Medical Officers under the Commissioners. By the terms of a new Order and Explanatory Letters issued by them in March 1842 it was evident that the Commissioners regarded Licences to practise Medicine and Surgery granted by the University and College of Surgeons in Edinburgh as inferior to those issued by various licensing bodies in England. Although at the time 'not . . . concerned as a body, either in the Education or Licensing of Practitioners in Edinburgh', the College of Physicians espoused the case of the Edinburgh trained doctors with vigour verging on fervour. In a Memorial sent to the Poor Law Commissioners it pointed out that individual Members of the College were concerned with duties in connection with the award of the University Degree of M.D. and in the granting of a diploma by the Royal College of Surgeons: and stated unreservedly that the degree and the diploma were 'decidedly superior, as a qualification for general Practice, to those which are prescribed by the Royal College of Surgeons and the Company of Apothecaries in London'. That being so, and after making due allowance for the monopoly of dispensing medicines unreasonably enjoyed by licentiates of the Apothecaries' Company, the College urged that the Commissioners should 'issue such modifications of their order, as will prevent an unmerited stigma being thrown on those ancient and well established schools of Medicine and Surgery'. A copy of the Memorial was sent to the Secretary of State for the Home Department.[51]

To say that the attitude of the College was not wholly magnanimous is not to belittle its sincerity of purpose. The fact remains, however, that, in formulating their policy the College must have been well aware of its bearing on the Bill on Medical Reform in course of preparation at the time. There is evidence of this in a letter sent to the Commissioners after receipt of their reply to the Memorial, stating that 'if there were anything in the present Law preventing the Commissioners from granting the prayer of the College, it was hoped this power would be given to them, in the Bill now brought into Parliament, to continue the Commissioners'.[52]

The reply of the Commissioners had a significance extending far beyond the realm of Poor Law administration. It consisted of a terse letter enclosing a copy of a 'Minute of the Poor Law Commissioners respecting the admissability of Scotch and Irish Medical Practitioners to Union Medical Offices in England, dated the 12th day of May 1842'. The Minute was as verbose as it was lengthy; as cautiously defensive as it was paternally apologetic; and a classic example of sustained circumlocution. The College had not been alone in its protestations. Other bodies who had voiced their like opinions included the Universities of Edinburgh and Glasgow, the Edinburgh Royal College of Surgeons, and the Glasgow Faculty of Physicians and Surgeons. To these was added a letter from the Lord Provost of Edinburgh to the Home Secretary.

HISTORICAL INCONSISTENCIES

Referring to their Order which had given offence, the Commissioners maintained that in drafting it they had the Poor Law Unions of England and Wales in mind, and that under the Statute Law they had no option but to declare 'an English license to practise to be a necessary qualification of a Medical Officer'. They specified the authorities 'competent to confer a license in England and Wales' as the College of Physicians (meaning thereby, of London), the Universities of Oxford and Cambridge, the College of Surgeons (again implying, of London), the Ordinaries of the several Dioceses in England and Wales, and the Court of Examiners of the Apothecaries Company—all of which authorities had expressly defined territorial limits, with the exception of the College of Surgeons. Pursuing their argument, which admittedly had legal basis, the Commissioners stated arbitrarily that 'a degree or diploma of a Scotch University . . . or other body having power to confer an authority to practice in Scotland . . . is no such licence to practice in England or Wales'. They quoted as further evidence a court case in 1833 in which the Queen's Bench ruled that whereas 'an English physician is exempt from the penalties of the Apothecaries Act . . . the Scotch diploma was held to confer no such exemption'.

As if that were not sufficiently conclusive the Commissioners went on to emphasize that in that particular court case no weight was attached by the court to the argument that under the Articles of Union between the Kingdoms of England and Scotland 'there shall be a communication of all rights which belong to the subject of either kingdom except where it is otherwise agreed in the Articles'. A vestige of expedient humility surfaced in a brief specific reference to Scotland in which the Commissioners allowed it was not within their province 'to enquire what may be the privileges conferred in Scotland . . . , by a degree or diploma in Medicine granted by a Scotch . . . University or College, or Medical Authority'. They concluded by saying that while they 'do not conceal from themselves that the present state of the law . . . is unsatisfactory . . . The remedy . . . can be applied only by the power of Parliament'.[53]

Tradition dies hard. Many years elapsed before a Ministry of Health assumed central responsibility for the administration of what remained of the old Poor Law. Less than thirty years ago the lists of medical staff in the Annual Reports of the Chief Medical Officer recorded the possession of Diplomas of Membership (or Fellowship) of the London College of Physicians; but no such recognition was accorded to the Fellowship, much less Membership of the Edinburgh College of Physicians in the case of whole-time medical officers on the establishment. Asked for an explanation, the Establishment Officer, with a history of long service, stated categorically that for official purposes the Department recognized London Diplomas only. The rich, broad West of Scotland accent of the Establishment Officer did not add to understanding of the ruling!

POOR RELIEF

Interest in another aspect of Poor Law was evidenced in the mid-nineteenth century when the Lords of the Treasury were memorialized by the College 'in regard to the distinction of medical grants' under that Law. The system in operation consisted in a total sum being apportioned to several Parochial Boards according to population and area of territory, each Board being empowered to claim its share on providing evidence of having expended double the amount on medical relief. Any Board distributing a lesser amount forfeited its quota which was then divided among other Boards. The College regarded the arrangement as fair in that it favoured those Parishes who in times of epidemic disease had been faced with abnormal expenditure. A different view had been taken by the Parochial Boards of Old Machar in Aberdeen-shire and the Memorial of the College aimed at countering it. An incidental point made by the College was that prior to the overall grant of the total sum distributed as described, relief of the Poor in Scotland had been 'much too parsimoniously afforded and they were consequently by much too independent on the unrequited services of the members of the medical profession'.[54] Actually about this time the Parliamentary grant of £10,000 represented about one quarter of the amount expended on medical relief, in contrast to the one half in the case of England and Ireland.[55]

THE HIGHLANDS AND NORTHERN ISLANDS

. . . a voice that hurled his salutations across two fields, he suggested the moor rather than the drawing room . . . He was 'ill pitten thegither' to begin with, but many of his physical defects were the penalties of his work, and endeared him to the Glen.

Ian Maclaren

There is no creature in Scotland that works harder and is more poorly requited than the country doctor, unless perhaps it may be his horse.

Sir Walter Scott

A 'deficiency in the number of Medical Men in the Highlands and northern Islands' was brought to the notice of the College by one of its members (Dr Coldstream) in 1850[56] and was the subject of a paper read at an Extraordinary Meeting. There can be no doubt that the subject was taken seriously by the College because it straightway appointed a Committee to enquire into the number of medical practitioners in the northern counties with particular regard to the Shetlands, Orkney, Caithness, Sutherland, Ross, Inverness, and Argyll including the Hebrides. Enquiries were directed also to the number of practitioners in relation to population and to the extent of country covered by individual practitioners. Authority was given the Committee to have questionnaires printed and distributed at the expense of the College.[57] An interim Report was submitted by the Committee within four months, stating that

H

the Board of Supervision had been asked to make available any information they might possess.[58]

Consideration as well as preparation of the final Report took a considerable time and the note struck by Council when referring it back to the College was one of judicious caution. Members were advised that the subject was beset with difficulties and that any recommendations they might make should be mindful of the need not to 'aim at any object which they are very unlikely to obtain'.[59] The final Report of the Committee was read at a Quarterly Meeting in August 1852 and a motion was passed that after a printed proof had been circulated among and approved by Council, the Report should be circulated as the Committee might direct.[60]

On 3rd August 1852 the College ordered the publication of what it termed *Statement regarding the Existing Deficiency of Medical Practitioners in the Highlands and Islands: being the substance of a Report presented to the Royal College of Physicians of Edinburgh by a Committee appointed to make inquiries on the subject*.[61] The substance was vividly revealing of prevailing conditions. Enquiries had been pursued in 170 parishes with the active co-operation of various parties, 'chiefly Ministers of Parishes'. Of the parishes at least 41 representing a population of over 34,000 were destitute of visits by any regular Practitioner, and in 93 inadequate medical help contributed greatly to suffering from disease and accidents. As evidence of the state of affairs the publication stated, 'the deficiency of duly-qualified Practitioners is compensated in many Parishes . . . by the Ministers themselves giving advice and medicine: while, in a few places, there are proprietors and factors on large estates, who, having studied medicine in their youth, benevolently exert their skill on behalf of their sick neighbours. In some remote districts, the Midwife is the only person who undertakes the treatment of disease.' Some parishes did not have a midwife.

And what of the doctors themselves?—their daily rounds ranged from 3 to 14 miles, their greatest distance from 10 to 100 miles. Most travelled on horseback, a few on occasion only by wheeled conveyance, and as many had to resort to boats daily. Many had reason to complain of the hardships and dangers in 'travelling great distances by sea and land in all weathers, over bad roads and in crazy boats'. Among other reasons for complaint were the intolerant and scarcely tolerable attitude of the parochial authorities, and the inadequacy of the remuneration received—the statement declared 'in some places, two-thirds of the people pay nothing, in others, the proportion of gratis to paying patients is at 19 to one'. By way of inducements to settle in remote localities, some of the larger landed proprietors allowed practitioners land on which a horse or cow could graze, together with a free house. It was pointed out also that by its method of operation the new Poor Law '. . . has . . . produced the anomaly of the very poor, who are recipients of parish-aid, receiving more attention than those who are in comparatively independent circumstances, although unable to pay for medical aid'. State aid coupled with inherited pride, whether under the guise of old Poor Law or new Welfare State, is prone to create such a situation.

A MORAL PROBLEM

One paragraph of the Statement needs quotation *in toto*, if only because throughout their history of almost 300 years, the College has in real practical terms had the interest of the sick poor at heart. By no stretch of imagination did the College stand to gain materially by espousing the cause of the Highlands and Islands. That it knew deep concern is undeniably evident in the following paragraph:

> 'This destitution is at once a consequence and a proof of the miserably depressed social state of the Highlands. With the economics of that state, a College of Physicians has not a direct concern; but, whether the physical well-being of the people at large be considered, or the interest of the professional brethren who share the privations of the poor Highlanders, and help them to the best of their ability, it is conceived that the simple facts now brought out afford a sufficient apology for the College having made this attempt to bring the subject under the consideration of the public.'[62]

CONSTRUCTIVE SUGGESTIONS

The Statement did not confine itself to revealing the facts of the situation. It contained among other practical suggestions 'Salaries for Medical Practitioners . . . in the districts now destitute'; the placing of Army and Navy medical officers 'now on half pay, in the destitute parishes'; the use of 'small steam-ships . . . in which the Practitioners might be conveyed to the more distant localities, at certain fixed times, where and when the sick, able to travel, might rendezvous to meet them'; 'small hospitals . . . in some of the more populous districts'; a benevolent Association for supplying 'medical aid . . . for the poor, not receiving parish relief . . . and training . . . as nurses and midwives'; and the formation of Mutual Assurance Societies for securing medical aid to their members.

If the Statement was vivid, its suggestions were visionary—visionary to the extent of only stopping short of air transport. One of the signatories was James Y. Simpson.[63]

LUNACY

That he is mad, 'tis true; 'tis true 'tis pity;
And pity 'tis 'tis true.

William Shakespeare

From a time relatively early in the history of the College the plight and care of the mentally afflicted were the subject of recurrent consideration and discussion. A Committee for the Lunatic Asylum was one of several instituted by Dr Andrew Duncan on assuming Presidential office. In February 1792 he informed the College that proposals for establishing an asylum were well advanced, trustees having been appointed and the time having arrived for the College to make a donation.[64] He had publicized the idea many years previously without success, and in the interval Thomas Wood, a Fellow of the Surgeons' College, had obtained the support of his College to institute an asylum for lunatics. There seems to have been an element of genuinely friendly rivalry between physician and surgeon. Wood withdrew his proposals in favour of Duncan's plan only to renew them on a modest scale when the latter's initial efforts were unsuccessful.[65] It is of interest that about this time (Sir) Alexander Morison, who was to achieve great renown in the field of mental disease and who was to be one of the College's most generous benefactors, was admitted a Licentiate in May 1800.[66]

Fourteen years after Dr Duncan's statement, Dr Thomas Spens, the President of the time, was able to announce that proposals for 'a Lunatic Asylum in this City' had received warm support from prominent citizens and that the Intended Managers had purchased a suitable piece of ground having further expectations of Government aid.[67] The expectations were realized when the Government appropriated £2000 from the Fund derived from the Estates forfeited after the Rising of 1745.[68] Subject to certain regulations the Managers of what had come to be known as the Royal Lunatic Asylum agreed in 1853 that the Institution should be available for clinical instruction.[69] Previously in 1850 the College had requested Fellows who were Directors of the Asylum to raise the possibility of this with the Managers.[70] At an even earlier date a letter from the Institution's Treasurer acknowledging donations from the College had concluded by saying that the donations would entitle the College 'to the perpetual right of presenting two patients to the Asylum, to be maintained at the lowest remunerating rate of Board'.[71]

THE PAUPER LUNATIC

As events proved, however, the Institution at Morningside did not cater for all needs in the Edinburgh district. The fact was brought home to the College by an unsolicited letter addressed to the President (Dr Davidson) by one of the Fellows—Dr Richard Poole. So impressed were the College that they ordered the letter to be permanently preserved.[72] A Committee was appointed, given full powers and instructed in the course of its activities to search for relevant documents in the possession of the College, obtain information from local authorities and public bodies and hold any necessary conferences.

Considerable weight attached to Poole's views in virtue of his holding the office of Manager of the Charity Work House on the nomination of the College. His letter declared that Edinburgh did not possess 'one Lunatic Asylum, of size and accommodation sufficient for public demand' and was 'absolutely surpassed, in this respect, by some minor towns of Scotland, and no less so by others in the sister Kingdom and on the Continent'. The statement, 'without deprecating' took full account of 'the Institution at Morning Side' and declared that the measure of relief which the Charity Workhouse at Bedlam, Teviot Road justly expected from it had not materialized. Continuing, it declared that a desperate need remained for an Asylum for the Pauper Insane and 'numerous unhappy individuals among the lower, or even the middle, classes of Society'. Quite apart from essentially medical considerations it was argued that 'a slight glance at . . . the receptacles in which they [patients] are confined . . . will dissipate every particle of hesitation to own the truth . . .'.

Paupers, afflicted with insanity in the City parishes, numbering on average 40 per annum were admitted to 'premises attached or contiguous to the Charity Work House'. Similar use of their own Work House was made by the Parish of St Cuthbert's, while the Parishes of Canongate and Leith having no Work Houses dispersed their insane as 'most convenient', paupers among them at times being admitted to Bedlam. Two sentences in the letter deserve quotation *in toto*, if only to consider their significance in relation to modern times. They are:

> 'It [Bedlam] contains . . . some patients, not paupers, but the friends of whom have recourse thereto in their behalf—for reasons of different kinds, including economy, the estimation of a Board of Managers under the public eye, and as I verily believe, the well-founded conviction, that, most objectionable as the locality and arrangements may be, it rivals any institution whatever in the proportion of cases recovered to usefulness.'

And the second sentence:

> '. . . without invidious surmise, I may safely say . . . an inquiry into the family circumstances . . . would disclose an amount of suffering and hardship scarcely less, and actually, in one sense, more pitiable than is endured by the patients themselves.'[73]

In the meantime a major step towards improved care of the mentally afflicted had taken place with the preparation of a Bill provisionally entitled 'Bill to repeal an Act made in the 14th year of the Reign of His present Majesty entituled "An act for regulating Mad houses"'. The Bill was laid before the College.[74] A recommendation was made that the Lord Advocate for Scotland and Lord Provost of Edinburgh might use their good offices to secure for the College of Physicians of Edinburgh the same powers for the Kingdom of Scotland as were proposed by the Bill for the College of Physicians of London for the Kingdom of England. At a later meeting a deputation waited on the Lord Advocate and additional to suggesting amendments, raised the question of a petition to the House of Peers should that be necessary.[75] Some ten months later having naively acknowledged the accidental possession of a printed copy of the Bill embodying certain alterations by the Lord Advocate, the President (Dr James Hamilton, jun.) gave it as the view of the College Committee that the proposed clauses would 'trench most materially in the Chartered Rights of the College'. In the circumstances, and having the necessary authority, the Committee wasted no time in presenting an appropriate petition to the House of Peers. Application to the House of Lords was necessary because of the already advanced stage reached by the Bill in the Lower House. Simultaneously letters on the subject were addressed to two members of the Scottish nobility.[76] This prompt action was successful in having expunged clauses which were causing the College concern.[77] The new Lunacy Bill for Scotland came up for consideration by the College in 1849 which remained 'Neutral, it not appearing . . . that the Bill affected the College or Medical Profession as a Body'.[78]

To be forewarned is to be forearmed: the College appointed a Committee as early as 1839 to enquire 'into the practical working of the Act of Parliament regarding the appointment of Four Inspectors of Houses for the reception of the Insane, from this College'. The Committee reported specifically on the powers and duties of the College in respect to the Act of 1815 'for regulating Mad Houses in Scotland'. Two main objectives of the Act were to create an efficient inspectorate of all public and private institutions, and establish an accurate Regisrty of 'the names, number and description' of those confined in houses kept for their retention. The Committee's Report made clear that for the purposes of inspection the College was concerned only with Institutions in Midlothian: and that by law the College was required to select from among its Fellows four Inspectors who, when required, were to accompany the Sheriff Depute or his substitute on visits of inspection. By the same enactment the Sheriff Depute was required, among other duties, to transmit to the College and to the Justiciary Court a copy of an Account to be laid before the Commissioners of Supply annually, stating the expenses incurred in putting the Act into execution. In the matter of inspection, the Committee were satisfied that the provisions of the Act were being rigidly enforced. The Sheriff accompanied by an Inspector who was usually a Physician from Morningside Lunatic Asylum, made regular biennial tours of inspection and invariably sent in reports to the College.[79]

The College was not dilatory in this respect: on being approached by the Sheriff of the County of Edinburgh to nominate four Fellows 'to Inspect every house . . . for the . . . confinement of furious or fatuous persons or Lunatics' it responded with alacrity.[80] The Committee on the other hand was highly critical of the laxity characterizing the efforts of Sheriffs to implement the provisions in the Act for Registration, and of the limited value of many of such returns as were made. Examination of the College Minutes bears ample testimony to the casual way in which returns were received by the College despite the attempts on the part of at least one President to get the situation remedied. Having approved the Report, the College resolved to send a Memorial to the Home Secretary indicating that owing to causes outside their control certain clauses of the Lunatic Asylum Act had been inoperative.[81] The action of the College only served to underline the persistence of a state of affairs to which the attention of members and Council had been emphatically drawn more than four years before. There is at least the possibility that Inspectors may at times have been undesirably restricted in their activities, because on one occasion when the subject of Lunatic Asylums was raised 'the matter dropped—it being understood that the Inspectors appointed by the College were not called upon to interfere unless some flagrant case of abuse were brought under their notice'.[82] No details are vouched but it is not unreasonable to ask, was the explanation excessive professional zeal in need of curbing, or administrative expediency overriding medical appraisal?

MEDICAL AND LEGAL OUTLOOKS CONTRASTED

When lawyers take what they would give,
And doctors give what they would take.

Oliver Wendell Holmes

In May 1862 the Council reported on a Bill to make further provision respecting lunacy in Scotland. Five years previously a Royal Commission report had revealed the literally appalling circumstances and conditions surrounding both the retention in asylums and 'the farming out' of lunatics. To remedy the situation an Act was passed by Parliament and received the Royal Assent on 25th August 1857. This Act constituted a General Board of Lunacy. The College Council Report of 1862[83] was concerned with a new Bill intended to modify the provisions of the Act of 1857. Profound exception was taken to some of the proposed modifications. In particular the Report condemned the intention to remove all medical representation on a new Board in favour of members of the legal fraternity 'whose ears are supposed to be more attuned to the cry of ratepayers than to that of humanity labouring under a disease which has little to alleviate or mitigate its sufferings'. The attitude of the lawyers who sanctioned the licensing of poorhouse wards 'for pauper lunatics who are not dangerous, and who do not require curative treatment' came in for similar condemnation by the Report which described the contemplated proposals as 'peculiarly repugnant'.

MEDICAL PRACTITIONERS AT RISK AND UNDERVALUED

In essence the Report deplored the belittlement of professional medical knowledge and advice and, referring to the medical profession, expressed the view that 'Their philanthropic and general liberality of sentiment are offensive to Parochial Boards'. Pleas were submitted also for some protection for medical men signing certificates required by the Act; special houses for dipsomaniacs; legal provision for voluntary entry into an ayslum; and arrangements whereby householders might be granted special licences for the reception and detention of pauper lunatics, not exceeding four in number. In pressing for these improvements the College were mindful of the background described in its own Report—'Lunatics insufficiently kept by their relatives . . . some even confined like wild beasts, not from cruelty, but to keep them out of mischief or [out] of the hands of the Parochial Boards'. The Parochial Boards actuated 'by a miserable economy, either retained the poor sufferers . . . or farmed them out to persons who made a living by keeping them', without regard as to the suitability of the place of detention, or to overcrowding which was almost universal as a profit could only be made out of large numbers.[83]

How true those words of Robert Burns:

Man's inhumanity to man
makes countless thousands mourn.

PUBLIC HEALTH PROBLEMS

SCOTLAND AND ENGLAND CONTRASTED

In 1847 the College turned its attention to public health problems. The sequence of events resembled in many ways that described in connection with Lunacy and Care under the Poor Law. Knowledge of a Bill being prepared for application in England came to the notice of the College, which then appointed a special Committee to consider what action was necessary to promote comparable legislation to deal with the situation in Scotland. *Sanatory Regulations of Towns* was the subject of the English Bill in this instance.[84] A notably comprehensive Report on the proposals was given at an Extraordinary Meeting based upon a detailed study of 'the Drafts of two Bills, the one entitled a Bill for improving the Health of Towns in England, and the other a Bill for consolidating in one act certain provisions . . . for paving, draining, cleaning, lighting and improving Towns . . .'.[85] Among conditions dealt with in the Bills were the laying out of streets with particular reference to ventilation and drainage; the removal of nuisances; the regulation of slaughter houses, burial places, fairs and markets; the lighting of, and supply of water to towns; and the regulation of lodging houses for the poor, baths and places of public recreation. It was the opinion of the College Committee that there was room for material amendments were a bill to be drafted for the peculiar needs of Scotland.

After careful consideration, the Committee's Interim Report expressed their conviction as to the great value of the proposed measures. At the same time, without entering into details, they stated that the contemplated 'measures are even more demanded by the present Sanitory condition of the Towns of Scotland than of those of England, particularly as the extension of contagious fevers have been of late years much greater in some of our Scotch towns than in any of the English Towns'.[85] After approving the Interim Report the College decided that the Report should be printed and circulated in such quarters as the Committee might think expedient.[86] A second Report was submitted to the College after an interval of over a year—this too was approved and ordered to be printed, copies to be sent, among others, to the promoters of the Bill, and the Parliamentary Members for the City. The second Report vied with the first in its thoroughness of observation, logical development of arguments, rational justification of recommendations and overall lucid presentation despite the complications inseparable from the subject under analysis. Together the two Reports provide exemplary models for those of succeeding generations.

In the interval between the separate issue of the two Reports there had been certain highly relevant developments. Thus, in so far as England was concerned, the *Health of Towns Act* and the *Towns Improvement Clauses Act* had been put on the Statute Book; and in Scotland, the same applied to the *Edinburgh Police Act* which contained a number of clauses dealing with the maintenance of sanitary standards. Furthermore two general Bills applicable to Scotland had been laid before Parliament—the *Public Health (Scotland) Bill* and the *Police of Towns (Scotland) Bill*. The College Report advised that in so far as these two Bills were concerned, special attention should be paid to sanitary regulations to be made under them, the mode of bringing them into operation, and to the choice of authority to administer them. Cordial approval was expressed in the second Report of the inclusion in the *Edinburgh Police Act* of a number of regulations in the *English Health of Towns Act* relating to nuisances and cleansing of the streets. Clauses in that Act dealing with lodging houses came in for particular mention. Criticism was directed towards the failure to provide for the appointment of an Officer of Health, and to regulate the breadth of streets and the height to which houses could be carried. It was stated, however, that deficiences had been partially made good in the Bills still awaiting Parliamentary approval. None the less the College Committee considered that room remained for improvement of regulations dealing with new buildings, the use of cellars as dwelling-houses, and the extension of water supplies throughout Scotland.

CENTRALIZATION OPPOSED

In the matter of administration the Committee found ample grounds for misgivings. After drawing attention to a certain amount of overlapping liable to follow insufficiently considered apportionment of responsibilities as between Local Boards and the Board of Police Commissioners, the Report wasted neither time nor words in stringently condemning the intention to vest ultimate superintendence and control in the General Board of Health in London. Such an arrangement the Report went on to say 'would not work satisfactorily either to the medical profession or to the public' in spite of the supposed advantage expected to accrue from national uniformity. Full concurrence was expressed by the College Committee with a statement of the Committee of the Police Commissioners that 'harmony should exist between the General and the various local Boards; and that this is much more likely to be secured by having a general Board for Scotland, and having at that Board persons conversant with the Law of Scotland, and the habits and character of the Scottish population'. As an instance of the absurdities that could arise, it was pointed out that under the provisions of the Public Health (Scotland) Bill, appointment and removal of an Officer of Health would rest with the Local Board of the Scottish Town concerned, but direction of his duties would be the responsibility of the General Board in London.

Then came the coup de grâce. With dignity the Report continued:

'the Committee will take the liberty of adding, that although they have a high respect for the individual members of the General Board of Health in London, yet the confident expression of opinion which these gentlemen have officially made on several important questions touching the diffusion of epidemic diseases, which the Committee regard as very difficult and doubtful—and on which they know that some of the most experienced practitioners in Scotland hold very different opinion—have by no means tended to increase their expectation of the efficacy of measures, applicable to Scotland, for restraining the diffusion of epidemics . . . If it be thought necessary that a central authority should regulate and controul [sic] the proceedings of all Local Boards . . . such a Board can be easily formed in Scotland itself . . . the Board of Supervision in Edinburgh is quite competent, or might very easily be made competent (as, e.g. by the addition to its Members of the Presidents of the Royal Colleges of Physicians and Surgeons, or of members chosen from each of these bodies . . .)'.

The cynic might wholly unjustifiably say 'Nationalistic rhetoric'. The reaction of the College Committee to ill-inspired excess centralization was no different to that of bluff, rugged north of England deputations who in modern times have returned rebuffed by Whitehall, or of suppliant management committees shewn the door by omniscient regional hospital board officials. Far from being rampant nationalists the College Committee were realistic, factual, forthright and far-seeing.

It would have been strange indeed had the College not lent its full support to the

Committee's Report. With the two Committee Reports as basis, a Petition was prepared and submitted to Parliament 'in reference to the Public Health Bill for Scotland'. The Petition embodied the majority of points contained in the Reports. In addition it took the opportunity to emphasize that epidemic diseases are 'better known by experience to some of the medical men of the Great Towns in Scotland, than to any of those in London': and that in 'the publications of the Board of Health in London . . . the importance to the Community of early separation of the Sick from the Healthy, in the case of Epidemic Fever, appears . . . to have been very much overlooked, and in the case of Epidemic Cholera, has been absolutely and confidently denied'. These considerations, the Petition maintained had convinced 'those who have studied the subject by actual observation in Scotland . . . that . . . the Board of Health in London are not masters of the facts, on which the results of any measures, that can be devised to check the diffusion of Epidemic diseases in the Great Towns of Scotland, must chiefly depend'.[87] With the sudden withdrawal of the Bill the work of the indefatigable College Committee was terminated—or presumed to have terminated.[88]

FURTHER SUGGESTIONS

That was in 1849. In the following year acting on unsolicited advice the resuscitated Committee decided to concentrate attention on the 'Police and Improvement Bill', in respect of which they prepared a Petition for submission to Parliament. On this occasion they went even further than previously. Having outlined a number of constructive suggestions in the Petition they enlisted the professional help of lawyers to draw up the suggestions in legal terms suited for insertion into the Bill as 'actual amended clauses'. Simultaneously with transmission of the Petition and 'clauses for insertion' to the House of Commons copies were sent to the Lord Advocate and all Scottish Members of Parliament. The Petition made clear the College's appreciation of the *Police and Improvement Bill* for Scotland, but suggested that its value in improving the sanitary condition of the towns of Scotland would be enhanced were certain modifications introduced. In furtherance of this it was recommended that parts of the *Public Health (Scotland) Bill* then before the House of Commons could with advantage be transferred to the *Police and Improvement Bill*. The parts mentioned included those relating to the appointment of an Officer of Health, provision and maintenance of sewers, street construction, and the regulation of lodging houses. Among omissions drawn attention to were, the absence of reference to deprivation of water necessary for flushing sewers owing to the demands of mill races, and the regulation of byres with particular reference to disposal of urine. Stressing the injurious effects on pigs and cows of 'ill regulated' accommodation as a cause of disease, the signatories to the Petition emphasized that disease of animals leads to the exposure for sale of a large quantity of diseased meat.[89]

LODGING HOUSES

The City of Edinburgh Sexcentenary volume refers to a pamphlet published by Dr George Bell in 1850. On a number of his exploratory investigations Bell was accompanied by Professors J. Y. Simpson and Goodsir and he described how they found the lodging houses to be the worst of all dwellings. In one such place it was the practice of the owner to 'pack each room or cellar' with men and women behind locked doors.[90] Bell goes on to say:

> 'the black hole of Calcutta . . . has been described, and the hold of a slave ship: but no description has, because none can be given of the interior of a low Edinburgh lodging house. It defies the graver of Hogarth, the pencil of David Scott so familiar with nightmare horrors, the pen of Dickens, and the tongue of Guthrie.'[91]

For those averse to the drama of fervid evangelism there is instead the stolid, calculated and even more convincing version of Dr W. P. Alison of our College who in his Lectures on Medical Police advocated the licensing of Lodging Houses which he maintained should be watched with a jealousy no less than that characterizing the supervision of 'ships or military depots' of navy and army.[92]

The attitude of the College was clearly outlined in the legal clause submitted by them for insertion into the Bill:

> 'That all keepers of such lodging houses, in the event of any person in their respective houses becoming ill of fever or any other disease, forthwith make intimation thereof to one of the magistrates of Police or the Officer of Health, in order that the nature of the complaint . . . may be ascertained, and the proper medical attendance and treatment procured.
>
> '. . . if at any time the Officer of Health, or if for the time being there be no Officer of Health, any two surgeons or physicians, or one surgeon and one physician, certify, under his or their hands . . . that any infectious or contagious disease exists in any lodging house, the Commissioners shall have the power to order the keeper of such lodging house to shut it up, and to prohibit him and any other person from re-occupying it, until it and the furniture contained in it be cleansed and purified . . .'

In their prolonged studies of sanitary problems successive College Committees had consistently insisted that lodging houses 'had been found . . . to be the foci whence epidemic diseases most frequently diffuse themselves among the poor of large towns'.[93] Within less than two months the Convener of the Committee was able to tell the College that with one exception the substance of the proposed clauses for insertion had been introduced into the Bill.[94]

At the Quarterly Meeting in November 1851 it was reported 'we succeeded in getting almost everything that we wished inserted into the *Police and Improvement Bill*, which is now law'. Success only served to stimulate the inexhaustible College Committee into further activity. The act was an adoptive Act and it was important that its effect should not lapse for lack of momentum. A decision was arrived at to circulate the Sheriffs in Scotland drawing their attention to the new powers they possessed for the purpose of improving sanitation—and in particular the powers regulating Lodging Houses, the height of streets and 'cleaning and draining'.[95] To read the communication is to realize that atmospheric pollution and the construction of 'lofty lands or piles of buildings' were problems of the nineteenth no less than the twentieth century. Due regard was paid to the propriety of the College communicating with the Sheriffs but none the less the receipt of gratuitous advice on the discharge of their judicial duties must have been something of a novel experience![96]

PRISONS IN IRELAND

The caption may encourage wild imaginings—prisons, Ireland, the College—what have they in common? The fact remains that in the first quarter of the nineteenth century a Bill was introduced into Parliament, one clause of which proposed the appointment of surgeons to the exclusion of physicians from attendance on the Jails.[97] The offending Bill was entitled *An act for consolidating and amending the Laws relating to Prisons in Ireland*. The duties of the surgeon were to entail thrice-weekly visits, prescribing for those in need, and examining the condition of the hospital. There were two caveats concerning physicians. A physician appointed prior to the Act coming into force was to continue in office, and 'the City of Dublin, in which more extensive Medical assistance has been found to be necessary' was authorized 'to appoint with the approbation of the Court, a regular bred Physician in addition to . . . a Surgeon'.[98]

In the eyes of London, Dublin apparently was as much in need of tutelage as Edinburgh!

Correspondence passed between the Royal College of Physicians of Edinburgh and the King's and Queen's College of Physicians, Dublin and eventually separate Petitions were submitted by both Colleges. The Edinburgh Petition to Parliament stressed that 'the diseases which occur in Prisons for the most part require medical and not Surgical treatment'. It concluded with the following words—'to give the sanction of legislative authority to the appointment of Surgeons to duties which are purely of a medical nature, would be highly injurious to the reputation and interests of the medical profession in general, and to the Fellows of this College, who reside and practise in Ireland'. The judiciously chosen words precluded any official protest of unwarranted officiousness.[99]

POLICE SURGEONS

Passing from Ireland to Scotland and leaving prison for the 'beat'—the question of the duties of police surgeons was raised with the College by the Edinburgh Commissioners of Police. Separate copies of proposed Regulations were sent for the opinion of the two Edinburgh Colleges.[100] In the summarized views sent to the Commissioners, our College criticised the proposed duties of a surgeon of police as too numerous and diversified: and expressed the fear that the importance of the office was not fully appreciated. Had the College acquired modern terminology it would have described the suggested salary of £155 per annum as derisory. Instead it referred to the £800 per annum being paid the recently appointed Officer of Health at Liverpool.

The duties of a police surgeon were reviewed according to whether they were essentially medicolegal, of an ordinary medical nature, or involving work at night. Because of the 'very rough work, especially . . . at night' it was recommended that an assistant medical officer should reside in the Police Office, and importance was attached to the frequency with which post-mortem examinations had to be undertaken. Then followed recommendations which might well help candidates appearing for interview for a medical post of any kind today! Referring to the discharge of medicolegal duties by a medical man—the College described how in addition to possessing the medical qualifications he must have

> 'an accurate acquaintance with the fundamental correlative sciences of medicine, much discretion, and urbanity and cultivated manners, as the officer is often brought in contact, in somewhat delicate circumstances, with his professional brethren, who

may be, and frequently are, in a superior professional position to his, and with whom it is necessary he should cordially co-operate'.[101]

ANATOMY: MATERIAL FOR TEACHING

Critics! appall'd I venture on the name,
Those cut-throat bandits in the paths of fame,
Bloody dissectors, worse than ten Monros;
He lacks to teach, they mangle to expose.

Robert Burns

burke, v.t. smother; hush-up . . .
(*Concise Oxford Dictionary*)

Credit for the first dissection of human bodies for demonstrations must be given to Alexander Monro *primus* who, at first closely associated with the Incorporation of Surgeons, was admitted to the Fellowship of the Royal College of Physicians, Edinburgh in 1756. Monro acquired skill in dissection in London under the tutelage of Cheselden. Before leaving London in 1718 to continue his studies in Paris, he sent a number of his dissections to his father, John Monro in Edinburgh. Writing of himself quixotically in the third person Monro *primus* left on record 'The Father vain of his Son's Performances showed them to many curious people who asked to see them and at the sollicitation of the College of Physicians and Board of Surgeons made A Present of many of them to these Societies to be put in their Repositories'.[102]

While lecturing in the theatre at the Edinburgh Surgeons' Hall Monro found safety for his own person and for his anatomical preparations in the University when crowds, incensed by the practice of body-snatching, threatened him. Violation of graves for the purpose of dissection had resulted in surgeons and their apprentices becoming the object of the wrath of the populace. In 1721 a clause was inserted in the indentures of apprentices with the object of preventing this form of desecration, but body-snatching continued more or less throughout the century and gave rise to periodic rioting. There is on record the account of the rescue from marauding apprentices of the body of a supposedly executed woman. The rescuers discovered that the woman was not dead, and she survived many years to enjoy her acquired name of 'Half-hangit Maggie Dickson'. That was in 1724.

'Body-snatching' as it was termed certainly persisted and was not limited to the cities. Samuel Smiles (1812–1904) the nineteenth-century sociologist, remembered how when he was scarcely of teenage 'there were many prejudices about doctors' and how even before the exposure of Burke and Hare regular watch was kept over the parish burying ground in his native Haddington. 'I remember going with my father', he wrote in his autobiography, 'when he was on the watch, to take the first turn with him round the churchyard. There were three or four men . . . supplied with some old muskets, mounted with bayonets, to give the resurrectionists a warm reception.'[103] As elsewhere there were 'watch houses' in a number of East Lothian cemeteries. Martine—the father of a local general practitioner—described how the one still extant at Oldhamstocks in the Lammermuirs was erected by the wife of a minister of the parish. Cut on the original dedication stone there were the following words from Jeremiah xxxi, 40:

> 'And the whole valley of the dead bodies, and of the ashes . . . shall be holy unto the Lord; it shall not be plucked up, nor thrown down any more forever.'[103a]

Even more gruesome is the existence in intact state to this day in Crail kirkyard of a stone structure commonly referred to as 'the Dead House'. Above the door there is the original inscription on the lintel 'Erected for securing the dead 1826'. Professor Dow, a Fellow of our College, wrote a short historical account of relevant local events. He described how the Body Snatchers 'entered the Church Yard by the Back Style, robbed the graves, transported the bodies across the Forth to Edinburgh and sold them to the Anatomists . . .'. Mort-safes proved no deterrent and the Public then proceeded to build a Watch House which came to be known locally as the Dead House. Bodies were placed in the building for safety, 'and watchers armed with guns, whisky and cheese, were on guard at night'. The first body to be lodged in the Watch House was that of one of the main contributors to the building fund for the House. Ironically his body was stolen and the coffin filled with stones. According to Dow, the dead man's son was Lord President Inglis, the eminent Court of Session judge who took a prominent part in the trial of Madeleine Smith.[104]

Progress in the teaching of anatomy was rapid under the stimulating pioneer leadership of Monro *primus*, and was so advanced after the turn of the century that grave difficulty was experienced in obtaining the material required. With the citizens in general understandably suspicious, fractious and obstructive to any proposals for meeting the situation, an impasse was reached. In 1828 certain members of the Royal College of Physicians asked that a Petition for Parliament's consideration be drawn up.[105] A form was agreed upon and forwarded to London, together with a confidential letter to the Home Secretary (Sir Robert Peel). Having briefly outlined the importance of anatomical instruction to all in the medical profession, and having expressed understanding of the particularly formidable prejudice in Great Britain against anatomical dissection, the Petition stated that the College, aware of its responsibilities under its Charter, considered itself 'called upon to aid the representations of their professional brethren in other parts of the country'. The Royal College of Surgeons were among those brethren, but neither College made specific reference to the other in their submissions to Parliament. The Petition from our College made no constructive suggestions but contented itself with allusions to its conviction that adequate remedies could be devised. In contrast the letter to the Home Secretary, signed by Alexander Monro, was particular and dealt with such issues as intrusion into premises in which bodies are retained for educational purposes; means of satisfying Excise Officers; enablement of local authorities to grant for dissection certain bodies in special circumstances; and legislation of bequests, during life, of dead bodies.[106]

A letter was later received from the Chairman of the House of Commons Committee appointed to deal with Facilities for Anatomical Dissection. Understandably he asked indirectly for permission to include in the Minutes of his Committee the nature of, and means of granting facilities as they had been enumerated in Monro's confidential letter to Sir Robert Peel.[107] A Bill passed through the House of Commons with greater speed than expected. It far from satisfied the College who, faced with an urgent situation adopted the expediency of submitting a further petition, this time to the House of Lords. Words were not minced. The Bill was criticized as being partial—seriously restricting facilities for Scottish Universities and in particular that of Edinburgh, in contrast with those for anatomical schools in London and English provincial cities; exploiting centralization by concentrating officials concerned in London; and being inadequate in that it did not extend to Ireland. Of the two signatories, one was Alexander Monro *tertius* who inserted 'Prt' after his name although at the time Vice-President.[108]

Withdrawn because of unsatisfactory details and unpopularity with the public, the Bill was reintroduced a few years later following an attempt to repeat the Burke and Hare episode in London.[109] The new Bill was laid before the College in January 1832[110] and considered at several meetings.[111, 112] Correspondence was exchanged with Mr Warburton about changes made in the draft of the third Bill, which when passed into Law dealt with most, but not all, problems of the anatomists at least for the remainder of the century.

REFERENCES

EPIDEMIC DISEASE

(1) College Minutes, 25.x.1721.

(2) Ibid., 31.x.1721.

(3) Ibid., 17.xii.1781.

(4) Ibid., 23.iii.1785.

(5) Ibid., 15.iii.1796.

(6) Ibid., 30.i.1817.

(7) Ibid., 6.v.1817.

(8) Ibid., 28.x.1817.

(9) Ibid., 1.viii.1843.

(10) Ibid., 16.iv.1771.

(11) Ibid., 6.viii.1771.

(12) Ibid., 7.v.1771.

(13) Ibid., 6.xi.1781.

(14) Ibid., 2.viii.1791.

(15) Ibid., 1.xi.1791.

(16) Ibid., 7.ii.1792.

(17) Ibid., 7.viii.1792.

(18) Ibid., 6.xi.1792.

(19) Ibid., 26.xi.1806.

(20) Ibid., 1.v.1821.

(21) Ibid., 2.viii.1831.

(22) Ibid., 27.x.1831.

(23) TAIT, H. P. (1957) The Cholera Board of Health, Edinburgh 1831–34. *Medical Officer*, **98**, 235.

(24) ABERCROMBIE, J. (1832) *Suggestions Submitted to the Medical Practitioners of Edinburgh, on the Character and Treatment of the Malignant Cholera*, 2nd Edition. Edinburgh: Waugh & Innes.

(25) College Minutes, 6.xi.1832.

(26) Ibid., 1.viii.1848.

(27) Ibid., 12.x.1848.

(28) Ibid., 7.xi.1848.

(29) Ibid., 7.xi.1854.

(30) Ibid., 6.v.1817.

(31) Ibid., 16.v.1817.

(32) Ibid., 22.x.1817.

(33) Ibid., 28.x.1817.

(34) Ibid., 19.xii.1818.

BILLS OF MORTALITY

(35) Ibid., 2.viii.1791.
(36) Ibid., 1.xi.1791.
(37) Ibid., 4.ii.1806.
(38) Ibid., 7.viii.1810.
(39) Ibid., 5.xi.1811.

REGISTER OF BIRTHS, DEATHS AND MARRIAGES

(40) Ibid., 3.xi.1840.
(41) Ibid., 26.ii.1846.
(42) Ibid., 23.iii.1847.
(43) Ibid., 4.v.1847.
(44) Ibid., 2.v.1854.
(45) Ibid., 9.v.1854.
(46) Ibid., 26.v.1854.
(47) Ibid., 1.viii.1854.

CARE UNDER THE POOR LAW

(48) Ibid., 4.ii.1840.
(49) Ibid., 5.v.1840.
(50) Ibid., 23.vi.1840.
(51) Ibid., 3.v.1842.
(52) Ibid., 16.v.1842.
(53) Ibid., 15.vi.1842.
(54) Ibid., 3.ii.1852.
(55) RIVINGTON, W. (1879) *The Medical Profession*, p. 178. Dublin: Fannin & Co.

THE HIGHLANDS AND NORTHERN ISLANDS

(56) College Minutes, 21.vi.1850.
(57) Ibid., 16.vii.1850.
(58) Ibid., 5.xi.1850.
(59) Ibid., 4.v.1852.
(60) Ibid., 3.viii.1852.
(61) R.C.P.E. (1852) *Statement Regarding the Existing Deficiency of Medical Practitioners in the Highlands and Islands*. Edinburgh: Royal College of Physicians.
(62) Ibid., p. 6.
(63) Ibid., p. 7.

LUNACY

(64) College Minutes, 7.ii.1792.
(65) CRESWELL, C. H. (1926) *The Royal College of Surgeons of Edinburgh. Historical notes from 1505 to 1905*, p. 164. Edinburgh: Oliver & Boyd.
(66) College Minutes, 6.v.1800.
(67) Ibid., 6.v.1806.
(68) Ibid., 5.viii.1806.
(69) Ibid., 3.v.1853.
(70) Ibid., 7.v.1850.
(71) Ibid., 9.ii.1841.
(72) Ibid., 4.xi.1834.
(73) R.C.P.E. (1834) *General Correspondence*, 1.xi.1834.
(74) College Minutes, 18.xii.1813.
(75) Ibid., 6.vii.1814.
(76) Ibid., 2.v.1815.
(77) Ibid., 3.vii.1815.
(78) Ibid., 5.iv.1849.
(79) Ibid., 5.xi.1839.
(80) Ibid., 3.vii.1815.
(81) Ibid., 5.xi.1839.
(82) Ibid., 13.ii.1855.
(83) Ibid., 6.v.1862.

PUBLIC HEALTH PROBLEMS

(84) Ibid., 2.ii.1847.
(85) Ibid., 14.v.1847.
(86) Ibid., 19.ii.1848.
(87) Ibid., 1.v.1849.
(88) Ibid., 7.viii.1849.
(89) Ibid., 7.v.1850.
(90) EDINBURGH. City corporation (1929) *Edinburgh, 1329–1929.* [Sexcentenary], p. 23. Edinburgh: Oliver & Boyd.
(91) Ibid., p. 23.
(92) BROTHERSTON, J. H. F. (1952) *Observations on the Early Public Health Movement in Scotland*, p. 52. London: H. K. Lewis.
(93) College Minutes, 7.v.1850.
(94) Ibid., 21.vi.1850.
(95) Ibid., 4.xi.1851.
(96) Ibid., 3.ii.1852.

PRISONS IN IRELAND

(97) Ibid., 26.v.1825.
(98) Ibid., 4.iv.1826.
(99) Ibid., 11.iv.1826.

POLICE SURGEONS

(100) Ibid., 20.vii.1854.
(101) Ibid., 1.viii.1854.

ANATOMY: MATERIAL FOR TEACHING

(102) ERLAM, H. D. (1954) Alexander Monro, *primus*. *University of Edinburgh Journal*, **XVIII**, 2, 81.
(103) SMILES, S. (1905) *The Autobiography of Samuel Smiles*, ed. by T. Mackay, p. 28. London: John Murray.
(103a) MARTINE, J. (1894) *Reminiscences and Notices of Ten parishes in the County of Haddington*, Edited by E. J. Wilson, p. 205. Haddington: Wm. Sinclair.
(104) DOW, D. R. (1967) Bygone days in Crail. *Karail*. (Crail Parish Church magazine: February issue.)
(105) College Minutes, 15.iv.1828.
(106) Ibid., 17.iv.1828.
(107) Ibid., 26.v.1828.
(108) Ibid., 23.v.1829.
(109) CRESWELL, C. H. Op. cit., p. 205.
(110) College Minutes, 4.i.1832.
(111) Ibid., 15.iii.1832.
(112) Ibid., 11.i.1832.

Chapter X

MUTUAL DISTRUSTS PERSIST

Greed's envy's auldest brither;
Scraggy wark they mak' thegither.

Proverb

Muted mistrust to the point of veiled antagonism characterized the attitude of the College towards the apothecaries. To a large extent this was a legacy from the days when the apothecaries combined the practice of venturing diagnosis and prescribing with the running of druggists' shops. Understandably relationships were not improved by the alliance of apothecaries with the surgeons which produced the forerunner of the general practitioner. Nor was the power retained by the Society of Apothecaries in England involving victimization of Scottish trained doctors practising in the south, calculated to dispel the mistrust. Likewise, as events proved, the authority granted to the College in its Charter to supervise the shops of apothecaries in Edinburgh, no matter how well intended, proved to be very much of a mixed blessing. Seen from the pharmacist's point of view the Edinburgh pharmacists in the seventeenth century were described as 'striving towards that desirable situation where the doctor would prescribe and the druggist dispense'. By the 1730s, medicine and pharmacy were acquiring their separate identities.[1]

PHYSICK AND PHARMACY

So modern 'Pothecaries taught the art
By Doctor's bills to play the Doctor's part,
Bold in the practice of mistaken rules,
Prescribe, apply, and call their masters fools.

Alexander Pope

TRIAL OF INTRANTS

An Act of the Privy Council, dated 21st November 1684 and signed Will. Paterson, appointed the President and others of the College of Physicians to visit the apothecaries' shops and the Act was engrossed in substantial measure in the Charter of Ratification of 16th June 1685.[2] The Act ordained that the College should at least twice yearly visit all apothecaries' shops and chambers within Edinburgh with the concurrence of one of the Baillies or magistrates: and that 'no persons who have not already been examined and admitted by the Fraternity of Apothecaries be suffered . . . to keep any apothecaries' shops . . . except such as allenarly (only) as shall be tried and approved by the President and Censors of the . . . Royal College'.[3] Not surprisingly the edict stirred emotions in a number of quarters. The problem of executing the policy came up for consideration in the College on several occasions early in December 1864 without the result of deliberations being recorded except in so far as it was remitted to a Committee instructed to revise the Laws of the College. This is the more to be regretted in view of the loss of College Minutes between 22nd December 1684 and 21st March 1693. For their part, the Fraternity of Apothecaries were apprehensive lest the 'tryall of intrants for the art of Pharmacie' rendered 'voyd' their own 'rights and priviledges' dating back to their virtual erection into a Fraternity by the Town Council in 1657.[4] They accordingly petitioned the College for its interpretation of the Act.

Although no Minutes were available, Poole discovered a paper headed 'Explanation of the Act for trying intrant Apothecaries by the Royal College of Physicians. 1684.'[4] There can be little if any doubt that this constituted the College's reply to the Fraternity. It was admirably conciliatory in tone and was tantamount to a total reassurance. 'The President Censors and remanent Members' were at pains to declare that they had never contemplated encroaching on the Fraternity's 'just priviledges' and that they were still resolved to 'support them in all their lawfull designes'. Picturesquely it was said 'all jealousie of any such invasion . . . may be taken off'. Then followed the Explanation proper. The College undertook not to take 'tryall of any of the intrants' who had not been previously examined by the Fraternity and recommended to the College for further 'tryall': and 'notwithstanding thereof, they shall again submitt these intrants to the Fraternity . . . without imposing upon the . . . Fraternity to admit . . . untill they be fullie satisfied . . .'.[5]

SYMPATHY FOR SIMPLE APOTHECARIES

That the sympathies of the College were with the simple apothecaries there can be no question. This view is substantiated by another manuscript unearthed by Poole, and with no corresponding reference in available Minutes. It had marked on the back 'Act of the College of Physicians anent the simple apothecaries 1684' and dealt with the Decreet of Separation of those practising surgery and pharmacy. 'The Colledge of Physicians' the document declared 'having soon after their erection, taken into their consideration, the great importance of this Separation . . . did harmoniously resolve to concurr with the Apothecaries in getting their Decreet of Declaratour made effectual'. Then followed a most colourful if slightly unctuous declaration on the part of the College!! 'Seeing the Indulged Chyrurgeon–Apothecaries do still make a noise and clamour as if they were able to withstand authority, and render the foresaid Decreet elusory, and for that end falsely pretend that some Members of the Colledge of Physicians joyn with them: Therefore the Colledge . . . for the vindication of their own honour and interest especialy for the safety and security of the Practice of Medicine . . . DO declare that they do adhere to the foresaid Decreet . . . and that they will endeavour by all just and legal means to render the said Decreet effectual . . .'.[6]

APPOINTMENT OF VISITORS—SUBTLE TACTICS

The situation was not helped when in 1684 the surgeons gave notice of their intention to continue admitting intrant apothecaries and, with the connivance of the Town Council, secured the appointment of a surgeon as 'sole Visitor' for the purposes of the Apothecaries Act. The College of Surgeons and Town Council did not desist and in 1687 a chirurgeon–apothecary was again nominated for the post of Visitor. According to Eccles, after considering a petition by the apothecaries the Lords of Session discharged the persons nominated by the Town Council and appointed a simple apothecary as Visitor.[7]

Then in 1699 an agreement between the College and the apothecaries of Edinburgh was approved whereby certain named apothecaries were 'obleidged ilk ane of them to pay to the colledge . . . for the tyme the soume of Ane Thowsand punds Scotts money and a rent yrof yrin sped if at any tyme any of the sds persons shall enter into or aggrie with the Chirurgeons for ther fredooms'. The President of the College was bound 'in twelve Hundreth merks of penaltie', and each of the apothecaries 'in ane Hundreth punds Scotts of penaltie in caice of faylzie by and attour performance of the sd. aggriement'. As was his due the President was assured by the College of indemnification for any loss or expense he might sustain. Legally the agreement was based on 'the decreit of separation prounced [sic] by the Lords of Counsell in . . . 1682'.[8] In August 1701 the President and Censors were instructed to visit 'the Appothecary's Shops',[9] a recommendation which was repeated four years later.[10] Seemingly all did not go smoothly because the next year a Committee was appointed by the College 'to Consider and give theire opinion upon some things relateing to the Visitatione of the apothecaries Shopes'[11]; and within two weeks, at the next sederunt, the Committee were urged 'to meet again alsoone as they can conveniently and give their opinion what is the most proper method of visiteing the apothecaries shopes'.[12] A report was forthcoming in 13 days and once more the President and Censors were recommended to carry out visits, but on this occasion 'alsoone as they can conveniently with the Concurrence of a Magistrat and such tuo apothecaries as shall be appoynted to go alongst with them.'[13]

An early outcome was that the President and the two Censors obtained advice from an Advocate which was submitted for study by a specially appointed Committee.[14, 15] Although instructed to report to the next sederunt the Committee is not recorded as having done so.[16] The questions put to the Advocate concerned 'maintaining of the priviledges of the Colledge, the visiteing the apothecaries shops and other concerns of that nature'. It is more than probable that the Advocate's advice gave rise to a resolution passed by the College in the following year to the effect that 'the Rights and Priviledges granted to the Physitians by King and parliament are totaly evacuated and virtually rescinded They Doe therefor Resolve and each man for himself sincerelie promeis and Declair That they will stand by one another In Defence of the honor of their professione and the Rights and priviledges of their Societie'.[17]

SURGEON–APOTHECARIES ON THE OFFENSIVE

After an interval of many years a joint meeting of the College and the Chirurgeon-apothecaries 'for Regulateing of Pharmacy In this place' was arranged.[18] A report was not produced in the time ordained. Indeed the College seemed to be too absorbed with the perplexities of the Cold Bath! However a complication was not long in arising with the submission to the Town Council by the Surgeon-apothecaries 'craveing That non for the future Should Exercise the apothecarys art within the

Citty of Edgr. . . . But such as were or should be only tryed and Examined by them.'[19] No notice of this manoeuvre had been given to the College. Legal advice was got without delay and a true Representation of the Rights and priviledges of the College was transmitted to the Town Council. There followed a meeting between the lawyers representing the College and apothecaries. No agreement was reached.[20] The College then adopted another line of approach, directing the former Committee 'to Inquyre when the act uniteing Churgerie and Pharmacy comes in to be Considered by the Toun Councill . . . That the said Committee attend the Councill and there In the name of the Colledge To Declair That they adhere to their Representatione formerly given in . . .'.[21]

In a number of respects the position of the College of Physicians was invidious. Historically the physicians based their claim to undertake the visitation of apothecaries' shops on their Royal Charter whereas the surgeons based theirs on a series of Acts of the Town Council dated from 1641 to 1657. The Court of Session decreeing separation of the arts of surgery and pharmacy had ruled that these acts should be rescinded in so far as skilled, as opposed to apprentice apothecaries were concerned.[22] Understandably the attitude of the apothecaries was conditioned by the Court of Session ruling. To add to the complexity of the situation, from the year 1702 apothecaries had received training from Instructors at the College of Surgeons in chemistry and later in pharmaceutical processes. Nor did this cease when the Royal Public Dispensary, founded in 1776 largely as a result of the persistence of Dr Andrew Duncan of our College, organized classes in pharmacy which in the course of time assumed the status of a School of Pharmacy. This school acquired a national reputation and ultimately became a constituent member of the Heriot-Watt College— now the Heriot-Watt University.[23]

FELLOWS WARNED

And still the sultry atmosphere persisted. Twenty-six years later a member, at a Quarterly Meeting of the College, represented that a custom had developed of taking a 'Degree of Doctor of Medicine to Exercise likewise the Employment of Surgeons or appothecarys or both'.[24] An act was passed declaring 'That no person who is a member of the Corporation of Surgeons or apothecarys, Or who keeps a Shop for Dispensing of medicines Shall hereafter be admitted a fellow of the Colledge'. At the same time it was decreed that any Fellow of the College who 'enters' with the Corporation of Surgeon–apothecaries or 'sets up' a shop for dispensing of medicine, the thing being 'notour' would forfeit all the 'priviledges and Immunitys' of a Fellow and have his name 'Expunged out of the Roll of fellows'. The phraseology certainly conveys a sense of impressive determination. Moreover it was further ordained that every Licentiate, when admitted a Fellow, should have the act read to him 'That he may not pretend Ignorance therof'.[25] Not wholly satisfied, the College passed yet another act in the course of about three and a half years with the avowed object of preventing the abuse by any Fellows or Licentiates of keeping or setting up an apothecary shop. This interdict applied not only to a Fellow or Licentiate but also to his partners or servants: and it was required of any applicant for a licence regardless of the source of his Degree that he first 'enact and oblige himself' to adhere to the demands of the act. Any applicant who was practising Pharmacy had to cease the practice and give the same undertakings before his application received consideration. From the preamble to the act it is evident that the practice of combining 'Physick with Pharmacy' had developed significantly among physicians licensed by the College.[26]

A NOVELTY FAILS TO MATERIALIZE

The apothecaries did not always indulge in guerrilla tactics. In 1754 they made an undisguised frontal counter attack when they informed the College of their intention 'to Erect a dispensary for Supplying themselves with medicines of the Best kind both Chymical and Galenical'. The information was contained in a memorial from the Incorporation of Surgeon–apothecarys and commenced with a homily on 'the Low State of Pharmacy in this Country'. Coupled with this admission was a diplomatic 'desire to Cultivate that harmony and Relation that naturally Subsists Between the Royal Colledge of Physicians, and the Community' of surgeon–apothecaries; astutely followed by a protestation that they would never contemplate embarking on the Dispensary project 'without first Communicating their designe to the Colledge'. Then and only then was the design unfolded! Ingredients of every 'Compounded medicine' were 'to be faithfully prepared . . . according to the Pharmacopiea of the Royal Colledge'; and the College was assured it would not be 'at a Loss thro the want of any particular or Rare medicine' as it was proposed to supply 'Such of these as are not Commonly to be found in the Shops'. To complete the cajoling the Dispensary undertook to 'observe the Smallest hint from any member of the Colledge, with Regard to any particular medicine they Incline to use'.[27]

The College decided that it should 'make ane answer thereto, Lest their Silence might be Interpret to be ane approbation of their Intended Scheme'. Both gracious-ness and subtlety characterized the opening sections of the reply sent! Allowing great interest in the subject, the College admitted to success in Physick being con-siderably dependent upon 'the goodness and faithful preparation of the medicines' prescribed: and indicated that in giving 'advice and Countenance' they would employ their powers 'To Incourage and Inforce the Regular practise, and to Restrain the abuses Committed' in the important art of pharmacy. The surgeon–apothecaries were then advised that medicine and pharmacy should be developed separately and 'that Pharmacy alone, is Sufficient to occupy the appothecarys whole time and attention'. In their discouragement of the scheme the College commented upon the disadvantages to apprentices no matter 'how Convenient or usefull . . . to the mas-ters'.[28] Not to be outdone in the matter of conventional courtesy the Incorporation of Chirurgeon–apothecaries said they 'should be exceeding sorry if the proposition they have made . . . should occasion any difference or misunderstanding betwixt them and the Royal College, for whom they have all the Regard due to that Learned Body'.[29]

LEST THERE SHOULD BE MISUNDERSTANDING!

Means of effectively separating the practice of physic and pharmacy were for long a matter of active concern to the College, and in 1761 a decision was arrived at to publish their views in the local newspapers. This was largely actuated by recognition of the fact that implementation of the College Act of 11th April 1754 (Chaps. XIX and XXVI) had been ineffective.[30] The 'advertisements' as they were misleadingly called, outlined in cryptic terms the responsibilities of the College to the inhabitants of Edinburgh, gave the views of the College concerning pharmaceutical practice and its relations to physic, and referred to action taken to date by the College. Finally it was stated that to prevent 'abuses for the future, the Said Royal College, do hereby Certifie all whom it may Concern That they are Resolved to prosecute, as their Patent authorizes and directs them to do, all Such who without their Licence . . . shall . . . assume the title of Doctor of Physick, and prescribe for the Internal diseases of the Inhabitants of Edinburgh . . . and that they have unanimously determined, not to Consult with, or otherwise Consider Such unlicenced practitioners, as Physicians, and that it may be known who are at present Fellows of their College, or Licenced by them to Practice Physick, a List of Both is hereunto annexed . . .'. The list gave the names of twenty-eight Fellows and six Licentiates. Only the places of residence were missing![(31)]

The Act of April 1754 came up for review in 1764 when it was decided that no alteration with regard to its application to Licentiates was called for because the regulatory powers of the College did not 'extend beyond the Libertys of the City of Edinr.'. At the same time expression was given to the view that in so far as Fellows were concerned 'on accot. of Particular Circumstances it may be allowable for them to keep shops or Practise Pharmacy, abroad, Especially in the plantations'. The embargo on such activities by Fellows within Great Britain or Ireland still held good.[(32)]

Some years later the College were faced with a novel and at the same time legally puzzling problem. A request was received from a practising apothecary and druggist to be examined on his knowledge and skill in Pharmacy and if found sufficiently qualified to be given 'a licence to Continue in the practice of that Branch of Medicine'. He also asked that 'a visitation of his Shop and Laboratory' be made by appointment.[(33)] Beginning from strength and terminating in weakness, the reply from the College asserted its statutory right 'To visit the Shops and Chambers of the appothecarys and all others who vend and dispense Drugs within the City', but that with regard to the other specific points raised in the apothecary's petition 'the further Consideration thereof Should be delayed untill the College think of some more effectuall methods of Regulating the Practice of Pharmacy according to the Rights and privileges of the Royal College of Physicians'. Lacking venturesomeness maybe, the reply was none the less wise.[(34)]

The question of 'examination of Apothecaries and their Medicines etc' was raised by a member in November 1787 and subsequently considered at several meetings.[(35)] On more than one occasion final discussion was postponed for 'still further deliberation'.[(36)] Eventually a Committee was appointed but it cannot be said its report contributed much to any clarification of policy. Formal visitation of shops was considered to have detrimental rather than beneficial results, but importance was attached to the practice of pharmacy in the shops being inspected and to the prosecution of 'delinquents'.[(37)] It was about this time that the College was instrumental in introducing 'glass measures and Laudanum vials' of their own choice to apothecaries' shops.[(38)] Some nine years later in the course of discussion at a Quarterly Meeting of Dr Harrison's plan for medical reform (Chap. XI), a motion was proposed that the Royal College of Surgeons should be asked to co-operate in carrying out the examination of apothecaries' shops as required by Act of Parliament.[(39)] At a later meeting, although the existence of abuses was acknowledged, it was considered inexpedient to proceed with the motion.[40] Eventually some degree of finality was reached in connection with the oft-quoted Act of 1754. On 6th May 1823 the part of that Act relating to the practice of Pharmacy was altered to read as follows:

> 'If any Fellow or Licentiate of the College shall, by himself, or copartners, or servants, keep a public Apothecary, Druggist or Chemist shop, he shall ipso facto forfeit all the rights and privileges which he does or may enjoy as a Fellow or Licentiate of the said College, and his name shall be expunged from the List.'[41]

In 1826, the progress through Parliament of a Bill presented by the Apothecaries of London was observed with considerable misgivings by the College.[42] Consideration was given to submitting a Petition but there is no evidence of its having materialized.[43] On the other hand a petition was sent by the Royal College of Surgeons to Parliament, and a copy to the Royal College of Physicians. The Surgeons' petition took grave exception to the monopoly acquired by the Society of Apothecaries of London under the Act of 1815 enabling them to insist on all who practised as apothecaries in England and Wales being licensed by them. It submitted that Licentiates of the Royal College of Surgeons, and others in possession of testimonials or Diplomas from different public bodies should be exempted from application of the monopoly rights of the Apothecaries Company.[44] There is no note of any report which may have been made by the Committee appointed by the College of Physicians to study the position, nor indeed any evidence that the College of Surgeons' note received acknowledgement. Dealing with mutual distrust, it is perhaps not unreasonable to ask—was the College of Physicians concerned that the case of apothecaries as distinct from surgeons should have been so vigorously espoused by the Surgeons?

An Extraordinary Meeting of our College was called in April 1833 to consider the Apothecaries Act with particular reference to clauses limiting the dispensing of medicines in England and Wales to those having the Licence of the Apothecaries Company of London. The College was informed that the Senate of the University and other medical bodies were striving to secure amendment of the Act.[45] A decision to send a petition was arrived at, but before agreement was reached there were conflicting opinions as to the form to be adopted.[46] Subsequent developments over the Apothecaries Act became increasingly involved in the whole question of Medical Reform dealt with in Chapters XI and XII.

BREAKING THE SABBATH DAY

What might be termed a local swan-song in miniature among these persisting differences between physicians and apothecaries took place in 1839 when some of the latter in Edinburgh decided to shut their shops during the time of Divine Service. The College took exception to this and declared that 'one qualified person should be in attendance . . . at all hours, Sundays not excepted'.[47] Something of a furore among the medical profession in general resulted from the action of the apothecaries,[48] who eventually adopted proposals put to them by a Joint Committee of the Colleges of Physicians and Surgeons and of practitioners not Members of either College. The proposals contemplated closure of the shops all day but with an assistant available inside, it being accepted that many druggists would find it adequate to provide even this degree of accessibility at certain hours only.[49] Little can the College have expected one outcome of their involvement in the problem of Sunday closure! A memorial was received from, of all people—the Druggists' Assistants and Apprentices in Edinburgh and Leith, outlining the excessive hours worked and their inability to attend to their studies. Inexpert in arbitration, the College in its undoubted wisdom felt obliged 'to decline interfering in the matter betwixt the Petitioners and their Employers'.[50]

MEDICINE AND SURGERY

We [Physicians and Surgeons] are certainly a most amiable brotherhood . . . Yet, whatever the majority of us may be, I am afraid we are not all perfect angels.

James Gregory

When account is taken of the crudely disparaging attitude adopted towards the surgeons in the early unsuccessful petitions for a College of Physicians, and of the remorseless attempts at every turn of the surgeons to thwart the ambitions of the physicians, it is not to be wondered at that the mutual antagonism between the two bodies persisted for many years. Youthful factions today might argue that it is not yet wholly resolved.

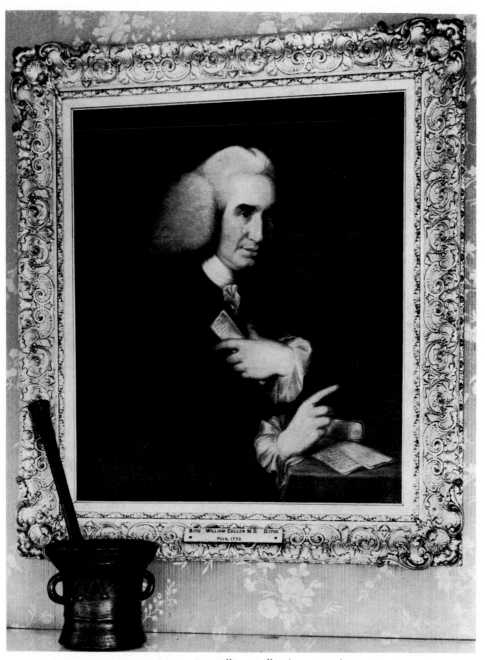

PLATE 19   Dr William Cullen (1710–1790)
Reproduced from a copy in the College of original portrait by William Cochrane;
photograph by George B. Alden

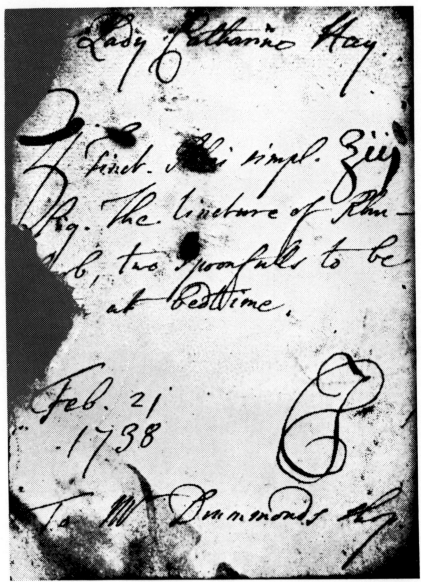

PLATE 20   Eighteenth–century prescription for Lady Catherine Hay of the Tweeddale family bearing
the initials 'J.C.' of Dr John Clerk (1738)
Reproduced from manuscript in the College

THE SURGEONS SEEK A CHARTER

Without doubt antipathy towards the College was favoured by events preceding the year 1681, and the part played by individual physicians in the separation of the two callings of surgery and pharmacy did not help matters (Chap. III). The Court ruling at that time was that surgeons were not to compound medicines to be taken inwardly by mouth, although permitted to buy and sell 'simples' and compound drugs necessary for surgical and external application. In 1686 the Surgeons endeavoured to get a new Charter.[51] According to the records of the Surgeons a 'signature' or writing ready for the seal of Royal Warrant was on the instructions of the Secret Council to be sent to the Physicians and other persons interested. Inevitably much trouble ensued and the 'signature' instead of being sealed was consigned to the archives.[52] King James VII granted a signed patent but Parliament failed to ratify it in 1693.

It is uncertain if the 'signature' was seen by the College of Physicians. That they knew of it there can be no question because, at a Sederunt on 9th December 1686 with the President (Sir Andrew Balfour) in the Chair it was resolved unanimously that 'the Colledge should pursue for a reduction of the said Patent of Chirurgions . . . before the Lords of Session'. Poole provided the information, commenting at the same time that 'this minute, of course, is not in the Books now extant, being within *the blank period*'.[53] He also quoted from a letter written in 1686 which 'is marked on the back, in a later hand, as follows: "Copy of a Letter written by order of the College to the Secretary . . . at London, petitioning about a Reduction of the Surgeons' Patent, and seems to have been wrote before the Ratification of the said Patent in Parliament".' According to Poole 'the Patent objected to is that of Windsor 25 Sept[r] 1686, which was not ratified'.[54] The letter was long and subservient in its appeal that the King might be persuaded to support the plea of the College of Physicians. The phraseology was mellifluous in the extreme recalling how 'justice and equitie' had 'been alwayes most resplendent in all his [the King's] actions, and a considerable part of that character whereby Kings so much resemble God'. With delightful delicacy Poole commented at this stage, 'The writer was quite in fashion!' Fortunately or unfortunately, the document was a copy and unsigned—but there is reason to believe the writer was Sibbald.[55]

A second attempt made by the Surgeons in 1694 was successful and the resulting patent reunited the arts of surgery and pharmacy, and confirmed all the grants in favour of the surgeon–barbers and the surgeon–apothecaries. No opposition was offered by the Physicians who according to one historian 'had established more

I

friendly relations with the surgeons'.[56] Subsequent events at an early stage scarcely bore this out. A College Minute dated 27th September 1694, from which it appears the initiative came from the Surgeons, stated: 'The Deacon of the Chirurgeons had proposed to severall members of the Colledge his earnest Desyre for ane accomodatione betwixt the Colledge and there calling anent some Differences that may fall out betwixt them'. Almost certainly, although not specified, the question of a Charter being obtained by the Surgeons was in the mind of the Deacon. The Surgeons' informal approach was favourably received and certain Fellows of our College named 'to meet and receive any proposalls from the Chirurgeons'.[57]

AMNESTY AMIDST CONFUSION

In May of the following year the College were informed of the Surgeons' intention to secure early ratification of their Patent. Rancour came to boiling point on the instant and a Committee was charged with employing all possible means to stop the ratification. The College's determination was given practical expression by instructing the Treasurer to advance money to the Committee which was empowered to disburse it and 'to chuse Lawyers'. At the same meeting Dr Dickson, a Fellow, was instructed to attend the Secretary and 'give him thanks for his obleidging Letter and to crave his countenance and protectione'.[58] As there is no previous reference to the letter it is difficult to be certain as to whose interests the Secretary represented. If he was one of the Surgeons, then the tone of the College Minute is out of character. Unrepentant, on 5th July (1695) the College reaffirmed their intention to pursue their course of obstruction.[59] Then within four days there is engrossed another curiously contradictory record. 'The Qlk day the colledge have appoynted dr Dicksone to meet with the chirurgeon Apothecarys and fully conclude all differences betwixt the Colledge and them concerning the Chirurgeons ratificatione . . .'.[60]

The next Minute is dated 14th September 1695, on which day it was recorded that the sederunt 'mett at the Presidents ledgeings being denyed the keys of the Colledge by doctor Stevenston'.[61] There is no trace of any kind, nor any mention of the obliteration of any record for the month of August, and yet Creswell referred unhesitatingly to 'Minutes of the Royal College of Physicians (6th August 1695)'.[56] Accepting his information as being entirely accurate, the Minutes in question had an unmistakable significance. They were to the effect that Dr David Dickson having been commissioned to negotiate with the surgeon–apothecaries was satisfied that all the rights and privileges of the physicians were reserved, and agreed not to oppose ratification. According to the same source, there was manifest approval of Dr Dickson's action in a Statement made to the College by its President.

There is confirmation of Creswell's statement in three documents in the Archives of the College. Of these the first is the Commission of the College to Dr Dickson on action to be taken on their behalf concerning the ratification of the surgeon–apothecaries. The Commission was brief and to the point, signed by the President (Dr Trotter), and dated the 9th Day of July 1695.[62] The second document gave the text of Dr Dickson's agreement verbatim. It was as follows:

> 'I David Dickson, Doctor of Medicine, by vertue of a Commission from the Said Cole. am content and satisfied that the ratification given in by the Sur^n Apoths. to the present session of parl^t shall pass in the terms following—viz: Providing alwayes that the present ratificatione shall be noe ways prejudiciale to a former patent of erection of the R. Coll. P. at Edin: in Novr 1681 years, but that all their liberties priviledges and immunities contained in their said patent be reserved intire to them such like as if thir presents had never been granted. And furder more in name of the C. of P. I shall take up and pass from the petitione given in to the parl^t by the said Colledge against the ratificatione of the Surgeon–Apothecaries patent. In witness whereof &c. &c. (dated 11th July 1695 and subscribed etc.)'[63]

The third document purported to be a reproduction of the 'approbation' of Dr Dickson's declaration by the President of the College, Dr Trotter.

> 'I undersubscribed doe declare in name of the Coll. that whereas we have ridd marches with the Surgeons of Edin: we will not anie manner of way oppose the re-uniting of Surgery and Pharmacy; and seeing Dr. Dickson was fully empowered by us to settle with the Surgeons, I doe by this homologate what he hath done in this business in name forsaid. Att. Edin: this 22nd of July 1695 years (sic subscribitur &c.)'[64]

As Poole commented, Dr Trotter went 'beyond Dr. Dickson' when he declared 'we will not &c oppose the re-uniting of Surgery and Pharmacy' for which neither the Commission to nor the consent of Dr Dickson gave authority.

Had the College's tactics been those of 'Brinkmanship'? To judge by the tenor of the records this is unlikely, and it is more probable that the College deliberately and courageously made a Churchillian change of course requiring neither excuse nor apologia. Certainly the desired hope of peace between the two callings was fulfilled for a period of several years, only to be broken when the College fined the Surgeon Nisbet for practising medicine (Chap. VIII). A succession of court actions followed, involving the Lord High Chancellor, the Earl of Seafield. In March 1707 the College decided to accede to a proposal made by the Lord Chancellor 'that the Earle of Leven should meet and commune for the Colledge with such other persone as the Chirurgeons should appoynt' for a friendly agreement between the College and the chirurgeons.[65, 66] None the less the College was obviously consumed with apprehension because it unanimously recommended to the President and every member of the Society 'to use their outmost diligence . . . and to Informe the members of parliat. that justice may be done to the Colledge'.[67]

HOSPITAL RIVALRY

Another situation arose in 1737 capable of creating misunderstanding. The Infirmary at that time was known to Surgeons as the Physicians Hospital because association of Surgeons with it was as individuals, and not as a body. Because in their view the Infirmary was unable to meet the demands being made upon it and because they wished to participate in the charitable work of the city, the Surgeons established a hospital for surgical patients only—known as the Surgeons Hospital. There were the makings of an explosive situation. Fortunately, however, difficulties were effectively if slowly resolved (Chap. XXI).

ACADEMIC ASPIRATIONS

A few years later the Incorporation of Surgeons reinforced their attitude by publicly advertising their approval of highly successful private systematic and clinical lectures in surgery given by a surgeon named James Rae, who was elected their Deacon in 1764.[68] At the time, in accordance with established custom, surgery was included in the University anatomy course given by Monro *secundus* who was a physician with minimal if any knowledge of practical as distinct from theoretical surgery. In 1776 the Surgeons considered a proposal to seek a regius chair of surgery in the University. A Committee appointed by them reported 'That as the Professors of Anatomy and Midwifery have of late connected themselves with the Royal College [of Physicians], the members should also have in their view by a proper direction of their Studies to qualify themselves for supplying future vacancies in these different professions which seem naturally to arise from the College of Surgeons . . .'.[69] The Professor of Anatomy referred to was Monro *secundus* who became a Fellow of the College of Physicians in 1759: and the Professor of Midwifery, Dr Thomas Young who had been Deacon of the Incorporation in 1756 and was elected a Fellow of the Physicians College in 1762. Despite their apparent reasonableness the proposals did not come to immediate fruition, but a University chair in Clinical Surgery was eventually founded in 1803.

MIDWIFERY POSES A PROBLEM

Although not involving the College of Physicians directly the concern of the Incorporation of Surgeons to establish their legal position in relation to the practice of midwifery had some interesting sequellae. In 1769 the Incorporation took the advice of Counsel upon privileges contained in their Charter of 1694 touching on the boundaries between the physicians and surgeons. In particular the question arose as to whether midwifery did not belong exclusively to surgeons, more especially as physicians by their Charter were excluded from performing any sort of manual operation which it was argued must be interpreted as including midwifery. Counsel to whom the question was directed gave it as his opinion 'that if midwifery did exclusively belong, either to the Physicians or the Surgeons, it does seem more naturally to belong to the art of the latter than that of the former'. He amplified his opinion on the same question by concluding 'there is no room for entering into a discussion to settle the boundaries betwixt the Physicians and Surgeons as to this point . . .'.[70]

Midwifery again necessitated the former Incorporation, now College, of Surgeons to obtain legal advice in the following century. The Surgeons' College took exception to a Licentiate of the College of Physicians advertising his midwifery lectures as entitling those attending to appear before the College of Surgeons for a diploma. The point at issue was that lecturers had to be members of one of the Colleges and being a Licentiate did not constitute membership. Interestingly, the Licentiate involved was the one who was advanced to Fellowship only on the third occasion of balloting (Chap. VIII). His altercation with the Surgeons was followed by a not altogether dissimilar case which accelerated the College of Surgeons in their search for a legal view. A significant answer was given by Counsel to the question—is a Licentiate of the College of Physicians of Edinburgh to be considered a Member of that body? It ran:

'. . . If in common speech a licentiate of the College of Physicians was styled a member of the College . . . the term licentiate must be taken in that acceptation.'

Referring to the position of the Colleges of Physicians in London and Dublin the reply continued:

> '. . . I think it is clear that the licentiates of the College of Physicians of Edinburgh must be held to have been placed upon the same footing.'[71]

VILLAINY OF SURGEONS DECLARED!

The year 1817 found the College considering the *Bill for the Regulation of Surgery*, which was the subject of a Report eventually transmitted to the Attorney General. Previously on 17th May 1815 the President (Dr James Hamilton, jun.) had occasion to write the Marquis of Douglas and Clydesdale. The letter was concerned with the practice of medicine by the surgeons in a way with which 'Brethren of London' had not to contend. Amusing if decorative analogies were employed. Lunacy not being a surgical disease, surgeons it was avowed had 'no more title' to be employed than the Faculty of Advocates! Surgeons the letter declared, were practising illegally and if they had acquired the confidence of the public as medical practitioners, they resembled others dealing in 'contraband goods' who had won public favour! Attention was drawn to the potential advantage to the surgeons of having a Deacon in the Town Council: and a complaint was voiced that the surgeons had 'managed to impress the minds of the people here, that it is impossible to separate the two departments of the profession'.[72] The undeclared fears of the physicians were ill-concealed!

Admittedly the Report of 1817 was repetitive and used to ventilate chronic grievances, but none the less was of interest in that it revealed the attitude of the physician to other disciplines. Essentially the Report aimed at the extension of the Bill's provisions to all branches of the profession, and more especially to the practice of Medicine. Some surprising statements were made in support of this objective. Thus it was said that of all maladies calling for professional treatment '19 out of 20 are medical and do not require any surgical aid': 'Surgical aid is certainly not more frequently needed in the practice of midwifery than in the practice of medicine': and 'all the most celebrated accoucheurs have been and are at this moment Physicians'. Discussing what today is referred to as general practice it was maintained that 'the most ignorant person' may enter it and could 'practice in every respect, as 99 Surgeons out of 100 practise at this moment, without coming within the reach of the proposed Law'. Then followed an unexpectedly comprehensive profession of honesty:

'The Medical Man administers his remedies, often unknown, for inward diseases, and it is frequently impossible to distinguish between the effect of the Medicine and the natural progress of the Malady, hence his ignorance escapes detection . . .'

Nor did the surgeon escape scatheless in the Report which declared:

'the awkwardness and want of skill of the Operator in Surgery instantly betray themselves, and banish all confidence in the future.'

But, throughout the Report there is a subtlety which, when recognized, implies a distinct difference between 'the Medical Man' and the Physician. Suggesting that legislation should embrace medicine as well as surgery, 'and all persons engaged in the exercise of the profession' it emphasized the necessity of everyone being submitted to examination *excepting* those who have obtained the Degrees of M.B. or M.D.'. And what of the proposed examination?—'as the practice of Phisic would necessarily constitute the far greater part . . . at least an equal share in the business . . . should fall to the Colleges of Physicians'. But all was not acquisitive in the Report. There was even a hint of delicious self-appraisal as witness—'. . . one effect of the present Bill would be to give a weight and consideration as well as revenue to the Royal College of Surgeons of which the Royal College of Physicians of Edinburgh conceive that the place they have for a Century and a half held in the estimation of the public entitle them to at least an equal share'. An interesting subsidiary recommendation was that as thinly populated areas do not provide for 'a well educated Man of the Profession', authority should be given to those who have not obtained the Testimonials required by the Bill, to practise in those areas.[73]

ADULTERATION OF DRUGS

Almost two decades later the Surgeons expressed concern over the adulteration of medicines by both wholesale and retail dealers, and asked that the College join with them in 'putting a stop to the nefarious practice'.[74] This the College agreed to do and referred the matter to their Pharmacopoeia Committee, the Report of which was ordered to be published but does not seem to be mentioned again in the records.[75, 76] Two things may have contributed to this. A minority of members considered that criticism of the retail dealers was too severe, and the Committee involved was actively engaged in producing a new edition of the *Edinburgh Pharmacopoeia* to which they would almost certainly give priority.[77, 78]

Nevertheless (Sir) Robert Christison who was Secretary of the Committee and personally responsible for the Appendix accompanying the College Report[79] did express satisfaction with the eventual outcome. In his biography he is quoted as saying that 'the College Report, the simultaneous inquiries of Dr. Pereira in London, and the efforts of the newly founded Pharmaceutical Society of Great Britain, soon greatly abated the practice of adulterating drugs'.[80] Considered in retrospect the College Report is interesting. It expressed conviction that adulteration was carried out on a considerable scale, a strong case existed for the better education of pharmacists, and that improvement would follow methodical visitation of public shops.

Each of these and other points were dealt with in considerable detail in Christison's Appendix. After giving concrete instances of adulteration which covered drugs in common usage (e.g. iodine, spirit of nitric ether, hydrocyanic acid, strychnine, opium and laudanum) the Appendix outlined how, depending upon the source and method of distribution, adulteration might be attributable to the foreign producer, the merchant abroad, and in England—the drug-broker, wholesaler and retailer. In keeping with his forensic ability Christison gave an unmistakable impression of his views without exposing himself or the College to the risk of actions for libel. At the same time he pointed out how unscrupulous action on the part of some could be traced to insistence on uneconomic prices by the ultimate purchaser.

Of greater historical interest are Christison's constructive suggestions accepted by the College. Two have already been mentioned. On the subject of 'visitation of public shops' he commented 'It is true that the Colleges of Physicians of London and Edinburgh possess the right of visitation, and that this right has been long abandoned by the latter College, and is practised by the former with no material good effect'. Pursuing his argument and drawing on continental experience, he broached the possibility of visiting being made the responsibility of the most eminent members of a body equivalent to the Pharmaceutical Colleges of France and Germany. Christison also suggested that visitations should embrace the warehouses of wholesale druggists.

By the time of publication of the Report effect had already been given to another of Christison's recommendations. This consisted of an addition to the College *Pharmacopoeia* drawing the attention of practitioners and druggists to 'the most simple and accurate criterions for determining the requisite purity of drugs, and their freedom from certain known impurities'. Christison in the Appendix commented that an alteration along these lines had already been resolved upon by the Edinburgh College and been proposed 'to the sister college of London in the course of certain negotiations towards the establishment of a conjunct or National Pharmacopoeia'. Disinclined to change at first, the London College had later, again to use Christison's words, 'endeavoured to adopt it [the proposal] in the late edition of their Pharmacopoeia', but in a way which left him in some doubts.[80]

CONCERN ABOUT THE FUTURE

Initiative was again shown by the Surgeons when their Royal College (with a Charter dating back to May 1778) communicated with the Royal College of Physicians seeking a Conference with Committees of the College and Medical Faculty of the University, on the present state and future prospects of the Profession. The request had particularly in mind a meeting of those representing the same interests four years previously when the medical curriculum of the University was discussed,[81] and of a recent meeting representative of the three Royal Colleges of Surgeons. The Joint Committee had its first meeting within four days.[82] This may be regarded as one of the early moves to achieve professional unity with Medical Reform looming on the horizon.

REFERENCES

(1) DRUMMOND, C. G. (1953) *Pharmacy and Medicine in Old Edinburgh*, p. 7. London: Pharmaceutical Press.

PHYSICK AND PHARMACY

(2) POOLE, R. (1838) *Preparatory Notes for a History of the College*, p. 49. (Ms.)
(3) Ibid., p. 50.
(4) Ibid., p. 53.
(5) Ibid., p. 54.
(6) Ibid., p. 55.
(7) [ECCLES, W.] (1707) *An Historical Account of the Rights and Priviledges of the Royal College of Physicians, and of the Incorporation of Chirurgions in Edinburgh*, p. 18. [Edinburgh: Privately printed.]
(8) College Minutes, 19.vi.1699.
(9) Ibid., 25.viii.1701.
(10) Ibid., 30.viii.1705.
(11) Ibid., 29.i.1706.
(12) Ibid., 12.ii.1706.
(13) Ibid., 25.ii.1706.
(14) Ibid., 18.vi.1706.
(15) Ibid., 25.vii.1706.

(16) Ibid., 5.viii.1706.

(17) Ibid., 19.ii.1707.

(18) Ibid., 4.vi.1723.

(19) Ibid., 4.ii.1724.

(20) Ibid., 14.viii.1724.

(21) Ibid., 8.xi.1724.

(22) CRESWELL, C. H. (1926) *The Royal College of Surgeons of Edinburgh. Historical notes from 1505 to 1905*, pp. 119–20. Edinburgh: Oliver & Boyd.

(23) GILMOUR, J. P. (1938) Phases of pharmacy in Edinburgh. *Quarterly Journal of Pharmacy and Pharmacology*, **XI**, 358.

(24) College Minutes, 6.ii.1750.

(25) Ibid., 6.xi.1750.

(26) Ibid., 11.iv.1754.

(27) Ibid., 7.v.1754.

(28) Ibid., 6.viii.1754.

(29) CRESWELL, C. H. Op. cit., p. 143.

(30) College Minutes, 4.viii.1761.

(31) Ibid., 3.xi.1761.

(32) Ibid., 1.v.1764.

(33) Ibid., 7.viii.1770.

(34) Ibid., 21.viii.1770.

(35) Ibid., 6.xi.1787.

(36) Ibid., 1.ii.1791.

(37) Ibid., 2.viii.1791.

(38) Ibid., 7.ii.1792.

(39) Ibid., 4.xi.1806.

(40) Ibid., 3.ii.1807.

(41) Ibid., 5.xi.1822.

(42) Ibid., 4.iv.1826.

(43) Ibid., 11.iv.1826.

(44) Ibid., 14.vi.1827.

(45) Ibid., 8.iv.1833.

(46) Ibid., 16.iv.1833.

(47) Ibid., 13.iii.1839.

(48) Ibid., 3.iv.1839.

(49) Ibid., 7.v.1839.

(50) Ibid., 5.ii.1839.

MEDICINE AND SURGERY

(51) CRESWELL, C. H. Op. cit., p. 116.

(52) Ibid., p. 119.

(53) POOLE, R. Op. cit., p. 62.

(54) Ibid., p. 64.

(55) Ibid., p. 67.

(56) CRESWELL, C. H. Op. cit., p. 121.

(57) College Minutes, 27.ix.1694.

(58) Ibid., 17.v.1695.

(59) Ibid., 5.vii.1695.

(60) Ibid., 9.vii.1695.

(61) Ibid., 14.ix.1695.

(62) R.C.P.E. (1695) *Miscellaneous papers*, no. 85, 9.vii.1695.

(63) R.C.P.E. (1695) *Miscellaneous papers*, no. 86, 11.vii.1695. [Transcript.]

(64) R.C.P.E. (1695) *Miscellaneous papers*, no. 87, 22.vii.1695. [Transcript.]

(65) College Minutes, 5.iii.1707.

(66) Ibid., 7.iii.1707.

(67) Ibid., 13.iii.1707.

(68) ROYAL COLLEGE OF SURGEONS OF EDINBURGH. *Minutes*, 27.viii.1772.

(69) ROYAL COLLEGE OF SURGEONS OF EDINBURGH. *Minutes*, 30.x.1776.

(70) CRESWELL, C. H. Op. cit., p. 168.

(71) Ibid., p. 177.

(72) R.C.P.E. (1815) *General Correspondence*, 17.v.1815.

(73) College Minutes, 25.ii.1817.

(74) Ibid., 2.ii.1836.

(75) Ibid., 2.v.1837.

(76) Ibid., 6.ii.1838.

(77) Ibid., 16.ii.1838.

(78) Ibid., 2.iii.1838.

(79) R.C.P.E. (1838) *Report of the Royal College of Physicians of Edinburgh on the Adulteration of Drugs. 2d March 1838*. Edinburgh: A. & C. Black.

(80) CHRISTISON, Sir R. (1885) *The Life of Sir Robert Christison, Bart.*, vol. 1, p. 297. Edinburgh: Blackwood.

(81) College Minutes, 5.iii.1834.

(82) Ibid., 8.x.1838.

Chapter XI

MEASURES FOR MEDICAL REFORM GAIN MOMENTUM: A MULTINATIONAL PROBLEM

Some are bewildered in the maze of schools,
And some made coxcombs nature meant but fools.

Alexander Pope

With the passing of the Medical Act of 1858 the College was faced with problems which were as fundamental as they were far-reaching. Major readjustments had to be made, representing the beginning of a new phase in the history of the College. For a proper understanding of the background to the new legislation an appraisal of the situation prevailing in the early years of the nineteenth century is essential. Nor can appraisal ignore the position as it obtained at the time south of Tweed because, of those who crossed the border a large proportion were Licentiates of the Royal College of Physicians of Edinburgh.

NATIONAL AND INTERNATIONAL CONFUSION

Of Authorities conferring degrees or licences there were seven in Scotland, seven in England and five in Ireland. They consisted of: in Scotland—the Royal College of Physicians of Edinburgh, the Royal College of Surgeons of Edinburgh, the Faculty (now Royal College) of Physicians and Surgeons of Glasgow and the Universities of St Andrews, Glasgow, Aberdeen and Edinburgh; in England—the Royal College of Physicians of London, the Royal College of Surgeons of England, the Apothecaries Hall and the Universities of Oxford, Cambridge, Durham and London; and in Ireland—the Royal College of Surgeons, the King's and Queen's College of Physicians in Ireland, the Apothecaries Hall of Ireland, the University of Dublin and the Queen's University. Each of these institutions possessed rights and privileges which dated back to their original Charters and which each regarded as its bounden duty to preserve intact, regardless of changes in the world around. Conflict of interests was inevitable—some national, some parochial; others academic and many material; and others again concerned with status.

The Universities saw grave threat in the ambitions of the Colleges, and the Colleges saw reasons for resentment in each other's overlapping activities. National animosities were not dampened by the entrenched imperiousness of the oldest Universities and the senior Corporations in the South. Simmering jealousies knew little immediate influence from the Treaty of Union. The nearest approach to accord was in the subjugation of quacks and mountebanks. All is comprehensible if not pardonable when account is taken of the welter of inherited conflicting privileges: many already become archaic, and some not wholly dissociated from ecclesiastical history. Nor can the unedifying internal dissensions known through the centuries to Universities and Corporations alike, both north and south of Tweed, be ignored. They have impeded, not hastened progress. A further complication was that by an Act of 1533-4 authority was vested in the Archbishop of Canterbury to grant Lambeth degrees in medicine, an authority which was used from time to time to confer a licence to practise[1] and which applied to the whole of England.

TRADITIONAL JURISDICTION OF OUR COLLEGE

As already described (Chap. III) the jurisdiction of the Edinburgh Royal College of Physicians extended 'to the City of Edinburgh, its suburbs, and privileges' and territorially was measurably less than those of the Edinburgh College of Surgeons or the Glasgow Faculty. Moreover graduates of any University who practised in Edinburgh did so without being required to submit themselves to examination or incurring the risk of fines. This limitation of the College's powers was imposed by the terms of its Charter. In marked contrast doctors holding Scottish degrees were prohibited by law from practising in England until such time as they had graduated at an English University or become Licentiates of the College of Physicians of London. That which applied to Scottish graduates applied also to Licentiates of the Edinburgh College of Physicians wishing to practise in England. The following is an excerpt from the Act of Parliament 14-15 Henry VIII c. 5:

> 'And where that in Dyocesys of England out of London it is not light to fynde alway men liable to sufficiauntly examyne after the Statute such as shall be

admitted to exercise Physyke in them that it may be enacted in this present
Parliament That noo person from hensforth be suffered to exercyse or practyse in
Physyke through England until such time that he be examined in London by the
said President and three of the said Electys (of the College of Physicians). And to
have from the said President or Electys Letters Testimonialae of their approving
and examination Except he be a Graduat of Oxford or Cantebrygge which hath
accomplished all thing for his fourme without Grace.'[2]

At first little recourse was made to this clause by the London College. In the
course of time however free use was made of the powers contained in it when licensing physicians in the provinces. The clause proved a useful instrument in repelling
invaders from the north. It is not without significance that the Edinburgh and London
Colleges of Physicians were alike in that, in their endeavours to establish and maintain
the pre-eminence of the physician, each preferred to utilize such statutory powers as
they had at their disposal to contain the Surgeon and the Apothecary rather than to
eradicate the mountebank and quack. The London College exercised authority
locally in a way partly but not wholly analogous to that of the Edinburgh College.
In and within seven miles of London the practice of physicians was legally restricted
to Fellows and Licentiates although the privilege was generally extended as a
courteous gesture to graduates of Oxford and Cambridge.[3] The net result was that,
subject to the provisos mentioned, Scottish graduates were legally precluded from
practising in England, while graduates from English Universities had unrestricted
rights to practise in Scotland elsewhere than in Edinburgh and Glasgow. Within its
limited area of jurisdiction the College of Physicians of Edinburgh could not exclude
graduates of the Universities of Oxford, Cambridge and London but could place an
embargo on all other English physicians. The particular position of London University in this connection was explained by the Medical Graduates Act of 1854
whereby it was empowered to grant to its graduates a licence to practise medicine in
any part of the United Kingdom other than within seven miles of London. Thus the
University of London was placed almost on a par with those of Oxford and Cambridge. The authority conferred by the degrees of Oxford and Cambridge Universities to practise 'per universum Angliae regnum' was not questioned.[4]

General Practitioners

In the field of general practice involving the dispensing of medicines, the Scottish
licentiate or graduate who wished to pursue his profession south of Tweed was at a
particular disadvantage. By Law, examination by the Apothecaries' Society was a

prerequisite, and for admission to that Society an applicant had first to serve a five years' apprenticeship with an apothecary.[5] The jurisdiction of the Society, at first applicable only to London, was extended to the whole of England by the Apothecaries Act of 1815 (q.v.). It has been written by a Southerner of 'this exclusive system':

> 'This great and glaring injustice was especially hard upon the many Scotch graduates . . . and affected the interests of a greater number of persons than did any other act of provincial legislation under which the profession laboured.'[6]

The Southerners in general were not lacking a champion: the flaw in their defensive armament was spotlighted by the *Lancet* in no uncertain self-congratulatory terms. In a leading article dated 17th May 1828 it declared:

> 'The *Lancet* is the first and only medical journal which showed that the pretensions of the Scotch doctors to superior attainments were founded in delusion, and that the public have in reality no security whatever for the competence of Scotch medical graduates, as such, because the *Lancet* is the only English medical journal free from Scotch influence and not subjected to Scotch control.'[7]

Scottish provincial legislation did not simplify the situation. In 1694 the exclusive privilege of practising surgery and pharmacy previously enjoyed by the barber–surgeons of Edinburgh was extended to include the three Lothians and the Counties of Fife, Peebles, Selkirk, Roxburgh and Berwick. The exclusive rights were retained on a nominal basis latterly and then, only until 1858. This so-called 'Edinburgh District' was counterbalanced by a 'Glasgow District' comprising Lanark, Renfrew, Ayr and Burgh, and the barony of Dumbarton under the medical jurisdiction of the Faculty of Physicians and Surgeons of Glasgow. The Faculty relinquished its authority in 1850. During such time as these two Corporations exercised their rights, transfer by a practitioner from one district to the other necessitated first obtaining the Licence to practise of the Corporation with authority over the area into which he intended moving.[8] The policy of the College of Physicians of Edinburgh was exceptional in that it did not require its members to forfeit their membership of other professional bodies.[9]

Single and Double Qualifications

Although not directly involved in the affairs of the Barber–surgeons' 'district', the Edinburgh College of Physicians certainly had an interest where illegal practice or practice with a single qualification was concerned. The Licence issued by the Edinburgh College of Physicians served as a qualification to practise medicine only, and in this respect resembled licences issued by the Society of Apothecaries and the University of Durham in England, and the Society of Apothecaries in Dublin. Licences qualifying to practise surgery only, were obtainable from the Edinburgh College of Surgeons, the Glasgow Faculty of Physicians and Surgeons, and the Universities of Durham and Dublin. Membership of the English College of Surgeons conferred a similar right. The only comprehensive licence conferred by one Corporation entitling the holder to practise medicine, surgery and midwifery throughout the United Kingdom was that of the London College of Physicians. Furthermore those holding this licence were able both to compound and dispense medicines for their patients.[10]

Of practitioners in England anxious to acquire a double qualification, a number obtained the Membership of the English College of Surgeons and the Licence of the Apothecaries' Society. The Licence of the London College of Physicians later came into increasing favour after modification of the Regulations attached to it. Nevertheless for many years both in Scotland and England, many members of the profession conducting general practice possessed only one diploma; medical in the case of some, and surgical in the case of others. Indeed, as events turned out, the Medical Act of 1858, of which the background is being considered did in fact admit practitioners with only one qualification to the Medical Register. The attraction of the Licence of the Apothecaries' Society has been ascribed to the fees for it being less than for medical licences obtainable elsewhere in Scotland and England, and to the examination involved being less exacting. At a later date a similar explanation was vouchsafed for a surge of popularity enjoyed by the double qualification conferred by the Colleges of Physicians and Surgeons in Edinburgh.[11]

While on the subject of the relative values of different qualifications the experience of Samuel Smiles is worth mentioning. To quote from his *Autobiography* he 'matriculated in November, 1829, and attended the lectures of Dr. Duncan for Materia Medica, Dr. Hope for Chemistry and Mr. Lizars for Anatomy . . . In the following year, I . . . attended the lectures of Liston on Surgery and Dr. Fletcher on the Institutions of Medicine.' Smiles was a fellow student in Dr Fletcher's class of the future Dr John Brown and author of *Rab and his Friends*.[12] Eventually the time arrived for the inevitable examinations. These Dr Smiles continued, were 'conducted *viva voce*, and without any written papers . . . There was Dr. Huie, a difficult examiner, Dr. Simson, Dr. Begbie, Dr. Maclagan and others. First, there was a paragraph of Gregory's *Conspectus* in Latin to be construed, or a passage of *Celsus*. Then

Materia Medica, when the method of preparing Antimonial Powder and Calomel had to be explained. Then Anatomy, when the arteries, nerves and muscles at the base of the scull, had to be described.'[13]

Having obtained his Diploma, of which Edinburgh College is not clear, and served his apprenticeship in Haddington where he afterwards practised for some years, Samuel Smiles left for Leyden in 1838 to obtain his degree of M.D. There he says 'In due course of time I submitted myself to an examination by Professor Van der Hoeven, Dean of the Faculty of Medicine, and other gentlemen. It was by no means so thorough as the one at Edinburgh some years before.'[14]

The Medical Act 1858 sought to secure justice for those in need of medical aid while at the same time endeavouring to reconcile the many, varied and often undisguisedly opposed claims of other interested parties. Innumerable, almost interminable consultations among those interested and with the legislature were unavoidable, and the background of sundry personalities, susceptibilities and jealousies gave rise to inordinate delay in drafting a succession of Bills before a tolerably effective enactment eventually evolved.

Legislation was designed to cover Scotland (and Ireland) as well as England. Herein was a further complicating factor in so far as the relations between Universities and the Licensing Corporations were concerned. In no small measure due to the inborn national dedication to learning the Scot set great store by the acquisition of a University degree. This was evident long before the creation of medical faculties but, with the conferment of medical degrees first on the continent and subsequently at home, soon extended to those intent on becoming doctors. That this should have occurred in no way disregarded or in any way belittled the fact that in Edinburgh the erection of the Royal College of Physicians preceded the creation of a medical faculty in the University by over forty years; and that through the agency of its Fellows the College contributed largely to the early forms of education and examination instituted by the University. Such was the eventual attraction of academic qualifications that in the course of time a very real but healthy rivalry developed between the medical Corporations and the University.

This rivalry applied particularly to the training offered to those planning to equip themselves for general practice. A Southerner chose to write more especially for the benefit of the Irish, 'Scotch University degrees are as plentiful as blackberries; and it is open to grave doubt whether they are a whit superior to the licences of the Colleges'.[15] Ignoring this incidental evaluation by an observer from the periphery the statement pointed to the recognized greater number of Scottish than English medical degrees. The point of significance is that the position of Corporations *vis-à-vis* Universities in this particular field differed markedly from that obtaining in England.

Medical Degrees of Scottish Universities

There can be no denying that the medical degrees awarded by Scottish Universities, with the exception of the University of Edinburgh, were in disrepute at one time, because of their being given 'in absence'. Writing in 1754 to William Cullen from London, William Hunter said: 'You no doubt know how contemptuously the College of Physicians here have treated all Scotch degrees indiscriminately . . . We are very inclinable to think that the prostitution of degrees . . . is indeed sometimes with justice, but often insidiously, thrown out against all Scotch graduates here, does not appear in that light to the authors of this evil . . . who may be . . . abused by some people here, who pass by the name of Brokers of Scotch Degrees.'[16]

The overall position was the subject in 1774 of a Memorial submitted by William Cullen to the Duke of Buccleuch at the instance of the latter, who was Chancellor of the University of Edinburgh and an Honorary Fellow of the College. Cullen was President of the College at the time, and before coming to Edinburgh University had held a Chair at the University of Glasgow. The following were opinions contained in his Memorandum:

> 'The Universities of St. Andrews and Aberdeen have frequently given degrees in absence . . . upon a certificate of two physicians . . . very often obscure persons' and it is 'commonly believed, that little else than the payment of the usual fees is necessary to obtain such a degree.'
>
> As to the University of Glasgow, 'though they do not commonly give degrees in absence, yet they often give degrees, without requiring any certificates of the candidate's previous study.'
>
> 'The abuses complained of are particularly a hardship upon the Royal College of Physicians of Edinburgh who are obliged by their charter to grant licences, without examination, to any person who has obtained a degree from any of the Universities of Scotland.'[17]

It is not claiming over much for the College to say that it was largely instrumental by its initial tutelage in encouraging the University of Edinburgh to refrain from the award of degrees *ad eundem*. Unfortunately in 1766 the University gave a Medical Doctorate to an illiterate tradesman of the name of Leeds. Dr John Fothergill, although a fellow Quaker and prominent Fellow of the Edinburgh College, warned the London Hospital not to give an appointment to Leeds. The warning was effective but Fothergill had to defend himself at Law.[18] It was the Leeds case which prompted the Duke of Buccleuch to require a memorandum from Cullen.[19]

A further but not wholly unrelated difference between the two countries at the beginning of the nineteenth century, concerned the type of practice undertaken by physicians, surgeons and apothecaries. In England the work of physicians consisted in the main of attending to the wealthier members of the community and of philanthropic activities in hospitals and elsewhere: the majority of the surgeons were occupied even more in general practice than strictly surgical activities: and to an increasing extent the apothecaries were assuming the role of general practitioners. Over and above these there were large numbers of practitioners with Scottish and Irish University qualifications. In addition, constituting a motley and largely irresponsible group on their own, were those who could claim a semblance of apprenticeship but no formal professional training, and those who were no more than thinly disguised impostors.[20]

'Pure' Physicians

As to physicians, interpreting the term to connote consulting physicians—or, as they were sometimes decorously referred to, 'pure physicians' practising medicine only—their number in Edinburgh was still infinitesimal two decades after the passing of the Medical Act of 1858. It was written at this time that 'Scarcely any of the medical men in Edinburgh are exclusively occupied with either medicine or surgery. Perhaps about half-a-dozen connected with the two Colleges of Physicians and Surgeons are pure physicians or pure surgeons.'[21] The term 'pure' is neither italicized nor in quotation marks in the original article which went on to declare that 'In Scotland an intermediate class between general practitioners and physicians has long existed. This class practises physic, to which some add minor operations of surgery, and a few add midwifery, but none practise pharmacy.' Dr Begbie (without distinguishing between James Begbie or his son Warburton Begbie) and John Abercrombie were instanced as examples of general practitioners who became consultant physicians.[22] Writing of a colleague a few years later Christison described him as belonging 'to the highest class of general practitioners in the city [Edinburgh]— those who practised physic and surgery as family medical attendants, but not either pharmacy or midwifery', and added 'Edinburgh has long been famous for this class of professional men . . .'.[23]

Others have followed the same course in the present century and the 'pure physician' of the future, no matter how ultra-specialized he may be expected to become, will be the better the closer the insight he has had into general practice. The demands on time, the prevailing urge to haste, and the mesmerism of drama are the deterrents to progress along these lines. Without such progress there is a danger of a resurgence of confusion akin to that which the Medical Act of 1858 was designed to unravel.

PROBING TOWARDS REFORM

Recognition of the need to reform was not confined to any one section of the medical profession. This held good despite the fact that the eighteenth century had witnessed an unprecedented rise in the population of both Scotland and England due to a rapid fall in the death rate. According to Trevelyan this remarkable statistical development 'was the outcome of improved conditions of life, and of better doctoring, a science in which Scots in the reign of George III were already able to instruct the English'.[24]

Latham's Proposals

One of the first significant proposals for reform was advanced in 1804 by Dr John Latham, a Fellow and later President of the Royal College of Physicians of London. It was submitted to that College under the title '*Outline of a Plan, for an intended Bill for the better Regulation of Medical Practitioners, Chemists, Druggists and Venders of Medicine*'. Medical Practitioners included surgeons and apothecaries. The plan contemplated the division of the country into districts—16 for England and 8 for Ireland. Scotland evidently posed a problem because for it 'the number was left blank'.[25] Each district was to be administered by a District Physician with extensive authority to regulate the practice of physicians, surgeons and apothecaries. The qualification to practise as a physician was to be a degree of an English, Irish or Scottish University obtained after a comprehensive course of study. It was not intended that the Corporations should lose their control. The degrees of Scottish, Oxford, Cambridge and Dublin Universities were associated with rights to practise in prescribed territorial areas, and the Royal Colleges of Physicians and their surgical counterparts were to be empowered to admit a doctor or bachelor for any other part. Among the responsibilities to be attached to the District Physician were the inspection of parish poor-houses and places for the reception of the insane. For some strange reason the proposed terms of his appointment suggested a need for protection from excessive influence by a University or professional College.[26]

Harrison's Recommendations

While Latham's proposals were still under consideration a new approach to reform emanated from another source. At their annual meeting in 1804 the *Lincolnshire Benevolent Medical Society* arranged that one of their members, Edward Harrison, a Doctor of Medicine of Edinburgh University, should enquire into the state of medical practice in Lincolnshire. In his report he maintained that unqualified out-numbered qualified practitioners in the ratio nine to one. At the instigation and with the help of the Society's Patron, the then President of the Royal Society, Harrison made contact with many leading members of the London Colleges. Personal difficulties arose which probably prevented collaboration between the London College of Physicians and Harrison[27] but the latter, not without influential support, pursued his plan and in 1808 a Bill for reform was drafted. This Bill envisaged the annual registration of physicians, surgeons and apothecaries and suggested the qualifications necessary for entry into each of the three divisions of the profession. For a physician it was intended that he should have attained the age of 24 years; be a medical graduate of any University in the United Kingdom; and have completed five years of study in a University 'or other respectable school or schools of physic', two of the five years having been spent in the University at which he obtained his degree. It came to naught, but not for want of trying. Mr Pitt is credited with having said 'I have had so many communications on this subject, that I am quite convinced something is wanting; and I will try to carry it into effect'.

Pitt died and Harrison was granted an interview with his successor. A Committee formed of Harrison's well-wishers did not find favour with the London College of Physicians possibly because 'it was not a body representative of the whole profession but a gathering of the discontented and the critical'.[28] Frustrated, Harrison and his supporters then sought the advice of a legal authority who among other things would not accept that Scottish doctors had any right to practise in England.[28] An incidental occurrence during the time of discussions was the issue by a sympathizer of a pamphlet which, intended to rouse the general public to an appreciation of Harrison's objectives, criticized the shortness of the courses provided in Edinburgh. Ultimately Harrison's proposals assumed the form of a draft *Bill for the Improvement of the Medical and Surgical Sciences* which on being submitted to the London College of Physicians was rejected out of hand.[29] That proved to be the end of Harrison's effort to secure reform, but the events which followed cast a light on the atmosphere of the times. Defeated, Harrison continued practising in Lincolnshire but in 1817 came to London where 'of all living physicians he was the most notoriously unqualified to practise in London but he was left in peace for ten years'. Then came the summons from the London College. And the response?—tantamount to a 'wha daur meddle wi me?!' A court case eventuated and Harrison was acquitted on the grounds that he had practised surgery, not medicine.[30]

The Apothecaries Act, 1815

To add to the variety the next move towards reform arose from quite unpredictable causes. The cost of the Napoleonic War resulted in the imposition of a heavy tax on glass which in turn seriously increased the operative costs of apothecaries. A protest movement won the support of doctors of standing and there evolved the London Committee of Associated Apothecaries and Surgeon–Apothecaries of England and Wales. The Committee was instrumental in introducing into the House of Commons a Bill intended for application to the whole of England and Wales, including London. This Bill and two which followed were not successful but paved the way to the passing in 1815 of the *Apothecaries Act*. By the terms of the Act the Society of Apothecaries became the administrative authority and were required to establish a Court of Examiners which had to examine those proposing to practise as apothecaries in England and Wales. A prerequisite to examination was the completion of a five years' apprenticeship with an apothecary. Successful candidates became Licentiates of the Society of Apothecaries. As a result of the Act the Society of Apothecaries assumed control of the education of a very considerable body of general practitioners in England and Wales. Coupled with this were the powers vested in the Society enabling them to impose penalties for irregular practice.

A Home Secretary's Conception

The next important Bill was introduced in August 1844 by the Home Secretary, Sir James Graham. It was promoted '*for the Better Regulation of Medical Practice throughout the United Kingdom*'. In many major respects the Bill was revolutionary, and not conducive to placation of the Colleges, Universities, the Society of Apothecaries or general practitioners. A central administrative body overweighted by members outside the profession, was proposed to supervise and co-ordinate the work of the various licensing bodies numbering 19 at that time. General practitioners were to be alone in not being associated with one of the Colleges, and the Society of Apothecaries was to be divested of its power of licensing practitioners. With creditable candour the *History of the Royal College of Physicians of London* tells of how 'Scotch graduates, and others who had long been untroubled in their practice, found that they were expected to pay £25 for nominal membership of a College which they detested'.[31] The Bill was withdrawn in January 1846.

Sundry Unsuccessful Bills

With the withdrawal of Graham's Bill and a change of government, private members were alive to the improved prospects of Bills which they might themselves promote. At least 18 Bills concerned with the medical profession were tabled in Parliament during the period 1840 to 1858.[32] As early as 1840 Thomas Wakley, a member—but a critical radical member—of the London Royal College of Surgeons, and both founder and editor of the *Lancet*, sponsored a Bill for medical reform in company with a fellow Member of Parliament of the name of Warburton. These two individuals submitted a second Bill of a more ambitious nature in 1847. Wakley and Warburton aimed at the establishment of three Medical Registers—one each for Scotland, England and Ireland, an annual registration fee to be exacted from those legitimately included in the Registers: the creation of three Medical Councils, again—one for each country in the United Kingdom: and the erection of a College of Medicine. Their second Bill was referred to a Select Committee which published three reports but no Act eventuated.

Other Bills laid before Parliament but eventually withdrawn included three (1855, 1856 and 1857) sponsored by a barrister named Headlam and two (1856 and 1857) by Lord Elcho. The former advocated a Central Board representative of the licensing bodies and of the Government but not of the Universities, whereas the latter submitted a proposal for a Governing Board to be appointed by the Board of Health and the Privy Council. Lord Elcho also suggested the creation of a new board of examiners, the Universities to be responsible for nominating members to examine in the collateral sciences and the Corporations to nominate those to examine in the practice of medicine. Irrespective of its merits or demerits, Lord Elcho's Bill started with the initial disadvantage of portraying the views of the Scottish Universities and being reputedly 'as from the University of Edinburgh . . .'. It was 'wholly objectionable' in the opinion of the London College of Physicians.[33]

About this time a Bill for the registration of practitioners was introduced by a private Member (Mr Brady) who was a surgeon by profession, but met with no success.[34] Another unsuccessful Bill, to which no reference appears in the Minutes of the Edinburgh College but which is mentioned in the history of the London College, was associated with the name of Duncombe. It was a *Bill to Define the Rights of the Medical Profession and to Protect the Public from the Abuses of the Medical Corporations* and has been described by Clark as 'a mere voice from the past'.[35]

To read the progress, if such it can be called, of medical reform as conducted by the politicians conveys a bewildering impression of confusion worse confounded. That the view was shared by the three London Corporations was amply demonstrated by their decision 'to act for themselves'. To quote from Clark's *History*, 'They agreed on the principles of a Bill, and set out to bring the Universities in with them. Oxford, Cambridge and Trinity College, Dublin, came into line . . . But London and the Scottish Universities were not persuaded. This flicker died out.'[36]

The British Medical Association's Contribution

Any review of professional disentanglement would be incomplete without reference to the contribution of the British Medical Association. Originating as the *Provincial Medical and Surgical Association* at Worcester in 1832, it assumed its present name in 1856. Among its original purposes was removal of the disadvantages experienced by provincial medical practitioners attributable to isolation and lack of co-operation. From its inception the Association showed a deep interest in the question of medical reform and a desire to encourage public interest in the subject. In 1852 the Association appointed a Medical Reform Committee. Various attempts to promote legislation were unsuccessful and in 1853 a deputation seeking support for a Bill drafted by the Association was received by Lord Palmerston. The deputation did not succeed in its task any more than did another deputation two years later to Sir George Grey (Home Secretary). However when the way to legislative success was opened by an amended new Bill introduced by Headlam and considered by the House of Commons in 1858, many of the recommendations of the Association were dealt with effectively.[37] Sir Charles Hastings of the Association made a major contribution to co-operation when he finally jettisoned an oft-repeated demand for one uniform qualification for all branches of medical practice.[35]

Approaching Resolution

In 1858 Lord Elcho withdrew his last Bill on medical reform *To Alter and Amend the Laws regulating the Medical Profession*; and with the rejection of Duncombe's Bill the way was cleared for the final passage of the successful Bill, which received the Royal Assent on 2nd August 1858. Best known as *The Medical Act*, it was legally entitled 'An Act to regulate the Qualifications of Practitioners in Medicine and Surgery' and took effect from 1st October 1858.[38]

REFERENCES

NATIONAL AND INTERNATIONAL CONFUSION

(1) CLARK, Sir G. (1964) *A History of the Royal College of Physicians of London*, vol. 1, p. 78. Oxford: Clarendon Press.

(2) 14 and 15 Henry VIII, c. 5 (1523).

(3) RIVINGTON, W. (1879) *The Medical Profession*, p. 100. Dublin: Fannin & Co.

(4) CHAPMAN, J. (1870) *The Medical Institutions of the United Kingdom*, p. 19. London: John Churchill.

(5) RIVINGTON, W. Op. cit., p. 101.

(6) CHAPMAN, J. Op. cit., p. 22.

(7) Leading article (1828) *Lancet*, **ii**, 211.

(8) CHAPMAN, J. Op. cit., p. 21.

(9) Ibid., p. 30.

(10) RIVINGTON, W. Op. cit., p. 46.

(11) Ibid., pp. 46–7.

(12) SMILES, S. (1905) *The Autobiography of Samuel Smiles*, ed. by T. Mackay, pp. 34–5. London: John Murray.

(13) Ibid., p. 45.

(14) Ibid., p. 67.

(15) RIVINGTON, W. Op. cit., p. 49.

(16) THOMSON, J. (1859) *An Account of the Life, Lectures and Writing of William Cullen, M.D.*, vol. I, p. 660. Edinburgh: Blackwood.

(17) Ibid., pp. 468–9.

(18) CLARK, Sir G. Op. cit., vol. 2, p. 568.

(19) THOMSON, J. Op. cit., vol. I, p. 468.

(20) POLLAK, K. (1968) *The Healers; the doctor, then and now.* In collaboration with E. Ashworth Underwood, p. 157. London: Nelson.

(21) RIVINGTON, W. Op. cit., p. 52.

(22) Ibid., p. 53.

(23) CHRISTISON, Sir R. (1885) *Life of Sir Robert Christison, Bart.*, vol. I, pp. 173-4. Edinburgh: Blackwood.

PROBING TOWARDS REFORM

(24) TREVELYAN, G. M. (1944) *English Social History*, p. 462. London: Longmans, Green & Co.

(25) CLARK, Sir G. Op. cit., vol. 2, p. 626.

(26) Ibid., p. 627.

(27) Ibid., p. 628.

(28) Ibid., p. 631.

(29) Ibid., p. 632.

(30) Ibid., p. 665.

(31) Ibid., p. 710.

(32) POLLAK, K. Op. cit., p. 183.

(33) CLARK, Sir G. Op. cit., vol. 2, p. 725.

(34) Ibid., p. 723.

(35) Ibid., p. 727.

(36) Ibid., p. 725.

(37) RIVINGTON, W. Op. cit., p. 252.

(38) 21 and 22 Victoria, c. 90 (1858).

Chapter XII

COLLEGE PARTICIPATION IN MEDICAL REFORM

It is one of the consolations of middle-aged reformers that the good they inculcate must live after them if it is to live at all.

H. H. Munro

Every reform was once a private opinion, and when it shall be a private opinion again it will solve the problem of the age.

R. W. Emerson

LONDON INITIATIVE

The first intimation the College had of Dr Latham's proposals was on 7th August 1804. On that day the President (Dr Thos. Spens) announced that he had received 'a printed letter' from 'the Register of the College of Physicians, London offering a copy of a proposed plan for the better regulation of Medical Practitioners in the Country Districts of the United Kingdom, which it was intended application should be made for an act to Parliament to that effect'. There had been no delay in communicating with the President because a decision to print Dr Latham's proposals had only been decided by the London College towards the end of the previous June.[1] The copy of the proposed act was laid on the Library table in the Edinburgh College for inspection by members until the next meeting and a Committee appointed in view of the 'mature deliberation' required by the subject.[2] A note accompanying the plan made it clear that there was to be no precipitate approach to Parliament 'in order that the several Royal Colleges may have to view it in all its different Bearings'.

CAUTION IN THE ABSENCE OF INFORMATION

In his interim letter of acknowledgment the President expressed the view that implementation of the plan would involve considerable difficulties, and that it did not seem right that the Universities of St Andrews and Aberdeen, which granted degrees without residence or examination, should be put on the same footing with the other Universities of the United Kingdom.[3] As a reply was still awaited to a request for further information it was decided at the next Quarterly Meeting that the previously appointed Committee should consider corresponding with the individual members of the London College before drafting any recommendations.[4] In August of the next year another letter was received from London indicating that the plan to proceed with a Bill was temporarily in abeyance but 'that when the subject shall be resumed, the College will have pleasure in communicating with the University of Edinburgh thereupon'. Enclosed with the letter was an amended plan.[5] The last reference in the Minutes to the Latham proposals appeared in May 1808, and consisted of an explanation for the delay in reporting by the responsible Committee.[6]

PROVINCIAL INITIATIVE

But there was to be no respite. In August 1806 a letter addressed to the President was received from Dr Edward Harrison writing on the instructions of his Committee and enclosing a copy of resolutions passed by them of a Plan 'for better regulating the Practise of Physic in the different Branches'. At the same time as seeking the support of the College the covering letter went out of its way to emphasize that Harrison's Committee thought it 'highly desireable to maintain and perhaps to extend' the rights and privileges of incorporated medical Bodies.[7] A business-like letter of acknowledgment courteously allowed of the College's awareness of abuses in the practice of Medicine and of its desire that 'the Profession might be rendered more useful as well as more respectable': and pointedly concluded with 'When you shall communicate your plan, the College will be enabled to take the subject into more particular consideration.'[7] Within less than three weeks an 'Outline of a Plan of Medical Reform' was received with an attached short printed circular letter which concluded with a 'P.S.' asking that 'circular letters should be distributed as generally as possible . . . to . . . practitioners . . . in order to give publicity to the undertaking.'[7]

MORALIZING IN RESPONSE TO HARRISON

A Report[8] submitted by a Committee appointed to consider Dr Harrison's communications was adopted unanimously by the College which was careful when writing to Dr Harrison to do so in terms of 'resolutions . . . for the consideration of the Gentlemen in whose names he has sent this plan'. The reply was lengthy and comprehensive. Accepting that a need for reform existed it maintained with canny patriotism that 'the same abuses do not prevail or at least not in the same degree in Scotland as in England', and thereupon adjured that any regulations should be enacted in the interests of the community at large and not merely for the emolument or respectability of the medical profession. Moralizing maybe—but moralizing in a way appropriate to the succeeding century. The College took exception to restriction of physicians to those with United Kingdom degrees, maintaining that good surgical and medical training was procurable in some foreign universities but not at all those in the United Kingdom. Could the College with its Leyden ancestry think otherwise? Whereas Harrison advocated that no one should practise as a physician until 24 years of age, the College was satisfied that given proper education a person 'may be qualified to enter on the practice of Medicine at the time of life they are entitled by law to manage their own affairs'. The operative word is 'entitled'—but would the patient of today welcome an attendant entitled to practise in virtue of being given voting powers at 18 years?! In similar vein the College considered that three years at a University and not five as suggested by Harrison were adequate provided strict and impartial examinations conditioned the award of degrees.

DETERRENTS TO RECRUITMENT

Comments in the reply concerning surgeons and apothecaries were particularly interesting. Aspiring surgeons should have instruction in medicine additional to anatomy and surgery, and the same should apply to apothecaries who 'as well as surgeons are not very generally engaged in the practice of medicine'. There was consistency also in the College's declared view that 'as Men-midwives are employed in the cure of the Complaints and diseases of women and children as well in cases of pregnancy', they too should have studied the different branches of medicine and should be examined as to their eligibility on the basis of practical ability. Harrison urged that apprenticeship for chemists or druggists should be of five years duration;

the College was satisfied that two years would suffice. While Harrison wished that those already legally engaged in practice should not have new restrictions imposed on them the College, anxious to avoid discouragement of recruits to the profession, maintained that comparable safeguards should be extended to students preparing for any of the branches of the medical profession.

DOUBTS *RE* REGISTRATION

Two other opinions recorded in the College's reply to Harrison's Committee deserve mention—one surprising; the other not surprising. The first was disagreement with the suggestion that there should be a register of medical practitioners: and the second, opposition to fines on admission to any register. The term 'fine' to modern ears suggests 'culpability' or being 'agin the government'. Even allowing for changes in connotation, the College were rightly always on the alert lest the insidious introduction of registration fees and the like should contribute to the continually increasing expenses incurred by those entering practice.[8]

Consideration of Harrison's contemplated measures for Reform did not cease at this stage in so far as the College was involved. A letter was received from the Secretary to the Lords of the Treasury concerning a Petition and a proposed Act of Parliament submitted by Doctor Harrison. A request was made for an early opinion on these, the request being signed by Geo. Harrison not to be confused with the petitioner Edward Harrison who was no relation.[9] George Harrison's letter from the Treasury Chambers had enclosed a sketch of his namesake's *Bill for the Improvement of the Medical and Surgical and Veterinary Sciences*. Before submitting a Report the Council of the College, to whom the subject material had been remitted as a Committee,[9] obviously expended much time and labour in discussion.

From their Report, approved by the College as a whole, it is obvious that the attitude of the College had undergone a measure of modification. Thus it categorically expressed approval of the registration of members of the medical profession and went so far as to say that together, registration and a requirement that a licence to practise should be subject to previous examination, would prevent 'many of the abuses, now existing in the practice of Medicine'. Earlier in the Report existing abuses were attributed to the practice of medicine by educationally unqualified persons; the daily deceptions of 'advertising Empyrics' . . . ; and, 'the incompetence of existing authorities to prevent these abuses'. Having stated which, the Report then declared that 'the Legislature is above competent to prevent these abuses' and that the basic need is for 'a Temperate Reform'.[10]

BOARD OF COMMISSIONERS UNDESIRABLE

The Report, however, did not lack trenchant criticism. It disapproved unreservedly of the proposal to create a Board of Commissioners with powers to levy large sums of money from the medical profession, establish medical schools, appoint professors and build hospitals. Criticism was justified on the grounds of the ability of existing medical institutions to carry out the functions of such a Board, the pecuniary burden which would be imposed on the profession of medicine, and the infringement of the rights and privileges of existing establishments which would follow the assignment of the intended responsibilities of the proposed Board.

Another point which proved irksome to the College was less fundamental. It related to names on the doors of houses occupied by members of the profession. While not objecting to name-plates bearing the title of 'Dr.' as an indication of the branch of medicine practised, the College thought 'it unnecessary and degrading that they, or any other practitioner in medicine, should be obliged to exhibit their names in such large and permanent characters as to have the appearance of a Sign-post'.[10] It is tempting to visualize the fleeting relaxation of expression on the part of the first Treasury civil servant to read this reply! None the less a matter of principle and professional deportment was involved—a matter of principle and professional deportment which should not be ignored today with the temptations of name-plates replaced by those of newspapers, radio and television.

How wise Bernard Shaw was when in his Preface to *The Doctor's Dilemma* he wrote:

> *Make it compulsory for a doctor using a brass plate to have inscribed on it, in addition to the letters indicating his qualifications, the words 'Remember that I too am mortal'* [11]

The Report concluded as it had begun in terms of carefully guarded, if conventional, diplomacy! 'If a Bill be brought into Parliament which may in some measure meet the ideas of the Royal College of Physicians of Edinburgh, they will most readily assist in adapting its particular provisions to the local circumstances of this Country.'[10] With increasing maturity the College had learnt the art of countering civil service expertise by the employment of multiple caveats.

REPERCUSSIONS OF APOTHECARIES ACT, 1815

There is no evidence that the College was involved in events leading up to the Apothecaries Act of 1815. It is possible that this reflected the rather different position obtaining at the time in Scotland and more particularly in Edinburgh as compared with England. A pharmacist writing of Edinburgh has described how the druggist, having escaped from the overlordship of the surgeon, later acquired in the eighteenth century 'that separate identity which has characterised medicine and pharmacy in the capital'.[12] Referring to the 'more complete fractionation of pharmacy from medicine in Edinburgh than in some other urban parts of Scotland', another pharmacist ascribed 'the remarkable development of professional pharmacy' to 'quasi-academic specialisation of function' contributing to a professional etiquette which in turn viewed the 'doctor's shop' with disfavour.[13]

In subsequent years, senior Fellows of the Edinburgh College of Physicians although not directly concerned, regretted that the London College had not taken advantage of an offered opportunity to undertake the licensing of general practitioners in England. The offer came in the form of a suggestion for a statutory authority consisting of the President and Censors of the London College, the Master and Governors of the Royal College of Surgeons, the Master and Wardens of the Society of Apothecaries and some London practitioners. The authority was to appoint and superintend district committees, one of whose functions was to be registration.[14] To the Edinburgh College with its close association with general practitioners and anxious to discard application of the name Apothecaries to medical practitioners, it seemed that London reluctance had encouraged the policy of entrusting the licensing of general practitioners to a trading Society of Apothecaries. By doing so it was felt 'the name of Apothecary, as that of a Medical Practitioner, was legalised, instead of one of the time-honoured names—Physician or Surgeon'.[15]

Although in no way involved in the passing of the Apothecaries Act of 1815, the College was directly concerned with subsequent measures for amendment of the Act. In 1827 the Edinburgh College of Surgeons invited the co-operation of its sister Edinburgh College, together with that of the University, in 'an application to Parliament to have the injurious effects of that Bill removed'.[16] The Petition which the Surgeons proposed to submit to Parliament drew attention to their diploma being recognized as a qualification to practise surgery and pharmacy; and to the Act procured by the Apothecaries Society of London without the knowledge of the Edinburgh College of Surgeons, whereby those of their Diplomates practising in

England and Wales have had to be licensed anew by the Society of Apothecaries. A plea was advanced for the abolition of this monopoly.

No action was taken at this stage by the Physicians but six years later an Extraordinary Meeting was called with the express purpose of considering the Apothecaries Act, and more particularly those clauses of the Act dealing with the limitation of dispensing medicines in England and Wales to holders of the Society of Apothecaries' Licence.[17] A draft Petition was considered but another Extraordinary Meeting was required before agreement was reached about the form the Petition should take.[18, 19] Copies were eventually sent to the Duke of Buccleuch and the Lord Advocate for presentation to Parliament and to 'all the Peers connected with Scotland'. That to the Lord Advocate was accompanied on the instructions of the College by a letter which can only be described as voluminous and verbose in the extreme and, as the signatory spontaneously allowed, 'written . . . in a hurry . . . and possibly, though most unwittingly, in a manner at variance with ceremony'.

The gist of the letter consisted in a review of the College's past record in the exercise of its powers more especially in relation to apothecaries and their shops: evidence that in these respects the College had 'virtually and essentially abandoned its exclusionary power' and willingly relinquished the odious spirit of monopoly: criticism of the Apothecaries Act as having proved 'vexatious and oppressive' more especially having regard to the calibre of doctors trained by Scottish Universities and Corporations: and, 'the prayer of the College' that the Apothecaries Act should be amended to 'exempt from its operation all who have been regularly educated and found duly qualified, to practice Medicine'.

The Bill to amend the Apothecaries Act made provision for the extension to Scotland of the freedom of practice intended for England but contained no vestige of mention of the Royal College of Physicians of Edinburgh despite 'the general nature' of the Bill being in accord with recommendations of the College. Manfully if not very diplomatically the writer of the letter suggested to the Lord Advocate: 'Beyond all doubt, your Lordship if a friend to the Bill—or, if not, on the score of justice and impartiality—would say, in the premises, the College of Physicians ought equally to be sanctioned by the contemplated enactment.'[20]

Action of an unprecedented character followed in the course of a few days. On the requisition of two members (Drs Davidson and Renton) an Extraordinary Meeting of the College was called to consider 'the propriety of one of the Fellows going to London immediately, to watch over the interests of the Royal College, before the Committee of the House of Commons now deliberating about the Apothecaries Act, or before the House of Lords when the Bill comes before that branch of the Legislature'.

K

The Fellow who initiated the move referred to action along these lines having already been taken by the Edinburgh College of Surgeons: and inferred that the Lord Advocate may not have presented 'as he was requested, and promised he would' the Petition of the Edinburgh College of Physicians.[21] The College as a whole was not entirely convinced of the immediate urgency of the situation and obtained the opinion of a local Member of Parliament who replied to the effect that the College had 'done most wisely in delaying to dispatch any of your Body to London'.[22]

RETURNS REQUIRED BY PARLIAMENT

New and wider considerations entered into the picture with the arrival, from the Home Secretary, of a requirement 'in pursuance of a Resolution of the House of Commons', that returns be made to him of the regulations and bye-laws under which graduates in physic had been admitted Fellows and of the number of persons prosecuted by order of the College.[23] Of necessity compliance with the Home Secretary's demand involved transmission of a lengthy document which bore the obvious legal imprint of an expert Clerk to the College. By way of introduction the document emphasized that the College's Laws and Regulations were not codified until 1788; and then presented *seriatim*, alterations made between 1st January 1771 till 4th November 1799, the Laws and Regulations as ratified on 4th November 1788, and alterations made between 4th November 1788 and 31st December 1832.

That part of the College's reply to the enquiry about prosecutions was brief, and because of its historical significance justifies quotation. It was as follows:

> '. . . there is no instance of any persons having been prosecuted, by order of the Royal College, for Mal-practice, or for refusing to apply for their Licenses to practise, during the period from the 1st day of January 1771 till the 31st December 1832, the last example on the latter account, being in 1754, when Dr. Martin Eccles,★ who tried the power of the College in that respect, was defeated—He afterwards voluntarily became a Licentiate, namely in 1771, and was chosen a Fellow in the following year.'[23]

While the information required by the Home Office undoubtedly had a bearing on the workings of the Apothecaries Act it is equally evident that it furnished details invaluable to a government department pondering over the immensely wider issues of possible medical reform. The motives of civil service questionnaires are not always apparent on the surface.

★ See p. 139.

THE COLLEGE TAKES THE INITIATIVE

Discontent with the Apothecaries Act persisted without any significant action being taken until, in 1837 the President (Dr W. P. Alison) and a number of Fellows waited on a Member of Parliament for the City of Edinburgh. The Member for the City was satisfied with the informal case presented by Fellows of the College and acting on his advice the College decided to approach another Member of the House—Mr Warburton, with whom the College of Surgeons were communicating separately. Essentially the gravamen of the communication was the need for relief of Fellows and Licentiates of the two Colleges from restrictions selectively imposed on them in England.[24] This same need was re-emphasized two years later in a Memorial to the Home Secretary based on the conclusions of a conjoint committee on medical education on which the College was represented.[25]

A Memorial submitted in 1840 deplored governmental unresponsiveness to professional and public representations; admitted the delay may have been due to the comprehensiveness of the government's unrevealed intentions; and suggested that a limited measure might straightway be introduced and confined to determination of a minimum course of education, granting appropriate equal privileges to medical and surgical practice throughout the Empire, and preventing medical degrees being conferred without study or examinations. The Memorial did not conceal the fact that the medical institutions of Scotland would stand to benefit from any such measure.[26]

LONDON MONOPOLIES: FIRM PRESIDENTIAL LEAD

That was in 1840, and although in some respects strangely lacking in specificity, the Memorial manifestly had in mind redress of grievances from the Apothecaries Act, and the rumoured grand-scale preparations of the Home Office in the matter of medical reform. In 1848 with the complete agreement of the College the President (Dr Robert Christison) wrote a note of firm protest, as unmistakably emphatic as it was strictly courteous, to the Home Secretary. The subject of the protest was the publication of draft New Charters. It was represented to the Home Secretary 'that the dissatisfaction, which has for so many years prevailed throughout the medical profession in Great Britain, originally arose in a great measure from the want [sic] and exclusive spirit, in which the London College of Physicians and the London Society

of Apothecaries, the Monopolies conferred upon them by their existing Charters';
and that 'the Universities and Royal Colleges of Scotland have in particular had great
reason to complain, and have repeatedly complained to the legislature of the spirit in
which their exclusive privileges have been exercised against Scottish Graduates,
Fellows and Licentiates'.[27]

This was no case of the pot calling the kettle black. Abundant recorded facts bore
testimony to the validity of the complaint. With admirable logic the President
presented the case for justice in the form of freedom for qualified Scottish doctors to
practise in England unfettered by restrictions embodied in the charters of metropolitan licensing corporations: and for equitable reciprocity in the matter of privileges, derived from Charters granted to licensing bodies in Scotland and England.
The bases of reciprocity were detailed. Essentially the letter was directed towards
preventing extension of the Charter advantages of the London licensing bodies.
Written as it was by a man of the eminence and integrity of Robert Christison, it
would not be lightly ignored. Furthermore as he indicated in his letter, Christison
was genuinely in favour of the Government's efforts 'to attempt the organisation of a
general measure for regulating the medical profession'.[27]

The two Edinburgh Royal Colleges and the Glasgow Faculty returned to the
charge with undiminished determination in 1850 when, after considering the Bill of
the Provincial Medical and Surgical Association, they memorialized Sir George Grey
once again. The basis of representations was a reiteration of the iniquities of the
Apothecaries Act of 1815 because of the restrictions imposed on 'general practice in
England of gentlemen educated in Scotland' in a way 'unjust, inconsistent with the
union between the two Countries and injurious to the Interests of both, but especially
the former'. It was indicated that the Colleges and the Faculty were prepared to form
a Conjoint Board of Examiners and the Memorialists, who included the Dean of the
Medical Faculty of the University of Edinburgh, stated that they found 'their exertions impeded by the regulations of the Society of Apothecaries in London'.[28]

AN ENCOURAGING GESTURE

Then the unexpected took place. On 28th June 1850 a letter was published in the
Times addressed to the Home Secretary (Sir George Grey) and signed by the Master
of the Society of Apothecaries suggesting certain amendments in the Apothecaries
Act of 1815. Even more surprising were the profound changes advocated in relation
to certain clauses of the Act. Thus it was proposed that the service of an apprenticeship

by students should no longer be insisted upon. Even more unpredictable was the proposal that holders of British University degrees and licences or certificates of Scottish and Irish Colleges should be admitted to the medical register without further examination on payment of a small registration fee.

Straightway a meeting was held of the Joint Committee representative of the two Edinburgh Royal Colleges and the Edinburgh University Medical Faculty who then wrote to the Home Secretary. After deploring the dilatory progress of legislation in the matter of medical reform, the communication expressed 'peculiar satisfaction' and 'general concurrence' in the suggestions made by the Master of the Apothecaries' Society: and advanced the view that 'a measure' framed in accordance with the suggestions 'would go far to remove the most material of these grievances under which Practitioners of Medicine educated and licensed in Scotland have so long labored'. In all probability the 'peculiar satisfaction' referred to might reasonably be interpreted as elation, because no time was lost in carefully depositing the Society of Apothecaries' Memorial under lock and key in the Archives of the College.[29]

Apparently the sister College in Edinburgh was more cautious and perhaps more volatile in their impatience because, in 1854, they sent a copy of recent resolutions to the College of Physicians. These stated that the Surgeons were satisfied that there was no reasonable prospect of relief from persisting grievances being obtained through any measure of Medical Reform. They went on to give as 'an easy and effectual mode of redress', amendment of the Apothecaries Act to exempt Scottish graduates and licentiates from penalties under the Act.[30] The Surgeons' remedy did not appeal to the College of Physicians as being too limited and associated with difficulties of adoption even greater than those facing a more comprehensive measure.[30]

The trend of events both in and out of Parliament pointed to growing public interest in the state of the medical profession and its work. Concern was less focussed on the preservation of competitive interests and more on the infinitely wider ranging issues of medical reform as a national necessity. The conception underlying Graham's Bill was designed on a scale intended to deal with just such a problem. Preparatory participation by the College entailed an immense amount of work and were complete justice to be done to it, a volume would be required for the subject alone.

A DELEGATE GOES TO LONDON

While rumours had been current for some time, the first reliable information vouchsafed the College was in 1842. It took the form of a statement by the President

(Dr Robert Graham) that in sifting out facts from rumours he had approached the Home Office and been given in confidence some indication of the Government's intentions.[32] At an early date, following the example of the College of Surgeons and the University, a delegate was appointed in the person of Dr Renton 'to attend to the interests of the College in the construction of a Bill at present preparing'.[33] Previously Professor Christison and Mr William Wood had been appointed in similar capacities by the University and the College of Surgeons. Curiously another 'clash' of names occurred at this time calling for care to avoid confusion in consulting papers: the President of our College was Dr Robert Graham and the Secretary of State for the Home Department Sir James Graham. The heads of a proposed new Bill were communicated confidentially to the President by Sir James and laid before the College Committee on Medical Reform. In their Report the Committee expressed gratification that the provisions embodied the three principles—efficient education of all qualified medical men, a uniform plan of examination, and complete reciprocity of the right to practise in all parts of the United Kingdom. At the same time the Report remarked on the fact that some of the provisions betrayed ignorance of the nature and constitution of the Medical Schools and Corporations in Scotland.

A visit to London was necessary to clarify a number of points. Dr Renton, Mr Wood and Professor Christison proceeded south and throughout acted in unison and complete mutual understanding to the benefit of the three bodies they represented. They had an interview with, among others, Sir James Graham who suggested another meeting at which in view of the unanimity among the Edinburgh representatives only one need attend. On their return to Scotland these three representatives, by request, submitted to Sir James suggestions known to be agreeable to the London College of Physicians, a Committee of which they had met. One suggestion was to the effect that the Edinburgh Colleges should be endowed with the same privileges as those of London and remodelled if found necessary; another that any Central Council of Health should include one person connected with Scotland among non-professional members, and one physician and one surgeon from Edinburgh or Glasgow among professional members; and a third suggestion that the names of those receiving the degrees of M.D. and Bachelor of Medicine and Surgery of Edinburgh and Glasgow Universities should be included in the Medical Register. As to examinations in Edinburgh for general practitioners it was recommended that these should be conducted by a joint Board of Examiners from the two Colleges in equal proportions. A section of the Report dealt with suggestions applicable only to the Universities. Other points dealt with were the perennial problems of provincial cousins' travelling and subsistence allowances involved in visits to London.[34] The interim results obtained by the representatives of the two Colleges and the University were the subject of an appreciative letter from the College of Surgeons.[35]

In 1844 Dr Christison was adopted as a delegate for the College, he having spontaneously declared that although acting in a similar capacity for the University he would inform the College should his dual function involve any conflct of interests.[36] First introduced into the House in 1844, the Bill, slightly amended, was introduced a second time in the following year. After prolonged consideration of the amended Bill, the College in another Petition expressed their high approval 'of its leading principles and general provisions' and made certain suggestions about minor details.[37]

During a subsequent visit to London, the College delegate was impressed with the need for continuing observations 'on the spot' lest the College be injuriously affected by still further amendments. He was apprehensive that the interests of the three Medical Bodies might not be regarded as one and the same, and that legislation for one might be attempted at the expense of the others.[38] The College Committee on Medical Reform took exception to certain of the latest amendments and reiterated their views after detailed consideration of the Bill of July 1845. They objected in particular to the lack of assured medical representation on the Council of Health, and of the probable inadequate number of those representing Scottish interests; to proposals for the transfer of rights 'hitherto exercised' by Scottish Universities in the field of licensing to the Royal Colleges; and to the preservation of the privileges of Oxford and Cambridge as being inconsistent with the general principles of the Bill.[39] In February of the following year the College learnt that the Bill had been withdrawn.[40]

Within about 14 months the College was considering yet another Bill and on this occasion was recommended by its very favourably impressed Reform Committee to accept it without change, modification or delay. This the College did.[41]

INTER-CITY ACRIMONY

The next development was the receipt of instructions requiring the attendance of a member of the College for examination by a Committee of the House of Commons. Dr Renton was detailed off for this purpose. On his return he indicated that difficulty had occurred in arranging matters with the Glasgow Faculty which it had been suggested might be settled by amalgamating the Glasgow Faculty with the Edinburgh Colleges. Following discussion the College of Physicians resolved that it 'was prepared to receive, either as non-Resident Fellows according to the present charter or as members under the proposed new charter, without examination or Ballot, all Doctors of Medicine who may be members of the Faculty of Physicians and Surgeons of Glasgow'. Arrangements for agreement as to mode of tenure of properties were suggested and reference to the Lord Advocate considered in the event of arbitration being required. Copies of the resolution were sent to the Lord Advocate, the Registrar of the London College of Physicians and Mr William Wood of the Edinburgh College of Surgeons.[42]

An early outcome was a conference with a Committee of the Glasgow Faculty followed by the exchange of countless communications but with no discernible prospect of a satisfactory agreement being reached.[43] Negotiations dragged on, unseemly dissension was not lacking, correspondence became less and less edifying and eventually the College of Physicians declared 'the Committee for a junction between the Royal Colleges and the Glasgow Faculty to be at an end, and the proposals made by the Committee on the part of this College to be finally and entirely withdrawn'.[44] In the following year an attempt to reopen serious negotiations again failed.

EXASPERATION

Proceedings in general, and not merely those involving the Glasgow Faculty, were conducted in a new atmosphere at the turn of the half century. Quite obviously prolonged frustration was giving place to anger, hitherto successfully restrained. Years of plodding progress had apparently produced no more than a complete impasse. Prospects of overcoming this appeared negligible with so many interests embroiled in bitter irreconcilable disagreement. At an Extraordinary Meeting of the College in April 1850 recent events were subjected to a chronological review. Driven far beyond the point of exasperation the Medical Reform Committee had reported that 'the hopes . . . that the formation in the year 1848 of the Medical Reform Committee of the different classes of the Medical Profession in England would have led to the improvement of the Medical Polity of Great Britain, have been entirely blasted'.[45] In incisive but rather more temperate terms a Conference Committee reported to the Home Secretary that the plan for medical legislation which had won considerable favour among the profession could not be put into effect 'on account of the impossibility of reconciling the claims of the Royal College of Surgeons and those of the promoters of the intended new Royal College of General Practitioners, as to the examination in Surgery of General Practitioners'.

Amidst all this emotional turmoil one common desire transpired, that 'the Medical Bodies of Scotland should, so far as possible, act harmoniously together' with as one main objective the 'relief from the grievances under which Medical Men, educated or licensed in Scotland, now labour'. No semblance of humour enters into any of the proceedings. This is perhaps regrettable because for the silent Scot in the audience, the English medicopolitical stage provides something akin to a repertory of Falstaffian tragi-comedies. It is a measure of the intensity of Scottish resentment at the obdurate obstructionism of certain English interests that despite the disagreeable outcome of attempts to secure mergence of the Edinburgh and Glasgow Medical Corporations a new approach was considered. On this occasion the initiative was taken by the Edinburgh College of Surgeons which enquired from the Glasgow Faculty as to the practicability of forming a Conjoint Board to examine Candidates for licence as general practitioners. Happily an agreement was reached. Despite having been outpaced the College of Physicians gave the arrangements its blessing, after cautious deliberation.[46]

There is little doubt that in many respects the College shared genuine regret at the withdrawal of Graham's Bill. This is patently evident in resolutions passed in 1851 and prompted by consideration of yet another Bill, on this occasion for the Incorporation of General Practitioners. The College reacted strongly to a number of proposals under consideration for inclusion in the new Bill, and lost no time in writing to the Secretary of the national institute which was sponsoring it. Points selected for particular criticism included the suggestion that a proposed College of General Practitioners should control curricula of study and standards of examination of all licensing bodies 'out of London'; the suggested course of study over 'at least five years'; the implied requirement that all Scottish licentiates proposing to practise in England should first become members of the proposed College of General Practitioners; and the exclusion of the Colleges of Scotland from rights and privileges conceded to those in England.[47]

PHYSICIANS AND PHARMACISTS

Another Bill which came up for consideration by the College about this time aimed at Regulating the Qualifications of Pharmaceutical Chemists. While not objecting to druggists uniting in one body the College were concerned that the timing of the Bill might prove contrary to the interests of medical reform, and anxious lest there might be a reversal of prevailing trends were exclusive privileges granted to any new corporation. In support of the latter point the College drew attention to the way in which it had ceased to exercise its power of inspecting druggists because public competition had proved to have a more salutary influence. Rightly, rational nationalism demanded that the College should argue that nomination of parties to carry out the objects of the Bill in Scotland should be made 'on the spot' and not by a Board in London. Proposals to inflict penalties were condemned as obsolete except where a title had been fraudulently assumed. Looking to the future there was foresight in the objection of the College to exclusion of the medical profession from registration as pharmaceutical chemists because of the dependence of the public in remote districts unable to support a druggist. Once again the indefatigable Dr Renton was called upon to go as delegate to London where he joined forces with representatives of the Edinburgh College of Surgeons and the Glasgow Faculty.[48] The joint deputation and the College of Physicians were reassured by the amendments made to the Bill before it passed into Law.[49]

SEVERANCE OF INTER-CITY RELATIONS

Mention of the Medical and Surgical Association's Bill has already been made (q.v.). January 1852 saw publication of the first draft to which official representatives of the two Edinburgh Colleges quickly raised strong objections. Despite consequent amendments a letter signed by the Conveners of the Medical Reform Committees of the two Colleges and the Glasgow Faculty was sent to Mr (Sir) Charles Hastings, framer of the Bill. Much of the consultation between the three Scottish Medical Corporations was conducted on a semi-informal basis and most unfortunately this led later to undisguisedly acute disagreement, involving personalities which had official cognizance.

Two points were at issue between the Committees of the Colleges and the Glasgow Faculty. The first concerned the inclusion of the College of Physicians in an Examining Body proposed by the Bill. Whereas the Glasgow Faculty contended that it was not committed to any such policy, the Edinburgh Colleges maintained it was. Again there were opposed views as between the Glasgow and Edinburgh Councils in the matter of University representation on the new Board. At this late date, it would be pointless to adjudicate as to the rights and wrongs clouded as they were by mutual suspicions of misinterpretation, misrepresentation and even astute manipulation. Press Relations Officers were not known in those days—nor were centrally sponsored arbitrators. The upshot was that the correspondence which passed to and fro rarely achieved its declared intention of avoiding prolixity and reached a veritable crescendo. Consultations were broken off but information continued to be exchanged.[50]

Eventually the Edinburgh Colleges, aware that the possibility of one Examining Board for Scotland had been set aside, offered suggestions for the constitution of an Examining Board in Edinburgh 'leaving the constitution of one for Glasgow for future consideration in the proper quarter'.[51] Meanwhile a Report on the Bill of the Provincial Medical and Surgical Association by the Committees of the two Edinburgh Colleges had been transmitted to those drafting the Bill. Among recommendations made by it were that the title of Licentiate should follow and not precede registration, and that proof of age should be required before acceptance for examination. Possible constitutions for a Medical Council and an Examining Board for Scotland were submitted and it was urged that an Examination should be necessary for admission to all grades conferred by the Scottish Corporations and that 'one examination or set of Examinations should serve for every purpose'.[52]

A LEAK TO THE PRESS

About this time and wholly unexpectedly a spanner was thrown into the erratically grinding machinery for medical reform. There appeared, at the instance of the Provincial Medical and Surgical Association, an article entitled 'The Medical Reform Bill' in the *Lancet* and other medical journals. The Edinburgh College of Surgeons took immediate umbrage, and unintentionally and temporarily unmindful of its policy to co-operate with the sister College of Physicians, sent independently and without further ado the strongest of protests to the Secretary of State for the Home Department. There followed a prolonged series of communications between the two Colleges, and weighty deliberations in the College of Physicians. A Report submitted to the latter by its Medical Reform Committee stated that the publicized form of the Bill contained some but by no means all the Amendments recommended by them and previously accepted by the Association. The omissions seriously prejudiced the interests of Scottish Institutions. Acting on the advice of its Committee, the College noted that despite the error of having prematurely published the terms of the Bill the promoters were willing to introduce further amendments, and decided to delay final judgment 'in the present circumstances of the several Bills, relative to Medical Reform'.[53]

HESITANT OPTIMISM

While still engrossed with the situation created by the Provincial Association's Bill, the College had occasion to consider yet another Bill—that of Mr Brady—on 'the Registration of qualified Medical Practitioners, and for amending the law relative to the practice of Medicine in Great Britain and Ireland'. The Bill had little appeal for the College which forwarded a petition to the Home Secretary criticizing it on the grounds that it contained no provision for uniformity of medical education for candidates seeking licence to practise, and none for uniformity of examination by the licensing medical boards. It further took exception to the perpetuation of 'the obnoxious privileges in respect of practice' possessed by existing Medical Corporations, and expressed the hope that the Bill would be prevented from passing into Law.[53] When in fact Brady's Bill passed a second reading the College in the persons of the President (Dr T. S. Traill) and two members redoubled their efforts to oppose it by personally approaching the Lord Advocate and several Members of Parliament.[54] There followed a direct approach to the Home Secretary and Lord Advocate by the College representative (Dr Renton). This involved a visit to London during which Dr Renton took part in a meeting of the various medical bodies of the United Kingdom called to consider Medical Reform in general terms. As an indication of the difficulties of those holding a watching brief on behalf of the College, the concluding sentence in one of their Medical Reform Committee's Reports was illuminating.

> 'The committee being well aware that the Expectations of the College have been so often disappointed . . . are very unwilling to excite hopes on the present occasion . . . They however consider it their duty, in the present aspect of affairs, not to appear lukewarm or indifferent . . .'.[54]

However unconsciously, their attitude could not have better reflected that of others anxious for reform.

Having dealt with Mr Brady's Bill in so far as was within its power, the College had of necessity to turn its attention once more to the Provincial Association's Bill. After considering correspondence exchanged between Dr Renton and Mr Hastings of the Association, the College determined that it would not support the amended Bill because, among other reasons, there was no provision for reciprocity upon equal qualification throughout the Kingdom, and passage of a qualified doctor from one division of the Kingdom to another would involve additional examinations and expenditure.

UNIVERSITIES: A SOURCE OF INCREASING CONCERN

Constantly concerned to further general as distinct from fragmented medical reform, the College saw just cause for apprehension in the tabling in the House of Commons of a Bill intended to lead to 'The University of London Medical Graduates Act'. A Petition sent to Parliament opposed the Bill because it proposed, while excluding all other Universities, to grant to London University medical graduates privileges enjoyed for questionable historical reasons only by those of Oxford and Cambridge Universities. The extension of the privileges was seen not without reason as 'a gratuitous increase of the anomalies of Medical qualification, the prevalence of which is the chief source of the evils requiring correction in the exercise of the Medical Profession'. With equally good reason tribute was paid to the University of Edinburgh standing 'second to none as a Medical School [which] preceded . . . by many years every other University of the Empire in the establishment of a complete system of Medical Instruction and in making that instruction imperative for the attainment of Medical Degrees'.[55] To have mentioned in the protest the extent to which the University's auspicious achievement was contributed to by the College would have been inappropriate, and perhaps in those days unethical (Chap. XVII).

Distractions were not far to seek, nor long awaited. Fast on the heels of the London University Bill came one sponsored by a Colonel Dunne 'to extend the rights enjoyed by the Universities of Oxford and Cambridge in respect to the practice of physic of the Graduates of the Universities of Ireland and Scotland'. There was considerable discussion, revolving around the College view that a University medical degree should be evaluated as an honorary distinction; and that the legal right to practise should be 'derived from the license or letters testimonial of a Body composed of Gentlemen actually engaged in the practice of Medicine'. Some members saw in the Bill an endeavour to remedy an anomaly by placing the graduates of all Universities in the United Kingdom on an equal footing. Eventually the Bill was condemned by the College and the successful motion drew attention to the objectionable situation at Durham University which 'does not even profess to have any arrangements to the public teaching of Medical Science within its walls'.[56] It was decided that a Petition against the Bill should be sent.

Simultaneously a short Memorial was submitted outlining the effect Dunne's Bill and the London University Graduates Bill if passed, would have on prospects of medical reform.

Exception was taken by Dr Christison to the implied criticism by the College of the legal privilege of graduates to practise, and to the liability of dissension being created between the College and the Universities.[57] As events turned out, acting on instructions the Secretary to the Senatus Academicus of the University of Edinburgh transmitted to the College a copy of a highly condemnatory Senate minute, accusing the College of conducting negotiations liable to prove detrimental to the privileges of Edinburgh graduates.[58] The College for its part maintained that its concern had been that University Degrees should not become the subject of legislation until Parliament had considered the overall question of Medical Reform.[59]

The list of proposed enactments was well-nigh interminable. It is to the immense credit of the College that despite the variety of emphases and aims of successive Bills, and despite altercations with friends and foes alike, they did not deviate from their long-term objective of securing comprehensive overall medical reform while at the same time preserving the rightful interests of Scottish medicine. This consistency prevailed for over 50 years. To stigmatize the College as repetitious because of its many memorials and petitions would be entirely unwarranted. Such repetitiveness as was evident was a measure of the consistency which enabled the College to salvage and preserve professional principles threatened with submergence in a legislative quagmire.

Headlam's Bill followed that of Dunne and was considered by the College in May 1855, the draft copy having been obtained from the Home Department on application by the Secretary of the College Reform Committee. This Committee heartily endorsed proposals for a uniform system of qualification for general practice, complete reciprocity for practice throughout the Kingdom, the creation of a supervisory Medical Council to be nominated by the Crown, and the establishment of a medical register. In marked contrast they disapproved of the proposed recognition of University degrees of Doctorate of Medicine as a legal title to practise medicine, and so strong were their feelings that they maintained that the provision vitiated the entire Bill.

This problem of University degrees was to be a thorny one for a number of years. Christison in particular was a redoubtable champion in College *sederunts* of the case for the University. After lengthy discussions the College expressed its general approval of Headlam's Bill while reserving the right to suggest any desirable modifications of details at a later stage. At the same time they showed both tact and tactical skill in deciding not to enter on the delicate questions involved in 'the Edinburgh University Bill'.[60] As described by Grant, the inflammable question of University patronage was being debated[61] and the politicians were talking in terms of a Central University for Scotland which would involve the abrogation by existing

Universities of their individual existences and the suppression of ancient corporations linking Scotland with her ancient past.

HEADLAM WINS EVENTUAL FAVOUR—WITH RESERVATIONS

The next development was the receipt from the Home Secretary of a copy of Headlam's 'Bill for Amending the Laws relating to the Medical Profession' with a request for the College's assessment.[62] In arriving at their opinion the College had available, additional to that of its own Reform Committee, the Reports of the Edinburgh College of Surgeons and the Glasgow Faculty together with independent statements from Drs Christison and Alison.[63] Deliberations were numerous and detailed. Final resolutions expressed doubt about the size of the proposed Medical Council which would, if meetings were to be frequent, possibly give undue influence to those 'who from locality . . . may find it most convenient to attend with regularity'. This long-standing bogey had basis. A case was made out for a Secretary who should also be Registrar for Scotland to avoid 'the impediment of local business' from centralization in London. Agreeing that examination of the surgeon should be conducted by both Royal Colleges in Edinburgh, our College indicated its willingness to implement a similar plan for the examination of physicians and 'a joint Board for the two Colleges for all purposes of Examination'. As to powers being conferred on Corporations including the College, to remove a medical practitioner's name from the General Register, the College was insistent that such powers should be vested in the Crown, and the Crown alone. Other resolutions drew attention to the need to keep the expenses of study, licence and registration to a minimum in order not to discourage recruitment which would leave the field wide open to 'unlicensed pretenders'.[64] It emphasized also, the plight of the Highlands and Islands. These views formed the basis of representations made by the President (Dr James Begbie) and Secretary who went to London to promote College views among those concerned, including appropriate Members of Parliament. About this time the returns relating to medical licences were made in conformity with a resolution of the House of Commons.[65] Subsequent amendments met with the approval of the College which thereupon agreed to petition in favour of the Bill, and the petition was presented by a Member for Edinburgh, but all to little avail.[66] Unexpected opposition in Parliament and the lateness of the Parliamentary Session combined to compel withdrawal of the Bill.[67]

CO-OPERATION AMONG CORPORATIONS

Belatedly there was frank admission that disagreement among representative bodies of the profession was a major factor in impeding progress in medical reform. This was recognized in a Report by Council in February 1857 which ventured

> 'there is a reasonable prospect of the eight Medical Incorporations of the United Kingdom concurring in their views of Medical Reform to an extent never before witnessed in the long period during which this subject has been agitated'.

Several developments justified this happier outlook.[68]

In 1856 the three Royal Colleges of Surgeons and the Glasgow Faculty had come to an agreement to promote the formation of a Council composed of representatives of all the medical incorporations with a view to creating a Register of qualified Practitioners, regulating medical and surgical education, and securing uniformity and reciprocity of privileges 'of members of each division of the profession in the United Kingdom'.[69] In due course our College joined in the agreement 'on the distinct understanding' that they were to be left 'quite unfettered thereby in regard to any medical Bill' that might later be brought before Parliament.[70] At a subsequent meeting with the Edinburgh College of Surgeons and another in London it was considered reasonable that medical practitioners not being physicians should be enrolled in a College of Surgeons, and registered as surgeons and practitioners in medicine and midwifery: and that the Edinburgh College of Physicians should endorse the Diploma of the College of Surgeons with 'Letters Testimonial' certifying merely examination, provided examiners from the College of Physicians were admitted into the Examining Board appointed by the College of Surgeons.[71]

With the full agreement of Council two representatives then joined a meeting in London attended by delegates of all the medical incorporations to discuss medical reform. Agreement was reached on a form of 'Amended proposals for a Medical Bill', and a decision made that there should be established 'a Committee for Correspondence' in each Division of the United Kingdom. These Committees came to be referred to as the Scottish, English and Irish 'Branch Conferences'. The proposals met with the general approval of the College.[72] They provided for the continued separation of the three Scottish Incorporations without precluding the possibility of amalgamation into two Royal Colleges for Scotland should it be desired at any future time. A proviso was that there should always be an Examining Board both in Edinburgh and Glasgow, and that our College should supply examiners to the Glasgow Examining Board and endorse the Glasgow testimonial with its own letters testimonial. A proposal at the Conference that a degree in Arts should be an essential preliminary to one in medicine was rejected. The desirability of a National Pharmacopoeia was endorsed, as was a proposal to prepare a draft Bill and send a deputation to Lord Palmerston. The Report of the Edinburgh delegates to the London visit was approved. It was then decided that the time had come for the College Reform Committee to be dissolved and for full responsibility for all negotiations to revert to the Council of the College.[73]

Following this decision the first Report by the Council confirmed the agreement already contemplated with the Glasgow Faculty, and referred to two draft Bills submitted to it—one from the English Branch Conference and another from the Irish counterpart. A meeting in London of the eight medical corporations to discuss the first of these was attended by the Council's Secretary. Final adjustments were made to the draft Bill which was entrusted to three Members of Parliament, including Mr Headlam, to bring it before the House. Unfortunately the Bill had to be withdrawn because of the anticipated Dissolution of Parliament.

CORPORATIONS AND THE UNIVERSITIES

A feature of this last London meeting of the medical Corporations (at which there were no delegates of the Scottish Universities) was the support in principle given to the draft Bill by two University representatives—those of Oxford University and Trinity College, Dublin. This was not without significance. Although preceding years had seen some considerable degree of mergence between Scottish and English attitudes, physicians and surgeons, and competitive medical licensing bodies, no clear understanding had been arrived at between the Corporations and the Universities. Influenced by the proceedings at London, the views expressed by Oxford University, and a 'Statement issued by a majority of Scottish Universities' the Scottish Branch Conference submitted a number of resolutions to the Scottish Universities. One was to the effect that the Scottish Universities should be represented on the General Council by two members. Another was that the title to Registration as Physician should consist of a certificate of examination in a series of specified subjects including 'the Practice of Medicine by the College of Physicians'; a Degree of Doctor of Medicine from a University; and a Licence to practise from the College of Physicians.

This second resolution was not intended to interfere in any way with the rights of Universities to grant degrees. An analogous resolution dealt with Surgeons.

All the resolutions of the Scottish Branch Conference were sent to the English and Irish Conferences who indicated general approval; and after being seen by the Council of the College were forwarded to the Scottish Universities whose reactions were not known for some time. Obviously the Council, with its eye to both present and future relations with the Universities, was in a difficult position and it is recorded that 'while the Council consented to the transmission of the Resolutions to the Universities . . . they expressed their regret that they were as they conceived, inadequate for effecting a compromise'.[74] If the position of the Council was difficult that of individual Fellows who were also University Senators must have been invidious at times, no matter the dignity with which it was faced.

On 12th May 1857 a meeting took place of representatives of Edinburgh University, Glasgow University and Marischal College, Aberdeen with the delegates of the Scottish Medical and Surgical Corporations. From the outset it was clear that the views of the Corporations and Universities were widely at variance. For the Universities it was explained that the 'Statement' (q.v.) was an expression of what the Universities would wish if preparing a draft Bill independently of the Corporations. Discussing examinations for the degree of M.D. a representative of the Corporations maintained that licence to practise medicine should 'proceed from the Profession itself' as in the case of licence to practise in 'the Legal and Clerical Professions'. As to the privileges of the holders of University Degrees there was agreement that under the proposed Bill the degree of M.D. would be evaluated as indicative of a physician. The position was different in so far as the proposed degree of M.B. was concerned. Those with the M.B. would, according to the University, be entitled to act as ordinary general practitioners not practising pharmacy, but would not be entitled to hold surgical appointments in all circumstances. With minimal delay the Edinburgh College of Surgeons recorded their inability to agree to the proposals, and declined to countenance them.[75]

CLASH OF RESUSCITATED BILLS

Once again there was a plethora of Bills. A Report on two was submitted by the Council on 22nd May 1857. One was Lord Elcho's Bill, differing little if at all from his Bill of the previous year; and the other Mr Headlam's Bill, closely resembling the draft Bill produced at the London Conference four months previously, and differing only in the matter of the constitution of the Council. Which of the two Bills should be supported? That was the dilemma confronting the College; a dilemma compelling the Council to refrain from offering advice 'thinking it to be more advisable that such proceedings . . . should originate in the College itself'. As was to be expected discussion was long and as the subject deserved, profound, necessitating more than one Extraordinary Meeting. One issue around which discussion revolved particularly was the interests of the Universities. Headlam's Bill made no attempt to propitiate the Universities in Scotland and England most interested in medical legislation, but was unquestionably more favourable to the Corporations.[76]

A PERPLEXITY OF CONSCIENCE

The College found itself in the equivalent of a cleft stick. It had exclusively exerted its influence in favour of Headlam's Bill before the resuscitation of Lord Elcho's Bill. The last named contemplated removing the responsibility of licensing the general practitioner entirely from the licensing Corporations, a proposal which was inflexibly opposed by all Medical Corporations except the Edinburgh College of Physicians. No success attended determined attempts to persuade the other Corporations to make concessions to the claims of the Universities. No less entrenched opposition was shewn by the members of the Irish and English Branch Conferences. Consistency and indeed integrity pointed to the need to continue pressing the claims of the Scottish Universities on the other promoters of Headlam's Bill. Undoubtedly persistence along these lines involved risk of antagonizing all the Corporations, and of a completely isolated negotiating position. Eventually at the same time as deciding to negotiate in the further stage of Headlam's Bill, the College resolved to endeavour by every means in their power to 'secure a due recognition for such claims of the Scottish Universities as have been admitted to be reasonable'.[77] Not blatantly courageous in cold print perhaps, but no graduate of the University of Edinburgh can read the Minutes of the College without warming to the persistence with which the College lent its weighty support to many of the claims of the University. Grant, the Principal of the University, indulged in an unqualified critical judgment on the attitude of the Corporations towards the institution of a Degree of Bachelor of Medicine after the passing of the Medical Act of 1858, specifically mentioning our College.[78] Scant recognition indeed for the unpopularity incurred by the College on behalf of the University!

ALACRITY WHEN INDICATED

At times the College may have seemed ponderous in deliberation but there were occasions when it could act with alacrity. One such situation occurred in connection with Headlam's Act. The College was approached to support it at extremely short notice in anticipation of a deputation from the London College of Physicians waiting on Sir George Grey. At this late stage it was found that a 'mischievous and unexplained interpolation, totally at variance with the principle of a uniform reciprocity of license to practise within the three Kingdoms' had been effected. It transpired that an invitation to send a representative with the deputation had been received from the London College of Physicians but insufficient time was given in which to take advantage of it. To obviate misunderstanding or misconstruction in the event of the acknowledgment not reaching London in time, a confirmatory Telegraphic Message was sent. By general consent the interpolated passage from Headlam's Bill was withdrawn and news to that effect was again conveyed by Telegraphic Message to the President (Dr David Maclagan).[79]

A TEMPORARY VACUUM

On the 1st July 1857 after discussion of the two Bills before the House, Headlam's Bill was carried by the surprising majority of 147—225 votes 'for' and 78 'against'. At a meeting on the following day to discuss amendments considered desirable for introduction by Mr Headlam in Committee, the College delegate found that attempts by him to obtain improved terms for the Universities met with intensified opposition. This he attributed to irritation following speeches in the House the previous evening on behalf of Lord Elcho's Bill. Nevertheless an important concession was obtained in that preliminary examinations were to become the sole responsibility of the Universities, the conduct of the strictly professional examinations remaining that of the College. Again the circumstances of Parliamentary business compelled withdrawal of the Bill without it passing through the committee stage. As Lord Elcho's Bill had also been withdrawn no measure relative to medical reform remained before Parliament.[80]

COWPER JOINS THE FRAY

At an Extraordinary Meeting of the College on 9th April 1858 it was reported that in the new session of Parliament Lord Elcho's Bill had been revived and that another Bill had been introduced by Mr Cowper. As to the Elcho Bill it was not expected to differ from its predecessor except in so far as a representative medical council might be considered instead of a Council to be elected by the Crown.[81] Cowper's Bill had already been considered by the Scottish Branch Conference and they were of the opinion that it embodied important principles repeatedly approved by the College. Discussion by the College devoted much time to the position of the Universities as potential licensing authorities. One curious outcome was realization that whereas at one time the College had been opposed to University degrees conveying a right to practise, resolutions in support of Headlam's Bill implied anxiety to secure better terms for the Universities.[81] To some extent this apparent paradox may have been attributable to delegation by the College Council of powers to negotiate to its representatives on the Scottish Branch Conference.

A representative attended a Conference of Corporate Bodies in London when Cowper's Bill was studied clause by clause, after which, in a way curious to those uninitiated in lobbying procedures, those at the Conference made contact with Mr Headlam who had sponsored the Corporation's Bill of the previous session. Headlam's advice was that the delegates should outline their precise objections to the Bills of Lord Elcho and Mr Cowper to the Prime Minister and Secretary of State; and endeavour to have brought forward a modified form of the recent Corporations' Bill. He was opposed to amendment of Cowper's Bill being made because of the number of alterations which would be required. Representatives of all the Royal Colleges, the Glasgow Faculty and the Society of Apothecaries were later received by Mr Walpole who ruled that attention be confined to Mr Cowper's Bill, Lord Elcho's having been put aside. Convinced that there was little likelihood of the Government's introducing a Bill, the delegates returned to the Conference where it was decided to revise and improve Mr Headlam's Bill of the previous Session and to be guided in future procedure by Mr Headlam.[82] Later the College approved a report by its delegate at a subsequent Scottish Branch Conference which, having been informed that the English Branch intended to wait on the Prime Minister and urge the introduction of a modified Bill of the Corporations as a Government measure, had expressed its cordial concurrence with the objective.

A DIVIDED COUNCIL

Disagreement of a distasteful kind then surfaced in the College deliberations. Essentially the division of opinions related to University degrees and the privileges to be associated with them, but a major disturbing factor was doubt about the procedure whereby instructions to College delegates were issued directly by the Council. A strong body of opinion considered that instructions should emanate from the College itself, having regard to 'the divided state of the Council'. It was accordingly decided until the next election meeting, 'to transfer the management of the whole matter from the Council to a special Committee who shall be instructed to carry out the former decisions of the College but not to originate any new plan or to concur in any plan so originated without coming to the College for farther instructions'. Pioneer delegates were not discarded—Drs Renton, Seller and Wood were included in the Committee.[83]

PROTESTS IN ABUNDANCE

All was not set fair for the newly launched Committee. In response to a requisition signed by a number of Fellows an Extraordinary Meeting was held. At this meeting protests were heard concerning the irresolute attitude of the College and its delegates, and the 'hostility' of the College 'to the Scottish Universities, and more especially to the University of Edinburgh its most natural and respectable ally'. These protests were linked with an objection to the restitution of a Medical Reform Committee. Among signatories to the protest were such prominent Fellows as (Sir) Robert Christison and (Sir) J. Y. Simpson. Troubles did not come singly. At the same meeting another protest also coupled with a request for an Extraordinary Meeting was considered. This concerned 'the infringement of Collegiate action involved in a Memorial addressed to the Honourable W. J. Cowper and signed by certain Fellows of the College'. The names of signatories to the protest included those of two members who had been untiring in their efforts as College delegates—Drs Robert Renton and Alexander Wood.[84]

Within six weeks another Extraordinary Meeting was called in response to a request from half a dozen Fellows to consider steps to be taken in connection with 'the exclusion of Medical Graduates from voting in the University Council under the Lord Advocate's Universities Bill'. After considerable discussion and careful drafting a Memorial was submitted by the College to the Lord Advocate giving reasons for regarding the selective exclusion of medical graduates as 'alike indefensible and unjust': and urging that appropriate amendments be introduced into the Universities Bill.[85] The College throughout had adopted the widest of interpretations of medical reform, and it was rational to view the Universities Bill as it affected graduates in medicine in the context of medical reform.

SOBER OPTIMISM

On 20th July 1858 the College received a Report from the Committee on Medical Reform. Without being ebullient or ecstatic it was cheerfully optimistic about prospects 'of a very speedy settlement of the much vexed question of Medical Reform'. Mention was made of the numerous meetings of the General Conference held in London during the preceding four weeks. Obviously conscious of the criticism of extravagance directed by a few Fellows against the previous Medical Reform Committee, the Report elaborated how attendance at all meetings was not considered vital and how delegates 'were unwilling to draw too largely . . . on the Funds of the College'. Despite limited resources an endeavour was made however, 'to maintain its [the College's] position among the other corporate Bodies, and to retain that amount of influence which it has hitherto possessed in the deliberations of the Conference'. Considering that the culmination of years of effort on behalf of medical reform was near at hand, and that in the absence of their delegate the interests of the College were looked after by 'delegates of the other Scottish and Irish Bodies who were more frequently and assiduously in London'—this aspect of the Report makes distressing reading.[86]

RESERVED APPROVAL OF SUCCESSFUL BILL

By the end of June (1858) the successful passage of Cowper's Bill was a more or less foregone conclusion and the Conference had been successful in securing one or two last minute amendments. An attempt to insert a clause preventing the Universities from acquiring licensing powers failed, but two clauses which had been omitted were inserted—one enabling separate bodies to unite to form a joint complete examining board, and the other giving Fellows of the Edinburgh College *ad eundem* admission to the Sister College in London. Amendments intended to secure to Colleges the licensing power were lost by an overwhelming majority in Committee. On 12th July 1858 the General Conference resolved to offer no further opposition to the progress of the Bill. Having considered and approved the Report of their Reform Committee the College resolved 'to take no farther action regarding Mr. Cowper's Medical Practitioners Bill, and in the event of that Bill becoming Law, remit to the Committee to report to the College fully in regard to the new Charter and other changes required . . . '.[86]

The Bill passed into Law on 2nd August 1858 and the first recorded reference to it as an Act is in the Minutes of 26th August when it was agreed that the Reform Committee's final Report (q.v.) when complete should be printed for the private and confidential perusal of the Fellows of the College.[87]

ACT TO AMEND THE MEDICAL ACT

Having regard to the prolonged confusion which characterized Parliamentary proceedings prior to the passing of the Medical Act of 1858 it is not surprising that the need for amendments was soon recognized. In 1883 the College remitted to Council to watch progress of a Medical Act Amendment Bill which was in course of preparation. Council was empowered to take all needful steps to safeguard the interests of the College.[88]

An early step taken was the calling of a Conference of the Councils of the two Edinburgh Royal Colleges. The Conference instructed the President of our College (Dr George Balfour) to write Mr Gladstone, First Lord of the Treasury, with the object of securing his influence to have the new Medical Act Amendment Act modified in view of its 'influence . . . on the Scottish Medical Corporations and Universities'. Acting on instructions the President communicated also with the Chairman of the Midlothian Liberal Committee who thereafter served as intermediary for transmitting correspondence. Two letters were sent by the President which referred to the preponderance of University influence on the Medical Board for Scotland, and described the proposed measures as being essentially English in conception and based upon jealousy of the success attained by the Scottish Universities and Corporations. Predictably, Mr Gladstone's response was in accordance with established Parliamentary non-committal procedure. 'He', wrote his Midlothian agent, 'will at the present . . . confine himself to saying that all the Representations in the Medical Act Amendment Bill . . . made by these important Scottish Corporations will be sure to engage the careful consideration of Her Majesty's Government.'[89-92]

The Medical Act Amendment Act passed into Law in June 1886. By its enactments examinations could be conducted by universities, combinations of corporations, combinations of universities, and combinations of universities and corporations; and passing of an examination in medicine, surgery and midwifery was made a condition of registration. The Act also increased the number of members of the Medical Council from twenty-three to thirty of whom one was to be elected by the profession in Scotland, one by the profession in Ireland, and three in England and Wales.

REFERENCES

(1) CLARK, Sir G. (1966) *A History of the Royal College of Physicians of London*, vol. 2, p. 625. Oxford: Clarendon Press.
(2) College Minutes, 7.viii.1804.
(3) Ibid., 5.xi.1805.
(4) Ibid., 6.xi.1804.
(5) Ibid., 5.xi.1805.
(6) Ibid., 6.v.1806.
(7) Ibid., 4.xi.1806.
(8) Ibid., 3.ii.1807.
(9) Ibid., 7.viii.1810.
(10) Ibid., 22.ii.1811.
(11) SHAW, G. B. (1911) *The Doctor's Dilemma*. (Preface on doctors.) London: Constable.
(12) DRUMMOND, C. G. (1953) *Pharmacy and Medicine in Old Edinburgh*. London: Pharmaceutical Press.
(13) GILMOUR, J. P. (1938) Phases of Pharmacy in Edinburgh. *Quarterly Journal of Pharmacy and Pharmacology*, **XI**, 361.
(14) CLARK, Sir G. Op. cit., vol. 2, p. 646.
(15) R.C.P.E. (1925) *Historical Sketch and Laws*, p. 63. Edinburgh: Royal College of Physicians.
(16) College Minutes, 14.vi.1827.
(17) Ibid., 8.iv.1833.
(18) Ibid., 16.iv.1833.
(19) Ibid., 7.v.1833.
(20) Ibid., 29.vi.1833.
(21) Ibid., 2.vii.1833.
(22) Ibid., 8.vii.1833.
(23) Ibid., 24.viii.1833.
(24) Ibid., 1.viii.1837.
(25) Ibid., 5.xi.1839.
(26) Ibid., 4.ii.1840.

(27) Ibid., 1.v.1848.
(28) Ibid., 1.ii.1853.
(29) Ibid., 6.viii.1850.
(30) Ibid., 2.iii.1854.
(31) Ibid., 30.iii.1854.
(32) Ibid., 1.ii.1842.
(33) Ibid., 16.v.1842.
(34) Ibid., 15.vi.1842.
(35) Ibid., 2.viii.1842.
(36) Ibid., 17.iv.1844.
(37) Ibid., 27.iii.1845.
(38) Ibid., 6.v.1845.
(39) Ibid., 4.xi.1845.
(40) Ibid., 3.ii.1846.
(41) Ibid., 11.v.1847.
(42) Ibid., 17.v.1848.
(43) Ibid., 1.v.1849.
(44) Ibid., 7.viii.1849.
(45) Ibid., 16.iv.1850.
(46) Ibid., 16.iv.1850.
(47) Ibid., 4.ii.1851.
(48) Ibid., 4.v.1852.
(49) Ibid., 3.viii.1852.
(50) Ibid., 11.iii.1853.
(51) Ibid., 13.iv.1853.
(52) Ibid., 11.iii.1853.
(53) Ibid., 20.iii.1854.
(54) Ibid., 2.v.1854.
(55) Ibid., 26.v.1854.
(56) Ibid., 20.vii.1854.
(57) Ibid., 1.viii.1854.
(58) Ibid., 3.viii.1854.
(59) Ibid., 7.xi.1854.
(60) Ibid., 15.v.1855.
(61) GRANT, Sir A. (1884) *The Story of the University of Edinburgh*, vol. II, p. 93. London: Longmans, Green & Co.
(62) College Minutes, 7.viii.1855.
(63) Ibid., 15.v.1855.
(64) Ibid., 18.iii.1856.
(65) Ibid., 6.v.1856.
(66) Ibid., 16.vi.1856.
(67) Ibid., 5.viii.1856.
(68) Ibid., 3.ii.1857.

(69) Ibid., 18.x.1856.
(70) Ibid., 5.viii.1856.
(71) Ibid., 8.ii.1857.
(72) Ibid., 4.xi.1856.
(73) Ibid., 3.ii.1857.
(74) Ibid., 5.v.1857.
(75) Ibid., 19.v.1857.
(76) Ibid., 22.v.1857.
(77) Ibid., 2.vi.1857.
(78) GRANT, Sir A. Op. cit., p. 110.
(79) College Minutes, 2.vi.1857.
(80) Ibid., 4.viii.1857.
(81) Ibid., 9.iv.1858.
(82) Ibid., 4.v.1858.
(83) Ibid., 7.v.1858.
(84) Ibid., 11.v.1858.
(85) Ibid., 22.vi.1858.
(86) Ibid., 20.vii.1858.
(87) Ibid., 26.viii.1858.
(88) Ibid., 1.v.1883.
(89) Council Minutes, 9.vi.1883.
(90) Ibid., 26.vi.1883.
(91) Ibid., 3.vii.1883.
(92) Ibid., 14.vii.1883.

Chapter XIII

MEDICAL REFORM AS LEGALLY
INTERPRETED:
THE MEDICAL ACT, 1858

Quaestio fit de legibus, non de personis.

Officially entitled *An Act to regulate the Qualifications of Practitioners of Medicine and Surgery*, the Medical Act of 1858 took effect from the first day of October that year.[1] Today the preamble reads strangely giving as reason for the enactment that 'it is expedient that Persons requiring Medical Aid should be enabled to distinguish qualified from unqualified Practitioners'.

MAJOR RELEVANT FEATURES

For administrative purposes a General Council, or to give it its full name 'The General Council of Medical Education and Registration of the United Kingdom' was created, together with three Branch Councils—one each for Scotland, England and Ireland. It was ordained that the General Council should consist of twenty-three individuals. Of these one each was to be chosen by the College of Physicians of Edinburgh; the College of Surgeons of Edinburgh; the Faculty of Physicians and Surgeons of Glasgow; the University of Edinburgh and the two Universities of Aberdeen collectively; and the University of Glasgow and the University of St Andrews collectively. English Bodies to have one representative each were the Royal College of Physicians of London; the Royal College of Surgeons of England; the Apothecaries Society of London; the University of Oxford; the University of Cambridge; the University of Durham; and the University of London. The Irish Bodies each to have one representative were the King's and Queen's College of Physicians in Ireland; the Royal College of Surgeons in Ireland; the Apothecaries

Hall of Ireland; the University of Dublin; and the Queen's University in Ireland. In addition the Crown on the advice of the Privy Council nominated six individuals of whom one was appointed for Scotland, four for England and one for Ireland. The General Council was to elect its own President. For no discernible reason, the Edinburgh Colleges of Physicians and Surgeons were alone among Royal Colleges mentioned in the crucial fourth clause, in not being credited with their centuries old historical 'Royal' designation. Elsewhere in the Act and its Schedules there is no such discriminatory omission.

The Branch Council for Scotland consisted of those members of the General Council chosen by the Medical Corporations and Universities of Scotland, together with the Crown nomination for Scotland and the President of the General Council who was a member of all three Branch Councils. Comparable arrangements were established for the other Branch Councils. It was stipulated that representatives of the Medical Corporations on the General Council had to be qualified for registration under the Act. Appointment of any member of the General Council was not to exceed five years, but reappointment was not precluded. Acts of the General Council were to be decided by a majority vote of those present, eight constituting a quorum and the President having a casting vote 'in case of an Equality of Votes' additional to his vote as a member of the Council. Power was vested in the Council to appoint an Executive Committee of which a quorum was not to be less than three. In common with the other Branch Councils that for Scotland was required to appoint officers including a Registrar, who was to act also as Secretary to the Branch Council and as Treasurer in addition if considered desirable.

The duties of the Branch Council Registrar included the keeping of Registers up to date in respect of the addresses, qualifications, retirements and deaths of those on the Register: and in the fulfilment of his duties he was authorized to write making enquiries of any registered person and in the absence of any reply to have his name erased after an interval of six months (§ XIV*). Names entered into the local register by the Registrar of the Branch Council for Scotland required to be sent to the General Council for insertion in the General Register (§ XXV). The annual publication of a Register was made the responsibility of the Registrar of the General Council (§ XXVII). It was also made incumbent upon any College or Body which in virtue of legal powers possessed by it removed one of their number from its list of members, to report such action to the General Council. Should the General Council see fit the Registrar could erase from the Register the qualification granted by the College in respect of the member concerned, subject always to the proviso that 'the Name of

* Roman figures refer to Sections of the Act.

no Person shall be erased . . . on the Ground of his having adopted any Theory of Medicine or Surgery' (§ XXVIII). Registrars of Deaths were under obligation to keep the Registrars of the General Council and appropriate Branch Council informed by post of the death, together with time and place, of any medical practitioner. To ensure reliable returns the Registrar of Deaths was told he might charge the cost of certificates and transmission as 'an Expense of his Office' (§ XLV).

Those eligible after payment of a fee to inclusion in the Register were persons who possessed one or more specified qualifications. These qualifications, given in Schedule A of the Act, were:

> Fellow or Licentiate of the Royal College of Physicians of Edinburgh.
> Fellow or Licentiate of the Royal College of Surgeons of Edinburgh.
> Fellow or Licentiate of the Faculty of Physicians and Surgeons of Glasgow.
> Fellow, Licentiate or Extra Licentiate of the Royal College of Physicians of London.
> Fellow or Licentiate of the King's and Queen's College of Physicians of Ireland.
> Fellow or Member or Licentiate in Midwifery of the Royal College of Surgeons of England.
> Fellow or Licentiate of the Royal College of Surgeons in Ireland.
> Licentiate of the Society of Apothecaries, London.
> Licentiate of the Apothecaries Hall, Dublin.
> Doctor, or Bachelor, or Licentiate of Medicine, or Master in Surgery of any University of the United Kingdom; or Doctor of Medicine by Doctorate granted prior to passing of this Act by the Archbishop of Canterbury.
> Doctor of Medicine of any Foreign or Colonial University or College, practising as a Physician in the United Kingdom before the First Day of October 1858, who shall produce Certificates to the Satisfaction of the Council of his having taken his Degree of Doctor of Medicine after regular Examination . . . (There was provision also for dispensation in exceptional circumstances.)

The Registrar was entitled to accept periodic lists received from Colleges and Bodies for the extraction of details intended for insertion in the Register on payment of the requisite fee. A provision of particular importance (§ XVII) was that any person who was actually practising medicine in *England* before 1st August 1815, could on signing a declaration to that effect on payment of a fee be registered by any one of the three Branch Councils.

Equally important in an entirely different connection was the authority given the General Council to require information about courses of studies, examinations, the ages of students, and qualifications awarded: and to arrange for members or representatives to be present at examinations (§ XVIII). Subject to the agreement of the General Council two or more Colleges mentioned in Schedule A were permitted to co-operate in conducting qualifying examinations. In the event of courses of study and examinations leading to qualifications not satisfying standards considered desirable, the General Council were empowered to report to the Privy Council. Representations along these channels, if not successful in remedying the situation, could withhold recognition for the purpose of registration of qualifications conferred by the offending College or Body (§§XX and XXI). Attempts to impose restrictions on the practice by candidates of any particular theory of medicine or surgery were declared unacceptable and if persisted in, involved the risk of the offending Body being deprived of authority to grant qualifications registrable under the Act (§ XXIII).

Sundry sections of the Act dealt with situations in which Licentiates and to a lesser extent Fellows of the Edinburgh College of Physicians found themselves in their land of licentiateship or in England. Thus—provided they registered—medical officers in the employ of the Poor Law Commissioners or Poor Law Board were not subject to disqualification: and registered practitioners were exempted from service on a jury or in the militia. All public appointments including those of medical officers of health, service as medical officer in whatever professional capacity in the fighting services, and those involving attachment to hospitals, asylums, work-houses and poor-houses, could be held only by practitioners registered under the Act (§ XXXVI). In like manner a Certificate required under any enactment was valid only if signed by a registered practitioner. Fraudulent attempts to represent registration under the Medical Act, and fraudulent use of the titles Physician, Doctor of Medicine, Licentiate in Medicine and Surgery, Practitioner in Medicine, or an Apothecary were punishable at Law. A false claim to registration was politely termed a Misdemeanour in England: and a forthright Crime or Offence in Scotland. No matter: English Misdemeanour and Scottish Crime were alike in that, on conviction, the accused ran the risk of imprisonment 'for any Term not exceeding Twelve Months' (§ XXXIX). The Act was at pains not to prejudice in any way the lawful activities of Chemists, Druggists or Dentists (§ LV): and the General Council were under instructions to publish, and reissue as often as they considered desirable, a 'British Pharmacopoeia' (§ LIV).

The terminal sections of the Act were no less important than the earlier ones in so far as the Edinburgh Royal College of Physicians was concerned. Section XLVII declared that a new Charter might be granted to the Corporation of the Royal College of Physicians of London to enable modifications in the constitution to be made, and alteration of the Corporation's name to 'The Royal College of Physicians of England'. As stated in the Medical Act 1858 acceptance of the new Charter would involve surrender of certain earlier charters. The Act proceeded 'nevertheless, that within Twelve Months after granting of such Charter to the College of Physicians of London, any Fellow, Member or Licentiate of the Royal College of Physicians of Edinburgh . . . who may be in practice as a Physician in any Part of the United Kingdom called England, and who may be desirous of becoming a Member of such College of Physicians of England, shall be at liberty to do so, and be entitled to receive the Diploma of the said College, and to be admitted to all the Rights and Privileges thereunto appertaining, on the Payment of a Registration Fee . . . to the said College' (§ XLVII).

Of equal if not greater significance were sections XLIX and L. The first of these declared that 'It shall be lawful for Her Majesty to grant to the Corporation of the Royal College of Physicians of Edinburgh a new Charter, and thereby to give to the said College of Physicians the Name of "The Royal College of Physicians of Scotland", and it shall be lawful for the said Royal College of Physicians, under their Common Seal to accept such new Charter, and such Acceptance shall operate as a Surrender of all Charters heretofore granted to the said Corporation' (§ XLIX).

There followed in section L the statement 'If at any future Period the Royal College of Surgeons of Edinburgh and Faculty of Physicians and Surgeons of Glasgow agree to amalgamate, so as to form One united Corporation, under the Name of "The Royal College of Surgeons of Scotland", it shall be lawful for Her Majesty to grant, and for Such College and Faculty under their respective Common Seals to accept, such new Charter or Charters as may be necessary for effecting such Union . . . and in the event of such Union it shall be competent for the said College and Faculty to make such Arrangements as the Time and Place of their Examinations as they may agree upon . . .'.

And then there loomed on the horizon fears again of a revival of Corporation power! The Charters—be they contemplated for Edinburgh or Glasgow were not to contain new restrictions: '. . . nothing herein contained shall extend to authorize Her Majesty to create any new Restriction in the Practice of Medicine or Surgery, or to grant to any of the said Corporations any Powers or Privileges contrary to the Common Law of the Land or to the Provisions of this Act, and that no such new Charter shall in anywise prejudice, affect or annul any of the existing Statutes or Byelaws of the Corporations to which the same shall be granted, further than shall be necessary for giving full Effect to the Alterations which shall be intended to be effected by such new Charters . . .' (§ LII).

A century later, the Act of 1858 might well have been known as the 'Medical Relations Act'!

Background Considerations

What in broad terms were the objects of the Medical Act? They certainly were much more than the enablement of the public to distinguish qualified from unqualified practitioners, as stated in the preamble. A second major purpose, essential if the first was to be achieved, was the creation for the United Kingdom as a whole of some degree of uniformity in the education and examination of those training for medical practice. Considered from the point of view of the Medical Corporations and to a lesser extent the Medical Faculties of Universities, the imposition of central supervision allied to elements of control was a new phenomenon, far removed from but destructive of many cherished charter rights. By the Act, Medical Corporations found themselves shorn of their centuries-old right to confer the right to practise. Their diplomas provided the means whereby an aspiring medical might seek inclusion in a Register, which, being the responsibility of the General Council, alone conferred legal authority to practise. Although permitted—and the very word permitted has a deep significance—to conduct examinations the College's activities in this sphere were to be subject to the General Council's observation, suggestions and in some circumstances, direction. Always too, the image of the General Council and its functions had for background the austere authority of the Privy Council.

The very terms of the Medical Act betray a veiled continuing anxiety concerning the historical conflicts, animosities and jealousies which it was intended to dispel finally by a form of compromise machinery. Chaos was to be replaced by organization. In retrospect it can be seen that one of the most profound innovations in the attempted process of mediation was the introduction in the form of the General Medical Council of a governmentally sponsored Body able to exercise limited disciplinary control over certain aspects of professional activities. In reality the civil service had secured a first entry into a new sphere of influence, its hold upon which has intensified with each succeeding decade.

These were aspects of the Medical Act involving all medical corporations. There was, and is, another: the dominant influence of London upon policy planning. Understandably this arose in part from the massive concentration of population in that territorially relatively small area of the United Kingdom. Two other factors were of no less importance. Of these the first was the unchallengeable seniority of the London College of Physicians—the oldest Medical Corporation in the country. The second was the physical proximity of that College to the seat of Government. There were no serious problems of distance or communication to discourage direct

L

approach to Government Departments, personal contact with Ministers, or seemingly fortuitous encounters in the Athenaeum. Proximity and accessibility in this context were valuable in furthering objectives, overcoming misunderstandings and ensuring consultation. As centralized organization has won increasing favour, these advantages from being valuable have become invaluable.

Scottish Corporations were at a disadvantage in this respect and in the opinion of some still are. Remote central departments can on occasion betray woeful ignorance and prove administratively inept when dealing with what they regard as peripherally provincial. This was particularly true of the protracted events leading up to legislative medical reform. Our College certainly was indebted on occasion for support from the London College. That did not alter the fact that during the first two hundred years of its existence the Royal College of Physicians of Edinburgh was subject directly and indirectly to the dominating influence of the more advantageously situated older sister College in London.

Before considering in detail the situation faced by the Edinburgh College with the passing of the Medical Act, it is interesting to know how the London College reacted. Clark sums this up.

> 'Nothing could deprive the College of Physicians of London of its seniority among the professional bodies, nor could any of the others emulate its formal dignity; but its primacy was decidedly reduced when its representative had to take his seat among the rest, the rest including the universities, several of which were older than the College, while in their way the universities as such were more influential in politics and in the country than the professional corporations.'[2]

REPORT OF THE COLLEGE COMMITTEE ON MEDICAL REFORM

On 21st September 1858 the Secretary of our College laid before the meeting a *Report on the position of the College of Physicians of Edinburgh under the New Medical Act and on the course which the College should follow regarding it.*[3] The Report had been compiled by the Committee on Medical Reform and was one of several urgent subjects, consideration of which had prompted the calling of an Extraordinary Meeting. Copies of the Report had been previously circulated among the Fellows of the College.

The Report, more especially in so far as the preamble is concerned, was somewhat discursive. There was obvious disappointment that 'the Act is not an Act, such as the College was entitled to expect, and that the more its Clauses are examined, the less these will be found to be of a Character to have deserved from the College an unqualified support'. It pointed out that although never a teaching body, having been debarred by a clause inserted in its Charter at the instance of the Universities, the College had for two reasons always been 'deeply interested' in the academic institutions. Fellows included a number of professorial status in the Scottish universities and a further considerable number who were teachers in the Extra-Academical School. As to the licence to practise conferred by the College it was explained that this had applied only to Edinburgh and certain suburbs, and had been sought because the College Bye-laws required that any candidate prior to being balloted for the Fellowship should have been a Licentiate for at least one year. Because of the excessive stamp duties involved, the Bye-law had been abolished in 1829 and thereafter no applications for Licences had been received. Reasons given for Edinburgh practitioners wishing to become Fellows were social benefits, the excellent library and reading room and the status held by Fellows. The number of these resident Fellows was described as smaller than that of 'non-resident Fellows, chiefly from England'. Between 1829 and the end of 1857 admissions numbered 70 resident and 82 non-resident Fellows. With the acceptance under the Act of a University Degree as constituting a licence to practise the Committee foresaw an initial increase in applicants among non-residents 'in the expectation that the London College will give effect to the 47th Clause of the Act' (q.v.); but considered that termination of this increase would be followed by a virtually complete cessation of further applications for the non-resident Fellowship from England. Figures were given for the admission of resident Fellows during the inclusive period 1847–57. They totalled twenty-one. In the matter of financial repercussions of the Act the conclusion was arrived at that 'There is . . . no cause for solicitude as to the pecuniary consequences to the College.' This view was based on the assumption that loss in fees would be more than compensated for by the certain considerable diminution on 'charges for deputations'.

Referring to the obligation imposed by Charter on the College to confer its licence without examination or ballot on any graduate of a Scottish University applying for it, the Report maintained no good reason remained for perpetuation of the compulsory clause with the right to practise now allowed to a medical graduate. They none the less recommended that consideration of the compulsory clause be left open.

Rightly the Report gave as the first duty devolving upon the College the election of a Representative to the General Council, and recommended that, as election would require to be made soon after 1st October (1858), the College should determine in advance the procedure for election to be adopted. This was no straightforward task because the office involved was an entirely new one in the history of the College. The Committee pointed out that 'the genius of the Charter' was that 'while the College elects the Council, the Council elects the Office-bearers', and that 'with the exception of the Councillors the laws of the College make no provision for the direct election of any office-bearer'. Wisely the Committee went on to recommend with conviction that in the altogether exceptional circumstances, election to this previously non-existent office should be left 'in the hands of the General body of the Fellows'.

The Report then proceeded to the second duty imposed on the College by the Act—whether or not to apply for a new Charter. Previous information gleaned from the London and Irish Colleges indicated that new charters were not favoured by either. Nor were the Committee particularly enamoured of the idea in so far as the Edinburgh College was concerned. They considered that the only benefits that might accrue from a new Charter were a change of name to the College of Physicians of Scotland; abolition of restrictive clauses; abolition of the name of Licentiate and substitution by that of Member; enablement to examine all applicants for the Membership or the Fellowship, or failing that power to submit Members as well as Fellows, to the ballot; and, vestment without reservation in the College of powers to suspend and expel.

On the question of the College giving an independent licence, the Committee conceded that together, lack of power to award a degree and prohibitive stamp duties would prove a possibly insurmountable handicap. None the less they recommended that regulations for conferring their licence should be framed, and that the College might review possibilities of reviving co-operation with the Glasgow Faculty. At the same time the opinion was expressed that the question of licensing was not one 'of vast importance to the College' and that it might prove possible to confer upon 'Licentiates (i.e. Members) . . . a Status ranking probably above that of a University graduate under the risk which the latter must henceforward incur of being forced into the field as the competitor of the ordinary general practitioner'.

Finally, admitting to the immensity of the problems involved, the Report outlined ways in which the study of Scientific Medicine might be given greater encouragement by the College in the absence of an Academy of Medicine in Scotland. This it was argued 'would be of signal credit and advantage to our College and to the Country at large'. The recommendation was the more noteworthy considering the almost totally negligible consideration given to medical science as such by those who over so many years had been intent on securing medical reform.

Reception of the Report was followed by considerable discussion. Eventually a motion was moved and carried in the face of an amendment by 19 votes to 4, there being one abstention. The successful motion was to the effect that 'the College approve generally of the Report . . . and order it to lie on the Table': and 'that the College approve of the proposal in the Report as to the mode of electing a Representative to the General Medical Council . . . and direct a Meeting to be summoned on an early day . . . to elect a Representative'. Any resolution as to applying for a new Charter was postponed: and any formal resolution to give the College a new scientific character was regarded as unnecessary at the time, although the importance of the suggestion was acknowledged.

The defeated amendment was proposed by a Fellow who 'disapproved entirely' of the Medical Reform Committee's Report and who with his three supporters was anxious 'to draw the College . . . in closer alliance to the Universities'. A fundamentally different policy in reference to the new Medical Act was put forward as desirable, and discussed in general terms before rejection of the Amendment.[3]

REFERENCES

(1) 21 and 22 Victoria, c. 90 (1858).
(2) CLARK, Sir G. (1966) *The History of the Royal College of Physicians of London*, vol. 2, p. 729. Oxford: Clarendon Press.
(3) College Minutes, 21.ix.1858.

Chapter XIV

COLLEGE ACTION CONSEQUENT ON THE MEDICAL ACT

Necessarily the passing of the Medical Act meant that the College had to make a number of adjustments—some major, some minor: and some with the minimum of delay, others after due deliberation. That College business in no way diminished is borne out by the fact that additional to the four Quarterly Meetings there were fifteen extraordinary Meetings during the year ending February 1859.[1]

REPRESENTATIVE ON THE GENERAL MEDICAL COUNCIL: FIRST APPOINTMENT

Priority was given to the appointment of a representative to the General Council. This was not altogether easy because early in the year, before publication of the Medical Act, the Laws of the College had been under general review and those related to the election of office-bearers under particular scrutiny. Division of opinion led to reference of the subject to a Committee appointed for the purpose.[2] The Committee recommended the use of election papers prepared before the Annual Election Meeting; the nomination of three Scrutineers (not members of Council) by the President; and that Fellows should present their voting lists on being called. Because of doubts entertained by some Fellows the Report was remitted to the Committee for amendment to exclude any suggestion of alteration of the existing Laws.[3] Apart from making minor changes the Committee adhered to their original recommendations maintaining that their suggestions in no way ran counter to the spirit of the Law. Approval being given on this occasion, the motion was adopted as a temporary regulation pending receipt of the full sanction of the College.[4]

An Extraordinary Meeting was called on 12th October 1858 for the purpose of nominating and choosing a Member of the College for 'the General Council of Medical Education and Registration of the United Kingdom'. Proceedings commenced with the Secretary reading relevant clauses of the Act, and rules suggested by the President (Dr D. Maclagan) as desirable in the event of voting being necessary. Discussion followed but eventually the President's suggestions were approved with the proviso 'that it be understood that the present occasion does not form a precedent'. The Vice President (Dr Begbie) having already nominated a Fellow was himself proposed by a third party but declined to accept nomination. Dr Alexander Wood thus became the first representative of the College on the General Medical Council.[5] At the next Quarterly Meeting a technical hitch was set aright. In nominating Dr Wood notice had not been taken of the words of the Act—'The Members of the General Council Shall be chosen and nominated for a term not exceeding five years'. One Fellow of outstanding ability but inclined to be punctilious drew attention to the failure to specify that nomination had been for the full term of five years. He had already written to the Secretary to the same effect. Functioning in an age when cyclostyled admonitions from central departments were unknown, the Council of the College pontifically declared they did not share the feelings of apprehension; and covered themselves by saying that, if on further enquiry it should appear that there had been any informality in Dr Wood's election, the necessary steps should be taken to rectify it.[6] Officialdom was baulked of an early opportunity to assert itself.

A NEW CHARTER

Next in importance of major issues for consideration was the desirability or otherwise of applying for a new Charter. The subject was raised in December 1858. Acting on the advice of the Secretary the draft of a new Charter previously considered in 1845 was accepted as the basis for initial discussion.[7] The circumstances which had led to consideration of a new Charter earlier in the century are of significance.

The terms of the original Charter in 1681 have been outlined (Chap. III). For many years these terms conditioned the discharge of its functions by the College apart from the fact that exclusive rights conferred on it concerning supervision of apothecaries and their shops had fallen into abeyance by disuse.[8] Certain restrictions imposed by the Charter of 1681 had become increasingly irksome with the passage of years. This applied particularly to the requirement that all Scottish University Graduates applying for admission to the College's Licence had to be admitted without examination and without ballot. A sense of discouragement arose also from the clause prohibiting connection of the College with a medical teaching school. A third factor contributing to a certain sense of ineffectiveness was lack of powers to suspend or expel 'unworthy members'.

Although the subject of a new Charter was repeatedly discussed, any sense of urgency was discouraged by the tantalizingly erratic and inconclusive progress in the matter of medical reform. Attitudes changed however as legislative proposals acquired more concerted form; and, when prospects for Graham's Bill appeared more favourable, the College arranged for a draft new Charter to be prepared in 1843. At the time this seemed eminently desirable more especially as with each new legislative measure it became apparent that the Charters of other Corporations would probably be altered. With the aid of a Government official the draft was produced in final form in 1845 only to be consigned to the archives with the abandonment of Graham's Bill.[9] Interest in the draft Charter revived nine years later when it was referred for consideration and amendment[10] to the College Medical Reform Committee which reported in the following year. Events in Parliament so dominated medical affairs at this time that it was only in September 1858 after the passing of the Medical Act, that the question of a new Charter was again raised.[11] The views of the Medical Reform Committee at that time have already been outlined (Chap. XII).

Opposed Views

A decision to apply for a new Charter was arrived at on 21st December 1858.[12] This was at an Extraordinary Meeting. Two further such meetings in the same month followed in sufficiently rapid succession not to coincide with Hogmanay.[13, 14] A relatively lengthy lull followed, but discussions on a new Charter were resumed in February and March.[15, 16] Discussion over three months was prolonged and profound. Throughout, a sobering respect was shewn for verbal accuracy and the legal desirability of trying to cover all eventualities, foreseeable and unpredictable. Legal niceties of expression were not allowed to cloud issues of principle. Consideration of these last brought to light considerable differences of opinion, which genuinely reflected conflicting convictions.

Debates were characterized by acute awareness of the seriousness and far-reaching implications of the subject under discussion, with the result that emotions were contained and argument remained temperate throughout. On only one occasion did procedure give rise to difficulty. A proposal to exclude from any future Charter restrictions relating to establishing a teaching school and granting degrees prompted a motion for adjournment to allow of adequate consideration. The motion was rejected. In the course of continued discussion a small minority of Fellows took exception to the College's decision to exclude the clause in question. Eight of their number went the length of submitting a Protest, regretting the implied hostility to the University and the inevitable alienation of University professors by the support given by some Fellows to the 'private School of Medicine patronized by the Royal College of Surgeons'. Suggestions that a Board of Examiners composed of extra-academical teachers might confer the title of Physician on students having no degree, were condemned out of hand. It was maintained that by favouring an inferior class of practitioner under the guise that a College licence alone conferred a status 'ranking above that of a University Graduate' would only serve to degrade the College in the estimation of the profession at large. After what might be called the alteration of a procedural error the Protest was received by the College.[17] Signatories to the Protest were Drs Hughes Bennett, Robert Christison, Thos. Traill, Robert Bowen, John Myrtle, William Cumming, Robert Malcolm and Alexander Peddie. The President, Dr Alexander Wood, was in the chair. Council in reply to the Protest did not accept that Licentiates and Fellows should be exclusively derived from the Universities; that the College should be reduced to dependence on the goodwill of the Universities; or that a University by its degree of M.D. has any more power 'to make a Physician, than it can by that of LL.D. create a Lawyer'. Strong exception was taken by Council to a reference to Licentiates as 'falsely called physicians', and by way of counterblast it was declared that in the opinion of many members of the medical and legal profession 'it is only association with a College of Physicians which can constitute a Physician'.[18]

Terms 'Resident' and 'Non-Resident' Discarded

Having been remitted to Council,[19] the draft new Charter was brought before the College again on 1st March (1859).[16] In the interval a legal opinion had been obtained as to the powers of the College to make Bye-laws dividing the Fellows into two classes viz. resident and non-resident. It had been explained to Counsel that non-resident Fellows had no privileges 'except that of paying a smaller Admission fee', and that when applying for a new Charter the College wished 'to have only two Classes mentioned . . . Fellows and Licentiates—But at the same time . . . to have the power of dividing the Fellows into Resident and Non-Resident'. Counsel in reply gave it as his opinion that the original Charter did authorize distinction between resident and non-resident Fellows by Bye-laws: but pointed out that within the meaning of the Charter the status of a 'Collega' and 'Sodalis' was not conferred on non-resident Fellows who to become ordinary members had to go through a new election. This, he argued, pointed to the desirability of a new Charter taking express powers as to Bye-laws to define precisely the conditions appertaining to various classes of Fellows. Accordingly the Council of the College removed the words 'resident' and 'non-resident' from the draft Charter. This was approved, as was the inclusion of a new clause granting the College authority to make rules, bye-laws and acts for among other things 'the subdivision of the individuals composing the Body Corporate . . . into such orders . . . as the College may from time to time determine'. On the motion of Dr Seller seconded by Dr Duncan, full power was entrusted to the Council by the College 'to obtain the Grant of the Charter as now adjusted' withdrawal of an amendment (moved by Dr Wilson and seconded by Dr Macdonald) to the effect that final approval should be delayed 'and that whatever other conditions may appear in the Charters obtained by other Bodies, shall be first submitted to the College before their definite enrolment in the Charter'. Although the amendment was withdrawn it was agreed that should 'any material change be proposed by the Government' it would be submitted to the College for consideration.[16] A further clause which was inserted aimed at enabling the College to hold property in its corporate name.

Designation

Almost two years elapsed before the position with regard to a new Charter was again brought by Council before the College. Dubiety had arisen from study of Clause XLIX of the Medical Act of 1858 (Chap. XIII). Although the terms of that clause contemplated a New Charter taking the name of The Royal College of Physicians of Scotland, they made no provision for the retention by the College of rights and privileges enjoyed by it as the Royal College of Physicians of Edinburgh. Not being alone in their apprehensions, the College agreed with the London and Dublin Colleges to co-operate in the introduction of a Bill intended to abolish the offending clause of the Act of 1858.[20] A change in the situation followed the passing of the Medical Act (1858) Amendment Act.[21] This Act, which received the Royal Assent on 6th August 1860, ensured that a change in designation of the College involved no change in rights and privileges already possessed; and left it to the

College to decide whether to retain or change the existing designation. To change or not to change? This question was laid by the Council before the Laws Committee of the College for consideration, and the Committee expressed the view that the designation under which the College had been known since its foundation should be retained. The relevant minute of 5th February 1861 continued 'With this expression of opinion the Council concur, and they now beg to recommend to the College that no change in the designation of the College should be made, but that the New Charter be applied for in favour of the Royal College of Physicians of Edinburgh'. The College concurred with Council, the President at the time being Dr Alexander Wood.[22] Surprisingly, references to the subject in the Minutes of Council and of the Laws Committee are of the scantiest.[23]

The New Royal Charter of Incorporation under the Designation ' "The Royal College of Physicians of Edinburgh", dated 16th August and sealed 31st October 1861' was laid before the College on 5th November of that year. By unanimous agreement, it having 'for some days been patent to the Fellows of the College', a motion was passed declaring acceptance of the New Charter and directing that the College seal be appended to the Minute of Acceptance.[24]

LICENTIATESHIP: REVIVAL IN NEW FORM

In September 1858 the College Medical Reform Committee submitted to Council a *Report on the position of the College of Physicians of Edinburgh under the New Medical Act and on the course which the College should follow regarding it*.[25] Recommendations related to the granting of a Licence to practise were somewhat non-committal. Authority to issue Licences dated back to the time of the original Charter of 1681. In 1763 'doubts and questions' having arisen 'with Respect to the time in which any Licentiats of ye College may be admitted Fellows after they have obtained their Licence' an enactment was passed 'for obviating all debates and questions thereanent for the future'. This Act ordained that 'no person . . . shall be admitted a Fellow . . . Sooner than one full year after the day he has obtained his Licence'. It decreed also that 'any proposal . . . for admitting any Licentiat . . . a Fellow of the College . . . shall allways be made at a Quarterly Meeting . . . and shall Ly upon the Table till next Subsequent quarterly meeting to be then Considered'.[26] These requirements regularized a procedure whereby the Licentiateship became a necessary stepping stone to the Fellowship.

It soon transpired that the procedure involved payment of two taxes, and applications for licence to practise declined in number. A Committee appointed to revise the Laws and Regulations recommended in November 1828 that the College should consider the direct admission of Fellows without Licences.[27] The proposal was incorporated in the Revised Form of Laws and Regulations finally approved.[28] As a result the original form of licence ceased to exist in 1829. At no time had a licence been granted to other than a University graduate.

A Source of Growing Concern

In reviewing its Laws and Regulations the College was concerned to improve the status of the profession and to secure proper recognition in England of practitioners holding the licences of Scottish Corporations and the degrees of Scottish Universities. Unfortunately there was foundation for the suggestion that some of the Universities of Scotland made 'a shameful traffick of degrees in physic'. Thus the Universities of St Andrews and Aberdeen frequently gave degrees without examination on the certification of often obscure, ill-qualified referees; and when candidates were required to submit themselves to examination, the examinations were neither strict nor rigorous. Compelled as it was by Charter to grant licences to any applicant in possession of such a degree, the College was sensitive to the implied condonation of the abuses.[29]

The undeserved reflection on the College prompted Dr William Cullen when President to take action by approaching a recently elected Honorary Fellow, the Duke of Buccleuch, with a view to arousing governmental interest. This was in 1773.[30] An early outcome was the compilation by Dr Cullen of a Memorial at the request of the Duke who sent it for observations to his one-time tutor Adam Smith, then engaged in writing his *Wealth of Nations*. Cullen favoured a Royal Commission as a means of correcting academic irregularities, and among recommendations he made was one for compulsory attendance for two years at an appropriate University, a recommendation taken 'from a late regulation of the Royal College of Physicians at London, who have made it a condition with respect to the licentiates they are to admit'.[31]

Adam Smith wrote Cullen at some length. He considered that any monopoly of medical education established in favour of the Universities would be hurtful to their lasting prosperity, and in the matter of the College's particular problem he mischievously commented 'What the physicians of Edinburgh at present feel as a hardship is, perhaps, the real cause of their acknowledged superiority over the greater part of other physicians . . . The unworthiness of some of your brethren may, perhaps . . . be in part the cause of the very eminent and superior worth of many of the rest. The very abuse which you complain of may in this manner, perhaps, be the real source of your present excellence.' Well might Smith conclude his letter to Cullen, 'Adieu, my dear Doctor . . . I am afraid I shall *get my lug* (ear) *in my lufe* (hand), as we say, for what I have written.'[32]

The Memorial produced no practical results. Those holding discredited Scottish degrees and suspect College licences continued to increase in number south of the border and gave rise to an ever-deepening prejudice against doctors from the north. This attitude was prevalent at the time the College reviewed their Laws and Regulations—and was not discouraged by medical organizations in the south.

With the passage of the Medical Act of 1858 the College was faced with a completely new situation. The Report focussed attention on the fact 'that now that a simple University Degree seems by Law, admitted to be a sufficient license to practise, there may not be the same inducement for resident Fellows to join the College and that the most effectual way of keeping up their number will be by encreasing the advantages of entrance and rendering the terms easy and liberal'. As to non-resident Fellowship, the Report anticipated that after an initial large increase in number, applications would ultimately cease completely.[25]

College and University

The giving of an independent licence by the College was regarded as impracticable in the absence of authority to award degrees and in the continuing presence of exorbitant stamp duties. Mention was made of the possibility of reviving discussions with the Glasgow Faculty for joint action. Optimistically the Report did not consider the question of licensing as 'of vast importance', if only because Licentiates might possibly have conferred on them 'a Status ranking probably above that of a University graduate under the risk which the latter must henceforward incur of being forced into the field as the competitor of the ordinary general practitioner'. Notwithstanding a strong case was advanced for the abolition of the Charter requirement that Scottish graduates be awarded the Licence without examination or ballot, should the Medical Council decide that Degrees of M.D. confer a licence to practise. The Report was the subject of keen debate; a considerable proportion of the Fellows took exception to its attitude to the Universities with which they sought closer alliance.[25] Understandably the anger of the University Professors was roused, and won the support of a number of non-academics.

Curriculum of Study: and Examinations

Despite having frequently debated the question of revival of the Licentiateship the College appeared to be caught unawares when a letter dated 13th January 1859 was received from the General Medical Council requiring 'a Statement of the courses of Study and Examinations to be gone through in order to obtain' the Licence and Fellowship of the College. The last Report of the Reform Committee was still on the Table having not yet been considered *in toto*.[18]

The Council of College presented their Report on the 'Curriculum of Study and on Examination for the License of the College' at an Extraordinary Meeting in March and it was agreed to unanimously. By way of preliminary introduction Council gave it as their view that only those possessing the degree of M.D. should be admitted Fellows: and that all holders of University Diplomas of M.D. or Bachelor of Medicine should be admitted as Fellows and Licentiates respectively without examination provided that the College was satisfied with the curriculum of study and examination undergone. They further recommended that the College should 'secure a due preliminary examination', a University Degree of M.A. conferred after an examination being accepted *in lieu*.[33, 18]

As evidence of the need to take constructive action the Council referred to probable developments which would follow application for a new Charter by the London College of Physicians. An article in the medical press foretold that in future general practitioners would continue to acquire their surgical qualifications from the English College of Surgeons and that they might well be able to get their medical qualifications from the London College of Physicians in preference to the Apothecaries Society. A sentence of particular significance in the article quoted, was—'We have repeatedly shown, that by making itself the great Medical licensing body for the General Practitioners of the kingdom, the College [of Physicians of London] might repair the error made in 1815, and become a rich, useful, and powerful body. The Charter Committee have seen the importance of this position . . .'[34] In Edinburgh, the College of Physicians was with good reason advised by its Council that 'if Edinburgh is to continue as heretofore to be the great centre of Medical Education it is of essential importance that the Students frequenting her seats of learning should have facilities equal at least to those of England for obtaining a license to practise

Medicine'.[18] The argument was logical, realistic and in no sense open to the charge of narrow mindedness.

One further point was emphasized by Council. The London College were proposing that Doctors of Medicine of any British University and certain foreign graduates not practising Pharmacy could, within twelve months after acceptance of the College's new Charter, be admitted members of that College at a reduced fee. The Edinburgh College was recommended to adopt a similar procedure by their Council.[18]

Discussion of possible Regulations for any revived form of Licence was protracted. It was on the agenda at nine successive *sederunts* and almost a year elapsed before a final decision was reached as to the qualifications to be required of applicants for a Licence. The number and length of the meetings afforded an indication of the acute differences of opinion which prevailed. Investigations by the Council of the College established that the only course of study 'distinctly sanctioned' by the College as preliminary to the issue of a Licence or Letters Testimonial had been the 'course' embodied in an agreement in 1842 with the University and the Royal College of Surgeons of Edinburgh concerning the training of general practitioners. The course in question had dealt comprehensively with Medical Education and provided the basis of the return made in response to the requirement of the General Medical Council.

'The Year of Grace'

One proposed Regulation was to be the cause of great discomfiture to the College. It ran:

> 'For one year after the passing of these regulations the following Classes of Applicants may be admitted Licentiates of the College without examination provided that they do not derive any profit from the Sale of Drugs or Medicine and that they produce Certificates of Character and professional qualification satisfactory to the Council:—
> *First*—Gentlemen who have been 15 years in actual practice.
> *Second*—Licentiates of any of the Existing Licensing Boards.'[33]

This particular regulation came to be associated with the term 'Year of Grace'. What was its prime purpose? It was a direct result of the combined effects of the Medical Act and the Universities (Scotland) Act—both of 1858. The effects of the Medical Act have already been discussed. Despite opposition from the Medical

Corporations described by Grant as 'of a very selfish character',[35] the Commissioners appointed under the Universities Act decided that the award of a University Degree in Medicine was to confer license to practise. At the time these changes were due to come into effect there were throughout the country a considerable number of men of mature age and experience practising as general practitioners. Of these many had commenced their professional life as Surgeons and Apothecaries and were licentiates of an apothecary society or other licensing body which required of their Licentiates an education and examination equal to any and superior to that of some, of the Scottish Universities. To be compelled by the terms of the Charter of 1681, so artfully conditioned by the Universities of the day, to admit to the Licentiate without examination graduates with such background, had always proved mortifying to the College. By this essentially temporary measure the College aimed at providing many practitioners of unquestionable experience and proven worth with the opportunity at a relatively late and certainly crucial stage in their professional careers, to become directly linked with a Corporation of high professional standing. Put another way, a suitable applicant was enabled to change his designation of Apothecary to Licentiate of a College of Physicians.[36] In essence, the College might be said to have offered a bridging reinforcement for general practitioners at a time of fundamental medical transition.

Regulations for Conferment

Before being finally adopted the Regulation was the subject of further lengthy discussion at several successive Extraordinary Meetings.[37-40] On 5th April 1859 the College by a majority of one resolved to admit for its Licence, candidates who had no previous Medical Degree or Qualification, one member having declined to vote and two having left the Meeting before the vote was taken.[38] Those who opposed the narrowly successful motion included Professors of the University and a number of Fellows not directly connected with the University.

At another Extraordinary Meeting ten days later the College agreed to an alteration of the proposed Regulation concerning admission without examination.[39] The alteration after further amendment was incorporated in new 'Regulations for the conferring of the License of the College'. In final form the particular Regulation involved referred only to 'Licentiates of any of the existing Licensing Boards' and contained no selective mention of 'Gentlemen who have been fifteen years in actual practice'. Furthermore it was laid down that Petitions and Testimonials should be submitted to Council prior to being reported to the College: information concerning applications was to be circulated in advance of the College Meeting at which applications were to be considered and that 'the College shall then proceed to ballot on each application a majority of two-thirds of those who vote being necessary to declare the applicant duly elected a Licentiate'. The Regulations being approved by the College were 'forwarded to the General Council under the Medical Act' and thereafter publication was authorized by the Council of the College.[40]

Dr Christison was consistently outspoken in his criticism and summarized the reasons for his attitude in the form of a written Protest signed by himself and ten co-signatories. The Protest—the second in the course of a few months—took exception to the creation of 'a new order of general Practitioner' which was not in the interests of the public or the College; to a measure likely to 'engender estrangement on the part of the Graduates of Universities' to whom the College was greatly indebted; and to a resolution certain to give umbrage to other Medical Corporations, and 'more especially just cause of offence to the Royal College of Physicians of London with whom this College has hitherto acted harmoniously in organising its constitution'. Christison knew full well that there was foundation to his last remarks. Astutely he prevailed upon the President (Dr Alexander Wood) to have the order of business altered in order that correspondence with the London College should have first attention. The sequel is described in Chapter XIX.[41]

The Regulations for the Licence of the College finally approved on 20th April 1859 and forwarded to the General Medical Council, stipulated that those admitted to the Licentiate had to be not less than twenty-one years of age. Applicants had to produce evidence of having attended classes, which were specified, over a period of four years at a University or recognized medical school; and of having attended the practice of a public hospital of not fewer than 80 beds over a period of not less than two years. Those not exempt had to satisfy examiners in preliminary education of competence in ordained subjects. In the event of examiners in preliminary education not being Fellows of the College, a Fellow of the College had to be present. It was decreed that 'the Examination shall be conducted partly *viva voce*, partly by written papers, and, whenever practicable, shall consist in part in the actual examination of persons suffering under disease'.[40] Records of examinations 'with the State of the vote' were to be given to Council—those relating to successful applicants, but not those of unsuccessful applicants, being then laid before the College.

Under the Medical Act, Licentiates of the College could claim inclusion in the Register and practise Medicine throughout the British Empire.

As from October 1884, the College ceased to give the Licence as a single qualification to practise except to candidates who had passed an examination in surgery which already entitled them to registration.[42] Previously in 1874 a decision had been made to require all candidates to pass an examination in surgery before the examiners of the College, if they had not already done so before some other Licensing Body.[43]

Mutual Esteem: a Happy Gesture

Of University protagonists in this difference of opinion within the College (Sir) Robert Christison was without doubt the most formidable and effective. Whether by written or spoken word, he expressed his views with judicial lucidity and imperturbable conviction. Notwithstanding, he won the regard and affection of the College which at a later date arranged for his portrait to be painted and hung in the Hall. 'This', said Sir Robert at a public dinner given in his honour, 'would have been a great honour in any circumstances; but it was a double honour to me,—and, I may add, highly honourable too to my fellow members,—because for a good many years . . . the opinions of the majority in the College and mine, in regard to an important measure of medical reform, in which the interests of the College and those of the University were deeply concerned, on several occasions were much opposed to one another'.[44]

THE DOUBLE QUALIFICATION

In June 1859 a request was received from the Edinburgh College of Surgeons for 'a conference on the subject of granting Medical Qualifications'.[45] This was arranged and attended by five representatives of each of the two Colleges on 20th June 1859. There was agreement that were a double qualification embracing medicine and surgery practicable it would be permissible by law, beneficial to candidates and not entail interference with the independence of either College. The College of Physicians gave general approval to the Report received, encouraged further discussion with the Surgeons, and on a motion by a Fellow decided to approach the University Senate as to the possibility of establishing a Joint Board of Examination to award a Triple Qualification by one Examination from the University and the two Edinburgh Colleges.[46] As the Colleges of Surgeons had anticipated events by having a meeting on their own with University representatives, the Physicians decided to adopt a similar independent approach.

Negotiations between the two Edinburgh Colleges continued and, by the end of July, formulae agreed between representatives of the two Colleges were accepted by the Physicians who asked their representative to support their adoption by the Medical Council.[47] The proposals, submitted by the two Edinburgh Colleges on 6th August and approved on 8th August by the General Council of Medical Education and Registration were as follows:

'1. By Clause 19 of the Medical Act, "any two or more of the Colleges and Bodies mentioned in Schedule (A) may, with the sanction and under the directions of the General Medical Council, unite or co-operate in conducting the Examinations for Qualifications to be registered under this Act." Hence it is quite competent for a College of Physicians and a College of Surgeons to combine, in order, by a Joint Examination, to give a Double Qualification, embracing Medicine and Surgery.

2. Co-operation between a College of Physicians and a College of Surgeons being legal, as stated above, the Colleges of Physicians and Surgeons of Edinburgh propose, with the sanction of the General Medical Council, to make an arrangement for the purpose of granting, by a series of Examinations, Preliminary and Professional, their respective Licences in Medicine and Surgery, so as to constitute a Double Qualification.

3. It is proposed that the Preliminary Examination in Literature and Science, and also the Examinations on those professional subjects which are common to Medicine and Surgery, shall be conducted conjointly by a Board formed of Examiners in equal proportions from the two Colleges.

4. It is proposed that the Examinations in *Medicine* shall be conducted exclusively by Examiners from the College of Physicians, and the Examinations in *Surgery* exclusively by Examiners from the College of Surgeons.

5. It is proposed that the decision as to the competency of the Candidate, in all the branches except Medicine and Surgery, shall rest with the conjoined Board of Examiners from the two Colleges; but that the decision as to his competency in Medicine and in Surgery shall rest entirely, in the one case with the Examiners from the College of Physicians, in the other case with the Examiners from the College of Surgeons.

6. It is proposed that, having passed through the final Examinations, the Candidates shall receive two separate Diplomas—one from each College—signed by the Office-Bearers of each respectively, so that he may be enabled to produce them to the Registrar under the Medical Act, and to register two separate Qualifications—viz., L.R.C.P.Ed., and L.R.C.S.Ed.

7. The Colleges wish it to be clearly understood, that such co-operation is not to interfere in any degree with the right of each College to grant its Diploma separately, as heretofore, to those who may wish a Single Qualification, or with the right of each College to make similar arrangements with other Licensing Bodies, if deemed expedient, and if sanctioned by the Medical Council.

8. For the purpose of carrying out the objects stated above, the Colleges have prepared a Series of Regulations, which they beg now to submit to the Medical Council for their consideration.'[48]

In 1884 the College resolved not to grant the Licence as a single qualification except to those individuals who already possessed a registrable Diploma in Surgery.[49] This became effective, after appropriate alteration of the Regulations for the Licence, on 11th October 1884. On the same day effect was given to a recommendation of Council that all applicants for the Licence 'should be required to pass a written as well as an oral and clinical examination'.[50]

While negotiations between the two Edinburgh Colleges were in progress, the President of the College of Physicians received a letter from his opposite number in the Glasgow Faculty. It suggested that a deputation from the latter might meet the Committee of the Edinburgh College of Physicians 'with the view of making an arrangement under which [the] College might confer along with that Faculty a double Qualification'. Agreement was given to the suggestion.[51] The Faculty, like the Edinburgh College of Surgeons had the right to license in Surgery; and had in common with both Colleges the desire to meet the newly promulgated demands of Army and other Boards that candidates for their services should hold diplomas from two separate licensing authorities. Discussions between the Edinburgh College and the Glasgow Faculty could not have been more harmonious. Such was the rapidity with which progress was made that within a week of negotiations being opened the College sent copies of the proposed regulations resulting from conferences with the Glasgow Faculty, to the Medical Council 'with the understanding that they had not been finally sanctioned'.[49] The President was able to announce at an Extraordinary Meeting in August 1859 that the General Medical Council had sanctioned the co-operation agreed to by the College, the Royal College of Surgeons of Edinburgh, and the Faculty of Physicians and Surgeons of Glasgow for the purpose of granting a Double Qualification in Medicine and Surgery.[52]

THE TRIPLE QUALIFICATION

The 'Double Qualifications' attracted a large number of candidates and the College was responsible for conferring the right (subject to registration) to practise Medicine on a numerous and increasing body of general Practitioners.

At an Extraordinary Meeting in March 1884 consideration was given to a scheme of examination which had been discussed provisionally over a period of months by the College, with the Royal College of Surgeons of Edinburgh and the Faculty of Physicians and Surgeons of Glasgow. The scheme contemplated an examination to be conducted conjointly by the three Corporations.[53] Proposed Articles of Agreement were approved by the two Colleges and the Faculty: obtained the approval of the General Council of Medical Education and Registration on the last day of the month[54]: and came into operation on 1st October 1884.

It was about this time that Licensing Bodies throughout the country received a letter from the General Medical Council warning them of the existence of forged Diplomas and urging that certain precautionary measures should be taken in any case of doubt concerning the genuineness of foreign Diplomas presented to them.[55] Although in no way linked to the G.M.C. warning, accuracy requires admitting that in 1896 'the President explained that on going to the College of Physicians he found a large number of Diplomas in the officers hands and was astonished to discover that they were blank in respect of the recipient's name'. He found also laxity in the matter of safe storage.[56] There was however no evidence to suggest that the situation had led to any abuse in the issue of Triple Qualification Diplomas.

By the new agreement, a Licence to practise was conferred in association with the other two Scottish Corporations as a Triple Qualification, the two Double Qualifications being superseded. The following are among the agreed conditions of the scheme:

'I. That each of the said three Medical Corporations of Scotland—namely, the Royal College of Physicians of Edinburgh, the Royal College of Surgeons of Edinburgh, and the Faculty of Physicians and Surgeons of Glasgow, while reserving to itself liberty to confer its Higher Qualification or Qualifications as it may deem proper, resolves, That on and after the 1st day of October 1884, it shall abstain from the exercise of its power of granting its Licence separately and independently, except only in the cases herein provided for:—That is to say, the Royal College of Physicians of Edinburgh may, notwithstanding this Agreement, grant its Licence to Candidates already possessed of one or other of the Surgical Qualifications mentioned in Schedule (A) of the Medical Act, 1858; and the Royal College of Surgeons of Edinburgh, and the Faculty of Physicians and Surgeons of Glasgow, may each grant its Licence to Candidates already registered Licentiates of one of the Colleges of Physicians of the United Kingdom, or Graduates in Medicine of a British or Irish University mentioned in Schedule (A) of the Medical Act.

II. That the three Medical Authorities above mentioned shall co-operate to form an Examining Board to conduct their Examinations in combination; and that from the date to be fixed for the commencement of this Scheme, the Agreement or Convention at present subsisting between the Royal College of Physicians of Edinburgh, and the Royal College of Surgeons of Edinburgh, by which, under Section XIX. of the Medical Act, 1858, these two Colleges conduct Examinations in combination, and the similar Agreement or Convention at present subsisting between the Royal College of Physicians of Edinburgh, and the Faculty of Physicians and Surgeons of Glasgow, by which these two bodies conduct Examinations in combination, shall cease and terminate; and the provisions of this present Agreement, in respect to Combined Examinations, shall alone be valid.

III. That each of the co-operating Medical Authorities shall elect two Members of a Committee, herein called the Committee of Management. Of this Committee of six Members three Members shall retire annually, that is to say, one elected by each of the Authorities; but they shall be eligible for re-election, but shall not at the same time hold office as Examiners. To the Members of this Committee reasonable remuneration shall be paid for attendance at the Meetings.

. . . . .

V. That each of the co-operating Medical Authorities shall elect its own Examiners to examine on special or allied subjects, each of these Authorities determining the number to be elected on each subject, and the period for which they shall hold office; and notification of the names of the Examiners, with the subjects for which they are appointed, shall be duly made to the Committee of Management.

VI. That the Examination on the Principles and Practice of Medicine (including Clinical Medicine) and in Therapeutics, and except only so far as is provided otherwise in the note appended to this Article, shall be conducted wholly by the Examiners on these subjects appointed by the Royal College of Physicians of Edinburgh; that the Examination on the Principles and Practice of Surgery (including Clinical Surgery) and on Surgical Anatomy shall be conducted wholly by the Examiners on these subjects appointed by the Royal College of Surgeons of Edinburgh, and by the Faculty of Physicians and Surgeons of Glasgow; and that in all the other subjects the Examinations shall, subject to the provisions of Article VII., be conducted by the Examiners of the three co-operating Authorities.

Note.—At the Examinations to be held in Glasgow, the Examination in Clinical Medicine shall be conducted by Examiners of the Faculty of Physicians and Surgeons of Glasgow, being hospital Physicians, and by the Examiners of the Royal College of Physicians of Edinburgh.

. . . . .

VIII. The Examinations shall be held in Edinburgh and in Glasgow, it being arranged that at every third period they shall be held in Glasgow, and at the other periods in Edinburgh.

IX. That there shall be three Professional Examinations, named herein the First, the Second, and the Third Examinations.

X. That the Subjects of the First Examination shall be—
 Chemistry.
 Practical Chemistry.
 Elementary Anatomy and Histology.
That the Subjects of the Second Examination shall be—
 Anatomy.
 Physiology.
 Materia Medica and Pharmacy.
That the Subjects of the Third Examination shall be—

Principles and Practice of Medicine, including Therapeutics, Medical Anatomy, and Pathology.

Clinical Medicine.

Principles and Practice of Surgery, including Surgical Anatomy, Operative Surgery, and Pathology.

Clinical Surgery.

Midwifery and Diseases of Women.

Medical Jurisprudence and Hygiene.

XI. That a Candidate on passing the Third Examination shall be admitted and receive the Diplomas; as

Licentiate of the Royal College of Physicians of Edinburgh.

Licentiate of the Royal College of Surgeons of Edinburgh.

Licentiate of the Faculty of Physicians and Surgeons of Glasgow.

.   .   .   .   .

XV. That this Agreement shall come into operation on the said 1st day of October 1884, and remain in full force and effect for the period of five years from and after that date; but declaring that the same shall come to an end and shall cease and determine on the said 1st day of October 1889, provided one or other of the said parties shall have given to the said first, second, or third parties one year's previous notice in writing of their intention that the said Agreement shall be so terminated; and, failing such notice, the same shall continue in full force and effect from and after the said 1st day of October 1889, until the expiration of one year after such notice shall have been given as aforesaid.'[53]

In 1921 the National Board of Examiners, U.S.A. intimated that possession of the Triple Qualification would entitle candidates to admission to a practical examination for licence to practise in the United States.[57, 58]

Reports of the Visitors

Medical Reform brought a new experience to the College in the form of the occasional appearance of Visitors from the General Medical Council to approve or disapprove examination procedures as occasion demanded. In reality the term Visitor, then as now, was a polite euphemism for Inspector. In February 1875 the Council informed the College of the inspectorial comments following a recent visitation. The conduct of the examinations had met with general approval but exception had been taken to the absence of a surgical examination, and to a deficiency of dissected preparations. Both criticisms had been dealt with in advance of the College meeting. In the matter of surgery the Council had arranged that 'no Candidate can in future obtain the Licence . . . unless he has passed an Examination in Surgery before the

Examiners of the College, or before another Qualifying Body. The Surgical Examination . . . has been entrusted to a Board consisting of Three Fellows of the College of Surgeons, all of whom are Hospital Surgeons.'[59]

A report by more Visitors some three years later found that 'Final Examination in Medicine and Midwifery of the Conjoint Board in Scotland is "sufficient" ' and the examination in medicine was 'specially reported as "sufficient to guarantee the knowledge and skill requisite for the efficient practice of medicine" '. There were minor criticisms concerning the methods of marking and details of the clinical examination. They were in fact the kind of points that ultra-efficient inspectors seem compelled as a routine to make on the eve of departure. In this the Visitors were showing early evidence of the civil service image detectable in so many established governmental Inspectors.[60]

THE GOVERNMENT TAX ON LICENCES OF THE CORPORATION

By encouraging co-operation between licensing authorities the Medical Act of 1858 certainly contributed to the restoration of the Licence issued by the Edinburgh College. It did nothing whatsoever to mitigate the burden imposed by taxation on those obtaining a Licence to practise. By law in 1815 a tax of £15 sterling was imposed on a Diploma for Licence and £25 on a Diploma for Fellowship. A period of licentiateship being an essential preliminary to Fellowship, the taxation on each Fellow amounted to £40 additional to £10 already paid on his University degree if a British Graduate.

The Chancellor of the Exchequer, the Right Honourable Benjamin Disraeli, M.P., was reminded of these facts in a Memorial sent to him by the College in 1859, seeking abolition of stamp duties on their Diplomas. In the Memorial it was pointed out that as a result of the heavy taxation many students had chosen to graduate at Universities abroad; and that the College's effort to assist a Fellow to avoid treble taxation by dispensing with the Licentiate had been ineffective. Referring to the Medical Act, the Memorial focussed attention on how union or co-operation between Corporations would be rendered nugatory by a tax system which levied 'on the joint diploma a tax from which the bodies conferring the surgical diploma are exempt'. It was pointed out also that closer international contacts in the promotion of medical science were discouraged by the inability of the College to confer an honorary diploma on a distinguished Foreign Physician without subjecting him to the Stamp Duties. Not without good reason the College took exception to Corporations continuing to be subject to taxation of this kind at a time when 'other bodies which are not taxed at all while by the Medical Act they are put on an equality so far as licensing is concerned'.[61]

Previously, the whole subject had been under discussion by the General Medical Council at a meeting at which the representative and President of the Edinburgh College of Physicians (Dr Alexander Wood) submitted a motion summarizing the injurious effects on the Universities diplomas of M.D., and on the Licentiates and Fellows of the Colleges of Physicians by the prevailing form of taxation: and remitting to the Council's executive committee to prepare a Memorial to be sent to the Treasury.[62] Dr Wood meantime endeavoured to bring the several interested parties together and one outcome was that the London College of Physicians proposed a joint deputation to the Chancellor of the Exchequer to pray for relief from the stamp duties.[61-36] Those taking part were to be the Colleges of Physicians of Edinburgh, Dublin and London but to the surprise of the Council [of the Edinburgh College] the President of the London College drew back and communicated his opinion that it would be better for each body to go forward alone.[64]

Neither daunted nor discouraged by the procrastination of the Executive Committee, Dr Wood raised the matter again in the General Medical Council. There were no immediate results. Memorials and letters were apparently ineffective but at the express desire of the General Medical Council Dr Wood obtained an interview with the Secretary of the Treasury (Sir Stafford Northcote) on 20th May 1859 from whom he learned that his communication to the Lords of the Treasury had been taken up. In point of fact the Treasury had committed to writing their readiness 'to propose to Parliament the remission of the Stamp Duty . . . imposed on Licentiates to practice' but were opposed to 'alteration in the Stamp Duty on Fellowships or the higher Degrees of Medicine'. The information was confirmed in a letter to the President of the Medical Council who sent a copy to the Council of the Edinburgh College. The letter stimulated a delightful comment, with an appeal to all generations of all professions, in the College Minutes—'The Council are glad to find that as a Treasury Minute it will stand good even under a change of administration.'![64] Retrospective legislation was not yet in vogue! Reporting on his interview with Sir Stafford Northcote, Dr Wood declared him to be obdurate in the matter of remission of the tax on Fellowship.

A copy of a Bill introduced into Parliament for the removal of Stamp Duties on Diplomas was examined by the College in August 1859, which on advice tendered by the College Solicitors in London authorized them to try to secure 'a slight addition' to the Bill.[65]

DELAYED RECOGNITION OF LICENCE BY GOVERNMENT BOARDS

With the abolition of the stamp duty, all was not yet set entirely fair for the Licence of the College. There remained the need to have the Licence recognized as adequate qualification by the English Poor Law Board and the Army Medical Board.

Poor Law Board

There was evidence of uncertainties prevailing in a unique occurrence considered by College Council in 1858. Information had been received that the Medical Officer to a parochial board had been dismissed for 'having opened the body of a Pauper who had died in the workhouse'.[66] According to Ferguson,[67] death had been sudden and unexplained. The Medical Officer was violently criticized and unreserved disapproval of his action was expressed in the Annual Report of the Board of Supervision (1859). Previously separate Memorials couched in strong terms had been submitted by our College and the Glasgow Medical and Chirurgical Society to the Home Secretary (Mr Walpole) who replied to the effect that he had no authority to interfere.[68]

In February 1859 the Council of the College was in receipt of a Memorial from seven Poor Law Medical Officers all of whom held appointments with Berwick Unions or Unions in Northumberland, and all of whom were graduates of Edinburgh University and Licentiates of the Royal College of Surgeons of Edinburgh and Faculty of Physicians and Surgeons of Glasgow. The Memorial pointed out that under the consolidated order of the Poor Law Board of London no Medical Officer could hold a permanent appointment unless in possession of one of four qualifications, viz.:

> 1. A diploma or degree as Surgeon from a Royal College or University in England, Scotland or Ireland together with a degree in Medicine from a University in England legally authorised to grant such a degree or together with a diploma or Licence of the Royal College of Physicians of London.
>
> 2. A diploma or degree as Surgeon from a Royal College or University in England, Scotland or Ireland together with a Certificate to practise as an Apothecary from the Society of Apothecaries of London.
>
> 3. A diploma or degree as Surgeon from a Royal College or University in England, Scotland or Ireland such person having been in actual practice as an Apothecary on the 1st day of August 1815, or

4. A warrant or Commission as Surgeon or Assistant Surgeon in . . . [the] Navy, or . . . [the] Army or . . . The Honourable East India Company dated previous to 1st August 1826.

There was no questioning either the Memorialists' interpretation of the order of the Poor Law Board, or their assertion that they themselves held office 'merely by sufferance as their Scotch degrees and diplomas do not render them duly qualified'. The Memorialists had added reason for anxiety in that the Poor Law Board had decreed that although the qualifications of their Medical Officers were to remain the same, 'registration under the New Medical Act will be required in addition'. This be it noted more than a century and a half since the Act of Union and less than three years after the passing of the Medical Act designed to secure, among other objectives, professional reciprocity. And the victims: domiciled almost within hailing distance of the Border![69]

Correspondence between the College and the Board eventuated but as it 'was not of a satisfactory kind', the President (Dr Alexander Wood), no doubt anxious to cut red tape, requested an interview with the Chairman of the Poor Law Board, the Earl of March. This was granted and took place on 21st May (1859). Undaunted by the presence of several permanent officials, the President indicated that his object was to have the licence of the Edinburgh College of Physicians 'put on the same level' as that of the London College. Early and full consideration was promised by the Board's Chairman. On the last day of the month a letter as encouraging as it was gracious was sent by the Board, indicating that the General Medical Council was being consulted.[70] On 28th February 1860 the President was in a position to announce that the Poor Law Board in England had 'agreed to recognise the Licence of this College as a Qualification for Appointments under the Parochial Boards in all parts of the country'.[71] Time must have been required for news of changes in central policy to reach the periphery because almost a year later the Clerk to an English Board of Guardians objected to the reappointment as Medical Officer of a College Licentiate on the grounds that his qualifications were Scottish.[72]

War Office

In the following year when in conflict with the War Office over the recognition of Corporation licences, a joint letter was sent by the Presidents of the two Edinburgh Colleges seeking information from the Poor Law Board about the conditions applying to appointments of their Medical Officers. The reply could not have been more helpful or gratifying. It explained that in so far as the Regulations of the Poor Law Board were concerned

> 'it is not material . . . by what examination or examinations the Diploma is obtained, or whether more than one can be obtained. If there be one it will suffice if it certify to the proficiency of the Candidate in Medicine and Surgery; or if there be two Diplomas, there may be one certifying as to the proficiency in medicine and the other certifying as to the proficiency in Surgery . . . It will not, however, in opinion of the Board be requisite that the Candidate should shew by what curriculum or courses of study, or after what examinations, he obtained his Diploma.'[73]

In effect the Poor Law Board recognized the Double Qualification as equivalent to a Degree in Medicine.

Recognition of the College Licence by the Fighting Services gave rise to not dissimilar problems but more aggressive exchanges. An article which appeared in the issue of 9th October 1860 of the *Medical Times and Gazette* stimulated, or perhaps goaded would be the more correct word, the College into immediate action. The following is an extract from the offending article:

> 'We believe that, in consequence of the large number of candidates who have been attracted to the Army and Medical Service by the new Warrant, it has been decided that gentlemen who possess Degrees in Medicine and Diplomas in Surgery will be preferred to those who only possess a Licence to practise either Medicine or Surgery.'

The article went on to advise those contemplating a career in the Army Medical Service to shape their course of study with a view to obtaining a recognized Degree in Medicine, in addition to a Diploma in Surgery.[74] The wrath and ire of the man— Dr Alexander Wood—who had only recently been the mainstay in converting the Poor Law Board can well be imagined. Losing no time—three days to be precise— he sent to the Director General, Army Medical Department, a copy of the offending paragraph with a covering note enquiring 'for the information of the Fellows of The Royal College of Physicians of Edinburgh whether any new Regulation has been promulgated by the Army Medical Board and if so, what its provisions are'. As no reply was forthcoming a reminder was sent within a week. There followed a wordy correspondence in which the army authorities relied more on verbal manoeuvres than heavy armour. The President was informed by the Director General that 'the Secretary of State for War has decided that a preference may be given to men having Medical Degrees and Surgical Diplomas over those who possess mere Licences to practise medicine and surgery'. This the Director General considered would afford him 'an opportunity of selecting the men, prima facie, the best educated . . . for admission to the competitive examinations'.

A letter from the President (Dr Alexander Wood) putting the relative requirements for the College Licence and a University degree in perspective, produced from the Director General a bald statement of inability to reassure the College and a reminder that the Secretary of State had made his decision. Thereupon the College Council memorialized the Secretary of State for War with the object of securing reconsideration of his preference for men with medical degrees and surgical diplomas. The Memorial included mention of the arrangements entered into with the Royal College of Surgeons of Edinburgh with the sanction of the General Medical Council and, it was emphasized, with the prior knowledge of the Director General in office at the time. Receipt of the Memorial was acknowledged by a member of the Secretariat who curtly concluded on behalf of the Secretary of State for War with the words: 'he regrets therefore his inability to reverse the former decision on this subject'.

The acknowledgment was dated 7th November 1860. On the 11th of February a joint deputation of the Edinburgh Colleges of Physicians and Surgeons waited on the Secretary of State for War and afterwards at his request sent him on 12th February a memorandum of the points on which the two Colleges desired information. The memorandum consisted of a recapitulation of Corporation views interspersed with occasional pointed questions. Perhaps it was too lengthy to have much chance of influencing a well entrenched élite establishment. Certainly the response obtained was lofty to the point of patronage and wholly unconstructive. It was dated 19th February 1861.[75]

There was an allied problem in connection with the Indian Medical Service. Regulations determined the letters which could be affixed to the names of Officers but made no reference to the Fellowship of the College. In April 1897 the Secretary ((Sir) Robert Philip) wrote to the President of the Medical Board, India Office asking that the omission be 'rectified and the Royal College of Physicians of Edinburgh placed on the same footing as the F.R.C.P.Lond. and the F.R.C.P.I.'.[76]

Royal Navy

The College had been confronted earlier in the century with a situation involving the Royal Navy. At a Quarterly Meeting in November 1848 a Memorial from a group of Assistant Surgeons was read seeking assistance in remedying specified grievances.[77]

Satisfied that a reasonable case had been advanced, the College forwarded a Petition signed by the President (Sir Robert Christison) to the First Lord of the Treasury. A plea was submitted that greater attention should be paid to the standard of accommodation provided for Assistant Surgeons on board ship: an unfavourable comparison was drawn with arrangements in the Army: and a recommendation was embodied that 'a suitable place for study and for the accommodation of Books should be provided'. How many Hospital Management Committees have had to deal with similar representations from Junior Medical Officers since 1948?!

In April 1849, it was announced by the President (Dr Seller) that the College Petition had been presented to both Houses of Parliament[78] and a year later he was able to point to the success of a Bill on the subject in the House of Commons.[79]

SUING FOR PROFESSIONAL FEES

Under Section 31 of the Medical Act (1858) any College of Physicians was empowered to pass a bye-law prohibiting their Fellows or Members from suing for fees. According to Cooke the clause was inserted in response to a request submitted by the London College, and 'the chief effect of the rule seems to be, as in Roman Times, to foster in persons subject to it feelings of dignity and superiority over other professional men'.[80]

The Edinburgh College of Physicians has never invoked the powers in question. Judging by the number of enquiries made by Licentiates from different parts of England there was considerable doubt among them on this score. Replying to one such enquiry in 1886 the Secretary ((Sir) Robert Philip) gave the position of the College as follows—'there is no law against your suing for them [fees] in Court, but the College does not encourage its Licentiates to do so'.[81]

THE PHARMACOPOEIA: A NEW LAMP FOR AN OLD

By the terms of the Medical Act (1858) the general Medical Council was under a legal obligation to accept responsibility for the periodical publication of a British Pharmacopoeia. Use of this was made obligatory in Scotland, England and Ireland. This involved the replacement of the Pharmacopoeia published by the Edinburgh College of Physicians, by the British version. The College agreed formally on 11th July 1862 to the introduction of a Parliamentary Bill with this change as its objective.[82]

First published in 1699 the College Pharmacopoeia ran to 14 editions, the last being in 1841.[83]

INSTITUTION OF AN ORDER OF MEMBERS

Under the terms of the Charter of 1861 powers were conferred on the College to institute an order of Members who should be intermediate in rank between the Licentiates and the Fellows.[84] By a Law passed in the following year the qualifications for the Membership were that the candidate should be a Licentiate of a College of Physicians, or Graduate of a British or Irish University; that the College should be satisfied with his knowledge of Medical and General Science; that he should have attained the age of 24 years; that he should present satisfactory testimonials as to his social and professional status; and that a motion for his election should be made and seconded by Fellows at a Quarterly Meeting and carried by a majority of not less than three-fourths of the Fellows voting.[85]

With experience of a growing number of Members being admitted, an increasing proportion of Fellows came to share the view that the conditions of admission were unsatisfactory. The desirability of instituting an examination to be sat by all candidates was discussed periodically *in sederunt*, but action was postponed pending anticipated major governmental measures for Medical Reform. Eventually, anticipation not having been realized, a College Committee was appointed in 1880 to consider the Laws relating to admission to the Membership.[86] Considerable differences of opinion were evident when the Committee's Report came up for discussion,[87, 88] but agreement was reached on an amended Report at the first Quarterly Meeting in 1881, necessitating revision of the Laws.

In accordance with the amended Laws candidates for the Membership were now required, before being balloted for, to pass an examination on the principles and practice of Medicine including Therapeutics: and another examination on one of the following subjects (to be selected by the candidate)—Pathology including Morbid Anatomy; Medical Jurisprudence and Public Health; Midwifery and the Diseases of Women; Psychological Medicine. There was however an exemption clause applicable to a candidate aged 40 years and over. Such a candidate if he had been a Registered Practitioner for not less than ten years and if able to produce evidence of distinction in virtue of 'Scientific attainments or eminence as a Medical Practitioner', could be exempted by the Council from the whole or any part of the prescribed examination.[89]

Consideration was then given by Council to the form which the examination should take. Uncertain as to the likely number of candidates, they submitted tentative proposals only. These proposals deserve quotation if only to compare them with present-day procedure.

> 'The Candidate shall appear in the morning at the Royal Infirmary, and shall have a case submitted to him, for the examination of which one hour will be allowed. He shall then be conducted to the College where he shall write out a full account of the case with a commentary thereon, and shall answer in writing questions in Therapeutics; for the written examination three hours shall be allowed. At four o'clock of the same day he shall appear for oral Examination, which shall last one hour, and shall be conducted by two Examiners, one being the Clinical Physician from whose ward the cases were selected, the other an Examiner appointed by the Council.
>
> Should the Candidate be successful at this Examination he shall on the following day appear for examination in the other subject selected by him. This shall be conducted by writing and orally by two Examiners selected by the Council, three hours being assigned for the written, one for the oral Examination.'[90]

At two subsequent meetings Council advised that owing to the small number of candidates a case did not exist for the appointment of a permanent Board of Examiners.[91, 92]

As experience of the Examination increased further changes were made. The basis of the Examination remained the Principles and Practice of Medicine including Therapeutics: but the number of subjects from which a Candidate could select for the second examination was increased. Thus there were added 'One or more Departments of Medicine specially professed' and Diseases of Women in 1891[93]; Diseases of Children, and Tropical Medicine in 1904.[94]

The original Laws relating to Membership and Fellowship had determined that no one should be eligible for elevation to the latter until he had been at least one year a Member of the College.[95] This probationary period of one year was extended to three years following a review carried out by a Committee appointed in 1896. In due course an impression gained currency that the extended period placed aspiring physicians at an unfair disadvantage having regard to the fact that Fellowship of the sister Surgical College did not involve any probationary period. Another Committee was appointed in 1913 to consider the position, and suggested that as a preliminary step the Managers of the Infirmary might be asked to consider the eligibility of Members of the College for appointments to the Honorary Staff of that hospital.[96] Further discussion of the subject was rendered impossible with the outbreak of war,

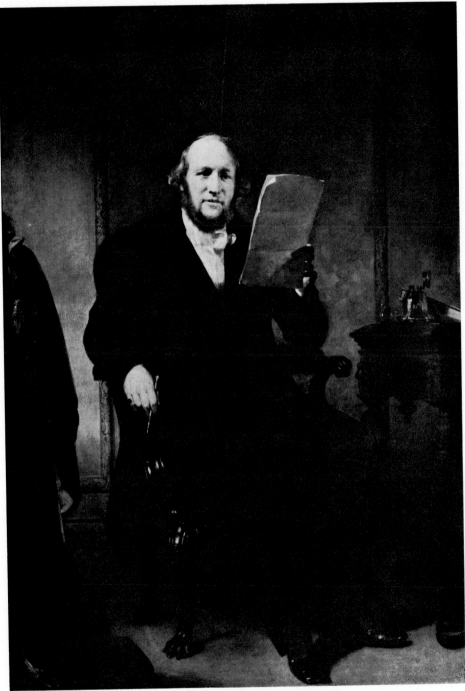

PLATE 21 Dr Alexander Wood (1817–1884)
Reproduced from portrait in the College by Sir John Watson Gordon, P.R.S.A.;
photograph by Tom Scott

but in 1922 it was mutually agreed by the Infirmary and College that Members as well as Fellows were eligible for Staff appointments.[97]

With hostilities ended, the Council again reviewed the overall situation. It was appreciated that young aspirants to the Fellowship included a number of those of proven high professional attainments in special branches of medicine, who were not in a position to devote the additional time necessary to study general clinical medicine of the increasingly high standard demanded of candidates. This aspect of the problem was the subject of discussion at a number of College meetings. Eventually Council were authorized to exempt candidates of high scientific attainments from part or the whole of the examination. Exemption of candidates on the ground of age was discontinued.[98] In 1922 the length of the probationary period came up for review but was not altered.

In 1938 an anomaly in the Laws relating to the Membership was removed. For some 200 years the College had prohibited the dispensing of medicines by Fellows and Members. Dr Edwin Bramwell explained that in many parts of England 'the practice of dispensing medicines for their patients was the almost universal custom among medical practitioners': and maintained that the existing College Laws 'by prohibiting this practice involved much hardship on many of the Members and acted as a deterrent to young practitioners from coming forward for the Membership'. He moved an amendment which while permitting a Member to dispense would require of him 'a written undertaking that in the event of his being elected to the Fellowship he will under no circumstances dispense medicines, and that should he subsequently do so he will immediately surrender his Diploma of Fellowship'. Dr Bramwell pointed out that the London College of Physicians had expressly altered their rules some ten years previously in order to admit of 'such dispensing as he now proposed'; and that as a result the number of their members had very materially increased. An amendment was moved by Dr W. T. Ritchie who considered the original motion represented a complete reversal of policy and if passed would 'bring the taint of commercialism upon the profession'. Seconded by Dr Gilchrist, Dr Bramwell's motion was carried with one dissentient.[99, 100]

THE TRIALS OF OFFICE BEARERS

No account of College activities leading up to and subsequent to the passing of the Medical Act of 1858 would be complete without tribute being paid to Dr Alexander Wood. The list of Fellows of the College contains the names of many illustrious physicians. To mention all or indeed many by name would not only be impracticable but would ignore the spirit of community fellowship which through the centuries has maintained a corporate sense of binding good will. Justification for making an exception in the case of Alexander Wood lies in his immense contribution in safe-guarding the interests of the College at a crucial stage in its history. Sometimes referred to as Alexander Wood *secundus* to distinguish him from his surgical great-uncle ('Lang Sandy'), he was the first to perform subcutaneous injections. His biography was written by a brother-in-law.[101-104] Elected President of the College in 1858 he held that office for three years, having previously been Secretary for six. While in office he was directly involved in negotiations for the new Charter, the revival of the Licentiateship, the retention of the rights of the Extra-Mural School, the repeal of stamp duties, and for the recognition of the double qualification by central government departments. When Secretary he kept a firm grip of all that was going on as evidenced in a letter from him to Dr Renton, well known for his tireless enthusiasm as negotiator and delegate on behalf of the College. Occasionally he overstepped the mark in the eyes of Wood and was castigated accordingly.[105] At a time when he was not in office a motion initiated by Wood implied criticism of the competence of two College delegates at a London Conference in connection with Medical Reform. The delegates were the Secretary (Dr William Seller) and Dr Renton. Both resigned.[106, 107]

Where the interests of the College were concerned Wood refused to accept defeat. When paper Memorials proved ineffective he did not hesitate to adopt the line of direct approach. For him, no cringing subservience to senior civil servants, high ranking service officers or powerful members of metropolitan sister corporations. Travelling long distances and at short notice had no terrors for him. To him railway sleeping cars were unknown—they did not appear on the Edinburgh–London route until April 1873; and as for artificial illumination on trains, flickering gas jets were the only source until the mid-1880s.

With the Medical Act on the Statute Book, Wood was elected the College representative on the General Medical Council on which he functioned for 14 years during which he was Chairman of 13 Committees of the Council.[108] His mastery of any problem under consideration was matched by his indefatigable industry and self-effacing determination.

Not that there were not times when he knew complete exasperation—as for instance when the Clerk to the College asked for assistance. In his bold long-hand Wood wrote on 14th February 1851, '. . . I began for the first time to keep a copy of all the letters written on College matters. The first is dated 5th April 1850 and I am already at the 201 page of the book. In all this I have no assistance from the Clerk farther than copying over my dfts. aftar they have been corrected by the Council—I need not say how unspeakably it would lighten my labors had I a person to whom I could send when a long letter or memorial had to be written to make him write to my dictation....'[109] Little did Wood realize what was in store for one of his successors after the passing of the Medical Act of 1858. In the College Letter Book for the year 1859 there are the carbon copies of no fewer than 3290 letters in the long-hand of the Honorary Secretary, Dr Daniel Haldane, over 96 per cent of them referring to applications for Licences. Six years were to elapse before the office of Registrar was created to deal with Licence applications.[110]

In the twentieth century Wood's administrative services to the medical profession would have made him an automatic choice for national committees and inevitably earned for him publicity and honours. It is to the credit of the College that it was neither slow nor grudging in showing appreciation; after occupying the Presidential chair for the customary period he was elected for a third year, at the end of which he was presented with a full-length portrait painted by the President of the Royal Scottish Academy of the day. The College had stipulated that 'on the condition of adequate eminence the choice of the artist [should] lie with Dr. Wood himself'.[111] Today this happily inspired tribute hangs in the College for Fellows, Members and guests of succeeding generations to see.

REFERENCES

(1) College Minutes, 1.ii.1859.

REPRESENTATIVE ON THE G.M.C.

(2) Ibid., 9.ii.1858.
(3) Ibid., 3.viii.1858.
(4) Ibid., 21.xi.1859.
(5) Ibid., 12.x.1858.
(6) Ibid., 2.xi.1858.

A NEW CHARTER

(7) Ibid., 28.xii.1858.
(8) R.C.P.E. (1925) *Historical Sketch and Laws*, p. 35. Edinburgh: Royal College of Physicians.

(9) College Minutes, 6.v.1845.

(10) Ibid., 9.v.1854.

(11) Ibid., 21.ix.1858.

(12) Ibid., 21.xii.1858.

(13) Ibid., 28.xii.1858.

(14) Ibid., 29.xii.1858.

(15) Ibid., 18.ii.1859.

(16) Ibid., 1.iii.1859.

(17) Ibid., 1.ii.1859.

(18) Ibid., 8.ii.1859.

(19) Ibid., 29.xii.1858.

(20) Ibid., 29.iii.1860.

(21) 23 and 24 Victoria, c. 7 (1860).

(22) College Minutes, 5.ii.1861.

(23) Council Minutes, 25.i.1861.

(24) College Minutes, 5.xi.1861.

LICENTIATESHIP: REVIVAL IN NEW FORM

(25) Ibid., 21.ix.1858.

(26) Ibid., 1.xi.1763.

(27) Ibid., 4.xi.1828.

(28) Ibid., 4.viii.1829.

(29) THOMSON, J. (1859) *An Account of the Life, Lectures and Writings of William Cullen, M.D.*, vol. I, p. 468. Edinburgh: Blackwood.

(30) College Minutes, 2.xii.1773.

(31) THOMSON, J. Op. cit., p. 471.

(32) Ibid., pp. 480–1.

(33) College Minutes, 8.iii.1859.

(34) The new charter of the College of Physicians (1859) *Medical Times and Gazette*, **18**, 61–2.

(35) GRANT, Sir A. (1884) *The Story of the University of Edinburgh*, vol. II, p. 110. London: Longmans, Green & Co.

(36) R.C.P.E. (1925) *Historical Sketch and Laws*, p. 59. Edinburgh: Royal College of Physicians.

(37) College Minutes, 29.iii.1859.

(38) Ibid., 5.iv.1859.

(39) Ibid., 15.iv.1859.

(40) Ibid., 20.iv.1859.

(41) Ibid., 26.iv.1859.

(42) Ibid., 5.ii.1884.

(43) Ibid., 4.viii.1874.

(44) CHRISTISON, Sir R. (1872) *Report of Proceedings at the Public Dinner . . . on Friday, February 23 1872*, p. 20. Edinburgh: Privately printed.

THE DOUBLE QUALIFICATION

(45) College Minutes, 14.vi.1859.
(46) Ibid., 24.vi.1859.
(47) Ibid., 26.vii.1859.
(48) R.C.P.E. (1925) *Historical Sketch and Laws*, pp. 66–7. Edinburgh: Royal College of Physicians.
(49) College Minutes, 5.ii.1884.
(50) Ibid., 6.xi.1883.
(51) Ibid., 19.vii.1859.
(52) Ibid., 19.viii.1859.

THE TRIPLE QUALIFICATION

(53) Ibid., 18.iii.1884.
(54) R.C.P.E. (1925) *Historical Sketch and Laws*, p. 68. Edinburgh: Royal College of Physicians.
(55) College Minutes, 4.xi.1884.
(56) R.C.P.E. (1896) *Letter Book*, 6.ii.1896.
(57) R.C.P.E. (1925) *Historical Sketch and Laws*, p. 168. Edinburgh: Royal College of Physicians.
(58) College Minutes, 19.vii.1921.
(59) Ibid., 2.ii.1875.
(60) Ibid., 17.x.1888.

THE GOVERNMENT TAX ON LICENCES OF THE CORPORATION

(61) Ibid., 18.ii.1859.
(62) Ibid., 14.vi.1859.
(63) R.C.P.E. (1925) *Historical Sketch and Laws*, p. 124. Edinburgh: Royal College of Physicians.
(64) College Minutes, 14.vi.1859.
(65) Ibid., 2.viii.1859.

DELAYED RECOGNITION

(66) Council Minutes, 5.viii.1858.
(67) FERGUSON, T. (1948) *The Dawn of Scottish Social Welfare*, p. 252. London: Nelson.
(68) Council Minutes, 17.ix.1858.
(69) College Minutes, 8.ii.1859.
(70) Ibid., 14.vi.1859.
(71) Ibid., 28.ii.1860.
(72) Council Minutes, 1.ii.1861.
(73) College Minutes, 7.v.1861.
(74) *Medical Times and Gazette* (1860) **2**, 339.
(75) College Minutes, 7.v.1861.

(76) R.C.P.E. (1897) *Letter Book*, 2.iv.1897.
(77) College Minutes, 7.xi.1848.
(78) Ibid., 5.iv.1849.
(79) Ibid., 16.iv.1850.

SUING FOR PROFESSIONAL FEES

(80) COOKE, A. M. (1972) *A History of the Royal College of Physicians of London*, vol. 3, p. 807. Oxford: Clarendon Press.
(81) R.C.P.E. (1886) *Letter Book*, 27.iii.1886.

THE PHARMACOPOEIA

(82) College Minutes, 11.vii.1862.
(83) R.C.P.E. (1925) *Historical Sketch and Laws*, p. 55. Edinburgh: Royal College of Physicians.

INSTITUTION OF AN ORDER OF MEMBERS

(84) Ibid., p. 74.
(85) College Minutes, 11.vii.1862.
(86) Ibid., 24.ii.1880.
(87) Ibid., 3.viii.1880.
(88) Ibid., 2.xi.1880.
(89) Ibid., 1.ii.1881.
(90) Ibid., 2.viii.1881.
(91) Ibid., 1.viii.1882.
(92) Ibid., 7.viii.1883.
(93) R.C.P.E. (1891) *Historical Sketch and Laws*, p. 130. Edinburgh: Royal College of Physicians.
(94) R.C.P.E. (1904) *Charters and Laws of the Royal College of Physicians of Edinburgh*, p. 80. Edinburgh: Royal College of Physicians.
(95) R.C.P.E. (1867) *Historical Sketch and Laws*, p. 86. Edinburgh: Royal College of Physicians.
(96) R.C.P.E. (1925) *Historical Sketch and Laws*, p. 76. Edinburgh: Royal College of Physicians.
(97) Ibid., p. 77.
(98) College Minutes, 4.xi.1919.
(99) Ibid., 19.vii.1938.
(100) Ibid., 1.xi.1938.

THE TRIALS OF OFFICE BEARERS

(101) MOGEY, G. A. (1933) Centenary of hypodermic injection. *British Medical Journal*, **2**, 1180–5.
(102) WOOD, A. (1855) New method of treating neuralgia by the direct application of opiates to the painful points. *Edinburgh Medical and Surgical Journal*, **82**, 265–81.

(103) WOOD, A. (1858) Treatment of neuralgic pains by narcotic injections. *British Medical Journal*, 721–3.

(104) BROWN, T. (1886) *Alexander Wood, M.D., F.R.C.P.E.: A sketch of his life and work*. Edinburgh: Macniven & Wallace.

(105) R.C.P.E. (1852) *Letter Book*, 3.xi.1852.

(106) R.C.P.E. (1857) *General Correspondence*, 6.ii.1857.

(107) R.C.P.E. (1857) *General Correspondence*, 19.v.1857.

(108) WOOD, T. Op. cit., p. 130.

(109) R.C.P.E. (1851) *Letter Book*, 14.ii.1851.

(110) R.C.P.E. (1859) *Letter Book*.

(111) College Minutes, 1.v.1860.

Chapter XV

NEW CHARTERS

Mention has been made of how rather desultory consideration of a new Charter by the College over a number of years assumed a more formative character at the time Graham was pressing ahead with his Bill for Medical Reform. Following withdrawal of the Bill, the draft of a new Charter which had almost reached the stage of finality was put into storage. Nine years passed before its existence was remembered. Having been unearthed it was referred to the College Committee on Medical Reform for review and amendment. Progress, however, was slow and erratic as a result of the prior claims on the Committee's time of events preceding the passing of the Medical Bill into Law in 1858. The Report by the Committee presented to the College in September of that year has been described in some detail (Chap. XIV). It made out a convincing case for obtaining a new Charter under the terms of the appropriate clause of the Medical Act. A new Charter could give a wider designation to the College; abolish certain embarrassing restrictive clauses in the original Charter; enable a new order of Members to be established; and give authority to the College to examine candidates for the Licence including University Graduates. In the event of power to examine not being granted, authority to apply the ballot was considered as an alternative; and it was hoped the College would have the undoubted power to suspend or expel unworthy members.[1] The decision to apply for a new Charter was made on 21st December 1858[2]; it was obtained dated 16th August, and sealed and registered on 31st October 1861.

As a preliminary step the College participated in a conference with the London and Dublin Colleges of Physicians, called with the object of securing some uniformity in the Charters being sought by the three Corporations.[3] One outcome was agreement by the three Colleges to co-operate in an endeavour to introduce into Parliament a Bill aiming at the abolition of Clause XLVII of the Medical Act.[4] The clause in question involved the probable surrender of privileges possessed by the Colleges at the time the Medical Act was passed.

Among specific points referred to in the preamble of the new Charter were that by the *Medical Act of 1858* it had been enacted that the College might be given the name of 'The Royal College of Physicians of Scotland':[5] but that by the *Medical Act (1858) (Amendment Act)* the College might alternatively retain the name of 'The Royal College of Physicians of Edinburgh'.[6] Specific reference was made also to the authority given under the *Medical Act (1858) Amendment Act of 1860*[7] to the addition of the term 'Member' to the Qualifications in the Schedule of the *Medical Act (1858)* in reference to the College. By the terms of another Amendment Act (*The Medical Act, Royal Colleges of Physicians, 1860*)[8] it was decreed that any new Charter granted could be given to the College 'by and in' its original name or 'by and in' the name of the Royal College of Physicians of Scotland: and that the College was to retain all existing rights and to hold property notwithstanding a change in name. On 5th February 1861 the College approved the Council's recommendation based upon the Law Committee's views to retain the name of the Royal College of Physicians of Edinburgh.[9]

By the terms of the new Charter the existing Fellows were constituted the first Fellows of the newly incorporated College, and the College was given power to admit new Fellows and Members, and to grant Licences. Decision as to regulations and fees for new Fellows and Members were left to the discretion of the College. Subject to the consent of three-fourths of Members present the College was empowered to censure, suspend or depose any Fellow, Member, or Licentiate of the College who had obtained admission by false pretence, or violated any of the Bye-Laws. The new College, Fellows, Members and Licentiates were given all the powers enjoyed by the old College, and the new College was enabled to make Bye-Laws for promoting and ordering the practice of the Science of Medicine and for the government and direction of the College.

Previous to the Charter of 1861 the term 'Member' was reserved for Fellows only. This fact was drawn to the attention of a Licentiate who in 1823 had described himself as a Member in a handbill. A letter from the Clerk of the College informed him that by the Regulations of the College 'the term "Member" can be applied to Fellows . . . exclusively, and no Individual not a Fellow is entitled to assume the designation . . . "Licentiates shall be designated by the name of Licentiate only".'[10]

Other provisions in the Charter were that the College was empowered to elect
its President directly, and not through the intervention of the Council; and that the
Council of the College should consist of the President and six of the Fellows resident
in Edinburgh, or within seven miles of the General Post Office in Edinburgh. Fellows
were to have powers to make Bye-Laws but any alteration of Bye-Laws, Rules or
Regulations were required to be approved by an Ordinary or Extraordinary Meeting
of the Fellows. A further decree was to the effect that the College was enabled to hold
property in its corporate name.

Following acceptance of the Charter the Offices of Censors and Fiscal were dispensed with—the duties of these offices having long been in abeyance.

In June 1860 the College were advised that by the terms of the proposed new
Charter, the Laws of the College required to be submitted to and approved by the
Secretary of State; and that the same would apply to any subsequent amendments.
This being the case the College appointed a Committee to revise and alter the
Laws.[11] Within five months almost to the day amended Laws proposed by the
Committee were laid on the Table and ordered to be circulated among the Fellows.[12]
After a second reading at the November Quarterly Meeting in 1861[13] the proposals
were discussed at four subsequent sederunts,[14-17] and at the last of these 'the College
declared that these Statutes and Bye-Laws of the College were the Statutes and Bye-
Laws of the College by which it should be governed . . . and . . . directed the Council
to have the printing of these Laws completed and Copies issued to the Fellows . . . .'.
Fellows present at this meeting numbered 29. The magnitude of the task of redrafting the Laws at this critical juncture in the history of the College needs no
elaboration except in so far as account should be taken of the other demands being
made on Fellows. Over and above routine business, prolonged and detailed study was
being given to major Bills concerned with Lunacy, Vaccination and Public Health.

Certain inclusions in the new Laws and Bye-Laws are of particular interest in the
light of the College's experiences over the preceding two centuries. Henceforth the
College was to consist of Fellows and Members, the discriminatory classification of
'Resident' and 'Non-resident' being discarded.[18] For election a Fellow had to have
attained the age of 25 years; been a Member for at least one year; and been supported
by at least three-fourths of Fellows balloting.[19] Fellows resident beyond five miles
from the Edinburgh General Post Office were to have the option of inclusion in the
Roll of Attendance with its liability to an annual contribution and fines. Discussing
eligibility a section of the College wished to limit Fellowships to those with a University Doctorate of Medicine, but were out-voted.[20]

To some extent the new laws relating to Fellows reflected a certain degree of liberalism. That this was desirable was evident in a requisition sent to the Secretary of the College by four non-resident Fellows from a London address in January 1859. The communication commenced with a reference to the right of non-resident Fellows of the Edinburgh College of Surgeons to sit and vote at meetings. The same was asked for non-resident Fellows of the College of Physicians together with an abrogation of the special privileges of resident as compared with non-resident Fellows. Continuing, the requisition urged that the President and Council should be elected by the direct votes of all Fellows and that the name of the College should be changed to that of the Royal College of Physicians of Scotland. Of the signatories one had been a non-resident Fellow for 18 years, another for nine and two for one year each.[21] The new Laws dealt rather belatedly with some of their pleas.

As to Members—those eligible were to consist of Licentiates 'of a College of Physicians, or Graduate of a British or Irish University, with whose knowledge of Medical and General Science the College may be satisfied' provided they were aged 24 years. Election was dependent on a petition being proposed, seconded and determined by a three-fourths majority in the course of balloting.[22] An aspiring Licentiate had to be 21 years of age, of good moral character, not under articles of apprenticeship and able to provide evidence of having 'fulfilled all the requirements that were in force at the date when he commenced his Medical studies'. A Curriculum of Study and Plan of Examination subject to annual review was laid down. Provision was made for a modified Examination limited to Medicine and Pathology, Materia Medica, Midwifery and Medical Jurisprudence in the case of applicants from among Licentiates of the London and Dublin Colleges; graduates in medicine of British and Irish Universities; Licentiates in Surgery of a Royal College or the Glasgow Faculty, of five years' standing; or Licentiates of an Apothecaries Company of five years' standing. Applicants satisfying the Examiners were later to be the subject of a ballot, a two-thirds majority being necessary for election.[23]

Forfeiture of all official connection with the College was to be the penalty for keeping a public shop, removal from the Register or infamous conduct. Unbecoming or unprofessional conduct was to involve the risk of censure, or deprivation of rights and privileges.[24] At an early stage the College had taken the precaution of obtaining legal advice as to the nature and extent of disciplinary measures to which they could resort should occasion arise.[25]

Other requirements, though possibly apparently minor in themselves had none the less a historical flavour. Mindful of the days of Sibbald, Stevensone and Pitcairne, there was reason in the instructions to the Secretary; he was required to keep College Minute Books, Letters and Papers in the College-Safe; could have the current Letter book and Minutes of Council in his own house, but 'the Minute-Book of the College is, on no account whatever, to be removed from the Building'.[26] The Clerk had to call the Roll 'at the commencement and close of each Meeting'— thereby being in a position to register the fines against the perennial late-comer and absentee.[27] Protests were dealt with in tolerant but precise terms. Those drafting the Laws cannot but have had visions of a Gregory resurrected, when they decreed— 'The College may reject any document, protest or instrument, the language of which may be considered objectionable, until amended to the satisfaction of the College.'[28] On at least one occasion a Treasurer had been unequal to his task and it was required that the annual accounts should be subject to annual audit by a chartered accountant.[29]

SUPPLEMENTARY CHARTER: 1920
(Appendix O)

The terms of section 4 of the Charter of 1861 precluded the election of women to the Membership or Fellowship of the College. This interpretation hinged on the use in the section of the word '*viros*'. At a Quarterly Meeting of the College in November 1918 a decision was arrived at 'to take steps to have the Constitution of the College altered or amended so as to permit of Women being admitted Members and Fellows of the College'. It was considered, were effect given to the recommendation, that the work of the College would be enhanced and the advancement of medical learning and science encouraged.[30, 31] Representations were favourably received. A Supplementary Charter dated 8th January 1920[32] was granted enabling persons of the female sex to be admitted as Fellows or Members of the College with 'the same powers, functions, rights, and privileges' and eligibility to election as office bearer; and, 'subject . . . to the like jurisdiction of the Fellows of the . . . College as if they were of the male sex'.

SUPPLEMENTARY CHARTER: 1950
(Appendix P)

This Charter deals with eligibility for election as a member of the Council of the College.

Article XI of the Charter dated August 16th 1861 provided that:

> 'Concilium Collegii constituendum esse ex Praeside et sex Sociis Edinburgi habitantibus ut intra septem millia passuum a domo, vernaculo sermone, "the General Post Office of Edinburgh", appellata, per proximam viam publicam.'

At a Quarterly Meeting of the College on 1st February 1949, it was resolved that steps should be taken to have Article XI altered in such a way as to remove the residential qualification. Such alteration would, it was considered, promote and facilitate the work of the College.[33]

The Charter of 15th March 1950 gave effect to the desire of the College by ordaining and declaring that:

> 'The Council of the College shall consist of the President and six of the Fellows.'[34]

Few would take exception to the view that implementation of this Supplementary Charter was overdue. Not many years had elapsed since a distinguished Fellow who had been nominated for election to the Council was declared to be ineligible on account of his living beyond the mileage limit prescribed in the Charter of 1861.[35] Technically the excess in mileage was minimal. The loss was the College's. The Supplementary Charter had not long become effective when a Fellow domiciled in Glasgow was elected to the Council.[36] Distance certainly did not curb his effective enthusiasm as a Councillor.

SUPPLEMENTARY CHARTER: 1959
(Appendix Q)

A Quarterly Meeting in May 1959 resolved that steps be taken to seek alteration of the Charter of the College with the object of making lawful the granting of diplomas in special subjects of medicine; and of enabling the College to hold lands, heritage, personal estate etc. of a value greater than that laid down in Article I of the Charter of 1861.[37] A Supplementary Charter was granted on 21st December 1959 whereby it was decreed that:

> 1. Article I of the Charter of 1861 constituting the College 'shall have effect as if the words "fifty thousand pounds" were substituted for the words 'Ten Thousand Pounds',
> 2. it shall be lawful for the College by themselves or in conjunction with any other Royal Scottish Medical Corporation having power to do so to grant to

persons who shall have passed such examinations as may be prescribed by the College by themselves or in conjunction with any other Royal Scottish Medical Corporation having power to do so diplomas in special subjects in medicine, . . .

3. the expression 'special subjects in medicine' shall mean psychological medicine and such other subjects as the College may from time to time prescribe by bye-laws by themselves or in conjunction with any other Royal Scottish Medical Corporation having power to grant diplomas in special subjects in medicine.[38]

SUPPLEMENTARY CHARTER: 1964
(Appendix R)

On 26th February 1964 a further Supplementary Charter was granted which determined that:

1. Article V of the Charter, constituting the College, shall have effect as if the words 'and Diplomates' were inserted after the word 'Licentiates' where that word first appears in that Article.

Article VI of the Charter shall have effect as if

(i) the words 'or diploma' were inserted after the word 'licence' in that Article; and

(ii) the words 'Licentiate or Diplomate' were substituted for the words 'or Licentiate' wherever such last mentioned words appear in that Article.

Article XX of the Charter shall have effect as if the words 'Licentiates and Diplomates' were substituted for the words 'and Licentiates' in that Article.

Article XXIII of the Charter shall have effect as if the words 'Licentiates and Diplomates' were substituted for the words 'and Licentiates' in that Article.

2. Article XII of the Charter shall have effect as if

(i) the words 'Vice-President' were inserted after the word 'President' in that Article; and

(ii) the words 'and for the election of Fellows to serve on the Fellowship Committee, the Library Committee and other Standing Committees of the College' were inserted after the word 'Council' in that Article.

Article XVI of the Charter shall have effect as if the words 'Vice-President' were inserted after the word 'President' in that Article.

Article XVII of the Charter shall have effect as if the words 'Vice-President' were inserted after the word 'President' wherever such last-mentioned word appears in that Article.

Article XIX of the Charter shall have effect as if the words 'Vice-President' were inserted after the word 'President' wherever such last-mentioned word appears in that Article.

3. It shall be lawful for the Fellows (as defined in Article XXIII of the Charter), to provide by bye-laws (as so defined) that a Fellow who has signed the Promissory Obligation referred to in bye-law 14 in Chapter II of the bye-laws, and is unable to

attend the Annual Meeting of the College, shall be entitled to vote by post for the election of Members of the Council of the College and the Charter shall be construed accordingly.[39]

REFERENCES

CHARTER OF INCORPORATION, 1861

(1) R.C.P.E. (1925) *Historical Sketch and Laws*, pp. 34–8. Edinburgh: Royal College of Physicians.
(2) College Minutes, 21.xii.1858.
(3) Ibid., 28.ii.1860.
(4) Ibid., 29.iii.1860.
(5) 21 and 22 Victoria, c. 90 (1858)
(6) 22 Victoria, c. 21 (1859).
(7) 23 and 24 Victoria, c. 7 (1860).
(8) 23 and 24 Victoria, c. 66 (1860).
(9) College Minutes, 5.ii.1861.
(10) R.C.P.E. (1823) *General Correspondence*, 7.v.1823.
(11) College Minutes, 5.vi.1860.
(12) Ibid., 6.xi.1860.
(13) Ibid., 5.xi.1861.
(14) Ibid., 19.xi.1861.
(15) Ibid., 20.xii.1861.
(16) Ibid., 4.ii.1862.
(17) Ibid., 11.vii.1862.
(18) Ibid., Chap. I, Law 1.
(19) Ibid., Chap. II.
(20) Ibid., 20.xii.1861.
(21) Ibid., 8.ii.1859.
(22) Ibid., 11.vii.1862. Chap. III.
(23) Ibid., Chap. IV.
(24) Ibid., Chap. VI.
(25) Ibid., 4.ii.1862.
(26) Ibid., 11.vii.1862. Chap. VIII, § 7.
(27) Ibid., Chap. VIII, § 10.
(28) Ibid., Chap. XI.
(29) Ibid., Chap. VIII, § 3.

SUPPLEMENTARY CHARTER: 1920

(30) Ibid., 5.xi.1918.
(31) R.C.P.E. (1925) *Historical Sketch and Laws*, p. 282. Edinburgh: Royal College of Physicians.

(32) R.C.P.E. (1920) Supplementary Charter.

SUPPLEMENTARY CHARTER: 1950

(33) College Minutes, 1.ii.1949.
(34) R.C.P.E. (1950) Supplementary Charter.
(35) College Minutes, 2.xii.1943.
(36) Ibid., 30.xi.1950.

SUPPLEMENTARY CHARTER: 1959

(37) Ibid., 5.v.1959.
(38) R.C.P.E. (1959) Supplementary Charter.

SUPPLEMENTARY CHARTER: 1964

(39) R.C.P.E. (1964) Supplementary Charter.

Chapter XVI

THE EXTRA-MURAL SCHOOL OF MEDICINE

Everybody who is incapable of learning has taken to teaching.
Oscar Wilde

The Faculty of Medicine in the University of Edinburgh was founded in the year 1726. Instruction in some aspects of medical education was available long before that date. When in 1505 the Barber–Surgeons successfully applied for a Charter of Incorporation the Town Council granted a request for anatomical material. Permission was given for one cadaver once a year, subject to 'ilk ane' of the Surgeons should 'instruct utheris'. In the course of time apprentices received instructions from their master, and more anatomical material was somehow obtained for the purpose.[1] Initially teaching consisted in the main of anatomy and James Borthwick who, originally an apothecary, had been admitted to the Craft as a surgeon, was appointed teacher for the purpose in 1647.[2] Nine years later the Incorporation developed a Physic Garden and this was used to instruct students in botany and the elements of pharmacy. Those engaged in teaching knew great encouragement when in 1697 an anatomical theatre was built by the Surgeons with the express purpose of conducting public dissections in it. In the same year a surgeon and former teacher of anatomy leased accommodation under the main hall where he organized a course of instruction in chemistry. Those who carried out dissections included Archibald Pitcairne who on being expelled from the Royal College of Physicians in 1695 had been admitted without fees being required of him, to the Royal College of Surgeons six years later. Our sister College was not long in learning the ways of the stormy petrel admitted to their ranks. They soon had occasion to fine him for 'blasphemy'.[3] This, however, may not have been so very grave or uncommon a crime because it has been said of the old Minutes of the Glasgow Faculty that one 'can hardly open them, without being struck with the frequency with which a crime known as "blaspheming" prevailed'.[4] Significantly Robert Elliot (1669–1715) who held the office of public dissector at the College of Surgeons had been a pupil of Pitcairne's in Leyden.[5]

With the opening of the Infirmary in 1741 clinical instruction became a practical proposition and its development led to the gradual decline of the apprenticeship system.

PRIVATE TEACHING POPULAR

Extra-mural teaching grew apace and did not suffer set-back with the creation by the University of a comprehensive course of instruction. At first extra-mural instruction was provided by teachers acting in an individual capacity, but with time, a number of schools developed, each being run by a group of teachers. One such school was exceptional in that it did not function for more than two years despite encouragement from Alexander Monro *primus*, a possible reason being resentment because the promoters were St Andrews graduates.[6] According to Lindeboom the promoters were William Graeme and George Martine; both had matriculated at Leyden, but Graeme was an alumnus of Rheims, not St Andrews.[7] This was in 1726, the College of Surgeons having appointed their first Professor of Anatomy in 1705. In the next 61 years additional courses available included Diseases of the Teeth; the Practice of Medicine and Materia Medica by Dr Andrew Duncan, a Member of the College of Physicians; and Midwifery.

Another unfortunate school was the Queen's College which, organized some 115 years later by a group of teachers on both medical and non-medical subjects, survived only a few years. The effect of the failure of some schools was not to discourage extra-mural instruction but to stimulate teaching by individuals rather than by groups of individuals. Between 1834 and 1878 the student was given new opportunities with additional courses in Physiology, Medical Jurisprudence, Public Health and Diseases of Children. Other subjects dealt with which were not in the University curriculum at the time, were insanity conducted by (Sir) Alexander Morison, Tropical Diseases, Diseases of the Ear, Nose and Throat and Diseases of the Skin.[8]

For eight years (1857–65) a course of lectures on the History of Medicine was given by Dr J. Warburton Begbie who was also an extra-mural teacher in Medicine. The son of a former President of the College, Warburton Begbie was one of Scotland's most highly respected and popular physicians. His influence was not limited to his native city or country. There could be no greater testimony to him than the following words taken from an address by Sir Mitchell Banks to the students of the Yorkshire College, Leeds in 1892: 'If ever I pictured myself as a great physician', said Sir Mitchell, 'when I looked closely into that picture, it was the portrait of Begbie that I saw . . . As a teacher he had no rival in Edinburgh when I was a student . . . When he entered a ward a new light seemed to shine in the faces of the sick . . . there stood our master, who had seen much human suffering; who had had not a few trials to bear himself; and every day he taught us not only lessons in medicine, but lessons in courteous and considerate demeanour to the poor . . . I have always striven in the hospital ward and in the clinical theatre to imitate his example.'[9] Could finer tribute be paid to any clinical teacher even in these administratively dominated days when 'Salmonised' nurses are numbered like the keys in the reception office of any hostelry?

By coincidence, in 1835 a request was received on behalf of the Leeds School of Medicine asking that the College of Physicians should confer upon the lecturers of that school 'the honor of recognition as Teachers in their respective Branches of Medical Science, and that Certificates of attendance on the Lectures delivered at their School may be considered as qualifying Pupils for examination'. The impracticability of complying with the request was explained to the surgeon originally submitting it.[10]

UNIVERSITY RECOGNITION

Until 1840 no teaching other than its own was recognized by the University of Edinburgh. Although teaching at other Universities was now accepted it was not until 1855 that extra-mural instruction was recognized, and students were allowed to attend half their classes extra-murally. In the words of the Goodenough Report 'the validity of courses by such [extra-academical] teachers . . . was . . . forced upon the University of Edinburgh by the Town Council of that city'.[11] This was the ultimate outcome of an appeal in 1840 by the surgeon Syme to the Town Council as patrons of the University, to require recognition of extra-mural classes on the grounds that 'one of the professors . . . was so comparatively inefficient that many Students, after paying him his fee and obtaining his certificate of attendance, went to learn his subject elsewhere'.[12] The Town Council took appropriate action. Regulations, however, only came into operation in 1855 after a prolonged duel in the Courts between the Town Council and the University. The case was eventually determined in favour of the Patrons. 'Extra-Academical rivals to the Medical Professors were started . . . without however bringing ruin on the University.'[13]

With the placing of the *Medical Act (1858)* on the Statute Book the Licences or diplomas of the Royal Colleges of Physicians and Surgeons conferred the right to practise, associated also with the Doctorate of Medicine of Universities. Moreover the recognition of extra-academical teachers was continued as a permissive power granted to the Courts of Universities in the Universities (Scotland) Acts of 1858 and 1899.[14, 15]

This recognition was only achieved after determined opposition on the part of the Edinburgh University Senate. The opposition did not have the support of the Governing Body of the University—the Town Council. All credit is due to the College of Surgeons for their persistent pursuit of Syme's objective and for their consistently co-operative attitude in keeping the College of Physicians fully informed. A move, distinctly parochial in outlook, to discriminate unfairly in the interests of the London and Dublin Colleges and to the detriment of the Edinburgh Colleges was successfully overcome. Thereupon the Senate urged that fees due to extra-mural teachers should not be less than those drawn by academic staff professing the same subjects. However the Town Council conceded on both issues provided that the two Royal Colleges raised their standards of medical instruction. The Senate which had not been directly involved in the drawing up of regulations following the Town Council's decision, raised an action against the Town Council which went in favour of the latter when taken to the House of Lords.[16]

The unnamed Professor singled out for Syme's criticism was Alexander Monro *tertius*. Apocryphal accounts have not added to his reputation. Whatever his inadequacies, the fact remains that (Sir) Robert Christison, a one-time pupil of his, recalled that 'Monro gave a very clear, precise, complete course of lectures on anatomy when I attended him; and certainly I learned anatomy well under him'.[17] Anyone ready to pass judgment should have regard to Sir Arthur Keith's appraisal in his Struthers Anatomical Lecture delivered before the Royal College of Surgeons in Edinburgh:

> 'If we accept the verdict of his contemporaries, that he was an incompetent teacher, and that his dullness was the virtue which gave Edinburgh the great extra-mural school of Barclay and Knox, we shall show but a meagre understanding of either the man himself or of the events which were shaping then in anatomy. The truth is, he had outlived his period. He had ideals. From the numerous researches and books which he published we can see that he studied the anatomy of the human body with two objects: (1) in order that surgeons might operate on it with dexterity; (2) to note the disturbances caused in it by disease, so far as these could be brought to

light by knife and forceps. These were the ideals which Allan Burns of Glasgow and Matthew Baillie of London had made popular in Monro's more youthful days. It was not because of his ideals he failed, it was because he was content to play the local tunes of his younger days while Knox was setting the youth of Edinburgh agog with a music which was then thrilling Europe. He failed in the first duty of a professor, the duty of bringing students in touch with the best movements of the time.'[18]

SUPERVISION

Already by the mid-nineteenth century the two Edinburgh Colleges had taken steps to supervise extra-mural teaching, and those applying for recognition as extra-mural teachers were required to satisfy certain standards. In April 1847 the College was advised that a copy of new Regulations adopted by the Town Council as Patrons of the University with regard to extra-academical lecturers had been received. The Regulations related to lecturers whose courses of lectures were to qualify for the Degree of M.D. in the University of Edinburgh. Recognition of Fellows of the two Edinburgh Colleges as lecturers was to be dependent upon their qualifications having been tried by examination before a Board appointed by the College of which they were members. Exemption was granted in the case of lecturers on subjects constituting a part of the course of study for surgical qualifications. No lecturer was to teach more than one prescribed subject 'excepting . . . where professors in the University are at liberty to teach two branches'. A fee was to be paid for every ticket intended as evidence of attendance with a view to graduation, the 'fee [being] of the same amount with that exigible by the medical Professors in the University'. Lecturers on Chemistry and Natural History who were not required by the University School of Medicine to be Fellows of the Colleges, or to possess medical status, were to be examined by a joint board equally representative of the two Colleges.[19]

A Report from a Committee appointed 'to draw up Regulations for an examination of Candidates to teach any of the branches of Medicine' was considered by the College in May 1847. Obviously the Committee, while agreed as to the constitution of the examining body, were unable to decide on detailed recommendations as to the form examinations should assume.[20] The Report occasioned intense discussion and was subject to considerable amendment before Regulations were finally drafted and approved in November 1847.[21-23] They made allowance for most of the requirements of the University: and decreed that intending lecturers should pass an examination, satisfy the examiners as to their competence to teach, and give evidence of having in their possession the means necessary for illustrating their lectures.

CHARTER FOR SCHOOL OF MEDICINE

Tribute is paid in the *History* of the University to the great experience and professional distinction of many of the extra-mural lecturers whose courses attracted a considerable number of students towards the end of the nineteenth century.[24] The number of private schools increased at this time and in the College Minutes it is recorded that in 1883 consideration was given to applications from the extra-mural teachers praying to be associated under the name of 'The Medical School of the Royal Colleges of Physicians and Surgeons'.[25] Because of 'the existing position of Medical Legislation' the College decided that action by them was contra-indicated.[26] There was formed, however, an *Association of Extra Mural Teachers*—the first surviving Minute of which was dated 8th July 1892.[27]

In 1895 the College after deliberation deferred consideration of a Memorial received at the hands of the School of Medicine. The Memorial sought the recognition of non-qualifying lecturers, that all recognized Lecturers should form the teaching staff, and most fundamental of all, that the School should be governed by a Board representing the Colleges and Lecturers.[28] Within two months a constitution for the School of Medicine was agreed and adopted,[29] and a Charter was obtained which vested responsibility for government of the School in a Governing Board along the lines suggested in the original Memorial. An *Annual Calendar* was first published in 1896 and appeared regularly until 1947–8, and Messrs E. & S. Livingstone published independently *Edinburgh Medical School Calendar and Guide to Students* for the years 1880–1, 1884–5 and 1895–6.

WOMEN STUDENTS AND WOMEN LECTURERS

The obstructions put in the way of women studying medicine are well known. Colleges and the University were alike in their obdurate conservatism. Efforts to secure emancipation in this field are inseparable from the names of Elizabeth Garrett and Sophia Jex-Blake—eventually Dr Garrett and Dr Jex-Blake. In 1862 Miss Garrett submitted a petition asking to be allowed to pass the Preliminary Examination with a view to taking the Licence of the College.[30] Her request was rejected after a division. Continuing in their attitude the College decided to oppose a Bill amending the *Medical Act (1858)* to make possible the Registration of Women possessed of a Doctorate of Medicine conferred by a Foreign University.[31] A grudging melting of hearts took place in the following ten years and on 2nd February 1886 with suitable dignity the College resolved to give its consent to the Admission of Women to the Examinations for the Conjoint Qualification.[32] In this the College of Surgeons concurred. At first women attended separate classes at the Extra-Mural School but by 1870 there were 'mixed classes'. Accounts as to how the male elements reacted are contradictory. According to Jex-Blake's biography the women were welcome,[33] but the College of Surgeons received protests from 65 males who asked for 'the removal of their grievances'. The Surgeons took the view that the format of classes was the responsibility of the lecturers but did later express understanding of the students' views.[34]

The need for separate accommodation became obvious. Three women including Miss Jex-Blake bought premises in Surgeons' Square which had previously been a medical school of long standing, won the co-operation of Leith Hospital (1887) by being granted clinical facilities, and obtained the services of clinical lecturers. In theory a School of Medicine for Women was established but not officially recognized as such. The lecturers however were recognized as individuals. In 1888 Dr Jex-Blake was declared by the College to be duly qualified to lecture on Midwifery and given authority to lecture on the subject. Previous to this she had been required to deliver a lecture before the Conjoint Board of Examiners who put questions to her and 'examined her Museum and Appliances'.[35] During the ten years the 'School' ran, it met an undoubted need and its success prompted the rise of competitive opposition classes with lesser fees.[36] According to Turner, the Anatomy Department of Minto House was handed over to the Women's School of Medicine in 1895.[37]

STUDENT NUMBERS AND STAFF DISTINCTIONS

The largest number of students in any one year at the Extra-Mural School was 1317 in 1897–8 when there were 44 lecturers. Enrolled students exceeded 1000 each subsequent year until the outbreak of hostilities in 1914. When the school ceased to function in 1947–8, the number of students was approximately 350. From about the middle of the nineteenth century the Physicians in Ordinary at the Royal Infirmary combined to give a joint course in clinical medicine, and the professorial staff with ward responsibilities followed suit in due course.[38] There was always a considerable number of extra-mural lecturers in Medicine and Surgery who never lacked pupils because University students attended courses in these particular subjects twice, and many elected to take the second course extra-murally. This obtained despite the fact that beginning in 1932 the University ceased to grant recognition to extra-academical teachers and also declared its resolve not to grant recognition in the future. On the other hand, with advances in medicine after the turn of the century the trend was for the number of extra-academical teachers to diminish gradually. Simultaneously the number of such teachers who attained academic professorial status declined, but it is deserving of record that over the years, of extra-mural lecturers a total of 35 eventually occupied chairs in the Medical Faculty of the University of Edinburgh, and 26 in the Medical Faculties of other Universities.[39]

POSTGRADUATE TEACHING

The beginning of instruction intended for postgraduates consisted of lectures, demonstrations and courses given by individual extra-mural lecturers. Postgraduate teaching on an organized basis was started in 1905 in accordance with an agreement reached between the University and the School of Medicine of the two Edinburgh Colleges. A joint Committee representative of the two Colleges and the extra-mural teachers was formed and arrangements made with the hospitals for clinical facilities. Courses and lectures were arranged to take place in the long vacation and these assumed an increasingly specialized character on resumption after World War I (Chap. XXX).

ENVOI

Incorporation of the School of Medicine of the Royal Colleges of Edinburgh by Charter took place in 1895. The school ceased to function 53 years later, in 1948. As to the circumstances surrounding, indeed ultimately compelling, the demise of the School—these are best given by reference to the section entitled *The Future of the Non-University Medical Schools* in the Goodenough Report. Not all were, or are, in agreement with all the findings in that Report but impartiality requires reproduction of relevant sections no matter their length.[40]

'THE FUTURE OF THE NON-UNIVERSITY MEDICAL SCHOOLS

38. The adoption of our recommendation that, in future, undergraduate medical training should be conducted only in university medical schools will involve either the absorption of the four existing non-university schools by the appropriate universities or the cessation of undergraduate training by those schools. It is, therefore, desirable that we should report on our inquiry into these schools.

The extra-mural schools in Scotland

39. The Scottish extra-mural schools are the Anderson College of Medicine, and St. Mungo's College, in Glasgow, and the School of Medicine of the Royal Colleges in Edinburgh.

42. The School of Medicine of the Royal Colleges is a corporate body consisting of lectures recognized by the Royal College of Physicians of Edinburgh and the Royal College of Surgeons of Edinburgh.

43. These three extra-mural schools have played an important part in the development of medical education in Scotland. Their greatest service was rendered during the last century. In those days, owing to the nature of the training and the methods by which it was conducted, the extra-mural schools were able to parallel successfully the courses of training provided by the university medical schools. Their fees were lower than those of the universities and they attracted to their service many able and ambitious young graduates. The medical curricula of the universities allowed considerable freedom in the arrangement of classes and it was quite a common practice for students of the university medical schools to attend some courses of instruction in the extra-mural schools, either instead of, or in addition to, the corresponding courses in the university schools.

44. At that time, in both the university and extra-mural schools, the basic form of teaching in most subjects of the medical curriculum, apart from simple laboratory work in chemistry and biology, work in the dissecting room, and the mixing of medicines, was the formal lecture. As a rule, the lectures were carefully prepared and ably expounded. The professor himself did almost all the teaching, departmental lecturers and assistants being very few.

45. Conditions nowadays are very different. In the university medical schools in Edinburgh . . . , as in the schools in other parts of the country, the university professor, who did almost all the teaching in his subject, has been replaced by a department consisting of a professor with a team of lecturers and assistants. To show the difference from the position in 1858 let us note the staff in the faculty of Medicine of the University of Glasgow in the current academic year. Instead of only ten professors and three assistants for which provision was made in 1858, there are now twenty professors, seventy-three lecturers and fifty-five assistants. The professors and the other members of the staff of the university schools are encouraged to undertake research work and are provided with facilities for doing so. One result of the growth of these university departments has been that, nowadays, the abler of the young medical graduates tend to seek appointments in the university schools in preference to teaching in the extra-mural schools.

46. During the present century the pattern of the medical curriculum has become more closely ordered and we recommend an ever closer integration. Under these conditions the use of the extra-mural schools by university students has been very much reduced and will continue to decline. The present enrolment of these students is chiefly for courses in such subjects as ophthalmology, dermatology, and oto-laryngology in which a series of clinical demonstrations in the appropriate hospital is associated with a short course of lectures. A certain number of students, who have failed in university examinations in pre-clinical subjects and

been required to produce evidence of further study before re-appearing for examination, may make use of extra-mural classes. If such revision courses are necessary, they should be provided by the universities.

47. The courts of the Universities of Edinburgh and Glasgow have already taken steps to curtail the recognition of "extra-academical" teachers . . . the future of the extra-mural schools must be considered from exactly the same angle as any other medical school, namely from the stand-point of the medical students who take the whole of the course of training under their aegis. There is no doubt that, looked at from this angle, the extra-mural schools are of a lower standard than other schools in the country.

(a) Teachers

48. The memorandum of evidence of the Royal College of Physicians of Edinburgh states that after 1918 the competition for teaching in the extra-mural school of that city became less keen. This change soon led to difficulty in finding staff.

50. If a fellow of the Royal College of Physicians of Edinburgh wishes to teach in the school on a subject of medical interest he applies to the College for permission to do so. He is then required to attend for formal interview by a committee appointed by the council of the College. At this interview he gives the necessary particulars concerning his premises (he need not necessarily teach on the school premises), his equipment and the arrangements he proposed to make for teaching. He may also be required to give a short exposition of a medical subject. If the applicant is a fellow of the Royal College of Surgeons of Edinburgh the same procedure is followed by that College. Should the candidate not be a fellow of either College he has to apply to both bodies, who appoint a joint committee, the procedure thereafter being the same. Vacancies are not advertised. Once recognized by the Colleges, a teacher automatically becomes a member of the Board of Management of the School of Medicine. Each teacher pays rent for the premises he uses for teaching purposes, provides his own teaching material and is remunerated out of the fees of students who attend his classes. At times in the past there have been several competing teachers in the same subject, but at the present time there is only one lecturer recognized in each subject. From August, 1941, students have had to attend the Dick Veterinary College in Edinburgh for instruction in physiology.

51. The witnesses who met us on behalf of the extra-mural schools stated categorically that these schools were interested only in the teaching of students and were not interested in medical research. We have already stated our views on the necessity for a combination of research and teaching in medical schools.

(b) Students

52. The number of students of the extra-mural schools has fluctuated widely since the beginning of the century. During the first fifteen years or so a large number of university students attended courses at the schools either in substitution for or in addition to the corresponding courses in the university schools. At the end

of the war of 1914–1918 both the extra-mural and the university medical schools were crowded with men demobilized from the Forces. When this wave of students had passed, the entries to the extra-mural schools declined greatly. By 1926 the entry to . . . the School of Medicine, Edinburgh, [was] forty a year. In the period 1931–38 the number increased enormously. In 1936 new entrants to . . . the School of Medicine in Edinburgh [numbered] ninety-five. The very inadequate accommodation and equipment . . . must have been severely overtaxed to provide an efficient pre-clinical training for such large numbers. The organized teaching clinics in the teaching hospitals were overcrowded and great difficulty was experienced in securing satisfactory provision in pathology and clinical midwifery for the normal number of university students, as well as for the extra-mural groups. This inflation in the entries to the extra-mural schools was the result of a movement in the United States of America to raise the standard of medical education in that country by reducing the number of entrants to the American schools and thereby securing higher standards. The authorities in the United States had to take steps to close this Scottish back-door to the medical profession in the United States. Their measures were just becoming effective in 1939.

53. On average the quality of students in the extra-mural schools does not seem to be as high as in the university schools. A small number of students who fail to keep their places in the latter transfer to the extra-mural schools . . . While the rules for the Scottish Triple Qualification indicate a standard of education for admission to the study of Medicine not lower than university matriculation, special concessions appear to be secured more easily from the Triple Qualification Board of Management than from the Joint Entrance Board of the Scottish Universities.

54. We have received evidence that in those classes in which extra-mural students meet university students on equal terms, such as the class of pathology and the clinical classes, the former are almost invariably of lower merit than the latter . . . While the qualifying examinations for the extra-mural students are conducted by the Board of Management of the Triple Qualification and not by the schools, it is common knowledge that university students who have repeatedly been unsuccessful at the university final examination often pass the final Triple Examination at their first attempt. There is no doubt that the less able student finds the Triple Qualifying Examination easier than the university examination.

55. Only a relatively small number of the extra-mural students after qualification secure resident hospital appointments, even in the teaching hospitals of Edinburgh . . . in which they receive their clinical training . . .

56. The representatives of the extra-mural schools laid great stress on the point that these schools could provide for students who, because they had been educated in other countries, or because they decided fairly late in life to study Medicine, were unable to secure a certificate of fitness from the Universities Joint Entrance Board and therefore were debarred from entry to one of the Scottish university medical schools. We are not able to attach much importance to this point. Relaxations in educational requirements do not help to maintain a good standard of medical education. The only sound policy is to apply the same standards to students from overseas as are applied to students educated in Great Britain. Further it is seldom difficult for a person of good general education to secure a certificate of

fitness from the Scottish Universities Joint Entrance Board under the special rules for persons of mature years, and, as appears from the statistics . . . many more students from overseas parts of the British Commonwealth and Empire were admitted by the university medical schools than by the extra-mural schools.

(c) *Accommodation and Equipment*

57. The buildings and equipment of the School of Medicine of Edinburgh . . . are out-of-date and entirely inadequate.

58. The provision and maintenance of equipment, particularly in the laboratory sciences, has become a very heavy charge on the funds of all medical schools. The funds which each of the extra-mural schools has for the purchase of equipment appears to be solely or largely an annual grant of £100 from the Carnegie Trust. Apparently, the provision of other material for teaching purposes, such as diagrams, models and specimens, is the responsibility of the individual teachers and not of the schools. The endowments and financial resources of the schools are very scanty. They do not receive government grants through any channel and the Scottish Royal Medical Corporations which conduct the qualifying examination for the extra-mural students do not make any contribution towards the expenses of the schools. The teachers pay to the schools a percentage of the fees which they receive, either personally or through the school, from the students enrolled in their classes.

(d) *Conclusion*

59. The conclusion to which we have been forced is that although they did good work in time past, these three schools cannot meet the modern requirements of medical training efficiently. They are not able to provide a comprehensive course of training satisfying the conditions which we have set out in chapter I of our report. If they continue, they will inevitably do so as schools of a lower standard than the other medical schools of Great Britain. Although, undoubtedly, lack of financial resources has been a great handicap to them, they could not be made the equals of university medical schools by being given increased financial aid. We cannot recommend that they should receive any grants from public funds.

60. The right possessed by these schools to use the same teaching hospitals as the university medical schools for the clinical training of their students has created difficulties for the university medical schools in arranging for the adequate clinical training of their students and will prove an obstacle to the development in Edinburgh . . . of medical teaching centres organized on the lines that we have recommended.

61. The whole conception of an organized medical teaching centre and of a correlated course of training is dependent upon the teaching hospitals of the centre being inter-locked in administration, policy and educational work with a *single* medical school.

62. In our opinion the three extra-mural schools in Scotland should cease to train medical students. In the absence of new legislation giving specific authority to close medical schools in certain circumstances, and no such authority exists at the present time, the decision rests with the governing bodies of the schools. Should

they continue, grants from public funds should not, in our opinion, be made in respect of either the teaching work of the schools or the provision of hospital facilities for students of the schools.

63. . . . We have no doubt that the buildings of . . . the Edinburgh extra-mural school could be put to other uses . . .

64. The closing of the extra-mural schools will probably lead to the disappearance of the Scottish Triple Qualification, since over 90 per cent of the candidates for that qualification are trained in these schools. There would be little loss as a consequence to the recruitment of doctors for service in Scotland, since only a very small proportion of practitioners who qualify by virtue of the Triple Qualification decide to practise in Scotland.'

MEMORANDUM BY THE ROYAL SCOTTISH MEDICAL COR-PORATIONS ON THE REPORT OF THE INTERDEPART-MENTAL COMMITTEE ON MEDICAL SCHOOLS, APRIL 1945

A sequel to the eventual publication of the Goodenough Report was the drawing up of a Joint Memorandum by the Scottish Corporations for dispatch to the Secretary of State for Scotland with a request for interview 'to enable them to elaborate certain matters'.[41] The signatories were Dr Fergus Hewat, Professor R. W. Johnstone and Mr W. A. Sewill, Presidents of the Edinburgh Royal College of Physicians, the Edinburgh Royal College of Surgeons and the Royal Faculty (now College) of Physicians and Surgeons of Glasgow respectively.

No words were wasted in the Memorandum but the indignation of the Colleges gained from the employment of patrician prose reminiscent of earlier professional writings of Professor R. W. Johnstone. It was only too obvious that the Corporations were alarmed by the gravity of the Interdepartmental Committee's recommendations. Immediate exception was taken to the proposal that only university medical schools should conduct graduate teaching. After all, the three Scottish Medical Corporations had co-operated for many years to form a qualifying board under the Medical Acts. Arguments advanced against the proposal were that it was beyond the capacity of the country's Universities to train all the medical students even when allowance was made for the Committee's somewhat nebulous suggestions for the incorporation of the London hospital medical schools in the University of London. With some justification the comment was made, 'It is not easy to see why the London hospital medical schools, with minor alterations in their constitutions, are to be allowed to continue, while the Scottish extra-mural schools are condemned to extinction'. Attention was drawn to ways in which the student had been helped by the Scottish extra-mural schools, and to the fact that Scottish students who might find themselves compelled to go south for their medical education would no longer be eligible for financial assistance from the Carnegie Trust for the Universities of Scotland. Only those *au fait* with Scotland's educational past can appreciate the pride known to so many Scots in voluntarily and spontaneously repaying assistance received from that Trust. Another point made in the Memorandum was that abolition of the medical schools would necessarily result in a reduction of students of medicine coming from overseas.

Otherwise the Memorandum dealt with specific criticisms of the extra-mural schools made by the Interdepartmental Committee. To detail argument and counterargument at this stage would serve no useful purpose. Suffice to record that certain of the criticisms were pin-pointed as being what was euphemistically called erroneous, and others were summarily refuted as being based on misrepresentation and misinterpretation. Precise figures were given which convincingly discounted the Committee's contention that university students 'who have repeatedly been unsuccessful at the university final examination often pass the final Triple Examination at their first attempt'.

Legitimately the Memorandum expressed the pride known to the extra-mural schools in having preserved an independent status: they had never received any government grant, but on the other hand had benefited from recent substantial benefactions from Licentiates—benefactions which would be available for the structural improvement and reconstruction of accommodation criticized by the Committee.

Government appointed Committees or Commissions are in an advantageous position to pontificate. The hazard is that those implementing recommendations may assume omniscience. Unprejudiced evaluation of considerations which are neither economic nor material is no easy task. The Corporations in their Memorandum adhered strictly to facts, and realistically concluded by urging, albeit in vain, that 'the extra-mural schools should participate in Government grants provided for medical education'. Recommendations concerning Staffing and Staff Training received attention in the 1947 Report of the Medical Advisory Committee (Scotland).[42]

More than a quarter century has passed since the School of Medicine was wound up, and it is now possible to review events less emotionally but without loss of admiration for those who contributed to the renown of its peak period. The School succumbed to the combined pressures of technical advances and economic necessity. An admirable summary of the course of events has been given by Sir Derrick Dunlop.[43] Referring to the period in the nineteenth century when the College was an important undergraduate teaching school competing with the University and possessing a research laboratory, he described how 'the systematic teaching of medicine demanded no more than a lecture room, some wall diagrams and bottled specimens, a skeleton and a teaching personality'. The situation changed, however, with the increasing complexity of medicine necessitating 'well staffed and equipped teaching departments' with ready-to-hand research laboratories of a calibre and scale which only a state-aided University could provide. It may even be said that the School of Medicine ran the risk of having its deservedly great reputation tarnished by continuing to function in an increasingly technical age.

Is the present-day scarcity of truly great human personalities in medicine the result of the precipitate application of science? Or is it but a figment of contemporary imagination? The answer may be in part that, as Bertrand Russell maintained, 'The cult of the hero is anarchic and retrograde, and does not easily fit in with the needs of a scientific society'.[44]

REFERENCES

(1) CRESWELL, C. H. (1926) *The Royal College of Surgeons of Edinburgh; Historical notes from 1505 to 1905*, p. 298. Edinburgh: Oliver & Boyd.

(2) Ibid., p. 34.

(3) GAIRDNER, J. (1860) *Historical Sketch of the Royal College of Surgeons of Edinburgh*, p. 15. Edinburgh: Sutherland & Knox.

(4) DUNCAN, A. (1896) *Memorials of the Faculty of Physicians and Surgeons of Glasgow, 1599–1850*, p. 66. Glasgow: Maclehose.

(5) LINDEBOOM, G. A. (1968) *Herman Boerhaave: the man and his work*, p. 368. London: Methuen.

(6) GUTHRIE, D. (1965) *Extramural Medical Education in Edinburgh and the School of Medicine of the Royal Colleges*, p. 11. Edinburgh: E. & S. Livingstone.

(7) LINDEBOOM, G. A. Op. cit., p. 372.

(8) GUTHRIE, D. Op. cit., pp. 14–21.

(9) BANKS, W. M. (1892) Introductory address on the popular idea of the doctor two hundred years ago and now. Delivered at the Yorkshire College, Leeds. *Lancet*, **II**, 819.

(10) College Minutes, 5.v.1835.

(11) SCOTLAND. Dept. of Health (1944) *Report of the Inter-departmental Committee on Medical Schools* (Goodenough report), p. 56. London: H.M.S.O.

(12) GRANT, Sir A. (1884) *The Story of the University of Edinburgh*, vol. II, p. 69. London: Longmans, Green & Co.

(13) Ibid., p. 74.

(14) 21 and 22 Victoria, c. 83. (1858).

(15) 52 and 53 Victoria, c. 55. (1889).

(16) CRESWELL, C. H. Op. cit., pp. 298–301.

(17) CHRISTISON, Sir R. (1885) *The Life of Sir Robert Christison, Bart.*, vol. I, p. 68. Edinburgh: Blackwood.

(18) KEITH, Sir A. (1912) Anatomy in Scotland during the lifetime of Sir John Struthers (1823–1899). [First Struthers anatomical lecture: Royal College of Surgeons of Edinburgh, 17th November, 1911.] *Edinburgh Medical Journal*, **8**, 11–12.

(19) College Minutes, 2.ii.1847.

(20) Ibid., 4.v.1847.

(21) Ibid., 11.v.1847.

(22) Ibid., 14.v.1847.

(23) Ibid., 3.viii.1847.

(24) TURNER, A. L., ed. (1933) *History of the University of Edinburgh, 1833–1933*, p. 101. Edinburgh: Oliver & Boyd.

(25) College Minutes, 1.v.1883.

(26) Ibid., 7.viii.1883.

(27) GUTHRIE, D. Op. cit., p. 23.

(28) College Minutes, 7.v.1895.

(29) Ibid., 6.viii.1895.

(30) Ibid., 20.vi.1862.

(31) Ibid., 4.v.1875.

(32) Ibid., 2.ii.1886.

(33) TODD, M. (1918) *The Life of Sophia Jex-Blake*, p. 277. London: Macmillan.

(34) CRESWELL, C. H. Op. cit., p. 302.

(35) College Minutes, 7.viii.1888.

(36) TODD, M. Op. cit., pp. 497–502.

(37) TURNER, A. L., ed. Op. cit., p. 107.

(38) Ibid., p. 150.

(39) GUTHRIE, D. Op. cit., p. 43.

(40) SCOTLAND. Dept. of Health. Op. cit., pp. 54–60.

(41) Royal Scottish Medical Corporations (1945) *Memorandum . . . on the Report of the interdepartmental committee on medical schools.* [Edinburgh: Privately printed.]

(42) SCOTLAND. Medical Advisory Committee (1947) *Report of the Medical Advisory Committee (Scotland)*. Edinburgh: H.M.S.O.

(43) DUNLOP, Sir D. M. (1972) Personal communication.

(44) RUSSELL, Sir B. (1952) *Impact of Science on Society*, p. 75. London: Allen & Unwin.

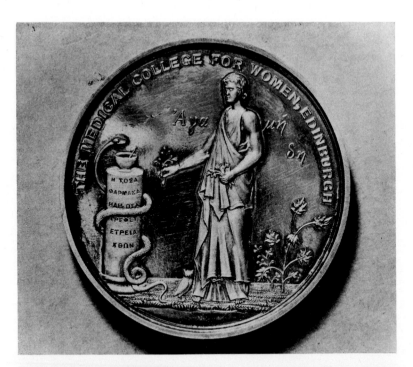

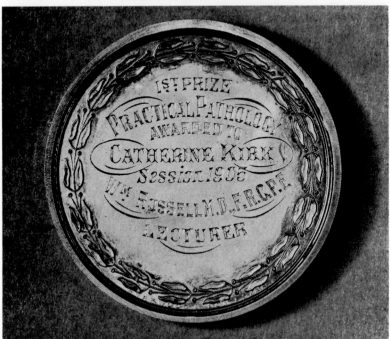

PLATE 22　Extra-mural School of Medicine for Women: Class Medal (1905)
Reproduced from the original in the College Library by Tom Scott

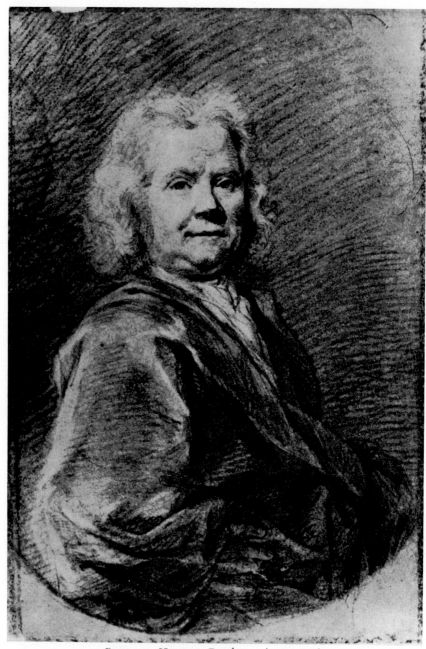

PLATE 23   Hermann Boerhaave (1668–1738)

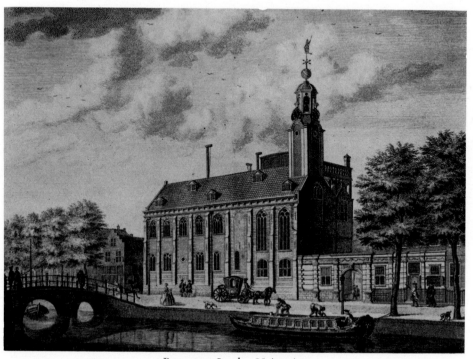

PLATE 24   Leyden University
Plates 23 and 24 reproduced by permission from Rijksmuseum voor de Geschiedenis
der Natuurwetenschappen, Leyden

Chapter XVII

EARLY HISTORICAL LINKS WITH SOME UNIVERSITIES

Thus the Greek spirit in Medicine, revived at the Renaissance in Bologna and Padua and borne across the Alps to Leiden and Edinburgh, spread overseas to enrich the medical schools of the New World.

A. Logan Turner

Mighty are the Universities of Scotland, and they will prevail . . . The greatest of them is the poor, proud homes you come out of, which said so long ago: 'There shall be education in this land'.

Sir J. M. Barrie (*Rectorial Address at St Andrews University*)

The College has never pursued its activities in isolation. It has known close associations with the University Medical Schools as well as the various Medical Corporations. Three Universities in particular hold honoured places in the history of the College— in chronological order they are the University of Leyden, the University of Edinburgh and the University of Pennsylvania. Edinburgh medical teaching exerted some influence also on the medical school in Montreal which was eventually incorporated in the Medical Faculty of McGill University. More recently Fellows of our College have been actively concerned in the foundation and development of the Medical Faculty in the University of Baghdad.

THE UNIVERSITY OF LEYDEN

Boerhaave lectured five hours a day: his hospital contained only twelve beds, but by Sydenham's method he made of it the medical centre of Europe.

Sir Andrew MacPhail

N

The Universities of Leyden and Edinburgh both had in common that they were products of the renaissance period—Leyden being founded in 1574 and Edinburgh (as the Town's College) in 1582. By the seventeenth century Leyden had acquired the reputation of being one of the leading centres of medical education, a reputation shared with Paris and Montpellier. Students from all countries went to Leyden, many but not all in search of training as doctors. The attraction to medical students was the association of Leyden University with such names as Franciscus de Le Boë [Sylvius] (1614–72), Boerhaave (1668–1738) and Gaubius (1705–80).

BOERHAAVE

To this day the name of Boerhaave is revered by his countrymen of which members of the Edinburgh College of Physicians are respectfully conscious on the occasions when they participate in periodic meetings arranged between the medical faculties of Leyden and Edinburgh Universities. He has been criticized on the score of his ineffective experimentation. Who among the great in medicine is not a victim of delayed retrospective criticism? None today can deprive Boerhaave of his prowess as a teacher and his skill as a chemist. Famous as a sound clinician he has been credited with being the first to establish the anatomical site of pleurisy and the spread by contagion of smallpox. His humbleness, kindness and dignity were in keeping with his professional eminence. By far his greatest contribution to medicine however was his realistic conception of instruction around the bedside where he emphasized *ad nauseam* the basic importance to practical medicine of anatomy, physiology, physics and chemistry, and where he demonstrated the supreme value of clinical observation and clinical interpretation. *Simplex veri sigillum* was his declared motto—and might well be that of the teacher of the medical student of today. An admirer of Sydenham, and follower of Boyle, Newton and Bacon,[1] his stimulus and example constantly revealed themselves in those of his pupils who were later to be associated with the College of Physicians and the University in Edinburgh. Monro *primus* was one of these pupils and according to Inglis many patients who came from Scotland to consult Boerhaave were put under Monro's care.[2]

After his death, the following reference to Boerhaave appeared in an English magazine:

'Dr. Boerhaave was a religious and modest Man, and so far from giving into the silly Affectation of Freethinking, which Pitcairn and some English Physicians valued themselves on, that he never made mention of the Supreme Being but to admire and exalt him in his Works . . .'.[3]

The Leyden tradition was admirably illustrated by the way in which John Ruther-ford, another pupil of Boerhaave, introduced his lectures at the Edinburgh Infirmary. 'I shall examine every patient appearing before you', he explained, 'that no circum-stances may escape you: I shall give you the history of the disease, enquire into the cause of it, give you my opinion as to how it will terminate, lay down the indications of cure which will arise or, if any new symptoms happen, acquaint you of them that you may see how I vary my prescriptions: If at any time you find me deceived in giving my judgment, you will be so good as to excuse me, for neither do I pretend to be, nor is the Art of Physic, infallible . . .'.[4]

To Rutherford credit is due for being the first in Scotland to teach students using the English language and not, as had been the previous custom, in the Latin tongue.[5]

There were many Scots among those who went to Leyden to study medicine, and no fewer than seven of those practitioners who tried unsuccessfully in 1656 to obtain a charter for a College of Physicians had been there. Four graduated M.D. Leyden—their names being David Balfour (1634), Henry Henrison (1653), George Hepburn (1648) and Thomas Glegg (1652). The three who attended without graduating were James Beaton (1627), John Sydserf (1644) and Alexander Yeaman (1649). Much the same position obtained among the 21 Fellows in the Original Patent at the time of the founding of the College: of them 11 had been at Leyden. The pilgrimage to Leyden continued for a number of years and in all, between 1680 and 1784, 85 Fellows including 16 Honorary Fellows had been to Leyden of whom 24 had been awarded the M.D. of the University there. Among Honorary Fellows were Pieter Camper (1722–89) whose original drawings for Smellie's obstetric text book are in the College Library: Hieronymous Davidius Gaubius (1705–80), successor to Boer-haave and author of *Praelectiones Chemicae* a copy of which is in the possession of the College Library: Albrecht von Haller (1708–77) the master physiologist and student of Boerhaave, born in Switzerland: the Scot, George Martine (1700–41) belatedly renowned for his study of clinical thermometry: Richard Mead (1673–1754) a fellow student of Boerhaave and successful London physician: and Gerard van Swieten (1700–72), the progressive re-organizer of the Vienna medical school—a copy of whose *Praelectiones Pharmaceuticae* is in the College Library.

Reference to one or two early ordinary Fellows who had been at Leyden is justified. John Boswell (1707–80), M.D. Leyden 1680, was the last British student promoted by Boerhaave; and David Campbell, M.D. Leyden 1771, was the last

Leyden graduate to become a Fellow of the College. Alexander Monro (Monro *primus*) (1697–1767), first of the Monro trio, presumed to have been sent to Leyden by his father, himself a Leyden alumnus, with the specific objective of establishing a similar medical school in Edinburgh: Alexander Monro (Monro *secundus*) (1733–1817), successor to Monro *primus*: and John Rutherford (1695–1779), Professor of Medicine in Edinburgh, promoter of clinical teaching at Edinburgh Royal Infirmary and grandfather of Sir Walter Scott—were among them. The case of Archibald Pitcairne requires special mention. He accepted an invitation to occupy the chair of medicine at Leyden University but within less than two years resigned of his own volition if pressure from 'in-laws' can be considered such. During Pitcairne's tenure of office, Boerhaave may have attended his inaugural lecture.[6]

Dutch references to Pitcairne's departure are characterized by typical national courtesy. Thus Lindeboom at the same time as describing Pitcairne as 'a skilful and learned man', told of how he returned during the vacation of 1693 to Scotland and 'having been a widower for several years he married again there'. That the Curators of Leyden University were taken aback can scarcely be wondered at, more especially as Pitcairne was slow to inform them of his intention not to return. In the circumstances the Curators showed great magnanimity when 12 years after his death and 32 years after his departure from Leyden they decided 'that the salary of 750 Dutch guilders which were still due to him, should be paid to Pitcairne's widow at her request'.[7]

SIBBALD AT LEYDEN

Another student to visit Leyden was Robert Sibbald. He described events in his *Autobiography*:

> 'I obtained the consent of my parents thereto, and went upon the twenty-thrid day of March 1660, from this in a dutch frigate to Holland. I stayed at Leyden ane yeer and a half, and studied anatomie and chirurgie, under the learned Professor Van Horne. I studied the plants under Adolphus Vorstius, who had been then Botanick professor 37 years, and I studied the institutions and practice, under Sylvius, who was famous then. I saw twentye-three human bodies dissected by him in the Hospitall which I frequented with him. I saw some dissected publickly by Van Horn. I was fellow student with Steno, who became famous afterwards for his wrytings. He dissected in my chamber sometymes, and showed me there, the ductus salivalis superior, he had discovered. I frequented ane apothecaryes shop, and saw the materia medica and the ordinary compositiones made. I studied Chimie, under a German . . .

'My father died about that tyme, and I considered I could not stay long abroad, so I applyed myself to my studie with great diligence. In September 1661, I went from Leyden for Paris . . .'.[8]

EXAMINATIONS

Sibbald's stay in Holland was relatively short and not graduating there, he does not describe the procedure required to obtain a medical degree at the University of Leyden. A description by Dr Charles Goodale is however quoted by Bower. It runs as follows:

'Whenever any student hath spent a competent time in that university, or any foreigner comes over to take his degree, he first makes his application to the dean of the faculty, who examines him one hour in the theoretick and practick part of physic; and if he finds him not well accomplished in either, he interdicts him making any further progress, in order to taking a degree, till he be better fitted for so great an undertaking; but if he gives a full and satisfactory account of his proficiency in both, he is sent to visit the rest of the professors of that faculty, who, appointing a convenient time, do all meet together and examine him two hours. And if he be then approved, they give him two aphorisms of Hippocrates to discourse of next day a quarter of an hour; and then they oppose that explication for three quarters of an hour. After this, he is to make and print certain theses upon what subject he pleaseth; which he sends to all the professors of the university, who meet him at an appointed hour, and are judges of his abilities in the defence of those theses against the four professors of physick, who, each man in his place, acts the part of an opponent till an hour be spent. Then is he admitted by the dean of the faculty, having obtained the approbation of the *rector magnificus*, and of the rest of the professors of the University, to the degree of doctor, and receiveth their diploma as a testimonial of his due performance of all the forementioned exercises. This, in short, is the manner in taking degrees privately; but if more publickly, the person that takes his degree is opposed by non-graduates in that faculty, in their publick schools; and the professors of physick, with the rest of the professors, sit by as judges.'[9]

Even in the absence of more detailed information there is a recognizable resemblance between the examinations at Leyden and those for Licentiates at the Edinburgh College. From the outset the examination for Licentiates consisted of three parts—the first on 'material questions', the second on aphorisms and the third and last in the presence of the assembled College on 'caices'. The Edinburgh practice differed from that at Leyden in terminating with a clinical examination and not a discussion of thesis: but resembled the Leyden procedure in that final decision concerning a candidate's proficiency rested not with an individual but with all present.

After some years the Edinburgh examination was modified in two ways. The examiners instead of being appointed before each examination were appointed for a year: and the first part of the examination, dealing with anatomy and physiology, was given the title of 'Institutions of Medicine'. Ritchie considered that both changes are to be ascribed to Pitcairne on his return from Leyden where professors were *ex officio* permanent examiners. His argument concerning the 'Institutions of Medicine' is more problematical and is based on the term having been used in Holland but not apparently in Leyden. This however does not in any way invalidate the accepted view concerning the conditioning of the examination procedure of the College by the previous experience of Fellows at Leyden. Were further supporting evidence required, it exists in the fact that of the Fellows involved in examining, nine were matriculated students of the University of Leyden.[10, 11]

Boerhaave and the early Medical School at Edinburgh was the subject of an Address delivered by Dr J. D. Comrie when, in 1939, he represented the University of Edinburgh at Leyden on the occasion of the bicentenary of Boerhaave's death.[12] In 1967 the College were proud to receive the gift of a reproduction of an old map of Leyden from visiting members of the Faculty of Medicine of Leyden University.[13]

The Leyden influence still continues—admittedly less potent, challenged as it is by the ruthless ascendancy of scientific medicine and in an age when history has lost some of its immediate appeal. Fortunately, although often belatedly, realization comes to most men of the overwhelming wisdom in Winston Churchill's words addressed to the Royal College of Physicians of London in 1944—'It is only from the past that one can judge the future'.

THE UNIVERSITY OF EDINBURGH

Any young man who can afford to wear a decent coat and live in a garret upon porridge or herrings may, if he pleases, come to Edinburgh and pass through his academical career just as creditably as is required or expected.

J. G. Lockhart (*Peter's Letters to his Kinsfolk*)

The Edinburgh 'Town's College' was opened in October 1583 and on 8th November of the same year the Town Council resolved 'that all the students . . . shall nightly lie and remain in their chambers within the same, and that they all shall have and wear gowns daily; and such as want gowns and will not lie therein to be put forth thereof'.

The intention apparently was to develop a residential institution in a true Collegiate spirit as appropriate today as in 1583. But as Grant, that master of isolated whimsical expression said, the Town Council 'were set to make bricks without straw. They had not the means of providing adequate lodging . . .'.[14]

A NEBULOUS FACULTY

More than a hundred years passed before the first steps were taken to promote a Medical School within the jurisdiction of the University. With a rare and refreshing generosity Grant declared that 'the origin of this new order of things was quite external to the [Town] College and its patrons: it rested with a small galaxy of accomplished, energetic, and some of them rather eccentric physicians, who having been bred in foreign schools, were now congregated in Edinburgh'. In marked contrast to Bower's version (q.v.), he named Sibbald as 'chief and leader among them' and Pitcairne, Balfour, Burnet and Archibald Stevensone as associates.[15]

The move to stimulate a new outlook towards medicine in Edinburgh derived impetus from the establishment of the Royal College of Physicians in 1681, and within less than four years three Fellows of the College were appointed by the Town Council to be Professors of Medicine in 'the University of this Cittee' as it was called for the first time.[16] Those appointed were Sir Robert Sibbald and Doctors James Halket and Archibald Pitcairne, but no directions were given as to their respective duties and it was left to them to arrange any division of labour among themselves. The professors received no salary. They delivered no lectures: whether *ad* or *propter hoc* is an open question. Grant described the situation succinctly.

> 'They [the Town Council] were, in fact, establishing a Faculty of Medicine in the College, but they were as unconscious of what they were doing as Columbus was when he discovered the islands off the coast of North America.'[17]

A FACULTY EVOLVES

Fellows of the College of Physicians were, indirectly, largely responsible for eventual recognition by the Town Council of the need for a Medical Faculty in the University and all that was entailed. The sequence of events was as follows. In 1724 Drs John Rutherford, Andrew Sinclair, Andrew Plummer and John Inness asked leave of the Town Council to keep and use the garden of the Town College with a view to cultivating pharmaceutical plants. The request was granted and in 1726 the selfsame four Fellows recommended to the Town Council that the Profession of Medicine should be instituted in the Town College and 'craved' that they, the four Fellows, should be appointed to teach and profess the subject. Never venture never win appeared to be their motto, and certainly on this occasion proved to be correct. Drs Sinclair and Rutherford were appointed Professors of the Theory and Practice of Medicine; and Drs Plummer and Innes Professors of Medicine and Chemistry. Authority derived from an Act of 1726 was given the four professors 'to profess and teach Medicine in all its branches, to examine candidates, and to do every other thing requisite and necessary to the graduation of doctors of medicine'. This Act of 1726, by creating four Professors of Medicine additional to an already existing Chair in Anatomy established the Medical Faculty of the University. Recognition of the medical professors by, and admission to the Senatus Academicus followed.[18]

From this time systematic courses of instruction were provided but have been described as lacking originality 'as they were entirely a reproduction of the system of Boerhaave'. To some extent there was support for this view in an 'advertisement' in the *Scots Magazine* in 1741. It ran:

'Professors of Medicine

Dr. Charles Alstone, Professor of Botany and Materia Medica. He gives lectures on the Materia Medica and Methodus praescribendi; and, in summer he teaches Botany in the town's physic-garden.

Dr. Andrew Plummer, Professor of Chemistry. He gives a course of Chemistry, Theoretical and Experimental.

Mr. Alexander Monro, F.R.S., Professor of Anatomy. He gives a course of Anatomy, Human and Comparative, Chirurgical Operations and Bandages.

Dr. Andrew St. Clair, Professor of the Theory of Physick. He teaches the Theory or Institutions of Physick, by explaining the *Institutiones Medicae* composed by Dr. Herman Boerhaave.

Dr. John Rutherford, Professor of the Practice of Physick. He uses as a text Dr. Boerhaave's *Aphorismi de cognoscendis* and *Curandis morbis*.[19, 20]

These five professors had matriculated in their day at Leyden University as also had Professor William Porterfield, John Innes and Alexander Monro *primus* although only Plummer graduated at Leyden.

Dr John Rutherford was Sir Walter Scott's maternal grandfather, a fact referred to in the latter's autobiographical notes.

'In April 1758', Scott wrote, 'my father married Anne Rutherford, eldest daughter of Dr. John Rutherford, professor of medicine in the University of Edinburgh. He was one of those pupils of Boerhaave to whom the school of medicine in our northern metropolis owes its rise and a man distinguished for professional talent, for lively wit, and for literary acquirements. Dr. Rutherford was twice married . . . My grandfather's second wife was Miss Mackay by whom he had a second family of whom are now (1808) alive, Dr. Daniel Rutherford professor of botany in the University of Edinburgh.'[21] Scott said also 'I was an uncommonly healthy child, but had nearly died in consequence of my first nurse being ill of a consumption, a circumstance which she chose to conceal . . . she went privately to consult Dr. Black, the celebrated professor of chemistry who put my father on his guard.' When about 18 months old Scott developed fever for three days. On the fourth they discovered he 'had lost the power of my right leg. My grandfather . . . , the late worthy Alexander Wood, and many others of the most respectable of the faculty were consulted . . . when the efforts of regular physicians had been exhausted without the slightest success . . . the advice of my grandfather Dr. Rutherford, that I should be sent to reside in the country . . . was first resorted to . . .'.[22]

SURGICAL AND CIVIC SUPPORT

While the College of Physicians played a major part in promoting a Medical School in the University, full recognition must be accorded the Edinburgh College of Surgeons, awarded a Royal Charter in 1778. In 1705 the Surgeons appointed a Keeper of their College Museum, whose successors ultimately came to be officially referred to as 'Professors of Anatomy in the City and College', who undertook teaching in the new anatomical theatre recently built by the Surgeons. Other surgeons and physicians commenced teaching in the City but outside the Town College and so further added to the pressure for better organised facilities for instruction in medicine.

But no individual effort among the Surgeons could compare with that of their President in 1712–13: Dr John Monro, father of the renowned Alexander Monro *primus*. John Monro, a pupil of Boerhaave, and Army Surgeon of distinction, communicated to the Physicians and Surgeons 'a plan which he had long formed in his own mind, of having the different branches of Physic and Surgery regularly taught at Edinburgh, which was highly approved by them'.[23] There is no reliable evidence that John Monro was a Member of the College of Physicians.[24] His son (Alexander) sent by his father to Leyden 'became a favourite and admiring pupil of the great Boerhaave'[25]: was elected a Fellow of both Edinburgh Colleges: and after a probationary period, was made professor of anatomy in Edinburgh *ad vitam aut culpam*—being the first medical professor to be appointed for life. His chair of anatomy was transferred physically from the College of Surgeons to the University as a safety measure at the time of civil disturbances given rise to by body-snatching in Greyfriars

Churchyard. The transfer was permanent and the chair of this 'city and college' became the Chair of Anatomy in the University. The indefatigable personal efforts of Alexander Monro *primus* earned for him recognition by many as the founder of the Medical School. In all his activities he was fortunate to have the interested advice and close friendship of Edinburgh's eminent civic dignitary George Drummond.

PROFESSORIAL ACROBATICS

The College of Physicians was, on occasion but not always, involved in academic appointments. In November 1723, on being advised that Dr Porterfield among their number intended to 'give Colledges upon the Instituts and practise of Medicine Provyded That he get suteable Incouragement', the College rose to the occasion with a handsome tribute. Incorporated in the tribute was an outlook of surprising breadth and wishful foresight. It was indicated that serious consideration had been given to, 'the great Losse our youth sustain from their not having Medicine in all its parts taught in this place, and the great advantage that would Redound to such of the Inhabitants of the Good Toun of Edenburgh as have Sons who are to follow medicine by having them Compleatly Instructed in that Science at home . . . as also that in the event good numbers of Students not only from all parts of our oun Country, But Lykewise from England and Ireland might be Induced to come here for their Improvement in Medicine and Spend that money amongst us which otherwayes they are oblidged to carie abroad to forraigne universities.'[26] Dr Porterfield was successful in his application, and was appointed Professor by the Town Council subject to agreeing to lecture regularly. There is no evidence that he did ever lecture and in this he conformed to the pattern set by Sibbald, Halket and Pitcairne towards the end of the previous century. Within 18 months two successors to Porterfield were appointed, without there being any known record of why the vacancy occurred. Neither Bower nor Grant was able to afford a convincing explanation.[27, 28]

An equally complex but different series of events had occurred previously in April 1713. Dr Crawford, a graduate of Leyden and the Secretary of the College, asked to be relieved of his duties as he was going abroad for what might be a considerable time. His request was granted[29] but he continued to attend meetings until November when he was the subject of a letter received by the President from the Principal of the Town's College of Edinburgh. The letter asked about Dr Crawford's suitability for a chair in Medicine which the University were contemplating. By way of reply 'a very ample Character' was provided and at the same time thanks were given 'to the Princl. and Masters of the said university for their Civility to the Colledge'.[30] Commenting pithily on the sequel, Ritchie wrote 'And of course by this time Dr. Crawford was at home again, and at the following Election . . . resumed his position of Secretarius and Bibliothecarius'.[31]

EXAMINATION EXPERTISE

Crawford's name comes up again in connection with University examinations for the Degree of Doctor of Medicine, but other events in this context require first mention. In April 1705 the College considered a petition from a Mr David Cockburne 'to take tryall of his qualificationes and progres in the study of medicine which way and manner as they [the College of Physicians] shall think fitt, and to Reporte their opinion to the principall and masters of the University of Edgr That he may have the degrie of Doctor of Medicine conferred upon him'.[32] The petition was acceded to and Mr Cockburne submitted to an examination in three parts conducted over a period of three weeks. Examinations covered the 'Institutiones', the 'aphorisms of Hippocrates' and two clincial cases: and were conducted by six physicians in the presence of the assembled Fellows. Cockburne satisfied the College, and a recommendation was submitted to the University in favour of a degree being conferred on him. The University acted accordingly and the College, very much alive to the situation, reminded Cockburne of his need to petition for admission as Licentiate 'after he has got his degrie befor he practise'.[33] Cockburne was the first candidate for the Degree of Doctor of Medicine in the University of Edinburgh.

Five years later the College participated in dealing with another application. The approach was made by that great university Principal, William Carstairs, and related to a Mr Jonathan Harley. By way of explanation the Principal wrote '. . . we are not haveing at present a ffacultie of that usefull science [medicine] Doe Desyre the favor of your honorable societie to take such a method as they shall think fitt for knowing how he is qualified for haveing the Degrie that is Desyred, which upon yor Recommendatione we are all heartilie willing to bestow upon him'.[34] Examiners were appointed but with what result is not recorded.

After rather more than two years Principal Carstairs wrote again, this time concerning a Revd. Mr Threlkeld and concluded with 'we Relye so much on your kyndnes as not to Doubt of yor Granting our Desyre . . .'.[35] As in the case of the two previous candidates, the examination was carried out in the College Hall and the form of examination remained unaltered. Mr Threlkeld was awarded his Doctorate on the recommendation of College.

A few years later and without forewarning there were whisperings of a wind of change—a semblance of aspiring academic protocol. Principal Carstairs had been followed by William Wishart who in November 1718 wrote the College 'the ffacultie here haveing appoynted ane Professor Doctor Crawfurd To Examine a Young Gentleman in order to his receiving the Degree of Doctor of Medicine, and there being no other Physitian in the university at present, it is humbly Desyred by the ffaculty That yor Royall Society may be pleased to appoynt one or more of their number to joyn with Doctor Crawfurd in the said Examinatne in the Library of this university. The tyme for it may be either to-morrow, or ffryday, or any other tyme that may be Judged most Convenient, only you will be pleased to acquaint me that I may advertise Dr. Crawfurd.'[36] This constituted an unmistakable departure from the procedure adopted in the examination of at least three previous candidates for the Degree. Ironically the Professor who was so meticulous in his requirements of co-examiners was the same 'physician' who had failed to appear at Dr Kello's examination for licence to practise (Chap. VII) and who was, to say the least, somewhat cavalier in his regard for the dignity customarily associated with the office of Secretary to the College. It may be that Crawford was a victim of his own erudition—because not only was he Professor of Medicine and Chemistry, but in 1719 took on the additional not inconsiderable duties of Professor of Hebrew.

There was another unusual feature—the candidate on this occasion was the son of a Fellow and Past President of the College. Whatever the intended significance in the change of meeting place from the College to the University, it was of no real importance except in so far as it appears to have involved dispensing with clinical cases as part of the examination. Of unquestionably greater significance was the examination of the candidate by three physicians in the seclusion of the University Library instead of by six physicians, two at each of three sessions, before the Fellows assembled in their College Hall. With the changes there was an accompanying transfer of emphasis from practical to theoretical considerations, which contrasted with the form of examination to which Candidates for its Licentiateship were submitted by the College.

By March 1719 the wind of change had become more evident. A new form of approach was adopted by the University. A College Minute recorded that 'the President [Dr Wm. Cochrane] reported to the Colledge, That Dr. Crawfurd, Professor of Medicine in the university of Edinburgh, and soume of the Professors yrof, had acquainted and signified to him That there was a young Gentleman named

[Robert] Stoddart . . . That had applyed to the Princill and other members of the said university to have the Degree of Doctor of Medicine Conferred upon him, and that the sd Doctor Crawfurd being present acknowledged the samen.' Dr Crawford then apparently asked 'in name of Prinll. and professors . . . that the President and Members of the Colledge of Physitians might appoynt one or more of their number, to joyne' with him 'in the Examinatne of Mr. [Robert] Stoddart . . . within the bibliotheck' of the University. There was no communication from the Principal, but an assurance was given that he 'wold wryte a Letter to the president yr.anent.' Whether in fact the letter did arrive is not known. Two Fellows were appointed to meet Dr Crawford. A further resolution was arrived at to the effect that 'in caice of the like occasione . . . the president by himself appoynt one or tuo physitians . . . without the necessity of Calling a meeting of the Colledge, he always giveing ane account of the name and Designates of such persones as so Desyre to be examined . . . with the Physitians names . . . appoynted to be Examinators . . . the samen may be recorded in the Colledge sederunt book, and this to Continue until next election day'.[37]

A RESPONSIBILITY DISCHARGED

The College continued to co-operate with the University in the award of medical degrees—or, to put it more correctly in the words of Grant, degrees continued to be awarded by the University 'on the recommendation of the College of Physicians'. The arrangement ceased to operate in 1726, twenty-one years after the first degree had been awarded. In all, twenty-one degrees were conferred on the recommendation of the College during that time, two being admissions *ad eundem* granted to Doctors of other Universities. Intimation of termination of the arrangement was conveyed to the College on 1st November 1726.[38]

On that day the President 'Represented that Mr. Stewart and Mr. Drummond Regents* in the university of Edr. were Commissionat by a General meeting of the said university To give thanks to the Colledge of Phisitians for sending some of their members To joyne with ye professor for trying and Examining those who were to Receive the Degrees of Dr. of medicine from their university And that now there was a sufficient number of Professors of medicine To make a faculty of medicine And

* The equivalent of Professors.

that they would not trouble the Colledge any more upon that head But were thankfull for what favours they had Received and Desired to Live in good Correspondence with the College'. Concluding, the relevant Minute stated 'This Commission was Delivered by the @ named Gentlemen to the President [Dr John Drummond] And Desired to be reported to the Colledge at the first meeting which accordingly was done as above'.[39]

Criticism has been voiced in after years at the apparent peremptory method of intimation and insufficiency of appreciation of the College's assistance. This scarcely seems justified. A perennial handicap of administrators in all spheres is their discomfiture when called upon as beneficiaries to express gratitude. Legal phraseology, more especially when employed by a para-judiciary body, is often incapable of giving expression to even constrained emotion. Hence possibly the ponderous embarrassment evident in the intimation. Nor would it be charitable to grudge the University a sense of pride at having at long last after many extraordinary vagaries established a stable and functioning Faculty of Medicine. If Dr Crawford and his colleagues were very conscious of newly acquired trappings of power, they were but human in a way only too prevalent to this day. At least it was not puppet power of which they were conscious, as borne out by the outstanding achievements and stature of the Edinburgh School of Medicine in subsequent decades.

Far from feeling discarded at the action of the University, the College had good reason to be gratified. Nobody could deny that the College had been largely instrumental in fostering the University Faculty which was now declaring self-sufficiency and independence. The University historians, Bower and Grant, were alike in the credit they gave to the College, but unalike in their evaluation of the relative contributions made by individual members of the College. What cannot be gainsaid is that the filling of academic chairs by Fellows of the College resulted in the best of Leyden traditions being inherited by the University Medical School in its earliest days. This was evident both in the matter and manner of teaching but also in the form and conduct of examinations.

In the particular sphere of examinations the College exerted a very special influence. It can fairly be claimed in no spirit of prudery, that the attitude, practice and principles of Fellows of the College in their associations with the University served to save the University from the pitfall of trafficking in medical degrees in the way adopted by certain competitive academic bodies in Scotland. The College was entitled to be gratified, conscious that its influence had been in the interests of the academic body which in the previous century had unsuccessfully opposed the creation of the College but successfully precluded it from teaching activities.

THE UNIVERSITY OF PENNSYLVANIA AND THE COLLEGE
OF PHYSICIANS OF PHILADELPHIA

Genealogically we might speak of our College and of the University as children of Edinburgh and grandchildren of Leyden.

S. Weir Mitchell

The above quotation referred to the College of Physicians of Philadelphia and the University of Pennsylvania and were words spoken by Dr Weir Mitchell in the course of an address at the Centennial Celebration of the founding of the former.

Similar sentiments were expressed in 1939 by Dr Henry Sigerist on the occasion of the second centenary of the death of Boerhaave. 'If the faculty of Edinburgh could be called a daughter of Leiden', he wrote, 'then the faculty of Philadelphia can with equal right be called a daughter of Edinburgh, and therefore, a grand-daughter of Leiden. No wonder that the spirit of the new clinical medicine was fully alive and that Boerhaave's influence was strongly felt.'[40]

PHILADELPHIAN BACKGROUND

It was in Philadelphia that the first hospital was founded (1751), the first public medical library was started (1763) and the first medical school established (1765), in what the historian refers to as the British Colonies. The hospital was the Pennsylvania and the medical school the College of Philadelphia. According to MacDermot, clinical teaching after the Edinburgh pattern was a feature of instruction given at the College from the outset, but was interrupted by the War of Independence. Resumption of the tradition took place when Osler went to Philadelphia in 1884.[41]

In 1779 the Charter and privileges of the College of Philadelphia were transferred arbitrarily by law to a new institution with the title of the University of the State of Pennsylvania. Ten years later (1789) the College of Philadelphia had its Charter and rights restored but in 1791 it was united with the University of the State of Pennsylvania to form the University of Pennsylvania.

The College of Physicians of Philadelphia was founded in 1787.[42] To quote Weir Mitchell once again, 'Who first suggested the formation of this College is unknown, but, as many of our Fellows were educated in Edinburgh, it is likely enough that the success of its Society . . . may have led them to imitate it here'. Referring to the founders of the Philadelphia College of Physicians he said, 'As to their medical education, the best of them had been educated in Edinburgh'.[43]

YOUNG AMERICANS ABROAD

According to Packard there have been in the history of American medicine well-defined periods in the migration of young medical men going abroad to study. He stated categorically that 'during the Colonial period and down to 1800 the majority went to London and Edinburgh, partly for the obvious reason that they regarded Great Britain as their mother country, but . . . more especially because at that time London and Edinburgh were at the zenith of their fame'.[44] He expressed the view that at this time 'although there were many excellent physicians in London . . . the opportunities for the study of "physic" . . . did not compare with those to be got in Edinburgh'[45]; and stated that 'the Edinburgh degree of M.D. was held in much higher esteem than that obtainable anywhere else in the United Kingdom, ranking with that of Leyden'.[46]

RECEPTION IN THE UNITED KINGDOM

Young American doctors coming to the United Kingdom were fortunate in being able to make ready contact with those in a position to give them valuable help. First and foremost among these was their fellow countryman Benjamin Franklin, who at different times made three protracted stays in London where he became friendly with John Fothergill, and Fothergill's close friend and fellow Quaker John Lettsom. Fothergill was a graduate of Edinburgh University and Fellow of the Edinburgh College: Lettsom took out some of his studies in Edinburgh but obtained his M.D. at Leyden. Franklin knew also Sir John Pringle, the founder of modern military medicine, a one-time student at Edinburgh, an M.D. of Leyden and Fellow of the Edinburgh Royal College. Advising a friend on the medical education of his son, Franklin seems to have evinced surprise at the popularity of the teaching available in Edinburgh. Having referred to the excellence of facilities in London he wrote in a letter 'and yet the general run is at present to Edinburgh; there being at the Opening of the Schools, when I was there . . . a much greater number of medical Students than had ever been known before. They have indeed a Set of Able Professors in the several Branches, if common Opinion may be rely'd on. I who am no Judge in that Science, can only say that I found them very sensible Men, and agreeable Companions.'[47] At a later date, when in Scotland, Franklin made the acquaintanceship of Sir Alexander Dick—another Fellow of the Edinburgh College.

Of Sir John Pringle in London, Franklin wrote that 'he admits young Physicians and Surgeons to a Conversation at his House, which is thought very improving to them'. He expressed his evaluation of Pringle's advice most delectably if realistically— 'There is more valuable knowledge in Physic to be learnt from the honest candid Observations of an old Practitioner, who is past all desire of more Business, having made his Fortune, who has none of the Professional Interest in keeping up a Parade of Science to draw Pupils, and who by Experience has discovered the inefficacy of most Remedies and Modes of Practice, than from all the formal Lectures of all the Universities upon Earth.'[47] Solace indeed for those relegated to cobwebbed shelves! No matter that, according to a critical cleric—Alexander Jupiter Carlyle, 'Dr. Pringle, afterwards Sir John, was an agreeable lecturer, though no great master of the science he taught." !'[48]

FOTHERGILL'S STATURE

Fothergill, a Fellow of the Edinburgh College and Licentiate of the London College, was something of a rebel in the latter where he probably forfeited his chances of elevation to the Fellowship by being too ardent, although decorously so in pressing the claims of Licentiates. This did not prevent him developing a rewarding practice rivalling that of the renowned Mead, an Honorary Fellow of the Edinburgh College. Doubtless it was with tongue in cheek that Benjamin Franklin writing to Fothergill in 1764 asked—'Does your conscience never hint to you the impiety of being in constant warfare against the plans of Providence?'[49] None would appreciate the sally better than Fothergill!

A Quaker and son of a Quaker preacher who had visited the American colonies, he was always interested in America and it was natural that he should be especially drawn to Pennsylvania where William Penn founded a Quaker colony in 1682. Fothergill's interest took many forms. Indirectly he was instrumental in Franklin being awarded the Copley Medal by the Royal Society. By sending the hospital managers of the Pennsylvania a book entitled *An Experimental History of the Materia Medica* by William Lewis, F.R.S. 'for the benefit of the Young Students in Physic who may attend under the Direction of the Physicians', he unwittingly stimulated the medical staff to establish a hospital medical library at their own expense. Another gift Fothergill made to the hospital was a collection of anatomical drawings by van Rymsdyk who was responsible for most of the illustrations in William Hunter's *The Gravid Uterus*.[50]

Of special historical interest was an approach to Fothergill by Thomas Penn as to the desirability of the Medical Society in Philadelphia applying for a charter of incorporation as a college of physicians. Writing on 4th February 1768 Fothergill replied:

> 'I think however their application . . . is rather too early. I know not that it would be usefull to the promotion of medicine. The skillfull Physicians will always be found out. And the unskillfull deserted, however he may be invested with external dignitys . . . Unanimity is necessary for such an institution. There is a College of Physicians at Edinburgh, at Paris, in London and other places. Experience does not clearly prove they have been of much utility. The pretence of founding these Societys was to countenance and support the regular Physician: to suppress Quackery: but the effect has generally ended in a sort of monopoly. A few have got into the management of these Societys, who have gradually found means in order to raise themselves, and lay others, not less knowing, able or honest, under great difficultys. All the advantages of a medical Society may be obtained without a Charter.'[51]

Fothergill had no axe to grind. Sheer professional skill had won for him rich reward and envied status. Rebuttal by the London College had left his dignity unimpaired and bred no resentment. He was well equipped to pronounce impartial judgment. The words quoted contain more than a grain of common sense. They serve as warning to our College, spared as it has been from abuse by over ambitious aspiring egotists within its ranks, of the dangers of direct involvement in mighty mergers at present in favour. Other warnings are to be found in government, local and central; in industry and in the Universities.

In the words of Adam Smith 'monopolists very seldom make good work'[52]: and of Bertrand Russell 'The tyranny of officials is one of the worst results of increasing organization . . . .'.[53]

MIGRATION TO EDINBURGH

Absence of complete records makes it impossible accurately to estimate the number of young Americans who studied in Edinburgh. This applies to records on both sides of the Atlantic. There is the further complication that while the names of a goodly number are known, there is no information to indicate which of them studied at University classes, extra-mural classes or at classes of both kinds. The facts are only clear in the case of those who acquired a Doctorate of Medicine at the hands of the University. A number of the students came to Edinburgh for part of their training; some had first studied anatomy and surgery in London under the Hunters and Cheselden, and others who had studied for a time in Edinburgh before proceeding to Leyden or some other continental University or before returning home for economic reasons.

According to the American Wilson of Chicago, Edinburgh had on its roll of M.D.s prior to 1765 fifteen names of men from almost all the American Colonies.[46] Thomas Jarvis who graduated M.D. at Edinburgh University in 1744 was the first American colonial to do so, coming from Antigua. In the succeeding twenty years there was almost invariably at least one American graduate each session: and in the hundred years beginning in 1764, 650 students from the Americas graduated at Edinburgh. Comrie estimated that the total number of Americans studying in Edinburgh during that period was probably twice as great if allowance is made for those who took out a limited number of classes.[54]

THE FIRST AMERICAN LICENTIATES

Mention has already been made of the first two American Licentiates of the Edinburgh College of Physicians—John Morgan and Benjamin Rush. These two men together with William Shippen, another Licentiate, were among those who came to Edinburgh in the 1760s. All three graduated M.D. at the University and later played major parts in the development of the College of Philadelphia. While in London Benjamin Franklin sent Morgan to Fothergill on whose advice he undertook 'practical work' in London before proceeding to Edinburgh. In London he was a pupil of William Hunter, and in Edinburgh of William Cullen to whom he had been introduced by Franklin, and whose kindness to students left a lasting impression on him. When in Edinburgh Morgan was entertained by a former President of the College, Sir Alexander Dick at Prestonfield House, was a frequent guest of Lord Provost Drummond, and met James Boswell. At a later date (1763) Sir Alexander Dick received a letter from Morgan describing how he had met Sénac, the physician to the French King at Fontainebleau and how Sénac 'was very inquisitive about the College of Physicians' at Edinburgh.[55]

Future events were to reveal that other activities of Morgan in Edinburgh were to have long-lasting results of even greater significance. While still a student there, he took part in a money-raising campaign on behalf of the College of Philadelphia. At the same time he joined forces with other American students in an effort to promote the dignity of the profession by adopting Edinburgh standards and refusing to practise surgery or sell drugs. This evangelical decision reflected the prevailing policy of the Edinburgh College. The students then organized a club, admission to which required applicants to sign a pledge 'not to degrade it [their profession] by . . . mingling the trade of apothecary or surgeon'.[56] Morgan for one was certainly as good as his word. On his return to Philadelphia he launched out on his career as a physician by announcing that he would neither dispense medicines nor practise surgery; but, that he had brought over from Britain a man who was qualified to practise surgery and pharmacy and whose services were available to such of Morgan's patients as might desire them.[57]

Meanwhile, Morgan had been preparing details for a plan to develop a medical school in connection with the College of Philadelphia. In this he collaborated closely with Shippen and received a great deal of valuable advice from Dr William Cullen with whom he had come to share a friendly relationship. Eventually his plan took shape in the form of a 'Discourse' intended in the first place for the trustees of the Philadelphia College. Both Fothergill and William Hunter helped him in the preparation with criticisms and suggestions. The 'Discourse' was eventually accepted by the Board, won universal approval and in the words of Packard 'it shows how thoroughly Morgan was imbued with the Edinburgh tradition'.[58] Morgan and Shippen were the principal founders of the College of Philadelphia: Morgan held the first Chair in the Practice of Medicine and Shippen the first Chair in Surgery and Midwifery. There can be no doubt about the extent to which Morgan's views reflected the influence of his Edinburgh experiences. In another 'Discourse' upon the Institution of Medical Schools in America he said 'we must regret that the very different employment of a Physician, Surgeon, and Apothecary, should be promiscuously followed by any one man, however great his abilities. They certainly require very different talents.'[59] It has been said of Morgan by a fellow countryman that he 'persuaded the College of Philadelphia to set up a medical faculty . . . and so introduced the Continental–Scottish tradition of a university-college'.[60]

When Shippen went to the Pennsylvania Hospital he took with him drawings and casts, the gift of Fothergill.[61, 62] With the gift Fothergill sent a note to the Board of Managers to the effect that, 'In the want of real subjects these will have their Use and I have recommended it to Dr. Shippen to give a Course of Anatomical Lectures to such as may attend. He is very well qualified for the subject and will soon be followed by an able assistant, Dr. Morgan, both of whom I apprehend will not only be useful to the Province in their Employment, but if suitably countenanced by the Legislature will be able to erect a School of Physic amongst you.' Sixteen years elapsed before Shippen was elected to the hospital staff, but during them and after, he used Fothergill's illustrations for courses of private lectures. These lectures have been described as 'directly in line with the Edinburgh policy of extra-mural schools . . . conducted outside of the University curriculum'.[63]

In later years Fothergill acted as agent in London for the purchase of books for the Pennsylvania Hospital Library, a duty subsequently undertaken by Lettsom.[62]

Morgan lacked neither ambition nor determination from his earliest days. Anxious to be made a member he submitted papers to the Royal Academy of Surgery but was awarded the lesser title of 'correspondent'. Shortly afterwards he applied for 'Membership' of the Royal College of Physicians of Edinburgh, and was made Licentiate without examination. According to his biographer, Morgan did not relish waiting indefinitely for election as a Fellow, and possibly a sense of injured vanity and urgency moved him to protest. When elected a Fellow in 1765, he became the first American to be enrolled. Shippen was the second being elected in 1768 one year after being made a Licentiate.[64]

Another who studied in Edinburgh, where he obtained his M.D. at the University, was Benjamin Rush. He was influenced by Cullen more than any other and wrote of him in his Scottish Journal, 'It is scarcely possible to do Justice to this great man's Character either as a scholar, a physician, or a Man.'[65] None the less according to Garrison he disapproved of Cullen's classification of diseases.[66] The pity is that no stimulatingly worthy biography has been written of Cullen. Playfair said of him 'Chemistry owes but little to Cullen as a discoverer, but much to him as a clear and philosophical expounder.'[67] Numbering 17 at first, Cullen's students rapidly increased to 145.[68] At the time of his death many 'heads of him . . . out of respect to his memory were instantly set up as signs for druggists' shops'.[69]

While in Edinburgh Rush was exposed to the same risks and indignities as the natives. Writing in 1784 to a friend in Philadelphia about his experiences he said 'The inhabitants, although they live together in their human hives are entire strangers to [one] another. There is a family living above me and another immediately below me, and yet I know no more of their names or persons than you do. This way of living subjects the inhabitants to many inconveniences, for, as they have no yards or cellars, they have of course no necessary houses and all their filth of every kind is thrown out of their windows. This is done in the night generally, and is carried away next morning by carts appointed for that purpose. Unhappy they who are obliged to walk out after ten or eleven o'clock at night. It is no uncommon thing to receive what Juvenal says he did, in his first satire, from a window in Rome. This is called here being *naturalized*. As yet I have happily escaped being made a freeman of the city in this way . . .'.[70] Doubtless his last remark was an allusion to his 'naturalisation' in more gratifying circumstances in 1767: it was on 4th March of that year that the City of Edinburgh had conferred on him and another its freedom as 'Burgesses and gild brothers . . . in most ample form'.[71]

AMERICAN DECLARATION OF INDEPENDENCE

On his return to America Rush became Professor of Chemistry in the College of Philadelphia and later Professor of the Institutes of Medicine and of Clinical Medicine in the University of Pennsylvania. He together with three American surgeons was allowed to cross the British lines and treat those of their own seriously injured who had not been removed from the battlefield of Brandywine.[72] Rush was a signatory of the American Declaration of Independence and it was his future father-in-law who presented John Witherspoon with minutes of his election as President of the College of New Jersey, Princeton.[73] Witherspoon (1723–94) was born in the East Lothian parish of Yester and there is today a plaque near the former manse, which was his birthplace, situated twenty miles from Edinburgh. A graduate of Edinburgh University he was a minister in Paisley when he received the invitation to go to America. From all accounts he was slow to come to a decision and Benjamin Rush was asked to bring pressure to bear. This he did by letter, but a visit to Paisley proved necessary before Rush successfully discharged his future father-in-law's instructions.[74] Witherspoon took up the post of President of Princeton College, later became the first Moderator of the Presbyterian Church of America and was the only cleric to sign the American Declaration of Independence in 1776.[75]

Among Americans who studied at Edinburgh there are three others who qualify for special mention. One was John Redman (1722–1806), the first President of the College of Physicians of Philadelphia, who graduated at Leyden, and who while President sent to our College several copies of a pamphlet published by the Philadelphia College on *The nature and origin of the pestilential fever*.[76] The other three were Adam Kuhn (1741–1817) who occupied several chairs in Philadelphia, having graduated M.D. at Edinburgh after studying under Linnaeus at Uppsala, and in London; and Philip Syng Physick (1768–1837) who graduated M.D. at Edinburgh having previously worked under John Hunter at St George's Hospital, London, whose principles he is credited with having implanted in America; and Caspar Wistar (1761–1818) who obtained his Edinburgh M.D. in 1768, assisted Shippen in anatomy, and was a renowned botanist after whom was named the wistaria vine.[77]

Physick pioneered gastric lavage in children who swallowed poison. After publishing his first case, he learned that Monro *secundus* had previously suggested the procedure without practising it. Greatly to his credit, in a second report Physick straightway gave Monro the recognition due him.[78] That contact between the Edinburgh and Philadelphia Colleges persisted, is evidenced by the receipt in 1818 by our College of a copy of Dr Wistar's *Eulogium on Dr Shippen* with an accompanying letter from the College of Physicians in Philadelphia.[79] It is of interest too that when a scheme was being drawn up for the Pennsylvania Hospital a study was made by those concerned of the plans of the 1738 Edinburgh Royal Infirmary building and its methods of management.[80] There is further reason for gratification in the fact that Benjamin Rush delivered a *Eulogium in Honor of the Late Dr. William Cullen* before the College of Physicians of Philadelphia on 9th July 1790; and that Rush's son named tracts of land which he owned in western Pennsylvania, after two British physicians— one on Loyalist Creek, he called, Fothergill; and the other on Sugar Creek, Lettsom.[81] Another interesting fact is that Cullen's name appears as a European member in the first volume of *Transactions of the American Philosophical Society held at Philadelphia*—published in 1771.[82]

Nor is it out of place to mention in passing that James Graham of Temple of Health notoriety included Philadelphia (and other American cities) as well as Edinburgh in his itinerary. Indeed it has been said that Graham's use of electricity in his Temple of Health, and it will be remembered on the young Walter Scott (Chap. I), can be traced back to meetings with Franklin, firstly in Philadelphia and later in Paris.[83, 84] Graham was described as a frequent if not habitual inhaler of ether, by Professor A. J. Clark[85]—a great-grandson of Sir Robert Christison.[86]

Such then was the influence of Edinburgh medicine, largely inherited from Leyden, upon the practice and teaching of medicine in their beginnings in Philadelphia. To attempt to differentiate how much of that influence was derived from the College and how much from the University would be unworthy of the subject. Robert Whytt, William Cullen, Monro *secundus* were among great names remembered by the American doctor on return to his home country: all men of stature with dual allegiance to the Edinburgh College of Physicians and their University. In addition, there was the influence of such men as Fothergill and Pringle with past ties with Edinburgh but pursuing their vocations elsewhere. According to Shryock, the King's

College Medical School established in New York in 1768 (later to become the Medical School of Columbia University) incorporated many of the features introduced by Morgan to Philadelphia.[87]

Within comparatively recent years the College of Physicians of Philadelphia honoured Sir Thomas Grainger Stewart and Sir Thomas Fraser by electing them Associate Fellows. At a still later date the same College awarded Dr Chalmers Watson its Alvarenga Prize for physiological studies under the supervision of Professor Sharpey Schafer.[88]

Although, inevitably, a history of the College reflects corporate pride, it must be seen in the context of the overall contribution of these islands to American medicine at the time under consideration—a contribution which owed much to such outstanding London men as Cheselden and the Hunters, and the Fellows of the Royal College of Physicians of London. This in no way detracts from the just claim of the Royal College of Physicians of Edinburgh to have played an important and especially significant part.

THE UNIVERSITY OF McGILL

Scottish influence extended to Canada and according to MacDermot 'the channel through which the Scottish tradition flowed most directly in Canada was medical teaching, and the school in which this was first exemplified was the Medical Faculty of McGill University'.[89] This Faculty was originally a private medical school established in 1823 by four medical men who composed the medical staff of the Montreal General Hospital founded four years previously. All four men (William Robertson, William Caldwell, John Stephenson and A. F. Holmes) had 'had training' at Edinburgh and two had obtained the degree of M.D. at the University there. From the time the Hospital opened they gave clinical teaching at the bedside and advocated the establishment of a School of Medicine.

In a Memorandum submitted to the Hospital Board these four pioneers described how they had been 'encouraged to attempt the formation of a medical seminary, when they reflect that the Medical School of Edinburgh, the basis of which they would adopt for the present institution, now justly considered the first in Europe, is of comparatively recent formation, it being little more than one hundred years since medical lectures were first delivered in that city. And the early history of the Royal Infirmary of Edinburgh is not dissimilar to that of the Montreal General Hospital.'[90]

Following lengthy negotiations the members of the original private medical school were 'engrafted on the college' as its medical faculty. The college was the University of McGill College which owed its existence to the beneficence of James McGill, a native of Glasgow who became a leading Montreal merchant.[89]

It is not suggested that the Edinburgh College of Physicians contributed in any direct way to what has been described as 'the first attempt at medical education in Canada'. What can be said however is that in their capacity as teachers such individual Fellows as Gregory, Home and Duncan were instrumental in setting the Edinburgh standards adopted by those of their students who later found their vocation in the University of McGill.[91]

A point of incidental interest is how, in many respects, the versatility of one of McGill University's outstanding nineteenth-century Principals resembled that of our own Sir Robert Sibbald two hundred years previously. The Principal in question was Sir William Dawson. Like Sibbald his interests provided the bases for contributions to the scientific literature and included chorography, geology, palaeontology, botany and fauna. In his younger days Dawson studied chemistry at the University of Edinburgh.[92]

THE UNIVERSITY OF BAGHDAD

During the period 1921–63 there were four British Professors of Medicine at the University of Baghdad. All four were Fellows of our College. They were: Sir Harry C. Sinderson, Pasha, K.B.E., C.M.G., M.V.O. (1921–46), Sir Robert M. Drew, K.C.B., C.B.E. (1946–51), Major General W. H. Hargreaves, C.B., O.B.E. (1951–9), and Major General R. M. Johnstone, M.B.E., M.C. (1959–63).

The success of the Medical School at Baghdad led to the establishment of Medical Colleges at Mosul and Basra which now train their own medical graduates.

THE UNIVERSITY OF TEHERAN

(Sir) Ian G. Hill was Visiting Professor of Medicine for one academic year (November 1970–July 1971) his remit being to develop a British style medical teaching unit in a newly commissioned hospital. The post involved the giving of lectures and bedside instruction in English, and being prepared to deal with questions posed in French or German.[93]

HAILÉ SELASSIÉ I UNIVERSITY, ADDIS ABABA, ETHIOPIA

Approached by the Inter-University Council for Higher Education Overseas, (Sir) Ian Hill followed his period in Teheran by taking up the duties of Dean of the Medical Faculty at the Hailé Selassié I University in November 1971. He continued in office for almost two years.[93]

THE INSTITUTE OF POST-GRADUATE MEDICINE, DACCA

See Chapter XXVII, p. 642.

REFERENCES

THE UNIVERSITY OF LEYDEN

(1) LINDEBOOM, G. A. (1968) *Herman Boerhaave; the man and his work*, p. 329. London: Methuen.

(2) INGLIS, J. A. (1911) *The Monros of Auchinbowie*, p. 58. Edinburgh: Constable.

(3) *The Gentleman's Magazine* (1738), **8**, 491.

(4) TURNER, A. L. (1937) *Story of a Great Hospital; the Royal Infirmary of Edinburgh, 1729–1929*, p. 133. Edinburgh: Oliver & Boyd.

(5) THIN, R. (1927) The old Infirmary and earlier hospitals. In *The Book of the Old Edinburgh Club*, vol. xv, p. 157. Edinburgh: Constable.

(6) [PENDRILL, G. R.] (c. 1963) *Leyden University and the Royal College of Physicians of Edinburgh*. (Typescript.)

(7) LINDEBOOM, G. A. Op. cit., pp. 31–2.

(8) SIBBALD, Sir R. (1833) *The Autobiography*, pp. 15–17. Edinburgh: Thomas Stevenson.

(9) BOWER, A. (1817) *The History of the University of Edinburgh*, vol. II, p. 217. Edinburgh: Oliphant, Waugh and Innes.

(10) RITCHIE, R. P. (1899) *The Early days of the Royall Colledge of Phisitians, Edinburgh*, p. 99. Edinburgh: G. P. Johnston.

(11) Ibid., pp. 165–8.

(12) COMRIE, J. D. (1939) Boerhaave and the early medical school at Edinburgh. In *Memorialia Herman Boerhaave*, pp. 32–9. Haarlem: De Erven F. Bohn N.V.

(13) College Minutes, 25.vii.1967.

THE UNIVERSITY OF EDINBURGH

(14) GRANT, Sir A. (1884) *The Story of the University of Edinburgh*, vol. I, p. 138. London: Longmans, Green & Co.

(15) Ibid., p. 217.

(16) EDINBURGH. City council archives (1954) *Extracts from the records of the burgh of Edinburgh, 1681 to 1689*, ed. by M. Wood & H. Armet, p. 140. Edinburgh: Oliver & Boyd.

(17) GRANT, Sir A. Op. cit., p. 226.

(18) Ibid., pp. 308–15.

(19) A short account of the University of Edinburgh, the present Professors in it, and the several parts of learning taught by them (1741) *Scots Magazine*, **III**, 371.

(20) GRANT, Sir A. Op. cit., p. 315.

(21) LOCKHART, J. G. (1908) *The Life of Sir Walter Scott*, p. 9. London: Dent (Everyman's Library).

(22) Ibid., p. 12.

(23) GRANT, Sir A. Op. cit., vol. I, p. 298.

(24) RITCHIE, R. P. Op. cit., p. 292.

(25) STRUTHERS, J. (1867) *Historical Sketch of the Edinburgh Anatomical School*, p. 21. Edinburgh: Maclachlan & Stewart.

(26) College Minutes, 21.xi.1723.

(27) GRANT, Sir A. Op. cit., vol. II, pp. 307–8.

(28) BOWER, A. Op. cit., vol. II, pp. 200–3.

(29) College Minutes, 14.iv.1713.

(30) Ibid., 23.xi.1713.

(31) RITCHIE, R. P. Op. cit., p. 285.

(32) College Minutes, 10.iv.1705.

(33) Ibid., 1.v.1705.

(34) Ibid., 26.xii.1710.

(35) Ibid., 6.i.1713.

(36) Ibid., 4.xi.1718.

(37) Ibid., 24.iii.1719.

(38) GRANT, Sir A. Op. cit., vol. I, p. 311.

(39) College Minutes, 1.xi.1726.

THE UNIVERSITY OF PENNSYLVANIA AND THE COLLEGE OF PHYSICIANS OF PHILADELPHIA

(40) SIGERIST, H. E. (1939) Boerhaave's influence upon American medicine. In *Memorialia Herman Boerhaave*, p. 44. Haarlem: De Erven F. Bohn N.V.

(41) MacDermot, H. E. (1959) The Scottish influence in Canadian medicine. *Practitioner*, **183**, 88.

(42) Packard, F. R. (1932) How London and Edinburgh influenced medicine in Philadelphia in the eighteenth century. (The S. Weir Mitchell oration.) *Annals of Medical History*, **4**, 241.

(43) Ibid., pp. 220–1.

(44) Ibid., p. 222.

(45) Ibid., p. 223.

(46) Ibid., p. 224.

(47) Franklin, B. (1772) Letter, 1772 Feb. 5, to Dr. Thomas Bond. In Pepper, W. (1910) *The Medical Side of Benjamin Franklin. University of Pennsylvania Medical Bulletin*, **23**.

(48) Carlyle, A. (1910) *Autobiography of Dr. Alexander Carlyle of Inveresk, 1722–1805*, ed. by J. H. Burton, p. 54. Edinburgh: Foulis.

(49) Franklin, B. (1764) Letter, 1764 March 14, to Dr. John Fothergill.

(50) Packard, F. R. Op. cit., pp. 226–7.

(51) Bell, W. J., jun. (1965) *John Morgan; continental doctor*, p. 139. Philadelphia: University of Pennsylvania Press.

(52) Rae, J. (1895) *Life of Adam Smith*, p. 274. London: Macmillan.

(53) Russell, B. (1952) *Impact of Science on Society*, p. 48. London: Allen & Unwin.

(54) Comrie, J. D. (1932) *History of Scottish Medicine*, 2nd Edition, vol. II, p. 734. London: Baillière, Tindall & Cox.

(55) Bell, W. J. Op. cit., p. 78.

(56) Ibid., p. 71.

(57) Packard, F. R. Op. cit., p. 230.

(58) Ibid., p. 231.

(59) Morgan, J. (1765) *A Discourse upon the Institution of Medical Schools in America . . .* , p. 40. Philadelphia: W. Bradford.

(60) Shryock, R. H. (1960) *Medicine and Society in America, 1660–1860*, p. 24. New York: New York University Press.

(61) Bell, W. J. Op. cit., p. 107.

(62) Malloch, A. (1946) *Medical Interchange between the British Isles and America before 1801*, p. 65. (Fitzpatrick Lecture, 1939.) London: Royal College of Physicians.

(63) Packard, F. R. Op. cit., p. 233.

(64) R.C.P.E. (1925) *Historical Sketch and Laws*, p. 4. Edinburgh: Royal College of Physicians.

(65) Binger, C. (1966) *Revolutionary Doctor; Benjamin Rush, 1746–1813*, p. 35. New York: W. W. Norton & Co.

(66) Garrison, F. H. (1929) *An Introduction to the History of Medicine*, 4th Edition, p. 379. Philadelphia: W. B. Saunders Co.

(67) Grant, Sir A. Op. cit., vol. II, p. 395.

(68) Ibid., p. 394.

(69) Cockburn, H. (1910) *Memorials of his Time*, New Edition, p. 7. Edinburgh: Foulis.

(70) Packard, F. R. Op. cit., pp. 243–4.

(71) Ibid., p. 236.

(72) Cantlie, Sir N. (1974) *A History of the Army Medical Department*, vol. I, p. 147. Edinburgh: Churchill Livingstone.

(73) BINGER, C. Op. cit., p. 44.

(74) Ibid., p. 45.

(75) [MONRO, G. D.] (1970) *Yester Church and Parish.* [Yester: Privately printed.]

(76) College Minutes, 7.v.1799.

(77) MALLOCH, A. Op. cit., p. 69.

(78) PACKARD, F. R. Op. cit., p. 239.

(79) College Minutes, 4.viii.1818.

(80) PHILADELPHIA MUSEUM OF ART (1965) *The Art of Philadelphia medicine.* [Exhibition catalogue], p. 106. Philadelphia: The Museum.

(81) PACKARD, F. R. Op. cit., p. 227.

(82) GRAY, J. (1952) *History of the Royal Medical Society, 1737–1937*, p. 47. Edinburgh: Edinburgh University Press.

(83) MALLOCH, A. Op. cit., p. 71.

(84) GARRISON, F. H. Op. cit., p. 387.

(85) CLARK, A. J. (1938) Aspects of the history of anaesthetics. *British Medical Journal*, **2**, 1031.

(86) GRAY, J. Op. cit., p. 132.

(87) SHRYOCK, R. H. Op. cit., p. 25.

(88) College Minutes, 7.v.1946.

THE UNIVERSITY OF McGILL

(89) MacDERMOT, H. E. Op. cit., p. 86.

(90) MEAKINS, J. (1920) The influence of Edinburgh on McGill University and American medicine. *Edinburgh Medical Journal*, **24**, 7.

(91) MEAKINS, J. Op. cit., p. 9.

(92) RATTRAY, W. J. (1882) *The Scot in British North America*, vol. III, p. 820. Toronto: Maclear & Co.

THE UNIVERSITY OF TEHERAN

(93) HILL, Sir I. G. W. (1975) Personal communication.

Chapter XVIII

COLLEGE, GOWN AND TOWN

Yet in practice, all schools alike are forced to admit the necessity of a measure of accommodation in the very interests of truth itself.

John Morley

The Royal College of Physicians of Edinburgh and the Medical School of the University of Edinburgh have in common that they were established for the furtherance of medical science. In many respects the progress over the centuries of these two institutions ran parallel courses but not without periodic 'collisions'. There have been periods of close co-operation and periods of intense antagonism. Many Fellows of the College were in their day on the staff of the Medical School. Dual loyalties frequently presented problems and opinions were not always devoid of partisanship. Difficulties were both personal and corporate.

SIMILAR EXPERIENCES

The Medical School, no less than the College, had its domestic problems and allowance should be made for them when considering the relationships between College and University in the early years. There were problems of Town and Gown as well as College and Gown. Earliest efforts to found a Town's College in Edinburgh experienced obstruction from the Universities of St Andrews, Glasgow and Old Aberdeen of a nature closely similar to that later meted out by the University of Edinburgh when a College of Physicians was first mooted in the city. Strangely too, University and College of Physicians had a similar experience in the loss of valuable historical papers relating to crucial periods of their existence. The loss of Sederunt Minutes by the College which occurred in the last years of the seventeenth century has already been mentioned. Early in the following century, 1704 to be precise, the Town Council acting as Patrons and bent on exercising disciplinary authority removed the Town's College Records to the City Charter-house. The Records were not returned and were eventually lost by the Town Council in circumstances described by Grant with the result that valuable information about the Town's College for the period 1645 to 1703 was lost for all time.[1]

MEDICAL EDUCATION LAGS

In Hannay's words, the Town's College remained 'for many years an institution confined in scope to the Faculties of Arts and Divinity'.[2] Gradually an administrative concept of University as distinct from Town's College evolved as Professors replaced Regents with the disbandment of the tutorial system. 'Faculty', in the minds of the Patrons, was incompatible with their conception of a Town's College as it implied the unwarranted usurpation of authority by academic staff. It was while this and similar attitudes pervaded the Town's College that the slow indefinite beginnings of an as yet undefined medical school began to take shape. Grant in his *History* makes it unequivocally clear that 'the origin of this new order of things was quite external to the College and its patrons'.[3] He gave prime credit to Sibbald, and described his activities and those of Balfour and Sutherland in developing a Physic Garden which the Town Council incorporated into the Town's College in 1676. Nineteen years later Sutherland was appointed Professor of Botany by the Town Council in their capacity of Patrons of the Town's College.[4]

RESIDUAL CHAGRIN AND ROYAL UNDERSTANDING

Although successful in obtaining their Charter of Incorporation, there is evidence that the concessions made by the College of Physicians to meet the opposition of the Universities continued to rankle. Apparently a letter dated 6th July 1686 was sent to the Earl of Perth (who had become Lord Chancellor in 1684) and another on 18th July of the same year to Lord Melfort, Secretary of State and brother of the Earl of Perth. Available copies of the letters are unsigned but their method of expression and references in them point almost conclusively to their having been written by Robert Sibbald. Both letters were couched in the most florid of ingratiating terms, and with open acknowledgment of the fact that the College owed its erection 'in a great pairt' to Perth. In effect the letters consisted of petitions in favour of the College that they might be granted power to refuse Licences to Scots Graduates, unless upon examination. Mention was made in the letter to the Lord Chancellor (but not in that sent to Lord Melfort) of 'the enclosed Memorandum [which] will serve for informing the Lord Secretary and contains a true narrative of the case'.[5]

This Memorandum is of considerable significance in the light of relations at the time between the College and the Universities. Dated 1686 it was entitled 'Memorandum for the Royal Colledge of Physicians, that all who apply for a licence to practise Physic in Edinburgh should be previously examined by the College'. After the customary prosaic, almost pious preamble appropriate to the period, the Memorandum referred to the conditions of the Charter whereby graduates of the Universities of St Andrews, Glasgow, Aberdeen and Edinburgh should be licensed by the College 'to practise medicine [in Edinburgh] without any previous or antecedent tryall, But merely upon production of their patent on Graduation to the President'. This the Memorandum contended, was 'contrair to the practice of other nationes where Colledges are erected and particularly of England, where the Graduats of Oxford and Cambridge are not admitted to the Colledge of London without a new examination'. It continued 'And it being presupposed and understood the tym of granting the said patent that the Universities within this Kingdom should take a serious and exact tryall before Graduation, and that the samen should be by a *duly constitute faculty of Medicine as is usual* in the Universities of other nationes, whereas most of the Universities of this Kingdom had *no professor of Medicine and some only* which cannot constitute a faculty. Notwithstanding they conferr degrees in medicine without any tryall, or at leist the samen is only perfunctorious and for a show and thereby sordid vile and illiterat persones without any education or knowledge are made doctors of medicin, to the great scandall and disgrace of that honourable profession, and whom the College of Phisitianes are ashamed to licentiat or admitt into their Society and thereby the great designe of their erection is frustrat.'

To prevent this, the Memorandum pleaded that 'His Majesty . . . ordaine that all persones . . . in any tym coming, wherever they be Graduat either at home or abroad, shall be . . . tryed and examined by the said Colledge, to the effect that they may be admitted if they shall be found sufficiently qualified, or otherwise that they may reject them (That) notwithstanding of any clause or provision contained in the patent and erection of the said College.'

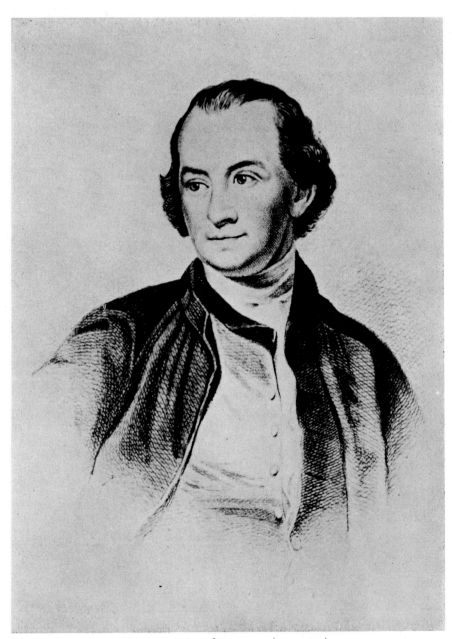

PLATE 25   Dr John Morgan (1735–1789)
By courtesy of the College of Physicians of Philadelphia

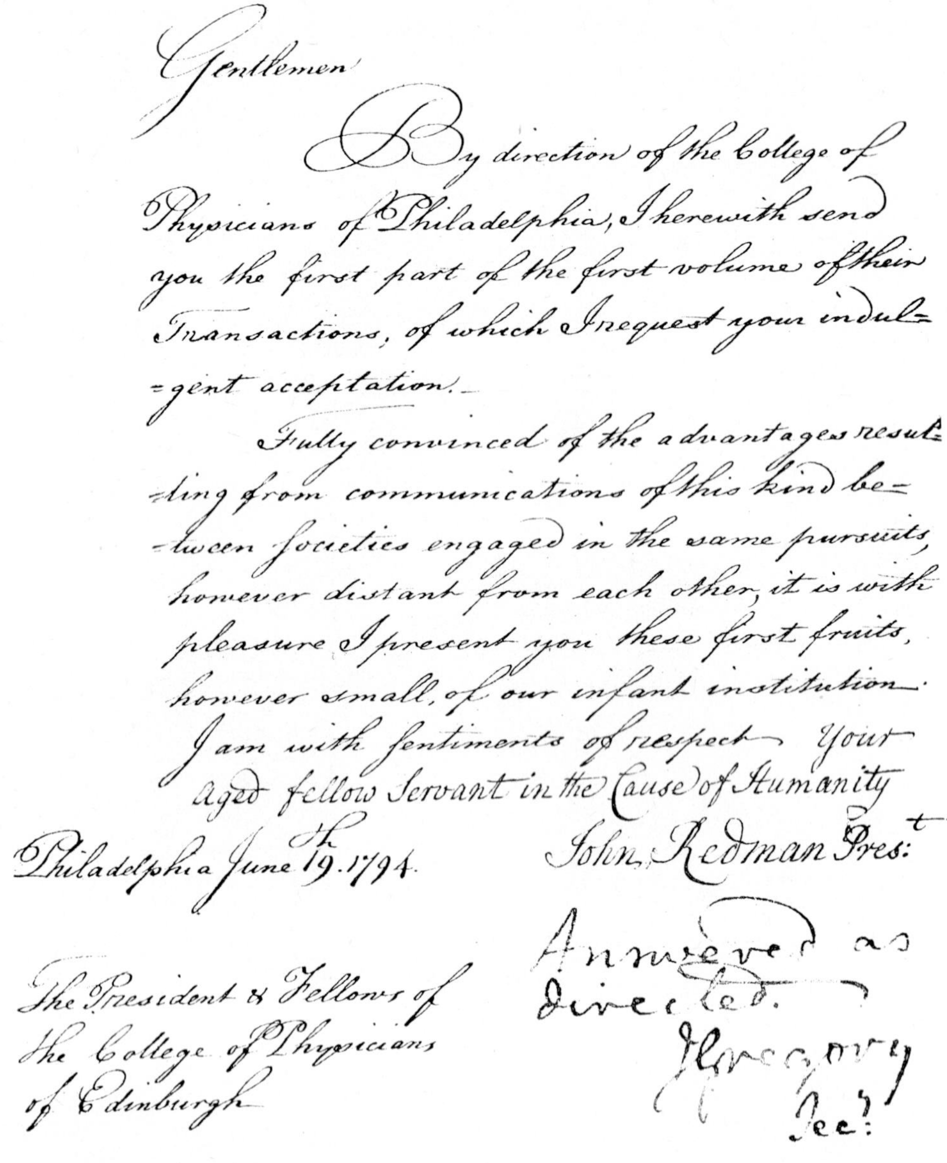

Gentlemen

By direction of the College of Physicians of Philadelphia, I herewith send you the first part of the first volume of their Transactions, of which I request your indulgent acceptation.—

Fully convinced of the advantages resulting from communications of this kind between societies engaged in the same pursuits, however distant from each other, it is with pleasure I present you these first fruits, however small, of our infant institution.—

I am with sentiments of respect Your aged fellow Servant in the Cause of Humanity

Philadelphia June 19. 1794.   John Redman Pres.t

The President & Fellows of the College of Physicians of Edinburgh

Answered as directed.
Gregory
Sec.y

PLATE 26   Letter from Dr John Redman as first President of the College of Physicians of Philadelphia. (Acknowledged by Dr James Gregory, Secretary of the Royal College of Physicians, Edinburgh, 1794.) Reproduced from the College General Correspondence

It would appear that the Memorandum met with success, but whether as a result of the extravagance of its introduction or the directness of its concluding plea is an open question. Doubtless my Lords Perth and Melfort added the weight of their recommendations. No matter; there was drawn up a 'Warrant for a Grant in favor of the Colledge of Physicians in Edinburgh authorizing them to try and examine Graduates in Medicine before their being allowed to practise there'.[5]

The Warrant commenced with what was in essence a recapitulation of the case presented in the College Memorandum. There followed 'Therefore His Majesty ordaines a Letter to be made and past under his Majesty's Great Seale . . . Ordaining and Requiring that no Person wheresoever Graduated shall presume to practise Physick in the said City of Edinburgh or Liberties thereof untill they be first tryed and examined by the said College of Physitians.' Then came authorization of the College to pursue 'offendors' in accordance with their powers of jurisdiction granted by King Charles the Second; but, significantly the Crown reserved 'full power . . . to revoke, alter or change any Power, Liberty or priviledge whatsoever hereby granted'. None the less the Warrant was submitted to the King and issued as being 'given at the Court at Whitehall the 19th day of November 1686 and of his Majesty's reigne the 2nd year.'[5]

Anticlimax followed. The circumstances are wreathed in uncertainty. There is no mention of the Warrant in surviving College Minutes, it having been issued during the so-called 'blank period'. According to Dr Richard Poole the Warrant 'was never acted on, because though judicious, an Act of Arbitrary power soon afterwards set aside'.[6] A sad if perhaps fortunate outcome of what Poole described as 'one of the very few really good deeds of the unhappy King'.[7] The King was James VII of Scotland.

In retrospect it would seem that the view of the College had sound basis. This is especially the case if credence is to be attached to the following statement in the letter addressed to the Lord Chancellor—'It is the clause concerning the Universities' power of graduation which the Colledge of Physicians doe not pretend in any sort to infringe; bot in regard that a facultie of Medicin cannot consist of lesse than three professors who ought to be constant residentes and teachers of the several pairts of Medicin for the instructing of youth in that study; and seeing there is no such constitution in any of our Universities—nay not so much as one professor of Medicin in any of them except a single one in Aberdeen who neither has publick nor private lessons. Therefor the Colledge of Physicians does humbly conceive oure Universities cannot regularly confer any degrees in Medicin untill they be provided of a sufficient number of professors to constitute a facultie of Medicin . . .'. A fear was also expressed

o

that unless the situation were remedied 'all the Apothecaries and Surgeons wee have will goe and be graduat at Aberdeen . . .'.[8]

Accepting that the College had a case for remonstrance, there remains the difficulty of understanding the timing of its initial petition having regard to early developments already taking shape in University circles with the knowledge of Fellows (q.v.).

COLLEGE INFLUENCE

In 1685, almost four years after the erection of the College of Physicians, three prominent Fellows of that College were appointed Professors of Medicine at the Town's College by the Town Council. Excerpts from the relevant Acts of the Town Council are of interest. That of 24th March 1685 reads—'The Council considering that the College of this City being . . . erected into a University, and endowed with the privilege of erecting professions [professorships] of all sorts, particularly of medicine, and that the Physicians have procured from his late Majesty, a patent erecting them into a College of Physicians, and that there is therefore a necessity that there should be a Professor of Physic . . . unanimously elect, nominate and choose the said Sir Robert Sibbald to be Professor of Physic in the said University.'[9]

Another Act of the Town Council in September 1685 declared that Sir Robert Sibbald having 'compeared and accepted his office and made faith . . . there is a necessity for more Professors of Medicine'; and elected Dr James Halket and Dr Archibald Pitcairne 'to be joined with Sir Robert Sibbald'. Although provided with 'convenient rooms in the College' they were to have 'no salarie from the good Town nor from the said University'. Discussing the phraseology of the Acts, Grant commented on the Town Council's usage for the first time of 'University' in preference to 'Town's College'; and suggested that the explanation may be that the new phraseology 'was an echo of the language used in a petition of the College of Physicians for the appointment of Sir Robert Sibbald as Professor'.[10] It was pointed out by Bower that Pitcairne enjoyed an intimate friendship with Principal Carstares which did not falter with years despite their 'very different political sentiments'.[11] Bower maintained also that Pitcairne received encouragement in his mathematical leanings from a close friendship with Professor David Gregory[12] and that despite Pitcairne's friends being reluctant to accept that he was author of the stingingly derisory criticisms of Sibbald's *Prodromus* and other publications, clear proof existed that Pitcairne was in fact the critic.[13]

APPROACH OF THE UNIVERSITIES: COLLEGE INITIATIVE

Early in the eighteenth century the College took the initiative in promoting co-operation with the Scottish Universities. On 13th July 1704 the President (Dr Alexander Dundas) informed sederunt that he had spoken to the Principals of the Edinburgh and Glasgow Colleges 'anent ane agriement betwixt the Colledge of Physitians and the ffour universities'. An immediate outcome was the appointment of three Fellows additional to the President to confer with the two Principals, or failing them their Deputies.[14]

There was no further mention of the proposed meeting but on 19th July 1705, Dr James Halket now being President, a Committee of six Fellows (including Sir Robert Sibbald and Dr Dundas) was appointed with as object 'to sie what agriement they can make with the universities of the Kingdome upon the terms of the proposalls formerly made to the said universities, and Lykewayes to take in to their consideratione some other things relateing to the order of the Societie'.[15]

Poole has recorded finding a number of documents with unquestionable bearing on the subject despite several of them being undated.[16] Such is the importance of the documents for present purposes that the reproduction of excerpts is warranted. Of these the first is:

> 'Proposalls for ane agrement betwixt the Universities of St. Andrews, Aberdeen, Glasgow and Edinburgh on the one parte and the Royall Colledge of Physicians in Edr. on the other parte.
>
> .   .   .   .   .
>
> 'The Universities as well as those that have received there degrees from them contend, that none graduated by them can be constrained to pay anie thing to the coledg of physicians, because by there charters of erectione from former Kings confirmed in Parliament prior to the erectione of the colledg of physicians they have the power to giv degrees to practise per totum terrarum orbem, so that no subsequent right granted to the coledg of physicians can derogate from or invalidate anie former right of which they were in ane uninterrupted possessione.
>
> 'This being the state of the questione . . . it may be thought reasonable to take away anie occasione of difference . . . in all time coming to propose. 1. That the Royall Coledg of physicians shall admit none to be of there number but such as shall receive there degrees in one of the above named universities. 2. That the Universities shall confer no degrees to anie that may practise within the bounds and priviledges of the said Royal Colledg of Physicians but to such as shall be recommended by the said Coledg of Phys[s] to one of the said Universities. 3. That to such as may pretend that they are not to live or practise within the priviledges of said coledg, there either may be a restrictive clause . . . excepting the priviledges and

rights of the coledg of physicians if they shall ever come to live and practise within there bounds, or else to take ane obligation from them to be liable to the coledg in the soume of . . . in the case forsaid . . . That the Universities shall not exact above the soume of for conferring such degrees. 4. That both parties shall be bound to the performance under the penalty of . . .

. . . . . .

'And to evince that it is the intrest of the universities, of the coledg of physicians, and of the nation in generall, it is to be considered that, 1. By this means, the money that is thrown out abroad in graduation may be saved, and therby the honor and reputatione of our owne universities rais'd. 2. The Universities' advantage thereby is most conspicuous, when they are put in minde, that there is not one admitted to be sociu of the coledge but such as have been graduated in foreign universities, which by the proposalls above narrated will be quite otherways; and that it will be certainly to the honor and advantage of the coledg of physicians (though more to the particular intrest of the Universities) if they be instrumental both in saving the money that was thrown out upon foreign graduations, and in retriving the reputatione of degrees conferr'd by our own universities which will redound to the honour of the nation in generall.'[16]

What action followed drafting of the proposals in unknown. Nor is it certain to whom the final proposals were sent but it is probable, or at least possible, that the following letter from St Andrews, dated 25th July 1704 and addressed to Dr Dundas 'at his lodging' might refer to them.

'Sir
I communicat yours to the Masters of our University who desired me to give you this returne that they particularly agree to your proposals untill a publick profession of Medicin be established in our University which is an objection I suppos you will not much regaird since (for what I know) that may be ad Callendas Graecas and this is the needfull from
Sir
Your most humble servant
(signed) Robert Ramsay.'[17]

Dr Dundas was in receipt of another letter dated 28th July 1704 from Principal Carstares of Edinburgh University. It ran as follows:

'Sir
I no sooner had a proposal made by you to this Universitie in the name of the Colledge of Physitians, when I took the first opportunitie of calling the Professors together, who after deliberating upon what was proposed to them about conferring the degree of Doctor of Medicine, did desire me to signifie in their name to the Colledge of Physitians . . . that they are ready to agree with the proposal as made, untill Medicine be taught in the Colledge of Edin[r]., provideing allways the

Candidates apply to the Universitie first, who are to remitt them to the Colledge of Physitians for examination: and further that they want to have it explained what that expression in their Proposalls (in each of them) means. This is Sir what I am desired to give in return to your letter, and doubt not but it will shew how willing this Universitie is to keep up a friendlie correspondence with the Colledge of Physitians. I am without complement

Sir
Your most humble servant
(Signed) W. Carstares.'[18]

Obviously the Principal's letter was concerned with the subject of the College sederunts in the two weeks before he wrote. Nor can there be serious doubt that the troublesome case of Dr Drummond (Chap. VII) was in the back of the minds of all concerned.

In this connection there was yet another document which unfortunately being undated cannot be linked with any chronological certainty. The document in question was entitled 'Proposal by the Colledge of Physicians at Edinburgh to the Universitys of Scotland', the tenor of which closely resembled that of the other 'Proposals' already quoted, except in so far as there was more specific reference to the University of Edinburgh. It read as follows:

'That in case the Universitys will admit none graduats of Medicine at any of their Universitys untill they have professions of Medicine of their own, but such as come from the Colledge of Physicians with a recommendation and declaration of their being tryed by the said Colledge and found qualified, that then the Colledge of Physicians will oblidge themselves to admit none either Licentiate or Fellow of the said Colledge but those that have taken their degrees at one of the Universitys at home, and will joyne their interest with the Universitys' to obtain ane Act of Parliament that none shall be capable to practise Medicine but such as have their degrees at one of the foresaid Universitys; and when the foresaid Universitys, or any one of them, have got a profession of Medicine, then the said Colledge of Physic[ns] shall be upon the same terms with that University as the Colledge of Physicians at London are with the Universitys of Oxford and Cambridge; viz. they examine all their graduats that come to reside with (within) the said Colledge's libertys before they are allowed for practise physick therein; and least the University of Edinburgh, as being the nearest to the Colledge of Physic[ns] should have most advantage of this proposal, therefore it's proposed to the Universitys that they agree amongst themselves that the whole emoluments be divided equally amongst them or any other way they think fitt.'[19]

So far as is known there is no available evidence as to whether this proposal was submitted, but without question the sentiments contained in it correspond to those which conditioned the arrangements eventually implemented jointly by the College and the University of Edinburgh. Poole arrived at the conclusion that the applications which were subsequently submitted by the Principal of the University '*did* arise out of such an agreement as was suggested by the Coll.'. In support of his contention Poole drew attention to implementation of the condition required by the University that candidates should 'apply to the University first'.[20]

Whatever the gaps in available information, it can be said that the College showed initiative and the University of Edinburgh readiness to co-operate in furthering the interests of medical education.

An element of mystery surrounds the possession by the College of a document headed 'Generall Letters wherein the patent granted by King James VI to the Physicians and Surgeons of Glasgow is further narrated'. The document is dated 4th April 1673 and consists of a summary of the Charter granted to the Faculty of Physicians and Surgeons of Glasgow by King James VI, 'the penult day of November 1599, which will be found at large in "Record & Appendix of Documents in the conjoined Processes etc. between the Faculty and University of Glasgow" 1833 pp. 31–33; and also of the Ratification thereof by Parl^t 11th September 1672 ....'.[21] The quotation is from Poole who commented 'how and why this document was in possession of the College it is impossible to discover. My conjecture is that, however obtained, it was employed as one of the materials out of which the founders of the College drew arguments for their own design. But I admit that it may have been used for a different purpose, namely in relation to Proposals for an agreement between the College and the Universities of Scotland—the Faculty of Glasgow being in a state somewhat analogous to that of the former *quoad* these privileged bodies.'[22]

Poole scribed those words in or around 1838. No further enlightenment has been forthcoming in subsequent years. Whatever the whys and wherefores, the fact remains our College sought assistance from the experience of the Glasgow Faculty. Regardless of how the document was procured, belated acknowledgment of the fact is surely due our sister College in Glasgow in 1974!

THE STIMULUS OF MONRO *primus*

Bower was an unrestrained admirer of Pitcairne. Discussing what he termed 'The foundation of the medical school' he gave first attention to Pitcairne's insistence on improving anatomical teaching which 'most or all anatomists have neglected, or not known, what was most useful for a physician'.[23] Pitcairne's activities, in the face of discouragement from the College of Surgeons and at first in collaboration with Alexander Monteith and Robert Elliot, were seen as a prelude to Alexander Monro's (*primus*) espousal of the anatomical cause. Elliot's titular status was curious in that in the College of Surgeons he was 'Keeper of the Museum', but in the Town Council acted as a 'Professor of Anatomy'. In this there was evidence of the early peripheral influence of extra-academical medicine. As described by Grant the trend of events was 'successful practice or teaching had grown up outside the [Town's] College, and then the practitioners or teachers were dignified by the Town Council with the title of Professors, and were given a more or less close connection with the [Town] College or University'.[24] Without being tortuous, application of the machinery was to say the least illuminating. In Chapter XVII the support of the College of Physicians of Dr James Crawford is described. It was not mentioned that, returned from Leyden and impressed by Boerhaave's teaching, Crawford suggested to the Town Council that he should be allowed to teach chemistry. The upshot was that he was given the title, together with appropriate accommodation in the Town's College, of Professor of Physic and Chemistry. He gave few lectures and those irregularly.[25, 26]

Monro *primus* illustrated the trend to better purpose. Returned from his intensive training on the Continent and after examination by the College of Surgeons, he was on the recommendation of that College appointed in 1720 'Professor of Anatomy in this City and College' by the Town Council. It is recorded of the Town Council that in August of that year 'having heard a representation from the Royal College of Physicians, as also from the Incorporation of Chirurgeon Apothecaries of this city, both setting forth the necessity and usefulness of encouraging a school of anatomy and chirurgery . . . do authorize and give power to the present magistrates to give such encouragement to Mr Alexander Monro . . . as they shall think convenient . . .'.[27] Among assured benefits was a supply of anatomical material.[28]

For some years Monro delivered his lectures in the Surgeons Hall. Those who attended his inaugural delivery included 'The Lord Provost accompanied by his friends in the magistracy, the President and Fellows of the College of Physicians, and the President, accompanied by the members of the College of Surgeons.'[28] In 1725 Monro transferred his work to the Town's College where he was given a theatre for public dissections intended for students being given supervised instruction. As a result, the Chair of Anatomy while titularly still of 'this City and College', became a University Chair in fact and in practice. The notable part played by Monro in collaboration with George Drummond in founding the Edinburgh [Royal] Infirmary has been outlined (Chap. XX). In 1756 he had the degree of Doctor of Medicine conferred upon him by the University of Edinburgh, and in the same year he was licensed by and elected a Fellow of the Royal College of Physicians, taking his seat as Fellow on the same day as his friend William Cullen.[29]

He was the 'first Professor of any kind who drew great attention to the University of Edinburgh from without, and gave it the beginnings of its celebrity'.[30] Such was Sir Alexander Grant's appraisal of Monro *primus*. As a student Oliver Goldsmith described him as 'the one great professor'.[31] Truly Monro *primus* was a great man and no tribute would have appealed to him more than the description of his family by one of his medical sons (Dr Donald Monro) embodied in a preface to the Collected Works of his father:

> 'All that a child can owe to the best of fathers, a pupil to his tutor, or a man to his friend, they owed to him. In their youth he not only superintended their education, but was himself their master in several branches; and when they grew up he made them his companions and friends.'[32]

About the time he transferred to his Town's College theatre Monro *primus* together with leading physicians and surgeons in the City endeavoured to persuade the patrons of the Town's College to supplement the existing instruction on Anatomy and Surgery with systematic teaching of Medicine. In this they were successful. In 1724 the Town Council passed an Act 'wherein "considering the great benefit and advantage that would accrue to this City and Kingdom, by having all the parts of medicine taught in this place; and likewise considering that hitherto the Institutes and Practice of Medicine, though the principal parts thereof, have not been professed or taught in the said College. Therefore they hereby institute and establish the aforesaid Profession of the Institutes and Practice of Medicine in their said College and do elect, nominate and choose Mr. William Porterfield, Doctor of Medicine in Edinburgh" to be Professor.'[33] Porterfield had the support of the College of Physicians.[34, 35] Known principally for *A Treatise on the Eye*[36] (published in 1759) Porterfield was not a success as professor and in a way which has mystified historians quietly disappeared from the academic scene.[37, 38]

With his characteristic aptitude in the use of metaphors Grant writes 'We find four members of the College of Physicians, Drs. John Rutherford, Andrew Sinclair, Andrew Plummer, and John Innes, pressing forward into the breach'. He explained how these four sought and were allowed to use, for rearing pharmaceutical plants, the neglected Town's College garden which had once belonged to the old Kirk o' Field.

This move Grant quoted as 'indicative of the enterprising spirit of the Physicians in Edinburgh of those days' even although it had as ulterior motive bringing 'the four

Physicians into prominence, and into a sort of relationship to the [Town's] College, which very soon became closer'.[39]

A MEDICAL FACULTY

Doctors Sinclair (St Clair) and Rutherford were appointed Professors of the Theory and Practice of Medicine, and Doctors Plummer and Innes, Professors of Medicine and Chemistry. According to Bower, 'To Dr. St. Clair was allotted the theory, and to Dr. Rutherford the practice'.[40] The vital importance of the Acts of 1726 was that they translated into action a previous declaration of intent that in the Town's College 'Medicine in all its branches be professed . . . by such a number of Professors of that science as may by themselves promote students to their degrees, with as great solemnity as is done with any other College or University at home or abroad'.[41] In realistic practical terms the appointment of the four new professors signalized the birth of a Faculty of Medicine: but still reluctant to concede unrestricted authority to the Principal and Professors 'to deliberate and vote on the affairs of general concern to the [Town's] College', the Town Council stipulated that of the four new professors 'two only shall at one time have the privilege of voting'.[42]

John Rutherford, maternal grandfather of Sir Walter Scott, was the first to give clinical lectures in the Infirmary, arrangements being agreed to by Drummond when, after Culloden, prospects of civil peace improved. Cullen writing about the time of Rutherford's resignation said, 'When I first applied to the study of physic I learned only the system of Boerhaave; and, even when I came to take a Professor's chair in this University, I found that system here in its entire and full force.'[43] Plummer, appointed at the same time as Rutherford, had been a student of Boerhaave and had developed a special interest in chemistry. His name was associated with a pill of antimony and mercury named after him, and with his analysis and advocacy of the therapeutic waters of Moffat.[44, 45]

POLICY WITH REGARD TO M.D. EXAMINATIONS

Another and intended result of the creation of a Faculty was the discarding of direct dependence on the College of Physicians for assistance in examining candidates for the degree of M.D. The fact remains however that the College continued to serve as an intermediary in conveying to the newly born Faculty the Leyden outlook in so far as teaching and examining were concerned. Both Plummer and Innes were *alumni* of Leyden. So also was Crawford.

In its newly acquired enlightened mood the Town Council once again succumbed to external pressure and decided to appoint a Professor of Midwifery. The title was conferred on a Surgeon of the name of Gibson who was supported by recommendations from Fellows of the College of Physicians and members of the sister Surgical College. Impressed by the novelty of the new chair and by the procedure adopted in creating it, Bower was prompted to record 'This Institution, like every other connected with the history of Medicine in Edinburgh, originated with the colleges of physicians and surgeons.'[46]

Both Bower and Grant described the type of examination to which the candidate aspiring to a degree of Doctorate of Medicine of Edinburgh University had to submit himself.[47, 48] A study of the *List of Graduates in Medicine* shows that from 1726 to 1748 less than six graduated each year: the number had doubled by the mid-century and trebled by 1770.[49] *Statuta Solennia* were enacted in 1767 for the ordering of medical degrees. Basically, apart from minor changes at irregular intervals, the *Statuta Solennia* remained unaltered until 1833. There was no escaping the influence on the main features of procedures laid down in the *Statuta Solennia*, of previously established practice in the College of Physicians. Thus:

The first examination dealt with a candidate's general literary attainments, and his proficiency in the different branches of Medicine. Until 1811 this phase of the examination was conducted in the privacy of a professor's house. Then followed the necessity to submit a Medical Thesis. The third phase consisted in more minute examination by two professors in the presence of the Faculty on different branches of medicine. Next the candidate was required to answer in writing and defend before the Faculty, answers to questions attached to two case histories. Finally, previous hurdles having been surmounted, printed copies of his Thesis had to be sent to each member of the Medical Faculty by the candidate who before receiving his Doctorate Degree had to defend the Thesis on graduation day.[50]

Such is Grant's description. There can be none who fail to appreciate the close resemblance of procedure with that of the College (Chap. VII). Discussing the preliminaries to conferment of a medical degree Bower stated that 'with slight variations, the form adopted at Leyden . . . was preferred'.[51] All that was lacking was live 'clinical material' in lieu of 'clinical histories'. There was virtually no discrepancy between Grant's account and Bower's, except in so far as, writing of an unspecified but unquestionably earlier period, the latter recorded that at the third examination when being examined by two professors, the candidate had one of the

Aphorisms of Hippocrates assigned to him.[52] Latin was employed in the course of both oral and written examinations—until 1833. This and the presentation of statutes 'couched in not unclassical Latin' struck Grant as being quite in keeping with the symbolic wigs and gold-headed canes of members of the Medical Faculty.[53] In this these gentlemen did not differ from Fellows of the Physicians' College. James Hamilton (the Younger), adorned with a three-cornered hat, was the last to visit patients in a sedan chair—doing so until 1830.[54] Nor did Fellows, except at times of isolated fracas, lack 'the air of old-fashioned dignity' of the University Medical Faculty to which Grant alluded, albeit whimsically—a form of dignity which if restored in part at least, would be to the advantage of patient, physician and profession today.

MEDICALS IN A RESTIVE SENATE

Acknowledgment by the Town Council of the existence of the Senate eventually materialized in 1772. Absence of any definition of the powers of the Senate was to prove a source of disagreement among members of the Faculty of Medicine, in which some Fellows of the College were involved.[55] In 1809 a decision on the part of the Senate to raise the fee for diplomas in medicine was resisted by the students who appealed to the Town Council. Largely as a result of the advice of the Professor of Scots Law the Senate was dissuaded from pursuing their objective.[56] Six years later Dr Duncan, jun. was, through no fault of his own, involved in difficulties in connection with his duties as Librarian. Senate took exception to an enactment of the Town Council determining that finance to increase the Librarian's salary should be withdrawn from a library fund originated by the Senate to purchase books. An element of gymnastic expediency succeeded in solving matters to the satisfaction of all concerned.[57]

There then arose a major source of disagreement with the application by Dr James Hamilton, Professor of Midwifery, for his subject to be made an obligatory one for graduation. The reaction of the Town Council was favourable: that of the Senate antagonistic. Hostilities, for such they were, persisted for over nine years; considerable legal fees were incurred by both contending parties; the Senate's claim to exclusive rights based on a century and a half's custom was shewn to be at fault in law, and the Courts declared that the legal right of making Regulations rested with the Town Council. Attendance on the class of midwifery was made compulsory after 1833.[58] Four Professors, all Fellows of the Physicians' College offered to lend the Senatus a sum adequate to meet the bill of £610 for legal expenses. The offer was accepted, the Senate giving binding assurances as to repayment.[59]

While the legal battle was at its height a visit was paid to the University by a Royal Commission under instructions to undertake a Visitation of the Universities and Colleges of Scotland. Application for a Royal Commission of Inquiry had been made by the Senate in 1826.[60] The Commission had wide terms of reference and in general their activities are not the concern of this history. Of significance however were certain sections of a 'Scheme of Studies' submitted by the Commissioners in so far as they had a bearing on medical education. Thus it was recommended that Surgery should be separated from Anatomy and erected into a separate chair; there should be a Chair of Mental Diseases; examinations in the Medical Faculty should be conducted in English; there should be a degree in Surgery, but only one degree in Medicine.[61] A draft of the Scheme of Studies was sent to Senate by the Commission but with no reference to the constitution or government of the University. This was the more unsatisfactory because in the words of Grant—'The whole quarrel with the Town Council had arisen from the proud unwillingness of the Medical Professors to accept external dictation upon a single point.'[62] Some of those who have had experience of municipal health services may on reading the quotation wonder if 'principles' not 'pride' were a root cause of the trouble.

There was, however, another rather extraordinary complicating aspect to the Town and Gown confrontation. The Town Council's College Committee had at one time among its members two Fellows of the College of Physicians and two members of the College of Surgeons.[63] A specific criticism of the Commissioners charged the Medical Faculty with increasing laxity in examinations for the M.D. The view arose from the fact that M.D.s 'had multiplied in a greater ratio than the medical students'; and was frankly admitted by Members of the Commission, after the winding up of the Commission, to be erroneous. But as is so liable to occur in such a sequence of events 'The error lives on—the correction dies out.'[64] A Parliamentary Bill based on the Commission's findings was dropped by the Government of the day.

RECOGNITION OF EXTRA–ACADEMICAL TEACHERS

A problem directly involving both College and University arose from the successful practice of private extra-mural teaching. After considering Professor Syme's letter (Chap. XVI) recommending recognition of extra-academical teaching, the Town

Council, regardless of the instinctive opposition of Senate, drafted a modified *Statuta* which provided for the recognition of four extra-academical classes as qualifying towards a degree. In due course the Senatus retaliated by sending to the Town Council a draft of alterations in the Senate Rules for medical degrees. The amended rules indicated preparedness to recognize the teaching at London medical schools and at the Dublin College of Surgeons school as equivalent to that of the University of Edinburgh. There was no mention of equivalent facilities in Edinburgh. A year passed and the Town Council issued their new Regulations. These Regulations added to the London and Dublin schools in the Senate proposals, the lectures 'of teachers of medicine in Edinburgh, recognized as such by the Royal Colleges of Physicians and of Surgeons in Edinburgh' as qualifying for graduation to the extent of one-third of all the subjects required, and of one year out of the four years' medical course. Fees were to be the same as those paid for the corresponding class in the University.[65]

The majority of the medical professors were adamant in their resistance, and they won the support of Senate. An interim order of suspension of the new Regulations was obtained from the Court of Session. Thereupon an action was lodged against the Town Council on the grounds that the sole power of enacting University graduation laws rested with the Senate and that the issue of Regulations by the Town Council had been illegal. It was contended by Senate that the extra-academic teachers were of 'spontaneous generation', lacked cohesion, were not subject to discipline, and were not limited as to the number who could teach on any one subject.[66] Court judgment went in favour of the Town Council, a decision which was confirmed when the Senate appealed to the House of Lords. The Town Council's Regulations came into operation in 1855, fifteen years after the receipt of Professor Syme's letter.

Without doubt the Senate had been worsted. Nor can it be said that the medical Senators showed up in the best of lights. Some of their number sensed possible serious rivalry. Their reaction to the Town Council proposals was that while 'they could bear the idea of accepting teaching that was given in London or Dublin as equivalent to their own', they were intransigently averse to any encouragement of rival teachers in Edinburgh. To quote Grant, they foresaw that 'any Student . . . might elect to walk across the street and get his teaching from some rising genius who had been recognized by the Medical Corporations of the City'.[67]

Inevitably personal animosities were rampant and Christison, one not given to veiled cynicism, described the lengths to which 'a small section of men belonging to the Extra-Academical School of Medicine' would go to insult any University man they might meet on a public occasion.[68] Offensive behaviour however was not limited to the extra-academics! Initially and for a considerable period of time, the customary designation of those giving instruction under other than academic aegis was 'private teacher'. According to Christison the change from 'private' to the 'sesquipedalian designation' of 'extra-academical' was a direct consequence of the deliberate humiliation embodied in a toast to a 'private teacher' at an annual dinner of the Royal Medical Society.[69]

A CRUCIAL BONE OF CONTENTION

Antagonism between College and Gown reached its zenith as measures for medical reform struggled to achieve an acceptable and at the same time reasonably practical solution. During the years that a plethora of Bills were being submitted to Parliament it became evident that legislators were becoming increasingly enamoured of a 'one portal system of examination and licence' and of proposals to create 'compulsory conjunct Boards'. Sharing an antipathy to such reforms the Scottish Medical Corporations and Universities for a period worked in greater harmony than previously. In the course of time, however, there developed an increasing insistence on the part of the Corporations to reserve to themselves the right to grant licences to practise. This view was shared by the English and Irish Corporations with the result that a quasi-alliance of the Corporations undermined the unity previously characterizing the relations between Scottish Corporations and Scottish Universities. It was the declared view of the Corporations that University degrees of Doctorate of Medicine were in the nature of professional honours and not associated with any conferment of right to practise.

On 2nd August 1858 the *Universities (Scotland) Act*[70] received the Royal Assent. In accordance with its terms a Commission was appointed to implement the Act in detail, and to frame ordinances for the regulation, among other activities, of studies and degree systems. Decisions of the Commissioners were subject to the review of Parliament and appeals to the Privy Council.

In the course of formulating regulations for degrees the Commissioners considered representations submitted by the Scottish Corporations and the English College of Surgeons but were not favourably impressed. At a later date the Corporations were given a hearing by the Privy Council but with no better result. Indeed Christison, a University man first and last in this particular matter, declared with undisguised exuberance, that the Privy Council on receiving the Corporations' report 'tore it to shreds'.[71] Confirmation if it were needed, of Christison's attitude was evident when he wrote 'I have published a little book . . . my inquiries do not leave the Medical Corporations as much as a toe to stand on in their late opposition to the Universities'.[72] A less emotional summation of the University point of view was given by Grant in his *Story of the University of Edinburgh*. It deserves full quotation. Referring to a Commissioners' ordinance of 1860 whereby medical degrees were divided into the three classes M.B., C.M. and M.D., he wrote 'This new arrangement evoked opposition from the Medical Corporations of Great Britain (among which were the Colleges of Physicians and Surgeons of Edinburgh) who wished to prevent degrees in Surgery being granted by the Universities. Their opposition was really of a very selfish character; it was an attempt to stamp University degrees as an insufficient qualification for general medical practice, which they would have been under the terms of the Medical Act of 1858, if the Universities, though examining their Students in Surgery as well as Medicine, gave them nominally only a degree in Medicine.'[73]

Despite the periodic acute difference of opinion between the College and University the former was not guilty of parsimony where support of new University projects was involved. At a meeting in November 1789 the College 'having taken under their consideration the subscription proposed to be set on foot for building a new College [University] in this City They are unanimously of opinion that it will be proper for them to contribute both in a corporate capacity and as individuals to this very desirable work . . . .'.[74] At a subsequent Extraordinary Meeting expressly called to determine the sum which the College should contribute it was agreed that in a corporate capacity £150 should be subscribed.[75] Rather more than eighty years later the President received a letter from the Principal of the University of Edinburgh (Sir Alexander Grant) submitting a Statement of a Scheme for extending the Scientific and Educational Buildings of the University, and requesting that the College should 'grant some assistance to a proposal for the maintenance in high efficiency of the great Medical School of Edinburgh, for the general improvement of the Educational Appliances of the Metropolitan University'. The communication was considered by the Council who by a majority recommended that the College should vote a sum of One Thousand Guineas for the purpose.[76] After discussion, the Council recommendation was approved by the College, the approval being confirmed at the next Quarterly Meeting. The final approval stipulated that payment of the 1000 guineas should be made 'in two Instalments, one half six months after commencement of the Buildings and the other in twelve months thereafter'.[77]

Not a little astonishingly, four years had hardly passed when the College received a communication from the Principal of the University which concluded 'You will observe that the Town Council of Edinburgh have repeated their subscription of One Thousand Pounds and I now venture to ask whether your wealthy and munificent College will be disposed to take similar action, in the cause of Medical Education and Science.' Notwithstanding the eminence of the writer—the letter was certainly not the product of a skilled professional beggar. Underlying all was fear of losing a conditional Government grant. Even so the College felt constrained to reply that they did 'not feel called upon at present to make any addition to the donation' previously voted.[78] However after an interval of time, in December 1884 the Treasurer moved 'That the College vote a Donation of Five Hundred Guineas towards the Fund for the completion of the New University Buildings, and Fifty Guineas to the Marine Station at Granton.'[79] The motion was finally agreed to on a second reading at the next Quarterly Meeting.[80]

Support was forthcoming from the College for the *Representation of the People (Scotland) Bill* which on receipt of the Royal Assent in 1868 empowered the Universities of Edinburgh and St Andrews to return jointly a Member to the House of Commons.[81-84] Previously, representations had been made by the College to ensure for medical graduates voting rights in the University Council on a par with graduates in other faculties.[85] A co-operative gesture was shewn by the College when in 1860 they allowed the use of the Hall to the University Senate for the purpose of entertaining the Chancellor of the Exchequer (The Right Honourable W. E. Gladstone) on the occasion of his Installation as Rector of the University.[86] At a later sederunt it was decided to entertain at Dinner the Chancellor of the University, Drs Watson and Sharpey of London, and Dr Stokes of Dublin upon whom the University proposed to confer degrees of LL.D.[87] When in 1884 the University attained its Tercentenary, the College forwarded an appropriately worded illuminated congratulatory address[88]: and took the opportunity of entertaining a number of distinguished medical guests of the University.[89]

None the less restiveness apparently persisted within the ranks of the College Council at least. Inflammatory views had not been entirely extinguished as evidenced in the following letter sent to the Secretary of the Royal College of Surgeons of Edinburgh on 10th February 1894:

'Dear Sir
   The Crown Patronage of Chairs in the Scottish Universities has been under the consideration of the Council, and I have been instructed to ask you to bring the subject before the Council of the Royal College of Surgeons, in order to ascertain whether it might be possible for the three Scottish Corporations to present a joint petition to Her Majesty, praying her to place her patronage in the hands of

Parliament with the specific object in view of transferring it by enactment to the
University Court of each University
                                        I am
                                    Yours faithfully,
                                        (Sgd.) G. A. Gibson Secretary.'

A similar communication was sent at the same time to the Secretary of the Glasgow
Faculty of Physicians and Surgeons.[90] There is no evidence that the subject came up
for discussion at any sederunt of the College. The motive underlying the Council's
action must remain a matter of surmise. Fortunately no serious developments took
place, but had Sir Alexander Grant been alive and had an opportunity to comment
upon events, his version would certainly have been vividly candid!

THE COLLEGE IN UNUSUAL RÔLE

In a little over a quarter of a century later, the College assumed the entirely different
function of potential mediator when difficulties arose between the University and the
Town Council. The latter terminated an arrangement whereby the Professor of
Tuberculosis acted as consultant to the City Tuberculosis Services and had access to
material for clinical teaching. Inevitably the position of the College was to some
extent delicate in that at the time the Professor concerned, Sir Robert Philip, was
President of the College.[91] This however did not deter the College from writing to
the University expressing willingness to give any assistance in its power. At the same
time the College was at pains to stress that Sir Robert being away had taken no part
in their deliberations and that the subject had come up for discussion 'without pre-
meditation and in particular without any suggestion on his part'.[92]

Having regard to Sir Robert's international eminence, that such a situation should
ever have arisen is scarcely credible. A general physician by training, Philip devoted
his professional life to the development and establishment of what came to be
known the world over as the 'Edinburgh Plan' for the recognition, treatment and
prevention of tuberculosis. The plan, together with trained staff for the follow-up of
contacts incorporated a Dispensary, Sanatorium, Sanatorium School and Colony.
These last were transferred by the Royal Victoria Hospital Tuberculosis Trust as a
free gift to the City of Edinburgh. A condition attached to the gift was that should
the University appoint a Lecturer in, or a Professor of Tuberculosis he should be
given facilities for teaching and research. Three years later, in 1917, Sir Robert was

appointed the first incumbent of a Chair of Tuberculosis towards the endowment of which the Tuberculosis Trust contributed £18,000.

Shortly after the end of World War I, Philip with the enthusiastic support of the Royal Victoria Hospital Tuberculosis Trust embarked on the development of Southfield Sanatorium Colony to which patients from all over Scotland were admitted. Provisions included facilities for research. Acutely aware of the prevalence of bovine tuberculosis in Scotland, Philip persuaded the Trust to establish Gracemount Farm where the practicability of establishing a tubercle-free herd was demonstrated. In 1950 the Farm was gifted to the University of Edinburgh, the Southfield Colony having been previously absorbed into the National Health Service in 1948.

Such then were some of Philip's concrete achievements during his lifetime. It is a measure of his greatness that, not content with accomplishing so much in the face of considerable scepticism his vision extended to the future with remarkable accuracy. He foretold the decline in mortality which took place; foresaw the employment of chemotherapy in tuberculosis along lines analogous to those already in use in syphilis; and was convinced that a national medical service 'in some shape or form' was inevitable. While not a prophet entirely without honour in his own country, recognition of his pioneer work was less hesitant in France, Belgium, Switzerland, Italy and the United States of America. Calmette was one of the first to adopt Philip's methods.

In 1913 Philip had gifted to him by grateful pupils a silver model of his monaural stethoscope which came into the possession of the College in 1962.[93] He was unique among British doctors in that his portrait was one of several appearing (1955) in a set of Belgian stamps with as theme 'Anti-tuberculosis and other Funds'.[94]

The National Association for the Prevention of Tuberculosis, in 1957 commemorated the centenary of Sir Robert's birth by publishing a book of memories contributed to by friends and pupils.[95] Those contributing included Drs Fergus Hewat and Christopher Clayson, both past Presidents of our College; and (Sir) Derrick Dunlop, Dr Charles Cameron and Dr David Marais. As to Philip's contributions to the College—they were many. He was one of the early workers in the College Laboratory of which he was Curator for no less than fourteen years. Noted for his culture, courtesy and diplomacy his term of Presidential Office afforded scope for these attributes as it did for his masterly skill in discharging the duties of Chairman. Secretary for ten years he had the unique distinction of being the first President since 1763 to hold office for five consecutive years.

To quote another Past-President, Dr Edwin Bramwell, Sir Robert Philip's name 'is to be included among the masters of medicine . . .'.[96]

A NOTABLE BICENTENARY

Happily a spirit of utmost good-will prevailed at the time of the Bicentenary of the Faculty of Medicine in the University of Edinburgh. This was in 1926. The College was able to be of some slight service to the Faculty. At the time Professor Lorrain Smith was Dean of the Faculty. Those who knew him will recognize his philosophy and unadorned graciousness in the following letter dated 16th June 1926 and addressed to the President of the College.

'Dear Mr. President
The Members of the Faculty at the last meeting gave me the very pleasing duty of expressing to the Royal College of Physicians their appreciation and thanks for the service the College rendered to the Faculty in the recent Bicentenary Celebration. That the College has contributed to the prosperity of the Faculty from the foundation in 1726 till now was realised anew by everyone who took part in the celebration and the gathering at dinner in the College on the evening of Friday, 10th June in maintaining and promoting the old established bonds was both memorable and pleasing.
Yours sincerely
(Signed) J. Lorrain Smith.[97]
Dean'

Truly there had prevailed the spirit of *Floreat res medica.*

A DISTINGUISHED VICE-CHANCELLOR

An event of equally delightful significance took place on 14th June 1972. On that day, having accepted an offer of Honorary Fellowship by the College Sir Michael Swann, Vice-Chancellor of the University of Edinburgh, signed the Promissory Roll. He was the first Vice-Chancellor of the University to be so honoured and, fortuitously but most happily, had been accorded the accolade of Knighthood only a few days previously. Signing of the Roll was followed by dinner with members of Council and a few other Fellows. Sir Michael replied to the President's toast of the newly admitted Honorary Fellows who included Sir Stanley Davidson and Lord Erskine of Rerrick. His felicitous speech dwelt upon the growth of ties which linked University and the College, was unmarred by a single historical inaccuracy, and revelled in not a few subtle sallies directed towards the medical profession, past, present and future![98]

In retrospect it can be said that none of the corporate bodies involved in the earlier events described have reason to be satisfied with, much less boastful of, their methods or all their accomplishments. Historical evidence points to the predominance of selfish vested interests over concern for the common weal of medical education and medical progress. In this the College can lay claim to no more innocence than those against whom they were arraigned for different reasons. This the vast majority of, if not all, Collegiate Fellows would acknowledge. The rights and wrongs are no subject for discussion in this day and age, least of all by one with long-standing loyalties to College, University and Town.

REFERENCES

(1) GRANT, Sir A. (1884) *The Story of the University of Edinburgh*, vol. I, p. 245. London: Longmans, Green & Co.

(2) HANNAY, R. K. (1933) The foundation of the college of Edinburgh. In *History of the University of Edinburgh, 1833–1933*. Turner, A. L., ed. p. 16. Edinburgh: Oliver & Boyd.

(3) GRANT, Sir A. Op. cit., p. 217.

(4) Ibid., p. 220.

(5) R.C.P.E. (1686) *Miscellaneous Papers*, no. 71.

(6) POOLE, R. (1838) *Preparatory Notes for a History of the College*, p. 76. (Ms.)

(7) Ibid., p. 73.

(8) Ibid., p. 71.

(9) GRANT, Sir A. Op. cit., pp. 223–4.

(10) Ibid., pp. 224–5.

(11) BOWER, A. (1817) *The History of the University of Edinburgh*, vol. II, p. 127. Edinburgh: Oliphant, Waugh & Innes.

(12) Ibid., p. 128.

(13) Ibid., p. 132.

(14) College Minutes, 13.vii.1704.

(15) Ibid., 19.vii.1705.

(16) POOLE, R. Op. cit., pp. 251–3.

(17) Ibid., p. 255.

(18) Ibid., pp. 255–6.

(19) Ibid., pp. 253–4.

(20) Ibid., p. 256.

(21) Ibid., p. 5.

(22) Ibid., p. 6.

(23) BOWER, A. Op. cit., vol. II, p. 149.

(24) GRANT, Sir A. Op. cit., vol. I, p. 296.

(25) Ibid., vol. II, p. 392.

(26) BOWER, A. Op. cit., vol. II, p. 126.

(27) EDINBURGH. City corporation (1720) *Town Council Register*, 24.viii.1720. Vol. XLVIII, p. 204.

(28) BOWER, A. Op. cit., vol. II, p. 178.

(29) COMRIE, J. D. (1932) *History of Scottish Medicine*, 2nd Edition, vol. I, p. 295. London: Baillière, Tindall & Cox.

(30) GRANT, Sir A. Op. cit., vol. II, p. 386.

(31) FORSTER, J. (1863) *Life and Times of Oliver Goldsmith*, 4th Edition, p. 33. London: Chapman & Hall.

(32) INGLIS, J. A. (1911) *The Monros of Auchenbowie*, p. 74. Edinburgh: Constable.

(33) GRANT, Sir A. Op. cit., vol. I, p. 306.

(34) BOWER, A. Op. cit., vol. II, p. 199.

(35) College Minutes, 21.xi.1723.

(36) PORTERFIELD, W. (1759) *A Treatise on the Eye*. 2 vols. Edinburgh: G. Hamilton & J. Balfour.

(37) BOWER, A. Op. cit., vol. II, p. 203.

(38) GRANT, Sir A. Op. cit., vol. I, p. 308.

(39) Ibid., pp. 309–10.

(40) BOWER, A. Op. cit., vol. II, p. 212.

(41) GRANT, Sir A. Op. cit., vol. I, p. 311.

(42) Ibid., p. 314.

(43) CULLEN, W. (1791) *First Lines of the Practice of Physic*, vol. I, Preface, pp. 28–9. Edinburgh: Bell & Bradfute.

(44) COMRIE, J. D. Op. cit., vol. I, p. 299.

(45) BOWER, A. Op. cit., vol. II, p. 216.

(46) Ibid., p. 257.

(47) Ibid., pp. 219–20.

(48) GRANT, Sir A. Op. cit., vol. I, pp. 330 f.

(49) UNIVERSITY OF EDINBURGH (1867) *List of the Graduates in Medicine in the University of Edinburgh, from 1705 to 1866*. Edinburgh: Neill.

(50) GRANT, Sir A. Op. cit., vol. I, pp. 331–2.

(51) BOWER, A. Op. cit., vol. II, p. 217.

(52) Ibid., p. 219.

(53) GRANT, Sir A. Op. cit., vol. I, p. 330.

(54) [STUART, W. J.] [1949] *History of the Aesculapian Club*, p. 22. [Edinburgh: Aesculapian Club.]

(55) GRANT, Sir A. Op. cit., vol. II, p. 7.

(56) Ibid., p. 9.

(57) Ibid., p. 14.

(58) COMRIE, J. D. Op. cit., vol. II, p. 487.

(59) GRANT, Sir A. Op. cit., vol. II, p. 55.

(60) CHRISTISON, Sir R. (1885) *The Life of Sir Robert Christison, Bart.*, vol. I, p. 322. Edinburgh: Blackwood.

(61) GRANT, Sir A. Op. cit., vol. II, p. 44.

(62) Ibid., p. 40.

(63) Ibid., p. 66.

(64) CHRISTISON, Sir R. Op. cit., vol. I, p. 323.

(65) GRANT, Sir A. Op. cit., vol. II, pp. 70–71.

(66) CHRISTISON, Sir R. Op. cit., vol. I, p. 329.

(67) GRANT, Sir A. Op. cit., vol. II, p. 71.

(68) CHRISTISON, Sir R. Op. cit., vol. I, p. 285.

(69) Ibid., p. 69.

(70) 21 and 22 Victoria, c. 83. (1858).

(71) CHRISTISON, Sir R. Op. cit., vol. II, p. 39.

(72) Ibid., p. 77.

(73) GRANT, Sir A. Op. cit., vol. II, p. 110.

(74) College Minutes, 3.xi.1789.

(75) Ibid., 13.xi.1789.

(76) Ibid., 4.ii.1873.

(77) Ibid., 6.v.1873.

(78) Ibid., 7.viii.1877.

(79) Ibid., 26.xii.1884.

(80) Ibid., 4.ii.1885.

(81) 31 and 32 Victoria, c. 48. (1867–8).

(82) GRANT, Sir A. Op. cit., vol. II, p. 167.

(83) College Minutes, 21.v.1866.

(84) Ibid., 7.viii.1866.

(85) Ibid., 22.vi.1858.

(86) Ibid., 29.iii.1860.

(87) Ibid., 14.v.1860.

(88) Ibid., 6.v.1884.

(89) Ibid., 18.iii.1884.

(90) R.C.P.E. (1894) *Letter Book*, 10.ii.1894.

(91) Council Minutes, 29.iii.1921.

(92) Ibid., 26.iv.1921.

(93) Ibid., 3.i.1962.

(94) WILLIAMS, H. (1974) Personal communication.

(95) NATIONAL ASSOCIATION FOR THE PREVENTION OF TUBERCULOSIS (1957) *Sir Robert W. Philip, 1857–1939: memories of his friends and pupils.* London: N.A.P.T.

(96) Ibid., p. 17.

(97) College Minutes, 20.vii.1926.

(98) Ibid., 20.vi.1972.

Chapter XIX

DISPUTATION, VITUPERATION AND, ON OCCASIONS, RECONCILIATION

The Demon of Discord with her sooty wings had breathed her influence upon our Counsels.
Tobias Smollett (*Roderick Random*)

O wad some Pow'r the giftie gie us
To see oursels as others see us!

Robert Burns

Essentially the physician is an individualist—even in an age of biochemistry and bio-engineering. Had it been otherwise some new, as yet unheard of discipline, far removed from the art of the physician, might be dominating the world of healing. Closely allied to individualism is the badinage beloved of the Scot. Badinage can stimulate, but when carried to excess or used as a means of expressing superiority it can lead to strife and on occasion to prolonged irreconcilable feud. These have been characteristics of the College over its approaching 300 years history. Throughout these years personalities outstanding for whatever reason have surfaced and not been submerged. Inevitably there have been violent disputations, and even physical broils: emotions in private have found expression in extreme form, usually to be followed by amnesty and reconciliation. Such events have always been seen out of perspective, and acquired undue prominence. Some were in a corporate sense internal in origin; others arose as a result of external factors. Incompatible personalities, administrative conflicts or both at times dominated the picture. Rarely disagreements and anim-adversions merit recording, not because of the persons involved, but because of the gravity or complexity of the reasons giving rise to them. Even they have to be seen in perspective—and should not be regarded as unique in any one Corporation's history. It is no exaggeration to say that major events of this kind have been recorded in the histories of every ancient medical Corporation.

SIMMERING CAULDRON OF THE 1690s

> . . . *Men began not to philosophise till they had experienced the Operations of Remedies, and till they could with Security, and at their Leisure, search into the Relations of things, and emulate each other in intellectual Endowments.*
>
> Archibald Pitcairne

> *Double, double toil and trouble;*
> *Fire burn, and cauldron bubble.*
>
> William Shakespeare (*Macbeth*)

Disagreements of a serious, even violent nature, occurred early in the history of the College—to be precise within ten years of the Charter being granted. Unquestionably opposed personalities entered the picture but retrospective judgments are prone to prejudice. This is only too evident in many of the studies of military and naval leaders in the two world wars. Considering events in the College towards the end of the seventeenth century, the situation is further complicated by the total absence of Minutes from 22nd November 1684 to 21st March 1693—a period of particular relevance to the disagreement under consideration.

THE BACKGROUND

Contributory factors were several and knowledge of the background is necessary for an understanding. While the College as a whole was involved, certain of the Fellows were more immediately implicated. These included Sir Archibald Stevensone, Sir Robert Sibbald and Drs Robert Trotter, Archibald Pitcairne, Charles Oliphant, George Hepburn and (Sir) Edward Eizat. With the exception of the last named all were Fellows in the original patent, Pitcairne being the youngest. The major part played by Sibbald in the establishment of the College has been described (Chap. III). He was the second President (elected in 1684). Trotter had two periods in office as President—being elected in 1694 and again in 1700. Stevensone, Sibbald and Trotter had in common that they had each studied in Leyden, Sibbald having previously attended University classes in Paris and Angers. A Master of Arts at Edinburgh

University, Pitcairne studied in succession divinity and law, and then took up medicine in Paris before obtaining a Doctorate of Medicine at Rheims University. Returning to Edinburgh he rapidly acquired an enviable reputation but in 1692 accepted an invitation to be Professor of Medicine at Leyden University, from which he resigned a year later for domestic reasons, and resumed practice in Edinburgh. According to the *Acta* of Leyden University, Pitcairne's letter of resignation prompted the academic authorities to dismiss him on the score of improper conduct and of departing for Scotland without notice or leave.[1] A son-in-law of Archibald Stevensone, Pitcairne had early in his career devoted much time to the mastery of mathematics which paved the way to his eventually founding with Borelli and others the iatro-mathematical or iatro-mechanical school of thought. Oliphant, Hepburn and Eizat were relatively junior Fellows having been elected in 1694, 1695 and 1696 respectively, the first named being on friendly terms with Pitcairne.

Treatment of Fever

There was another doctor who, although on the fringe, was very much involved. He was Dr Andrew Brown of Dolphinton in Lanarkshire, an admirer of Sydenham under whom he had studied for a number of months. Brown was certainly not a Fellow of the College and it is doubtful if he possessed their Licence which was not required in order to practise in his area. Despite his lack of connection with the College he managed to provoke discussion within its walls when he published a modest book entitled *A Vindicatory Schedule concerning the New Cure of Fevers*.[2] That was in 1691. Brown's ardent advocacy of evacuant remedies, especially blood letting, the use of active purgatives, and occasionally emetics stirred up professional controversy which was to persist for a number of years, more especially among those accustomed to employ 'diluents, . . . saline medicines, clysters [and] very gentle diaphoretics . . .'.[3] For Brown, vomiting had a value in eliminating poisonous material; and horse-riding in 'jogging the humours'.[4] In general the reaction of Edinburgh physicians was actively antagonistic[5]; his doctrines were strenuously opposed; and he himself was reproached with being an Aberdeen graduate. An element of jealousy may well have played its part because it was common knowledge that patients unable to see him in town travelled to Dolphinton for advice. Pamphlets and tracts appeared in abundance. There are in the College Library no fewer than fourteen pamphlets published between 1691 and 1700 either advocating or condemning Brown's recommendations. In terms of intemperate bitterness and vulgarity of language there was nothing to differentiate those issued by his opponents and those published by Brown[6, 7] and his supporters.

Stirring the Pot

This was the prevailing atmosphere when Pitcairne, returned from Leyden in 1693, added fuel to the fire with the publication within two years of a treatise on the *Treatment of Fevers*.[8] Evacuant remedies constituted the basis of his recommendations and while his theorizing had some originality the treatment he advocated differed little from that already associated with the names of Sydenham and Brown. Such attention as the treatise received was probably due as much to the eminence of the writer as to the clinical value of the material. Critics were not long in appearing. A particular target for their denunciation was Pitcairne's mathematical interpretation of physiological functions. This attitude was crystallized in the appearance of a pamphlet entitled *Apollo Mathematicus, or the Art of Curing diseases by the Mathematicks, etc. according to the principles of Dr. Pitcairn*.[9] Produced anonymously it was scathing in the extreme, but rendered ineffective by its uninhibited coarseness of expression. The author soon came to be recognized as Sir Edward Eizat.

Pamphlets and Personalities

Apollo Mathematicus prompted rapid retaliation not from Pitcairne, but from a recently elected Fellow and supporter of Pitcairne, Dr George Hepburn. Retaliation took the form of a pamphlet bearing the title *Tarrugo Unmasked*.[10] Publication was in 1695. The title was in the nature of a parody of a self-styled comic opera published in 1668.[11] Unmasking by Hepburn consisted in endeavouring 'to expose the cunning and address of Sir Edward Eizat in studying to attain his objects as a medical practitioner'.

College Authority Questioned

At a meeting of the College on 7th November 1695 it was reported that 'yr was a pamphlet written by a fellow of ye colledge wt out a license from ye colledge' and a Committee was appointed to investigate.[12] The following week the Committee gave it as their opinion that 'several positions in ye pamphlet' were 'censurable', a view with which the College agreed 'by plurality of votes'. The author was 'cited to appear before ym . . . to answer to what is libelled against him' on the 22nd of the month.[13] In the meantime at a meeting on 18th November a protest was presented by Pitcairne in his own name and that of others alleging incompetence on the part of the President and other Fellows to sit and vote as Fellows. Pitcairne's action has been interpreted as an attempt to call a halt to the emotional consequences of Hepburn's pamphlet.[14]

Hepburn appeared as directed, on 22nd November; acknowledged his authorship of the offending pamphlet[15]; and was ordered to be served with a libel in the following month when 'the Colledge yrupon did remove him as ipso facto suspended from siting or voting and so is to continue untill he satisy ye Colledge'.[16] Pitcairne had been previously suspended for totally different reasons on the fateful 22nd November. His protest had been adjudged 'a calumnious scandalous false and arrogant paper refuseing ye authority of ye president and colledge and contrair to the promissory engagement'.[15] The fact that a majority of Fellows present voted in favour of his suspension, forestalled Pitcairne's intention to cast doubts on the eligibility of the President and certain other Fellows to vote at the pending annual election on 5th December.

THE CAULDRON ERUPTS

In accordance with statute the Fellows met on 5th December to elect office-bearers. At a meeting two days previously the Treasurer (Dr Oliphant) was given precise instructions to disburse no funds except as required by the President.[16] The following day, the day before the annual election, Dr Oliphant was suspended for failure to produce his accounts: and it was carried unanimously 'yt noe person nor member qtsomever have liberty to vote in ye colledge till they own ye authority of ye president and colledge as presently constitute conforme to ye promissory Engadgement . . .'.[17] These measures were obviously intended to forestall trouble at the election meeting. They were further reinforced by the presence at the meeting of 'one of the Baillies, and one or more of the Town Officers' who as events turned out gave assistance in removing the suspended Pitcairne and his supporters intent on recording their votes. Proceedings were far from uneventful. In subsequent years they were referred to, by those present at the time, as the Riot in the College[18] and there can be little doubt that the scenes were violent perhaps even to the point of baillies' wigs

flying. Of necessity the meeting was held not in the College, but in the lodgings of
the President for the previous year, Dr Trotter. Mention in the Minutes is limited to:

> 'The qlk day the Colledge chosed Sr. Thomas Burnet Sr Robt Sibbald Drs Trotter
> Sinclair Cranstoune Mitchell Dicksone to be counsellors for this year and they
> removeing to another Room choose Dr. Trotter president, Drs Mitchell and
> dicksone censors, Dr Dundas secretary and Dr ffreir treasurer for the ensewing year,
> Robert Trotter wryter to the signet was chosen clerk, Robert Maisterton wryter
> in Edgr pror fiscall and Coline Scott was continewed officer.'[19]

No indication in that phlegmatic record that the simmering cauldron had erupted!
Evicted, Pitcairne and his friends had gone straightway to the dwelling of Sir
Archibald Stevensone and forthwith elected him President for the ensuing year. If
there had been any pretence at concealing the cleavage within the College this had
now been removed. There was in effect open warfare between two factions—on the
one side those constituting the majority included Sir Thomas Burnet, Sir Robert
Sibbald, Dr Trotter, Dr Sinclair and Dr Cranstone: on the other, Sir Archibald
Stevensone and Drs Pitcairne, Eccles, Dicksone and Oliphant among others.

Examinators: Bones of Contention

Quite apart from the litigious pamphleteering which accompanied prolonged controversy on the treatment of fevers the two factions within the College were in
direct opposition over another matter. This concerned the selection of 'examinators'
for candidates applying for the Licence of the College by examination. It had been
the original intention of the College that Examinators should be appointed as each
candidate presented himself. However during the years for which no Minutes are
available the custom had developed of nominating Examinators to hold office for an
entire year covering the period intervening between successive annual elections. The
subject was raised at a College meeting in September 1695—'it being put to the vote
whither the old Law anent the examination of intrants as it was at the first errection
or the new law appoynting examinators for a whole year together should be observed
in tyme comeing it was caried by the plurality that the old law should be observed
and the new abrogate'.[21]

Neither Stevensone nor Pitcairne was present at any of the three readings of the
Act.[20-22] These two excepted, the original Fellows were in favour of restoration of
the old order, whereas recently elected Fellows preferred yearly nomination of

Examinators. Stevensone was adamant in his attitude, doubtless being encouraged in his habitual obduracy by his pertinacious and abundantly confident son-in-law. It was at this time that Stevensone, who lived in the same building as that in which the College had its meeting place, 'denyed ye keyes of the College'. Alternative accommodation was found in Dr Trotter's lodgings and on 16th September 1695 the Act resuscitating the original method of appointing Examinators was read a third time.

At a later date Stevensone dealt with events in some detail as he saw them, almost certainly in emotionally prejudiced fashion. In his *Information* prepared for submission to the Courts in defence of himself 'and the other Physitians who adhere to him ... when they were pursued by Doctor Trotter before the Lords of His Majesties most Honourable Privy Council' he protested that he and those who joined him thought to have suppressed these 'angry Sparks ... before they should break out into a Flame'. Prevailing animosities were he maintained 'crystallised' by 'Dr. Trotter who has done the wrong, makes the loudest Complaint, and Dr. Stevinson most lesed makes least noise'. Continuing Stevensone stated that 'having signified in anno 1694, that he would continue no longer President, Doctor Burnet was proposed as the fittest person to succeed, both for his Age and Experience; but he declining the Offer made by Doctors Stevinson and Dickson in Name of the Colledge, Dr. Trotter came to be considered as next in Seniority, but Doctor Dickson having insinuate that he had good "Ground to believe that the making Doctor Trotter President might be displeasing to Authority", they had some thoughts to turn the Election another way.' Tortuous manoeuvres it would seem—without hint of Dr Trotter's sins of omission or commission and without specification of the 'authority' not to be offended.

No matter, anxious to protect Dr Trotter from 'Affront or Disappointment', Dr Stevensone claimed to have 'procured him to be chosen President' and from that moment Stevensone seems to have seen in Trotter something approaching the devil incarnate. According to Stevensone the meeting which culminated in 'the Ryot' was called 'on a Saturnday' entirely contrary to precedent: the meeting itself was 'pack't', implying thereby something akin to what in modern slang would be termed 'rigged': and 'there was never any Magistrat of Edinburgh present at any Election before'.

> The Declaration described also, how 'Dr. Pitcairn was Removed by the Town of Edinburghs Officers, after having protested against the Violence used against him, three other Members also pretended to be Suspended were pointed at, and the Bailie desired to Remove them, but they thought fit to prevent the hard usage their Colleague had mett with, and with the Plurality of the College did withdraw

to Dr. Stevinson's house, and there unanimously Elected him President in the usual form and manner, and did also Constitute the other Officers of the College.

'This Election being free and Legal, Dr. Stevenson with the Censors and others came to the Ordinary place of Meeting to Intimate the Election, but finding Dr. Trotter there and the other Physicians removed, the Chair emptie and the Books on the Table, Dr. Stevenson having signified to Dr. Trotter that he was Chosen President by the pluralitie of the Colledge, took Possession of the Chair by way of Instrument in the Clerks hands, and Dr. Trotter going about to carry away the Books, he was hindred, but without any Force or Violence, for some he let fall on the Floor, and others he threw down on the Table.

'This was no Ryot, for by an Act of the Colledge, the Books and other Evidents, are ordained to be keept in a Press there, but Dr. Stevinson not finding the Key, was obliged to cause carry them to his own House, to be keeped there until they should be Ordered to be delivered to the President and Members who should be found to have best Right thereto,

'This is the Ground of all this Clamour of a grievous and unaccountable Riot, . . .'.[23]

The crux of the legal problem posed was, who in law was President—Dr Trotter or Dr Stevensone?

Personalities

It is scarcely credible that disagreement over such a relatively minor point should create a conflict capable of rocking the very foundations of the College. There are those who consider such to be the case and they have support for their views in the baronially autocratic action of Stevensone. Others suggest that disagreement over fever therapy was the root cause of Collegiate troubles. True the literary polemics indulged in suggest an almost satanic mutual contempt, but it was after the manner of the time for pamphlets to justify themselves by vituperation disguised as wit. What appears more likely is that a simultaneous accumulation of provocative factors explained the storm which eventuated. For practical purposes the simmerings about fevers and those about examinations synchronized. Then, as now and ever, personalities tipped the scale from restrictive reason to fiery petulance. Sibbald and Pitcairne were the principal actors on the stage. While each respected the ability of the other, latterly there was no amity lost between them. Pitcairne was well aware of an intellectual advantage. Bower goes so far as to say 'the epigram on Sibbald, after his death, clearly demonstrates the contempt in which Pitcairn held him'.[24]

Not all Bower's statements concerning the two men are altogether accurate. Moreover Bower makes no effort to hide his admiration for Pitcairne and to that extent his opinions are open to question. For the sake of historical completeness rather than strict accuracy, Bower's appreciation of Sibbald must be mentioned. 'Sibbald' he wrote 'appears to have been open and undesigning; like all weak men, fond of flattery, but attached to science; and his labours in this respect were most indefatigable.'[25] There is further evidence of Bower's supposedly misinformed bias in his statement that 'Sir Andrew Balfour and Dr. Sibbald, whose exertions for the advancement of medical science deserve . . . to be mentioned . . . ; but their labours were not be be compared with those of Dr. Pitcairn'.[26]

Resentment at Sibbald's reasonably expressed doubts about Pitcairne's application of geometry to physic prompted the latter to attack Sibbald's *Prodromus Historiae Naturalis Scotiae* with characteristic invective.[27] Nor can differences in religious outlook be wholly ignored. Admittedly there is no recorded evidence to suggest that these were a source of personal conflict. None the less, in a country so subject to political and religious strife, it seems not unreasonable to wonder if personal relationships were not influenced on the one hand by Pitcairne's oft strongly avowed leanings to episcopacy and the Jacobite cause, and on the other by Sibbald's denominational vacillations and temporary espousal of Roman Catholicism. Certainly the circumstances surrounding Sibbald's sudden exit from Edinburgh in 1686 heralded a decline in his overall influence on the policy of the College.

Of Pitcairne, Chambers wrote that 'professedly an Episcopalian' he 'allowed himself a latitude in wit which his contemporaries found some difficulty in reconciling with any form of religion'.[28] Whatever his denomination he successfully petitioned for the 'seat in the Tron Kirk formerly possessed by Sir Archibald Stevenson'.[29] Although popular he could be ribald and scurrilous as an author. His custom was to meet doctors and see patients in a fashionable tavern in the neighbourhood of St Giles.[30] Whatever their incompatibilities both Sibbald and Pitcairne were intense individualists of the kind which sound medical teaching nourishes, which has contributed to the greatness of many teaching schools, but which has rarely jeopardized the spirit of Fellowship so symbolic of medical Corporations.

Regardless of the fundamental cause of the strife, the repercussions were serious for the College and its Fellows. The College had to enlist legal aid in order to compel Stevensone to hand over College property retained by him—including the key to the meeting house and papers among which was the manuscript of the Pharmacopoeia overdue, by no less than sixteen years, in being sent to the printers on the instructions of the College. Expense on an even larger scale was incurred in two Court of Session cases—one concerned with establishing the authority and rights of the College, the other in resisting a claim by Stevensone for a restitution of rights of which he and some of his supporters had been deprived. A Court decision in favour of the College was given in 1699.

These events were referred to in a Minute dated 6th November 1699. 'The said day the colledge taking into their serious consideration that Sir Archibald Stevensone, Master William Eccles, John Robertsone, John Smelholme and Andrew Melvill . . . having been found guilty of a Ryot about four years ago in a proces persued by the said Colledge against them before the Lords of his majestie's privie Councill In the prosecution of which process and of the colledges just right a great part of the public stock was consumed.' The Minute goes on to deplore the failure of the Fellows in question to respond to invitations to 'keep the meetings' and having referred to their 'manifest contempt' of the College Laws declared their suspension.[31] Towards the end of the same month the Treasurer was authorized to draw on College funds to pay outstanding debts incurred as a result of the Court proceedings.[32]

Peace Feelers

The New Year ushered in cautious promise of a return to harmony. On 31st January 1700 it was decided to lift the suspensions imposed in the previous November.[33] The name of Dr Oliphant, suspended previously and separately for contumacy of a different kind, was added to those offered reprieve. There was no mention of restitution for Dr Hepburn and it has been inferred that he had died an early death.[34] Removal of suspensions was conditional—'provydeing always the said persones compear and acknowledge the authority of the . . . colledge att any meeting yrof Betwixt and the 1st day of May next'.[33] But the time was not yet ripe for reconciliation. None took advantage of the proferred amnesty and on auld year's night 1702 the College were still seeking the advice of Advocates 'in defence of the Reduction and Declarator at Doctor Stevensone and oyrs yr instance against the Colledge'.[35]

Poole had an exceptional opportunity of studying College papers relevant to these times. He wrote in 1838 'A very considerable space would be needed for an exposition of the serious and really not creditable altercations which took place in the College between Sir Archd. Stevenson with his adherents on one side and Dr. Trotter with his on the other'. Then follows the exasperatingly tragic statement 'I have elsewhere gone somewhat fully into the matter for the information of Dr. Irving (Advocates' Librarian) with whom my notanda and some papers were temporarily deposited till he finished Memoirs of Dr. Pitcairn . . .'.[36] That Dr Irving was the Advocates' Librarian has been confirmed, and the existence of his Memoirs of Dr Pitcairn,[36a]

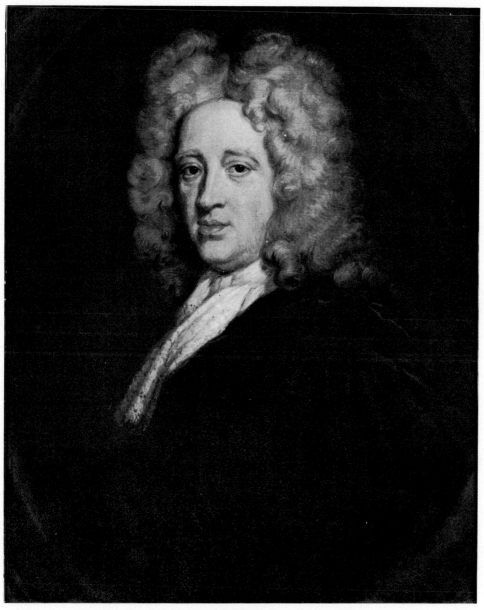

PLATE 27   Dr Archibald Pitcairne (1652–1713)
Reproduced from a copy in the College of original portrait by Sir John B. Medina;
photograph by Tom Scott

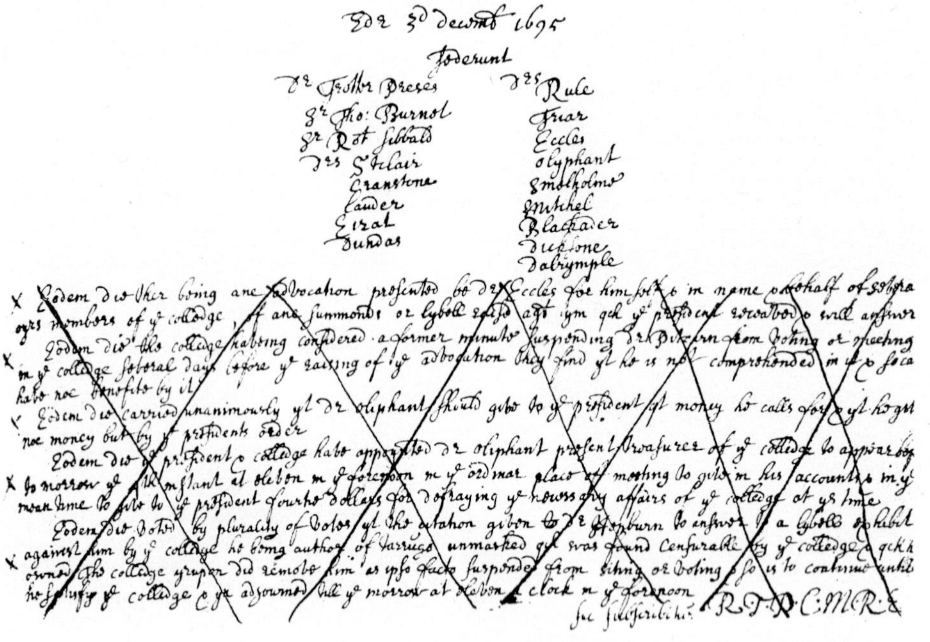

PLATE 28   College Minutes for 3rd December 1695 showing ineffective deletions
Reproduced from College Minutes

but no trace of the papers reputedly loaned by Poole has been found. There is an indication of the historical value of the papers in the following 'catalogue of documents' made by Poole at the time together with an added short memorandum:

'Charge. Dr. Oliphant
Letters of Horning by the Coll. against him 1696.
Information for Dr. Stevenson & others agt. Dr. Trotter and others.
Petition for Dr. Stevenson & others agt Dr. Trotter & others 1696.
Representation for Drs. agt. do.
Information for Drs. agt. Do. (printed paper)
Declaration by Sir Th. Burnet & Sir Robt. Sibbald against the present President etc. 1699.
Accompt of money disbursed &c for Dr. Stevenson &c.
Minutes of Lords in the debate etc. 1703.
Proposals for Dr. Stevenson and others etc.
  Memo. a few more left in hands of Dr. Irving (Advocates Librarn) with notanda [by Poole] . . . intended to aid his memoirs of Dr. Pitcairne etc. Mr. Small is aware of the fact and can claim for the College, when necessary.
        19.VI.1838.'[36]

Persistent bitter disharmony failed to dissuade the College from making a yet further attempt to restore unity in its ranks. On 7th January 1703 the Minutes recorded:

'The which day the Colledge of Physicians considering how desyrable a thing it is for the members thereof to leave in peace and unity and being sensible of the prejudice the Society has sustained by the late unhappy divisions and notwithstanding of the repeated offences committed against the said Colledge by the suspended members after named whereby the Colledge has been put to a vaste charge to assert its own priviledges yet to show to the world the Colledge's readiness to forgive injuries, and that nothing may be wanting on there part to restore the peace of the societie and in hopes the said suspended members by there after deportment will be ready upon all occasions to shew them selves more sensible of the obligations they lye under from the Promissory Ingadgement signed by all of them Thairfor the Colledge in consideratione of the premisis Doe hereby repeal the former acts of Suspensione made against Sir Archibald Stevensone, Maister Archibald Pittcairne, John Robertsone, William Eccles, Charles Olyphant, John Smelholme and Andrew Melville . . .'.[37]

'Ane act of oblivion'

Magnanimity did not reap immediate reward. For reasons unknown there is no record of another meeting for almost eleven months. This was not attended by any

P

Fellows who had been the subject of previous suspension.[38] The annual election meeting took place in December and those present included four prodigal members—Drs Robertsone, Eccles, Olyphant and Smelholme, of whom Drs Eccles and Smelholme were elected Councillors and appointed Censor and Treasurer respectively.[39] Reconciliation acquired momentum in the New Year. At the first meeting in 1704 a 'draught of ane act of oblivion' was presented by the President and accepted 'nemine contradicente'[40] being passed 'into ane act' by a unanimous vote at a subsequent meeting eight days later. By this Act 'to the end that no memory may remain of what is past' all Acts 'whereby any Censures were Inflicted' were 'not only Cassed and anulled, But lykewayes razed and Deleite out of the records'. A Committee which included Dr Eccles was appointed to revise the College records[41] and its recommendations were made 'patent in the Presidents Lodgeing for the satisfactione of any of the members that shall Desyre to sie . . .'.[42] The President reported in March that final effect had been given to the Committee's recommendations.[43]

Poole had some revealing comments to make. He recorded in 1838 'the Minutes relative to the context were ordered to be deleted, of course with a view to restoring and preserving harmony; but, notwithstanding crosses etc., they are legible enough in the old books, though not transcribed in Vol. III'.[36] Revision of College Minutes had not been accompanied by destruction of the original versions, as can be seen in the Minute Books (Numbers 1, 2 and 3) now in the College Library.

Does invocation of oblivion benefit the individual, or indeed posterity? As Sir Thomas Browne wrote 'the iniquity of oblivion blindly scattereth her poppy, and deals with the memory of men without distinction to merit of perpetuity'.[44]

UNITED AGAIN

St Andrew's Day, 30th November 1704 signalized reconciliation in its most convincingly tangible form. The occasion was the annual election day and was attended by twenty-four Fellows. The only absentees among those who had been suspended were Drs Hepburn, Melville and Smelholme.[45] As already mentioned, Hepburn was probably dead (q.v.). Smelholme who had returned to the fold a year previously, attended with Dr Melville at the next meeting on the day following the election sederunt.[46] Notable for their return on St Andrew's Day after prolonged absence for different reasons were Sir Robert Sibbald, Sir Archibald Stevensone and Doctor 'Pittcairne'. The two first named were among those chosen as Councillors as were Drs Eccles and Melville: and Dr Eccles was elected as one of the Censors and Dr

Smelholme as Treasurer. There is no evidence that past differences had been allowed to prejudice the interests and prospects of those banned until recently from participation in College affairs. One possible, indeed probable exception was the case of Dr Pitcairne. Some would say that he was at one and the same time the most able, the most impetuous and the most irreconcilably indiscreet in the ranks of Fellows—he was not appointed to any office at this time of reunion. No aspersion on Pitcairne is implied in saying that, in its efforts to consolidate restored stability, the College adopted a wise course.

Mention of Pitcairne would be incomplete without reference to a Harveian Oration delivered at Edinburgh in 1781 by a Dr Charles Webster on the subject of the *Life and writings . . . of . . . Pitcairne*. There is no reason to regard the Oration as in any way connected with the first centenary of the College. Indeed there is only one passing reference to the College from beginning to end of the speech. In the printed version for publication however, Dr Webster is described on the title page as 'Physician to the Public Dispensary, Of the Royal College of Physicians, Edinburgh: Of the Royal Society of Medicine, Paris etc.' The only Charles Webster appearing on the Roll of the College obtained his licentiate diploma only four years before, and was admitted as a Fellow of the College eight years after the date of the Oration. He was a graduate of the University of Edinburgh. These facts are given because no matter how impartial the reader may try to be, the Oration is impressive only in virtue of its superficiality and its sycophancy. Certainly some of the effusive praise bestowed upon Pitcairne was merited; but the opinions expressed concerning his attitude in Holland are markedly at variance with views held elsewhere, and limitation of any mention of the College to Pitcairne's name 'gracing the original patent', points to inadequate treatment of the subject.[47]

POLEMICS AND POWDER

Wisdom has taught us to be calm and meek
To take one blow, and turn the other cheek:
It is not written what a man shall do,
If the rude caitiff smite the other too!

Oliver Wendell Holmes

One of, if not the most unsavoury event in the history of the College was a period of open warfare between the College and one of its eminent members, Dr James

Gregory. The term 'open warfare' is no exaggeration. Indeed the words are those of Dr James Gregory himself who, admonished for his undisguisedly aggressive condemnation of the College, proclaimed 'Since the College will have war, they shall have war, and that not secret but open war.'[48] There is significance in his use of the term 'secret' because, for a period extending over a number of years prior to this outburst, Gregory had indulged in a series of vicious if clandestine guerrilla attacks on the College and on those of his collegiate 'brethren' who had undeservedly roused his personal animosity.

It is not for a history written almost two hundred years after the events to define Gregory's motives. His own explanations provide little evidence that is reliable because of the extent to which he gave rein to his unbridled emotions, indulged in rhetoric intended to confuse, and resorted to ingenious but inaccurate use of facts. This is not to deny he was a compulsive writer of immense versatility. His eruptive violence, his impetuosity and his apt use of biblical quotations for pungent purpose were on a par with those of the World War I personality First Sea Lord Admiral Fisher of Keddlestone. But whereas Fisher never forgot that brevity is the soul of wit, Gregory was prolix, verbose and discursive.

A COLLEGE DILEMMA

Of greater importance than Gregory's motives was the College's policy in restricting the professional activities of Fellows and Licentiates. This apparently was the initial subject of disagreement. It had long proved a thorny problem for the College anxious to consolidate the position and status of the physician as distinct from those of the surgeon, while at the same time aware of the widening general interests of the surgeon–apothecary. The problem was further complicated by the fact that members of the College at the time under consideration were of several kinds—Licentiates and Fellows, the Fellows for their part being resident or non-resident according as they were or were not on the College Roll of Attendance. Residence implied practising within the geographical area of jurisdiction of the College as defined in the Charter of Erection. Of Licentiates the majority practised outside Edinburgh, and the activities of many in Scotland and England were the equivalent of the general practitioners of later generations.

During the latter half of the eighteenth century the College passed a succession of relevant enactments, which almost without exception were passed only after long and lively debate. College perplexities were reflected in the hesitancy and indeed contradictoriness of some of the Laws in question. Initially an incisive, unequivocal line was taken when in 1750 an Act was passed ruling that 'no person who is a member of the Corporation of Surgeons or appothecarys, Or who keeps a Shop for Dispensing of Medicines Shall hereafter be admitted a fellow of the Colledge'. It was further decreed that anyone who after admission to the College infringed these particular regulations would 'forfeit all the priviledges . . . as a fellow . . . And his name shall be Expunged out of the Roll of Fellows.'[49] Over forty years previously an earlier Act passed to render effectual separation between physician and surgeon, had to be signed by all members, a practice which apparently fell into abeyance about 1756.[50, 51]

In 1754 yet another Act, which in years to follow was to be the subject of much acrid discussion was passed with the clearly declared object of preventing anyone from combining the professions of Medicine and Pharmacy. By way of justification the Act stated that 'ane Innovation and abuse has been Lately Introduced into the manner of practiseing Physick within this City whereby Some Physicians Licenced and authorised by the . . . Colledge to Practise Physick have also acted as apothecarys by keeping or Setting up appothecarys shops . . .'. To prevent this it was enacted that no member of 'the said Colledge, nor any Physician by them Licenced . . . to practise physick within the . . . City and its Libertys, Shall take upon himself, to use the Employment of ane appothecary, Or to have and keep ane apothecarys shop, by himself his partners, or Serts . . .'. At the same time it was declared that all applicants for a Licence to practise Physick in the City of Edinburgh and suburbs would be obliged to give an undertaking not to set up an apothecary's shop and 'not to practise Pharmacy by himself, Co-partners or Servants'.[52]

Hesitant Liberalism

Experience demonstrated the ineffectiveness of the Act of 1754 and Dr Cullen was instrumental in getting the College to appoint a Committee to investigate the position.[53] The Committee reported at the next Quarterly Meeting. Sixteen members were present and unanimously approved 'ane advertisement which they [the Committee] thought would be proper for the College to Publish', and 'appoint the Same to be published in each of the Edinburgh news papers for Two Several times'. With terse clarity the advertisement summarized the views and action taken by the College concerning the need for separation of the professions of medicine and pharmacy, and concluded with an intimation that the College 'are Resolved to prosecute . . . all Such who without their Licence shall . . . assume the title of Doctor of Physick, and prescribe for the Internal diseases of the Inhabitants of Edinburgh . . . and that they have unanimously determined, not to Consult with, or otherwise consider Such unlicensed practitioners, as Physicians'. Annexed was a List of 28 Fellows and 6 Licentiates.[54] Almost certainly the 'advertisement' of principles and purpose, and not of persons as the malevolent might suppose, would interest the reading public because in the interval between the passing of the 1754 Act and the insertion of the advertisement there had been two events of significance. The establishment of a dispensary by the College of Surgeons (Chap. X) and the rebuff administered to Mr—later Dr Eccles (Chap. VII). Meanwhile the attitude of the physicians to the surgeons showed no signs of relaxing and in 1763 without evident precise pretext it was ordained 'that no member of the Corporation of Surgeons in Edinr. while he Continues such shall hereafter be admitted a Licentiat or Fellow . . . And that if any Licentiat or Fellow shall become a member of the Corporation of Surgeons he shall forfeit his place of Licentiat and Fellow of the College'.[55]

And still the problem of conjoint medicine and pharmacy proved a source of uneasiness. Consideration by the Council had led to the conclusion that because the powers of the College to regulate the practice of medicine were limited to the City of Edinburgh there was no justification for modifying enactments relating to Licentiates. Fellows were regarded as entirely different and in so far as they were concerned they not only continued to be subject to the prohibitions contained in the Act of 1754 (q.v.), but they were subject in addition to an extension of the part of the Act prohibiting the practice of pharmacy 'within the three Kingdoms'.[56]

Restrictive policies continued to be applied with increasing vigour. Within about a year it was decided to debar from admission to the Fellowship any 'whose Common Business it is, either to practice Surgery in General, or midwifery, Lithotomy, Inoculation, or any other Branch of it'. At the same time it was decreed that any member convicted of practising 'any of these Lower Arts' after being received as a Fellow would be struck out of the Roll of Fellows. Again recourse was had to informing the public by advertisement in the newspapers of the College's Resolution.[57]

Four years later the prohibition of midwifery, lithotomy and manual operations of surgery already imposed on Fellows was extended to Licentiates, despite the registration in *sederunt* of dissent by among others, such senior Fellows as Drs William Cullen, Alexander Monro, John Gregory and Joseph Black. Those proposing the successful motion referred to 'abuse . . . Lately Introduced into the manner of Practiseing Physick . . . by Some Licenced Physicians who have acted Rather as

Surgeons than Physicians . . .'.[58] In 1765 the College had, when proposing new legislation, declared that one of their aims was 'to keep up that distinction which ought to be made between the members of the College and the Practitioners . . . of the healing art which have been allways esteemed the Least Reputable . . .'.[59] Continuing adherence to this attitude betrayed inadequate awareness of the clinical demands on many Licentiates. Cullen and his supporters formally presented their dissent to the Act of 1769 at a Quarterly Meeting on 7th November 1769.[60] Among reasons given for dissent were doubts concerning the economic position of Fellows and Licentiates who were practising surgery under powers previously conveyed by the College Licence; the impossibility of drawing 'an exact Line betwixt Physic and Surgery'; surprise with a policy which favoured joining the profession of surgery to the Apothecary rather than to the Physician; anxiety lest subspecialties be favoured to the detriment of general training; and failure to recognize the frequent inseparability of judgment in physic from the practice of midwifery. The dissenters regretted the prolonged nature of the dispute which they considered was contrary to the interest of the College. Little did they realize what lay ahead! The Committee to whom the Reasons for Dissent had been referred submitted lengthy Remarks in writing by way of reply.

At the meeting attempts were made to delay consideration of the Reasons for Dissent, but Dr Cullen with audacious deftness countered with a proposal that the Act which was the source of contention and which had been passed only nine months previously should be rescinded. Inevitably points of procedure were raised on the instant. The skill of the chairman (Sir Stuart Threipland—President) had already been put to the test earlier in the meeting and he did not conceal his chagrin at this second incident. None the less on a vote a decision to rescind was arrived at and the Law of 7th February 1769 declared 'void and null'.[60] Doubtless emboldened by this success Dr Cullen moved in the following year[61] that the Act of May 1765 (q.v.) be rescinded but the motion was rejected by a large majority.[62] In 1772 proposals were made on several occasions to repeal the law debarring the practice of midwifery by physicians and eventually the subject was remitted to a Committee. Although as a result the Law in question was amended, Fellows were still prohibited from taking part in surgical or midwifery practice.[63] Some fifteen years later the practice of midwifery again came up for special consideration.[64] A Committee appointed to study the matter admitted that restriction on midwifery practice 'has been so often transgressed without challenge as to lead to the opinion of its being obsolete'. Discussion in the College was lengthy and controversial but in the words of the Minutes 'a motion was at last made' and 'by a great majority' it was recommended that the

Resolution of 4th August 1772 should be repealed 'in so far as it prohibits the Members of the College from the practice of Midwifery'.[65] The recommendation became law in August 1788.[66]

What was the net result of the reviews and re-reviews of their Laws by the College in the years since the mid-eighteenth century? The practice of surgery continued to be prohibited, but that of midwifery was permitted. As to the practice of pharmacy the requirements of the enactment of 1754 (q.v.) remained effective. Additional to the atmosphere of uncertainty introduced into the College by interminable legal adjustments an element of querulousness had crept into proceedings without, however, any impairment of dignity or propriety in debate. An indirect result of repeated attempts to amend the Laws was an increasing tendency for debate to reveal an opposition of views as between senior and junior Fellows.

For a better appreciation of subsequent events it is, at this stage, worth asking where did James Gregory stand in this atmosphere of as yet politely but only partially muted conflict? In particular he was an enthusiastic advocate of the repeal of restrictions on the practice of midwifery and his vigorous support contributed considerably to the College decision in 1788 (q.v.).[67] Nor is it out of place to mention that Professor John Gregory, father of James and one time holder of the Chair of Medicine at Edinburgh University, had in his day shewn liberality in his support of those anxious to allow Licentiates to practise surgery and physicians to furnish medicines to their own patients.[68] It was the general opinion of the College that 'Dr. James Gregory was one of the most strenuous advocates for . . . relaxation of the acts 1750, 1765 and 1772' to which reference has already been made.[69]

To some extent the review of the 1772 Act was prompted by the findings of a Committee appointed in 1784 to review the standing Laws of the College with the ultimate objective of composing and publishing a Code of Laws.[70] The Committee's final Report was received in February 1787[71] and finally approved on 4th November 1788.[72]

The Fuse set Alight

On 2nd February 1796 Dr Thomas Spens moved 'that the Act of the College bearing date 11th April 1754 be repealed, in so far that every Fellow and Licentiate of the College may have it in his power to supply his own patients with medicines, or the patients of those with whom he may be conjoined in practice'.[73] After its third reading, the motion was adjourned to 'stand over untill some future contingency shall seem to render such a vote more necessary'.[74] There is little doubt that much disapproval of the motion was voiced in debate, and it is of interest that whereas the Minutes recorded that a vote was not insisted upon, the College *Narrative* stated that Dr Spens's proposal was 'supported by a majority of his Brethren'.[75]

Dr Spens was elected President on 1st December 1803.[76] In February of the following year he suggested that the Laws be reprinted and a Committee was appointed 'to revise the former Edition . . . and to make such alterations as might seem necessary'.[77] As a result of their deliberations on all the existing Laws of the College the Committee suggested amendments to the Act of 1754 (q.v.) among many other enactments. With regard to this particular Act the Committee reached a unanimous opinion only after a great deal of argument and counter-argument. They eventually concurred in 'thinking, that it might be expedient to permit the members, when they thought fit, to prepare and dispense medicines to their own patients, and also in doubting, whether the terms of this Bye-law, did actually debar them from so doing'. Rather than alter or repeal the Bye-law, the Committee preferred to deal with the element of dubiety by adding the following explanatory sentence viz. 'As doubts have been entertained respecting the purport and extent of the Act . . . , it is hereby declared, that the restrictions therein mentioned apply solely to such persons as keep or may set up Public apothecaries or druggists shops for the purpose of selling medicines by retail.'[78] A copy of the Laws and Regulations as revised by the Committee was laid on the table in August 1804[79] and was the subject of debate in November of the same year[80] and in February 1805.[81]

Rally of the Reactionaries

No matter the restraint exercised by those compiling the College *Narrative* there is no escaping the fact that opposition to this particular proposal was great, and the proceedings turbulent. The substance of the proposal was all too reminiscent of the motion submitted by Dr Spens in 1796, before his election as President. Such was the vehemence and intensity of the opposition that at the meeting in February 1805 the Committee 'having taken into consideration the wide difference of opinion which subsisted among the members' obtained leave 'once more to revise the Laws, in order to withdraw those parts of their Report which are likely to divide the College . . .'.[81] As events turned out the revised Report was never submitted to the College.[78]

'OPEN WAR'

Rather less than two months previously the Committee had made a point of advising those Fellows who had opposed the measure, of the Committee's intention to withdraw that part of their proposals which dealt with the Act of 1754 (q.v.). To quote the *Narrative* again—'As Dr. Gregory had expressed his disapprobation . . . in very decided terms, they took particular care to notify to him, that part of the report was to be withdrawn.'[78] Six weeks later towards the end of January 1805 Gregory unmasked his main armament and straddled his target—or rather his targets. His timing and tactics might well have provided a blue-print for Pearl Harbor almost a century and a half later. His ammunition consisted of what have been referred to as pamphlets. They were scarcely pamphlets in modern parlance. Both were printed on quarto paper. One entitled *Review of the Proceedings of the Royal College of Physicians in Edinburgh, from 1753 to 1804, both inclusive; with respect to separating the practice of medicine from the practice of pharmacy*'[82] extended to 32 pages: and the other entitled *Censorian Letter to the President and Fellows of the Royal College of Physicians in Edinburgh*[83] consisted of 142 pages. Later these publications were literally dwarfed with the appearance in 1811 of Dr Gregory's *Defence before the Royal College of Physicians, including a postscript protest and relative documents*[84] again on quarto, but on this occasion amounting to 700 pages. Distribution of the 'pamphlets' was Empire wide but probably not as extensive as Gregory had encouraged people to believe. Neither the College nor its Officials were favoured with official copies but some Fellows were given one in an essentially personal capacity. Distribution took place while revision of the Laws of the College were still under review.

Adroitness and the Unpardonable Sin

Gregory's accusations and insinuations were legion. He maintained that the Act of 1754 was a fundamental part of the College Constitution, that to repeal the Act would be contrary to the Law of the country, and that any relaxation of restrictions relating to dispensing would be immoral. No exception could be taken to a man of integrity adhering to such views no matter with how much tenacious conviction. The same cannot be said of the unrestrained criticisms levelled at the President and Committee revising the Laws on the score of their alleged falsehoods, duplicity, fraudulence, chicanery and manipulative unscrupulousness. Corporate Body and individual Fellows alike were deeply wounded by the allegation that modification of the Laws relating to pharmacy had been motivated by prospects of pecuniary gain. Nor was tolerance favoured by the nauseatingly unctuous attitude adopted by Gregory in his self-appointed task of incriminating those whom he continued to refer to glibly as 'brethren'. He did protest too much where the high-mindedness and purity of his own motives were concerned.

Nowhere was this more evident than in his *Censorian Letter*. The very use of the title is testimony to the artful alacrity of the author. It is true that in accordance with time-honoured procedure Dr Gregory had been elected Censor at the Annual Meeting in December 1803 and again in December 1804, but his interpretation of the functions of the office was certainly unique. The duties of the Censor, as described in the Charter of Incorporation consisted of ensuring that medicine was not practised in Edinburgh by anyone not in possession of a Licence from the College. Together the President and two Censors were authorized to sit as judges on unlicensed practitioners after giving notice to the Magistrates of Edinburgh who could then appoint a Baillie as assessor.[85] Dr Gregory presumed, in virtue of his office as Censor, to have authority to rebuke and arraign the College and its members. Overshadowing the whole unhappy series of events there was one irrefutable fact. In common with all Fellows of the College at the time of their election Dr Gregory had subscribed to a solemn Promissory Obligation to the effect that he would 'never divulge any thing that is acted or spoken in any meeting of the . . . College, or Council or Court thereof which' he thought 'may tend to the prejudice or defamation of the same or any Member thereof'.[86] The sin was the more heinous in that Gregory had held office as President of the College (1798–1801).

Ingenious Loyalty

Faced with an unparalleled dilemma the College was concerned to vindicate the characters of their injured brethren while at the same time betraying no official recognition of Dr Gregory's publications 'which were not regularly before them, having neither been sent to the College, nor to all the individual Members'.[87] At a Quarterly Meeting on 5th February 1805, attended by all members on the Roll with the one exception of Dr Gregory, a motion was approved by those present 'with the exception of one Member, who objected merely to the form of the motion'. The motion was to the effect that 'the College . . . are of opinion, however different the sentiments of the different members may be' upon the late revisal of the Laws, the

President 'has acted from the purest motives, and in the most honourable manner, and that he well deserves the thanks of the College'. A motion re-committing to the former Committee revision of the Laws for further review was then unanimously supported, thus making manifest the unimpaired confidence in which the Committee was held.[88] At a later date Gregory allowed that his absence from the meeting was deliberate,[89] and he adopted the view that far from being evidence of confidence in the President and the Reviewing Committee the motions were in effect an attack upon himself.

The amended Report of the Committee was debated at a series of meetings and finally approved in September 1805.[90] Adoption prompted one member to register a protest against confirmation of the Act of 1754 on among other grounds that combining the practice of medicine and pharmacy was not undesirable; the practice of pharmacy was not derogatory to the dignity of a physician; the Act imposed unwarranted restrictions on members; and that the function of bodies was not to confine members but to secure for them 'sole and exclusive exercise' of their calling.[91] There was further incontrovertible evidence of the feelings of the College towards the President when, in December 1805 they elected him for a third term of office—a procedure permissible only in the presence of special indications.

Circumspection and Confidence

'After the quarterly meeting in May 1805, Dr Gregory attended the Royal College as usual, and conducted himself at least quietly till towards the end of the year 1806.' These words are quoted from the College *Narrative*.[92] The lull was to prove a prelude to further storms. In the ordinary course of a Quarterly Meeting the President stated that 'he had by desire of the Council, to mention a circumstance, which the Council considered of much importance to the College, but which was not intended to have particular reference to what may have happened at any former period—The mention, out of doors, of what passes in any of the Meetings of the College, may be attended with most unpleasant and even prejudicial consequences both to individual members and to the College as a Body—The Council therefore take the liberty of recommending a strict observance of secrecy with regard to all such proceedings, and as they are convinced that any Gentleman must be sensible of the propriety and necessity of this measure, they trust that in future it will be rigidly adhered to.'[93]

The admonition was conveyed with complete dignity and without suggestion of specificity. No exception could be taken to the wording which had obviously been chosen with diplomatic correctitude and circumspection. And yet this exemplary presidential statement exposed the College to the full fury of a veritable hurricane. Gregory was not present at the meeting when it was made but at the next quarterly sederunt intimated that he had several queries which he wished to put to the College relative to the admonition.[94] It was soon unmistakably evident that he regarded the admonition as having been directed at him personally and as being part of a plot contrived by the Committee which had previously been the target for his own invective.[95] In actual fact, the comments made by the President at the instance of Council had no connection whatsoever with Gregory's past indiscretions and had been prompted by discussion by others of affairs connected with the visiting of apothecaries' shops.[92]

It is scarcely to be wondered at that about this time when writing to the Clerk concerning invitations to the College Breakfast, the President (Dr Charles Stuart) added a footnote that it would not under the circumstances be necessary to invite Dr Gregory![96]

A 'Kangaroo' Court in Reverse

The Minutes of 4th November 1806 record that after indicating that he had 'several queries . . . to put to the College relative to the admonition', Dr Gregory read them. Discussion followed and they were transmitted 'for consideration of the College, thro' the President and Council'.[97] There were sixteen queries in all. As an indication of their tenor reproduction of two will suffice:

> 'Query 6. Does the obligation of Secrecy extend and apply only to things positively dishonourable, done by this College, or acted or spoken by any of us individually in the meetings of this College, or Council and Court thereof?', and
> 'Query 16. Have our Office-Bearers contented themselves with thus endeavouring to bespeak the Secrecy and enforce the connivance, of the other Members of this College, with respect to things notoriously dishonourable?'

The sixteen queries were considered at a meeting in November and found to contain 'utterly groundless and unwarranted' imputations and accusations, and to be 'very disrespectful if not a direct Insult to the College'.[98] In the course of discussion and after himself referring to his *Review* and *Censorian Letter*, Dr Gregory denied all knowledge of any opinions expressed by the College about these publications. He continued to adhere to this after being shewn in the Minute Book the resolution passed on 5th February 1805.[99] Following his refusal to retract the offensive matters contained in the queries, Dr Gregory's indecorous and improper conduct was described as meriting 'very severe Censure from the College'.[100] As was to be expected Gregory protested against the vote of Censure and at the Quarterly Meeting on 5th May 1807 submitted a lengthy paper under the name of *Reasons of Protest*.[101]

Had the gravamen not been so serious, events thereafter might have been reasonably described as a burlesque. Deeply concerned for the dignity of the College, Members refused to be outraged by outrageous procedures and allowed the protester quite extraordinary latitude and consideration. The defendant for his part was his own worst enemy. He was incapable of halting either tongue or pen. His persistent malevolence was in keeping with a persecution-obsession and his incursions into astrology and metaphysics only served to introduce fantasy into the whole affair. Nor did he assist his case by the influence he seemed to exert on two Fellows both of whom, finding themselves awkwardly placed as witnesses, soon vanished permanently from the stage of College activities.

At the Quarterly Meeting in May 1807 Dr Gregory indicated that his protest was to be of two parts—one against the Admonition to Secrecy and the other against the vote of Censure, but that only the latter part was complete.[102] Three months later the Council was empowered by the College to obtain the advice of legal Counsel by whom they were to be directed. The response of Counsel to questions put to him may well have disconcerted the College. He considered an unequivocal answer to Dr Gregory in the first place might have prevented 'the agitation': and being hypothetical the queries chiefly giving offence 'arose from the nature of the Argument' and not with intent to insult the College. The concluding comment differed from the bewildering ramifications of modern legal presentation only in that punctuation was not lacking. Even so—it read strangely and unhelpfully:

> '. . . if he [Dr Gregory] . . . has shewn in the clearest manner, that the injunction itself, under every point of view, or, in every possible mode of interpretation, is better adapted to the Craft of a Corporation of Mechanics, than necessary as a rule of conduct to the Members of this College of Physicians . . . So far is his conduct in this respect from deserving censure, that on the contrary, it appears to me rather liberal and praiseworthy.'[103]

Ill-timed Burlesque

By his own testimony determined to lead the College into 'a trap', Dr Gregory attempted to do so in a way which would have done credit to an angler playing a salmon. In a letter read to the College in February 1807 he asked for and was granted extension of time until the next Quarterly Meeting before giving his reasons of protest.[104] By the date of the next meeting Gregory had indicated his intention to produce a second protest on the advice of his Counsel.[105] It was at this stage that the College were informed of their own Counsel's view (q.v.). At the Quarterly Meeting in November 1807 the President told of having received a letter of sixteen sheets from Dr Gregory only minutes before the Council Meeting; and a special meeting was arranged on a date specified to consider the letter and Dr Gregory's *Reasons for Protest*.[106] The day arrived; it was announced that the Council were unanimously of opinion that the 'length and prolixity' of the letter were 'such that to enter into a Minute consideration of it would be altogether inconsistent with the time which the meetings of the College should occupy and with the other engagements of its members'. Dr Gregory was 'desired in future to condense his arguments and to avoid the diffuse illustrations and the redundant expression with which his papers abound'. Having sat late considering Gregory's letter, the College arranged a further Extraordinary Meeting to hear his *Reasons of Protest*.[107] A meeting called by requisition on 5th December 1807 opened with a plea for adjournment by Dr Gregory who 'at same time put into the hands of the Clerk a sealed pacquet which he wished to remain unopened'.[108]

Eleven days later the College met 'according to adjournment' and after having by permission put questions to certain members, Dr Gregory stated he must submit his defence in writing for which he demanded many weeks. His expertise in framing questions would have won him laurels in the kangaroo courts of an age of industrial strife. The proceedings were described by Gregory in the presence of the College as 'a villanous Conspiracy against my fame and fortune, not by the College but by certain individuals'. He did however undertake to be ready with his defence at the Quarterly Meeting in February (1808) and not to indulge in the meantime in publications or appeals to the public.[109] At the Quarterly Meeting in question a letter was read from him stating that preparation of his defence was not yet complete although 'it was in considerable forwardness'. The writer was told 'his whole defence must be peremptorily given in on or before Saturday four weeks from this date'.[110] At a special meeting a month hence he explained his delay on the score of indisposition and urgent professional business, deposited copies of his defence to date promising the sequel and conclusions 'as soon as he was able to write them and get them printed'. For this last purpose he was granted some three to four weeks extension,[111] an 'indulgence' which later was extended for a further two months.[112] Prevarication continued and June 1808 found Dr Gregory 'very sorry to find himself again under the necessity of asking a week or two longer' while at the same time he transmitted 'no less than 112 additional pages' of his defence.[113] Surely a naïve form of olive branch!

Nevertheless although 'Dr. Gregory had already had no less than six months to prepare his defence, and that there had been six Meetings of the College during that period four of them Extraordinary Meetings for the express purpose, at each of which they expected to have received Dr. Gregory's defence complete, yet from the desire of shewing every indulgence to Dr. Gregory, agreed to grant the further delay requested'.[113] By way of climax to the burlesque, on 2nd August 1808 as the Council in solemn conclave, deliberated on what action to take to counter Dr Gregory's recurrent delaying tactics—a sealed packet and letter were received from him. The letter stated that copies of the concluding pages would follow. Such was the speed with which they arrived that the Council were still in session when the day's second sealed packet was deposited with them. Understandably 'several Members expressed very strongly their opinion of the hardship of being compelled to peruse such voluminous papers and the impossibility of bestowing sufficient time for that purpose consistently with their other avocations'.[114] Nor should it be forgotten that at the time the College was already considerably involved in national negotiations for medical reform.

Something approaching finality was reached on 13th September 1808. On that day the College, in the absence of Dr Gregory, at a special meeting passed a lengthy resolution declaring the conduct of Dr Gregory to have been 'highly immoral' and expressing the reprobation of the College, regretting 'that any one of their body should have acted so as to call forth an animadversion and censure of this nature'. Disapprobation was expressed concerning Dr Gregory's irrelevancies, misrepresentations, insinuations and 'the coarse, rude, and even sometimes grossly indecent language'.[115]

Towards the end of the sederunt and after lengthy deliberation the Council were instructed to draw up a 'narrative of the transactions alluded to by Dr. Gregory and of the conduct of Dr. Gregory'. This was felt 'indispensably necessary' to prevent the public being misled by the aspersions which had been cast on the College as a body and on members individually.[115] Publication took place in 1809. In February of that year Gregory reacted by sending a paper entitled *Protest*, dealing with the resolution of September 1808. The *Protest* showed no evidence of diminished hostility; repeated the previous contentions concerning selective victimization, coupled this time with the names of seven members who were unreservedly accused of combining 'to do me this new and most foul injustice'. There was a clear declaration of intent to resort to legal action against the College and those seven members. Dr Gregory's *Protest* was remitted to a Special Committee which recommended that it should be kept *in retentis* but not ingrossed in the Records. The Committee proposed also that Dr Gregory should be suspended 'till he shall make satisfactory acknowledgments'.[116] Suspension became effective on 13th May 1809, the relevant Minutes being noteworthy for their uniquely condensed abrupt form.[117]

Twenty-one years were to pass before all Minutes relating to the unhappy events of 5th December 1807 and 12th September 1808 were removed at the instance of Dr Hope, who in his day had been in succession a student, family friend, main target and critic of Dr Gregory.[118, 119]

There is in the College Library a copy, once in the possession of Dr Andrew Duncan, sen., of Gregory's *Review*. Dr Duncan was one of the listed 'seven'. The book was inscribed 'To Dr. Andrew Duncan from the Author'. Bound with the *Review* is *Dr. Gregory's Defence*. On the title page of this Dr Duncan has written in manuscript:

'Character of the Author, from S. Butler.
He was in Logic a great Critic,
Profoundly skilld in analytic,
He could distinguish & divide
A hair twixt South & South West side,
On either which he would dispute,
Confute, change sides, and still confute.'

Dr Duncan was one of the most socially amiable men to occupy the presidential chair. Doubtless many, if not most members at the time in question would have regarded the quotation as apt. But an almost Jekyll and Hyde contrast seemed to characterize Gregory in the College on the one hand, and in professional and social society in Edinburgh on the other. We have it on the authority of Cockburn that 'He was a curious and excellent man, a great physician, a great lecturer, a great Latin scholar and a great talker; vigorous and generous; large of stature and with a strikingly powerful countenance. The popularity due to these qualities was increased by his professional controversies, and the diverting publications by which he used to maintain and enliven them. The controversies were rather too numerous; but they never were for any selfish end, and he was never entirely wrong. Still a disposition towards personal attack was his besetting sin.'[120] This predisposition assumed extreme form when having belaboured a fellow senator with his stick in the street and been successfully sued for £100 in damages, his reaction was to declare his willingness to pay double for another opportunity![121]

In fairness it should be added that it has been said of his victim 'As a critic he seemed to be in his favourite element: and a snarling, unfair, unfeeling critic he was'.[122] None the less Cockburn rather relished independence in the medical ranks because, discussing proposed changes in the rota for professional visits at the Infirmary, he wrote '—most of the medical profession, including . . . even the two Colleges, who all held that the power of annoying the patients in their turn was their right, were vehement against this innovation . . . Dr. Jas. Gregory whose learning extended beyond that of his profession attacked this absurdity in one of his powerful, but wild and personal, quarto pamphlets. The public was entirely on his side.'[123]

An outstanding teacher and greatly appreciated by students Gregory was not lacking in eccentricity. Never failing to apologize he made a habit of keeping his hat *in situ* when lecturing. None other than Robert Christison described him as the most captivating lecturer he had encountered.[124] Eminently successful as a practitioner in Edinburgh, he acquired eponymous fame from the powder of magnesia, rhubarb and ginger which to this day bears his name.

> *If in doubt, 'lead with trumps', is counsel so old*
> *As never to fail with the game in a fixture;*
> *And medical men, in their doubt, I am told,*
> *Are safe when they lead with—Gregory's Mixture.*
>
> (From an Old Play)

Perhaps the Reverend Sydney Smith, a doctor and canon of the Church, had known benefit from the mixture when he wrote from Vienna to an intimate friend— 'What, in the name of Dr. Gregory, can you see in Germany of a therapeutic nature, which you cannot see better in Scotland?'[125]

Coming from an Aberdeenshire family uniquely distinguished for academic achievements, James Gregory was the only individual considered for the Chair of Institutes of Medicine at the University of Edinburgh,[126] at which at an earlier date his father John Gregory had occupied a different chair in the faculty.

In trying to reconcile James Gregory's attitude to the College with his popularity in Edinburgh circles, it is tempting to attribute some of his personality to inheritance of certain of his father's characteristics. Jupiter Carlyle of Inveresk shared lodgings with John Gregory at Leyden and wrote of him 'never contradicting you at first, but rather assenting . . . as it were, to your knowledge and taste, he very often brought you round to think as he did, and to consider him a superior man'.[127] Certainly, James the son was no respecter of persons. A close acquaintance of Robert Burns he accepted an invitation to criticize one of his unpublished poems. The criticism evoked from Burns 'Dr. G[regory] is a good man, but he crucifies me . . . I believe in the iron justice of Dr. G[regory]; but like the devils, I believe and tremble.'[128]

But Gregory's attitude was not solely one of destruction. There is extant an English translation of Cicero's *Select Orations* (London 1756) given to Burns by James Gregory. Inscribed on a blank page of the volume is the following:

> *Edin. 23 April 1787*
> *This book, a present from the truly worthy and learned Dr. Gregory, I shall preserve to*
> *my latest hour, as a mark of the gratitude, esteem and veneration I bear the Donor. So help*
> *me God*
>
> Robert Burns[129]

Gregory's acquaintanceship with Burns was both social and professional. It began when they met at one of the classic suppers arranged at Ochtertyre by Lord Monboddo[130]: and it is known that, in company with the surgeon Mr Alexander Wood, Gregory once attended Burns on account of a 'sprained knee'.[131] In passing, two other admittedly remote links of the College with Burns can be mentioned; Sir Douglas Maclagan (President 1884–7) was baptized by the same minister as Robert Burns[132]; and Fellows who subscribed to the first Edinburgh edition of Burns in 1787 included Andrew Duncan, James Gregory, James Hamilton, Alexander Monro and Nathaniel Spens.[133]

No clear indication exists to explain James Gregory's sustained animosity towards the College. It has been written of him that 'he was a man having authority impressed on every feature, radiant with affection for his friends, intolerant of enemies, asking his own way and getting his own way, loving, hating, thinking, speaking, feeling always with intensest ardour. Here was a man whom none of his associates could regard dispassionately; they either loved him as a friend or hated him as an enemy.'[134] There is no concealing that he himself could and did hate with white-heat intensity.

There was nothing to suggest cleavage between the interests of College and University. His opponents among Fellows of the College included fellow Senators who held him in the highest respect academically. No one was more diligent than Christison in striving to be fair when compelled to be critical. All he could say of Gregory's great quartos of controversy was 'very clever, no doubt, but biting, personal, and surely a misapplication of . . . genius . . . involving him in deadly, life long feud with many estimable brethren, both in and beyond the University'.[135]

Certainly Gregory was not lacking in self-confidence. In his own words 'I know I can make myself perfectly understood by lawyers . . . : for I happen to be, from choice and taste, as well acquainted with the principles of strict reasoning (or what is called logic) as they are professionally'.[136] And yet there was assuredly a wholly different side to him. To read his lengthy *Memorial* to the Infirmary on the iniquities of the rota system of visiting surgeons is as fascinating as it is bewildering. In it he devoted some three pages to a study of himself. He confessed to 'an unfavourable opinion of his own profession' and was impressed by the fact that 'with respect to physic, each successive age had much more trouble to unlearn the bad, than to learn the good, of those which went before . . . and still more to distinguish between the good and the bad which itself produced'. This from the pen of the reigning President of the College who none the less, writing in the third person, readily laid claim to 'such a genius for quarrelling with his professional brethren, that, without even the pretence of any differences in medical opinions, and purely on account of certain differences in morality, he has quarrelled with some of them irreconcileably, and refused ever again to consult with them.'[137]

A sensitive man prone to indulge in exhibitionism, could the reason be that the relatively small audience in the College was insufficiently responsive? He was of too great professional and academic stature for this to be likely. Temperamentally tempestuous and ill-equipped to conceal contempt even of colleagues, a more probable explanation is that he nursed a growing, prolonged and irrepressible embitterment towards one or more particular members. There is some justification for this view in his outburst in December 1807 attributing a conspiracy to certain individuals. The naming of seven members in his Protest of 1809 would seem to provide supporting evidence. If this surmise be correct the College of Physicians had not been the main target, if target at all—but without question the College suffered the most.

In an obituary notice of Admiral Fisher's death the *Times* referred to him as '. . . the great man, the great child, the ruthless foe, the whole-hearted friend, the dark schemer, the open fighter, the "ruthless, relentless, remorseless" tyrant . . .'.[138] In many respects the words might be applied to James Gregory. Without implying any disrespect, might it not be said that both men on occasions showed evidence of genius near to madness?

Philosophically the College adopted the attitude later advocated by Bower, that Gregory's various disputes 'occasioned much regret to the friends of both parties, and it is better, perhaps, that they should now be buried in oblivion'.[139]

In 1836 a nephew of James Gregory[140] was elected President of the College in the person of Dr William Pulteney Alison.

VAGARIES OF THE ESCALATOR MECHANISM
(1827–8)

But God is the judge: he putteth down one, and setteth up another.

Psalms, LXXV, 6 and 7

Traditionally hospital appointments have meant kudos and hopes for future advancement for physicians and surgeons alike. Procedure for the application for, and the award of hospital attachments became regularized in the course of years. The interests of patients, the governing bodies of hospitals, and the Corporations and Universities concerned with the fostering and maintenance of professional standards and privileges were all involved. More especially in the earlier period of its existence the College had occasion to assert its influence in securing recognition of the status of the physician. In doing so it had no option but to differentiate clearly the functions in hospital of the physician as distinct from those of the surgeon, and to ensure that those being appointed as physicians had had the necessary experience. Then as now, the pace of escalation did not please all: among seniors there were those who would have welcomed deceleration; among juniors there were those anxious for acceleration.

Relations between College and Infirmary

For historical reasons the College was peculiarly well placed to exercise a continuing beneficial influence on the affairs of the Edinburgh Royal Infirmary. On the eve of the opening of the Infirmary in 1729 the Fellows of the College of Physicians did 'unanimously agree to attend the Infirmary in yr turns for the Space of a fortnight, until Some Settled Method be agreed upon . . .'.[141] Fellows and Licentiates visited in the order of their seniority on the College Roll, each attending for a two weeks period. The roster exhausted, the procedure was repeated. Experience made it clear that largely because of the considerable number of physicians on the College Roll, the arrangement was not in the best interests of the patients or the consultants responsible for their care. To meet the situation the Managers of the Infirmary unanimously agreed that 'the attendance be performed . . . by such physicians only as are Fellows of the Royal College, that the College be acquainted with this resolution at their first meeting, and the continuance of the attendance of the Fellows be humbly desired in the name of the Managers . . .'.[142] Effect was given to the decision on 1st January 1738, on and after which date participation in professional visits was not permitted to Licentiates, with the exception of two who had attended from the time the hospital opened.[143] A direct result of the overall decision was confirmation of the fact that Fellowship of the Royal College of Physicians was a necessary qualification for appointment to the honorary medical staff of the Royal Infirmary.[144]

The position appeared to be unmistakably clear: relations between the College and the Infirmary were excellent; and were any uncertainties to arise, there were five representatives of the College on the Infirmary Board to assist in clarification. Despite this a major misunderstanding did result from the unorthodox use of the escalation machinery. The year was 1827.

Principles Threatened and Dignity Injured

At an Extraordinary Meeting of the College on 6th December the first item on the agenda was the admission as a Licentiate of the Royal College of Physicians of Dr William Cullen,* a Doctor of Medicine of the University of Edinburgh. This business completed, one of the Fellows adopted the unorthodox approach of saying he had a motion to submit 'but first was desirous to know for certain whether Doctor William Cullen was elected a Physician to the Royal Infirmary by the Managers of that Institution on Monday last the 3rd inst.' The fact that the election had taken place was confirmed by one of the College representatives on the Infirmary Board of Management.[145]

Despite the decorous tone of the Minutes it needs no stretch of imagination to appreciate the rapidity with which the atmosphere became charged with suspicion and resentment. And why? In the first place the unfortunate Dr Cullen was not a Fellow, and at the precise time of his election was not even a Licentiate. Secondly, prior to his election as physician to the Infirmary he had been acting in the capacity of Surgeon in that self-same Institution. Moreover another aspect which to College members added insult to injury was, that only a month previously an exchange of correspondence had taken place between the College and the Infirmary about the need for the appointment of two additional Ordinary Physicians, as the needs of the sick had increased in proportion with the tripling of Edinburgh's population in the previous 70–80 years.[146, 147] An Infirmary reply to a College Memorial indicated that the appointment of one additional Physician was contemplated and went on to

---

* Not to be confused with the eminent Fellow of the same name who was President in 1773.

say 'The Managers therefore are desireous that the Members of the Royal College should be informed ... that Gentlemen intending to offer themselves as candidates ... may have an opportunity of doing so.' The reply was dated 12th November 1827.[148]

Discussion in College sederunt about the sequence of events was lengthy. A second Fellow, who was one of the Managers of the Infirmary, assured the College that the Managers had intended no disrespect whatsoever, more especially as 'before the election took place the Managers were apprised that Dr. Cullen was immediately to become a Licentiate of the College and they therefore considered it of little importance whether the election should take place on the 3d. inst. as it did or that it should be delayed till the Monday following, after Doctor Cullen had entered with the College'.[149]

The explanation was not accepted as satisfactory and at another Extraordinary Meeting a decision was arrived at to Memorialize the Infirmary. It was maintained in the Resolution that the College had been unjustly treated by the appointment, contrary to the terms of the Infirmary Charter, of other than a member of the College; and disrespectfully treated having regard to the way in which the resolution of the Infirmary Managers on 19th December 1737 (q.v.) had been ignored. By way of conclusion the College resolution expressed 'a formal disavowal of any admission of, or concurrence in, the legality of the appointment in question, which might be thought to be implied by the acts of such of their Fellows as were, at the time, Managers of the Royal Infirmary'.[150]

Claim and Counter-claim

The Infirmary reply vied with the Resolution of the College in its orotundity, platitudes and protestations of injured innocence. From beginning to end the reply was concerned, being too dignified to use the strongest available language, with condemning the terminological inaccuracies of the College. While maintaining that they possessed full power to choose whom they wished as physician the Managers pointed out that they 'made it indispensable' to Dr Cullen's nomination that 'he should with all speed join the College of Physicians'. They insisted too that the College misinterpreted the terms of the Infirmary Charter and argued 'a most fearful enactment for the Royal College of Physicians it would have been had they been Ordained to Entertain and take care of the sick poor from every quarter'. How much more effective this castigation would have been had it had but one terminal exclamation mark! But the pedagogic-cum-magisterial tenor continued. The College it was suggested were unacquainted with the history of the Infirmary, and were informed that the ordinary Managers had power to appoint as they thought proper 'without any restriction as to their connexion with the Royal College as Fellows or Licentiates'. In support of their contention the Managers gave the appointment of another Dr Drummond in 1751 as a precedent. At the time of his appointment he was neither a Fellow nor Licentiate of the College.[151] Dr Drummond was the son of the Lord Provost of Edinburgh who perhaps more than anybody else was responsible for the successful founding of the Infirmary. Replying to the Managers' reference to the son, the College stated 'in the case of Dr. Drummond there can be no difficulty in saying, that special, and what may justly be called undue influence was employed, in favour of the son of one of the most zealous of the early benefactors of the Infirmary: and the circumstance of the College of Physicians not having thought fit to make any objection to his Election, cannot be held as proof that it was legally conducted'.[152]

'Bona fide in cursu'

The Infirmary reply was not calculated to assuage the ruffled sentiments of the College. Nor were they. Advice was sought from Counsel with results which must have gratified the College despite the caveats which interlarded the legal opinion received. Counsel gave it as their opinion that 'The Managers have not power to appoint any persons . . . Physicians . . . who are not of the Royal College of Physicians of Edinburgh' but elaborated this by saying there 'may be a question of some doubt whether some Gentlemen who are Licentiates . . . are eligible or not; and supposing Licentiates to be eligible it may be another question . . . whether there is any violation of the rights of the College in chusing a person who, tho' not a Licentiate or Fellow at the time, is *bona fide in cursu* of becoming a Licentiate before entering on the duties of his appointment'. In furtherance of Counsel's view there followed a paragraph which was as illuminating as it was picturesque. It read:

> '. . . taking it thus, the Institution over which the Managers preside can only be an Infirmary, in which the poor sick, being *entertained* by the Corporation (for we think, that a *comma* must be understood after the word *entertained*)* are to be "taken care of by the Royal College of Physicians of Edinburgh, and some of the most skilful Chirurgeons." This care we conceive manifestly to consist in *medical attendance*. We are therefore of opinion that according to the Charter, it is a fundamental point in the constitution of the Corporation that the Physicians who

* This refers to the terms of the Infirmary Charter.

are to have the care of the Sick *in* the Hospital shall be exclusively Physicians of the Royal College.'[152]

At this juncture Counsel's advice assumed an almost paternalistic air. Having allowed that the College 'cannot with safety to their own rights, acquiesce in the construction which is put on the Charter in the answers made by the Managers . . . and the assertion of right therein contained', the College were advised

> 'that they ought to submit a further representation to the Managers, stating their great desire to maintain a friendly understanding . . . in all things, and their willingness to acquiesce in the late appointment, if their rights otherwise shall be fully recognised, but, at the same time, expressing, in respectful terms, their entire dissent from the statements in the Answers, and the necessity they are laid under of maintaining the rights of the College; and praying for such an answer, as may enable them to bring the matter to an amicable conclusion.' Counsel unreservedly discouraged discussion of the difficulties at a meeting of Subscribers and considered that were amicable settlement with the Managers not achieved 'it is in a Court of Law *only* that the Memorialists [the College] can establish their rights.'[152]

Protestations of Good Will

Duly, if not dutifully, the College replied to the Answer of the Infirmary Managers. When doing so they enclosed a copy of the Opinion of Counsel, and in no uncertain terms emphasized that the Opinion 'pointedly contradicts the doctrine of the Managers, that they are at liberty to appoint Physicians to the Infirmary, whether belonging to this College or not'. They then referred to Counsel's opinion concerning the appointment of a gentleman 'who is bona fide . . . in cursu to become a Licentiate'. In the particular case of Dr Cullen the College claimed to speak advisedly when they said 'they cannot regard' him 'as having been regularly and *bona fide* even *in cursu* to become a Licentiate, at the time when he was appointed . . . ; having reason to believe, that his resolution to enter this College was in fact contingent on his receiving that appointment'.

Not surprisingly the College cited in further support of their contention the circumstances in which Doctor Cullen 'held the Office of Surgeon to the Infirmary up to the moment when he was appointed Physician to it'. The appointment was regarded as 'quite anomalous, in the history of this or any other Hospital, in which the distinction between Physicians and Surgeons is recognised', but conforming to the recommendation of Counsel the College declared that they had 'no wish to disturb the appointment that has already taken place, provided that their rights shall otherwise be distinctly recognised by the Managers'.[152]

The Infirmary replied by return. After professions of a desire to continue 'friendship and cordiality' the letter conceded 'the point of right in regard to the election of Physicians . . . being confined to the Fellows and Licentiates of the Royal College': and stressed that Dr Cullen had not been sworn into office till some time after his admission as a Licentiate. Slow to have suspicions allayed the College acknowledged receipt, admittedly 'with much pleasure' but indicated that they were under the necessity of communicating with their legal adviser before taking 'any further step in this business'.[153] The final opinion of Counsel had not been received by the time of the Quarterly Meeting on 6th May and was not expected 'for some time'.

Altogether the negotiations on the subject of Dr Cullen between College and Infirmary make sorry reading. The inescapable impression gained is of two Corporations each so obsessed in the dignity of their own status that they both unwittingly cast dignity aside when involved in dispute, one with the other. Much the same atmosphere is created within the National Health Service when mutual 'animadversions' occur between hospital management committees, between regional and teaching hospital boards, or even between hospital boards and Universities. In retrospect, the temptation might well be to regard the animadversions of the early nineteenth century between College and Infirmary as light comedy. Final events however made of the comedy, a tragi-comedy.

Fate Decrees

The escalator mechanism ceased to function. Dr William Cullen died. Six months to the day after admitting him a Licentiate, the College made arrangements to return 'to the friends of the late Doctor William Cullen, the fee so lately paid by him, to the Royal College, with the view to his admission as a resident Ordinary Fellow'.[154] On 9th June 1828 the Infirmary addressed to the President of the College a letter intimating 'that in consequence of the Death of Doctor William Cullen, a vacancy has occurred in the situation of one of the Physicians to the Royal Infirmary, which you will please communicate to the Royal College'. This evoked an acknowledgment from the President to the effect that 'the Letter having this day been laid before a

Meeting of the Royal College, I am directed to return the thanks of the College for your polite communication'.[155]

Grudging without doubt, but reconciliation did eventuate.

POSTSCRIPT

As a quizzical and sympathetic postscript, the experiences of Dr Poole during the six months of 'animadversion' are worth recalling. Dr Poole, a Fellow, had accepted responsibility for all the administrative and research work involved. His activities won him the admiration and gratitude of a sensitively disturbed College. In a letter addressed to the President and Council and dated 2nd February 1828 Dr Poole wrote:

> 'I beg to suggest, what, from the labours I have undergone . . . the expediency of collecting and arranging, with a suitable index:—all the laws and regulations enacted by the College, since its erection, whether repealed or in force . . .
>
> Farther, it occurs to me to inform you, with a view to some remedy, that the Minute Books are far from being in anything like a very creditable condition. I allude to such of them as are old more particularly—as they are quite invaluable . . . a fair copy of them ought to be made, so that the originals might be laid up, under an injunction to be kept *intact* . . . A copy was made of them from 1682 to 1725 . . . it is by no means . . . such as befits the regard which the College ought to manifest towards the transactions of their predecessors.
>
> I hazard another hint, namely, that it is desirable all the loose papers, regarding the College . . . should be carefully examined . . . Even among a few old accounts and receipts, I have already discovered some particulars, of, at least a curious nature.'[156]

Admirable advice—with only one omission. There should have been added that oft-used phrase beloved by so many of our earliest predecessors—'for all-time coming'!

Dr Richard Poole

Throughout this history frequent reference is made to Dr Richard Poole. There is no escaping the fact that he had a deep attachment to the College, and betrayed unswerving jealousy for its privileges and rights. A man of wide professional interests he was responsible for two noteworthy contributions to the literature in the Library.

He was convener of the College Committee which drew up the classic *Report on Examination of Medical Practitioners* in 1833. Study of the *Report* and comparison with other writings of Dr Poole suggest in an unmistakable manner that the *Report* was largely drawn up and composed by Poole himself.[157] The other noteworthy contribution was a letter sent by Dr Poole to the President (Dr Davidson) on 1st November 1834 urging study and improvement of the lot of the Pauper Lunatic. So impressed were Council that they required that the letter should be preserved permanently[158] (Chap. XX). History, and more especially the history of the College, had a particular attraction for him and so much so that after years of research in the College archives, he produced notes which he suggested might provide the basis for an Official History of the College. These notes have been freely drawn on in the present text. They afford evidence of immense industry, untiring extraction of detail, great care in collating facts, and not a little sense of wry humour. A point of particular importance is that Poole had access to documents relating to periods when records of sederunts were lost or expunged under Acts of Oblivion. Poole made good use of his discoveries. His notes are of great value and should be studied without fail by anyone particularly interested in the prolonged feuds between physicians and surgeons, the legal arguments involved in establishing the position of the simple apothecaries vis-à-vis physicians and surgeons, and the major Court of Session cases in which the College of Physicians was involved from time to time. It is nothing short of a tragedy, and to Poole it must have been a source of bitter disappointment that he was not encouraged by the College to pursue his project. Minutes of Council record how on being offered preliminary manuscript notes for a History of the College for his perusal the President (Dr Sellar) referred them to the Secretary[159] who three months later reported that he 'did not consider that its acquisition would be agreeable to the College, if it involved any payment worth the Author's acceptance'.[160] Poole had the material, the knowledge, the industry, the urge and the ability ready to be harnessed in the interests of the College: all that was lacking at that particular time was vision on the part of Council. In retrospect an example of forethought lacking foresight!

There is no escaping Poole's inveterate restlessness. It was said of him that his 'mind fitted him less for the toils and distractions of the general practitioner or physician than for the labours of the literateur': and that 'his fertile brain and pen were always engaged on some literary work'.[161] In the 1820s he gave his support to proposals for a new Infirmary in Edinburgh. The proposals were published in unsigned pamphlet form (*Proposals for the Establishment of a New Infirmary*)[162] and were the subject of criticism in a public letter from the President of the College (Dr Andrew Duncan, sen.) to Sir William Fettes in which Duncan urged as a preferable alternative 'the establishment of a Lock Hospital and Hospital for Incurables' at the existing Infirmary.[163] Poole countered with the publication of a lengthy letter entitled *A letter to Andrew Duncan Senior, M.D. & Prof., President of the Royal College of Physicians; one of the Managers of the Royal Infirmary etc. etc. regarding the Establishment of a New Infirmary*.[164] The letter compared unfavourably with Poole's memoranda on other subjects. It was interspersed with unctuous protestations and laced with garlanded phraseology, not atoned for by the concluding 'Dear Sir, Your greatly obliged and sincerely affectionate Pupil and Friend'!

Perhaps Poole's tempestuous evangelism was out of character on this occasion. He was in the throes of domestic trouble, and within a short time was to find himself imprisoned in Calton Jail, having stood surety for a defaulting son's debts.[165] Some ten years later, having previously unsuccessfully sought an academic post in Belfast, Poole was an intending applicant for a post at Ipswich.[166, 167] Apparently the proposition was not pursued because he was appointed Medical Superintendent of the Royal Lunatic Asylum at Montrose in 1838, which post he held for seven years.[168] Thereafter and to within a few years of his death in 1870 he conducted a small private asylum in Aberdeen.[169]

No matter if Poole was by nature exasperatingly persistent and perhaps eccentric in his enthusiasm, he deserves greater posthumous recognition than that accorded him to date. Without question his legacy of manuscripts merit binding and indexing in the interests of posterity. Additional to his work on behalf of the College Poole's publications included the outstanding *Memoranda regarding the Royal Lunatic Asylum, Infirmary and Dispensary of Montrose*; contributions to the *Encyclopaedia Britannica*; articles on insanity; and in 1843, a Scottish drama written in Lowland Scots and dedicated to the President of our College, Dr Robert Renton. Published anonymously, the drama was entitled *Willie Armstrong: a Scottish drama, in three acts. By a man wise enough to know that amusement, even though somewhat coarse, is at times as salutary as any article in the pharmacopoeia*.[170]

Poole was the second youngest in a family of eleven. Married twice, he had no fewer than seventeen children. His father came to Edinburgh from Lincolnshire about 1764, became a Burgess in 1786 and, according to the entry at Calton Burial Ground where he was interred, had been keeper of Poole's Hotel at number one Princes Street being 'the first that ever kept a hotel in Edinburgh'.[171]

An M.D. (1805) of St Andrews University, Richard Poole was admitted as a Licentiate in 1824 and elevated to the Fellowship of our College in the following year. He was a Vice-President of the Phrenological Society. In 1868 a bust of Richard

Poole was gifted to the College by his daughter who described her father's condition as being 'very frail in mind and body'.[172] He was in his 86th year at the time. Today his descendants have in their possession a snuff box with an inscription:

'To Richard Poole Esq., M.D., F.R.C.P.
from some of his brethren
of the
Royal College of Physicians Edinburgh
as a small token of their friendship for him
and in testimony of his valuable service
in (sic) behalf of the Royal College.

Edinburgh June 1828.'

THE CITADEL REPROVES

A big toun to be sae far south.
(Aberdonian on being advised as to the population of London)

. . . the Fellows of the Royal College of Physicians in London, who have at all times been distinguished for their learning, their talents, and their liberal manners; and who, very justly, regard themselves, and are regarded by others, as Beings of a higher nature than the Physicians of any other country on the face of the earth.

James Gregory (*Memorial to Managers of R.I.E.*)

Non Angli, sed Angeli

Attributed to Pope Gregory I

If you venture only to tread upon the hem of that garment of self-sufficiency in which the true Scotchman wraps himself, he is sure to turn round upon you as if you had aimed a dagger at his vitals . . .

J. G. Lockhart (*Peter's Letters to his Kinsfolk*)

Factiousness did not disappear overnight with the passing of the Medical Act in 1858. On the contrary, for a period, old rivalries became inflamed and the medicopolitical atmosphere was charged with intensified testiness.

Difficulties continued to arise from the confusion of a haphazard past. Writing in the late eighteenth century Adam Smith gave it as his opinion that 'the persons who apply for degrees in the irregular manner complained of are, the greater part of them, surgeons or apothecaries who are in the custom of advising and prescribing, that is of practising as physicians; but who, being only surgeons and apothecaries, are not fee-ed as physicians. It is not so much to extend their practice as to increase their fees that they are desirous of being made Doctors.'[173] In some respects this lay view was shared by James Gregory who writing in 1800 said '. . . it can be no secret, that in Edinburgh a great part of the business of those called Surgeons, is physic rather than surgery . . . three fourths at least, more probably nine tenths, of the proper medical practice is done by members of the College of Surgeons; who in fact, though not in name, are the ordinary physicians in every family'. Gregory went on to say that he had no doubt that the system would 'continue in Edinburgh as long as the Medical School . . . shall continue to flourish'.[174] In the circumstances it is perhaps not surprising that as measures for medical reform assumed some semblance of shape, those engaged in various forms of medical and surgical practice sought ways and means of consolidating what might be termed their professional respectability and status.

Assumption of the Title 'Dr'

With reason the Universities waxed indignant at the usurpation by Licentiates of the title of 'Doctor' which it was their prerogative to award. Licentiates of all the medical Corporations were involved. The misdemeanour was not without precedent in one form or another. Thus it had been the practice for the names of many Licentiates of the London College of Physicians who were not university graduates to be recorded as 'M.D.' in the Army and Navy Lists. A possible explanation may have been that in earlier times the London College had customarily referred to all its Licentiates as Doctors. This in turn could account for the fact that on his appointment as the Registrar to the General Medical Council, the former Registrar to the London College of Physicians at first gave the title of Doctor to Licentiates of the Edinburgh College on the receipt forms for their registration fees.[175]

Our College was in no way responsible. At the same time it did not burke the issue. There were many occasions when the Honorary Secretary had to reply to enquiries from Licentiates.[176] With unmistakable precision Council recommended to the College in 1860 that Licentiates had 'no right to the appellation of "Doctor" '[177] and that Licentiates 'not being graduates in Medicine of a University acquire no right to place "M.D." after their signature'.[178] The subject came up again for discussion by Council in 1875 with the appearance of a critical letter to the Press. On this occasion it was recorded that 'Council is of opinion the College is not called upon to infere [sic] under existing circumstances; and the more so as the present agitation is led by a Journal which has uniformly placed the most unfavourable construction upon the actions of the College'.[179]

The College continued to be worried and eventually in 1896, on the recommendation of Council, additions were made to appropriate Chapters in the Laws. The addenda made it abundantly clear that no Diploma granted by the College authorized the holder 'to assume the title of Doctor or the letters, M.D., or other abbreviation' suggesting possession of a University Degree of Doctor of Medicine.[180]

Another designation giving rise to considerable thought was that of 'Physician'. At one time Council regarded it as eligible for insertion in Schedule 'D', column 4 of the Register and unsuccessfully sought the concurrence of the London and Dublin Colleges.[181] Uncertainty concerning use of the term persisted as is evident in the following reply by the Secretary to an enquiry from a Licentiate in the South— '. . . you have a perfect right to style yourself a Physician. There is no legal definition of what constitutes a Physician, but the general opinion . . . is that no one can be correctly styled such, unless he holds a Licence from, or the Fellowship of a College of Physicians.' Then to clinch argument there followed—'I do not consider that a University Graduate who is not also connected with a College of Physicians, can properly style himself Physician'.[182] Surely—as water-tight as humanly possible.

Hurricane—'Year of Grace'

Whatever the repercussions to abuse 'of the appellation Doctor' they were as nothing compared to those given rise to by the *Regulations for the conferring of the License* approved by the Edinburgh College of Physicians on 20th April 1859.[183] Christison's Protest on 26th April of that year was akin to a warning of an approaching hurricane.[184]

Condemnation was focussed on the Regulation providing for exemption from examination in certain prescribed circumstances. Emotions, many of them irrational, entered into the picture: prejudices abounded. The fact that admission to the Licentiateship was subject to detailed scrutiny and to a two-thirds supporting majority at a ballot was regarded with scepticism. To quote from a former College *History*, these securities 'appeared to the College to be better tests of the fitness of men to be Licentiates . . . than the subjecting them to an examination framed for Students fresh from their studies. They were in strict accordance with the principles of an *ad eundem* admission which almost every Licensing Body at the time permitted.'[185] Scrutineering was effectively carried out. Applications from large numbers of young men

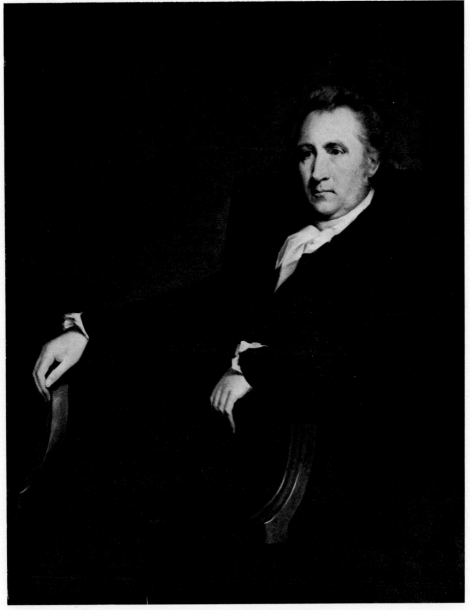

PLATE 29   Dr James Gregory (1753–1821)
Reproduced from a copy in the College of original portrait by Sir Henry Raeburn;
photograph by Tom Scott

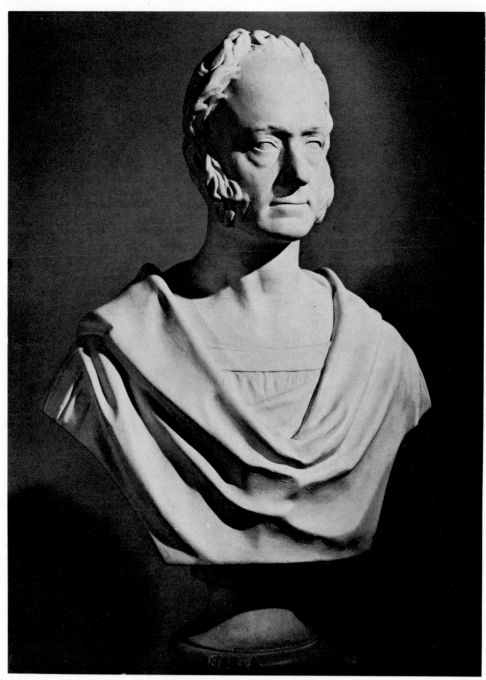

PLATE 30   Dr Richard Poole (1781–1870)
Photograph by Tom Scott

were a source of concern, but with few exceptions these applicants were informed that they must undergo an examination as the temporary Regulation providing exemption from examination applied only to practitioners of mature age.

The Bell Tolls

About this time the London College of Physicians had passed regulations which extended by one year the privilege of becoming Licentiates to all Graduates and Licentiates of Universities in Great Britain, requiring of them no more than the recommendation of three Fellows and the test of the ballot.[185] This did not prevent London brethren from voicing indignation over the action taken by the Edinburgh physicians. The same applied to the British Medical Association. Nor were certain members of the national Press slow to join in the hunt of the miscreant. The guilty party was the Royal College of Physicians of Edinburgh and its offence was variously described as 'manufacturing physicians for money payment'; 'providing an utterly unnecessary new source of obtaining a licence to practise'; and 'lowering the status of the physician, without elevating that of the general practitioner'. Much of the criticism, both vocal and written, was theatrical verging on the hysterical but amidst the confusion of remonstrances one protest tolled with all the compelling solemnity and ominous foreboding of the Lutine bell in Lloyd's.

The protest came in the form of a letter dated 19th April 1859 from the President of the Royal College of Physicians, London to the President of the Edinburgh Royal College. Commencing with punctilious politeness the communication wasted neither time nor words in informing the Edinburgh President that 'the following resolution was unanimously adopted at a Meeting of the College [London] held on Monday the 18th inst.:

> 'That the President and Censors be empowered to address in the name of the College, a strong and immediate remonstrance to the Royal College of Physicians of Edinburgh respecting the terms on which they have recently proposed to confer the License of their College.'

What followed might almost be described as a Censorian Letter, after the manner of James Gregory. It was maintained that the new Edinburgh Regulations would be 'injurious . . . on the character and status of British physicians and especially on the character and reputation of the London College of Physicians'. Having cast certain aspersions on the youth and qualifications of many of those licensed by the Edinburgh

Q

College, the Remonstrance viewed with the gravest foreboding the possibility of the London College being compelled by the recent Medical Act to admit into their body Edinburgh Licentiates who were practising in England. Such, it was declared, were the feelings of the London College that should Edinburgh persist in passing objectionable and injurious enactments, they 'would of necessity be compelled to abandon all present idea of seeking . . . a new Charter'.[186]

Ill-founded Unfavourable Comparisons

The Edinburgh President (Dr Alexander Wood), on his own initiative, arranged for a reply to be sent without delay on behalf of Council and himself. His letter was prompt, courteous but unapologetic. He expressed regret that the London College had not first communicated with Edinburgh 'before taking up the subject of the recent Regulations': and pointed out that had they done so they would have realized the inaccuracy of the information available to them and that a number of days prior to the London meeting at which the Remonstrance was decided upon, the Regulations had already been reviewed and modifications proposed. This was amplified by the significant remark that the Council 'have reasons to believe that an erroneous interpretation was put upon' one 'regulation by many of the Fellows of your College [London], and that a view of its intention and spirit at variance with that entertained by the Edinburgh College was submitted to the London College, by the mover of the Resolution, who was in communication with one of the dissentient minority of the Edinburgh College'. The reply concluded with an expression of regret 'that the manner in which some recent communications have been received by you has given but little encouragement to that free and friendly intercourse which the College of Physicians of Edinburgh have ever sought to maintain'.[186]

This reply was dated 22nd April and was, together with the original London letter, reported to the College which instructed the President to send a further communication on their behalf to the London College of Physicians. This second letter was both longer and more conciliatory in tone than its predecessor. Its subservience was out of national character. Surprisingly and without any obvious justification it tendered— 'tendered' be it noted—'thanks for the temperate terms' in which the remonstrance had been couched. There followed almost obsequious endeavours to placate. Then came the facts. The new Regulations respecting Licentiates had been 'made public before having been duly considered, according to practice' and had been subject to alterations before the time of premature publication. It was explained that among other things, these alterations required that Licentiates could only become such after subjection to a ballot, and that the professional examination should, instead of being single, consist of three series of examinations.

Next came an elaboration of the new Regulations relating to what later came to be referred to as the 'Year of Grace'. The relevant part of this second letter read as follows:

> 'During the year for admission the Licentiates without Examination, and without a University Degree, no one will be admitted without a Licence from some other Medical Corporation; and persons in practice for fifteen years without any License, who were admissible under the original resolutions, will not be allowed to apply for the license of the College at all.'

There are then reiterated the details of scrutinising candidates in terms of character, experience and a ballot approval by two-thirds.

David and Goliath

Continuing, the letter suggested that 'the only material difference' subsisting between the Regulations of the two Colleges related to the age of admission of Licentiates. This difference, it was contended, could be explained by the development in Scotland in a way 'comparatively little known in England' of a class of practitioner, charging 'fees . . . intermediate between those of the ordinary Class of general practitioners and those of consulting physicians' and to all intents and purposes discharging the functions of physicians although not legally accepted as such in England. This class of practitioner, which was well represented in the Roll of Fellows of the Edinburgh College, was described as including many of the most esteemed practitioners in Scotland and as deserving to 'belong to a College of Physicians quite as fairly as that Class who practise only as consulting physicians'. At this juncture the writer summed up courage to say 'Indeed, if this College has not been misinformed, there are not wanting practitioners of the same denomination in the London College of Physicians itself'. How the thrust contained in that apparently bold assertion was blunted by the terminal 'itself'—thereby adding a note of incredulity to a bare statement of fact!

On the matter of age the statement was made in the College reply, that it 'is not particularly wedded to the age of 21', but later, perhaps stimulated by awareness of Scotland's place in the world of education, asserted that the College deprecated any other rigorous rule as being calculated to obstruct the progress of talent and to interfere with the public usefulness of a College, whose purpose is to foster, and not to obstruct merit. Thereupon the London College is 'entreated to consider' that the views of the Edinburgh College 'in regulating the admission of its Licentiates rest on the organization of the Medical profession, and the practice of the other learned professions in Scotland'. Significantly and convincingly there followed the arbitrary statement that 'with a Medical Profession so organised as in Scotland a College of Physicians cannot now exist if it is to be composed only of consulting physicians, as the London College seems to desire'.

This written declaration—and declaration it was—deserves to be remembered and reconsidered in an age of big mergers and 'take-over bids' which have little if any respect for international boundaries. Medical Corporations will not be exempt from the trend; size and power are no assurance of professional or administrative efficiency. David can tender sound advice to Goliath. Doubtless those responsible for the drafting of this letter were of that opinion when they expressed the hope that the London College would be 'not unwilling to listen . . . to a suggestion, vizt. that it may be already full time to consider in England too, whether, under the operation of the Medical Act, a class of practitioners be not certain to arise, or be not already arising, akin to that which has been extensively established in Scotland, with great benefit to the nation . . .'.[186] With regard to its own particular position the Edinburgh College explained that the order of Licentiates had 'died out entirely' and that the 'College at present consists of Fellows alone. It desires to re-establish an order of Licentiates, and to constitute it in part of the practitioners in question. The College is unanimous in this desire.'[186]

The letters which were transmitted by the Edinburgh College at this time came in for mildly caustic comment in the recently published *History of the Royal College of Physicians of London*. 'The Edinburgh College replied' it is said 'in two pained letters, that together ran to thirteen foolscap pages . . .'.[187] 'Pained' is scarcely appropriate. Rather, reaction and counter-reaction reflected the lack of understanding prevailing between the two capital cities. The London attitude arose in considerable measure from fear of 'the prospect, or even the possibility, of an invasion by Scottish or Irish physicians with qualifications below the London standards'.[187] To some extent this was justified by the requirements of Clause XLVII of the Medical Act. As to the standard of qualifications—that was a different matter. None other than Sir Robert Christison, who was far from being antagonistic to the aspirations of the English Colleges, wrote of his experience in the South.

> 'I could thus easily understand subsequently' he said 'the superiority of the general practitioners educated at Edinburgh, where medicine proper held a prominent place in the system of hospital instruction, the preference in which they were held

in England, and their success and reputation, especially in most of the large English county towns.'[188]

Whatever the rights and wrongs of the arguments on one side or the other, the London College was determined to guard against any undermining of its influence or status. Towards the end of July (1859) a copy of a *Memorial* sent by that College to the General Medical Council was forwarded to the President of the Edinburgh College. The purpose of the *Memorial* was to direct the attention of the Council to a simultaneous consideration of the Medical Act and the implications of the new Regulations of the Edinburgh College having regard to existing bye-laws of the London College, and to the desirability or otherwise of the London College seeking a new Charter under the Medical Act. It was represented in the *Memorial* that under the new Edinburgh Regulations more than 190 persons had already made application for the Licence and with very few exceptions had been elected, 'almost all of whom are practising in England as General Practitioners, many possessing no other Qualification than that of Licentiate of the Society of Apothecaries and who, in the event of the College of Physicians of London obtaining a new Charter ... would be entitled ... to claim admission as Members of the College ...'. The London College maintained it could not 'accept a new Charter accompanied with a Proviso so detrimental to the interests of the Profession, and so degrading to the status of the English Physician'. The repeal of the offending clause (Clause XLVII) of the Medical Act was urged.[189]

At the same time as acknowledging receipt of a copy of the *Memorial* the Edinburgh College took the opportunity to declare 'concurrence in the proposal to get the suggested amendment made on Clause XLVII of the Medical Act'; and to represent that the statement of the London College that applicants for the Licence of the Edinburgh College 'have been with few exceptions admitted' to be 'founded on erroneous information'. As to other points in the *Memorial* about which a difference of opinion existed, the Edinburgh College preferred to withhold their explanation until the next meeting of the General Medical Council.[189]

Examinations for Licence Obligatory

At a meeting of the General Medical Council in August 1859 it was moved that 'any Degree or Licence obtained since the passing of the Medical Act without regular examination by the University or College granting such Degree or Licence, ought not to be placed upon the *Register*, excepting *ad eundem* Degrees, or Degrees or Licences in Medicine or Surgery, of any University in the United Kingdom, admitted to the Fellowships or Licentiateships of the several Colleges of Physicians and Surgeons'. The motion met with strenuous resistance. At the time the College was represented on the General Medical Council by Dr Alexander Wood who demonstrated the disadvantageous position in which graduates and licentiates of Universities would find themselves. Largely as a result of Dr Wood's exposition an amendment to the original motion was adopted to the effect that 'the General Medical Council are of the opinion that for the future, no Licence or Degree should be given by any of the Bodies in Schedule (A) of the Medical Act, without examination'.[190]

A Happy Outcome at Personal Level

At the personal level there was in the course of time a happy sequel to the General Medical Council meeting, at which Sir Dominic Corrigan had moved a resolution involving censure of our College. In February 1861 the Edinburgh College honoured Dr Alexander Wood by presenting him with his portrait and arranging a public dinner on his behalf. On reading of this in the medical Press Sir Dominic wrote Dr Wood in the following terms:

> 'No one . . . had more opportunity than I had of knowing how well you merited it . . . I cannot forget that when I brought forward a motion not to register licences granted without examination, my resolution was levelled at the College, and you will not be angry with me for still thinking that your College . . . deserved a whipping . . . it was your defence—one of the best pieces of argumentative reasoning and oratory I ever listened to—that saved your College as much as the reliance placed on your word . . .'.[191]

'The irony of it'

The interdict on the granting without examination of Licences to practise affected all examining bodies which admitted *ad eundem* Licentiates as well as the sister Colleges of Physicians in Edinburgh and London. No fair-minded person would begrudge the Edinburgh College a sense of chagrin at the course of events because in instituting admission without examination to its Licence the College had knowingly imitated its London counterpart. Ironically the London College had previously conceived of the idea of a Year of Grace, during which certain individuals had had Licentiateship conferred on them without examination. Unfortunately an immediate outcome in Scotland was that because of the different state of medical practice in that country as compared with England, admissions to the Edinburgh Licentiateship were on a considerably greater scale. The scale surprised the initiators of the scheme most of all.[192]

In this connection there was an interesting development later in 1860. Several Fellows submitted suggestions to Council for alteration of the Regulations. One proposal was 'to institute a Law similar to one which exists in the Glasgow Faculty and some other bodies by which Practitioners of some standing who may wish at a later period of life than usual to obtain the License of the College may, on application to the Council be relieved from Examination on such of the more elementary branches of Study as the Candidate may have previously been examined in by other Licensing Boards'.[193] A special Committee appointed to consider this among other suggestions were unanimous in recommending that 'in the case of duly qualified practitioners, of not less than five years standing, the Examination for the License should be limited to . . . Practice of Medicine and Pathology, Materia Medica, Midwifery and Medical Jurisprudence'.[194]

In so far as the Edinburgh and London Colleges of Physicians were at cross purposes it must be emphasized that there were within the Edinburgh ranks a certain number of Fellows who from the outset were anxious to avoid disturbance of prevailing friendly relations. As already described (Chap. XIV) the decision of the College not to restrict their Licence to University Graduates prompted an official Protest by ten Fellows. Dr Robert Christison was a prime mover in this dissent, and it was he who was largely instrumental in persuading the College as a corporate body to send a longer, informative and mildly suppliant communication by way of addendum to the letter sent by the President on 22nd April (1859) to his opposite number in London.[195]

Embarrassment from Within

Without question this group of dissentient diplomats proved to be an embarrassment. Nor were their harassing tactics always undeserving of criticism. If the impression conveyed by the Minutes is correct they had an unsavoury subterranean flavour, lacking the candour of a parliamentarian openly disobeying a three-line whip. This was evident in the acrid references to the sources of information available to the London College, made in the Edinburgh President's acknowledgment of the Remonstrance. It was evident also in the prior knowledge of the Remonstrance betrayed by some Fellows when they expressed concern at the delay in laying before the College a communication known by them to have been sent by the President of the London College. [195, 196] Indeed a protest signed by nine Fellows stated to three of their number having been informed by private letters of the transmission of the London communication. Additional to these unhappy developments a letter lacking 'the authority or sanction of the College or Council' appeared in the medical Press purporting to reply to the Remonstrance of the London College.[196] It is difficult not to regard these various unofficial actions as unfortunate, even if they cannot be unequivocally regarded as intrigue.

An Ungrateful B.M.A. joins the Fray

Not dissimilar difficulties arose in connection with the British Medical Association which discussed the new Regulations of the College at its Annual Meeting in July 1859. The discussion opened with attention being drawn to the admission as Licentiate of an individual who had practised homeopathy 'for a good many years' and who had been recommended by two homeopaths. Perhaps it was not without significance that the complainant was a practitioner in Bath. Even more perturbing was the complainant's action in reading to the assembled meeting a private letter he had received from one of the most eminent senior Edinburgh Fellows condemning recent proceedings of the College.[197] The letter was subsequently reported in the *Liverpool Mercury*.[198] Replying a few days later to a letter from the President asking for an explanation, the Fellow in question, who it should be emphasized was deservedly noted for his exemplary integrity, said, 'I beg to assure you of my sorrow and surprise, that Dr. ——— should have publicly used, and published in print, a letter, which as you correctly say, was evidently private, and which was intended by me for no other purpose than to satisfy his own mind as to enquiries addressed by him to me. I shall write . . . to desire that the publication of my letter may be stopped . . . That Graduates and Professors should have been led into correspondence on the subject was inevitable . . . but you will do me the justice to reflect, that, except in the College itself I have personally avoided all Public controversy on late College matters . . .'.[198] However sincere the explanation, and sincere it certainly was, an indiscretion had been committed—an indiscretion which might well have had more serious consequences in an age when retrospective legislation is acceptable as a matter of expediency.

Considered from the College point of view this was not the only unfortunate incident of the kind at the B.M.A. meeting. Another speaker argued that the College had opened their portals to any purchaser, whatever his mode of practice, or whatever pretensions he presented to them as a ground of claim: and he maintained he had it on the authority of a prominent Fellow of the College, whom he named, that the number of applicants and recipients of these licences very much corresponded.[197] The informant in this case was not the same Fellow as the one previously mentioned but had in common with him that he was a Professor at the University of Edinburgh. He differed in that he was not a Scot.

Not all the views expressed at the meeting were critical of the College. There were present a number ready to defend it from unwarranted insinuations but the meeting was determined to pass a condemnatory resolution. A motion was carried with five dissentients stating 'that in the opinion of this meeting, the conduct of the Edinburgh College of Physicians, in offering their licenses for a money-payment to all applicants having any medical or surgical qualification whatsoever, is reprehensible in the highest degree'. While agreeing with what had been said about the great want of caution which the College had shown Sir Charles Hastings maintained that the resolution was incorrect. Sir John Forbes deprecated the time spent on a subject which in former years would have been considered foreign to the objects of the Association and on his recommendation the motion was withdrawn.[199] A resolution was however adopted at the Annual Meeting by the Council of the Association. It declared 'That the recent proceedings of the Edinburgh College of Physicians, in the sale of their Licence without examination to gentlemen not already physicians, was not called for to meet any want in the profession; and that, inasmuch as it tends to lower the *status* of the physician, without elevating that of the general practitioner, it is calculated in every way to prove injurious to the body of the profession'.[200]

Misrepresentation born of Ignorance and Envy

To say that the College reacted with indignation to the attack upon it by the British Medical Association would be an understatement. The College knew deep hurt. Admittedly in its premature release of new regulations the College had shown a certain ineptitude and without doubt the actions, however innocent, of some of its Fellows were far from helpful. None the less these aspects of a confused situation did not justify imputing to the College disreputable and wholly mercenary motives. The College was concerned to advance the status of medicine in the light of prevailing conditions in Scotland and in anticipation of penalization of certain groups of practitioners consequent upon implementation of medicolegal reform. To suggest that the new Regulations represented a calculated attempt to improve the College finances was a travesty of the facts. What could be more sensible than that the College should review its resources faced with the inevitable changes being brought about by the Medical and Universities (Scotland) Acts of 1858? Because new proposals were drawn up was not justification for interested competitors condemning those proposals out of hand as lust for lucre. Those adopting that attitude were largely if not totally ignorant of the position in Scotland, and were wilfully blind to the continuing loyalty of the College to the principles embodied in the Charter of 1681.

The tragedy is that, to the detriment of medicine in general and the College in particular, genuine reconciliation was slow in being achieved. Emotionally charged misrepresentations continued to be bandied about indiscriminately for a number of years and to this day occasionally provide the misdirected, barbed reproof disguised as foolish ribald jests.

MALEVOLENT ANONYMITY

Few live exempt from disappointment and disgrace who run Ambition's rapid course.
                                                                    Tobias Smollett

Hard on the heels of troubles arising from the 'Year of Grace' the College was involved in another deplorably disreputable set of circumstances. The situation was most certainly not of the College's seeking and was in no way originated by the College.

After appointing the President (Dr Alexander Wood) of the Royal College of Physicians as his Assessor in the University Court, the Chancellor of the University received a number of anonymous letters containing grossly offensive references to the College, the President and another named eminent Fellow of the College. A fully attended Meeting of the Council of the College considered the matter and adjudged the letters to be 'false and calumnious' and were satisfied they bore evidence of intimate acquaintance with 'details of the affairs of the Royal College of Physicians and of the University, and . . . personal animosity towards Dr Alexander Wood and Professor Simpson'. News of events had already gained considerable currency because Members of Council were aware of reports circulating which attributed 'authorship and handwriting . . . to a Professor in the University' who was also a Fellow of the College. Council expressed their readiness to 'concur in any authorised enquiry'.[201]

That suspicion should so readily fall on one particular person was perhaps not surprising. The Professor in question had previously been involved in legal exchanges with the President before the time of election of the latter,[202-204] and had received a refusal on the part of the Council to accept a letter from him contradicting authorship of statements about the College in the medical Press which had appeared over the signature 'an Office Bearer' of the College. The reason for refusal was that no opportunity had been given for inclusion of a notice of the letter in the billet of the College Meeting.[205] Change in procedure did not account for the omission because six years previously as Honorary Secretary Dr Wood had had occasion 'to prevent any unpleasant feeling' to write to the individual concerned 'In the discharge of official duty I think it right to inform you, that if you have any motion to propose at the Quarterly Meeting . . . it will be necessary for you to give it to the Council in writing on or before their meeting.'[206] Personal antipathies prevailed before the events involving the University Chancellor.

A totally unprecedented step was then taken. The anonymous letters together with a 'known specimen of handwriting' were sent to be scrutinized by an official of the Bank of England and by the Post Office in London. The Minutes give no precise indication of the contents of the reports but the Secretary of the University Senate was advised concerning them.[207] By way of reply the Senate Secretary maintained that the subject did not come within the jurisdiction of the Senate who however were gratified to have received 'explicit denial of the authorship of the letters' from the Professor whose name had been linked with events.[208]

This prompted the Council to resolve that 'in the opinion of the Council the documents before them deeply concern the honour of a Fellow of the College named by the Senatus Academicus . . . : and that the Secretary be accordingly requested to convey to the Fellow in question the opinion of the Council, and to offer him the opportunity of such private reference of the matter as may tend to the elucidation of the truth as regards the handwriting of the letters . . .'. The resolution was communicated by an intermediary to Senate.[209]

Within a week a letter was received from the individual primarily involved, with enclosed a letter sent by him to the Chancellor. The response of the Council was to have transmitted by way of reply to the writer, a minute indicating that Council 'agree once more to press upon "him" the necessity of his joining with them in a farther inquiry . . . as a step required, equally for the vindication of "his" honour, and further protection of the College and the individual Fellows attacked in the anonymous letters'.[210]

And there, recorded references cease. Perhaps significantly, no mention is made of these particular events in Grant's detailed *History* of the University. There may however be an indirect clue to emotional undercurrents in Grant's description of the Professor concerned as 'a very keen, capable man, fond of controversy, and perhaps too stubborn an opponent of the recognition of extra-Academical teachers'.[211] Less kindly was the version to be found in the *Dictionary of National Biography*—'Critical and sarcastic remarks on the works of others did not make him a favourite among his professional brethren'.[212]

The drama—and drama there certainly was—is long since an event of the distant past. No final verdict was arrived at; not even an expedient one of 'Not Proven'. Was there reconciliation? Perhaps—in minor matters. Five months later the College Minutes recorded in incidental fashion that Library fines incurred by the once suspect Fellow were recommended for remission.[213] Graphologists would find an intriguing study in the contrasting signatures of the two main contestants!

Study of the major disputations in the history of the College compels realization of how they—with the exception of 'the Ryott' of 1695—did not result in creating administrative chaos or grave disruption of the College's other activities. Violent disputations were followed at the same meeting by cool consideration of pending legislation, sanitary problems, epidemiological challenges or more immediately domestic considerations such as extending library accommodation or even planning a new College Hall. In retrospect another feature is that seldom if ever did events of national importance appear to intrude on College business. There is for instance nothing in the records to jolt the reader into realization that as the College was indulging in intensive domestic bickering wars were being waged on the Continent culminating in such events as Corunna, Trafalgar and Waterloo. This alone illustrates the dangers of too dogmatic interpretation of Collegiate occurrences of almost three centuries ago.

REFERENCES

SIMMERING CAULDRON OF THE 1690s

(1) SMITH, R. W. I. (1932) *English-speaking Students of Medicine at the University of Leyden*, pp. 183–4. Edinburgh: Oliver & Boyd.

(2) BROWN, A. (1691) *A Vindicatory Schedule Concerning the New Cure of Fevers*. Edinburgh: J. Reid.

(3) R.C.P.E. (1898) *Historical Sketch of the Library of the Royal College of Physicians of Edinburgh*, p. iii. Edinburgh: Royal College of Physicians.

(4) COMRIE, J. D. (1932) *History of Scottish Medicine*, 2nd Edition, vol. I, p. 235. London: Baillière, Tindall & Cox.

(5) R.C.P.E. (1898) *Historical Sketch of the Library of the Royal College of Physicians of Edinburgh*, pp. iii f. Edinburgh: Royal College of Physicians.

(6) [BROWN, A.] (1692) *A letter written to a friend in the country, concerning Dr. Brown's vindicatory schedule. By Philander.* Edinburgh: Heir of A. Anderson.

(7) [BROWN, A.] (1692) *In speculo teipsum contemplare Dr. Black . . . a second letter . . . by Philander to his friend in the countrey.* Edinburgh: Heir of A. Anderson.

(8) PITCAIRNE, A. (1695) *Dissertatio de curatione febrium quae per evacuationes instituitur.* Edinburgh: (George) Mosman.

(9) [EIZAT, Sir E.] (1695) *Apollo mathematicus, or the art of curing diseases by the mathematicks.* Edinburgh:(James) Watson (younger).

(10) [HEPBURN, G.] (1695) *Tarrugo unmasked, or an answer to . . . Apollo mathematicus.* Edinburgh: n.p.

(11) SYDSERFF, Sir T. (1668) *Tarugo's wiles.* London: For Henry Herringman.

(12) College Minutes, 7.xi.1695.

(13) Ibid., 14.xi.1695.

(14) Ibid., 18.xi.1695.

(15) Ibid., 22.xi.1695.

(16) Ibid., 3.xii.1695.

(17) Ibid., 4.xii.1695.

(18) Ibid., 6.xi.1699.

(19) Ibid., 5.xii.1695.

(20) Ibid., 14.ix.1695.

(21) Ibid., 16.ix.1695.

(22) Ibid., 21.ix.1695.

(23) R.C.P.E. (1696) *Miscellaneous papers*, no. 98.

(24) BOWER, A. (1817) *The History of the University of Edinburgh*, vol. II, p. 132. Edinburgh: Oliphant, Waugh & Innes.

(25) Ibid., p. 131.

(26) Ibid., p. 148.

(27) RITCHIE, R. P. (1899) *The Early Days of the Royal Colledge of Phisitians, Edinburgh*, p. 178. Edinburgh: G. P. Johnston.

(28) CHAMBERS, R. (1949) *Traditions of Edinburgh*, p. 160. Edinburgh: W. & R. Chambers.

(29) EDINBURGH. City Corporation (1710) *Town Council Register*, 5.iv.1710. Vol. XXXIX, p. 182.

(30) STUART, M. W. (1952) *Old Edinburgh Taverns*, p. 40. London: Hale.

(31) College Minutes, 6.xi.1699.

(32) Ibid., 29.xi.1699.

(33) Ibid., 31.i.1700.

(34) RITCHIE, R. P. Op. cit., p. 181.

(35) Ibid., 31.xii.1702.

(36) POOLE, R. (1838) *Preparatory Notes for a History of the College*, p. 273. (Ms.)

(36a) IRVING, D. (1850) *Lives of the Scotish Writers*, vol. II, pp. 189-219. Edinburgh: Adam & Charles Black.

(37) College Minutes, 7.i.1703.

(38) Ibid., 24.xi.1703.

(39) Ibid., 2.xii.1703.

(40) Ibid., 4.i.1704.

(41) Ibid., 12.i.1704.

(42) Ibid., 19.i.1704.

(43) Ibid., 17.iii.1704.

(44) BROWNE, Sir T. (1835) Hydriotaphia. In *Sir Thomas Browne's Works*, ed. by Simon Wilkin, p. 492. London: William Pickering.

(45) College Minutes, 30.xi.1704.

(46) Ibid., 1.xii.1704.

(47) WEBSTER, C. (1781) *An Account of the Life and Writings of the Celebrated Dr. Archibald Pitcairne.* (Harveian Oration, Edinburgh.) Edinburgh: Gordon & Murray.

POLEMICS AND POWDER

(48) R.C.P.E. (1809) *Narrative of the Conduct of Dr. James Gregory towards the Royal College of Physicians of Edinburgh*, p. 39. Edinburgh: Hill, Manners & Miller and A. Constable & Co.

(49) College Minutes, 6.xi.1750.

(50) Ibid., 6.v.1707.

(51) R.C.P.E. (1925) *Historical Sketch and Laws*, p. 114. Edinburgh: Royal College of Physicians.

(52) College Minutes, 11.iv.1754.

(53) Ibid., 4.viii.1761.

(54) Ibid., 3.xi.1761.

(55) Ibid., 1.xi.1763.

(56) Ibid., 1.v.1764.

(57) Ibid., 7.v.1765.

(58) Ibid., 7.ii.1769.

(59) Ibid., 7.v.1765.

(60) Ibid., 7.xi.1769.

(61) Ibid., 6.ii.1770.

(62) Ibid., 5.v.1770.

(63) Ibid., 4.viii.1772.

(64) Ibid., 6.xi.1787.

(65) Ibid., 5.ii.1788.

(66) Ibid., 5.viii.1788.

(67) R.C.P.E. (1809) *Narrative of the Conduct of Dr. James Gregory*, p. 10. Edinburgh: Hill, Manners & Miller and A. Constable & Co.

(68) Ibid., p. 9.

(69) Ibid., p. 2.

(70) College Minutes, 2.xi.1784.

(71) Ibid., 6.ii.1787.

(72) Ibid., 4.xi.1788.

(73) Ibid., 2.ii.1796.

(74) Ibid., 1.xi.1796.

(75) R.C.P.E. (1809) *Narrative of the Conduct of Dr. James Gregory*, p. 3. Edinburgh: Hill, Manners & Miller and A. Constable & Co.

(76) College Minutes, 1.xii.1803.

(77) Ibid., 7.ii.1804.

(78) R.C.P.E. (1809) *Narrative of the Conduct of Dr. James Gregory*, p. 4. Edinburgh: Hill, Manners & Miller and A. Constable & Co.

(79) College Minutes, 7.viii.1804.

(80) Ibid., 6.xi.1804.

(81) Ibid., 5.ii.1805.

(82) GREGORY, J. (1804) *Review of the Proceedings of the Royal College of Physicians in Edinburgh from 1753 to 1804*. Edinburgh: Murray & Cochrane.

(83) GREGORY, J. (1805) *Censorian Letter to the President and Fellows of the Royal College of Physicians in Edinburgh*. Edinburgh: Murray & Cochrane.

(84) GREGORY, J. (1805) *Dr. Gregory's Defence*. Edinburgh: James Ballantyne & Co.

(85) R.C.P.E. (1789) *Regulations of the Royal College of Physicians*, p. 35. Edinburgh: Royal College of Physicians.

(86) R.C.P.E. (1852) *Statutes and Bye-laws of the Royal College of Physicians of Edinburgh*. Edinburgh: Thomas Constable.

(87) R.C.P.E. (1809) *Narrative of the Conduct of Dr. James Gregory*, p. 37. Edinburgh: Hill, Manners & Miller and A. Constable & Co.

(88) College Minutes, 5.ii.1805.

(89) R.C.P.E. (1809) *Narrative of the Conduct of Dr. James Gregory*, p. 52. Edinburgh: Hill, Manners & Miller and A. Constable & Co.

(90) College Minutes, 2.ix.1805.

(91) Ibid., 5.xi.1805.

(92) R.C.P.E. (1809) *Narrative of the Conduct of Dr. James Gregory*, p. 38. Edinburgh: Hill, Manners & Miller and A. Constable & Co.

(93) College Minutes, 5.viii.1806.

(94) Ibid., 26.xi.1806.

(95) R.C.P.E. (1809) *Narrative of the Conduct of Dr. James Gregory*, p. 39. Edinburgh: Hill, Manners & Miller and A. Constable & Co.

(96) R.C.P.E. (1808) *General Correspondence*, November 1808.

(97) College Minutes, 4.xi.1806.

(98) Ibid., 26.xi.1806.

(99) Ibid., 5.ii.1805.

(100) Ibid., 26.xi.1806.

(101) R.C.P.E. (1809) *Narrative of the Conduct of Dr. James Gregory*, pp. 40–1. Edinburgh: Hill, Manners & Miller and A. Constable & Co.

(102) College Minutes, 5.v.1807.

(103) Ibid., 4.viii.1807.

(104) Ibid., 3.ii.1807.

(105) Ibid., 19.v.1807.

(106) Ibid., 3.xi.1807.

(107) Ibid., 24.xi.1807.

(108) Ibid., 5.xii.1807.

(109) Ibid., 19.xii.1807.

(110) Ibid., 2.ii.1808.

(111) Ibid., 5.iii.1808.

(112) Ibid., 3.v.1808.

(113) Ibid., 8.vi.1808.

(114) Ibid., 2.viii.1808.

(115) Ibid., 13.xi.1808.

(116) R.C.P.E. (1809) *Narrative of the Conduct of Dr. James Gregory*, p. 95. Edinburgh: Hill, Manners & Miller and A. Constable & Co.

(117) College Minutes, 13.v.1809.

(118) Ibid., 2.ii.1830.

(119) Ibid., 4.v.1830.

(120) COCKBURN, H. (1910) *Memorials of his Time*, New Edition, p. 97. Edinburgh: Foulis.

(121) COMRIE, J. D. Op. cit., vol. II, p. 476.

(122) CHRISTISON, Sir R. (1885) *Life of Sir Robert Christison, Bart.*, vol. I, p. 86. Edinburgh: Blackwood.

(123) COCKBURN, H. Op. cit., pp. 96–7.

(124) CHRISTISON, Sir R. Op. cit., vol. I, p. 79.

(125) GRAY, J. (1952) *History of the Royal Medical Society, 1737–1937*, p. 98. Edinburgh: Edinburgh University Press.

(126) BOWER, A. (1830) *History of the University of Edinburgh*, vol. III, p. 200. Edinburgh: Oliphant, Waugh & Innes.

(127) CARLYLE, A. (1910) *Autobiography of Dr. Alexander Carlyle of Inveresk, 1722–1805*, p. 74. Edinburgh: Foulis.

(128) FINDLAY, W. (1898) *Burns and the Medical Profession*, p. 28. Paisley: Alexander Gardner.

(129) Ibid., p. 24.

(130) STEWART, A. G. (1901) *The Academic Gregories*, p. 129. Edinburgh: Oliphant, Anderson & Ferrier.

(131) FINDLAY, W. Op. cit., p. 25.

(132) TURNER, A. L. ed. (1933) *History of the University of Edinburgh, 1883–1933*, p. 123. Edinburgh: Oliver & Boyd.

(133) FINDLAY, W. Op. cit., p. 32.

(134) STEWART, A. G. Op. cit., pp. 127–8.

(135) CHRISTISON, Sir R. Op. cit., vol. I, p. 81.

(136) GREGORY, J. (1800) *Memorial to the Managers of the Royal Infirmary*, p. 119. Edinburgh: Murray & Cochrane.

(137) Ibid., pp. 221–4.

(138) MACKAY, R. F. (1973) *Fisher of Kilverstone*, p. 515. Oxford: Clarendon.

(139) BOWER, A. Op. cit., vol. III.

(140) COMRIE, J. D. Op. cit., vol. II, p. 610.

VAGARIES OF THE ESCALATOR MECHANISM

(141) College Minutes, 5.viii.1729.

(142) EDINBURGH ROYAL INFIRMARY. *Minutes*, 19.xii.1737.

(143) Ibid., 14.i.1738.

(144) TURNER, A. L. (1937) *Story of a Great hospital; the Royal Infirmary of Edinburgh, 1729–1929*, p. 55. Edinburgh: Oliver & Boyd.

(145) College Minutes, 6.xii.1827.

(146) Ibid., 6.xi.1827.

(147) Ibid., 10.xi.1827.

(148) Ibid., 17.xi.1827.

(149) Ibid., 6.xii.1827.

(150) Ibid., 13.xii.1827.

(151) Ibid., 26.xii.1827.

(152) Ibid., 2.i.1828.

(153) Ibid., 5.i.1828.

(154) Ibid., 6.vi.1828.

(155) Ibid., 20.vi.1828.

(156) Ibid., 5.ii.1828.

(157) R.C.P.E. (1833) *Report on Examination of Medical Practitioners*. Edinburgh: Neill.

(158) R.C.P.E. (1834) *General Correspondence*, 1.xi.1834.

(159) Council Minutes, 30.x.1857.

(160) Ibid., 29.i.1858.

(161) [*Montrose Standard*] (1870).

(162) [POOLE, R.] [1825] *Proposals for the Establishment of a New Infirmary*. [Edinburgh: n.p.]

(163) DUNCAN, A. (1825) *A Letter to Sir William Fettes . . . [on] the Establishment of a Lock Hospital, and an Hospital for Incurables . . . .* Edinburgh: Neill.

(164) POOLE, R. (1825) *Letter to Andrew Duncan, sen. . . . regarding the Establishment of a New Infirmary.* Edinburgh: Archibald Constable & Co.

(165) R.C.P.E. (1826) *Correspondence Relating to the Medical Provident Institution*, 22.xii.1826.

(166) R.C.P.E. (1828) *General Correspondence*, 5.vi.1828.

(167) R.C.P.E. (1829) *General Correspondence*, 16.iv.1829.

(168) *Medical Directory* (1870), p. 770. London: John Churchill & Sons.

(169) SCOTTISH LUNACY COMMISSION (1857) *Report by Her Majesty's Commissioners Appointed to Inquire into the State of Lunatic Asylums in Scotland*. Appendix, pp. 132–3. Edinburgh: Thomas Constable.

(170) HALKETT, S. & LAING, J. (1932) *Dictionary of Anonymous and Pseudonymous English Literature*. New & enl. ed. Vol. 6, p. 238. Edinburgh: Oliver & Boyd.

(171) POOLE, F. A. G. (1974) Personal communication.
(172) College Minutes, 5.v.1868.

THE CITADEL REPROVES

(173) RAE, J. (1895) *Life of Adam Smith*, p. 276. London: Macmillan.
(174) GREGORY, J. (1800) *Memorial to the Managers of the Royal Infirmary*, pp. 185–6. Edinburgh: Murray & Cochrane.
(175) R.C.P.E. (1925) *Historical Sketch and Laws*, p. 60. Edinburgh: Royal College of Physicians.
(176) R.C.P.E. (1850–63) *Letter Books*. 7 vols. (Mss.)
(177) Council Minutes, 26.vi.1860.
(178) Ibid., 3.vii.1860.
(179) Ibid., 24.iii.1876.
(180) Ibid., 28.i.1896.
(181) Ibid., 20.xii.1858.
(182) R.C.P.E. (1860) *Letter Book*, 9.x.1860.
(183) College Minutes, 20.iv.1859.
(184) Ibid., 26.iv.1859.
(185) R.C.P.E. (1925) *Historical Sketch and Laws*, p. 60. Edinburgh: Royal College of Physicians.
(186) College Minutes, 26.iv.1859.
(187) COOKE, A. M. (1972) *A History of the Royal College of Physicians of London*, vol. 3, p. 811. Oxford: Clarendon.
(188) CHRISTISON, Sir R. (1885) *Life of Sir Robert Christison, Bart.*, vol. I, pp. 193–4. Edinburgh: Blackwood.
(189) College Minutes, 2.viii.1859.
(190) R.C.P.E. (1925) *Historical Sketch and Laws*, pp. 62–3. Edinburgh: Royal College of Physicians.
(191) BROWN, T. (1886) *Alexander Wood, M.D., F.R.C.P.E: A sketch of his life and work*, pp. 126–9. Edinburgh: Macniven & Wallace.
(192) R.C.P.E. (1925) *Historical Sketch and Laws*, p. 62. Edinburgh: Royal College of Physicians.
(193) College Minutes, 1.v.1860.
(194) Ibid., 29.v.1860.
(195) Ibid., 26.iv.1859.
(196) Ibid., 10.v.1859.
(197) The Edinburgh College of Physicians (1859) *British Medical Journal*, p. 633.
(198) College Minutes, 2.viii.1859.
(199) Edinburgh College of Physicians (1859) *British Medical Journal*, p. 634.
(200) The College of Physicians of Edinburgh (1859) *British Medical Journal*, p. 704.

MALEVOLENT ANONYMITY

(201) Council Minutes, 11.vi.1860.
(202) Ibid., 24.xi.1857.

(203) Ibid., 4.xii.1857.

(204) R.C.P.E. (1857) *General Correspondence*, 17.xi.1857.

(205) Council Minutes, 14.vi.1859.

(206) R.C.P.E. (1853) *Letter Book*, 25.iv.1853.

(207) Council Minutes, 26.vi.1860.

(208) Ibid., 3.vii.1860.

(209) Ibid., 10.vii.1860.

(210) Ibid., 17.vii.1860.

(211) GRANT, Sir A. (1884) *The Story of the University of Edinburgh*, vol. II, p. 410. London: Longmans, Green & Co.

(212) *Dictionary of National Biography* (1885) Vol. IV, p. 245. London: Smith, Elder & Co.

(213) Council Minutes, 18.xii.1860.

Chapter XX

FOSTERING HOSPITAL AND OTHER CARE

The pioneering spirit has been to the forefront in many College activities. Nowhere was this more evident than in the promotion and sponsorship of hospital, dispensary and other services intended first and foremost for the benefit of the poor and necessitous.

THE ROYAL INFIRMARY, EDINBURGH

It may seem a strange principle to enunciate as the very first requirement in a Hospital that it should do the sick no harm.

Florence Nightingale

THE MONROS AND PROVOST DRUMMOND

'As Men and Christians we have the strongest Inducements, and even obligations to this sort of Charity, as it is warmly recommended and injoyned in the Gospel as one of the greatest Christian Duties: That Humanity and Compassion naturally prompt us to relieve our Fellow Creatures when in such deplorable Circumstances as many are reduced to, Naked, Starving, and in the outmost Distress from Pain and Trouble of Body and Anguish of Soul; That as the Relief of these is a Duty, so it is no less Advantage to a Nation, for as many as are recovered in an Infirmary are so many working Hands gained to the Country; That Students in Physic and Surgery might hereby have rather a better and easier Opportunity of Experience, than they have hitherto had by studying abroad, where such Hospitals are, at a great charge to themselves, and a yearly loss to the Nation: And as a Proof of the whole, they appealed to the good effects of the Infirmaries in all other Civilised Nations.'

The above words are taken from a pamphlet printed in 1721 which aimed at awakening the public to the need for an infirmary or comparable institution, and at promoting a fund to build and equip such an institution. There is general agreement that the words were inspired by John Monro and probably written by his son Alexander Monro *primus*.[1] John Monro, a one-time pupil of Pitcairne at Leyden,[2] had seen service in the Army under William of Orange and, on resigning his commission, joined the Incorporation of Surgeons of which he was Deacon in 1712.[3] Among his main purposes in life were the giving to his son every opportunity to follow him in his profession, and the creation of a 'medical seminary' in Scotland. His first ambition was achieved without set-back—Alexander being admitted into the Incorporation of Surgeons in 1719 prior to being appointed by the Town Council 'Professor of Anatomy in the City and College' in 1720. The son had in succession served as apprentice to his father, worked under Cheselden in London, and studied first in Paris and later under Boerhaave in Leyden. The first report of the Managers of the Infirmary was not published until 1730[4] and it was in response to a special request by Alexander Monro that the report contained an extensive quotation from the pamphlet of 1721.

COLLEGE TO THE FORE

Referring to the appeal of 1721 Turner recorded that it 'unfortunately met with no success and this effort on the part of the Monros, having failed to receive the support it deserved, was in consequence abandoned. But the seeds of a great idea had been sown which were to bear fruit at no distant date.'[5] He then went on to give credit to the Royal College of Physicians for initiating a second appeal in 1725.[6] First reference to the subject in the College Minutes appeared on 1st February 1726, but from the terms of the Minute it is evident that informal discussions had been proceeding for some time and were fairly far advanced.[7] Among those interested and promising support were George Drummond, the newly elected Lord Provost and friend of Alexander Monro. [6, 8] The President represented to the College 'That according to their desire, He and severall of the members had sett on foot a Subscription for Erecting, and Maintaining ane Infirmary or Hospitall for the sick poor and had pretty good Success, and Recommended to all the members of the Colledge To use their best endeavours To produce more Subscriptions for accomplishing So good and Charitable a work'.[9] There was no further reference to the project until 1st August

1727. On that day it was decided that an advertisement which was read to the College should be inserted in the newspapers.

The advertisement was to the effect that 'The Royall Colledge of phisitians Haveing allwayes shown such a particular Concern for the Sick poor That for severall years two of yr number have attended every week in yr Hall to give advice and also medicines to some proper objects Gratis and now Considering that yr is ane Hospitall for the Sick poor to be erected at Edgr. Therefor they for the Incouragement of Such a pious undertaking obleidge ymselves that one or more of their members Shall attend the said Hospitall faithfully and freely whout. any prospect of Reward or Sallary untill the Stock of ye sd Hospitall shall be so Increased that it can affoord a Reasonable allowance for one or two phisitians for yr proper use And the Colledge orders this advertisement Signed in yr name by yr president to be published . . .'.[10] At the next Quarterly Meeting it was confirmed that the advertisement had appeared in the Press after which the President (Dr John Drummond) 'Represented . . . that the first Subscriptions . . . was Compleated in due time, and the money was Comeing in And that it was the members of the Colledge that had sett this Charitable work on foot And had Contributed for it themselves and procured Contributions from other well Disposed persons, And Still hoped they would procure more Subscriptions for establishing the Infirmary that might be in some measure suitable to the necessitys of the Country'.[11]

THE KIRK

In an effort to stimulate further subscriptions the College decided to approach the General Assembly of the Church of Scotland. An address was prepared and three Fellows (Drs Rule, Riddell and Innes) appointed to attend 'ye Committee of Bills yranent'. In length the address vied with that of many a Scottish divine's sermon. It commenced with a reminder about the activities of the College in attending to the poor, and then emphasized 'yt ye advice given and ye medicines applyed often proved unsuccessfull, and Came short of their good effect, through the patients yr. wanting due Care taken of ym, and yr being Destitute of means for provideing a proper dyet and Lodgeing while under Cure'. The College proposals, influenced by 'ye example and practice of most oyr Countries and Cities' were then elaborated. Their purpose was to ensure that 'poor persons may not only have advice and medicine Gratis, But also (When ye physicians sees it necessary) be entertained at bed and board with proper serts. to attend ym during ye time of ye Cure'. Appropriately incidental comment was made on the Christian nature of the work involved.

The hope was expressed that realization of the project would result in 'many poor tradesmen, Servants, apprentices, journeymen, and Labourers, who Casually meet with fracturers Bruises, wounds, Dislocations or do fall into Sickness, by the Blessing of God, and the timeous application of proper medicines, be Recovered and Restored to health and Strength'.[12] Specific mention of 'Servants' is of significance because even moderate care of the many servants of the nobility and more well-to-do was precluded by the virtual total lack of suitable accommodation in the towering overcrowded tenement dwellings. This was a subject of a memorandum submitted by the physicians in 1738, but no action was taken until 1756 when twenty beds (ten for each sex) were reserved for this particular type of patient in the Infirmary.[13, 14]

The industrial age still lay ahead, but the economics of the situation were not forgotten in the Address to the Assembly. It was pointed out that want of help in the form of a hospital begat beggars and burdens 'upon yr. friends or the publict'; and that a hospital would 'be a Cheque upon many idle and Slothfull persons, who under pretence of some slight Lameness Sickness or weakness, give ymselves up to begging and become a burthen upon ye Countrey . . .'. Having already declared that 'some good progress' had been made in obtaining subscriptions and donations from 'some worthy Gentlemen and the Charitable Disposition of persons of all Ranks', a bold appeal was directed to 'the venerable assembly being in use to give Countenance to and forward all pious and Charitable undertakeings . . .'. With seemly deference the Assembly was asked 'To Consider the premisies and to Recommend A voluntar Contribution at ye Several parish Churches . . . in . . . Such manner As to ye venerable assembly Shall seem most Suitable'.[15]

The three emissaries to the Assembly succeeded in obtaining 'ane Act of ye assembly in favours of ye Infirmary', but on being informed to that effect the College, with an element of humility and seemly contrition quite out of character, confessed to ignorance of ecclesiastical protocol—'The Colledge not well knowing the forme of getting ye act made effectual So as to answer the designe yrby intended'. It was left to the President (Dr Francis Pringle) and one of the original emissaries (Dr John Riddell) to seek enlightenment[16] and in due course they were able to inform the College that the Depute Clerk had assured them that 'Circular Letters and Copys of the . . . act of the Assembly' would be sent to 'the moderators of the severall presbitrys whin. Scotland'.[17]

The first part of the Assembly Act consisted in large measure of a reproduction of the case submitted in petition form by the College. There then followed:

'The General Assembly having heard the said Petition and taking into their most serious Consideration the deplorable Circumstances of many industrous Poor of both Sexes, who while in Health and Firmness of Body do labour with Diligence, and maintain themselves and Families, yet when they fall into Sickness, or are otherwise disabled, are in the greatest Extremity of Misery, being not only destitute of Bread, but want the necessary Means of Cure and Recovery; against both which inconveniences a Remedy is proposed by this Pious and Christian Project. And the Assembly also considering that this Infirmary or Hospital will be of universal and common Use to the Poor of the whole Nation, they do therefore with the greatest Earnestness recommend a publick Contribution through all the Parishes of *Scotland* for advancing thereof, to be made upon such Lord's Days as the several Presbyteries or Ministers shall think most proper, after these Presents come to their Hands: And do exhort all well disposed Persons, especially those on whom GOD has bestowed the inestimable Blessings of Health and Strength, and any competent Measure of the other good Things of this Life, that they'll lay to Heart the Distress of such their fellow Christians as are deprived of them, and, according to their Ability, contribute chearfully to their Relief, by encouraging this so necessary and charitable a Design. And the Assembly appoints this Act and Recommendation to be published in all the Parish Churches of *Scotland*, upon the Lord's Day preceeding the Day to be appointed for the Collection, immediately after Sermon in the Forenoon; and recommends to the several Ministers who preach on the said Lord's Days, to enforce the same with suitable Exhortations; And appoints the Money collected in the several Parishes, to be put into the Hands of the Moderators of the respective Presbyteries, and by them to be carefully transmitted to *Edinburgh*, with the first Opportunity, to *David Spence* Secretary to the Bank of *Scotland*, who, at the Desire of the said Royal College of Physicians, has undertaken the Trouble of receiving the whole Contributions for this Charitable Work, and will give Receipts for the same, to be accounted for by him to the Managers of the said Infirmary, conform to his Obligation granted for that End.'[18]

As events proved, this method of approach did not meet with immediate success. Maitland offered an explanation but the stringency of his remarks may reflect the bias of an anti-cleric. He wrote that although contributions were earnestly and strenuously recommended by the Assembly in their Act and although copies of the Act were sent to incumbents of parishes throughout Scotland, 'Such was the amazing Indolence, Laziness and Obduration of the said Incumbents, to their eternal Reproach . . . few of them concerned themselves . . . many had not sent the Money collected'.[19] According to Arnot 'ten out of eleven of the whole established clergy of Scotland utterly disregarded' the Assembly Act.[20]

Turner in his account exercised greater tact and caution. According to him several Presbyteries had to be reminded of the Act and Recommendation of the General Assembly. Eventually response was forthcoming from all the parishes in Edinburgh and surrounding suburbs and from 72 others 'throughout the length and breadth of

Scotland'.[21] Contributions were received also from twelve Episcopal congregations. One aspect of the original Assembly appeal has assumed permanent significance. The origins of the Infirmary Sunday known to the present generation are to be traced to the Assembly's recommendation in 1728 that parish churches in Scotland should reserve a Lord's Day on which the initial collection should be made.[18]

Notwithstanding the lack of initial enthusiasm on the part of the Kirk, the College was encouraged by the continuing success of their appeal in other quarters, and decided to summon a General Meeting of the Contributors and make known the extent of the response to date. They therefore inserted an advertisement on 5th February 1728 in the *Caledonian Mercury* which had carried the previous notice. The terms of this later venture were as follows: 'The Subscribers or Contributors for erecting an Infirmary or Hospital for Sick Poor at Edinburgh are desired to be at a General Meeting on Monday, the nineteenth instant at 3 o'clock after Noon, at the Burrow-room; to direct and order what is necessary for carrying on that charitable work.' And then to conclude there came a sentence which must surely be regarded as the acme of purposeful diplomacy—'And the subscribers thereto who have not yet paid are intreated to pay up their Donations.'[22] Ironically the 'Assembly Ladies' who in the years ahead were to be a source of concern to Dr Beilby (Chap. IV) were among the most zealous in organizing subscription lists! The Society of Friends was particularly active.

The sequence of events was described as follows in the *History of the Royal Infirmary* (1778)—'The Subscription of £2000 was no sooner compleated, than the College of Physicians called the contributors together, who named twelve of their number, as a committee, for collecting the money subscribed, for obtaining more subscriptions, and for preparing a plan of management of the Infirmary.'[23] The Committee thereupon hired a small house for receiving the sick poor and appointed twenty managers to assume control. Members of the Committee included nine physicians, all on the Roll of the College—Doctors Drummond, Pringle, Clerk, Cochrane, Lowis, Innes, Plummer, Learmont and Dundas. Their surgical associates were Messrs John Kennedy, Alexander Monro and Robert Hope. Other bodies represented were the Town Council, Senators of the College of Justice, the Faculty of Advocates and the general body of subscribers. Meetings held at first in the Burgh Room were later transferred to St John's Coffee House in the corner of Parliament Close where they continued until 1742.[24]

Thin described how, construction eventually being started, gratuitous gifts and service were forthcoming from all quarters. '... the wrights made presents of window sashes ready made, the joiners gave windows, the quarries at Easdale provided slates which the slaters dressed and laid on. Timber was given by Leith merchants, while the Duke of Argyll's Duddingston tenants gave 6000 dales (planks). The brewers promised to supply . . . malt, the coal-masters . . . coals, farmers lent their carts, and . . . many workmen . . . gave one or two days' labour free.'[25, 26]

MEDICAL CARE

The house which was selected stood at the head of Robertson's Close and had accommodation for six patients.[27] In the interval, satisfied 'That the Infirmary is now in Readiness for Receiving patients And that it will be necessary they attend the Same' the College agreed unanimously 'To attend the Infirmary in yr Turns for the Space of a fortnight until Some Settled Method be agreed upon Anent their attendance'. It was left to the President (Dr Pringle) to appoint whomsoever 'he thinks fitt' and his first choice was Dr Drummond, whose attendance commenced on 6th August 1729[28] on which day the 'small hired house' was formally opened.[29] The President's authority in this connection was subsequently renewed for another quarter.[30]   Very appropriately the first Fellow to attend as physician, Dr John Drummond, had been President at the time the College set in motion the movement for the erection of an Infirmary.[31]

Arrangements for attendance on the Infirmary and Sick poor were modified in May 1730 to meet the situation whereby medical care for the poor was being provided at both the Infirmary and the College Hall. It was decided that 'in place of two phisicians who ordinarly attended the hall formerly, only one shall wait on And when the present Course is over, The Eldest phisician shall begin, And so in Course go on as formerly'. It was further ordered 'That when all the Fellows and Licentiats have gone through this Course at the Infirmary The Senior Phisician shall again begin and So to go on . . . And that all the Fellows and Licentiats shall be obleidged to attend both at the Hall and Infirmary in yr turns Or Send oyrs of ye Colledge . . .'.[32]

A CHARTER GRANTED

About this time consideration was being given to embarking on a larger hospital and to seeking a Royal Charter. With these objects in view Dr John Clerk, a Fellow of the College, wrote to his friend the Lord Advocate, Duncan Forbes of Culloden, impressing upon him that he 'could not certainly do a more charitable thing than to put us on a way or method to obtain the premisses'. Commenting on 'the looseness of our Society' he told of 'the generall Meeting' which gave 'management of the hospital to a committee, who pass under the name of managers (to shun that of directors) to be chosen annually'. How refreshing to read this of directorships but, how would the writer have expressed himself in an age when self-styled directors far outnumber managers, and their academic counterparts—professors! Whatever his views, Clerk abetted his argument by reminding his friend that 'The Crown has been in use to incorporate such charitable societies by Charter gratis, as particularly Q. Ann did the Society for propagation of Christian knowledge'.[33, 34]

Five years elapsed before the Infirmary was granted a Royal Charter[33] and ten before the first patients were admitted into a new hospital in Thomson's Yards not far removed from Robertson's Close.[35] The members of the Building Committee included Andrew St Clair, a Fellow of the College; Alexander Monro *primus*, professor of anatomy; a surgeon of the name of George Cunynghame; and the civic dignitary George Drummond.[36] According to Thin, Drummond relied at all stages on the advice of Dr John Clerk.[37]

SURGICAL CARE

While from the outset the medical care of patients in the embryonic Robertson's Close Infirmary had been established on a tolerably satisfactory administrative basis, the same could not be said of surgical provisions. Any suggestion that the Infirmary 'did not at first receive the support and assistance of the surgeons as an Incorporation' has been stoutly denied by Creswell.[38] He maintained that the undeniable fact that the surgeons as a body were not associated with the Infirmary until it had been functioning for nine years, was entirely attributable to rejection by the Infirmary of an offer made to them in 1729 by the Incorporation. According to the same authority, when it became necessary to appoint a surgeon two proposals were submitted in response to an invitation from the Managers—one by the Incorporation of Surgeons, and the other by Mr Alexander Monro in collaboration with five other surgeons.[39] The Incorporation offer contemplated the provision of medicines and operations gratis for two years, but again according to Creswell did not meet with favour because although supported by a majority of the Incorporation, in the opinion of the Infirmary Managers, no general Corporation Act could bind any particular member to a deed and service of charity. The Infirmary desired that members of the Incorporation willing to provide a surgical service to the hospital should sign an undertaking to that effect. Alexander Monro and his five colleagues accepted the Infirmary requirement and were appointed surgeons to the Infirmary.[40] Seen from the surgical point of view 'in this way the service in the hospital was performed by the attendance of the whole College of Physicians if they chose to do so, and by the six surgeons appointed in the manner above mentioned'.[39] Although not wholly accurate, the view is understandable in an atmosphere of embattled rivalries.[41]

Rejection of their proposal prompted the Incorporation of Surgeons to consider the erection of another Infirmary, to be called the Surgeon's Hospital in contra-distinction to the Infirmary in Robertson's Close, which was commonly referred to by the Surgeons as the Physicians' or Medical Hospital. In 1736 the Incorporation of Surgeons passed an Act to enable a Surgeon's Hospital to be erected.[40, 42] This second hospital was opened in College Wynd in July of the same year.[43]

Seemingly the surgeons were not without friends in the Church capable of 'stretching a point' to judge by the following minute of the Kirk Session of Kenmore Parish Church, Perthshire, for 18th September 1737:

> 'The Last Lord's Day an act of the General Assembly was read for a collection to the Chirurgeons at Edinburgh, and this being the Day appointed for the said Collection and the Session considering the smallness of the above Collection they thought it proper to appoint fortey six shillings and 6 pennies to be added to it.'[44]

Six months later a petition was received by the College of Physicians from the 'Surgeons Erectors of the Surgeons Hospital in Edinr.'.

> '... finding ymselves frequently at a Loss for want of furder advice Especially as to the use of Internal medicines Therefor Craveing That the Colledge would be pleased to Grant their assistance to ye petitioners in ye same Generous and Charitable way in which they served the Royal Infirmary which the petitioners heartily wish may florish or in any oyr Regular way of attendance which the Colledge in yr goodness and wisdom should think fitt, That the petitioners Can make no other Returns to the Colledge But yr Sincerest wishes for the Prosperity of the Royall Colledge and ane assurance That as the petitioners serve all Gratis that are able to Come to their Hospital to be drest besides those whom they accommodate in the house So they shall be most ready to assist in the same way such poor people in Chirurgical Cases as may Cast up to any of the Colledge at yr. hall or else where.'[45, 46]

No matter the temptation—comment would be immensely dangerous! Suffice to say the situation in which the College found itself could scarcely be more complicated considering the parties, alliances and past feuds involved—the managers of the

Infirmary, the Surgeons Incorporation, the College itself. How did the College react? The 'petition being read the Colledge delay the Consideration yrof till the [next] quarterly meeting . . . .'.[47]

At the next Meeting the College resolved 'That they are willing to give attendance to that Hospital when any of them are called upon. But refuse to bind themselves to give any Regular attendance.'[48] A more gracious word than 'refuse' might have been employed. And could there not have been courteous reference—no matter if implying refusal—to the offer of chirurgical assistance?

Without doubt the surgeons were acutely conscious of a sense of grievance. This is only too apparent in a statement made by them at this time in the course of debate to the effect that 'Everyone knows that the business of a surgeon . . . is not merely confined to surgical practice, or to the giving out of medicines as apothecaries, but they are employed as physicians-in-ordinary . . . It is only at extraordinary times that the assistance of the regular physician is required, and even that is very much confined to the higher and superior classes. Hence it has always happened that in this place, and indeed over Scotland, the great bulk of the practice is confined to the surgeons . . . if practice is so very essential to perfection in this profession, the chance of obtaining more skilful men was infinitely greater from the College of Surgeons than from the College of Physicians.'[49] How characteristic of strife arising from partition: an admixture of truth and misrepresentation! Whatever the rights and wrongs, the statement revealed the threatening cross-currents that were running. While understanding the opposed outlooks of physicians and surgeons sight should not be lost of the problems facing the Infirmary Managers or the impact on the welfare of patients in need of care. Fortunately resolution was achieved without too much bitterness. Nor should it be thought that Edinburgh Infirmary was alone with its staffing problems. They were known also to the Glasgow Royal Infirmary in the years to come.[50]

The Surgeon's Hospital was merged in the Infirmary after two years' separate existence.[51]

The Infirmary was incorporated by Royal Charter in 1736. Under the terms of the Charter, government of the Infirmary was vested in twenty Managers who were to include the President and four Fellows of the College, 'whereof two shall be of the Professors of Medicine in the University of Edinburgh'. Understandably, more especially in the light of practical experience gained in the interval, the Infirmary adhered to the policy of accepting professional services only from those willing to abide by regulations decided upon from time to time by the Managers. At a Quarterly Meeting in February 1738 the College was informed that a letter had been received stating 'That the managers had resolved That for the future the attendance of Physicians on the Infirmary be performed by such physicians only as are fellows of ye Royal Colledge And' by two named 'Licentiats . . . who in yr turns with the fellows . . . have attended ye Infirmary as Phisicians ever Since the first establishment yrof'. At the same time as conveying thanks to the College for 'good offices to ye Infirmary hitherto', the letter sought continuation of the services in question.[52] The purpose underlying the Managers' decision was to overcome the inconvenience consequent upon the large number of physicians, who consisted of all the Fellows and Licentiates on the Resident Roll of the College, involved in attending patients for short periods on a rotation system. In effect the new ruling established that in future none but Fellows of the Edinburgh College should act as Physicians, while at the same time making well-earned dispensation, involving no question of precedence, in the case of the two named Licentiates (q.v.). Without doubt the new arrangement favoured greater continuity of attendance to the ultimate benefit of patient, physician and pupils.[53]

A number of years later, in 1888 to be precise, the General Council of the University of Edinburgh approached the Infirmary Managers with a view to persuading them to recognise the degree of M.D. Edinburgh as an adequate qualification for election to the staff of the hospital. The reply of the Infirmary Board firmly indicated that 'both by the original Charter of 1736 and by subsequent resolutions of the Managers, the Board is absolutely bound to elect their physicians from the Royal College of Physicians of Edinburgh.'[54, 55] There could be no more convincing evidence of the way the understanding was respected than an enquiry received by the College from the Infirmary Managers as to the eligibility of a Fellow of the Royal College of Surgeons for the post of gynaecologist. No objection was raised by the College of Physicians. Indeed it is difficult to see how they could! They did however betray laudable astuteness in the light of the times by proscribing the designation 'Physician for Diseases of Women' and urging instead use of the term 'gynaecologist'.[56]

Reverting to the eighteenth century, a further and even more far-reaching adjustment in staffing arrangements was made in 1751, but in the interval the Infirmary had been transferred to a new building on a site belonging to the Trust for George Watson's Hospital.[57] The foundation stone of the new Infirmary was laid on 2nd August 1738 and in accordance with a resolution arrived at on the previous day the College met 'at yr own hall at three afternoon . . . to go in a body to witness the Laying'.[58] The Infirmary history recorded that 'The President (Dr. Robert Lowis) and Fellows of the Royal College of Physicians marched from their Hall in Fountain

Close'. In like manner the surgeons attended from their Hall in the immediate vicinity of Thomson's Yards.[59]

On the day of the event and presumably before 'falling in' for the march the College agreed to contribute to the ceremony 'Therty Guineas to be Levyed by voluntary Collection among the fellows'. The non-committal methods employed to ensure the target being reached were rather surprising. The Treasurer was 'ordered to give to the tresr. of the Royal Infirmary his note for the sd. Sum Instantly And if there is any deficiency in the said Collection the tresr. is allowed to make it up out of the stock of the Colledge, And if the Collection exceed the said Sum it is to be given in to the tresr. of the Infirmary'.[60] To complete the facts—the resolutions were passed at a sederunt attended by twelve Fellows none of whom is recorded as having opted for a fine and left early! This generosity did not reflect a passing mood. Four years later the Colledge decided that the twenty shillings formerly 'to be payed in to the dispensary by every member when admitted Socius Shall in time Comeing . . . be applyed for the use of the Poor of the Infirmary'.[61]

DISPENSARY—ADOPTION OF A COLLEGE CONCEPTION

There then occurred an event of considerable historic interest—more especially in retrospect. The Managers of the Royal Infirmary advanced a proposal 'That in place of the Colledge their giveing attendance upon poor patients at their own hall twice a week They will be pleased in time Coming in their turn to attend the poor out patients at the Infirmary upon Monday and friday weekly at three afternoon'. There could have been no greater tribute to the College than the implied recognition of the value of the attendance on the poor provided by the College from its earliest days. Furthermore the fact that the Infirmary Managers intimated their intention that 'out patients Shall get medicines gratis from the Infirmary Shop' was tantamount to accepting the Dispensary administered by the College as a model for imitation and development in the expanding Infirmary. Certainly this aspect of the Infirmary proposals greatly influenced the College in agreeing to them without demur.[62]

After medicines had been supplied for a number of years by the Infirmary shop the decision was taken that it involved 'too great expense upon the hospital charity'. The service was accordingly stopped, whereupon the College resumed the practice of giving medical relief to the Sick Poor in the Fountain Close Hall.[63, 64]

PENALTIES OF SUCCESS

Agreement having been decided upon there were presented to the College a 'Bound and titled' copy of the 'History and Status of the Royal Infirmary ... for the Library' and two dozen less elaborate 'Coppys of Said Statuts for the particular members of the Colledge'.[65] The statutes 'had been printed without any previous Concurrance of the Colledge'. Experience of them quickly revealed practical difficulties. It was 'found upon tryal very Inconvenient for the Same Physician to attend the Infirmary in the forenoon And the out patients in the afternoon'. To deal with the situation the College resolved 'That ... the attendance on the Infirmary and out patients shall be by two different physicians the one to attend the Patients in the Infirmary in the forenoon And the other to attend the Out Patients there on monday and friday afternoon'. Allocation of individuals to the different duties paid due regard to seniority, and to the conditions inseparable from a rotation system.[66]

Failure on the part of the Infirmary to consult the College prior to printing of the statutes was the subject of an apology,[66] and the arrangements as amended by the College were accepted by the Infirmary. It was arranged that the Clerk to the College should be made responsible for maintaining a list 'of Physicians who are to attend the wards', and another of those who are to attend out patients; and that the lists should be supplied 'To the Clerk of the Infirmary that the Physicians may be timeously advertised of the time of their attendance Respectively'.[67] The success of the arrangements was recorded at the next Quarterly Meeting[68]—the culmination of amicable negotiations which might serve as a useful pattern for clinicians and administrators at variance in the course of their N.H.S. duties. That was in 1750.

'FIXT PHYSICIANS'

In the following year effect was given to the major staffing change already mentioned. The College was written to by the Lord Provost 'in the name of the Corporation of the Royal Infirmary at a General meeting'. In it, mention is made of the 'Late Considerably Encreased' number of patients, the satisfactory state of the finances and prospects of 'Considerable future benefactions'—all pointing to the desirability of taking in 'Still a much greater number of distressed objects'. The Infirmary Corporation foresaw that as a result 'the trouble and attendance of the members of the Royal

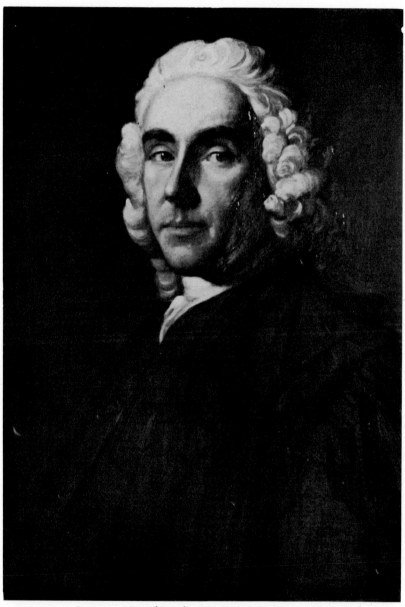

PLATE 31   Dr Alexander Monro *primus* (1697–1767)
By courtesy of the Royal College of Surgeons of Edinburgh

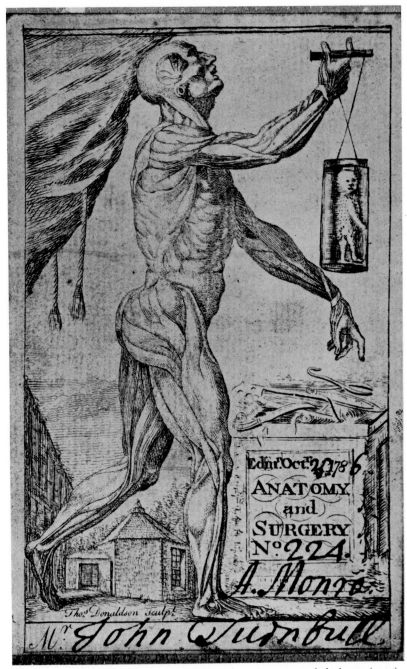

Edin Octr 20 1786
ANATOMY
and
SURGERY
N° 224.
A. Monro

Thos Donaldson sculp.^t

Mr John Turnbull

PLATE 32   Enrolment Card for Dr Alexander Monro *secundus'* classes (1786)
Reproduced from original in College Library; photograph by Tom Scott

Colledge who had the honour to give a Beginning to this useful undertaking . . . is Likely to be So much encreased'. As a remedy 'the managers have thought it yr duty' to appoint 'two fixt physicians for . . . the dayly attendance in the patients on the R. Infirmary under the Character of the physicians in ordinary thereto'. Claiming to have been suitably empowered the Managers stated their intention of naming the physicians on a day specified, and at the same time did 'Earnestly . . . Request of the Royal Colledge to Continue yr good offices . . . by appointing Some of their Number monethly by Rotation, Or in what other way They think proper, To visit the House Once or twice a week To give yr advice and assistance to the two ordinary physicians, When they judge it necessary to apply to them for ye Same'.

Dispersed throughout the letter were many genuinely sincere appreciative comments on the help given by the College in the past. To mention them all could well give a mistaken impression of misleading mellifluousness. One expression however does deserve selected quotation if only because of its deep significance, its manifest sincerity and its delectable phraseology. The writer of the letter said 'he was Commanded by the General Court of the Corporation . . . in yr name to Return their humble and hearty thanks for the great pains the Colledge have taken in nurseing this Child of their own from its earliest appearance till now . . .'.

Without doubt the College was moved: indeed was moved to the extent that the President (Dr Porterfield) replied on their behalf to the effect that they did most 'chearfully agree To what is . . . desired'.[69] Their response was the more significant as curtailment of their privileges was involved. Henceforth physicians nominated by the College were called extra-ordinary physicians and their duties became in the main those of consulting physicians.[70] The first physicians-in-ordinary to be appointed were Drs David Clerk and Colin Drummond, an innovation being introduced with the payment to each of an annual salary of £30.[71] Clerk had been qualified five years and was a Fellow of the College. Two years previous to his salaried appointment, at the request of the Managers he designed the Crest of the Infirmary from which a Seal was cut on steel and used as a stamp on official documents, until in 1914 an error in the original armorial bearings was corrected under the direction of the Lord Lyon King of Arms.[72] Circumstances in connection with the appointment of Drummond are mentioned in Chapter XIX.

Increasing attendances at the Infirmary amply testified to the value attached by the public to the services provided there. Problems arose from the growing demands being made on the medical staff. At a Quarterly Meeting in 1753 the statement was made that 'attendance . . . upon the out patients . . . is now very Burdensome . . . by reason of the Great number of patients which attend, who take up the Colledge time

R

for several hours twice every week'. A Committee was appointed to consider among other possibilities 'whether such as are fellows of the College Shall only attend the out patients or if the Licentiats of the Colledge Shall also attend in their turn'.[73] Reporting back in three months' time the Committee gave it as their unanimous opinion that Fellows only should 'Consult and advise in the Character of Physicians Either for the patients within the house or for the out patients, And that none of the Licentiats should be Imployed in this attendance except . . . [the] two Gentlemen' who as Licentiates had given 'good offices to the Infirmary in its Infancy'. The Committee further recommended 'That for the future it will be sufficient That each of the fellows and those two Licentiates in their turn attend the out patients only one day weekly viz Monday at three o'clock afternoon for the space of a moneth, but if the Physician attending Shall judge it necessary he may appoint a Second day in the Same week, for giveing advice to Such of the out patients, as he could not undertake on the Monday'.[74] A simple appointments system in reverse!

MONETARY SUPPORT

College support of the Infirmary did not relax and within the limits of available resources periodically took monetary form. Thus a donation of 50 guineas was made in February 1785.[75] In 1819 a similar sum was given in recognition 'of the very great increase of expenditure incurred by . . . the Infirmary . . . in fitting up the Establishment at Queensberry House for the reception of Fever Patients . . . and the increased number of Patients received into it and to the Infirmary.[76] In the year 1868 the Infirmary decided to transfer once again to a new site and a public subscription list was opened. A sum of £1000 was voted by the College 'for the New Buildings . . . provided that they are erected on the large scale proposed, and that the College agree to pay the sum in five yearly instalments the first instalment to be paid twelve months after the building is commenced'.[77] The College attended as a body at the opening of the new Royal Infirmary on 29th October 1879 having some five to six months previously contributed a sum in excess of £600 to furnish two medical wards.[78] With the end of World War I the Infirmary in common with other voluntary hospitals found itself in grave financial straits. To assist to meet the situation the College donated 1000 guineas.[79] It is only fitting that the College's indebtedness to the Infirmary many years previously for temporary library (Chap. IV) and laboratory (Chap. V) accommodation should not be forgotten.

INSTRUCTION AT THE BEDSIDE

The fame of Edinburgh as a medical centre owes an immeasurable amount to the early importance attached to clinical instruction at the bedside. The University, Fellows of the College combining clinical with teaching duties, and the Infirmary share the credit. A Fellow and President of the College, Dr J. Hamilton, has left the following account of the position in the Infirmary medical wards at the end of the eighteenth century.

> 'A clerk is attached to each physician. He is commonly a young gentleman, who is advanced in his studies. He resides in the Hospital and has a general superintendence of the patients, who are under the charge of the physician with whom he is connected. Besides other duties, it is his business to prepare a written account of the symptoms of those patients, who fall under the care of the physician . . . He inserts this account in the journal book, and reads it to the physician at the bedside of the patient, on the following daily visit.
>
> The physician either admits the account simply, or makes additions and alterations, as he may think proper.
>
> Regular reports of the subsequent state of the symptoms; of the remedies prescribed, and of the effects of these are given daily . . . These reports are the result of the accounts, which the patients give of themselves, or of the accounts which are received from the nurses, or both together; they are dictated by the physician to his clerk, who at the time, enters them into the journal book.
>
> All these proceedings take place in public, in the presence, and in the hearing, of a number of young gentlemen, who attend the Hospital . . .'.[80]

The description referred to 1800. It could well, and desirably, apply to any medical ward today, with as only amendment, reports of radiological and other laboratory findings! True, technical jargon and scientific intervention may have grown out of all bounds since 1800—but clinical observations remain the foundation of medical care.

In a material age the tendency is to focus attention on the architectural attraction and technical advances in a modern hospital. An enthusiastic vocational outlook among junior staff—medical and nursing—can too readily be looked at askance. Respect for, as distinct from deference to tradition is suspect. Be that as it may, the international greatness of the Edinburgh Royal Infirmary as a teaching hospital owes to this day an incalculable amount to the traditions established in the early eighteenth century. The spirit underlying the tradition and stimulating vocational enthusiasm is admirably delineated in Christison's description of his resident days in the Infirmary.

'I doubt', he wrote, 'whether any other medical school offers such a union of advantages as our resident Infirmary officers enjoy—ample materials for study; able superiors, engaged in teaching, and ever on a level with the times; a confidential position of much trust; companions from the ablest students of a populous University; museums and libraries freely open; professors and others, to whom it is a labour of love to foster diligence and talent; a city abounding with all sorts of rational amusement; and good society, easy of access.'[81]

It is an open question whether—considering hospitals in general—planners, seniors and juniors, lay and professional, are today always alive to the risk to themselves and patients that loss of these advantages involves.

THE N.H.S.

Administratively, the advent of the National Health Service involved what may reasonably be described as revolutionary changes in certain long-standing agreements between the Royal Infirmary and the College. Forewarning of this was given towards the end of 1947 when a College representative on the Management Committee of the Infirmary was invited by the President (Dr W. D. Small) to address the Fellows. He foretold that on the appointed day the new Infirmary Board would not inherit all the managerial responsibilities of their predecessor and would not deal with appointments. It was, he considered, more than likely that the Regional Hospital Board would appoint an Advisory Appointments Committee to deal with staff vacancies. Subsequent developments confirmed the accuracy of the forecast. A further regrettable change on both practical and historical grounds was that the League of Subscribers which during its twenty years of existence had collected over £1,000,000 was no longer represented on the Board of Management.[82]

Such then in bald terms is the part played by the College 'in nurseing the Child of their own Creation from its earliest appearance'. Records for the period convey a sense of quiet determination, readiness to deal with difficulties, willingness to co-operate with the Managers, and of unspoken reserved pride. Allowing that there was one major disputation (Chap. XIX) the relations between College and Infirmary were undisguisedly friendly, based on mutual indebtedness, trust, respect and endeavour. In this they contrasted pleasingly with the College's relations in some other spheres. There never was, nor ever could be, a hint of 'contumaciousness'.

FRAILTY—HUMAN AND INSTITUTIONAL

Nevertheless an unfortunate incident, reflecting discredit neither on the College nor on the Infirmary, took place in 1897. A doctor associated with the College understated his age when applying for a professional appointment at the Infirmary. His action was brought to the notice of the College by three Fellows and subsequently investigated, but without at first wholly satisfying the Infirmary.[83] Eventually the unfortunate affair was accepted as closed when the Council declared its sympathy 'with the zeal for the maintenance of the honour of the College and the profession shewn by the Fellows who have brought misstatements under the notice of the Council'; but at the same time stated that they had not found evidence of *muta fides* on the part of the gentleman in question.[84]

Again, early in 1915 there were the makings of misunderstanding between the College and the Infirmary. Fortunately they were transient. The trouble originated with a letter from the Treasurer and Clerk of the Infirmary Board informing the President of the College that the Hospital Managers had resolved to appoint a 'Temporary Assistant Physician'. This was followed by a statement that 'Candidates must be registered medical practitioners, but not necessarily Fellows of either Royal College . . .'. Possibly to mollify the College the letter went on to say that 'it is to be distinctly understood that the conferring of this office is not in any way to imply or to be regarded as giving the holder prior claim to consideration in any future election . . .'. The Secretary (Dr Dingwall-Fordyce) replied on behalf of the President (Dr Freeland Barbour) in terms which might have been expected—but none the less conciliatory. The Infirmary were reminded of long standing agreements, mildly reproved for 'going past' the Fellows of the College, and assured that the special circumstances being recognized, the College would offer every assistance in finding a suitable Physician. Twelve days later there came the comment 'As they had appointed a Fellow of your College to the post of Temporary Assistant Physician the Managers were of opinion that no action was necessary in connection with that communication'.[85]

There next appeared in the Minutes, copy of yet another letter from the Infirmary dated 29th September 1915—the first letter having been dated 8th March of the same year. Apparently there had been intervening correspondence, or inordinate delay understandable in war time. From the practical point of view the essential thing was that the College received an assurance that in the event of the post of Temporary Assistant Physician having to be advertised again there would be no suggestion that other than Fellows of the Royal College of Physicians would be eligible. Furthermore, the College were left in no doubt that the Infirmary Board would gladly avail themselves of the help offered by the College.[86]

A gratifying ending—but, without being oblivious to the interests of Fellows on active service, need such a misunderstanding ever have assumed these proportions at a time of mounting casualties in Flanders and of grave national crisis?

The year 1922 saw a major adjustment in arrangements agreed by the College and Royal Infirmary. Aware of the position of medical officers returned from the Services, and the situation created by intensified specialization, it was decided that additional to Fellows, Members should be eligible for appointment on the staff of the Infirmary.[87] Earlier in the century (1904) the College had agreed in principle to the imposition of an age-limit for members of the medical staff of the Infirmary.[88] When asked subsequently about the situation of university professors holding office 'ad vitam aut culpam' but dispossessed of beds, the College betrayed the agile evasion of experts.[89]

EDINBURGH LUNATIC ASYLUM

The body labours in this unhappy predicament until it is destroyed . . .
Sir Henry Halford (Evidence before a Select Committee on
Madhouses, 1816)

One of the very first actions of Dr Andrew Duncan, sen. after being elected President in 1790 was to recommend the appointment of a Committee to consider 'the establishment of a Lunatic Asylum—which is much wanted in this City'.[90]

MAN'S INHUMANITY TO MAN

Provisions in the city at this time for those suffering from mental derangement beggared description. They were limited to a branch of the Charity Workhouse named The City Bedlam which was subject to the superintendence and direction of the Workhouse Managers. In the words of an *Address* issued to the public at the turn of the century, it was 'scarcely possible to conceive a situation less adapted, either to promote recovery, or to confer that comfort which even the incurably insane are capable of enjoying . . . no degree of care, on the part of any Managers . . . or of those . . . under them . . . can ever, while the present circumstances exist, completely remedy the evils complained of . . .'.[91] Much earlier in the century when plans were being drawn up for the new Infirmary building, the architect—William Adam—included in his arrangements a small number of 'cells' for the accommodation of the insane. These cells formed part of the first section of the new building to be completed but their use for the originally intended purpose was discontinued about the end of the eighteenth century with the advent of special asylum institutions.[92]

There is reason to believe that towards the end of the eighteenth century a sadly slow and only very partially enlightened general awareness of the plight and needs of the mentally deranged was developing. It is possible that this may have arisen in part from the recurrent mental illness of George III, whose recovery from one of his most violent attacks was the occasion for a day of national rejoicing. At the time an Extraordinary Meeting of the College was called to consider an address of loyalty and thanksgiving which, having been approved, was duly sent through appropriate channels for presentation to the King.[93]

POET'S TRAGEDY

Whatever the factors disturbing public conscience, Andrew Duncan's compassionate interest in the subject was almost certainly stimulated by his experience when attending the Scottish poet Robert Fergusson in a professional capacity. Fergusson was in a delirious state of 'furious insanity', unsuited to being attended to any longer in his widowed mother's home. The only place to which he could be transferred was the City Bedlam. There he remained until death brought tragic but blessed relief, in a stone-floored cell with minimal ventilation and minimal natural light. It has been written of his decease '. . . who for but two years was to write Scots poems and songs of the truest ring, before Burns wrote them surpassingly . . . was to die in 1774 on the straw of a madhouse at the age of 24'.[94] Twelve years later Burns took the opportunity when in Edinburgh to visit Fergusson's grave in the Canongate Church Yard and to obtain from the Kirk Session permission to erect a tombstone to the poet's memory.[95]

Duncan's life and career testify to his sensitive humanism. It was but a natural course of events that he responded as he did to the circumstances of Fergusson's death. The College Committee for which he had asked (q.v.) reported back within six months.[96] They recommended 'the Establishment in the neighbourhood of Edinr.

of a Lunatic Asylum similar to that of York': and that 'Houses . . . kept by private persons . . . should be put under the same regulations with those in the neighbourhood of London and particularly that they should in the same manner be subject to a visitation of Commissioners appointed by the College of Physicians'. The Report expressed satisfaction that funds should be forthcoming 'provided a respectable set of Trustees were appointed'; and suggested the nomination of certain civic and legal dignitaries additional to the College President and Deacon of the Incorporation of Surgeons. A more debatable recommendation was that certain moneys bequeathed to the 'building a Foundling Hospital a species of Charity to which there are many strong objections would be much more usefully employed in building a Lunatic Asylum'. To implement this it was urged that some of the money in question might be appropriated by Act of Parliament.

THE COLLEGE PIONEERS

Having added two representatives of the Guild of Trades to the Committee list of suggested Trustees, the College sent the Report to the Lord Provost soliciting his active interest.[96] Six months later the President (Dr Andrew Duncan, sen.) was able to announce the acceptance of the responsibilities of trusteeship by all who had been approached; and then, evidencing a flair for charitable appeal, and having declared that 'the business now seemed to be in considerable forwardness', put it to the College that they should 'take some lead in subscribing' to the extent of twenty-five pounds.[97] Some years later, the *Address to the Public* was issued. Points emphasized in the *Address* were that the proposed asylum would promote the 'benefit of the Rich as well as of the Poor': and the expense to the public would be limited to the cost of the original erection. Assurance was given concerning professional superintendence: a list of Trustees, Managers and Office-bearers appended; and an appeal made on the grounds of urgent necessity, 'private humanity and a patriotic regard for the public good'.[98]

PUBLIC PARSIMONY

The proposals had the unanimous support of the Incorporation of Surgeons, but how did the lay public respond to the appeal? The answer to that is to be found in an illustrated pamphlet of 43 pages published in October 1812 and selling at 2s. 6d. per copy 'for the benefit of the Edinburgh Lunatic Asylum'. 'A subscription was set on foot' read the pamphlet '. . . But . . . made at that time very little progress. Although almost every member of the College of Physicians, and a great majority of the College of Surgeons, contributed something, yet from different circumstances, the subscription was almost entirely confined to them, in so much, that at the beginning of the year 1806, fourteen years after the subscription had been begun, the sum paid into the hands of the Treasurer . . . little exceeded £100.'[99]

Nevertheless a note of cautious optimism was evident when in May 1806 the College were informed by the President (Dr Thos. Spens) that 'he had great hopes of the Plan being now carried into effect'; 'The intended Managers . . . had lately had many meetings'; a piece of ground had been purchased; and that there were 'expectations of receiving considerable aid from Government'.[100] Expectations were fulfilled in so far as at the next Quarterly Meeting of the College it was announced that £2000 had been made available by the Government.[101] Credit was due to the Lord Advocate of the day who had obtained the sum in question, derived from the sale of Highland estates forfeited after the 1745 Rebellion.[102] A new appeal was issued to the public after a Royal Charter had been obtained in 1807 but again contrary to expectations subscriptions derived little impetus.

COLONIAL GENEROSITY

In a quite extraordinary way 'the undertaking . . . met with greater encouragement abroad than at home. In the East Indies . . . upwards of a Thousand pounds collected from different subscribers was remitted from that settlement.' A considerable number of subscriptions were remitted from Bengal and Ceylon, and some few were received 'from British Colonies both in the West Indies and in America'. These contributions, together with sums obtained as the result of church collections in Edinburgh and eastern Scotland, brought the total money paid in to the Honorary Treasurer to £7446 by November 1812. Whether in a spirit of disillusionment or sustained optimism is not evident, but the pamphlet went on to say that the advantage resulting from the anticipated reception of patients in 1815 'will give more convincing demonstration of' the Asylum's 'utility and more effectually arouse the attention of the Public, than any address either from the Press or the Pulpit'.[103]

Still determined to further the Asylum project which owed its origin to him, Dr Duncan, sen., now no longer President of the College, moved in July 1814 'that in order to afford to the Public convincing evidence of the necessity and importance of a proper Lunatic Asylum the College should subscribe Twenty Five Pounds sterling for carrying on the Buildings of the Asylum, as a second subscription'.[104] His motion was approved at the next Quarterly Meeting.[105] Interest in the 'Morningside' hospital lived long in the Duncan family. In 1886 Miss Elizabeth Bevan, a grand-daughter of Dr Andrew Duncan, sen., left a legacy of £13,000, the interest on which was 'to supplement the board of patients of the educated class'.[106]

CRAIG HOUSE

The subsequent development of the asylum now known as the Royal Edinburgh Hospital for Nervous and Mental Disorders was described in detail by Henderson. A larger building, West House, replaced the original small East House in 1839. In 1873 (Sir) Thomas Clouston was appointed Medical Superintendent and during his term of office the adjoining estate of Craig House was purchased and a new hospital department was built. Craig House was rich in history, which in one respect was remotely linked with that of the College. The name of King James VI will always be associated with his well-intentioned but unsuccessful efforts to found the College (Chap. II). Portraits of him and his wife Queen Anne are among those hanging in the College Hall. It was the father of a one-time owner of Craig House, a Captain John Dick, who was entrusted with the responsibility of escorting King James VI to Copenhagen on the occasion of his marriage to Anne of Denmark.[107]

The names of many eminent professional men have been associated with the Royal Edinburgh Hospital in one capacity or another. Clouston has been mentioned. Others were G. M. Robertson and (Sir) D. K. Henderson. All three were at one time Presidents of the College. Another President, (Sir) John Batty Tuke, who owned a private mental hospital collaborated with Clouston in founding the Pathological Laboratory of the Scottish Asylums. In the present age of fly-over bridges and 'snarling' if not 'snarled' traffic, there is almost pathos in an appeal made to the College in 1880 by Dr Clouston. A Bill was due for presentation to Parliament for 'an Edinburgh Suburban and Southside Railway'. Apprehensive that the close proximity of the proposed line would be prejudicial to the Asylum, Clouston asked that the College should petition against the proposal. To this the College consented.[108] Today, how many Fellows would sacrifice their private transport for a return of the old-time discarded suburban passenger service?!

SIR ALEXANDER MORISON

Although never directly connected with the establishment of mental institutions in Edinburgh, mention must be made of the name of Sir Alexander Morison. Having obtained his Doctorate of Medicine at Edinburgh University in 1799, he was elected to the Fellowship of the College in 1801. His petition for Licentiateship was heard and approved on 6th May 1800.[109] Election to Fellowship status was associated with a slight technical hitch. At a meeting in May 1801 it was pointed out that 'by an accident no mention had been made at last quarterly Meeting for balloting Dr Alexander Morison as a Fellow though he had already been twelve months a Licentiate'. It is of interest that it was Dr Andrew Duncan who raised the point and proceeded successfully to have 'the Law respecting the Election of Fellows . . . Suspended as to him'.[110] The College agreed, and an Extraordinary Meeting was arranged to set matters aright in five days' time. Morison was admitted a Fellow on 11th May 1801.[111] Duncan's evident interest in Morison may well explain one influence at least which led the younger man to take up a career in psychiatry.

It is known that while James Gregory favoured, Duncan was opposed to Morison's decision to go to London. As events turned out, his connection with Edinburgh was not completely severed and he had the altogether unusual experience of conducting lecture courses in both Edinburgh and London. In England Morison held appointments to numerous asylums including the Royal Hospitals of Bethlem and Bridewell.

Outstandingly and uninterruptedly successful in his career he failed in one thing. According to Henderson, Morison petitioned successively the University, the Town Council, the Morningside Asylum and the Royal College of Physicians for recognition but not one of them was prepared to afford him teaching facilities.[112] His organized course of lectures in Edinburgh was evidence of undismayed determination not to be thwarted despite multiple rebuffs. It is to this outstanding Fellow and President that the College is indebted for all time for the endowment of Morison prizes for long and faithful service to the insane, and of the Morison Lectureship. The endowment was made from the funds realized by sale of Morison's property of Larchgrove which he left to the College.

In his latter years Morison was frequently referred to as the Father of the College. A meeting of Council was held on 16th March 1866 'in consequence of the death of Sir Alexander Morison the father of the College': and it was agreed that they would attend his funeral 'from the position he had held in the College as well as from his eminence'.[113]

NEW CITY FEVER HOSPITAL

Permanent responsibility for the hospital care of patients with infectious diseases was first accepted by the City of Edinburgh in 1871, when the Municipality purchased the Canongate Poorhouse from the Canongate Parish Board. There was clear evidence of the harmonious relations prevailing between the College and the Public Health Department when in 1890 the former asked the Medical Officer of Health 'to set apart two wards for receiving cases of Influenza'. At the same time the College nominated a Committee of eleven Fellows to 'study any cases admitted'.[114]

By 1894 the need for more accommodation for infectious diseases patients became apparent and in May of that year the College were informed of a letter from the Convener of the City Public Health Committee asking for the College's opinion 'on the subject of the site' for an extension of existing Fever Hospital accommodation. A fundamental point at issue was whether the existing hospital should be extended, or whether a new hospital should be built in the suburbs. The need to take account of the usefulness of the hospital to the Edinburgh Medical School was emphasized by the Convener.[115]

An Extraordinary Meeting of the College was called but opinion as to desirable policy was divided. Dr Muirhead, a Fellow and holder of the City appointment of Consultant Physician to the Fever Hospital was all in favour of extension of the existing building. Others were anxious for a new hospital in the suburbs. The upshot was that a motion was carried for appointment of an exploratory Committee. Ten Fellows were nominated to serve and they reported in a little over two months. The Report opposed extension on the existing site; rejected 'a proposal to retain the present Hospital for certain of the Fevers, especially Typhoid Fever'; and recommended a new City Fever Hospital on a Southern Suburban site.[116]

Dr Muirhead, who was a member of the Committee, submitted a minority report. In this he focussed attention on 'the serious difficulties' in the way of movement of cases of enteric fever, and how 'a quarter of an hour's extra drive, however well appointed the conveyance plainly implies greatly enhanced danger to the subject of Enteric Fever'.[116] The two Reports were considered by the College, and that of the Committee was agreed to unanimously and thereafter forwarded to the Convener of the Public Health Committee. According to the College records, Dr Muirhead does not seem to have been present at the second College meeting.

The present Colinton Mains Fever Hospital was opened in May 1903, the first patient being admitted in the following October.[117] In the same year Sir Henry Littlejohn with the support of (Sir) Robert Philip won the City Council's support for a voluntary system of notification of pulmonary tuberculosis. Compulsory notification was introduced in 1907. To deal with increased demands for accommodation consequent upon notification, a pavilion was reserved in 1906 for cases of advanced phthisis.

The new hospital was superbly situated. In the days before the amoeboid spread of disenchanting suburban architecture it had an uninterrupted view of fields leading the eye upwards to the gently cosseted Swanston hamlet with its memories of Robert Louis Stevenson, thence to the 'T-Wood' and ultimately the unforgettable skyline of the Pentland Hills. Small wonder that Sir Henry Littlejohn used his influence in advising the Town Council to proceed diligently with the new hospital.[118]

ROYAL EDINBURGH HOSPITAL FOR INCURABLES

In the College Archives for the year 1790 there is a manuscript giving the recommendations of 'the committees appointed for considering what may be the best plans, for obtaining in the neighbourhood of Edinburgh institutions for the relief of incurables, and of convalescents in indigent circumstances'. The manuscript is unsigned and there are no records to indicate what action, if any, resulted from its submission or indeed to whom it was submitted. Nevertheless, the recommendations of the 'committees' are of interest as reflecting the views prevailing almost 200 years ago. They were as follows:

'1. That institutions for these purposes would afford very great relief to many individuals in circumstances of deep distress.

2. That if the benefit which the poor would derive from these institutions were known, funds for their support, might in time be obtained by donations or legacies from the marchalled humane.

3. That if the Lord Provost of Edinburgh with the Presidents of the Royal Colleges of Physicians & Surgeons were to become Trustees for superintending the proper application of any money given or bequeathed for these purposes, the chance of obtaining donations or legacies would be encreased.

4. That these establishments might also be somewhat forwarded, if the Trustees above mentioned, were to hold an annual meeting for considering the means of

promoting such institutions, & for directing such measures as may appear to them most likely for accomplishing that end, particularly by adding to their number, when they see reason for it, other proper persons to act as Trustees.'[119]

It was not until 1874 that 'The Edinburgh Association for Incurables' was founded having as first object 'the erection and maintenance of an Hospital for Incurables at Edinburgh'. The first Committee of Management appointed at the foundation meeting on 1st December, included Drs Douglas Maclagan and George Balfour of the College of Physicians and Mr Joseph Bell, F.R.C.S.Ed.[120] These names are of particular significance because they had appeared previously in a list of signatories to a Memorial published in May 1874 by leading members of the medical profession in Edinburgh dealing with desirable policy for the care of those with incurable disease. Other Fellows of the College who signed were (Sir) Robert Christison, Drs W. H. Lowe (President of our College at the time), Thomas Laycock, Grainger Stewart, Matthews Duncan and Claud Muirhead. Surgeons who signed included Messrs James Simson, Heron Watson, Thomas Annandale, Argyle Robertson, John Duncan and John Chiene of the sister College.

The Memorial referred to a scheme being considered to provide hospital accommodation for Incurables, by the erection of a single central institution for the whole of Scotland, and urged as a preferable alternative 'a number of smaller hospitals in different localities'. In support of their argument the signatories contended that the aggregation of large numbers of incurables would have a depressing effect on the inmates; emphasized the need for reasonable proximity of relatives and friends; and maintained that the time was unpropitious for an appeal for support of a vast undertaking in the face of competitive hospital and University ventures. It is possible at least that the Memorialists were influenced by the fact that the contemplated Edinburgh Association for Incurables was to be a branch of the Scottish National Association for the Relief of Incurables of which the Glasgow Branch was an exceedingly active component.[121]

With little delay the Committee purchased a house in Salisbury Place, Edinburgh, which after enlargement and alteration was opened for the reception of patients on 15th February 1875. There was accommodation for twenty patients, a number which rose to over 150 within fifty years.

Originally it was intended that admission was not to be limited to Edinburgh or its neighbourhood but in the course of time the constitution was so altered that the Edinburgh Association had as object 'the establishment of one or more Hospitals in or near Edinburgh'. In 1880 a large donation from the trustees of Alexander Longmore allowed of extensive rebuilding and from that time the hospital came to be referred to as the Longmore Hospital for Incurables. In 1903 a Royal Charter was granted, (Sir) James Affleck and Sir John Sibbald both Fellows of the College, being among the Petitioners.[122]

Dr George Balfour was the first to hold the position of physician to the hospital and continued to do so until 1877 when he was succeeded by Dr (later Sir) James Affleck. On the Management Committee from the outset, (Sir) Douglas Maclagan was joined by (Sir) Thomas Grainger Stewart in 1877 and (Sir) James Affleck four years later. Sir Thomas's last year on the Committee was 1882, the two others were still in office in 1889. At the time of his death in January 1882, Sir Robert Christison was a Vice President of the Edinburgh Association for Incurables—a post he had held since the founding of the Association.[123]

While the College can lay no claim to have functioned in a corporate capacity in the fostering of the Longmore Hospital, the erection and early history of the hospital bore testimony to the influence exerted by Fellows in their individual capacities.

CHALMERS HOSPITAL

Responsibility for administration of the bequest devoted to the erection of what was to become known as Chalmers Hospital was vested in the Faculty of Advocates. The Faculty in 1854 were 'advised by leaders of the medical profession'[124] and, although there is no evidence that the views of the College of Physicians were sought, it can be accepted that 'the leaders' included Fellows of the College. Dr Halliday Douglas was the first physician to be appointed to the hospital. His appointment in 1864 followed by a year his relinquishment of the office of Treasurer to the College, and he was President of the College during the time that he was physician to the hospital. In succession Drs George Balfour, J. Brakenbridge, Claud Muirhead, G. Lovall Gulland and Sir Byrom Bramwell succeeded Dr Douglas as hospital physician during the period 1887–1918.

DENTAL HOSPITAL AND SCHOOL

At an Extraordinary Meeting of the College in December 1894, explanations having been given, it was moved that a sum of two hundred guineas should be voted 'in aid of the Incorporated Dental Hospital and School'.[125] All did not go smoothly at first. The motion was twice negatived but subsequently renewed.[126] Approval was eventually obtained and receipt of the donation by the Dental Hospital prompted the offer to the College of 'the privilege of nominating one of your Fellows to be a Director of this Institution'. When accepting the proferred privilege the College decided that 'for the time being' they would be represented by their President.[127]

THE CHARITY WORKHOUSE

The main object for which the Commissioners had been appointed was the protection of private patients. Pauper lunatics were assumed to be already protected and provided for, in a manner appropriate to their station, by the local authorities . . .

An account has already been given of the inadequacy of measures for poor relief in Scotland in the sixteenth, seventeenth and eighteenth centuries and how begging, thieving and vagrancy were the inevitable outcome of widespread destitution. By 1632, a House of Correction constituted an established feature of measures in Edinburgh to deal with the worsening situation, and continued to function until 1748. The House of Correction, intended as a means of protecting the public, was in the nature of a prison admitting those who today would be regarded as 'petty offenders' and distraught persons euphemistically described in accordance with the custom at the time as 'distracted' or 'distempered'.[128]

About 1731 a Charity Workhouse was opened in the immediate vicinity if not within the curtilage of the original House of Correction. The erection followed an agreement reached between the Town Council and the Kirk Sessions to endow 'a Poor's House', and was of additional historical importance in that previously funds for the poor in Edinburgh had for all practical purposes been administered by the Kirk Sessions.[129] It was flanked on the East side by the offices of the Darien Company dating back to 1698.[130] The original Workhouse was replaced by a new Workhouse or Poorhouse in 1743 which Grant described as being 'four storeys in height, very spacious, but plain, massive, and dingy'.[131] Incorporated in the new Institution were a fifty-year-old building known as Bedlam, which, formerly used for housing lunatics, was now converted into an infirmary for the aged and infirm among inmates; a new building erected in 1746 consisting of 21 cells for the reception of

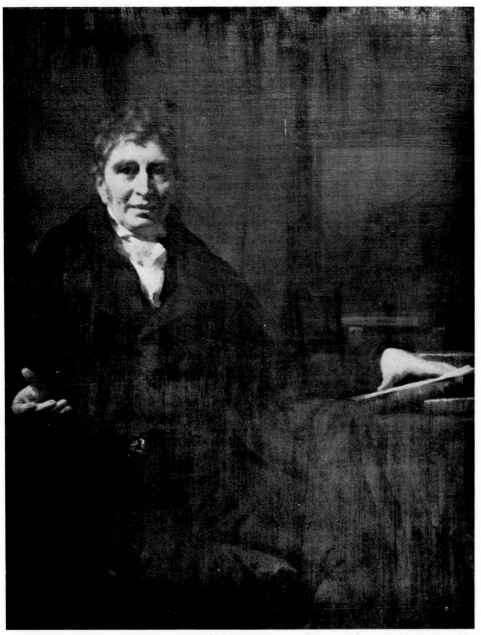

PLATE 33   Dr Andrew Duncan, sen. (1744–1828)
Reproduced from portrait in the College by Sir Henry Raeburn; by permission from *Scottish Field*;
photograph by George B. Alden

lunatics and used as a 'correction house'; and a section for the instruction of poor children in weaving.[132]

Association of the College with the Charity Workhouse certainly dates back to 1743 when the new Institution was opened, responsibility for administration being vested in no fewer than 96 Governors chosen from a number of City Corporations and Societies, representative of the Town Council, the Churches, the legal and other professions. Two of their number were Fellows nominated by the Royal College of Physicians. The task of the Governors can have been no easy one as according to one account there was 'persisting difficulty with contumacious offenders and criminals'.[133] A particularly acute problem was given rise to by those realistically if unsympathetically referred to as 'pauper lunatics'.

THE PAUPER LUNATIC

The problem was no new one, but had never been dealt with in other than desultory fashion. In 1681—the year of the College Charter—Fountainhall recorded that 'In Scotland we having no Bedlam commit the better sort of mad people to the care of and tameing of Chirurgeons, and the inferior to the scourge'.[134] The historically important letter sent by Dr Poole to the President (Dr Davidson) in November 1834 has already been mentioned (Chap. XIX). It gave a vividly intimate picture of the situation prevailing in the Charity Workhouse at that time, and of the glaring inadequacy of resources to meet public demands. Dr Poole's object in writing was to propose the formation of a College Committee to investigate 'the general condition of Lunatics in and around Edinburgh—more especially such as are Paupers or from the lower ranks of life—with a view to an extensive and a suitable establishment for their accommodation'.

While 'not depreciating the Institution at Morningside', Poole was sceptical about the design of the Institution and the likelihood of it ever fulfilling the intentions of the founders. His long-term objective was the creation of a Metropolitan or Midlothian Lunatic Asylum. He explained how, in his capacity of Medical Officer to the Charity Workhouses, he was compelled to adopt this idea after unsuccessful repeated negotiations to secure relief in terms of accommodation and finance from the recently established Morningside Asylum. Rightly he was convinced of the need for 'the entire removal of Bedlam' from the Charity Workhouse and was opposed to extension of existing provisions for the accommodation of lunatics within the curtilage of the Workhouse.[135] Poole was not alone in his criticisms and aspirations.

According to Robertson, a Dr Smith who was 'workhouse doctor' urged the transfer of mentally disturbed patients to Morningside without immediate success. There were acute differences of opinion about the originally intended functions and those realized in practice, at Morningside Asylum. Relations between the Town Council, the Charity Workhouse Governors and the Morningside Governors became severely strained. Contrary opinions on matters of finance also entered into the picture. If Robertson's account be accepted, influenced as it may have been by local authority considerations, Morningside Asylum was not proving altogether successful. This certainly applied to bed occupancy, and in 1836 Morningside agreed to provide accommodation for pauper lunatics.[136]

Thereafter the Charity Workhouse continued to function more in accordance with its designation until 1870 when the Craiglockhart Poorhouse came into existence.

How history repeats itself!—how often within recent times petty personalities, inter-hospital rivalry and unwarranted parsimony have bedevilled progress in hospital provision urgently needed by the community.

THE ORPHAN HOSPITAL

The Orphan Hospital was founded in 1733 for 'helpless Orphans and distressed Infants of indigent Parents',[137] being granted Letters Patent for a Royal Charter in 1742. Among those named in the Letters Patent were 'the Principal of the Royal College of Physicians', 'Dr. James Dundas, Physician' and 'Dr. James Boswal, Physician'.[138] These individuals were in effect Governors of the hospital which was incorporated as 'The Orphan Hospital and Workhouse at Edinburgh'. Shortly after the opening of the new Charity Workhouse in Edinburgh, city children in the Orphan Hospital were transferred to it. Children ineligible to benefit from the Workhouse were retained in the Orphan Hospital and included many from outside Edinburgh.[139]

A list of the original Governors of the Orphan Hospital makes specific mention of 'The Preses of the College of Physicians'; and in 1739 the name of Alexander Monro *primus* was among those added to the original list.[140] 'The Preses of the Royal College of Physicians' and 'The Professor of Anatomy' figured among members nominated by the Letters Patent in 1742.[141] During the first hundred years of the Orphanage's existence the following were among other eminent Fellows of the College at one time or another Governors—Drs Andrew Duncan, John Riddel,

James Dundas, James Boswell, John Hope, Gregory Grant, Charles Stuart, William Laing, Nathaniel Spens, John Abercrombie, James Buchan, William Beilby and W. P. Alison.

Those administering the Orphanage had not far to look for trouble. In 1809 an article written by a Continental author appeared in the local Press and cast grave aspersions on the running of the institution. Today our Parliamentary representatives would have vied with each other in championing the maligned Charity. With infinite wisdom the Managers invited the Principal of the University, the Lord Provost and the Presidents of the two Edinburgh Royal Colleges to investigate. This they did, and their Report which exonerated the Orphanage completely was published in the magazines responsible for the original libellous article.[142] From time to time, there were threats of other kinds. In 1774 the orphanage community was involved in the prevalent contagious fever and in 1780 despite the warnings of physicians, a slaughter house was erected in the near vicinity.[143] Dr Abercrombie was a party in 1823 to a recommendation to the Managers advocating transfer of the orphanage on health grounds. Referring to the recommendation, tribute is paid in the history of the Orphanage to Dr Abercrombie who it stated 'from the time of his becoming a Member of the Incorporation, had taken the warmest interest in the welfare of the children'.[144]

Under the terms of the present constitution of the Dean Orphanage and Cauvin's Trust one of the Governors continues to be the President of our College *ex officio* or a person appointed by him.

THE ROYAL PUBLIC DISPENSARY

From the teaching angle, and more especially from the viewpoint of what is now commonly referred to as Community Medicine, the gradual disappearance of public dispensaries is an irreplaceable loss. They provided invaluable opportunities of studying and developing the human relationship indispensable to patient and doctor alike—a relationship which regardless of economic class continues to bind rural neighbours to one another in ways unknown to their modern city counterparts.

Edinburgh was one of the first cities to establish dispensaries, the earliest being the Public Dispensary founded in 1776 and subsequently incorporated by Royal Charter in 1818. Dr Andrew Duncan, elected President of the College in 1790, was the prime instigator behind the movement and was granted temporary accommodation in the College Hall until the Dispensary acquired its own premises.

Relations between the College and the Dispensary were disturbed by a dispute over the possession of a portrait of Dr Andrew Duncan by Sir Henry Raeburn. The altercation started in innocent fashion. In 1827 the College received a request from one Lawrence Macdonald for a loan of Raeburn's work to enable him to execute a bust of Duncan on behalf of the Royal Dispensary.[145] The next communication was of a very different tone. It arrived in 1855 and consisted of a demand on the part of the Dispensary Management Committee that 'a portrait of the late Dr. Duncan presently suspended in the reading room of the College should be handed over to the Dispensary'. Council replied to the effect that they were not prepared to acquiesce 'until the Managers could prove a legal right'.[146] Things came to a head in 1912 when the Dispensary Managers intimated their determination to have the matter finally settled and suggested a conference with this end in view. The reaction of the College was to ask to see the documents on which the Dispensary claim was based. Study of papers convinced the College that the evidence was in their own favour but it was decided to obtain legal advice. [147, 148] Counsel advised the College not to recognize any claim to the portrait[149] but, a year having elapsed, the Dispensary indicated their intention to take the dispute to the Law Courts.[150]

There then followed a period of silence doubtless due to preoccupation with war-time conditions but the Dispensary returned to the fray by suggesting a conference in which the College Council unanimously declined to participate.[151] At this stage things became 'curiouser and curiouser'. A letter was read to the College in which the Directors of the Royal Public Dispensary requested 'that a plate be attached to the painting, stating that "the portrait had been painted for the Royal Public Dispensary"'. Thereupon the College Council appointed a Committee which in turn concluded from study of the various dates mentioned in relevant documents that the portrait could never have been in the possession of the Dispensary.[152] What would Duncan himself have thought of the almost 100 years bickering, so lacking in respect for his memory? As the saying goes 'There's nowt so queer as folk'.

The portrait continues to hang in the College Hall without any additional explanatory plate.

THE EDINBURGH MEDICAL MISSIONARY SOCIETY

Instituted in 1841, the Edinburgh Association for Sending Medical Aid to Foreign Countries had Dr John Abercrombie as its first President, the Vice-Presidents being

Dr W. P. Alison and the Reverend Thomas Chalmers, D.D. Dr John Moir was another who was active in the formation of the Association. In 1845, while President of the College, Dr William Beilby was elected President of the Missionary Society, and in 1858, by which time the Society had amalgamated with the Medical Missionary Society of the University of Edinburgh, premises were established in the Cowgate. There the training of medical missionaries was continued and dispensary services, including arrangements for domiciliary visits to the sick poor in the neighbouring district were provided. Throughout its existence to the present time Fellows of our College and of our sister surgical College have been active in their support of the Society.[153]

HERIOT'S HOSPITAL

George Heriot's Hospital, or School as it is better known, is one of the many ancient charitable foundations for which Edinburgh is famous.[154] The College was associated with the Hospital from the time of its erection in so far as one of their Fellows was the first physician to be appointed. The terms of his appointment were outlined in Statutes drawn up by the Reverend Walter Balcanquall, D.D. who had been appointed by George Heriot as one of the Overseers of his Will dated 12th December 1623. A Section of the Statutes was headed 'Of the Election and Offices of the Physician, Apothecary and Barber Surgeon' and ran as follows:

> 'There shall be appointed one Doctor of Physick, who for visiting and looking to all the sick in the Hospital, shall receive yearly from the Treasurer   . One apothecary, who shall be paid for all his Bills of Drugs, if they be subscribed with the Doctor of Physick his Hand. One Chirurgeon Barber, who shall cut and poll the Hair of all the Scholars in the Hospital: As also, look to the Cure of all those within the Hospital, who any way shall stand in need of his Art, and shall receive for his Wages yearly.'

The absence of any precise indication of remuneration was, Balcanquall explained, because he 'doth reserve unto himself full Power for the filling up of all Blanks in these Statutes, and all the Power which he now hath, for the determining of the Stipends, or Wages of all Persons'.[155]

Never one to mince his words, the historian Maitland condemned the Cleric responsible for the Statutes in unbridled fashion! The Statute dealing with the

Physician followed those relating to the appointment of a Butler, Cook, Caterer, Porterer and Gardener all of whom were forewarned that they would be instantly dismissed if convicted of immoral behaviour, drunkenness, being a 'common swearer', or wilful disobedience of the Master. Even the Master had to proceed warily! It was laid down that 'if at any time The Master shall marry, his Place shall be Void'. As if that were not warning enough, it was further stated that 'if . . . The Master . . . shall lie a whole Night out of the Hospital . . . without Leave of the Lord Provost' he would suffer public admonition by the Governors and forfeit a Quarter's Wages.[156]

In all the circumstances it is reassuring to find that any Fellow of the College appointed as Physician was not liable to pre-ordained disciplinary procedures!

The history of medical men attached to Heriot's Hospital in the first 150 years of its existence is not without interest. In 1687 the Governors received a petition from one David Pringle saying that his recently deceased father, a grand-nephew of the Founder, had held the appointment of surgeon and apothecary to the institution from 1660: and craving that he might be nominated as his father's successor. Young David Pringle was not dissuaded by the fact that he was not yet 21 years of age and had yet to go to France for 'further insight in the art of surgery and pharmacy'. Moreover he was emboldened to ask leave to employ a surgeon to officiate on his behalf pending his return and his attaining the age of majority. Pringle's prayer was unanimously granted.[157]

Perhaps fortunately the Governors differentiated between surgeon and physician. The former they regarded as one who 'makes regular visits to the Hospital', and the latter as one who 'does not attend except when the Surgeon specially stands in need of his consultation'.[158] David Pringle, sen. was the first surgeon to be appointed— in 1660; and Sir Archibald Stevensone the first physician—in 1666, 15 years before the College of Physicians was granted a Charter. Stevensone was followed by Dr George Mackenzie in 1705 one year after being elected a Fellow of the College. He was indebted for his appointment to Stevensone who had agreed to cancel a claim against the Hospital for £200 sterling provided Mackenzie was appointed to succeed him. An irrepressible Jacobite, and imprudent by nature, Mackenzie had his appointment rescinded and Dr Gilbert Rule, a Fellow of the College and Presbyterian minister was elected in his stead in 1711. Mackenzie reacted by publishing an obnoxious pamphlet but was reponed in 1713 by a Committee which insisted on his retracting strictures on the Church of Scotland contained in the pamphlet. Refusing to comply with the Committee's requirement, Mackenzie was dismissed a second time and once again replaced by Rule.[159] The fact that he was an Episcopalian may account for Mackenzie's having gone out of his way in a pamphlet to eulogize 'Dr.

Walter Balconquall' who was Dean of Rochester and who elsewhere was described as one of George Heriot's 'earliest and most attached friends'.[160]

There followed in succession in the long line of physicians Drs John Innes, John Smelholm, David Foulis, Colin Drummond, James Hamilton, James Buchan, John Abercrombie and in 1844 (Sir) Robert Christison—all Fellows of the College. Of them, Dr James Hamilton gave longest service and when, after 59 years as physician he asked for assistance in 1832 his request was granted, and as a token of respect the Governors arranged for him to 'sit for his picture' which was later painted by Dyce.[161] During his time in office Hamilton published an account in 1804 of an outbreak of scarlatina among the boys at the school. 'Upwards of fifty children' in a community of about 120 were involved. In the case of three, alarming symptoms prompted Hamilton to request 'Messrs. Alexander and George Wood, Surgeons to the hospital' to join him in consultation. The three cases had 'reported as unwell . . . in two or three weeks after discharge'. 'Within less than thirty-six hours, from the recurrence of complaint, the boys died, labouring under symptoms denoting ascites, hydrothorax and hydrocephalis.' Writing in 1806, Hamilton concluded his description in perplexed vein—'This termination' he commented 'was altogether new; I had never seen dropsy from scarlatina fatal.'[162] Another outbreak occurred in the years 1832–3 and was recorded on this occasion by the School Surgeon Mr William Wood.[163]

In 1842 the School Governors approved a series of questions to be answered by the medical attendants of applicants for admission to Heriot's Hospital, the answers to be delivered to the Medical Officer of the Hospital when boys were brought to him for examination. The questions dealt with a history of previous diseases and of 'swellings of the external glands, chronic sores, chronic ophthalmia, or . . . symptoms indicating internal disease of that nature, which is usually considered by medical men to depend upon a strumous tendency of the constitution'.[164] Dr John Abercrombie of the College, with outstanding experience of general practice, was Physician to the School in 1842 and it is unlikely that he did not take part in formulating the questionnaire.

In 1931 the Royal College of Physicians were granted power to appoint a representative to the Governing Body of George Heriot's Trust. The successive College representatives have been Drs Robt. Thin, A. Graham Ritchie and Alec. B. Walker.

SCHOOLS OF THE EDINBURGH MERCHANT COMPANY

In 1903 the Edinburgh Merchant Company saw fit to obtain the advice of the College concerning a proposal to institute medical examination and supervision at their schools. The Council of the College expressed cordial approval of the Company's intentions[165] and were later informed that it had been decided to establish a system of voluntary examination at the Company's schools for girls. Examinations were to be conducted by a lady Medical Officer.[166]

FETTES TRUST

By the terms of the 'Fettes College Scheme 1964 made under the Education (Scotland) Act 1962 and approved by Order in Council dated 14th May 1965' one of the Governors is a Fellow of the Royal College of Physicians. Other Bodies represented include the Bench, the Faculty of Advocates, Writers to the Signet, the University, the Church of Scotland, the Chamber of Commerce and Old Fettesians.

In actual fact the association of the College with the Governors of the Fettes Trust dates back to 1918 when Sir Robert Philip was appointed on behalf of the College. He was succeeded in 1942 by Sir Stanley Davidson, and thereafter by Drs J. K. Slater (1947), Fergus Hewat (1948), Lindsay Lamb (1958) and Neil Macmichael (1970).[167]

PUBLIC CHARITIES

In the summer of 1867 the College was invited to participate in an attempt to organize measures 'to simplify, economise and concentrate the action of the Public Charities of Edinburgh' and 'to improve the condition of the really deserving poor'. On the initiative of the Lord Provost a public meeting had been called and the Subcommittee appointed at the time approached the two Edinburgh Royal Colleges for their views. In particular the Committee sought advice as to the desirability of an amalgamation of the medical charities, Dispensaries and other Institutions connected with Medical Schools or Hospitals. Had they known it the Committee were foreshadowing the administrative ambitions of some hospital boards from sixty to seventy years later. The charities with which the Subcommittee were concerned included 'The Royal Infirmary, The Convalescent House, The Sick Children's Hospital, The Eye Dispensary, The Eye Infirmary, The Ear Dispensary, The Dental Dispensary, The Royal Dispensary, The New Town Dispensary, The Carrubber's Close Dispensary, The Edinburgh Lying-in-Institution for poor married Women, The Society for Relief of Poor Married Women of respectable character when in Childbed, The Royal Maternity Hospital, The Institution for Relief of Incurables, The Destitute Sick Society and The Society for training Sick Nurses'.[168]

A Report submitted by the Council some three months later was remitted to them by the College for reconsideration[169] and after an interval of three weeks an amended form was approved.[170] Having testified to the value of the charities in which the Lord Provost's Subcommittee was interested, the College Report made three suggestions viz:

> 1. Charities of the same or a similar kind should be amalgamated, subject to their situation within the City,
> 2. Charities capable of affording opportunities of teaching Students of Medicine should be placed as near the University and other Schools of Medicine as possible and 'when it can be advantageously done, the same management might be charged with the superintendence of several', and
> 3. '. . . such Charities as the Royal Infirmary, Convalescent House, Destitute Sick Society, Institution for the Relief of Incurables, Society for Training Sick Nurses, ought not to be interfered with.'

LYING-IN WARDS

These suggestions having been outlined, the Report then particularized. It maintained that improved efficiency would result 'were all the Eye Institutions . . . amalgamated: and were the general and special Dispensaries so placed together that the same roof and management would drive them all'. Without question the proposals were realistic and enlightened.

The same can only be said in part of the recommendation which followed to the effect that the Lying-in Institutions, The Children's Hospital and a Dispensary for General and Special Diseases should be 'connected with or attached to the Royal Infirmary'.[170] It was argued that better support and 'more important aids' would be enjoyed by lying-in wards were they connected with the Royal Infirmary. Whether physical connection was contemplated is not clear but in the following year in response to an enquiry from the Managers of the Royal Infirmary, the College replied that 'in accordance with the opinion formerly expressed by the College in a Report with regard to Medical Charities, the College recommend that the Maternity Hospital be combined with the Royal Infirmary and be placed under the managment of the Infirmary Board, but would strongly urge that it be placed in a separate building of the New Hospital'.[171] Many years were to elapse before the College recommendations in this connection were fully implemented. Immediate needs however were met with the erection in Lauriston Place in 1879 of the Royal Maternity and Simpson Memorial Hospital, successor to the Edinburgh General Lying-in Hospital of 1793 which during the times of its existence had occupied successively some six different buildings.[172]

PAEDIATRICS

And what of sick children? Without admitting it the College were, in this matter, on less sure ground. When submitting their Report on Medical Charities in 1867 they were not to realize that there was in Walker Street a lusty two year old of the name of John Thomson destined to become senior physician at the Children's Hospital and the pioneer and father of Scottish paediatrics.[173] The relevant section of the Council's Report requires full quotation. It stated:

> 'The Sick Children's Hospital should become a part of the Royal Infirmary, provided the Infirmary Buildings are extended sufficiently to afford the adequate accommodation.
>
> The Council recognise the great importance of a proper study of the diseases of Childhood, and know that Hospitals of this kind have sprung up in most large towns in this Country and especially on the Continent of Europe. But the Council feel that this want was in a great measure made up in Edinburgh by the necessity for the Students attending a certain period of Dispensary practice where the greater proportion of the cases of the poor seen at their own homes were the diseases of childhood. Seven years ago this Hospital for Sick Children was established having for its objects first the reception and treatment of the children of the poor, and second the advancement of Medical Science with reference to the diseases of childhood by affording the opportunity of these being studied when grouped in sufficient numbers and to provide for the more efficient instruction of Students in this essential department of Medical knowledge.
> [The underlining is in the original text.]
>
> The Council are willing to admit the success of the Children's Hospital, but the great object for Edinburgh in connection with the Medical School has proved a failure. The Students do not resort to it in sufficient numbers. The Council therefore recommend that this important establishment be joined to the Royal Infirmary . . .'.[174]

Restraint of comment is well-nigh impossible! To describe the section in question as arrant if well-intended nonsense would be no more libellous than certain of the insinuations contained in the section. Enlightenment was slow in being acquired. Inconsistence was slow in being discarded. When in 1881 the Directors of the Children's Hospital expressed an eager desire to have attendance of students at the hospital recognized for the Licence of the College, the Council replied to the effect that the hospital did not fulfil the necessary conditions, being 'of a special rather than a general character'.[175] Admittedly with hindsight, today the blindness of yester years is all too apparent.

DISPENSARIES

Proceeding from children's diseases to dispensaries the Council's Report considered that with the prospect of a new hospital being built advantage might be taken to attach to the Royal Infirmary one or other of the General Dispensaries. The reasons advanced were not a little naïve. It was suggested that such an association would induce students 'to attend to special diseases'. At this point the self-satisfied perennial hospital outlook, too common among 'pure consultants' came to the surface. 'For the Dispensary Physicians whose names might be connected with the Infirmary would gradually acquire the tact and experience as necessary for those who have to enter upon the important duties of Physician to the Royal Infirmary.'[176] Among the many today who would disagree with these arguments are those whose consultant activities were preceded by the educative experience of dispensary and general practice.

One of the unhappy developments has been the disappearance of dispensary attachments in student training in some if not most medical centres. Christison, it is true, referring to his work as a physician at the Royal Public Dispensary wrote 'I had been too long trained . . . to the precise and facile observation of hospital practice, not to tire very soon of the jejune weekly consultation-sittings, and the loose observation inseparable from the policlinical visits of the dispensary'.[177] In all respects Christison was of outstanding ability far above the average. His remarks have little bearing on the loss to average students in training as a result of closure of dispensaries. More especially when coupled with domiciliary visiting, dispensaries offered an ideal training ground in human relationships—*and* in the 'tact' which was mentioned in the Council's Report and which is sometimes lacking in present-day out-patient practice. Historically our College cannot afford to forget the example of Dr John

Abercrombie—in succession a successful family doctor in Nicolson Street, Edinburgh, with as his only public appointment attachment to the Royal Public Dispensary; a leading consultant in the City and Fellow of the College, awarded an Honorary M.D. by Oxford University; and eventually appointed physician to the King in Scotland and elected Lord Rector of Marischall College, Aberdeen.[178]

It is of interest that Abercrombie was one of ten individuals who on 3rd June 1822 attended the first meeting called to consider 'a Scheme for the Establishment of a School in the New Town of Edinburgh'. The Edinburgh Academy eventuated,[178a] and towards the end of the century was recognized for the purposes of the Triple Qualification of the Royal Colleges 'as a teaching institution where the subjects of Chemistry and Physics may be studied . . .'.[178b]

From a Minute relating to a Quarterly Meeting in February 1871, it is evident that a Joint Committee of the Colleges of Physicians and Surgeons prepared a Report on Medical Charities but without any specific form of action eventuating.[179] Indeed the subject of charities does not appear to have come up for discussion for some years, and then in relation to individual institutions rather than to the overall problem. An appeal in May 1874 on behalf of a proposal for the building of a new Maternity Hospital[180] was favourably received by the College who voted a sum of 100 guineas.[181] A similar amount was again voted in 1893.[182] In 1894, building proposals in connection with another hospital came to the fore—none other than the Hospital for Sick Children. The extent to which the College's faith in the hospital had been restored since 1867 was reflected in a donation of 100 guineas.[183, 184] Their faith was not misplaced. In 1900, von Pirquet described the Royal Edinburgh Hospital for Sick Children as the foremost in Europe.[185]

REFERENCES

THE ROYAL INFIRMARY, EDINBURGH

(1) TURNER, A. L. (1937) *Story of a Great Hospital; the Royal Infirmary of Edinburgh, 1729-1929*, p. 39. Edinburgh: Oliver & Boyd.

(2) COMRIE, J. D. (1932) *History of Scottish Medicine*, 2nd Edition, vol. I, p. 257. London: Baillière, Tindall & Cox.

(3) Ibid., p. 291.

(4) EDINBURGH ROYAL INFIRMARY [1730] *An Account of the Rise and Establishment of the Infirmary, or Hospital for Sick-poor, erected at Edinburgh.* [Edinburgh: n.p.]

(5) TURNER, A. L. Op. cit., p. 40.

(6) Ibid., p. 42.

(7) College Minutes, 1.ii.1726.

(8) BAIRD, W. (1911) George Drummond: an eighteenth century Lord Provost. In *The Book of the Old Edinburgh Club*, vol. iv, p. 15. Edinburgh: Constable.

(9) College Minutes, 1.ii.1726.

(10) Ibid., 1.viii.1727.

(11) Ibid., 7.xi.1727.

(12) Ibid., 7.v.1728.

(13) TURNER, A. L. Op. cit., p. 96.

(14) EDINBURGH ROYAL INFIRMARY. *Minutes*, 5.iv.1776.

(15) College Minutes, 7.v.1728.

(16) Ibid., 6.viii.1728.

(17) Ibid., 5.xi.1728.

(18) CHURCH OF SCOTLAND. General Assembly (1728) Act and recommendation for a voluntary contribution to be applied towards erecting an infirmary or hospital for diseased poor at Edinburgh. (11.v.1728.)

(19) MAITLAND, W. (1753) *The History of Edinburgh from its Foundation to the Present Time*, p. 451. Edinburgh: Hamilton, Balfour & Neill.

(20) ARNOT, H. (1779) *The History of Edinburgh*, p. 546. Edinburgh: Creech.

(21) TURNER, A. L. Op. cit., p. 48.

(22) Ibid., p. 45.

(23) R.C.P.E. (1925) *Historical Sketch and Laws of the Royal College of Physicians of Edinburgh*, p. 52. Edinburgh: Royal College of Physicians.

(24) TURNER, A. L. Op. cit., pp. 47–8.

(25) THIN, R. (1927) The old infirmary and earlier hospitals. In *The Book of the Old Edinburgh Club*, vol. XV, p. 154. Edinburgh: Constable.

(26) TURNER, A. L. Op. cit., p. 89.

(27) COMRIE, J. D. Op. cit., vol. II, p. 449.

(28) College Minutes, 5.viii.1729.

(29) EDINBURGH ROYAL INFIRMARY (1778) History and statutes, p. 8. Edinburgh: Balfour & Smellie.

(30) College Minutes, 4.xi.1729.

(31) TURNER, A. L. Op. cit., p. 56.

(32) College Minutes, 5.v.1730.

(33) TURNER, A. L. Op. cit., p. 69.

(34) WARRAND, D., ed. (1927) *More Culloden Papers, 1626-1745*, vol. III, 1725–1745, pp. 37–8. Inverness: Robert Carruthers & Sons.

(35) TURNER, A. L. Op. cit., p. 75.

(36) Ibid., p. 82.

(37) THIN, R. (1927) *College Portraits*, p. 39. Edinburgh: Oliver & Boyd.

(38) CRESWELL, C. H. (1926) *The Royal College of Surgeons of Edinburgh. Historical notes from 1505 to 1905*, p. 208. Edinburgh: Oliver & Boyd.

(39) Ibid., p. 210.

(40) Ibid., p. 212.

(41) TURNER, A. L. Op. cit., p. 57.

(42) ROYAL COLLEGE OF SURGEONS OF EDINBURGH. *Minutes*, 13.ii.1736.

(43) TURNER, A. L. Op. cit., p. 66.

(44) GILLIES, W. A. (1938) *In Famed Breadalbane*, p. 316. Perth: Munro Press.

(45) College Minutes, 18.i.1737.

(46) R.C.P.E. (1737) *Miscellaneous Papers*, no. 175, 17.i.1737.

(47) College Minutes, 18.i.1737.

(48) Ibid., 1.ii.1737.

(49) CRESWELL, C. H. Op. cit., p. 229.

(50) DUNCAN, A. (1896) *Memorials of the Faculty of Physicians and Surgeons of Glasgow, 1599–1850*, p. 138. Glasgow: Maclehose.

(51) CRESWELL, C. H. Op. cit., p. 218.

(52) College Minutes, 7.ii.1738.

(53) TURNER, A. L. Op. cit., pp. 116–17.

(54) Ibid., p. 55.

(55) EDINBURGH ROYAL INFIRMARY. *Minutes*, 26.xi.1888.

(56) College Minutes, 14.xii.1897.

(57) TURNER, A. L. Op. cit., p. 75.

(58) College Minutes, 1.viii.1738.

(59) TURNER, A. L. Op. cit., p. 85.

(60) College Minutes, 2.viii.1738.

(61) Ibid., 2.xi.1742.

(62) Ibid., 2.v.1749.

(63) Ibid., 4.ii.1755.

(64) R.C.P.E. [c. 1850] *Abstracts of the Minutes, AD 1682–1731*. By George Paterson. (Ms.)

(65) College Minutes, 2.v.1749.

(66) Ibid., 1.viii.1749.

(67) Ibid., 7.xi.1749.

(68) Ibid., 6.ii.1750.

(69) Ibid., 5.ii.1751.

(70) TURNER, A. L. Op. cit., p. 119.

(71) Ibid., p. 120.

(72) Ibid., p. 102.

(73) College Minutes, 7.viii.1753.

(74) Ibid., 6.xi.1753.

(75) R.C.P.E. (1925) *Historical Sketch and Laws*, p. 53. Edinburgh: Royal College of Physicians.

(76) College Minutes, 2.ii.1819.

(77) Ibid., 18.ii.1868.

(78) Ibid., 6.v.1879.

(79) Ibid., 15.vi.1920.

(80) HAMILTON, J. (1806) *Observations on the Utility and Administration of Purgative medicines in Several Diseases*, 2nd Edition, Preface. Edinburgh: James Simpson.

(81) CHRISTISON, Sir R. (1885) *The Life of Sir Robert Christison, Bart.*, vol. I, p. 181. Edinburgh: Blackwood.
(82) College Minutes, 4.xii.1947.
(83) Council Minutes, 25.vi.1897.
(84) Ibid., 6.vii.1897.
(85) College Minutes, 4.v.1915
(86) Ibid., 2.xi.1915.
(87) Ibid., 20.vi.1922.
(88) Ibid., 17.iii.1904.
(89) Ibid., 3.v.1904.

EDINBURGH LUNATIC ASYLUM

(90) College Minutes, 1.ii.1791.
(91) *Address to the Public, Respecting the Establishment of a Lunatic Asylum at Edinburgh* (1807) p. 4. Edinburgh: James Ballantyne & Co.
(92) TURNER, A. L. Op. cit., p. 97.
(93) College Minutes, 24.iv.1789.
(94) GRAHAM, H. G. (1899) *The Social Life of Scotland in the Eighteenth Century*, vol. I, p. 114. London: Adam & Charles Black.
(95) HENDERSON, Sir D. K. (1964) *The Evolution of Psychiatry in Scotland*, p. 22. Edinburgh: E. & S. Livingstone.
(96) College Minutes, 2.viii.1791.
(97) Ibid., 7.ii.1792.
(98) Address to the public. Op. cit., pp. 6 & 10.
(99) *Short Account of the Rise, Progress and Present State of the Lunatic Asylum at Edinburgh* (1912) p. 7. Edinburgh: Neill.
(100) College Minutes, 6.v.1806.
(101) Ibid., 5.viii.1806.
(102) HENDERSON, D. K. Op. cit., p. 23.
(103) *Short account . . . of the lunatic asylum at Edinburgh.* Op. cit., pp. 11–13.
(104) College Minutes, 6.vii.1814.
(105) Ibid., 2.viii.1814.
(106) HENDERSON, D. K. Op. cit., p. 60.
(107) Ibid., p. 57.
(108) College Minutes, 4.v.1880.
(109) Ibid., 6.v.1800.
(110) Ibid., 5.v.1801.
(111) Ibid., 11.v.1801.
(112) HENDERSON, D. K. Op. cit., p. 35.
(113) Council Minutes, 16.iii.1866.

NEW CITY FEVER HOSPITAL

(114) Ibid., 10.i.1890.
(115) College Minutes, 28.v.1894.
(116) Ibid., 7.viii.1894.
(117) TAIT, H. P. (1971) Personal communication.
(118) COMRIE, J. D. Op. cit., vol. II, p. 706.

ROYAL EDINBURGH HOSPITAL FOR INCURABLES

(119) R.C.P.E. [1790] *Miscellaneous Papers*, no. 226.
(120) ROYAL EDINBURGH HOSPITAL FOR INCURABLES (1874) *Report of Foundation Meeting*, 1.xii.1874.
(121) ROYAL EDINBURGH HOSPITAL FOR INCURABLES (1874) *Memorandum of Edinburgh Physicians and Surgeons*, May 1874.
(122) ROYAL EDINBURGH HOSPITAL FOR INCURABLES (1875–89) *Reports by the Committee of Management.*
(123) ROYAL EDINBURGH HOSPITAL FOR INCURABLES (1903) *Royal Charter of Incorporation.*

CHALMERS HOSPITAL

(124) BOOG WATSON, W. N. (1964) *A Short History of Chalmers hospital*, p. 9. Edinburgh: E. & S. Livingstone.

DENTAL HOSPITAL AND SCHOOL

(125) College Minutes, 19.xii.1894.
(126) Ibid., 15.i.1895.
(127) Ibid., 4.ii.1896.

THE CHARITY WORKHOUSE

(128) ROBERTSON, D. (1935) *The Princes Street Proprietors and Other Chapters in the History of the Royal Burgh of Edinburgh*, p. 279. Edinburgh: Oliver & Boyd.
(129) Ibid., p. 256.
(130) GRANT, J. (1882) *Old and New Edinburgh*, vol. II, p. 323. London: Cassell, Petter, Galpin & Co.
(131) Ibid., p. 325.
(132) ROBERTSON, D. Op. cit., pp. 287–8.
(133) Ibid., p. 293.
(134) LAUDER, Sir J., Lord Fountainhall (1759) *The Decisions of the Lords of Council and Session from June 6th, 1678 to July 30th, 1712*. [8.iv.1681.] Vol. I. Edinburgh: Hamilton & Balfour.

(135) R.C.P.E. (1834) *General Correspondence*, 1.xi.1834.
(136) ROBERTSON, D. Op. cit., p. 295.

THE ORPHAN HOSPITAL

(137) MAITLAND, W. (1753) *The History of Edinburgh from its Foundation to the Present Time*, p. 464. Edinburgh: Hamilton, Balfour & Neill.
(138) Ibid., pp. 465–6.
(139) Ibid., p. 467.
(140) ORPHAN HOSPITAL (1833) *An Historical Account of the Orphan Hospital of Edinburgh. Drawn up and printed by desire of the managers*, p. 44. Edinburgh: J. & C. Muirhead.
(141) Ibid., pp. 46–7.
(142) Ibid., p. 19.
(143) Ibid., p. 23.
(144) Ibid., p. 24.

THE ROYAL PUBLIC DISPENSARY

(145) R.C.P.E. (1827) *General Correspondence*, 3.ii.1827.
(146) Council Minutes, 28.vi.1855.
(147) Ibid., 9.vi.1913.
(148) Ibid., 8.vii.1913.
(149) Ibid., 28.x.1913.
(150) Ibid., 27.x.1914.
(151) Ibid., 6.vii.1922.
(152) Ibid., 29.iv.1924.

THE EDINBURGH MEDICAL MISSIONARY SOCIETY

(153) EDINBURGH MEDICAL MISSIONARY SOCIETY (1841–1972) *Annual reports*.

HERIOT'S HOSPITAL

(154) MAITLAND, W. Op. cit., p. 431.
(155) Ibid., p. 448.
(156) Ibid., p. 445.
(157) STEVEN, W. (1845) *Memoir of George Heriot; with the history of the hospital, founded by him in Edinburgh*, p. 105. Edinburgh: Bell & Bradfute.
(158) Ibid., p. 230.
(159) Ibid., pp. 111 f.
(160) Ibid., p. 35.

S

(161) STEVEN, W. Op. cit., p. 208.

(162) HAMILTON, J. Op. cit., p. 194.

(163) WOOD, W. (1835) An account of scarlet fever as it occurred in George Heriot's hospital, in the months of October, November and December 1832 and January 1833. *Edinburgh Medical and Surgical Journal*, **43**, 122, 32–49.

(164) STEVEN, W. Op. cit., p. 116.

EDINBURGH MERCHANT COMPANY

(165) Council Minutes, 23.vi.1903.

(166) Ibid., 16.v.1904.

FETTES TRUST

(167) MACMICHAEL, N. (1972) Personal communication.

PUBLIC CHARITIES

(168) College Minutes, 6.viii.1867.

(169) Ibid., 5.xi.1867.

(170) Ibid., 26.xi.1867.

(171) Ibid., 5.v.1868.

(172) COMRIE, J. D. Op. cit., vol. II, p. 664.

(173) CRAIG, W. S. (1968) *John Thomson; pioneer and father of Scottish paediatrics, 1856–1926.* Edinburgh: E. & S. Livingstone.

(174) College Minutes, 26.xi.1867.

(175) Council Minutes, 1.xi.1881.

(176) College Minutes, 26.xi.1867.

(177) CHRISTISON, Sir R. Op. cit., vol. I, p. 362.

(178) COMRIE, J. D. Op. cit., vol. II, pp. 489 f.

(178a) MAGNUSSON, M. (1974) *The Clacken and the Slate; the story of the Edinburgh Academy, 1824–1974,* p. 36. London: Collins.

(178b) ROYAL COLLEGE OF SURGEONS OF EDINBURGH (1896) *Triple Qualification Letter Book No. 10,* 2.xi.1896.

(179) College Minutes, 7.ii.1871.

(180) Ibid., 5.v.1874.

(181) Ibid., 4.viii.1874.

(182) Ibid., 2.v.1893.

(183) Ibid., 6.ii.1894.

(184) Ibid., 1.v.1894.

(185) RUSSELL, H. (1971) *J. W. Ballantyne, M.D., F.R.C.P.Edin., F.R.S.E., 1861–1923,* p. 33. Edinburgh: Royal College of Physicians (Publication No. 39).

Chapter XXI

SOCIO-MEDICAL PROBLEMS: COLLEGE INFLUENCE

The twentieth century will be remembered chiefly, not as an age of political conflicts and technical inventions, but as an age in which human society dared to think of the health of the whole human race as a practical objective.

Arnold Toynbee

Propaganda on health matters is apt to suffer from the disadvantage that in the necessary process of simplification most of the truth is apt to disappear.

H. C. Cameron

Socio-medical considerations have conditioned the activities of the College from its earliest days. They influenced the way in which the early College Halls were used for dispensary services and gave impetus to the College in their efforts to promote hospital services. Before Social Medicine and Community Medicine or their predecessors Public Health and Public Hygiene had established their claim to recognition as medical entities many Fellows of the College in their capacity as physicians had incorporated in their outlook and practice the first elementary principles of social medicine. As instances there were Lind in the Navy (q.v.), Pringle in the Army abroad and at home (Chap. XXVII) and Alison in civil practice (Chap. I). Nor in an age concerned with pollution and conservation should it be forgotten that almost a hundred years ago Sir Robert Christison declared, having carried out investigations on burning coal-gas, the discharge of acid from alkali works and other problems— 'Very early . . . I became satisfied that manufacturers of all denominations may, if they choose, greatly abate or altogether prevent the nuisances which they create'.[1] No one was more alive to this than Edinburgh's first Medical Officer of Health, Dr Henry Littlejohn, who in his famous *Report on the Sanitary Condition of Edinburgh* considered there would be 'no hardship in the Magistrates having the power, on consultation with such authorities as Professors Christison, Playfair and Maclagan, to prevent manufactories being established on sites that must lead to the annoyance of the inhabitants, and the impairment of the amenity of the city'.[2] All three of those named by Littlejohn were Fellows, and in their turn Presidents of the College. In this same Report, deploring the absence of all records of the cholera epidemic of 1832, Littlejohn recorded 'With regard to the second epidemic in 1849, I was more fortunate, as, in the library of the Royal College of Physicians, I found two large volumes of cholera returns from the city and county'.[3]

The nineteenth century witnessed the gradual evolution in recognizable progressive form of public health and mental health as subjects for study and advancement. Public health was not differentiated as a special function of local government until 1857 when Glasgow City created a 'Committee of Nuisances' under the *Nuisances Removal (Scotland) Act of* 1856.[4]

PUBLIC HEALTH: AN EXPANDING CONCEPT ACCEPTED

There is no kind of achievement you could make in the world that is equal to perfect health. What to it are nuggets and millions?
Thomas Carlyle (Rectorial Address, University of Edinburgh, 1866)

Of all the influences which tend to rob the citizen of the sense of his birthright, perhaps one of the strongest, and yet the most subtle, is that of officialism.
Wilfred Trotter

Kirk and State

'The Maker of the Universe established certain laws of nature for the planet on which we live; and the weal or woe of mankind depends upon the observance or neglect of those laws . . . the best course which the people of this country can pursue to deserve that the further progress of the cholera should be stayed will be to employ the interval which will elapse between the present time and the beginning of next Spring in planning and executing measures by which those portions of their towns and cities which are inhabited by the poorer classes, and . . . must most need purification and improvement, may be freed from those causes and sources of contagion which, if allowed to remain, will infallibly breed pestilence, and be fruitful in death, in spite of all the prayers and fastings of a united but inactive nation.'

Such was the reply of Lord Palmerston on receipt of an enquiry in 1853 from the Edinburgh Presbytery regarding a great religious fast in the hope of staying a threatened recurrence of epidemic cholera.[5] Compulsory fasting was a time-honoured resort in attempts 'for eschewing of the pest within this countrey'.[6]

A recent attempt to find the original Presbytery Minute[6a] was not without its amusing side. At first, a helpful if exasperated clergyman had to admit defeat, explaining 'Pam was not mentioned. The appeal was to God alone!'[7] Mechie however gave facts concerning events as they occurred and on the reaction of the Church. According to him 'The Synods of Lothian and Tweeddale of both the Established and Free Churches . . . appointed . . . a day of humiliation within their own bounds. In both some decidedly uncomplimentary things were said about the terms of the Home Secretary's letter.'[8]

Pioneers in Public Health

It was at this time that (Sir) John Simon then Medical Officer of Health for the City of London took the opportunity of his Annual Reports to expose publicly the degrading conditions under which vast concourses of citizens were compelled to live: and to foster awareness in the public of the dire association linking spread of cholera and other infectious diseases with the public health problems of a suitable water supply, effective drainage and competent sewerage. Together (Sir) Edwin Chadwick and (Sir) John Simon were the two incomparable mid-nineteenth-century pioneers of public health—the first a civil service administrator and the other a medical officer, at first in local authority and later central government employ. Their combined influence was immense and in the course of time extended to Scotland.

It has been argued that in the 1850s 'the star of Chadwick and his engineers began to pale before the light of Simon and his medical scientists'.[9] Such a view has scant regard for Chadwick's achievement, and does little credit when emanating from physicians or Colleges. Nor would everyone agree with the description of him as the first Englishman who aroused the common man's dislike of the bureaucrat.[10] How many bureaucrats of infinitely lesser ability within the medical profession and Corporations have earned the dislike of 'common' colleagues and 'common' patients? Scotland owed a debt of gratitude for the lead given by England in public health. (Sir) Henry Littlejohn was Edinburgh's counterpart to Sir John Simon, but credit for the first outstanding publication in English on the subject of public health must be assigned to Dr John Roberton, an Edinburgh practitioner and presumably a Licentiate of the College. His *Treatise on Medical Police* was published in 1809[11] and discussed the causes of diseases in the two capital cities of Edinburgh and London.[12]

He met with the frustration known to many pioneers in medicine of whom he was emboldened to write 'if he attempt to show the weakness of the fashionable system, or to introduce any alteration in the practice, the whole faculty are alarmed; their vanity is piqued in having opinions, which they thought perfectly established, brought into question . . .'.[13]

Naval Hygiene

While careful to acknowledge, Roberton quoted frequently from the naval hygiene pioneer of the previous century—James Lind. Son of an Edinburgh merchant and burgess, Lind married into a medical family one of whom—Dr John Smelholme—was elected a Fellow of the College in 1694.[14] Lind himself was admitted a Fellow in 1750[15] and elected Treasurer in 1756.[16] His experience was varied. After a period of apprenticeship to an Edinburgh surgeon he served ten years in the Royal Navy—mainly in the tropics. Then followed ten years in general practice in Edinburgh during which he published his *Treatise of the Scurvy* which was instrumental in his being offered the post of Medical Officer at Haslar naval hospital. Acceptance of the offer occasioned his resignation from the Treasurership of the College.[17] A letter to the College President (Sir Alexander Dick) from Lind written at Haslar was brimful of modest enthusiasm. He told of not having had above 1040 patients, and of prospects of further accommodation for an additional 500; and described the gratifying standards of hospital hygiene, patients being 'regularly shifted and kept quite neat clean and sweet at the Government's expence . . .'. Under Lind there were 2 master surgeons, 6 upper assistant surgeons, and 90 women nurses. Scarcely a staff-patient ratio in conformity with modern standards but one which did not prevent Lind from happily concluding 'Indeed no expence is spared for the regular management of the house . . .'.[18–20]

Civic Concern

Reverting to the situation in Edinburgh, public enlightenment and past experience had their impact on local administration. In 1866 the Magistrates and the Council of the City of Edinburgh resolved that the time was overdue for focussing attention on the sanitary condition of the City. Relevant civic minutes and papers were sent by the Lord Provost to the President of the College (Dr John Smith)—with the declared object of securing the opinion of the College. Before being introduced to the College for discussion at a special meeting the papers were laid on the Library Table for several days for perusal by Fellows.

Understandably the subject, on discussion, prompted references to Reports prepared by the College some years previously under the supervision of the late Dr Alison. While not prepared 'for the present' to offer opinions on 'the details of the Lord Provost's Scheme of Sanitary Reform' the College sought 'to lay down once more the principles which they have always maintained should guide those who endeavour to ameliorate the conditions of the dwellings of the working classes'. An enumeration of principles followed in the reply sent to the Lord Provost. They included stipulations concerning breadth of carriageways and heights of buildings; the flagging rather than 'causewaying' of footways; the use of incombustible materials for stairways; the prohibition of accumulations of 'dung or other filth . . . in any inhabited Court or Close'; the absolute necessity for a 'direct communication with the external air' of an inhabited house; periodic flushing of all sewers; and the devising of means to prevent overcrowding 'as far as possible'.

The communication ended with a wise plea for perspective—'The Royal College of Physicians is of the opinion that any comprehensive Scheme of Improvement will be successful in proportion as it fulfils these ends, and while it would not wish unduly to create expectation in regard to the effect of these or similar measures, yet it doubts not that they will gradually but materially improve the conditions of Edinburgh, tend to diminish the risk of epidemic disease, and lower the death rate in certain districts'.[21]

On this occasion there was no procrastination on the part of the civic authorities. Five weeks later the President was able to inform the College that the Town Council had decided 'to obtain and consider plans'. With the object of strengthening the Lord Provost's hand the College agreed the following motion:

> 'That the Royal College of Physicians have learned with satisfaction that the Town Council have resolved by a majority to proceed to consider plans for the amelioration of the Sanitary state of Edinburgh.
> 'The Royal College of Physicians will have pleasure in giving any further assistance to the Lord Provost in arranging the details of these plans.'[22]

Police and Sanitary (Scotland) Bill

Some years previously, when considering what was referred to as the *Edinburgh Paving Bill* the College had commented unfavourably on the state of the City streets and carriageways.[23] In the same year they passed certain strictures on the *Police and Sanitary (Scotland) Bill*. Exception was taken to the lack of provision for application of the *Nuisance Removal Act* to small villages; to a proposal 'handing over the whole of Scotland . . . to a Secretary of State or the Privy Council' for the purpose of dealing with certain petitions; and in particular to 'the absence of all power to appoint an Officer of Health'. The College Council noted with satisfaction, however, that Bills before Parliament for Aberdeen and Glasgow contemplated the possible appointment of such officers. Subject to the criticisms mentioned the College approved the *Police Improvement Bill* and instructed Council to prepare a petition in its favour for forwarding to Parliament.[24]

Public Health Bills

Within a month of delivering their note of appreciation to the Lord Provost, the College transferred attention from civic to national public health. The *Public Health (Scotland) Bill* had been introduced into Parliament and the College approved a motion to the effect 'that the College petition both Houses of Parliament in favor of the Public Health (Scotland) Bill, and it be remitted to the Council to take any steps that may seem to them expedient to secure the passing of the Measure'.[25]

As Ferguson pointed out, the College by adding their weight to criticism was partly responsible for withdrawal of an earlier Bill—the *Public Health (Scotland) Bill*, 1848. The criticism reflected Scottish resentment at the degree of centralization proposed, involving control from Whitehall.[26]

'STATE MEDICINE'

General Medical Council: Report on State Medicine

The College was requested by the General Medical Council to consider two series of documents viz. the *Resolutions of the General Medical Council and the Report on State Medicine* (1869)[27]; and the report to the General Medical Council of their State Medicine Committee. In March 1870 the College received from their Council a Report on the subject originally referred by the General Medical Council.

Manifestly the Council of the College had found itself placed in something of a quandary. For over a century the College had had amongst its members a number who were in the forefront of medico-social reform. The College as a corporate body had benefited from the individualistic efforts of these men and from its own support of them; and had been referred to for authoritative opinions by civic and governmental departments.

In the light of the times the College had legitimate reason for considering itself as equally well versed in social and environmental needs of the community as any other professional body. Not unnaturally it saw no rightful place for Chadwick's 'engineers' so indispensable today, and looked no less askance than many do now at the cult of 'multiple diplomatosis'.

The Report of the College Council doubted 'the policy of insisting on Examinations on branches of Study belonging to another profession'; was opposed to medical men overstepping the boundaries of their profession into branches 'so far removed from ordinary Medical practice as Engineering, Science and practice'; and was concerned that a class of engineers might be specially licensed to report on public health matters.[28] Who can blame the College? What percentage of knowledgeable citizens accepted with conviction predictions of planetary space flights before they were first attempted?

The Report of the G.M.C. State Medicine Committee commented upon the deficiencies of medical men as witnesses. Remembering that this was in 1869–70, the College with some justification reacted by stressing that accidents and unforeseen events occur in the practice of every Doctor and no 'amount of study or examination' can improve on the benefits of practical experience. As to the necessity for a special licence to qualify as Medical Officer of Health, the College was wholly unsympathetic. The duties of such men were not regarded as differing widely from those of general practitioners.

Without doubt the College and its Council were apprehensive about any proposal involving the 'placing' of a new qualification on the Medical Register. Not a few pitfalls were foreseen. To the College it appeared paradoxical that a new registrable qualification was being proposed by the self-same body which was endeavouring to abolish single qualifications. It was felt that a multiplicity of registrable qualifications was not in the interests of the public or the profession in that it encouraged specialism. Particular exception was taken to those proposals which seemed 'to draw an invidious distinction between the Universities and other Corporations and to assume that a University *ex proprio motu* and irrespective of its charter may create a new degree while the Corporations other than Universities are limited to those mentioned in their Charters'.

The College accepted its Council's report and in its reply to the General Medical

Council made clear its determination to resist any attempt to embody this particular suggestion in an Act of Parliament.[28]

VACCINATION

Jenner's discovery established not only the procedure of vaccination but also the science of preventive medicine.

L. Glendening

Coming nearer home the recurrent appearance of smallpox was a constant source of anxiety and presented physicians with an unsolved challenge. At the beginning of the eighteenth century Pitcairne had printed his recommendations for the management and treatment of the condition involving members of an aristocratic family.[29] Introduced into London in 1721, inoculation was given trial in Scotland some five years later[30] although Brotherston quoted from a medical paper of 1715 'in some parts of the Highlands . . . where they infect their children by rubbing them with a kindly pock as they term it'.

Progress with formal inoculation was erratic and opinions were divided as to its effectiveness in reducing mortality.[31] William Cullen was a protagonist of inoculation and there is in the College Library a letter from him dated 1771 to a medical practitioner outlining the method of choice.[32] Vaccination, introduced by Jenner in 1796, was not many years in being adopted in Scotland where it completely superseded inoculation[33] despite the disappointment experienced at the time of the 1817 epidemic when 'experience taught that immunity might wane and the vaccinated could develop smallpox'.[34] Alison had no doubts about the value of vaccination although aware of its limitations.[35] In his view use of inoculation made it 'impossible to root out or prevent the spreading of the disease'.[36]

The 'propriety of a Vaccination Act for Scotland' was the subject of a Memorandum submitted jointly by a Committee of the College of Physicians and a Committee of the College of Surgeons to the Lord Advocate. Measures suited to inclusion in such an Act were suggested. The Memorandum was dated 4th February 1860 and on 7th February the College was informed 'Beyond a simple acknowledgement of its receipt that they [the Committees] are not aware that the transmission of this Memorial has had any effect'.[37] When in later years (1871) the House of Commons formed a Select Committee on Vaccination Dr Alexander Wood of our College was the only representative from Scotland to appear as witness.[38]

Civic 'Suggestions'

In 1863 the President (Dr D. Craigie) at the invitation of the Magistrates and Town Council attended a conference on the subject of the prevalent smallpox epidemic and on the propriety of having a Vaccination Act for Scotland. Others present included the President of the sister College of Surgeons and the Chairmen of Parochial and other Boards. Giving a verbal account of the Conference to the College the President indicated that as a result of it the City Clerk and Medical Officer of Health [(Sir) Henry Littlejohn] had submitted suggested Heads of a Vaccination Bill, copies of which had been circulated by Council to Fellows. Resolutions on the proposed Act were discussed by the College after being moved by Dr Wood. The motion was agreed, the substance of which was as follows:

> 'The College were deeply impressed with the need for legislation which they had brought to the notice of the Lord Advocate four years previously without effect: were convinced of the necessity of compulsory vaccination, but deprecated any suggestion for the appointment of Special Vaccinators as every registered practitioner was competent to perform the simple operation: and that vaccination could be carried out efficiently by the existing machinery for the registration of births, deaths and marriages—the Parochial Boards 'taking care of the vaccination of those who cannot afford to obtain it otherwise.' The Council were vested by the College with powers to prosecute efforts 'to do their utmost, either singly or in combination with other bodies, to obtain an efficient Vaccination Act'.[39]

A Rampant Council

In preparing their Report, the Council certainly took the College at their word. They were hypercritical in substance and in tone—although constructive. In bald unmeasured terms the Report declared that the principle upon which the suggestions had been based was erroneous, put the Legislature in a false position, was an undue interference with the liberty of the subject, and an encroachment on the province of the medical practitioner. Certainly the manner of approach was not conducive to dispelling prospects of mutual suspicion which characterized relations between voluntary and statutory services in later years. Exception was taken to proposals for the gratuitous vaccination of every person applying, and emphasis was attached to 'leaving parties to choose whom they please' as vaccinator—gratuitous vaccination being reserved for paupers and those attested by an Inspector as being unable to pay a fee. This attitude is certainly open to criticism. By way of contrast another objection of the College was refreshingly realistic considered in the light of modern health services handicapped as they have been by a multiplicity of administrative bodies. 'To commit the supervision of any matter to two distinct Boards', said the Report, 'is to create a divided responsibility which is never found to work well in practice.' In the opinion of Council the Registration Act was capable of coping with registering all vaccinations; and existing Laws with securing facilities for 'vaccination of all'. For a Government to fix by Statute 'what is the due remuneration of a medical man for any part of his professional duty' was condemned as 'a most dangerous principle'. Still bellicose—there followed 'Those who drew up the suggestions do not seem to be aware that the plan of vaccination Stations has been already tried . . . and been found to be a complete and thorough failure'. Whether from exasperation, exhaustion or pique is not evident, the Report then recorded that 'the Council do not see any necessity for occupying the time of the College by commenting on such alterations of details as might be advisable'.

On the instructions of the College the Report was 'transmitted to the parties who issued the "Suggestions" '.[40]

Criticism of the First Bill

The next development took place in the following month. A *Vaccination Bill* for Scotland was introduced in the House of Commons. If the College were to exert any influence speedy action was necessary. As reported afterwards to the College, the Council prepared a Memorandum which embodied the views of the College and which was distributed to all Scottish Members of the House of Commons and Fellows of the College. The following were amongst views expressed in the Memorandum:

> 1. Regret that many of the proposed arrangements are to be placed under the charge of the Poor Law Boards which 'are surely not the fitting bodies to be entrusted with measures of sanitary police'.
> 2. Disagreement with proposals for vaccination districts and stations—experience of them in Scotland administered under the Board of Supervision having established their impracticability and the need for domiciliary vaccination in lieu.
> 3. Distrust of the suggestion to appoint Public Vaccinators involving the creation of a speciality in medicine, and the risk of giving unwarranted status to men of questionable professional standing, and
> 4. Preference for requiring vaccination before the age of one year and not as intended before the age of 3 or 4 months to minimise the dangers to infants of being brought to vaccination stations in inclement weather.

No exception can be taken to any of the above points of view, but even more impressive in terms of breadth of vision were the concluding criticisms of the Bill which were essentially practical and constructive, in no sense carping, and entirely lacking emotional bias. The criticisms dealt with the absence of provision for overtaking the existing unvaccinated population; for compulsory production of a vaccination certificate by all emigrants; for a reliable supply to medical practitioners of vaccine virus; and for securing the re-vaccination of the population at suitable intervals.[41]

Legal Admonitions

There then followed a somewhat confused state of affairs. Council were perturbed that in the course of the Committee Stage in the House of Commons 'every objectionable feature of the Vaccination Bill was retained and several new ones were added'. A meeting with representative members of the profession was 'well reported in the Daily papers' and copies of the *Scotsman* with the Report were sent to all Scottish Members of Parliament. Both the Home Secretary and the Lord Advocate were written to asking, or to be precise 'begging', that the Bill be delayed pending the proceedings of the Meeting being made known. A reply from the Lord Advocate in terms appropriate to the dignity of his office, chided the College for delay in making their views known and pointed out that to his knowledge the original 'suggestions' of the Clerk and Medical Officer of Health of the City of Edinburgh had been approved by the College of Surgeons in advance of receipt of the views of the College of Physicians.

Referring to the Memorandum from the College of Physicians the Lord Advocate read into it general approval of the Bill; expressed conviction with his proposals in respect of Parochial Boards but indicated his intention to suggest 'the employment of itinerant Vaccinators'; and stated that the College's objection to a Public Vaccinator was based on a misapprehension that 'Vaccination by him, has or was intended to have any other . . . effect than by an ordinary medical Practitioner': and gave as his opinion that the omissions which 'may or may not be important' were not valid reasons for delaying the Bill, had not been considered and were not being adopted. The Lord Advocate's reply to the College constituted a mild castigation wrapped up in exemplary legal equivocation, but diplomatically concluded with a conciliatory reference to the need for explanation because of 'the respect due to so distinguished a body'.[42]

A Warrior President

A doughty President (Dr D. Craigie) was equal to the situation! Replying he drew attention to the fact that he and the Vice-President had been informed at a meeting of the Promotors of the Bill that he—the Lord Advocate—'was already committed to all the principles contained in the "Suggestions" and that it was therefore too late to alter them'; and that this information had imposed upon the two representatives of the College of Physicians the necessity for disclaiming all responsibility for the Bill and withdrawing from the meeting. Apparently actuated by the belief that offence is the best form of defence the President retorted to the suggestion that ample time had been allowed for objections, by pointing out that committee proceedings had only been reported a day or two previously in the Edinburgh Press and that attempts to procure a printed copy of the amended Bill had proved fruitless. His argument gained momentum without loss of perspective. The Lord Advocate was reminded that following a College enquiry in 1860 he had been in receipt of 'an application . . . to introduce a Vaccination Act' and of a copy of a pamphlet entitled 'Small Pox in Scotland, as it is, was, and ought to be, with hints for its mitigation by legislative enactment'. 'If you will take the trouble of looking at the last few pages', his Lordship was advised, 'you will see many objections stated to portions of the English measure, which have unfortunately been introduced into your Lordship's Bill.'

At this point the President appears to have relaxed sufficiently to revert momentarily to conventional politeness, without implying undue deference. His Lordship was thanked for his 'full and explicit statement' of his—'his' be it noted!—difficulties and was thereupon invited by the President to bear with him while he endeavoured to put him 'in possession of our views'. The views in question related to the parsimony of the proposed rates of remuneration and the need to treat members of the medical profession as 'gentlemen'; the iniquity of 'mixing up the Poor Law Boards with vaccination' as proven by the workings of the English Bill; and to the error of depending, to the exclusion of indirect compulsion, upon fines or imprisonment for the effective application of the eventual Act. 'In respect to what the College regards as omissions in the Bill' the President accepted the Lord Advocate's 'explanation as to these forming with propriety part of another and more general measure', but did not refrain from clearly restating the risks attendant upon inadequate lymph supplies more especially at times of an epidemic when demands for revaccination reach peak level. The conclusion of the letter, couched in correct if not conciliatory terms, made clear the College's reservation to oppose the Bill, and the intention to have the letter published to correct current mistaken impressions that the College was in process of opposing a Bill which had previously had their support.[42]

To read the exchange of correspondence is to delight in a skilled warfare of words—although it is doubtful if either contestant would have accepted that description! The presidential College protagonist, Dr David Craigie, has been referred to as one who 'tried to affix to every disease a vernacular name'.[43] There is no evidence that he extended his inclination to administrative opponents! A victim of subacute rheumatism he was 'confined for years to a wheeled chair within doors for locomotion, and when at last he emerged from retirement, he could only walk a slow pace, with both the thighs and legs much flexed'.[43] As many years later, in the person of Philip Snowden when Chancellor of the Exchequer, notable courage in debate was allied to physical infirmity.

Two days after the President's letter was signed and presumably posted a Deputation consisting of two Fellows including the Vice-President (Dr Alexander Wood) left for London. There they had an interview with the Lord Advocate who maintained that 'he had been led to believe that the Colleges of Physicians and Surgeons and the Profession at large were in favour of the Bill' or 'he never would have introduced it'. Expressing concurrence with College views concerning the Poor Law Boards, the Lord Advocate said that raising the necessary funds presented difficulties. He regretted not having prior knowledge of College views about vaccination districts; and on the question of remuneration, declared the decision had been that of the Lower House and not his.

Permissible Manoeuvrings

The next item in the Deputation's programme was an interview in company with three Scottish Members of Parliament, with the Home Secretary who evinced some sympathy with the College's view but endorsed the Lord Advocate's statement that it was too late to alter the Bill in the House of Commons. He raised the possibility of a clause being inserted to terminate the Bill in two years. This the Deputation did not favour, as the Lord Advocate had made some concessions and had moreover undertaken in presenting the Bill to the Commons to do so in a way which would favour the later insertion in the House of Lords of clauses favoured by the College. The Lord Advocate went so far as to ask that anticipatory clauses might be framed without delay. However when, after invoking the aid of the College's London solicitors, the two College delegates presented the desired clauses next day, the Lord Advocate was taken aback at the number of alterations involved. None the less he was co-operative in many respects, and on their return the College representatives reported that while he 'would not pledge himself until he had consulted his friends, . . . if it could be managed he would secure the introduction of such clauses as should satisfy us in the House of Lords and if he resolved against that he would give us such timeous notice as would enable us to take our own way in obtaining modifications or even endeavouring to defeat the Bill'.

The Deputation's Report concluded with two statements, as significant as they were gratifying.

'We subjoin a Bill as altered by us for the Lord Advocate', and
'In all our proceedings we were assisted by the Glasgow Faculty who thoroughly enter into and sympathise with our views and who did all that was possible without having a Deputation on the spot.'[44]

Pledges Respected

When the subject next came up for consideration by the College, it was informed by the returned Deputation that the Lord Advocate had made a condition of his effecting the proposed alterations in the Bill that the threatened opposition in the House of Lords be withdrawn. The College arranged that the Resolutions of their meeting should be printed and circulated to among others each Representative Scottish Peer. Included in the Resolutions were two of especial significance—one relating to the dangers arising from the migratory unvaccinated population engaged in the construction of railways, canals and public works; and the other, the urgent need for an immediate adequate supply of vaccine.[45]

The Act

By the time of the Quarterly Meeting in February 1864, the *Vaccination Bill* had been placed on the Statute Book. The College was prompted to pass a series of eleven resolutions on the Act. Fellows, Members and Licentiates resident in Scotland were reminded of their legal obligations including the giving of a certificate to parents of infants as to the success or insusceptibility of vaccination. They were also advised against practising gratuitous vaccination or the gratuitous issue of duplicate certificates. One resolution deprecated 'the clamour that has been raised by some of these

Sir

I beg leave to inform you that having accepted of being Physician to his Majesties Royal Hospital at Haslar I am to leave this Country so soon as I have settled my private affairs, which I expect to accomplish in a few days.

It affects me much to think I am so soon to be deprived of the Society of the many worthy members of our Colledge in whose company I have so often met with entertainment & have always been improved ———— As I can no longer discharge the office of their treasurer, & am unwilling to occasion an unnecessary meeting of the Colledge upon account of my leaving Scotland if it is agreable; I shall put the papers in my Custody into the hands of Dr Boswell my Predecessor in office; to whom also I shall pay the Ballance of money in my hands viz £20:3:2½ — and Mr Woddrope Writer in Edinr my factor will transmit to me the proceedings of the Colledge upon my accounts

While due Compliments wait upon my fellow members I beg you'll be pleased to accept of my particular & sincere respects being truly

Sir a Sincere wellwisher to the prosperity of the Colledge of Physicians in Edr &
your most obedient humble Servan
James Lind

Edinr 18 May 1758

PLATE 34   Dr James Lind: Letter of Resignation, 18th May 1758
Reproduced from College General Correspondence

East India House
the 15th February 1821.

Sir.

     By direction of the Chairman and Deputy Chairman of the East India Company I had the honor in the early part of last Year, to transmit for your acceptance a Book printed at Bombay containing Reports made to the Medical Board at that Presidency on the nature and progress of the Malady generally known under the name of Cholera Morbus.

     Since that time another Book has been received from India being a Report on this Malady as it visited the Territories subject to the Presidency of Bengal in the Years 1817, 1818 and 1819; drawn up by order of the Supreme Government under the superintendence of the Medical Board at Fort William; and I have the Commands of the Chairman and Deputy Chairman to forward

The President of the Royal College of Physicians
in Edinburgh.

PLATE 35a   Cholera Morbus: Letter to College from East India Company, 15th February 1821 (page 1)
Reproduced from Royal College General Correspondence

forward to you a Copy of the said Work (which is accordingly herewith transmitted)# and to request your acceptance of the same.

I am, Sir,

Your most obedient humble Servant

[signature]

* Sent by the Mail Coach of this Night

PLATE 35b   Cholera Morbus: Letter (page 2)

officials [Parochial Vaccinators] against the limitation of their powers . . . under the Act'. It would seem that the College was not blind to the consequences of the mushroom-like proliferation of ill-defined para-professional activities so evident in the century to follow. A central depôt in Scotland for the issue of reliable vaccine was declared to be essential. The need to take advantage of any additional legislation for the furtherance of the College's views was stressed and in the meantime Fellows, Members and Licentiates and all Medical Practitioners were recommended to communicate to the College 'any suggestions which their experience in its working may lead them to make for the improvement of the Act'.[46]

Students and Proficiency

As a delayed sequel the General Medical Council in 1868 raised with their Scottish Branch the propriety of requiring students to obtain a special Certificate of proficiency in Vaccination. The suggestion did not meet with the unqualified approval of the College who advised the Branch Council that it would suffice were examiners at each examination on Practice of Medicine and Midwifery directed to satisfy themselves that 'each candidate . . . has a knowledge of the practice of Vaccination and of the progress of the vaccine vesicle'. It was considered unnecessary to require from a candidate a certificate from a 'Special Vaccinator'.[47]

TOWARDS A DIPLOMA IN PUBLIC HEALTH

Notification of Infectious Diseases

In July of 1874 an Extraordinary Meeting of the College was held to consider a communication from the Board of Supervision and Edinburgh Public Health Committee. The communication from the Board deplored difficulties encountered in administering the *Public Health (Scotland) Act* arising from the lack of early information on the part of Local Authorities as to the existence of infectious or contagious disease. It further argued that if Sanitary Officers were effectively to check 'spread' they must be provided with immediate information as to the existence of such disease; and that the necessary information could only be obtained from doctors practising throughout the country. To deal with the situation the Board gave it as its intention to issue an appeal to all members of the medical profession in Scotland to make returns to the local authority of all cases of infectious or contagious disease. With this the College were in full agreement and advised the Board accordingly.[48] Their reaction to a letter received about the same time from the Convener of the Edinburgh Public Health Committee was very different.[48]

The Convener's letter gave it as an accomplished fact that the Public Health Committee of the Town Council had approved of a recommendation to request the Government to add to the Public Health Act a clause making it compulsory for medical practitioners to report to the Local Authority all cases of infectious disease occurring in their practice. Anything savouring of compulsion was anathema to the College. No matter the rationality of subsequent public health measures as they evolved, the reaction of the College in no way differed from that of the average citizen finding himself in a comparable situation. Who today relishes a summons for immediate payment of Income Tax? In its wisdom the Council of the College declared that they 'most strongly object to the proposal to introduce into the Public Health Act' a compulsory clause along the lines just indicated. Perhaps College resistance acquired buoyant determination from awareness that Hogmanay was scarce forty-eight hours distant![48]

Events Determine the Pace

Developments were growing apace. It soon became evident that the momentum of events was giving rise to disquiet among the ranks of the College. In the wake of disquiet there was an unconcealed realignment of thought concerning the place of public health science within the general field of medicine. This was amply borne out by the Report of a Committee on State Medicine appointed by the College. Particular significance attached to the opening paragraph of the Report. It ran as follows:

> 'Your committee, considering the great and rising importance of State Medicine, or the Science of Public Health, its natural and popular distinction from the Ordinary Practice of Medicine, and the already great and quickly increasing number of important public health appointments, regard it as incumbent on the College to consider fully its position and duties in those circumstances.'

After referring to the part played in the past by the College in measures bearing on public health, the Committee did 'not hesitate to express it as their opinion, that the College should do what is in its power to encourage and direct the progress of this department of the profession'.[48] Could conversion have been more complete, and more frankly acknowledged? And yet was it complete? Contemplation conjures up memories elsewhere of pre-World War II conferences to plan emergency services—an impressive row of the most consciously eminent clinicians from famous teaching hospitals on one side of the table: on the other, a no less impressive row of leading medical officers of health jealously aware of their long established administrative expertise. Co-operation was assured in the face of the national crisis, but the initial atmosphere in which it would be secured, unpredictable. Every attitude had a background of inarticulate history.

Diploma in Public Health

To return to the College Committee Report, views concerning the establishment of a special qualification were defensively constructive. They were obviously conditioned by a dominant desire to protect the interest of medical corporations in general and the Edinburgh College of Physicians in particular. Convinced that 'a Qualification in State Medicine will, ere long, become necessary for all who desire Public Health appointments' the Committee recommended the establishment of a new qualification as a matter of urgency. They were influenced in this by a restriction imposed on candidates for the corresponding qualification conferred by the University of Edinburgh requiring that they must be graduates of medicine. The restriction obviously put Licentiates of the College and of other medical corporations at a distinct disadvantage.

Approval was given to the Committee Report and the College resolved to establish a Certificate of Qualification in State Medicine.[48] Regulations drawn up by the Council in connection with the new Certificate were finally approved in June 1875 and incorporated in the Laws of the College.[49] Under the regulations only candidates already on the Medical Register were eligible. While there was no insistence on a special course of instruction the attention of candidates was drawn to lectures on State Medicine and Analytical Chemistry; but candidates had to sit two examinations which were written, oral and practical. The first examination 'embraced' physics, chemistry and meteorology; and the second epidemiology, endemiology, practical hygiene, sanitary law and vital statistics.[49]

Fourteen years later the need arose to alter the regulations in order to comply with Resolutions passed by the General Medical Council. Among major alterations were that candidates could not appear for the Final Examination for the Diploma in Public Health until twelve months after receiving a registrable qualification; and evidence was required from candidates that they had 'worked in a Public Health Laboratory . . . recognised by the College' for a prescribed period and had 'for six months practically studied the duties of Out-door Sanitary Work under the Medical Officer of Health of a County or Large Urban District'. An interval of not less than six months between sitting the first and second examinations was made obligatory. Rules relating to study were not applied to registered medical practitioners who had for a period of three years held the position of M.O.H. to any County or to any Urban District of more than 20,000 inhabitants, or to any entire Rural Sanitary District. Holders of the Diploma were designated 'Diplomates in Public Health R.C.P.E.'.[50]

Then followed, what in retrospect is an illuminatingly amusing exchange of notes. In the autumn of 1890 the College of Surgeons informed the College of Physicians that 'having instituted an Examination for a Diploma in Public Health' the Surgeons considered that all Superintending County Health Medical Officers should be relieved from private practice 'so that they may be enabled to discharge their important duties without friction in their relations to the rest of the Medical Profession'. Upon receipt of which the College of Physicians seemed to have suddenly become acutely aware of their mature dignity. It is almost as if they wished to say with appropriate Victorian regal aloofness—'We are not amused'! Instead a copy of the following motion was sent to the sister College by way of reply:

> 'That the Royal College of Physicians of Edinburgh which has during the last two hundred years taken a deep interest in all matters connected with Public Health and has for many years conferred a Diploma in Public Health . . . having taken into consideration the numerous appointments of Medical Officers of Health made . . . would venture to urge upon the Board of Supervision the importance of relieving all Superintending County Health Medical Officers . . . from practice.'[51]

Conjoint Qualification in Public Health

Already there was obvious need for closer collaboration between the three Scottish medical corporations. Acting on a suggestion made by the General Medical Council, one representative from each of the corporations met informally 'to discuss the propriety of instituting a Conjoint Examination in Public Health'. Agreement was reached and on receiving a report from their representative the Edinburgh College of Physicians provisionally adopted the proposed scheme of amalgamation. The General Medical Council were kept informed.[52] Final agreement was formally reached when a motion was accepted and approved to the effect 'That after 31st July 1892 the Diploma in Public Health be granted as a Conjoint Qualification by the three Scottish Corporations'.[53]

Because of 'the changing aspects of Public Health and Industrial and Occupational Health in modern Medicine' Council of the College in 1966 'Resolved that the College should no longer award Diplomas in Public Health'.[54] Judging by the College records the decision was inevitable as there is no evidence of the services of an examiner being required after 1946.[55]

APPOINTMENTS OF MEDICAL OFFICERS OF HEALTH

Meanwhile the College had had an opportunity of expressing its views on certain important aspects of the terms of appointment of Medical Officers of Health. This arose when the *Burgh Police and Health (Scotland) Bill* came up for consideration. The College criticized the proposal that the appointment of a Medical Officer should be subject to annual election, in contrast with the terms of appointment of other officers. In the opinion of the College, a Medical Officer of Health should hold office *ad vitam aut culpam*. A further point of constructive criticism, certainly supported by subsequent experience was that, when advantage was taken of permissive powers to group Parishes, or Burghs and Parishes for the purpose of administration of Head Constables, a similar policy of fusion should apply to the appointment of Medical Officers. It was argued that such a policy would provide an adequate salary and so enable any appointee to dispense with private practice. On the instruction of the College, the Council embodied these suggestions in a Memorial which was submitted to Parliament.[56]

Early in the year 1891 the College received from the Board of Supervision a circular letter entitled 'Contribution from the Local Taxation Account to the cost of Medical Officers and Sanitary Inspectors of Counties and Districts of Counties'. It was accompanied by a request for the observations of the College.

In almost all respects the form of the Board's communication resembled that familiar to those who for better or worse have had dealings with twentieth-century civil service missives. A lengthy preamble summarized administrative principles for the benefit of the County and District Clerks to whom it was intended the circular would eventually be officially distributed. There then followed separate sections dealing with the conditions of appointment of Medical Officers and Sanitary Inspectors, with the inevitable decisions concerning salaries, travelling expenses and the apportionment of same between authorities sharing the services of an individual. Emphasis was attached to persons intended for appointment being of high standing in their profession and being possessed of 'scientific attainment and considerable practical experience'. Appointments for a 'limited' period were declared unacceptable. Mention of further details would be superfluous. Historically, however, the reply of the College to the Board is significant and of interest. It read:

> 'Having carefully considered the Circular . . . the Royal College of Physicians of Edinburgh expresses its satisfaction with the Circular as a whole and more particularly with those Sections in which the Board announce their intentions not to give their sanction to the appointment, as Medical Officers or Sanitary Inspectors, of persons who do not devote their whole time to the duties of such offices. The College desires to suggest to the Board that the area and population allotted to any Medical Officer or Sanitary Inspector should not be so great as to endanger effective supervision.'

Before a decision as to the nature of the reply to be sent was arrived at, all Fellows on the College Roll of Attendance had sent to them in advance of the Quarterly Meeting a copy of the Board circular letter, together with a report from the Council recommending that the College should express its satisfaction with the Circular as a whole.[57]

THE PROBLEM OF HABITUAL DRUNKARDS

As the end of the century came nearer, a novel approach to a far from novel socio-medical problem was made by Council. It was moved on behalf of Council 'that a Committee of the College be appointed to consider the expediency of petitioning Parliament with reference to legislation for Habitual Drunkards'. A powerful Committee was duly appointed with a remit to report back to the College.[58] It would seem that the subject was one which did not warrant ponderous deliberation. A report was forthcoming within less than five weeks but, in verbal not written form—an unusual procedure. Such was the determination of the Committee however that, having by word of mouth recommended that a Petition to Parliament was called for, the Convener without further ado laid before the meeting for approval by the College a form of Petition, ready in every detail for submission to Parliament. Approval was forthcoming without hesitation and with the additional recommendation that 'the petition should be presented to both Houses of Parliament and that copies . . . be sent to the other Licensing Bodies'. Seemly haste about an unseemly subject!

But what were the pleas contained in the petition?

In essence alteration and extension of the *Inebriates Acts* of 1879 and 1888 were sought to provide 'compulsory powers for the placing and detention of Habitual Drunkards in properly regulated houses', and treatment of those so addicted among the poorer and criminal classes at the public charge. Acknowledging the need to avoid 'anything that savours of interference with individual liberty', it was argued that those for whom legislation was being sought 'use their liberty in such a way as proves ruinous to themselves and their families and injurious to society at large'; and that the proposed measures of detention 'are the most likely means to restore to them the power of rightly using their liberty'. Existing measures it was stated involved those convicted being maintained at the public charge without any provision for their cure; and the Acts in force catered for 'persons of the better classes only, whereas . . . legislation should be available for dealing with . . . all classes of the community including paupers and criminals'. These conclusions were based upon the experience of Licensed Retreats which had been established under the Inebriates Acts and into which Habitual Drunkards were admitted on their own application and in which detention was limited to a period not exceeding twelve months. Treatment in these retreats had met with a measure of success, although Habitual Drunkards seldom voluntarily availed themselves of the opportunities of treatment.[59]

In 1908 an invitation was received from the Secretary of the Committee on the Inebriates Act for the College to submit evidence on the operation of the Act in Scotland. Dr Affleck gave evidence on behalf of the College.[60] Use of the College Hall for a lecture was granted to the Society for the Study of Inebriety in 1913.[61]

MENTAL HEALTH: IN THE VANGUARD OF REFORM

We are not ourselves,
When nature being oppress'd, commands the mind
To suffer with the body.

William Shakespeare (*King Lear*)

Nous avons des remèdes pour faire parler les femmes; nous n'en avons pas pour les faire taire.
Anatole France (in *La Comédie de celui qui épousa une femme muette*)

Elsewhere an indication has been given of the concern evidenced by the College in such measures as existed for the care of subnormal mentality and mental disease

(Chap. XX). In February 1854 there arrived in Edinburgh from the United States a pertinacious, philanthropic social worker of the name of Dorothea Dix. Her almost sole interest was betterment of the conditions of the insane. She already had a record of considerable accomplishment in her own country and in Canada[62] and at a later date was to carry her crusade to cities in Europe and Russia.[63] Originally intended to be a convalescent holiday her visit developed into an extension of her social-work activities. Convinced as a result of personal investigations that provisions in this country were no better than on the American Continent she decided upon action.

Wrongs to be Righted

Writing shortly after her arrival in Edinburgh to a friend she stated '. . . a few of the public institutions in the City and neighbourhood are pre-eminently bad. Of these none are so much needing quick reform as the private establishment for the insane. I am confident that this move is to rest with me . . . It will be no holiday work however; but hundreds of miserable creatures may be released from a bitter bondage which the people at large are quite unconscious of.' Her severest criticism was directed towards private nursing homes in the neighbourhood of Musselburgh[64] which thirty-eight years previously had figured in evidence given to a Select Committee of the House of Commons on Madhouses. Questioned about a private madhouse which he had visited in that town the Deputy Sheriff for Midlothian said of one of eleven inmates, chained by the leg, that 'It was indeed hardly possible to conceive of a human being in a more wretched condition . . .'.[65]

Paying no heed to convention and with indomitable determination Miss Dix informed the President of the College (Dr Traill), the Lord Provost of Edinburgh and the Sheriff of Midlothian of the deplorable state of affairs which she had encountered. Meeting civic as distinct from Collegiate obstruction and getting no satisfaction Miss Dix lost no time in taking train to London. There with an audacity which cannot have been far short of effrontery at times, she secured interviews with Lord Shaftesbury, the Home Secretary, Members of Parliament and the Queen's Physician. With a patronage rarely indulged in when visiting the sanctuaries of Whitehall, she—according to her own account—thanked the Home Secretary 'for his early attention to the subject and unprecedented alacrity in the annals of public affairs'. Her communications revealed an irrepressible missionary egotism, but no matter how irritating to the official mind, it certainly was an important factor in arousing public opinion and leading to the appointment of a Royal Commission 'to enquire into the state of the Lunatic Asylums in Scotland, and also into the present state of the law respecting Lunatics and Lunatic Asylums in that part of the United Kingdom'.[66]

The Lunacy (Scotland) Act 1857 was a direct result of the Royal Commission's findings. Previous Lunacy Acts were repealed; conditions for the certification and restraint of insane persons determined; and sustainment of a plea of insanity in a criminal case made a legal justification for detention 'during Her Majesty's pleasure'. It was decreed that a Board of Commissioners in Lunacy for Scotland, and District Boards of Lunacy should be established; and that district asylums should be developed which were to provide accommodation for lunatics previously housed in work-houses, hospitals and small private asylums.[67, 68]

A Report of the College Council referring to the Commission's findings gave some hint of the situation to be remedied by the new Statutory bodies:

'Lunatics were found insufficiently kept by their relatives; many of them insufficiently clad and insufficiently fed; some even confined like wild beasts, not from cruelty, but to keep them out of mischief or of the hands of the Parochial Boards. The Parochial Boards, Actuated by a miserable economy, either retained the poor sufferers in lunatic wards attached to the Poorhouse or farmed them out to persons who made a living by keeping them . . . ; while as the keepers of these houses could only make a profit out of large numbers, they were almost universally overcrowded, and the unfortunate patients were placed in a condition the most unfavourable for their health of body and in one very ill calculated to restore the tone of their mind.'[69]

The above is culled from the Council's Report to the College on the *Lunacy (Scotland) Bill* 'to make further provision respecting Lunacy in Scotland'. Introductory paragraphs in the Report are of interest in the mention made of experience under previous enactments. Previous to the Act of 1857 many Sheriffs of Counties habitually omitted to transmit to the President of the College of Physicians, as required by law, annual reports of asylums coming within the jurisdiction of the Sheriffs. Frequent complaints to the Legislature about these breaches of the law were consistently ignored. On the other hand, representations made to Parliament were successful in securing in the Bill now under consideration, provision for suitable asylums subject to adequate regulation. At the same time the College drew attention to the risk of exposure of medical men to legal action as a result of the Law's insistence on reception of a lunatic into an asylum in Scotland on a Sheriff's order founded on two medical certificates. Only partial success was achieved in so far as the proposed Act was modified so that in cases of emergency a patient could be received and detained for twenty-four hours on one medical certificate. The College also remonstrated unsuccessfully about the proposed form of medical certificate which made of the medical man a collector of evidence while vesting judicial functions in the Sheriff. Instances were known to have occurred of admission into an asylum on a certificate of emergency signed by two doctors being followed by wholly erroneous discharge next day by the Sheriff refusing his warrant.[69]

Professional Knowledge—Relative Values

Referring to the 1857 Bill the Council in their Report waxed wrathful on mention of the proposed abolition of the existing Board and replacement by a new one lacking representation of the medical commissioners and dominated by lawyers. 'It may be natural enough', Council maintained, 'for a legal functionary to take the view which, however, all experience contradicts that lawyers are not only competent to manage their own business, but that of all other professions, and that they are more able to decide the nature and extent of the treatment required than physicians who spend a long time in studying the characters and phases of insanity.' The 1970s have seen, not always without reason, comparable criticism levelled at the local and central authority administrators involved in National Health Service policies. Exclusion of medical representation on the proposed new Boards was 'peculiarly repugnant' to the Council, depriving as it did the Boards of 'fearless' professional information—'The whole profession know what lunatic wards in a poorhouse mean and openly express their disapproval of them'.

   Criticism by Council of the Bill was followed by unqualified approval of two features—extension from 24 to 72 hours of the protection provided by emergency certificates; and the power given to the Board to grant special licences to occupiers of houses for the reception and detention of pauper lunatics, not exceeding four in number subject to specified rules.

   Council concluded that there were 'provisions in the Bill which the College would desire to become law, there are others which they will probably be inclined to oppose'. The twenty-nine Fellows present at the Quarterly Meeting receiving the Report were more definite. They resolved that 'the College of Physicians . . . disapprove strongly of the measure in its present form and remit to the Council to take such steps as may appear expedient to them to secure its alteration in accordance with the views of the College, and failing the success of these to petition Parliament against the Bill . . .'.[69]

At an Extraordinary Meeting held about six weeks later the Council reported having requested a conference with the Edinburgh College of Surgeons and the Glasgow Faculty. The object was to secure agreement to a joint course of action, but this was not attained as evidenced in the decision 'to allow each body to pursue its own course in the matter'. There was disagreement not on the need for protection of the medical man, but on the form of protection.[70] Few practitioners had the alacrity of mind of Dr James Gregory who when, many years earlier, asked by eminent counsel to account for a supposedly insane patient's unusual skill at whist, replied on the instant 'I am no card player . . . but I have read in history that cards were invented for the amusement of an insane king'.[71]

In the interval between the Quarterly and Extraordinary Meetings another course of action had been pursued. Dr Alexander Wood, Vice-President and representative of the College on the General Medical Council, offered to use the opportunity of a visit to London on other business 'to press the views of the College' on Members of Parliament. This he did with the full support of Council.[72] His offer was to involve Dr Wood in an immense amount of work, and work under great pressure for a number of weeks. He was instrumental in engaging a Parliamentary Solicitor or Agent on behalf of the College with whom he was in frequent correspondence dealing with among other things lunacy wards in Poor Houses, the legal responsibilities of medical men, and voluntary confinement. Reinforcing an argument, one of his letters to the solicitor mentioned that a Fellow, Dr Skae, Medical Officer at Morningside Hospital had been written to by a clergyman of all people, saying he would hold him responsible for any consequences that might follow his discharging a dangerous lunatic. The patient in question had been removed despite pleadings and protestations on the part of Dr Skae.

For his part the Solicitor in London kept Dr Wood informed of progress in negotiations, and of the attitudes being assumed by different interested parties. If retrospective interpretation of correspondence is correct the Lord Advocate did not confine obduracy to his dealings with Miss Dix! This, however, did not discourage Dr Wood and the Solicitor from combining to redraft those amendments of the Bill which were a source of contention. Acute differences of opinion existed over the responsibility of medical men signing Certificates of Lunacy.[72]

Lords and Commons

In July 1862, the *Lunacy Bill* went through the Committee stage. It represented progress in so far as it allowed 'parties to be admitted on their own application' but the College was informed that the Lord Advocate had remained adamant in his refusal to accept an amended clause relating to medical responsibility. The solicitors explained that to press this second clause would have been inadvisable as it would have to have been taken up at a 'forenoon sitting, when the attendance is always limited, and the Government can therefore at all times command a majority'. But all was not so simple as that; the Lord Advocate had evidently astutely failed to give the 'precise nature of his objection', and it was cautiously inferred that he 'would not object' were the Bill on coming back to the Commons to have had an appropriate clause inserted during passage in the House of Lords. Such are the wiles of Parliament!

Dr Wood read in the letter sent to him '. . . if you can get any influential peer to take the matter up . . .'. A nod is as good as a wink. The Council of the College went into conclave and as a result of their deliberations Dr Wood was told to transfer his campaigning from the House of Commons to 'the other place'. 'In obedience to instructions' he proceeded to London, where a petition previously prepared by him and sealed and signed by the President (Dr D. Craigie), was presented to the House of Lords by the Duke of Richmond. The petition was exemplary in its concise brevity, and concluded:

> '. . . a simple remedy for the encreasing evils . . . would be to introduce a clause into the Bill . . . extending the same protection to Medical Men in signing such certificates as is extended to Witnesses in Courts of law: and if further protection to the public be thought necessary, providing that the Sheriff shall have power in all cases where he is not satisfied with the certificates presented to him to require additional certificates from Medical Men selected by himself.'

The petition was presented by the Duke of Richmond in the course of a second reading of the Bill stoutly supported by the Duke of Montrose. On 3rd July (1862) the House went into Committee.

About this time there was recorded in the College Minutes:

> 'Finding that mis-statements were being industriously circulated as to the real state of the Law in Scotland on the subject and that Noble Lords were being prejudiced by allegations that if the proposed clause were passed there would be no way of punishing unworthy Medical Men who might grant false certificates, the Delegate of the College prepared and circulated a Memorandum.'

By effectively quoting relevant portions of the Law in Scotland the Memorandum aimed at establishing that:

> (1) a medical man granting a Certificate of a person's insanity, as required by law 'has no protection whatever, but is liable to be sued for damages by every Lunatic who may imagine he has been unjustly confined', and
> (2) the Public would be sufficiently protected even were the proposed clause agreed to: anyone who considers the clause has been violated has the right of appeal to 'the Public Prosecutor, who is in Scotland bound to investigate any complaint, and to prosecute the offending party if he see cause'.[73]

A Scottish 'fashion'

The College Minutes went on to describe how Dr Wood had several subsequent conversations with the Lord Advocate who unexpectedly had conceded to the extent that he had arranged for a clause to be moved on behalf of the Government providing 'that prosecutions should not lie against Medical Men except for gross carelessness, dishonesty or malice in signing certificates'. In addition the College delegate found himself presented with something of a challenge by the Lord Advocate. The latter 'pledged himself, that if it could be shewn that Medical Men in England, in signing . . . Certificates had any protection which did not exist in Scotland he would extend the same protection to practitioners in Scotland'. Considered in true perspective—surely not so much a generous concession as an honest recognition of right! But alas! Dr Wood for reasons not elaborated, had the utmost difficulty in ascertaining what the law of England in this matter really was. Ultimately having consulted a member of the Common Law Bar he came to accept that 'the laws were identical in both countries, but that it seemed to be a fashion to prosecute the Doctors signing the Certificates in Scotland,—a fashion which had not yet been introduced in England'. Perhaps extension of the fashion was reserved for the supposed omissions of surgeons and anaesthetists in later years.

Unfortunately the clause which had the initial favour of the Lord Advocate did not retain government support largely as a result of influence exerted by, surprisingly, Lord Shaftesbury. Despite able support of the proposer, Lord Richmond, by the Duke of Montrose, the clause was finally rejected.[73] Unfortunate although this was, there is no questioning the fact that the prolonged strenuous effort on the part of the College and their delegate, Dr Wood, had effectively ventilated a serious and legitimate grievance with the result that there was increasingly general recognition of the need for protection of members of the medical profession involved.

In 1864 there were prospects of a new Lunacy Bill being introduced into Parliament. Anticipating events the President got in touch with other medical bodies with whom informal agreement was reached concerning the desirability of a clause in the new Bill to provide the protection required by doctors. Agreement covered the form of a proposed clause. The President (Dr G. M. Burt) then 'waited upon' the Lord Advocate who having been informed of the draft clause 'expressed himself favourable thereto, and . . . requested should a Lunacy Bill be brought into Parliament that a copy might be furnished to him'. On hearing the President's verbal report the College 'remitted to the Council to endeavour to have a clause similar to the one read embodied in any New Lunacy Bill'.

The draft clause proposed that a Sheriff in receipt of an application for the detention of a lunatic should, subject to certain conditions being satisfied, remit such a petition to two medical practitioners to be named by him, whose assessment of the lunatic's 'mental state or capacity' would determine the nature of any order to be made by the Sheriff. Reception of a patient by an asylum required production of a Sheriff's order, with the reservation that where a 'case is duly certified to be one of emergency by one qualified Medical Person', the patient might be detained for a period not exceeding three days.[74]

Need for protection of the certifying doctors was a continuing source of anxiety to the College. And in February 1864 an Extraordinary Meeting was called for the express purpose of considering specific recommendations drawn up by the Council. The two fundamental sources of conflicting views in society were fear on the part of the public that the right of detention would be abused, and of the medical profession that they would continue to be the victims of vindictive prosecutions. With justification the College claimed to have 'endeavoured . . . to establish a sound relation between the Profession and the Public in the matter of Certificates in Lunacy'. They were well aware of the painful nature of signing certificates in such circumstances but recognized that the signing of certificates was an indispensable part of medical practice. Furthermore the College was in favour of the section of the Lunacy Act providing for the imposition of 'a penalty not exceeding three hundred pounds' or of 'imprisonment for any period not exceeding twelve months' of any person wilfully and falsely certifying 'any person being a Lunatic'. None the less the College confirmed the motion of Council that 'the Legislature, which imposes by Statute on Medical Men the duty of signing Certificates in Lunacy, is bound to give them some protection in honestly endeavouring to discharge that duty'. Council were empowered to have publicity given to the resolutions. It is a measure of the depth of feeling among Fellows that one of their number had given notice previously of a motion 'with reference to the Fellows of the College resolving to refuse to sign Medical Certificates in cases of Lunacy, till they should have the same protection in the discharge of their duty as the Sheriff and Procurator Fiscal'. Permission was, as it turned out, given to the proposer to postpone his motion in the light of the resolutions of the College in respect of the Council recommendations.[75]

About two years later an Extraordinary Meeting of the College was called to consider the *Lunacy Acts (Scotland) Amendment Bill* before Parliament and a Memorandum prepared by the Council. The Memorandum expressed satisfaction with some clauses of the Bill, was highly critical of others and concluded with a recommendation that an additional clause to protect practitioners from unjust prosecutions similar to that shewn to the Lord Advocate two years previously (q.v.) should be inserted. Provisions for the admission of patients presenting themselves voluntarily were welcomed. Strong exception was taken to a reversion to arrangements whereby Parochial Boards were empowered to provide accommodation for the insane pauper poor. Attention was drawn to the undesirability of patients, not ready for discharge, being taken from asylums at the instance of relatives. Encouragement of patients to correspond *privately* with the Lunacy Board was deprecated as conducive to distrust and subversive of discipline.[76]

Humouring Bureaucracy

The College approved the Report and remitted to the Council for implementation so far as possible of the views of the College.[76] Council were unsuccessful in attempts to secure an interview with the Lord Advocate and therefore in the name of the College drew up a Petition which was presented to the House of Commons by one of the Members of Parliament for Edinburgh. In almost all respects the contents of the Petition corresponded closely to those of the Memorandum delivered by Council to, and approved by the College a month previously.[77] Knowing that a second reading of the Bill was due within three or four days, and aware that a meeting of Scottish Members of Parliament was to be held about the same time, Dr Wood was asked by Council once again to proceed to London with the object of encouraging acceptance of the College views. In London the College delegate got in touch with a Deputation from the Lunatic Asylums and from them learnt that a number of clauses of the Bill had been satisfactorily amended. Sound technical advice was obtained from the Solicitor General who suggested that the Medical Protection Clause advocated by the College should seek trial by the Lord Ordinary rather than by a jury—advice of which Dr Wood took full account when redrafting the clause in question.

Medical Diplomacy

Anxious to show tactical respect for conventional courtesies the College Delegate had at the outset of his visit endeavoured to see the Lord Advocate. This not having proved possible Dr Wood now wrote at some length, and an interview followed. The interview provided justification for encouragement, in that the Lord Advocate indicated agreement in principle at least, with regularization of the discharge of patients, and with the Solicitor General's suggestion concerning medical protection. As the Lord Advocate left to meet Scottish Members in another room, he asked that Dr Wood and an Assistant Commissioner of Lunacy should, there and then, co-operate in framing a clause dealing with the discharge of patients. This was done. What unexpectedly followed is best left to the following excerpt from the College Minutes and the imagination: 'At the close of the Meeting of Scotch Members, Dr Wood was called in to explain his views which he did as well as the confusion at the close of a Meeting would permit'!

Dr Wood had a final opportunity to see the Lord Advocate alone 'and went over all the points with him, when his Lordship saw no objections to any of his proposals'. Next day however there proved to be an exception. Through an intermediary the Delegate was asked to withdraw pressure for the clause relating to the discharge of patients because the Lunacy Commissioners were opposed to it, and because 'impediments thrown in the way of patients getting out of Asylums might lead to increase the unwillingness of friends to send them in'.[77]

Famous 'Opening Pair'

Demands on the time of the College by legislation for mental health lessened materially at this stage, but with the presentation to Parliament in 1886 of the *Lunacy Acts Amendment Bill*, the Council called for a Special Report. They were indeed fortunate in having among the Fellows, two so pre-eminent in this field of alienistic medicine as (Sir) Batty Tuke and (Sir) Thomas Clouston. The Report presented to Council was a model of lucid, factual presentation; and of unemotional, logical interpretation leading to incontrovertible conclusions.

Fears of Anglicization

The Report opened with a note of warning, having abundant historical justification. Emphasizing that the Bill applied to England and Wales the writers stressed 'There can be little doubt that if it passes into Law, a Bill containing similar principles may be introduced applying to Scotland'. Moreover it was argued that while certain features of the Bill could not under any circumstances directly affect Lunacy administration or the profession in Scotland, they might affect the large body of Licentiates of the College resident in England. In a way reminiscent of the Council's reaction to the proposed abolition of Boards in the Bill of 1867, the Report described the visiting Legal Commissioner as 'an entirely superfluous officer' and condemned an establishment of three Medical Commissioners for the proper inspection of 160 asylums (60,000 patients) as wholly inadequate. In Scotland two such officers were deemed necessary to visit 6500 patients.

With admirable precision it was declared that provisions should have been made for the licensing of Private Asylums to properly qualified persons only; and Council was urged to protest against the existence of any private asylum which was not the *locus* of the practice of a physician professing alienistic medicine. In so far as direct involvement of the profession in Scotland was concerned, attention was drawn to the complete absence of specific provisions to enable English, Scottish or Irish authorities to prosecute a medical man in a country other than that in which he lived. The net result, it was pointed out, would be that English or Irish certificates would not be acceptable in Scotland, and Scottish or Irish certificates would not be valid in England, and so on. Practical experience had convinced the writers of the Report that it was essential that the medical certificates should be operative in all three countries irrespective of that in which they were issued.

A final protest was made against clauses which placed the English Registered Hospitals entirely under the control of the Commissioners without any right of appeal. Concern was expressed at what might eventuate were similar provisions extended to Scotland where asylums were to a large extent charitable institutions owing their origin to local benevolent effort and to meet the needs of the lower middle class. Absolute bureaucratic power was unacceptable to those imbued with the age-old principles of Scottish democracy. Together the signatories to this stimulating if brief Report declared:

> 'the Bill as it stands is quite inadequate to procure . . . the same confidence in Lunacy administration as obtains in Scotland. Should this be the opinion of the Council, it might be advisable to make representations to Parliament showing the advantages this country has over England in matters connected with Lunacy administration'.[78]

It would have been strange indeed had the Report not been approved by Council and adopted by the College!

T

Courteous Advice to the Sassenach

This was not to be the end of the *Lunacy Act Amendment Bill*—much less of Drs Tuke and Clouston.[79] In 1888 Dr Tuke appeared to the fore again, moving that a Committee be appointed to consider the Bill with powers to frame a Memorial to Parliament. The College agreed and members of the Committee appointed included both Drs Tuke and Clouston. A Petition was duly drawn up and its adoption by the College was successfully moved by Dr Tuke and seconded by Dr Clouston. Veiled exception was taken in the Report to the Bill on the grounds that 'the principle of the Scotch procedure has been adopted, with somewhat fuller elaboration of details'. In the opinion of the College, impressed as it was by thirty years' experience of Scottish procedure, simplification not elaboration of legislation was needed. Again to quote the Petition—'In common with the whole medical profession the College objects most strenuously to the provisions by which the judge is encouraged to visit the patient, and to endeavour to find out personally what are medical facts'. In Scotland, the judge did not see the patient. Other differences between established Scottish practice and that proposed for England were criticized on the grounds that they were unfavourable to the latter. They included the proposed prohibition of treatment of mental disease by medical men in their own private houses; the failure to require as much medical evidence to prove the insanity of a pauper as a private patient; and the stringent 'hampering legal enactments' controlling the registration of hospitals.

Conviction Born of Experience

Concluding with fundamentals the College Petition put all modesty aside. 'The constitution of the English Lunacy Board is unlike that of the Scottish Board to the disadvantage of the former' it maintained. And again:

> 'In Scotland the Visiting Commissioners are medical men, they visit singly . . . The College believe that the more intimate personal knowledge of individual patients, and of the circumstances and character of each asylum, necessarily acquired . . . has greatly tended to the smooth working of the Scotch system and to the confidence of the public in that working.'[80]

It is not inappropriate to draw attention to similarities between the efforts of the College on behalf of public and mental health, and those already described in connection with medical reform. In all their activities the College was intent on securing realistic practical benefits for the nation, and more particularly for Scotland where the needs differed from those of England; on promoting and maintaining improved standards of socio-medical care; and on establishing for medical practitioners their rightful place in the social structure. From the time of its erection the College had not deviated from the objectives defined in the original Charter. Tribute is due to innumerable Office Bearers and other Fellows who over the years had spared neither time nor effort in furthering these objectives under conditions of communications and transport far removed from those obtaining today.

REFERENCES

(1) CHRISTISON, Sir R. (1885) *Life of Sir Robert Christison, Bart.*, vol. I, p. 305. Edinburgh: Blackwood.

(2) LITTLEJOHN, H. D. (1865) *Report on the Sanitary Condition of the City of Edinburgh*, p. 46. Edinburgh: Colston & Son.

(3) Ibid., p. 7.

(4) BROTHERSTON, J. H. F. (1952) *Observations on the Early Public Health Movement in Scotland*, p. 87. London: H. K. Lewis.

PUBLIC HEALTH

(5) WALKER, M. E. M. (1930) *Pioneers of Public Health; the story of some benefactors of the human race*, p. 103. Edinburgh: Oliver & Boyd.

(6) DUNCAN, A. (1896) *Memorials of the Faculty of Physicians & Surgeons of Glasgow, 1599–1850*, p. 10. Glasgow: Maclehose.

(6a) Scottish Record Office. CH2/121/24.

(7) Personal communication (1974).

(8) MECHIE, S. (1960) *The Church and Scottish Social Development, 1780–1870*, p. 163. London: Oxford University Press.

(9) CLARK, Sir G. (1966) *A History of the Royal College of Physicians of London*, vol. 2, p. 718. Oxford: Clarendon.

(10) Ibid., vol. 2, p. 674.

(11) ROBERTON, J. (1809) *A Treatise on Medical Police and on Diet Regimen, etc.* 2 vols. Edinburgh: J. Moir.

(12) COMRIE, J. D. (1932) *History of Scottish Medicine*, 2nd Edition, vol. II, p. 626. London: Baillière, Tindall & Cox.

(13) ROBERTON, J. Op. cit., vol. I, pp. XXXVII–XXXVIII.

(14) WALKER, M. E. M. Op. cit., p. 24.

(15) College Minutes, 1.v.1750.

(16) Ibid., 2.xii.1756.

(17) Ibid., 1.viii.1758.

(18) R.C.P.E. (1758) *General Correspondence*, 3.ix.1758.

(19) WALKER, M. E. M. Op. cit., pp. 26–7.

(20) COMRIE, J. D. Op. cit., vol. II, p. 440.

(21) College Minutes, 6.iii.1866.

(22) Ibid., 10.iv.1866.

(23) Ibid., 4.ii.1862.

(24) Ibid., 6.v.1862.

(25) Ibid., 7.v.1867.

(26) FERGUSON, T. (1948) *The Dawn of Scottish Social Welfare*, p. 147. London: Nelson.

'STATE MEDICINE'

(27) GENERAL MEDICAL COUNCIL [1869] *State medicine. Resolutions of the General Medical Council . . . ; together with the second report and appendix of the committee on state medicine . . . July 13, 1869*. London: [G.M.C.].

(28) College Minutes, 8.iii.1870.

VACCINATION

(29) PITCAIRNE, A. (1715) The method of curing the smallpox; written in the year 1704. For the use of the noble and honourable family of March. In *The works of . . . wherein are discovered the true foundation and principles of the art of physic*. London: E. Curll [and others].

(30) COMRIE, J. D. Op. cit., vol. II, p. 428.

(31) BROTHERSTON, J. H. F. Op. cit., p. 30.

(32) CULLEN, W. (1782) *Letter book*, 8.viii.1771. (Ms.)

(33) COMRIE, J. D. Op. cit., vol. II, p. 430.

(34) BROTHERSTON, J. H. F. Op. cit., p. 34.

(35) Ibid., p. 32.

(36) ALISON, W. P. (1821) *Medical Jurisprudence*, vol. II, p. 70. (Ms. Lectures.)

(37) College Minutes, 7.ii.1860.

(38) BROWN, T. (1886) *Alexander Wood, M.D., F.R.C.P.E. A sketch of his life and work*, p. 64. Edinburgh: Macniven & Wallace.

(39) College Minutes, 31.iii.1863.

(40) Ibid., 5.v.1863.

(41) Ibid., 23.vi.1863.

(42) Ibid., 7.vii.1863.

(43) CHRISTISON, Sir R. Op. cit., vol. I, pp. 120, 122.

(44) College Minutes, 7.vii.1863.

(45) Ibid., 16.vii.1863.

(46) Ibid., 2.ii.1864.

(47) Ibid., 4.ii.1868.

TOWARDS A DIPLOMA IN PUBLIC HEALTH

(48) Ibid., 29.xii.1874.
(49) Ibid., 8.vi.1875.
(50) Ibid., 21.xi.1889.
(51) Ibid., 4.xi.1890.
(52) Ibid., 3.xi.1891.
(53) Ibid., 23.xii.1891.
(54) Council Minutes, 18.x.1966.
(55) R.C.P.E. (1947) *Calendar*. Edinburgh: [Royal College of Physicians].

APPOINTMENTS OF MEDICAL OFFICERS OF HEALTH

(56) College Minutes, 1.v.1888.
(57) Ibid., 3.ii.1891.

THE PROBLEM OF HABITUAL DRUNKARDS

(58) Ibid., 4.ii.1890.
(59) Ibid., 3.vi.1890.
(60) Council Minutes, 3.xi.1908.
(61) Ibid., 12.vi.1913.

MENTAL HEALTH

(62) CHEYNEY, C. O. (1944) Dorothea Lynde Dix; servant of the Lord. *American Journal of Psychiatry*, **100**, 61.
(63) Ibid., p. 67.
(64) HENDERSON, Sir D. K. (1964) *Evolution of Psychiatry in Scotland*, p. 91. Edinburgh: E. & S. Livingstone.
(65) GORDON, S. & COCKS, T. G. B. (1952) *A People's Conscience*, p. 106. London: Constable.
(66) HENDERSON, Sir D. K. Op. cit., p. 93.
(67) Ibid., pp. 90–3.
(68) COMRIE, J. D. Op. cit., vol. II, p. 789.
(69) College Minutes, 6.v.1862.
(70) Ibid., 20.vi.1862.
(71) STEWART, A. G. (1901) *The Academic Gregories*, p. 139. Edinburgh: Oliphant, Anderson & Ferrier.
(72) College Minutes, 20.vi.1862.
(73) Ibid., 11.vii.1862.

(74) Ibid., 2.ii.1864.
(75) Ibid., 19.ii.1864.
(76) Ibid., 10.iv.1866.
(77) Ibid., 1.v.1866.
(78) Ibid., 25.v.1886.
(79) Ibid., 1.v.1888.
(80) Ibid., 1.vii.1889.

Chapter XXII

MEDICAL EDUCATION: 1860-1900, COLLEGE INVOLVEMENT

When a man has learnt his lesson very well it surely can be of little importance where or from whom he has learnt it.

Adam Smith

The contribution of the College to medical education has taken various forms. It played an important part in propagating the methods learnt at Leyden and in formulating the examination procedure for early degrees of Doctorate of Medicine and encouraging the creation of a Faculty of Medicine in the University of Edinburgh (Chap. XVII). To these activities must be added the teaching undertaken by the Extra-academical School of Medicine until its closure in 1948.

WITH THE UNIVERSITY

University Examinations

The whole situation acquired a new complexion with the passing of two Acts in 1858—the *Medical Reform Act*[1] and the *Universities (Scotland) Act.*[2] Chapters XI–XIV deal with the first named. By the terms of the second Act, Executive Commissioners were appointed to give detailed practical effect to the aims of the Act and to frame Ordinances for the regulation of many academic activities, including the system of awarding degrees. The Commission continued in office for more than four years, until December 1862. By July 1859 they had completed a draft of revised Medical Regulations, which despite the declared misgivings of an Edinburgh senatorial deputation were embodied in an Ordinance. In effect the Ordinance consisted of a modified version of the *Statuta Solennia* adopted by Senate in 1833.[3] This *Statuta* had replaced Latin by English as the language for both oral and written tests, and required that instead of being held in the private houses of the professorial staff the tests should take place within the precincts of the University. Examinations were divided into two stages, each consisting of both written and oral parts[4] and those on medicine and surgery were required as far as possible to include 'Clinical demonstrations in the hospital'.[5]

University Degrees

Hitherto it had been the practice of the University to award only one degree—a Doctorate of Medicine. The Commissioners now divided Medical degrees into three classes. Two of these, Bachelor of Medicine (M.B.) and Master in Surgery (C.M.) involved the passing of examinations in accordance with the modified *Statuta Solennia*. The third class of degree was that of Doctor of Medicine which a Bachelor of Medicine of at least two years' standing and of age not less than twenty-four years, could obtain if he had shown himself to have 'more general cultivation than the majority of his class' as judged by a knowledge of Greek and Logic or Moral Philosophy among other specified disciplines.[6]

The requirements concerning medical degrees were later modified after expiry of the Commission by Ordinances of the University Court in 1866 with Privy Council approval. As a result theses were no longer required from candidates for the degrees of M.B. and C.M., but had to be submitted on 'some branch of medical knowledge, which he may have made a subject of study' since graduating as M.B., in the case of a candidate for the M.D.[7] Still further changes followed the passing of the *Universities (Scotland) Act* of 1889. The two degrees now ranking for qualification were entitled Bachelor of Medicine (M.B.) and Bachelor of Surgery (Ch.B.), and two recognized higher qualifications consisted of Doctor of Medicine (M.D.) and Master of Surgery (Ch.M.).[8]

Inevitably, objections were voiced against the recommendations or rulings, for such they were in reality, of the Commissioners. The objections in the main arose from concern over relative status and vested interests and were not confined to the University or the College. One Ordinance in particular produced, to quote Grant, 'an expression on the part of the Senatus of their jealousy of the extra-mural teachers'. The focal point of the jealousy was that the Ordinance in question extended recognition to 'the lectures of such Teachers of Medicine in Edinburgh, or elsewhere' as should be 'recognised by the University Court'. The extent of recognition was that an attendance of one year, or at four departments of medical study under the supervision of the extra-mural teachers could be accepted as a part of a student's regular course of instruction. In actual fact the point at issue was identical to that which had already been the subject of a costly and prolonged legal action (Chap. XVIII) between the University and Town Council only ten years previously.[6]

WITH THE EXTRA-ACADEMICAL SCHOOL OF MEDICINE

Considering the other side of the question, and it must frankly be admitted there were two sides, what attitude did the Extra-academical Medical School adopt in the latter half of the nineteenth century? There is reason to think that despite their success the extra-mural teachers were alive to an air of uncertainty in the situation. A need to consolidate their position in the face of an academic resurgence became evident and it was the College which was looked to for encouragement and support—the College which included among its Fellows a number of distinguished and influential professors of the University. Co-operation between School, College and University was not, however, entirely lacking. In July 1863 the College was asked by the University about their reaction to a proposal to terminate the winter Session on 31st March.[9] Asked for the reasons underlying the proposal, the University explained that the advantages which the Medical Faculty hoped to secure were 'a rest between the Summer and Winter Courses as well as a month for examinations'. As to 'the rest', it is not clear whether the concern shewn was in the interests of teachers or pupils. There was no such dubiety in a succeeding sentence of the letter—'We all think that the Xmas holidays are not productive of good to students and that they might with propriety be given up.' Unanimously hard of heart, College and School of Medicine approved the University proposals and fell into line. One lone voice in sederunt, the voice of a realist and futurist expressed a doubt as to the practicability of compelling attendance of students at lectures during the Christmas holidays![10]

Class Examinations

At the Quarterly Meeting in November 1864 the College considered a Memorial from 'the Extra-Academical Lecturers on Medicine in Edinburgh' asking that account might be taken of class examinations conducted by them in the final examination of candidates for the Licence of the College. In support of their plea the Lecturers referred to the recent introduction by the University of Edinburgh of class examinations which in the event of a candidate performing creditably could possibly earn 'a certain remission . . . in the severity of the final or Pass Examinations'. According to the Memorialists an approach had already been made by them to the University asking that class examinations conducted by the Extra-academical lecturers might 'be put on the same footing as that of the Professors'. The reply from the University was thought to be favourable. General approval of the proposal was recommended by the Council and endorsed by the College 'if a guarantee was given that they [class examinations] were efficiently carried out'.[11]

Gloomy Prognostications

A number of years were to pass before another Memorial from the Extra-mural teachers was transmitted to the College. This in 1883 was of a much more far-reaching character, and was sent to both the Edinburgh Royal Colleges. It contained a proposal 'to constitute the present Teachers in a School under the auspices of the Royal Colleges: that, in short, the Colleges should add to their other functions that implied in the supervision of Medical education'.[12] Elaborating their argument the Memorialists pointed out that 'this function of teaching' belonged to one of the Colleges 'more than three centuries ago and, in so far as the Colleges determine admission to Lectureships and exercise a certain authority over the Lecturers, it has never been abrogated' (q.v.).

Tribute was then paid to the 'liberal policy of the University authorities in recognising Extra-Mural teaching'; and the argument advanced that, if Extra-academical teachers were to discharge their responsibilities efficiently, their position should compare more favourably with the Professors in the matter of resources necessary for appliances for teaching beyond the reach of individuals. 'Some palpable corporate connection . . . under the administration of the Colleges' might, it was thought, improve the situation. In conclusion the signatories to the Memorial expressed the view that their proposals 'would not be without its use to the Colleges'. 'The tendency of modern legislation' they rightly maintained 'is undoubtedly to diminish the value and power of the Medical Corporations'. Adoption of the lecturers' suggestions would, it was concluded, secure for the College 'a position of dignity and usefulness at least equal to any . . . hitherto held'.

A supplementary statement attached to the Memorial was even more outspoken. In the event of the *Medical Act Amendment Bill* becoming law it was foretold that 'the Colleges will sink into the position of Medical Clubs with gradually diminishing numbers and of little practical usefulness'. At the same time it was argued that 'by becoming great teaching corporations their dignity and position would be secured'.

The Memorial and Supplementary Statement were referred to a Committee for consideration.[12] They reported in a little over three months to the effect that it would not be expedient in the existing position of medical legislation to take any immediate steps 'upon the proposal to associate the Extra-Mural School of Edinburgh with the Colleges'.[13] The Committee's recommendation was accepted. It cannot be regarded as in any sense reactionary. For the College to embark on new measures which might well have been interpreted as conflicting with the terms of the original Charter, and to do so at a time of such uncertainty in the legislature, would have been impolitic in the extreme.

Accommodation Problems

Facilities for teaching were the subject of the next approach of the College in the form of a letter sent by a Fellow of the College of Surgeons on behalf of the general body of Extra-academical lecturers. Briefly a case was advanced for extensive improvement of existing lecture and laboratory accommodation and for financial contributions to any agreed scheme from the three Scottish Medical Corporations. The writer mentioned that the number of students attending the class in Practical Anatomy in the Winter Session had risen from 40 in 1884 to somewhere in the neighbourhood of 300 in 1889. Having carefully considered the letter, Council reported that in their view it would be inexpedient to entertain the proposal, and the College moved an appropriate motion without further ado.[14]

THE SCHOOL OF MEDICINE OF THE ROYAL COLLEGES

After an interval of almost twelve years the proposals contained in the Memorial of 1883 were again submitted in considerably modified form to the College. On this occasion submission followed a meeting of the Association of Lecturers, and sought closer connection with the Colleges without sacrifice of the School's 'freedom of teaching' and without prejudicing 'the impartial position of the Colleges towards teaching in the University, and other Schools preparing students for their Diplomas . . .'.[15] Accompanying the Memorial was a draft scheme which included a suggestion that government of the School should be vested in a Board consisting of five members from each of the Edinburgh Colleges and five elected by Lecturers in the School. 'Power of raising, controlling and expending funds' was to rest with the Lecturers and their General Business and Finance Committee.

In the opinion of the Lecturers their new proposal was 'no innovation, but merely the re-establishment of a connection of great advantage to the School, and of Credit to the Colleges'. By way of justifying this the Memorial included a section which because of its historical interest merits reproduction.

> '. . . Medical Teaching in Edinburgh was instituted by the Founders of the Royal College of Surgeons. When by Seal of Cause the Incorporation of Surgeons was instituted in 1505, provision was made that they should have—"Anis in the year ane condampnit man efter he be deid to make anatomea of quhair throw 'they' may have experience. Ilk ane to instruct uthers." After 1697 regular teachers of Anatomy were appointed by the College of Surgeons to give instruction in their theatre. When in 1722 Alexander Monro, their then Professor, was appointed Professor of Anatomy in the University, he remained also Professor in the College of Surgeons, and for some time gave his instruction in the Surgeon's theatre. Even after his removal to the Town's College, teaching was not discontinued in the College of Surgeons. In 1803 the College appointed a Professor of Surgery, and this Chair was continued till 1831. Not only did the College of Surgeons thus *appoint* teachers, but every Fellow had a right to deliver lectures which qualified for the Diploma of the College, and Fellows of the Royal College of Physicians had the same privilege. The close connection of the Colleges with the School is shown by the fact that the School advertisement was, so late as 1871, headed "Royal Colleges of Physicians and Surgeons, Edinburgh", and signed "By order of the Royal Colleges" by the two Secretaries. This was, unfortunately, discontinued, as the result of a slight misunderstanding between the Lecturers and the Royal College of Surgeons.'[15]

The Lecturers' proposals were placed before the College at a Quarterly Meeting in May 1895, but after discussion deferred for further consideration. At an Extraordinary Meeting two months later it was decided to refer 'the scheme . . . to the Council to act in conjunction with the Council of the Royal College of Surgeons with a view to carrying out the provisions in the Scheme'.[16] No time was lost. In the course of another month Council reported that agreement had been reached between them and the Council of the Surgeons' College to recommend the Scheme subject to acceptance of certain modifications suggested by the Surgeons in the first place. 'The Constitution and Regulations of the School of Medicine of the Royal

Colleges, Edinburgh', as amended, were thereupon adopted and accepted by our College. There had been inserted into the Regulations a clause absolving the Colleges from responsibility for, or liability in, expenses incurred by the Governing Board, the Lecturers or various Committees. It was laid down also, that each year the two Colleges should be given a statement of the number of classes, the number of students attending the School, and 'the mode in which the work of the School is being conducted'.[17]

WITH THE GENERAL MEDICAL COUNCIL

At a Quarterly Meeting in August 1863 it was moved by a Fellow and agreed by the College 'That a Committee be appointed to consider what improvements are required in Medical Education more especially in reference to facilities for Study, and to the different systems of Lecturing, Teaching and Examinations'.[18] In effect the Committee was concerned to deal with the situation brought about by the decision to issue, on 3rd June (1863), the resolutions and *Recommendations of the General Medical Council in reference to General and Professional Education*.[19] The College Committee was faced with a herculean task. Although conscious of a sense of urgency the Committee contented itself with an Interim Report which however emphasized that the College should direct immediate attention to those parts of the Report dealing with medical education. Embodied in the Report were indications that the General Medical Council were known to be contemplating a shortening of lecture courses and a reduction in the number of compulsory classes.

Provisionally the College Committee favoured a substitution of practical instruction for a proportion of lectures; the publication by Licensing and Examining Bodies of precise information distinguishing medical science subjects necessary for a pass examination from those which might earn honours; the provision in Universities of accommodation for practical study in each academic department; and the intention of the University of Edinburgh to appoint Tutors and Professors' Assistants. Particular value was attached by the Committee to the foundation of Scholarships and Special Lectureships.[20]

Intended to stimulate discussion the first Report was followed some months later by one of considerably greater length. What is described as 'Private Study' was advanced as a possible preferable alternative to lectures in some subjects, and a case was made out for greater opportunities for self-instruction at hospitals and medical schools. Significantly it was suggested that syllabi for the ordinary Diploma of

Licentiate or Practitioner should be 'less extensive' than those for the Degree of Doctor of Medicine. As a generality the Committee considered that medical education would be rendered less burdensome and more efficient were efforts made to limit the extent of each subject, rather than to exclude them.

There is an interesting reference to apprenticeship. A member of the Committee suggested that certain Fellows of the College 'might superintend the Studies of Young Men recommended to the guardianship of this College by their Parents ... so as to exercise something of the salutary supervision which was one of the benefits of the old system of Apprenticeship, now nearly obsolete in Scotland'.[21] It is fortunate that today the value of experience of general practice although not meriting the connotation apprenticeship, has come to be realized by the teaching schools; and unfortunate, that that other invaluable form of apprenticeship, introduction to medicine of a son by his father, is on the decline.

College Reply

Distribution to the College of the General Medical Council's Recommendations and Resolutions had been accompanied by an invitation to make comments. To assist in dealing with the situation another Report was prepared by the College Committee on Medical Education and on this occasion a detailed syllabus was incorporated. A great deal of discussion followed its presentation to the College which eventually, having added to the Committee membership, 're-remitted' the Report to Council and the Committee 'to frame an answer on behalf of the College to the Resolutions of the Medical Council'.[22] As stated by the President (Dr Balfour) at the May Quarterly Meeting, the Report had been transmitted on 26th March (1864). For all practical purposes it incorporated virtually all the recommendations contained in the two major Reports of the College Committee on Medical Education. In addition the transfer of certain specified subjects (e.g. Literature, Latin, Arithmetic and Geometry) from the curriculum of Professional to that of Preliminary Study was suggested; and a proposal to replace Pass by Class examinations was opposed.[23]

More G.M.C. Recommendations

The next development was the receipt by the three Scottish Corporations of *The Recommendations or Suggestions of the Select Committee of the General Council of Medical*

Education and Registration.[24] The Recommendations dealt with Registration; Age for Licence to Practise and Professional Study and Examinations.

Reactions of the Medical Corporations

Representatives of the two Edinburgh Colleges and the Glasgow Faculty met on three occasions to consider the Recommendations of the Select Committee. They in turn drew up a Report for submission to their respective Corporate Bodies. With certain reservations, the Report expressed general agreement with that of the Medical Council Committee. They approved the proposals for the Registration of Medical Students; and the recommendation that Licensing Bodies should refrain from examining candidates not on the Authorised List of Medical Students as having passed the Preliminary Examination in Arts, or not already on the Medical Register. A point was made of the need to insist that the Preliminary Examination should precede Registration in every case. It was accepted that the age of twenty-one years should be the earliest at which any Professional Licence could be obtained. Importance was attached to 'the extent and Duration of Courses of Lectures and Instructions' being left to the several Licensing Bodies. A Select Committee recommendation that 'no subject of Lectures be enforced by Regulation to be attended oftener than once' should, the Corporations' representatives maintained, be applicable only to 'systematic' lectures.

In the matter of examinations the Corporation representatives 'highly' approved the conception of Class Examinations, and went on to recommend that a prerequisite for award of a Certificate of Attendance should be evidence of having attended the Class Examinations. Approval was given to the division of the Professional Examination for any Licence into two parts: the First to embrace the primary or fundamental branches of Medicine, and the Second the Branches directly connected with the practice of Medicine and Surgery. It was agreed that 'the Professional Examinations be conducted both in Writing and orally: and that they be practical in all Branches in which they admit of being so'.[24]

Medical School: Definition

The Report of the General Medical Council Select Committee concluded by posing what they termed 'Suggestions for obtaining Information'. These particular suggestions were more in the nature of questions in search of enlightenment. Some of the answers agreed by the representatives of the three Scottish Corporations are of interest. They gave as definition of a 'Medical School' one 'which if qualified to grant a Degree or Licence, shall possess a General Hospital containing at least 80 beds for Patients, and in which regular Clinical Instruction is given; or which, if not qualified to grant a Degree or Licence, shall possess such an Hospital and shall give competent instruction in at least four of the branches required for the Medical Curriculum, of which Anatomy and Chemistry shall be two'. As to Apprenticeship or Pupilage, the representatives held that it 'should not be recognised as constituting the commencement of Professional Study' but with admirable if unwitting practical foresight saw 'no objection to these, under proper regulations, constituting a year of Study, but not at an earlier period than after the termination of the Second Winter Session'.[24]

Entry to Professional Study

With undisguised emphasis the representatives opposed any mode of study other than that at a recognized Medical School as a means of commencement of Professional Study. A suggestion that teaching of the fundamental sciences of medicine needed review and reform in the interests of subsequent practical application was refuted. Disapproving of the unnecessary multiplication of examinations the representatives considered that Registered Practitioners and Candidates who had passed the First Professional Examination by a Qualifying Body, could be admitted by another Body to the Second Professional Examination. A caveat was entered, however, that Candidates rejected by one Board should not be admitted to examination by another Board. Finally it was maintained that in the interests of medical students the Licensing Bodies in England and Ireland should adopt the practice already proving successful in Scotland of combining their Examinations as provided for in the *Medical Act*.

The signatories to the Report which was approved by the College included five representatives of the College, four of the Edinburgh College of Surgeons and four of the Glasgow Faculty.[24] The Report was later forwarded to the General Medical Council jointly on behalf of the three Scottish Corporations.

The Council Ruffled

Over three years were to pass before the College had another voluminous document from the Medical Council. This consisted of Recommendations on the Subject of

Medical Examinations and a Report of the Committee of the General Council on the Visitations of Examinations.

First consideration was given to it by the Council of the College whose advice to Fellows at a Quarterly Meeting in February 1868 was to use a good Scottish term 'decidedly testy'. Nor need they be condemned. Their reaction resembled that of a hospital management committee with detailed local knowledge being told its business by a near-omnipotent regional board. Purse strings were declaring their power in new spheres.

The College Council urged that the College should be divested of all responsibility in regard to the Preliminary Examination. Words of explanation were not minced! 'They have found that the Preliminary Education of many of the Candidates who present themselves for Professional Examination has been very defective, and they trust that in future the General Council will see that in this point a proper standard be enforced.'[25]

Still on the attack the College authorities criticized the Programme proposed by the General Council on the grounds that the multiplication of subjects was of less importance than requiring of Candidates 'accuracy of knowledge in essential branches and more particularly in English'. Exception was taken also to certain recommendations of the General Council relating to examination. The College made clear that they had confidence in the ability of their examiners to draw up suitable 'Written Questions'. As to the General Council's proposals for a 'Uniform Standard of Judging the Results of Examination' a nonplussed College Council admitted to being 'utterly unable to understand its meaning', and declared themselves averse to any system assuming 'an appearance of accuracy and uniformity in reality unattainable'. How, it is permissible to wonder, would the Council have reacted to computerization and multiple choice questions?! After limited discussion the College approved the Report and, adopting an impressive new terminology, instructed their Council 'to draw up a deliverance of the College' for transmission to the Registrar of the General Medical Council.[25]

Preliminary Examination

Seventeen years were to elapse before a formal motion was passed by the College to the effect 'That in the event of the General Medical Council recognising the Examination of the Educational Institute of Scotland as a qualifying Preliminary Examination, the Preliminary Examination at present conducted by the Royal Colleges of Physicians and Surgeons be discontinued'.[26]

College Replies—Old and New

In February 1870 an Extraordinary Meeting of the College was called to consider an amended Report of Council on the Report on professional education by the Committee of the General Medical Council. Salient features in addition to those in the previous Report of the College Council included an expression of doubt as to whether a special knowledge of botany was essential for the practitioner. The College was convinced that students required to attend a special course of lectures on, and to sit a separate examination in the subject acquire 'such knowledge as will enable them to pass, and forget the information obtained almost as rapidly as they had acquired it'.[27] To how many subjects might these words have been applied in the succeeding 100 years?

Instruction in the principles of elementary chemistry and in practical chemistry was considered essential, but it was agreed that zoology should not be regarded as obligatory. It was recommended that pathological anatomy might be substituted for general anatomy: and that while the student should be taught the physical and chemical characters of drugs early in the curriculum, his study of therapeutics should constitute part of his more advanced training. The view was expressed that practical midwifery deserved greater attention, and admission to the Final Examination should require the production of a Certificate that a candidate had attended at least twelve women in labour. In the matter of establishing a system favouring equality in examination, the College, although fully alive to the importance of the subject was 'not at present prepared to enter upon its consideration'. The College Report concluded with a repetition of views previously expressed concerning the practice of apprenticeship and the need for candidates admitted to the Final Examination 'having been engaged in actual attendance on the sick'.[27]

Another Extraordinary Meeting was called in ten days' time to consider a Supplementary Report by the Council of the College to be sent to the General Medical Council dealing with the formation of a Joint Board for Examination in Scotland.[28] The urgency which prompted summoning of the Meeting arose from information received by the College that a Bill or Bills intended for introduction into Parliament would probably contain clauses providing for the creation of an Examining Board for each division of the Kingdom.

'Equality of Medical Examination'

The Supplementary Report to the College Council commenced by explaining previous disinclination to express views on the inequality of the existing Medical

Examination as due to the need for consultation among the various affected Bodies. Attempts as far back as August 1869, to arrange a joint conference of Scottish Licensing Authorities had failed. A suggestion that the mass of the profession in Scotland were illiterate was rejected in downright terms, and the statement made that 'the more that is seen of Medical Practitioners over Scotland, the more surprise will be excited that men of their superior acquirements can be found to serve the wants of country districts, at the great expenditure of labour and the very small pecuniary returns which they receive'. The College was unquestionably allergic to uniformity of the examination system. 'Such Procrustean operations', they declared, 'have a tendency to dwarf intellect and arrest progress, and may prevent those improvements which have for years past been introduced into Medical Education and examination by rival Examining Bodies.'[28]

Administrative Intrusion

Blame was attributed to the University Commissioners for complicating the position in Scotland with regard to medical examinations, by enabling University Degrees to compete with Corporation Licences as qualifications for admission to general practice. A General Examining Board for Scotland based on co-operation between the Universities and other Licensing Bodies was suggested as a possibility worth considering. Having declared this, the College lost no time in enunciating that 'the Medical Profession depends upon its retaining the power of self-government': and that any proposal to subject the profession to State control, or a Board of supervision by the Minister of the day would be most objectionable. Nor did the General Medical Council escape castigation. According to the College that Council was not 'in a condition to determine this question' of amalgamating existing Boards to create any new Examining Boards. The question was one calling for mutual consultation among the Bodies interested.

This Supplementary Report of the Council of the College was approved by the eighteen Fellows present with instructions that it should be forwarded to the General Medical Council to arrive for the next meeting of that Body in two days' time.[28]

More Conferences

It now became the turn of the College Committee on Medical Reform to re-enter the picture. They presented a Report with the express object of briefing the College representative on the General Medical Council before his next attendance at that Council. The Reform Committee's Report dealt with Medical Reform Bills already before Parliament, some clauses in which dealt with Medical Education and Examination. Since their appointment the Committee had had several conferences with the other Scottish Medical Corporations, and one with representatives of the Scottish Universities. The Corporations considered that all subjects in the Medical Curriculum should be included in the Examination, whereas the Universities preferred that existing Boards should continue to examine as previously. Dealing particularly with Lord Grey's Bill (*The Medical Act (1858) Amendment Bill*) before the House of Lords, the Reform Committee confirmed that provision was made for the creation of a Central Examining Board for each Division of the Kingdom to be under the supervision of the Privy Council; and that it was intended that the General Medical Council should be empowered to draft Examination Rules intended to secure uniformity of examination by each of the three Boards. It was contemplated that in future General Examining Boards and not Medical Corporations should confer the title of Licentiate. The College Committee forewarned that difficulties might arise in connection with threats to Corporation Charter rights, and with financial adjustments. It also pointed out that throughout the Bill, 'future licentiates are designated "Persons" not Male Persons, obviously for the purpose of permitting Females to be admitted to the privileges of the Medical Act'.[29]

Conjoint Examining Board

Progress, if progress it could be called, was slow. A remit from the General Medical Council about the Establishment of a Conjoint Examining Board was discussed at a conference in Edinburgh of delegates from the three Scottish Medical Corporations and the four Scottish Universities. Agreement was reached that an Examination by a conjoint Board to test the ability of Candidates to practise was desirable in each division of the Kingdom; passing the Board Examination should be a prerequisite of admission to the Register; Examinations in the fundamental Medical Sciences should remain 'in the hands of the various Medical Authorities'; and that reception of the Examinations in the fundamental Medical Sciences by conjoint Boards should be reciprocal as between Scotland, England and Ireland. A suggested Committee of Management was to consist of an equal number of University and Corporation representatives.

The Edinburgh College of Physicians, in approving the agreement reached at the conference, instructed Council 'to continue negotiations with the view of completing arrangements' and authorized them should they see fit, to combine with the two other Scottish Corporations in forming a Joint First Professional Examination.[30]

More Recommendations and more Responses

In December 1884, there were laid on the Table before the Meeting extracts from *Recommendations of the General Council of Medical Education and Registration of the United Kingdom on age for the Licence to Practice and on Professional Education and Examination*. As with previous 'Recommendations', considerable space had been devoted to the format and content of both Curriculum and Examination. In a number of respects the new Recommendations took account of suggestions previously made by the College to the General Medical Council. A Certificate as to adequate knowledge and practical experience of performing (under supervision) vaccination was made obligatory. In future there were to be three Professional Examinations. These two requirements met with the College's unreserved approval. Further amendments of these latest Resolutions now suggested by the College included extension of the required curriculum to five years; and the inclusion of 'Mental Diseases' among subjects essential for qualification.[31]

WITH THE SCOTTISH UNIVERSITIES COMMISSION

As a result of the appointment of the Scottish Universities Commission, the College was faced with a situation which presented entirely new problems. In November 1889 a letter was received from the Secretary of the Commission asking if the College wished to lead evidence and if so, would they indicate 'the nature and amount of such proposed evidence'. Acting on the recommendation of Council, the College nominated a Committee to consider the communication from the Commission and to make contact with other Licensing Bodies. In view of the importance of the subject, the composition of this particular Committee is of historical interest. It consisted of Drs Peddie, Balfour, Peel Ritchie, Grainger Stewart, Muirhead, Wyllie, James, Bramwell, Gibson and Croom with Dr Peel Ritchie as Convener. The Committee was given power to co-opt.[32] Although the Committee had completed their Report by the time of the next Quarterly Meeting they postponed submitting it to the College until completion of discussions with the other medical Corporations.[33] Subsequent additions to the membership included Drs Tuke, Sibbald, J. A. Russell and Noël Paton. A Statement prepared by this enlarged Committee for presentation to the Universities Commissioners was submitted to the College in March 1890.[34] At the same time the College received a Minority Report. The Statement and Minority Report had been circulated among Fellows prior to the meeting.

Competitive Teaching

With Dr (Sir) Grainger Stewart in the Chair and fifty Fellows in attendance the Statement and Report of the Committee were discussed at length and after consideration of several amendments a form of Statement was agreed on for transmission to the Commissioners. Observations were confined to matters relating to the medical profession with special reference to the Medical Department of the University of Edinburgh. Concerned to maintain the standard of medical education and if possible to enhance the value of medical degrees, the College expressed disquiet lest the very success of the University Medical School might contribute to overcrowding of classes prejudicial to teaching, and to hurried examinations favouring inefficiency. They were particularly concerned about the effects of any such trends on instruction in the Clinical Departments. Encouragement of competition in teaching was regarded as a remedy which 'will always be most generally applicable', and to this end it was suggested that increased recognition might be accorded the teaching of Extra-academical Lecturers in Edinburgh. Value was attached to friendly rivalry between teachers which it was maintained could not 'be reasonably looked for within the University itself' but which could 'only be efficiently provided for by the adequate recognition of Extra-Academical Lecturers'.[34]

The attitude of the College contrasted with the views they had communicated to previous University Commissioners in a Report on Degrees in Medicine submitted in 1860. In that Report they had not hesitated to quote a communication by Sir William Hamilton to the University Commissioners of 1830. Referring to the Edinburgh Professors he said '. . . under their present system of conferring degrees, the number of students that flock to them for instruction is no more a test of the value of their lectures, than the resort of young couples to Gretna Green is a proof of the piety of the blacksmith who gives them his nuptial benediction'.[35]

Aware that the latest College view was in direct opposition to that of the Royal Commissioners who reported in 1878, the statement gave reasons for the College adhering to their opinion. A case was presented for recognition of the Extra-academical Lecturers being equivalent to that extended to any other medical school. The University of Edinburgh, it was pointed out, allowed Candidates who had studied at other Universities to present themselves for degrees in Medicine and Surgery after taking only one year in Edinburgh. That being so the College considered that 'a similar liberty of action' should be extended to students so far as the Extra-Mural Lecturers of Edinburgh were concerned.[34]

Edinburgh and Continental Systems Compared

It was common knowledge at this time that there were those in exalted administrative governmental posts who were enamoured of the German System. This the College Statement endeavoured to counter by underlining the advantages of 'the present dual system in Edinburgh' over that on the Continent which, however, it was allowed had its attraction. Under the German arrangements there were in addition to Ordinary Professors, Extraordinary Professors and Privat-Docenten all of whom taught within the University. The College Statement pointed out that 'In so far as the Privat-Docenten teach special subjects they are exactly represented at present in the University of Edinburgh by the recently appointed Intra-mural Lecturers on Insanity, Diseases of the Eye, and Diseases of Children. It is evident that in making these recent appointments the Universities have assimilated a most useful part of the German System.' None the less, the College regarded the German System as less elastic and more expensive involving remuneration of Extraordinary Professors by the State and submitted that 'in view of the great service which it [the Extra-Mural System] has done to the Edinburgh School where it had its origin, it is deserving of continued support and admiration'.[34]

Examiners and Examinees

When it came to dealing with Examinations, the Statement intended for the Commissioners betrayed a compassion for the Examiners no less than that for the Examinees! Examiners were depicted as absorbed during the day in conducting orals, and at night reading written answers not in their tens but in their hundreds, over a period of weeks. As to the student, compassion for him was mixed with an element of subtlety. He apparently might, despite the moral rectitude of Professors, be the victim of unintentionally biased tests had he studied under teachers other than

Professors. Certainly the College Statement cannot be suspected of guile in its naïve comment that in the circumstances the student 'may consider himself under the necessity of attending the Professor's class and any recognition of the Extra-Mural Lecturer granted by the University may thus prove to be a privilege of which the student cannot avail himself'. It was contended that the answer to the problem was for the University Court to appoint more Examiners. Surprisingly it was considered that two Examiners for every hundred Candidates would be adequate. Oral Examinations conducted by the University should, it was urged, be open to Members of the College Council in a way analogous to that applicable to oral examinations conducted by the three Scottish Medical Corporations.[34]

Clinical Medicine: Provisions Inadequate

The concluding section of the Statement dealt with improvements considered necessary by the College in the teaching of, and examinations in Clinical Medicine; the method of appointing Professors of Clinical Medicine; and the arrangement of Medical Classes. Certainly the College set their sights high, but at least they recognized the need to confine comments and criticisms to matters clinical! Not without reason a plea was submitted for important clinical appointments to be 'thrown open ... to ... all who are specially qualified to hold them' and for a Professor's duties to be limited to one department in view of the rapid growth characteristic of the various departments of medical study. Of changes urgently required in medical classes, the setting apart of additional time for senior students to undertake clinical work in the Infirmary was described as the one needing priority consideration. Acknowledging that 'very many students' did in fact voluntarily extend their time on the wards with, as one object, to get an insight into some of the Specialties, the College were wholly convinced that a fifth year of study devoted to the final and practical subjects should be made obligatory. Were effect to be given to this recommendation it was considered that examination in some of the more important Specialties should follow.

Having unburdened themselves, the College indicated its readiness to appoint representatives for interrogation by the Commissioners.[34]

Great credit is due to the College for its unfailing insistence whenever opportunity presented, in pressing for the highest standards in the clinical training of students. It cannot have been unmindful of the experience of Sir Robert Christison. He had told of how, during his attachment to a famous London teaching hospital, 'it was a frequent subject of wonder . . . so little use was made of the medical wards . . . for the purpose of instruction, and generally that education in medicine proper was almost entirely neglected . . . pupils . . . got no more information in medical practice than the few crumbs they might pick up now and then during the medical treatment of surgical cases'. Continuing his theme, Christison wrote 'I could thus easily understand subsequently the superiority of the general practitioners educated at Edinburgh, where medicine proper held a prominent place in the system of hospital instruction'.[36] Without doubt the College had an eye to improvement of their own position *vis-à-vis* the academic staff. They did not conceal the fact. Their self-interest did not detract from their genuine concern that the standards of clinical teaching in Edinburgh should continue to be in the forefront of medical education.

'Draft Ordinance—Edinburgh No. 1'

On 28th June 1891 the Commissioners issued their first Ordinance relating to Graduation in Medicine and Surgery in the University of Edinburgh. It ordained Regulations for Degrees in Medicine which implemented a number of recommendations previously made by the College, including the addition of a fifth year to the curriculum and the recognition of Physics, Insanity, Fevers, Diseases of Children and Disease of the Eye as subjects for study. To that extent the College were naturally gratified. Other sections of the Ordinance were however less pleasing and with the minimum of delay the College took it upon themselves to make representations to the Commissioners. Proposals for the teaching of and examination in Materia Medica and Pharmacy were described as giving the subject undue prominence. Perhaps it was loyalty to ancestral tenets which prompted the College to record that 'It seems as if it were the aim of the Ordinance that Graduation in Medicine of the University should be qualified to enter into competition with the retail druggists. It appears to be a retrograde step to devote such undue attention to the domain of the Pharmaceutical Chemist.' So indignant were the College that they stated that the proposal, if carried out, would 'entail the absolute wreck of the fifth year which has been wisely added to the Curriculum'.[37]

Another major complaint of the College concerned the preferential treatment given certain Provincial Schools of England to the disadvantage of the Edinburgh Extra-Mural School. Under the Ordinance, students seeking an Edinburgh degree would be able to take out many more classes in such provincial English Schools as Newcastle, Leeds and Liverpool than in the Edinburgh Extra-Mural School; this despite the English schools being affiliated to recently founded Universities and possessing equipment of inferior standard as compared with the Edinburgh Extra-Mural School. In seeking rectification of the anomaly the College gave it as their conviction 'that the Commissioners have at the present time an opportunity, such as will not occur again for many years, of welding together the different component parts of the Medical School, and of strengthening in this way the University of Edinburgh'.[37] Certainly there was much discussion and many amendments were required before agreement was reached on a final form of veiled protest for transmission to the Commissioners.[38] Nevertheless, reading the records it is difficult not to feel that a good case was ineffectively presented.

An Unsavoury Flirtation

About this time, what can only be described as an altogether extraordinary, and some might even go so far as to say disreputable development took place. Representatives of the College joined in a conference with delegates from the other Scottish Corporations and the University of St Andrews to consider the feasibility of an agreement whereby candidates who had passed the Triple Qualification might have the Degree of M.B. and Ch.B. conferred on them. On 23rd February 1892 the report of their representatives at the Conference was presented to the College at an Extraordinary Meeting. Sir Alexander Simpson, the President, was in the Chair and 57 Fellows were in attendance. After considerable discussion and rejection of an amendment moved as a direct negative, a motion was passed remitting 'to the Council to consider the lines upon which the alliance with the University of St Andrews should be carried out'.[39]

Protests were registered by Drs Byrom Bramwell and William Rutherford and their reasons for protest were submitted at the next meeting two weeks later. The reasons were emphatic in declaring that the proposed alliance would 'inflict serious injury upon the [Scottish teaching] universities . . . and therefore upon Medical Education in Scotland'; and would 'lower the value of the Medical Degrees of the Universities of Aberdeen, Edinburgh and Glasgow'. Those protesting were opposed to Licentiates of the Scottish Corporations receiving degrees from any Scottish University without having completed a Curriculum of Study in accordance with University Ordinances and without having studied for at least two years at the University or a School of Medicine affiliated to the University. Severe as these strictures were, the final one was even more outspoken maintaining 'that in desiring such an alliance ... the College is going beyond its legitimate sphere in seeking to increase its own prosperity without due regard to the injury that would be inflicted on the medical teaching Institutions of Scotland'.[40]

In due course the Council submitted its Report which recommended that the Conjoint Scheme for the Triple Qualification should continue for those not desiring to graduate; the University of St Andrews under conditions to be formulated should 'grant Degrees to the Licentiates of the Corporations and to them only'; and that Council should be empowered to support any Memorial from the University of St Andrews to the University Commission to this effect. The Report with a minor amendment was approved by a majority, Dr Bramwell again having unsuccessfully moved an amendment against adoption and being seconded on this occasion by Dr Clouston.[41]

The College was not to be dissuaded. The majority view prevailed. Notwithstanding, a feeling of unease existed. This was intensified when one of those present announced that there already lay on the Tables of the Houses of Parliament, Ordinances of the Scottish Universities' Commission 'providing for residence of Candidates for Medical Degrees in St Andrews University'. Urgent action was considered necessary by the College which suspended Standing Orders to discuss the situation, as a result of which Council was instructed 'to take immediately whatever steps they should consider most efficacious in preventing the disturbing Ordinances (No. 47 and Section 8 of Ordinance 45) of the Commission from becoming law'.[42] An early result was that in association with representatives of the two other Scottish Medical Corporations the Council of the College petitioned 'both Houses to present an Address to Her Majesty in Council, praying her Majesty to withhold Her assent' from specified parts of the Commission's Ordinances.

After reviewing the impact which the Commissioners' requirements would have upon the places and institutions at which intending candidates for degrees in Medicine at St Andrews University could pursue their studies, the College Petition outlined the case for the award of St Andrews degrees to holders of the Triple Qualification of the Scottish Medical Corporations. The Petition explained that the University of St Andrews had approached the Corporations with a view to submitting to the Commissioners a Scheme whereby, additional to granting Medical Degrees under conditions of residence, the University might continue to grant Medical Degrees without residence 'to properly qualified candidates'. It was explained that it was the desire of St Andrews University to confer Degrees without residence to candidates who held the Triple Qualification of the Scottish Corporations. Referring to the oft-quoted three divisions of the Kingdom, attention was drawn to the eligibility of non-residents to medical degrees at the University of Durham and at the Royal University in Dublin, and to the probability of comparable arrangements at London University in the near future.

'In these circumstances', the Petition concluded, 'the continuing of the privilege hitherto exercised by St. Andrews University under proper safeguards, and limited in its scope to Licentiates of the Triple Qualification, would be just and expedient, not only as regards that University, but as regards your Petitioners, and the extramural Medical Schools'.[43] For these reasons, the withholding of assent was sought, but without the desired result.

The Skeleton in the Cupboard

Further reference to the subject does not appear in the Minute Book. Whether from embarrassment or not is a matter for conjecture. Certainly had any Fellows at the time a knowledge of their predecessors' activities sixty years previously, they could be forgiven blushes of shame. On 28th December 1833 an Extraordinary Meeting had been called for no other purpose than considering 'if any or what steps should be taken by the Royal College in regard to the late Regulations of the University of St. Andrews on the subject of Degrees'.[44] Attendance was only moderate—the President (Dr J. H. Davidson) and nineteen Fellows, whether attributable to post- or pre-prandial factors is open to question. It did not however deter the College from forwarding to the Home Secretary a Memorial and Petition, with enclosed 'a Certified Copy of the Regulations of the University of St. Andrews'.

Memorials to those in high places are by tradition couched in terms as florid as they are laboured. They provide an opportunity for suppliant pomposity to verge on the ludicrous. On this occasion the College excelled itself. Apparently uneasy at intervening without solicitation 'beyond the limits to which their direct authority and power are extended', the Memorial stated that the College had 'established a claim to some regard' as evidenced by the frequency with which they had been consulted by 'Public Functionaries' and with which their many Memorials and Petitions had been well received by successive Royal personages. It was further claimed that prudence and delicacy had dissuaded the College from passing proposals for 'dispensing testimonials of competency' in advance of the anticipated Commission to be empowered by Her Majesty.

Having depicted the College as typifying all that was dutiful and exemplary, the Petition proceeded with supreme unctuousness 'to regret that similar deference and reserve have not been elsewhere observed'. Indeed, such is the regret that the Memorialists 'See cause to lament'. Then and only then did they get to grips with the subject of the Petition: 'one of the Universities of Scotland . . . has but lately announced certain regulations for granting the highest honors in Medicine and Surgery . . . supposing them to be legal, of exceedingly dubious propriety'. Reference was made to opinions expressed by the Commissioners to the Scottish Universities that Universities conferring medical degrees must regularly teach a certain proportion of medical classes, and ensure that the attainments of candidates can be adequately investigated. Whereupon, with an astuteness deriving much from indirectness, Her Majesty was asked 'to withold countenance from new or partial measures, whencesoever issuing at the present time'. The St Andrews Regulations aimed at offsetting their lack of facilities for clinical and other instruction by requiring a candidate to produce evidence of having 'regularly attended Lectures delivered by Professors in some University, or by resident Fellows of the Royal Colleges of Physicians, or Surgeons, of London, Edinburgh, Glasgow, Aberdeen, or Dublin, for at least Four complete Sessions during Four Years'. For conjoint examiners the Senatus Academicus appointed four Fellows of the Edinburgh College of Surgeons and William Gregory of the Royal College of Physicians of Edinburgh, any three of whom together with the Professor of Medicine in the University were to constitute a quorum.[44]

From a subsequent Minute it transpires that unmasking of the iniquities of St Andrews University had involved an element of collusion between the College and the University of Edinburgh. The College was indebted to the last named for an 'authentic copy' of the St Andrews Regulations, and also for a copy of the opinion of the Lord Advocate and Solicitor General as to the legality of those Regulations.[45] Mutual expressions of gratitude passed between Edinburgh University and the College, and the latter directed that their Memorial should be published in the Press. In arriving at this decision the College no doubt derived determination from the opinion of the two government legal experts who were 'decidedly against the propriety—and very strongly against the Legality' of the University of St Andrews' resolutions.[46]

The St Andrews Regulations were dated 9th December 1833 and the College Memorial to the Home Secretary 28th December 1833. Exemplary speed in pursuit of a permissible cause which none the less provided a quixotic background to the subsequent unsavoury flirtations of 1892.

REFERENCES

WITH THE UNIVERSITY

(1) 21 and 22 Victoria, c. 90 (1858).

(2) 21 and 22 Victoria, c. 83 (1858).

(3) GRANT, Sir A. (1884) *The Story of the University of Edinburgh*, vol. II, p. 108. London: Longmans, Green & Co.

(4) Ibid., vol. I, p. 333.

(5) Ibid., vol. II, p. 109.

(6) Ibid., p. 110.

(7) Ibid., p. 111.

(8) TURNER, A. L., ed. (1933) *History of the University of Edinburgh, 1883–1933*, p. 100. Edinburgh: Oliver & Boyd.

WITH THE EXTRA-ACADEMICAL SCHOOL OF MEDICINE

(9) College Minutes, 16.vii.1863.

(10) Ibid., 4.viii.1863.

(11) Ibid., 1.xi.1864.

(12) Ibid., 1.v.1883.

(13) Ibid., 7.viii.1883.

(14) Ibid., 4.ii.1890.

(15) Ibid., 7.v.1895.

(16) Ibid., 9.vii.1895.

(17) Ibid., 6.viii.1895.

WITH THE GENERAL MEDICAL COUNCIL

(18) Ibid., 4.viii.1863.

(19) GENERAL MEDICAL COUNCIL (1864) *Minutes*, 3.vi.1863. London: [G.M.C.].

(20) College Minutes, 3.xi.1863.

(21) Ibid., 2.ii.1864.

(22) Ibid., 22.iii.1864.

(23) Ibid., 3.v.1864.

(24) Ibid., 1.xi.1864.

(25) Ibid., 4.ii.1868.

(26) Ibid., 5.v.1885.

(27) Ibid., 12.ii.1870.

(28) Ibid., 22.ii.1870.

(29) Ibid., 25.iv.1870.

(30) Ibid., 29.xii.1871.

(31) Ibid., 26.xii.1884.

WITH THE SCOTTISH UNIVERSITIES COMMISSION

(32) Ibid., 21.xi.1889.

(33) Ibid., 4.ii.1890.

(34) Ibid., 7.iii.1890.

(35) R.C.P.E. (1860) *Opinions of the Council of the Royal College of Physicians of Edinburgh in relation to degree in medicine*, p. 28. Edinburgh: Murray & Gibb.

36) CHRISTISON, Sir R. (1885) *The Life of Sir Robert Christison, Bart.*, vol. I, pp. 193–4. Edinburgh: Blackwood.

(37) College Minutes, 4.viii.1891.

(38) Ibid., 3.xi.1891.

(39) Ibid., 23.ii.1892.

(40) Ibid., 8.iii.1892.

(41) Ibid., 3.v.1892.

(42) Ibid., 1.v.1894.

(43) Ibid., 28.v.1894.

(44) Ibid., 28.xii.1833.

(45) R.C.P.E. (1834) *General correspondence*, 1.ii.1834.

(46) College Minutes, 4.ii.1834.

Chapter XXIII

SOUTHERN MOVES TOWARDS
EMANCIPATION: THE COLLEGE REACTS

There is nothing makes a man suspect much, more than to know little.

Francis Bacon

In common with other medical Corporations, the College was sensitive to any threat to its privileges and the rights of its Fellows and Licentiates. Possible threats emanating from the South understandably resulted in developments being kept under close and, at times, suspicious observation. As medical reform got under way the situation arose in a variety of circumstances as illustrated by the following three examples.

THE UNIVERSITY OF LONDON

An Extraordinary Meeting of the College was called on Christmas Eve 1835 'relative to the contemplated Metropolitan University'.[1] To understand the confused evolution of London University is not easy, and is not made easier by such varied designations as Metropolitan University, Albert University and London University. Any concern shewn by the Edinburgh College of Physicians was indirect in nature and reflected the constant anxiety betrayed by all Colleges—medical or surgical, lest their privileges should be trespassed upon or overshadowed.

Phase one in the succession of events consisted of an entirely private venture in 1825 which assumed the designation University of London and which today is known as University College. It made claim to a faculty of medicine. Two petitions by University College for a Royal Charter were unsuccessful. A third attempt in 1835, however, succeeded in obtaining not one, but two Charters whereby the University of London and University College were incorporated as separate bodies. The new

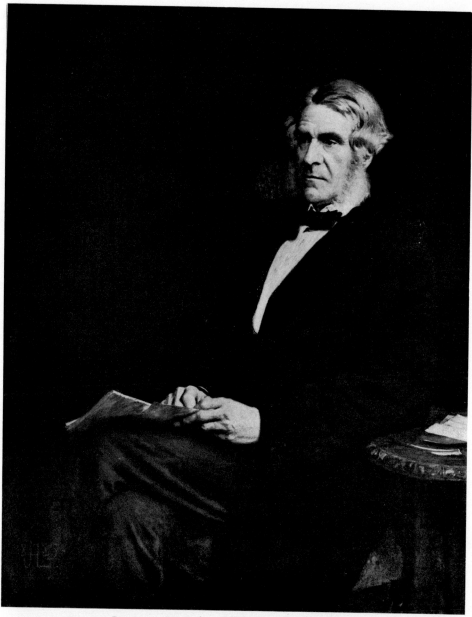

PLATE 36   Sir Robert Christison, Bt. (1797–1882)
Reproduced from portrait in the College by John H. Lorimer, R.S.A.; photograph by Tom Scott

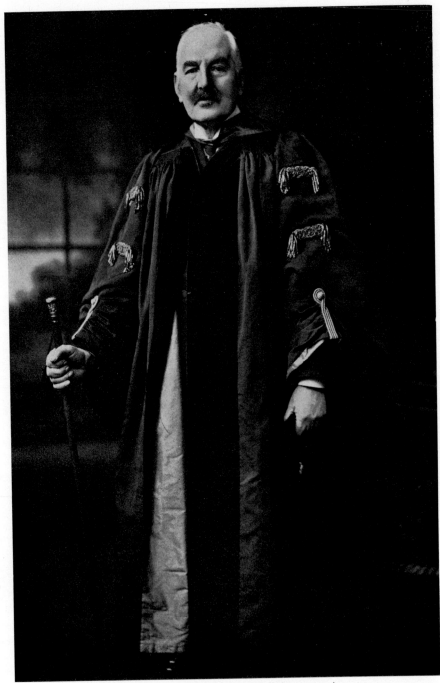

PLATE 37   Sir Byrom Bramwell (1847–1931)
Reproduced from photograph in the College by Tom Scott

University first conferred medical degrees in 1839. Meanwhile in 1829 King's College, a Church of England foundation intended to counter the influence of the non-sectarian University College, obtained a Charter.[2]

It was in the midst of these changes that the Edinburgh College became rather more than inquisitive, although there is no conclusive evidence that they were aware that in 1833 the London College of Physicians had drafted a petition seeking power to confer their own degrees.[3] Nevertheless as a result of the Extraordinary Meeting on Christmas Eve 1835 a Memorial was sent to the Secretary of State for the Home Department. Frankly it is difficult to grasp what the Memorandum was intended to achieve. Commencing with what Winston Churchill was wont to call 'platitudinous verbosity' the Memorandum was deferentially appreciative of Government action 'thus far' and suddenly became suppliant. The Royal College begged leave to express their deep anxiety that 'the very valuable privileges' contemplated for the proposed Metropolitan University 'may be extended towards other portions of Great Britain'. Although still verbose the Memorialists finally cast circumlocution aside and declared it to be 'their earnest hope that . . . the University and Medical School, with which they are more immediately connected, will be found, . . . worthy of participating . . .'.[1]

In a little over one year the College was warned against complacency by a Fellow who advised that their 'attention . . . should be fixed on the proceedings of the New University in London, and on the privileges to be conferred on them or by them on different Schools of Medicine . . .'.[4] Subsequent protracted devious events in London did not point to the need for instant action but certainly accentuated the desirability of continued remote observation. Classical medico-political manoeuvring for over half a century characterized efforts to establish a University of London possessed of powers to examine and confer degrees. Innumerable propositions involving close alliance between University College and the London College of Physicians came up for study. In 1884 the London College considered a suggestion that it might become associated with a University for the purpose of conferring degrees. The same College in the following year debated a resolution referred from the English College of Surgeons which had as a possible long-term objective the legal right of the two English Royal Colleges to give the title of Doctor to holders of the Physician's licence and the Surgeon's diploma. During discussion in *Comitia* of the Physicians' College one argument advanced against agreeing with the resolution was that 'the sister Colleges in Edinburgh and Dublin might apply for the same privilege'. The forecast was correct. The English College of Surgeons with minimal opposition and the London College of Physicians after considerable discussion, jointly authorized

U

their delegates to approach the Privy Council in an endeavour to obtain the necessary Charter. An immediate result was a declaration by the Scottish and Irish Medical Corporations that they would apply for similar Charters in the event of the London Colleges being successful.[5]

To complicate further the tangled situation University College and King's College now entered the political arena with a petition for a Charter enabling them to combine and function as a University with a medical and other faculties, and with power to confer degrees. Provisionally the University was to be known as the Albert University of London. This was in 1887. In the same year the London Royal Colleges lodged a petition intended to secure the incorporation of a Senate of Physicians and Surgeons empowered to grant degrees in medicine and surgery and to consist of the Presidents of the two Colleges and twenty-three Fellows from each College.[6] Herein is part explanation of a Petition proposing a Senate of Medicine for Scotland by the Scottish Medical Corporations (Chap. XXIV), a Petition which was referred to the Royal Commission considering proposals for an Albert University.[1]

The subject of the proposed Albert University came up for consideration by the Edinburgh College of Physicians in the middle of 1891. Privy Council deliberations on the Albert University 'prayer' had been delayed until settlement had been reached about the affairs of the University of London. It was felt that the Draft Charter of the Albert University contained provisions affecting the College, and Council were empowered to take any necessary action 'either simply or in conjunction with the other two Medical Corporations in Scotland'.[8] In due course a meeting was held with the Edinburgh College of Surgeons and the Glasgow Faculty. An immediate outcome was the preparation by a Joint Committee of the three Corporations of a Joint Memorial which was presented to the Privy Council. To strengthen further the Memorialists' case, the College's London Agents selected and instructed Sir Charles Pearson 'to appear in the joint interests before the Privy Council'. Sadly, the events which followed only served to confirm that 'the best laid schemes o' mice an' men gang aft a-gley'. Reporting on behalf of the Council at the August Quarterly Meeting, the Vice-President stated that 'without further reason being given Sir Charles Pearson was not permitted to address the Privy Council', on the score that the Colleges and Faculty had no *locus standi*. Peremptorily repulsed in this way the College Council was disinclined to take any further immediate action, more especially as there appeared to be little likelihood of further developments for at least six months in connection with the proposed Albert University.[9]

There, in so far as the Edinburgh College of Physicians was actively concerned, the story ended. Medico-political manoeuvring in the South continued unabated. A

Royal Commission was opposed to the Albert scheme as a means of creating a Teaching University in London. Nor was it in favour of the proposed English Senate of Physicians and Surgeons. In the opinion of the Commission a 'single-faculty' University was not desirable, and conferment of degrees by the Royal Colleges, possessed of no academical character, would be unwarranted. Cooke quoted Allchin as saying 'the pretensions of the Royal Colleges were dismissed in terms that as nearly approached the contemptuous as it was consistent with the dignity of a Royal Commission to employ'.[10] Allchin, a Fellow of the London College of Physicians, was at one time Assistant Registrar of that College and had been attracted by the idea of association with the University of London. Towards the end of 1889 the University Senate submitted a scheme more or less in accordance with suggestions emanating from the Royal Commission. 'The College's main aims were adequate representation on the Senate and to have its own examinations accepted for the pass degree of M.B. of the University'—so writes Cooke.[11] Although harmony was the objective, all was not harmonious! Agreement proved impossible between, among others, the two London Royal Colleges and University College and King's College on important points of parochial detail if such a term can be applied to England's metropolis. The Senate Charter was rejected by Convocation in 1891, but negotiations not devoid of wrangling persisted almost to the time of World War II. At the present time 'there is now no official connection between the [London] College and the University but many unofficial and personal contacts'[12]—the same it can be said as obtains in Edinburgh between College and University.

Lest what has been said may appear carping the following extracts from a Memorandum by Dr Edward Liveing prepared for a London College Meeting on July 28th 1890 serve to give a patently unbiased and admirably clear presentation of an otherwise somewhat unfortunate picture.

'. . . After all, what is the difference between the schemes of the two Royal [London] Colleges? . . . all the difference in the world. A distinguished Surgeon put the issue very clearly . . . "There are two totally distinct and different matters before us (1) One is the Reconstitution of the University; with that we desire to have nothing to do; we do not wish to become in any sense a part of the University. (2) The other is an arrangement for a conjoint Professional Examination by the University and Royal Colleges for the M.B. degree, covering also the Licence and Membership. We accept this 'crowning' of the Colleges' Examinations with a Degree, as a reasonable solution of the problem how to obtain London medical degrees for London students, and as affording the best security we can suggest for the maintenance of our own autonomy and the best protection for our diplomas."

'We of the [London] College of Physicians . . . have taken a wider view. We have never considered that the autonomy of the Colleges would be seriously compromised; and as regards the possible depreciation of our diplomas . . . we have been ready to accept . . . a greater loss than can possibly fall on our sister college. We have felt the occasion to be one of supreme importance . . . The occasion seemed to bring within sight the practicability of bringing together in one organisation, and for one purpose the independent Medical Institutions of London . . . ; it seemed to afford, in fact, an opportunity of shaping in and for London the greatest Medical Faculty in the World . . .'.[13]

What purpose is there in elaborating thus on repercussions from the policies of London University? Legitimately proud of its historical pre-eminence as a teaching centre it was only natural that Edinburgh should take wary cognizance of developments elsewhere. In this the Edinburgh College of Physicians was no less concerned than the University. Moreover there is no disguising the fact that the trend of discussions and negotiations opened up new, not necessarily desirable, vistas in the field of medical education. Remotely bastioned in its northern citadel the Edinburgh College cannot be blamed if with other Scottish Corporations it looked to the security of its defences. Nor, considering the changes in attitude dispassionately and in retrospect, can it be denied all was not altruistic. An analogy that comes to mind is that of a bevy of competing oil prospectors moving in their 'rigs' to stake sea-bed claims. Paradoxically the Edinburgh College was perhaps fortunate in that it was furthest removed from the spoils.

BRITISH MEDICAL ASSOCIATION

Ah me! What mighty perils wait
the man who meddles with a State.
                              Chas. Churchill (*The Duellist*)

Concern over Charters did not cease with the turn of the century. In March 1909 the Council reported to the College that to their knowledge a Petition had been presented to the Privy Council by certain officials of the British Medical Association. Notable omissions from the list of signatories were the names of the President, President-Elect and Past President of the B.M.A. From enquiries which they had made the College Council were satisfied that certain clauses of the Petition impinged on the legitimate rights of the College and those holding the College diploma; and would 'imperil' freedom of action on the part of individual members of the medical profession. Council submitted to the College a draft petition for transmission to the Privy Council.

The Petition suggested by its Council met with the unanimous approval of the College. It opposed unreservedly claims contained in the B.M.A. petition to publish registers of medical practitioners, promote the candidature of members of the B.M.A. for Parliament, and to establish a Central Ethical Standing Committee which might extend beyond membership of the B.M.A. and conflict with the authority of the General Medical Council.[14]

According to Little, the question of applying for a Royal Charter of Incorporation was dismissed by the B.M.A. 'in the years 1907–1910' after correspondence with the Privy Council.[15]

Happily, relations between the College and the Association have not suffered. Numerous evidences could be cited. Suffice to mention that in 1944 the President (Dr Fergus Hewat) accepted an invitation to attend meetings of the Scottish Committee of the B.M.A.[16]; and within five weeks nominations were being submitted by the College on request, for the Joint Committee on Consultants and Specialists under the National Health Service Scheme.[17] Some years later the College was informed that under the Constitution of the Scottish Council of the B.M.A. 'one member' was to be nominated by the College.[18] Largely as a result of the initiative of Dr J. G. M. Hamilton, a notably active B.M.A. member, and in his day Councillor and Vice-President of the College, consideration was given to ways in which the College and B.M.A. might co-operate in arranging scientific sessions.[19]

THE EDUCATION AND GRADUATION OF WOMEN IN MEDICINE

Tis known by the name of perseverance in a good cause, and of obstinacy in a bad one.
Laurence Sterne (*Tristram Shandy*)

A maiden at College, named Breeze,
Weighed down by B.A.'s and M.D.'s
Collapsed from the strain.
Said her doctor, 'It's plain,
You are killing yourself by degrees!'

Anonymous

'Gentlemen,

I purpose studying Medicine with the view of obtaining the Diploma of a Licentiate of the College, and I shall be obliged by your informing me whether I can be admitted to the preliminary Examination and to Registration as a Student of Medicine.

I have the honor to remain
Gentlemen,
Your obedient Servant
(signed) Elizabeth Garrett'[20]

The date of the application was 18th June 1862: the Gentlemen addressed—the Fellows of the Royal College of Physicians of Edinburgh. Reference by Council was *simpliciter* to the College. To have witnessed the first unspoken reactions at the sederunt must have been a unique and educative experience.

Prefacing his remarks with disapproval of the application, a Fellow moved 'the previous question'. This was followed by a motion by Dr Alexander Wood seconded by Dr Wright, to the effect 'That the College do not see it necessary at present to pronounce any opinion on the application of Miss Garrett as the arrangements of the existing Medical Schools in Great Britain do not at present admit of a Lady attending the full curriculum required by the College'.

Elements of cautious gallantry and foresight were not entirely lacking, however, because Dr Begbie moved an amendment to the original motion 'That the College receive the Petition of Miss Garrett, recognise the importance of securing a well educated class of women to be employed in the treatment of the diseases of Women and children, and remit to the Council to consider the best method of framing regulations on the subject . . .'. Dr Traill seconded the amendment. Thereupon there was evidence of qualified courage in a further amendment by Dr Balfour of the original motion 'That Miss Garrett be admitted to pass the preliminary Examination and that the College subsequently take time to consider what shall be done when she presents herself for examination'. Dr Struthers seconded. At this point the President (Dr Craigie) vacated the Chair and spoke in favour of Miss Garrett's Petition being granted. On the President resuming the Chair, it was agreed that the vote should be taken in the first place on 'the Previous Question' or not. Eighteen Fellows voted for and sixteen against 'the Previous Question', after which it was declared from the chair that the necessity to put the other amendments to the vote did not arise. One Fellow had left the Meeting before the vote was taken, and it is of interest that that arch-anti-feminist in the matter of medical education, (Sir) Robert Christison, was not present.[20] In his biography Christison's opposition to the education and graduation of women in medicine was described as almost violent.[21] He was not

alone in the strength of his opinions. A number of years later Sir William Jenner—
a future President of the London College of Physicians wrote the B.M.A. threatening
his resignation in consequence of 'Lady Members being permitted to attend the
meeting of the Association'.[22]

Nothing daunted, Miss Garrett sought 'permission to visit the female wards of the
[Edinburgh] Infirmary with any of the physicians and surgeons of the hospital who
may invite me to do so'.[23, 24] On the advice of the medical staff the suggestion wa
not acceded to, it being 'inexpedient to grant her request in the circumstances of th
hospital'.[25] How often these words 'in the circumstances' have been used, and are to
this day used, to circumvent in a fashion awkward situations raised by members
of the professions!

Miss Garrett met no better fate in London than in Edinburgh when, in 1864, she
submitted an application to be admitted to examination for the Licence of the London
College of Physicians. Rejection of the application was in accordance with legal
advice and despite the fact that by this time 'she was registered as a medical student
at the Apothecaries' Hall, had passed two examinations towards the Licence of the
Society of Apothecaries, and was well on the way to receiving a registrable qualification . . .'.[26] In point of fact Miss Garrett became the first woman to qualify when
she obtained the Licence of the Apothecaries' Hall in 1865, having received part of her
medical education under private auspices.[27]

The College and Infirmary were not the only objects of discomfiture. Miss Sophia
Jex-Blake's establishment in Edinburgh of an extra-mural medical school for
women has been described. In 1869 for the second time, Miss Jex-Blake endeavoured
to get the University to provide separate classes for her and her fellow female
students. Having agreed to admit women to study medicine in the University, the
Senate stipulated that not only should female students be instructed separately but
that instruction should be given only by those willing to provide it among professors
and recognized extra-academical lecturers. The decision was confirmed in turn by
the University Court and the General Council.

Inevitably, an early result was renewed pressure on the Infirmary to allow female
students to enter the wards. Again a refusal was forthcoming, albeit a polite refusal.[28]
As succinctly put by Logan Turner 'The hospital with the crest bearing the motto
"Patet omnibus" remained closed to . . . women students'.[25] In the course of a year
or two improvised arrangements, not to be regarded as constituting a precedent and
virtually precluding attendance in surgical theatres and post-mortem rooms, were
given a trial.[29]

About this time a letter was received by the College from the London School of

Medicine for Women asking to be recognized by the Edinburgh College of Physicians. Council's reply was to the effect that the situation could not arise as it had been decided not to admit women as candidates for the Licence of the College.[30]

There was further evidence of resistance to intrusion on the part of women in 1876 when the College decided to petition against the provisions of a Bill before Parliament in so far as it related 'to the Registration of Women who have taken the Degree of Doctor of Medicine in a Foreign University'.[31] However the late 1880s were to coincide with a series of decisions of greater moment than was probably realized at the time. In February 1886 the College consented to the admission of women to the Triple Qualification examination. The issue was raised following receipt at the office of the Triple Qualification of two applications—one from a lady in Liverpool and the other a Canadian lady temporarily resident in Birmingham. Considering the significance of the College decision the relevant minutes are surprisingly brief, whether as a result of pained surprise or a sense of decorum on the part of the Secretary is not evident.[32] Three years later, and three years before 'perfect equality between the sexes in the [British Medical] Association' had been attained,[33] the passing into law of the *Universities (Scotland) Act 1889* under powers granted by the University Commissioners, enabled the Universities to admit women to graduation in medicine. The University of Edinburgh took advantage of the Commissioners' Ordinance in 1894.

In the meantime the hesitant attitude of the Infirmary towards women had relaxed to a certain extent with the establishment of special out-patient sessions, ward rounds and post-mortem attendances.[34] The innovations were not without their growing pains. (Sir) Byrom Bramwell was the first to teach Clinical Medicine to women in the Royal Infirmary. He together with Mr J. M. Cotterill, F.R.C.S.E. were put in charge of new medical and surgical wards respectively, and male medical students knew resentment when they found that they could attend Bramwell's clinics on one day in the week whereas the women were privileged to do so throughout the remainder of the week! Such restrictions as remained disappeared during the years of World War I.

As recently as 1900 a lady licentiate was informed that by the terms of the Charter, Membership was not open to women.[35] During the years of World War I the College resolved to petition for an alteration in the Charter which would enable women to become Fellows and Members.[36] The necessary Supplementary Charter was granted and sealed on 8th January 1920.[37] Dr Ella Pringle was the first lady Member. Awarded her Diploma in 1925, she was created a Fellow in 1929.[38]

REFERENCES

THE UNIVERSITY OF LONDON

(1) College Minutes, 24.xii.1835.
(2) COOKE, A. M. (1972) *A History of the Royal College of Physicians of London*, vol. 3, p. 931. Oxford: Clarendon.
(3) Ibid., p. 396.
(4) College Minutes, 7.ii.1837.
(5) COOKE, A. M. Op. cit., pp. 942–4.
(6) Ibid., p. 945.
(7) College Minutes, 11.i.1888.
(8) Ibid., 12.vi.1891.
(9) Ibid., 4.viii.1891.
(10) COOKE, A. M. Op. cit., p. 947.
(11) Ibid., p. 949.
(12) Ibid., p. 971.
(13) Ibid., Appendix VII, pp. 1190–1.

BRITISH MEDICAL ASSOCIATION

(14) College Minutes, 30.iii.1909.
(15) LITTLE, E. M., comp. [1932] *History of the British Medical Association, 1832–1932*, p. 88. London: British Medical Association.
(16) Council Minutes, 14.iii.1944.
(17) Ibid., 18.iv.1944.
(18) Ibid., 2.vii.1958.
(19) Ibid., 26.ix.1967.

WOMEN IN MEDICINE

(20) College Minutes, 20.vi.1862.
(21) CHRISTISON, Sir R. (1886) *The Life of Sir Robert Christison, Bart.*, vol. II, pp. 43 f. Edinburgh: Blackwood.
(22) LITTLE, E. M. Op. cit., p. 92.
(23) EDINBURGH ROYAL INFIRMARY. *Minutes*, 16.vi.1862.
(24) Ibid., 23.vi.1862.
(25) TURNER, A. L. (1937) *Story of a Great Hospital; The Royal Infirmary of Edinburgh, 1729–1929*, p. 246. Edinburgh: Oliver & Boyd.
(26) COOKE, A. M. Op. cit., p. 832.

(27) COMRIE, J. D. (1932) *History of Scottish Medicine*, 2nd Edition, vol. II, p. 667. London: Baillière, Tindall & Cox.

(28) EDINBURGH ROYAL INFIRMARY. *Minutes*, 31.x.1870.

(29) TURNER, A. L. Op. cit., p. 248.

(30) Council Minutes, 30.x.1874.

(31) College Minutes, 2.v.1876.

(32) Ibid., 2.ii.1886.

(33) LITTLE, E. M. Op. cit., p. 94.

(34) TURNER, A. L. Op. cit., p. 251.

(35) Council Minutes, 30.i.1900.

(36) College Minutes, 5.xi.1918.

(37) Ibid., 3.ii.1920.

(38) Ibid., 16.vii.1963.

Chapter XXIV

OH! EAST IS EAST, AND WEST IS WEST, AND...

Nae mair shall Glasgow Striplings threap
Their City's Beauty and its Shape,
While our New City spreads around
Her bonny Wings on Fairy Ground.
                         Robert Fergusson (*Auld Reekie*)

. . . Glasgow and Aberdeen are Scotorum Scotissimi, particularly Glasgow . . .
                         Sir Robert Christison

Mergers are a feature of the present age, and can be associated with megalomania. They have attendant risks but sometimes achieve spectacular success. No section of society is free from their influence and national boundaries are no longer sacrosanct. Mergence may be offensive in that it seeks to acquire increased power, or defensive in that it aims to consolidate privileges and interests already acquired. Motives may be altruistic, wholly selfish or basically emotional.

In the course of their long histories the Medical Corporations of Scotland have from time to time, at widely spaced intervals, tentatively considered ways and means of joining forces in whole or part. A factor common to most attempts has been a desire to resist dominance from the South. It is to the credit of the Scottish Corporations that although a means of formal union among them has not been crystallized, relations between them have progressively gained in amicability. Inability to agree on union has in no way prevented the closest of co-operation in many matters of common interest—as for instance in the establishment of conjoint examinations.

The chapter heading has been borrowed from Rudyard Kipling. Perhaps the failure to date to achieve complete union among the Corporations may be explained by another quotation from the same writer provided that, in its application to Scotland, the term 'Asia' is not too literally applied to the East!

Asia is not going to be civilised after the methods of the West. There is too much Asia and she is too old.[1]

EARLY UNCERTAINTIES

In so far as the history of our College is concerned, the first phase took place when Charters were being sought but which were never ratified. The warrant issued by James VI (I of England) to the Commissioners and Estates of Parliament was indefinite in so far as it implied rather than specifically declared that the influence of the College when erected should extend to the whole of the Kingdom of Scotland (Chap. II). When required by the Privy Council in the reign of Charles I to 'submit heads' for the erection of a College, the Edinburgh physicians did not propose to exercise professional authority further than 24 miles beyond the City (Chap. II). The Commission of Physicians appointed by the Lords of Council to advise Cromwell, to judge by their documents, seem to have interpreted their brief as applying to Scotland in general rather than Edinburgh in particular. This may well be the explanation why the Charter sent north by Cromwell required the establishment of a 'Colledge of Physitians of Scotland . . . with power . . . in any pairts or place in Scotland' (Chap. II). Understandably, already possessed of a Charter, the Glasgow Faculty, foreseeing conflict with their established supervisory privileges in the West of Scotland, took an active part in the protests against the creation of a College of Physicians for Scotland. Equally understandably the Edinburgh Incorporation of Surgeons recognized a serious threat to their own activities in the proposed new College and added their weight to the opposition (Chap. II). Surgical fears were not allayed when George Sibbald started his campaigning in the time of James VI (I of England) but as already explained (Chap. III), the Charter eventually obtained in 1681 was notably less ambitious and less acquisitive than its ill-fated predecessors, and the objections of the Edinburgh Surgeons and Glasgow Faculty became less strident.

INTER-COLLEGIATE MANOEUVRINGS

Not to be outdone, however, the Incorporation of Edinburgh Surgeons decided to obtain a new Charter on their own account and went so far as to obtain a document ready for sealing as the warrant for a proposed Royal Charter. At this stage the document was read in the presence of the surgeons, only to have their aspirations damped by the announcement of the Deacon of their Guild that the Secret Council had decreed that the document should be sent to the physicians. The conclusion was straightway arrived at that in the circumstances nothing but endless trouble was to be expected. In the words of the history of the Royal College of Surgeons 'the deacon was right, for the "signature" [document] still lies in the archives of the college unsigned and useless'.[2]

Injured Dignities

It would be gratifying to feel that the surgeons' forebodings had been unwarranted, but it has to be admitted that it was a more or less established practice for any progressive measure by one Corporation to be obstructed by the others on any pretext whatsoever. In this the Edinburgh College of Physicians was no less guilty than its sister Corporations. There could be no better evidence of this than the attitude of the College on the receipt from the Lord Advocate in 1817 of a communication inviting a comment on a prayer by the Faculty of Physicians and Surgeons of Glasgow that they 'be erected into a Royal College'. It is no exaggeration to say that our College vouched not so much as a word in favour of the 'prayer', seeing in it no 'measure calculated to maintain and exalt the character of the Physician or advance the progress of medical Science . . .', but a development 'most prejudicial to their Patrimonial Interests'.[3]

The College submitted a number of specific objections of which some had a particular underlying significance. Exception was taken to there being two Royal Colleges of Physicians or Surgeons in one Kingdom, it being maintained that 'it has hitherto been considered that a single College of both descriptions is sufficient for each Kingdom of the United Empire'. The next reason for objection was that 'a conjoined College of Physicians and Surgeons is an anomaly' and that to judge by the proposed provisions the Glasgow College 'would be to all intents and purposes a College of Surgeons', and 'the physician would be thrown into the second rank, no provision whatever being made to secure his Status and Dignity'. A challenge to the *Edinburgh Pharmacopoeia* was foreseen, with resultant 'complexity and confusion and to the no small injury of the Lieges' if that second Royal College were also to publish a Pharmacopoeia. Then followed an arbitrary statement to the effect that 'The Royal College of Physicians of Edinburgh has uniformly been considered as the Royal College of Physicians of Scotland' as evidenced by the requirements of the original Charter appertaining to the right of medical graduates of Scottish Universities to admission as Licentiates, and the right of Professors of Medicine in those Universities to be *ex officio* Honorary Fellows. Attention was drawn to the pecuniary loss which the Edinburgh College would sustain were the number of non-resident associates to be reduced by the attractions of 'a Rival Establishment'.[3]

In particular, and with every justification in the light of the restrictions imposed by their own Charter, the Edinburgh College took the strongest exception to the projected new Glasgow College's intention to establish a medical school. Two claims made by the Faculty in their Petition came in for what can only be described as ridicule. Of these the first related to the highly creditable way in which students trained by the 'Petitioners' had discharged their duties in the fighting services—a claim which Edinburgh emphasized was not unique to the Glasgow Faculty. The second claim urged by the Faculty was described as 'if possible still more preposterous'. It obviously annoyed the Edinburgh Fellows that Glasgow in support of its Petition should declare 'That the utmost attention is paid by the Petitioners to the advancement of Medical Science'. In the letter of reply the Lord Advocate was advised that 'the Public as well as the Royal College of Physicians of Edinburgh have yet to learn in what respects the exertions of the Faculty . . . of Glasgow in the improvement of Medical knowledge have been so pre-eminent as to found a claim for a Royal Charter . . .'. Finally with a tactical ingenuity the more remarkable when account is taken of their attitude in subsequent years at the time of the Scottish Universities Royal Commission (Chap. XXII) the Edinburgh College focussed attention on the harm to the School of Physic in the University of Glasgow which would result were a rival School of Medicine established in that city. In conclusion the College declared 'the Charter Petitioned for by the Faculty . . . instead of answering any useful purpose would tend to the degradation of the Profession of Physic, and would materially injure certain existing Establishments . . .'.[3]

Amity in the Capital

Relations between the two Edinburgh Colleges were seemingly on a friendlier footing. Co-operation in London between the representatives of the two Corporations and Edinburgh University endeavouring to adjust provisions in Graham's *Medical Reform Bill* to the needs of Scottish Medical Institutions, could scarcely have been more harmonious. The College of Surgeons recorded their particular appreciation of Drs Christison and Renton for their 'Liberality, courtesy and frankness during the negotiations'; and expressed the hope that a successful outcome would ensure 'a new Bond of Union' among the three parties with enhanced identification of mutual interest.[4] It is interesting that some twenty years previously a Fellow of the Edinburgh College of Surgeons had published a pamphlet in which he developed an argument for a union between the two Edinburgh Colleges.[5] Not surprisingly his opinions did not meet with general approval and another pamphlet produced by a Fellow of the College of Physicians and intended as a reply to the first, whilst not decrying the idea of union, advocated waiting for a time as the 'most prudent proceeding'.[6]

The Lure of National Status

The Faculty of Physicians and Surgeons of Glasgow having failed with their Petition, contemplated making another attempt about the middle of the century. Circumstances and procedure were different on this occasion and our College was not directly involved. Ironically the initial source of trouble was the College of Surgeons of Edinburgh. This College had prepared a draft Charter with the primary objects of winding up their Widows' Fund and of securing separation from 'the Convenery'. Included in the draft Charter was a clause aiming at the elevation of the College to the status of a national College under the title of the Royal College of Surgeons of Scotland. According to Creswell 'the Physicians were to receive the same dignity', presumably meaning thereby that they too were to acquire national status. It was intended that a private Bill should be brought before Parliament and, in accordance with customary procedure, a statement of the intentions of the College of Surgeons appeared in the Edinburgh newspapers. An immediate result was that the Glasgow Faculty lodged a Bill with as its purpose, acquisition of the title of Royal College of Physicians and Surgeons of Glasgow. Concerned at the prospect of two Royal Colleges of Surgeons in Scotland, the Edinburgh surgeons avowed their intention to oppose the Glasgow Bill to their utmost. A compromise was reached. 'The Faculty withdrew their claim, but only on condition that the College of Surgeons gave up their aspiration to national distinction.'[7]

UNION A DESIRABLE ADJUNCT TO MEDICAL REFORM

Meanwhile events in connection with other Medical Bills before Parliament gave a new prominence to the possibility, indeed desirability for an amalgamation embracing the two Edinburgh Colleges and the Glasgow Faculty. In the course of evidence given before the Select Committee of the House of Commons on Medical Registration and Medical Law Amendment, a suggestion was made that amalgamation along these lines offered a way of removing 'the only important obstacle which at present impedes the satisfactory adjustment of a sound measure of Medical Reform, so far as Scotland singly is concerned'.[8] At the time Mr William Wood of the Edinburgh Royal College of Surgeons and Dr Weir of the Glasgow Faculty were in London acting as observers for their respective Corporations on progress in Parliament of the Medical Bills. There was a tacit agreement whereby in the absence of a representative of the Edinburgh College of Physicians Mr Wood might observe on behalf of both Edinburgh Colleges. Mr Wood and Dr Weir followed up the Select Committee proceedings by having an informal discussion in conjunction with Dr Burns, another Fellow of the Glasgow Faculty. Still on a strictly informal basis, the three delegates agreed on tentative arrangements which might win the favour of the Scottish Corporations for the creation of new Colleges to be called 'The Royal College of Physicians of Scotland' and 'The Royal College of Surgeons of Scotland'. Admirably intended although it was, the document drawn up by these gentlemen was later to prove a source of disagreement not devoid of recriminations and insinuations on the part of both Eastern and Western negotiators. Overmuch authority, whether or not from genuine misunderstanding or the demands of expediency is uncertain, was attached to the informal views recorded as having been expressed in London.

Briefly, the proposed arrangements contemplated that physicians who were Members of the Faculty should become an integral part of the proposed Royal College of Physicians of Scotland with the same privileges as existing Fellows of the Edinburgh College of Physicians; and that in like manner surgical Members of the Faculty would be integrated into the proposed Royal College of Surgeons of Scotland. Fellows of the two Edinburgh Colleges residing in Glasgow were to have the same privileges (other than those arising in connection with the Faculty Widows' Fund) as Members of the Faculty; and Fellows of the two Royal Colleges of Scotland residing in Glasgow were to form a Board of Examiners along with the Examiners in the University of Glasgow with 'power to examine Candidates and grant Licenses to the General Practitioner and the Surgeon and Physician . . .'. Finally it was proposed that Licentiates of the Faculty should enjoy the same rights in regard to practice and to enrolment as Fellows of the proposed Royal Colleges of Scotland, as those conferred on Licentiates of the Edinburgh College of Surgeons.[8]

Distrust Born of Informality

Of necessity the informal suggestions of Mr Wood and Drs Weir and Burns, having no background of authority, had to be referred to the Councils of the three Corporations. The authorities of the Royal College repudiated the document which had been drawn up by Mr Wood and Dr Weir 'the moment' it 'was brought before them'. The Council of the Edinburgh College of Physicians had the advantage of the observations of Dr Renton, a delegate who had recently visited London on the subject of medical legislation and who had met Dr Weir and Mr Burns. Dr Renton advised the College that the opinion in London was that certain privileges possessed by the Glasgow Faculty alone stood in the way of contemplated necessary reforms, and that amalgamation of the Faculty with the Edinburgh Royal Colleges might solve the problem.

A motion moved by Dr Renton and unanimously adopted resolved that the 'College is prepared to receive, either as non Resident Fellows according to the present Charter or as Members under the proposed new Charter, without examination or Ballot, all Doctors of Medicine who may be members of the Faculty . . . and who . . . are willing to come under an obligation not to dispense Medicine for profit'. Continuing, the resolution provided for the adjustment of 'the particulars relative to the amalgamations' to be undertaken by a body consisting of three delegates from the Glasgow Faculty and three from each of the two Edinburgh Colleges. Any differences of opinion were to be referred to the Lord Advocate and a Member of the House, specified by name. Copies of the Resolutions were sent to the Lord Advocate, Mr Wood and the Registrar of the London College of Physicians.[9] At a subsequent meeting the College was informed that the President had named as College Delegates—Drs Christison, Renton and Seller.[10]

Informal 'Agreement' as to Terms

The three delegates met their opposite numbers appointed by the Edinburgh College of Surgeons with whom they discussed and unanimously agreed terms to be submitted to the Glasgow Faculty 'for an amalgamation . . . under the contemplated Bill for Medical Registration etc.'. Provision was made for members of the Faculty to be admitted as Fellows to the appropriate Royal College of Scotland, except in so far as any Faculty member who kept an open shop, was to be admitted as 'Member only of the Royal College of Surgeons of Scotland, until he cease to keep such open shop';

and for existing Licentiates of the Faculty to be enrolled as Members of the Royal College of Surgeons of Scotland. An item of importance in relation to negotiations was that any agreement was not to be binding on either party in the event of the Bill before Parliament not passing during the current session.[8]

Additional 'claims' by the Glasgow Faculty

The 'proposals of Agreement' were accepted by the Faculty, and detailed reference to the other proposals is unnecessary. However, at the same time as accepting the proposals the Faculty to use their own word 'claimed' additional terms. These were three in number. Of them the first was that the admission fees of Members as well as Fellows resident in Glasgow paid to the Royal Colleges should be 'paid over' to the Faculty. Secondly, the Faculty claimed that there should be an Examining Board in Glasgow to obviate the necessity of students wholly or partly educated in Glasgow, having to travel to Edinburgh or London to be examined; and that students 'found qualified' by such a Glasgow Board should 'receive from the Royal Colleges of Scotland the same diploma granted by them to Students similarly examined in Edinburgh'. The third claim of the Faculty was cryptic but fundamental viz.: 'That their designation shall continue to be the Faculty of Physicians and Surgeons of Glasgow'.[8]

A Merited Glasgow Appraisal

The two Edinburgh Colleges were unable to accede to the first two claims. As to the third they did 'not think it expedient to retain the old name of the Faculty' but expressed their readiness to be guided by the Arbiters to whom the two other points of disagreement would be referred. The letter submitting the three points at issue to the Lord Advocate for arbitration was signed by representatives of all three Corporations. From this stage on there were pleas and counter-pleas, none of which was really creditable, much less elevating. Each party laboured under the misapprehension that it was being called upon to make not merely the greatest, but an inordinate sacrifice. Mutual understanding was not aided by a certain attitude of superiority on the part of the Edinburgh Colleges who, having professed anxiety not to prejudice 'minor medical corporations in provincial districts', had the temerity to record 'Among these provincial bodies the Faculty of Physicians and Surgeons of Glasgow must be viewed as not the least important, whether regard be had to their number, the extent of their jurisdiction, or their antiquity'.

It is not to be wondered at that the Faculty, with the Lord Advocate functioning in a sense as postal agent, objected 'to the general tenor and spirit of the Memorial of the Edinburgh Colleges'. With justification the Faculty retaliated in robust fashion. 'The Faculty', it asserted, 'as a licensing Corporation is equal in every respect to the College of Surgeons of Edinburgh and Superior to the College of Physicians. It is equal to the College of Surgeons as regards the antiquity privileges and extent of jurisdiction of their respective Charters, and not inferior in respect of ability numbers and wealth.' No one can denigrate the Clydesider with impunity—be he a shipwright or boiler maker; a Jimmy Maxton or Emanuel Shinwell; physician or surgeon. Nor can the reaction of the Faculty on this occasion be attributed to puerile pique of which too much prevails in professional circles. Factually the Faculty was at the time partially correct when it asserted that it was 'superior to the Edinburgh College of Physicians in as much as the latter body has no examining or licensing powers whatever, and only an absolute jurisdiction over a portion of the old Town of Edinburgh'. Furthermore, the Faculty with incisive precision exposed the flaw in the approach made to them when they stated 'The error . . . lies in the Edinburgh Corporations already assuming the Status of the Colleges of *Scotland*'.[8]

Amalgamation: Differing Interpretations

Crediting the Colleges with a genuine desire to see the establishment of Scottish National Colleges, there was justification for their contention that the wish of the Faculty to retain their designation was contrary to a correct interpretation of inter-collegiate relations within the ambits of the projected national colleges. Were the Faculty to retain their designation the implication would be that the Faculty was independent and not a Branch of the Royal Colleges. As to the Faculty claim that there should be an Examining Board for the examination of Glasgow Students, the Colleges could not accept the argument that 'the Medical School of Glasgow cannot exist unless there be in that City a Board empowered to examine Glasgow Students directly for the licence of General Practitioner upon the minimum qualification'. Nor did the Colleges find themselves in agreement with a Faculty suggestion that Aberdeen might 'prefer' to submit a similar claim. Although this would involve Aberdeen 'asking a new privilege, not of claiming the continuance of one long enjoyed' the Glasgow Faculty indicated that they would not be inclined to raise objection. Both Edinburgh Colleges agreed that any suggestion for more than one Examining Board involved the unquestionable risk of what was vaguely described as 'a diversity of Examination'.

Financial adjustments inevitably gave rise to a conflict of views which, however, to judge from the tenor of the Memorials addressed to the Lord Advocate and interchanged between the Colleges and the Faculty, do not seem to have been a major factor in ultimate disagreement. They do not call for further reference. Nevertheless, together the three claims of the Faculty would in the opinion of the Colleges result in 'an amalgamation merely in name, and scarcely even in name'. The Colleges were adamant and their Joint Committee concluded their Memorial dated 16th June 1848 to the Lord Advocate with 'they would think it preferable that the case of the Faculty . . . were taken up by the Legislature on its own basis, and independently altogether of the Royal Colleges'.

Further observations on the part of the Glasgow Faculty and a Supplementary Memorial from the Colleges followed, which were neither constructive nor conciliatory in spirit. The degree of acrimony is evidenced by the concluding remarks of a letter signed by the nine members of the Faculty Committee to the Presidents of the Colleges. 'You have no grounds to complain that your Committees have "carried too far the spirit of concession toward your Glasgow Brethren". The Glasgow Faculty think they have an equal right with the Edinburgh College of Surgeons to become a Royal College of *Scotland*. We therefore protest against the use of such terms as "concede" and "concession". It is one of just and gentlemanly arrangement [between] professional brethren. Such we desire that it should be—more we do not ask—less the despotic power of Parliament will alone force us to accept.'[8]

There is a suggestion in the above extract that disagreement was particularly evident among the surgeons of East and West. This may or may not have been the case. There is, however, some support for the view in Creswell's history of the Royal College of Surgeons of Edinburgh. Referring to a meeting called to discuss 'a proposal for amalgamation of the three bodies', Creswell stated, '. . . the surgeons demurred; the proposals had the approval of the delegates of the physicians'.[11]

RE-OPENING OF NEGOTIATIONS

A further complication now arose. In April 1849 the Council of our College sanctioned a proposal by those who had acted as their Delegates in conferences with the Glasgow Faculty, to open negotiations again with a view to the re-submission of differences to arbitration by the Lord Advocate. It was known that this would be in accordance with the Lord Advocate's wishes, despite the fact that the original proposals for arbitration were no longer binding as no Medical Bill had been brought before Parliament during the last Session.[12] An offer to this effect was transmitted to the Faculty, it being stipulated that procedure should be determined by the previous 'terms of agreement' and Statements already submitted, and that no further written pleadings should be produced by either party except at the request of the arbiters. The offer was declined on the grounds that the Faculty had 'especially Resolved that they will not submit to an Arbitration their claim to the formation of a Board in Glasgow'.

This information was contained in a letter dated 24th April 1849.[8] 'Out of the blue', it would seem, a further letter dated 1st June 1849 was received from the Faculty indicating that the College communication had been considered again, suggesting that there may have been misunderstanding, and expressing a willingness to refer to arbitration 'all the disputed points . . . with the exception of the existence of a Committee of Examiners in Glasgow . . .'. In reply the Colleges were dogmatic in their insistence on *all* disputed points being the subject of arbitration. Back came another communication from Glasgow, addressed this time to the Presidents and Fellows of the Edinburgh Colleges. Although lengthier than its predecessors this communication contained not a hint of 'concession' on the one major outstanding point at issue—an Examining Board in Glasgow. The Edinburgh Colleges then sent a letter reviewing the situation for the information of their Fellows, and copies to the Glasgow President.[8]

Mutual Obduracy Persists

Negotiations ground slowly to a halt, to the regret certainly of Fellows of the Edinburgh College of Physicians and of some at least of the Fellows of the Faculty, if reading between the lines of correspondence can be relied upon. The first Minute on the subject was recorded in May 1848[13] and the concluding one in August 1849. On the last named date, after hearing Dr Christison review the activities of the Joint Committee over the months, the College unanimously resolved 'That the College approves of the view taken by the Committee and hereby declares the Committee for a junction between the Royal Colleges and the Glasgow Faculty to be at an end, and the proposals made by the Committee on the part of this College, to be finally and entirely withdrawn'.[8]

Without pretence of hindsight it is difficult to escape the impression that persistence with round-the-table conferences might have succeeded where resort to the interchange of correspondence failed.

Friendly Informal Frankness

A letter in the College files dated 6th February 1857 clearly indicates that despite the decision of the Joint Committee, closer association between the Glasgow Faculty and our College continued to be the subject of informal discussion. It was sent to Dr Seller, the then College Secretary, by Dr Watson of Glasgow, who with Dr Douglas Maclagan of Edinburgh was joint secretary of the Conference of the Medical and Surgical Corporations Scotch Department. Couched in the friendliest of terms the letter was an unofficial response to a request from Dr Seller about the admission of Faculty Members as non-resident Fellows of the College. Exception was taken to the College claim to entry money beyond a small sum to cover expenses; and the point made that 'we consider ourselves as entitled . . . to a literal ad eundem admission'. The claim was substantiated by the statement that the Faculty 'had some fair pretensions to being a College of Physicians themselves' with a Charter conferring 'power precisely the same as the only one your body has to this time'. Dr Watson expressed a desire to smooth down 'the asperities of our present position'; legitimately stated a change of name of the Edinburgh College to one 'of Scotland' could not in justice be made in the absence of previous *ad eundem* admission, with a small fee, of Fellows of the Faculty; and asked 'could the matter not be compromised by admitting all Fellows . . . prior to the passing of the Act'. From beginning to end, Dr Watson's arguments were actuated by 'every sentiment of respect for your College and sincere desire for the most friendly connection between our two bodies'.[14]

Surgeons as Conciliators

In terms more characteristic of Surgeons than of Physicians, the Reform Committee of the Royal College of Surgeons told of hopes indulged in of improved 'Medical Polity' having 'been entirely blasted'. Harmonious action of the Scottish Medical Bodies was described 'of the utmost consequence' and it was recommended that the Glasgow Faculty should be sounded concerning their 'sentiments' for joint action. Copies of the eventual official document were sent to our College and the University.

There followed a meeting of the Medical Reform Committee of the College of Physicians attended, by invitation, by the College of Surgeons' President (Professor Syme) and four other Fellows and Members of the Surgeons' Reform Committee. Professor Syme made a weighty, reasoned pronouncement. 'The former negotiations between the Royal Colleges of Physicians and Surgeons of Edinburgh and of the Faculty of Physicians and Surgeons of Glasgow having been finally broken off, these Bodies', he argued, 'were at liberty to entertain any new proposals'. Because of this, he informed the Physicians' Reform Committee, the College of Surgeons had been in touch with the Faculty with the immediate object of forming a conjoint examining and licensing Board and with the ultimate aim of removing 'the restrictions under which Gentlemen, licensed in Scotland, at present labour in England'. Syme gave it as the view of the Surgeons' Reform Committee that the College of Physicians should be willing to conform 'to the agreement entered into in 1842 by the Representatives of the three bodies'. The College Minutes contain no record of this agreement. At the conclusion of the meeting the Physicians rightly refused to commit themselves and insisted on obtaining instructions from their Council. Council in their turn demanded information about details which when received were regarded as satisfactory. It is interesting to note that on this occasion when negotiating with Edinburgh Surgeons only, the Faculty suggested that students should 'have free choice of being examined in either City'. Still only peripherally involved, the Edinburgh Physicians' Reform Committee were authorized 'to carry out the negotiations . . . with full power to petition Parliament in favour of the Bill' before the House.[15]

CO-OPERATION REVIVED: THE DOUBLE QUALIFICATION

Time proved to be a slow, partial healer. In June 1859 the College received the Report of their Committee which had been discussing with a Committee of the Royal College of Surgeons of Edinburgh the possibility of 'an Union for Examination between the Colleges'. Initially the Surgeons submitted 'a series of propositions' upon which the Physicians wrote observations. 'A conference then took place at which the utmost harmony prevailed', as the well-nigh unique account in the Minute Book bears witness. General approval was given to the Report, but the Committee responsible was instructed to suggest to the Surgeons' Committee that the Colleges might confer with the University to see whether a Joint Board of Examination could be instituted for giving a Triple Qualification.[16] As the Surgeons had already had a meeting with a Committee of Professors of the University, it was decided that the

Physicians should go to the proposed meeting alone. No success attended the meeting[17]; the arrangements already provisionally agreed with the Surgeons were proceeded with; and in July Regulations for giving a Double Qualification along with the Royal College of Surgeons by a single examination were drawn up for the approval of the General Council of Medical Education (Chap. XIV).

At the same Extraordinary Meeting as that at which the Regulations were approved by Fellows, the College was given a verbal Report of a Conference held the previous day between the Committee of the College and delegates of the Glasgow Faculty.[18] At the conference the basis and principles of the arrangements agreed between the Colleges for a double qualification were explained and this was followed by a Statement of the Glasgow position with regard to a 'proposed Union with the Royal College of Physicians . . . to meet the recent enactments of the Army and other Boards'. The Faculty made certain stipulations of which the following were three:

(1) Applicants to the Faculty for Licence were to be examined in Glasgow. Examiners were to be appointed in equal numbers by the College and the Faculty—those appointed by the College to examine in Medicine and those by the Faculty in Surgery. (2) Successful candidates should be given a diploma from each Body. And finally (3) of particular interest in the light of experience a decade previously, 'The Union of the Edinburgh College and the Faculty of Glasgow shall neither prejudice nor interfere with any legal rights or privileges of either of the contracting parties . . .'.[18]

'Union': Whisperings

On this occasion the term 'Union' was employed in a greatly restricted sense as compared with previous years, and the Faculty was obviously still acutely concerned to protect their privileges from infringement. Those attending the conference had no authority to commit their Councils, but they did agree that 'so long as the Faculty of Physicians and Surgeons of Glasgow remain a separate Corporation so as to require for its examinations under the new Medical Act the admission of Examiners appointed by the Royal College of Physicians of Edinburgh (or Scotland) it shall be understood that the Royal College . . . prefer for that office those of its Fellows who are resident in Glasgow, and farther—That Fellows of the Glasgow Faculty . . . receiving Degrees in Medicine and being otherwise eligible . . . shall be admitted by the College . . . as non Resident Fellows on the Nomination of the Council of the Glasgow Faculty or on the nomination of the Faculty itself . . .'. The College, with certain minor reservations, approved 'the Report . . . with the interpretation of the

Delegates' and remitted it to the Committee with powers to arrange the details on the same basis as that arranged 'with the College of Surgeons of Edinburgh'.[18]

Early in August, Fellows were informed that 'the Co-operation of this College and the Royal College of Surgeons of Edinburgh and the Faculty . . . of Glasgow for the purpose of granting a double Qualification in Medicine and Surgery . . . had received the sanction of the General Medical Council'.[19] Later in the same month a meeting took place of representatives of the two Colleges and the Faculty. Details of arrangements were agreed and subsequently approved by the Councils of the three Corporations who in due course drew up 'an Advertisement announcing the Commencement of the system of the Conjoint Examination'.[20]

TOWARDS A DEFENSIVE ENTENTE CORDIALE

In 1887 a sudden flutter in the dovecots of the Scottish Corporations took place when it became known that the English Medical Colleges were seeking powers to confer degrees in medicine and surgery on their Licentiates and Members. In modern parlance, the 'doves' became 'hawks'. The first intimation to the Edinburgh College took the form of a letter from the Delegates of the Scottish Medical Corporations addressed to the Fellows of those Corporations, accompanied by a proposed petition to the Queen in Council. From the tone of the Minute it is obvious that the Council of the College took exception to the irregular method of approach and the delegates' 'report' was referred *simpliciter* to the College. Discussion revealed considerable difference of opinion as to what line of action should be adopted, but eventually it was decided that a Memorial should be submitted to the Queen in Council, and a Committee was appointed to prepare the Memorial.[21]

A few days later another Extraordinary Meeting was called at which Council showed a readiness to descend from its pedestal of high dudgeon. It was revealed that a request for a conference had been made 'by an informal meeting of Representatives of the College invited to meet the delegates of the Royal College of Surgeons of Edinburgh and the Faculty of . . . Glasgow'. The Council felt unable to accede to the request and referred it to the College. In the interval however the position had been regularized by the receipt by the President (Dr R. P. Ritchie) of personal communications from the Presidents of the two other Scottish Corporations 'requesting that the College would meet these Bodies in conference'. In the changed circumstances the College were recommended to co-operate and this sequence of events, worthy of interdepartmental manoeuvring in Whitehall, concluded with the appointment of delegates. It was arranged that the conference should be held in the College's Hall and prior to the meeting those attending were provided with copies of the Memorial which it was intended to present to the Queen in Council and which had been amended since it was originally drafted.[22]

There was an element of confusion at this stage. The delegates did meet colleagues from the other two Corporations but the meeting evidently did not rank as a conference. Having been assured that the earlier attitude adopted by the Edinburgh College had not been 'a slight intended to them', the representatives of the Edinburgh Surgeons and Glasgow Faculty then repeated their request for a conference. This was agreed to, together with a decision to postpone consideration of the projected Memorial to the Queen in Council.[23] The meeting was held on 9th January when adoption of the Memorial as a Petition of the three Scottish Corporations was agreed. The Petition as finally determined incorporated an additional valuable clause suggested by the College of Surgeons and the Faculty.

'Your Petitioners', the Memorial declared, 'had no desire to take any step to disturb the existing arrangements whereby the Universities alone had the privilege of granting Degrees in Medicine, but in consequence of the action of the Royal College of Physicians of London and of the Royal College of Surgeons of England they have been constrained to apply for powers similar to those sought by these Royal Colleges'. In essence the three Corporations sought powers 'to unite and co-operate not only in conducting examinations for the purposes of the Medical Act, but also for the purpose of conferring Degrees in Medicine and Surgery . . .'. A proposal was submitted that a Senate of Physicians and Surgeons should be constituted. This Senate was to consist of the President and six other Fellows of each of the three Corporations; 'persons chosen by Graduates of the Senate when the number of such Graduates shall have attained to two hundred'; the Lord Provosts of Edinburgh and Glasgow; and the Chairmen of the School Boards of those two Cities. The new Body it was suggested should officiate 'under the name and style of "The Senate of Physicians and Surgeons of Scotland"'.[24]

Four months later the Secretary verbally reported to the College that the subject of the proposed Senate together with the proposed Albert University had been referred to a Royal Commission.[25]

SCOTTISH UNIVERSITIES COMMISSION: THE COLLEGE PREFERS INDEPENDENT ACTION

An account has been given in the previous chapter of the various representations made by the College to the Scottish Universities Commission (Chaps. XXII and

XXIII). The College had decided 'to go it alone'. Policy in this connection was determined after receipt of a Report by Council and a Committee appointed to consider Conjoint Qualification with the Council—a Report which dealt with the powers of the Conjoint Committee. The Report expressed the view that 'seeing that there is no probability of an increase being made to the number of Representatives of the College on the Conjoint Committee of Management, the Council and Committee of College . . . are of opinion that it would be best to represent to the College the inexpediency of discussing with Representatives of the other Corporations any proposition which might be calculated to extend the powers of the Conjoint Committee. They hold that important interests of the College should not be committed to a Body in which they can only command one-third of the votes.'[26]

Was this evidence of realism, or lack of faith? Perhaps those reporting were aware of Tacitus' account of the failure of the northern tribes to arrest Agricola's advance into the Highlands through inability to co-operate in defence.

1946. A NATIONAL COLLEGE: COLLEGE INITIATIVE AND FAILURE

The Charter intended by James VI for the Edinburgh physicians may well have contemplated a Royal College of Scotland; and such certainly was the intention of Cromwell. In the mid-nineteenth century a National College might well have materialized had Union of the Corporations not been prevented by the susceptibilities of competing local interests. The new Charter granted the College in 1861 provided an opportunity to assume the designation of Royal College of Physicians of Scotland (Chap. XV). Subsequent legislation gave assurance that the change involved no loss of privileges or rights and yet advantage was not taken of the opportunity. Thus on four occasions over a period of 180 years a Royal College of Physicians of Scotland was within the realms of possibility.

In 1946, eighty-five years later, the possibility momentarily came nearer being a probability. For the sake of completeness, however, it must be mentioned that in 1905 the College Council on being approached by the Secretary of the Glasgow Faculty regarding *ad eundem* admission of Fellows of the Faculty to Membership of the College, declared themselves opposed to the suggestion and unable 'to take part in a conference between the Faculty and the Colleges'.[27] At an Extraordinary Meeting of the College on 4th June 1946 (Sir) Stanley Davidson proposed a motion designed to give Council a mandate to explore the formation of a College of

Physicians of Scotland. The motion had been considered previously by Council who decided on its referral *simpliciter* to the College. In advising the College of this the President adopted an attitude of caution which was later to prove ominous. He gave a review of the historical background of the Scottish and English Corporations; quoted legal opinion to the effect that it was not now competent for the College to assume a designation refused by them at the time of the Medical Act of 1858; and elaborated on the geographical distribution of Fellows of the College—151 resident in Scotland, 79 in England and Wales, and 82 overseas.

According to Davidson, he was satisfied that any proposal to establish a National Royal College would have the widespread approval of physicians in Scotland. To his knowledge Fellows living in Glasgow, unable to attend the meeting owing to the short notice given, were very much in favour of the project and had asked to be kept informed. He gave as reasons for creation of such a Body the need for central authoritative representation of the consultants in Scotland; a greater supply of teachers and lecturers; and the enhancement of the College's prestige at home and abroad. With candour Davidson gave it as his view that 'the College as at present was not a representative body, but a local body . . . and the London Diploma was considered more useful than the Diploma of the Edinburgh College'; and that the disadvantage might be offset were there a National Body of Scotland. Seconding the motion (Sir) J. D. S. Cameron, drawing on his extensive experience abroad, allowed that he had 'considerable doubt as to the present status and prestige of the College overseas'. Those present consisted of the President (Dr D. M. Lyon) and 44 Fellows, and ensuing discussion was considerable and conflicting. It is reasonable to say that broadly speaking youth and age were in opposition. Those who considered that no change was called for were in the main among senior Fellows present, whereas those most concerned to invigorate College activities, while recognizing that the formation of a National Corporation would entail sacrifice, were mostly junior Fellows. The original motion had been 'That the Council be authorised to examine the project and consider whether a Royal College of Physicians of Scotland be practicable and desirable'. With the approval of the mover, and by a majority of 45 to 1, the meeting finally approved an amendment—'That the President be authorised to appoint a Committee to examine the project . . .'. A Committee was forthwith nominated and consisted of six Fellows additional to the President, the Council, the Treasurer and the Secretary.[28] Six months later discussion on the future of the College took place but does not appear to have given rise to any constructive conclusions.[29]

Meanwhile the Committee had held a meeting several months previously.[30] An Extraordinary Meeting was eventually called in April 1947.[31] According to the

President the Committee appointed by him had been unable to agree on a Report. Confronted with this situation he explained that he had 'taken upon himself the responsibility of preparing the Memorandum' which had been sent out with the billet calling the Meeting. He emphasized that his Memorandum was not for discussion but contained 'all the available information which he thought the Fellows should have before them' including the different views expressed to the Committee.

Objectives of Proposal

(Sir) Stanley Davidson thereupon introduced his motions by explaining there would be three—the first a general outline of the main objective, the second a broad indication of the plan to attain the objective, and the third a proposal to appoint a suitable executive committee. Dealing with the first motion Davidson referred to the probable functions of a National College as educational, medico-political and social. He saw educational activities as concerned with examinations, ensuring high standards in connection with Diplomas, the development of postgraduate work and the extension of clinical conferences already in demand. Concluding his supporting argument, he stated 'that the idea of a National College was supported by leading Physicians throughout Scotland'; referred 'to a Meeting of the Faculty in Glasgow at which a motion was passed on 28th January 1947 agreeing that such a College was desirable'; and indicated that 'he believed the President had received a letter . . . on behalf of the Physicians in Aberdeen and a letter written on behalf of the Physicians in Dundee both agreeing that the foundation of a National College was desirable'. Because he considered the Physicians in the East of Scotland should express their views, he moved:

> 'That in the interests of Scottish Medicine a National College of Physicians is desirable.'[31]

Administrative Attractions

Seconding the motion Dr Gilchrist focussed attention on the mutual advantages to teaching hospitals and the College; while Sir Andrew Davidson (C.M.O. Scotland) saw great benefits in the proposal which would simplify negotiating machinery between Government Departments and consultants, particularly where National Health Service planning was involved. By way of contrast and in a way reminiscent of the nineteenth-century negotiations with the Glasgow Faculty, one Senior Fellow and member of the special Committee delivered himself of the opinion that 'he regarded the College as already the National College of Scotland . . . [and] the existing College was quite capable of fulfilling the functions of a National College'. Interspersed were some unwarranted references to the Glasgow Faculty which drew an immediate and deservedly condemnatory riposte from a physician who was a Fellow of both the Edinburgh College and Glasgow Faculty. He made it abundantly clear that those in the West did not regard the College as national in any sense of the word, nor did they consider it capable of fulfilling that function. Another in the ranks of the conservative senior Fellows was unable to see how a National College would simplify negotiating machinery with the Home and Health Department, and predicted indifferent attendance by any Members of Council from as far afield as Aberdeen and Dundee. However when it came to voting by card, the motion was carried by 56 votes for, to 22 against.

(Sir) Stanley Davidson then introduced his second motion, which he went out of his way to underline was concerned with general principles and not details which would require negotiation. His motion was to the effect that:

> 'The College believes that this objective can be most effectively achieved by the Royal College of Physicians of Edinburgh obtaining a new Charter which *inter alia* authorises the College to change its name to the Royal College of Physicians in Scotland.'[31]

Dr Gilchrist seconded and in doing so reminded the College that the traditions and Library would remain inviolate. He was supported by (Sir) Derrick Dunlop who discouraged comparison with the London College whose authority was unchallenged by any other College in England; and who emphasized the manifest need for closer co-operation between the Teaching Schools in Scotland.

'Alienation of Property': a Stumbling Block

At this juncture a Fellow intervened in his capacity of Trustee for the College to stress that Chapter XIV of the Laws of the College had been specifically designed to prevent precipitate action in regard to College property; and to ask the President for a ruling as to whether the motion before the Fellows should not be dealt with under Chapter XIV paragraph 1 of the Laws. Having read out the Law in question, the President gave it as his ruling that the Motion before the Fellows was one which tended to alienate the property of the College and that, therefore, it would require to be passed by a three-fourths majority of those voting. There were not lacking those who challenged the ruling, but to them the President replied that he had already taken Counsel's opinion on the particular point. Of Fellows present many were dumbfounded. The reaction was aggravated by the fact that there had been no mention of this in the Memorandum circulated to Fellows by the President prior to the meeting, which had commenced in a spirit of free open discussion. Action from the Chair had savoured of a guillotine motion, but a guillotine motion without the customary forewarning.

Discussion was keen and prolonged. Those opposing the motion took the line that 'the College had been undersold' and that the strength of the College lay in its individual Fellows. A leading antagonist, commenting on the impartiality shewn by the Chairman at meetings of the Committee and College, asked that the President should state his views. Maintaining that his Memorandum had been presented without bias, the President considered that no concrete scheme had been 'set forth' and he 'could see nothing in favour of the change of name'. Before voting took place, one Fellow submitted a plea that the matter was urgent in that it affected not only the College but the survival of Scottish medicine as an independent body. Replying to the discussion (Sir) Stanley Davidson suggested that the question before the Fellows was whether they were to remain a local College and, if they did not wish a national College and preferred to remain a local College, then Fellows should vote against the motion.

Voting was by card: the result—42 for the motion; 28 against. In announcing the result the President declared that the motion was not carried, there not being a three-fourths majority of those voting. With the permission of the Chair, (Sir) Stanley Davidson withdrew his third motion. The meeting then terminated.[31]

The Minutes of the meeting are frigidly factual. There is no suggestion of a revival of Gregorian vitriolism or a return to the blasphemies of Pitcairne. Nor is anything recorded which is likely at some future date to prompt recourse to the age-old expediency measure of erasing Minutes under an Act of Oblivion. None the less it is known that feelings ran high at the meeting and unsavoury memories were nursed by many for a long time. The many included representatives from not one but from all four Scottish cities. No one could envy the President in the position in which he found himself. On him rested the onus of interpretation and execution of existing Laws. It was his misfortune that in carrying out his Presidential duties it should fall to his lot to function in the role of executioner. Whether efficient or inefficient and whether willing or unwilling, an executioner cannot escape incurring a measure of odium.

INFORMAL INTER-CITY CONTACTS

No mention appears in the records of the many exploratory discussions and visits undertaken in Glasgow, Aberdeen and Dundee. From the Edinburgh point of view, (Sir) Stanley Davidson was the irrepressible advocate on these occasions of a College of Physicians of Scotland but he was always careful to visit in company with a colleague or colleagues known to be luke-warm in their attitude. A not infrequent topic of conversation on the many inter-city railway journeys was the possible creation of a Scottish Academy of Medicine. According to a participant, enthusiasm had invariably evaporated before arrival at the journey's destination. Those with personal recollections of these contacts do not disguise the fact that a certain air of supercilious superiority, akin to that one hundred years previously, prevailed among the unenthusiastic Edinburgh representatives. To these last, the College of Edinburgh was as inviolable as the castle dominating the sky-line of the City bearing the same name. This fostered doubts and suspicions, even antagonism, in the course of several unrecorded informal meetings to the ultimate detriment of the project for a National College.

Two months after the rejection of (Sir) Stanley Davidson's motion the College were invited (June 1947) to send a deputation to the sister College of Surgeons to take part in a preliminary discussion of a committee report on the desirability or otherwise of establishing a Royal College of Surgeons of Scotland. The Committee had been appointed in October 1946 by the Surgeons on receipt of a letter from an informal group of Physicians and Surgeons drawn from Edinburgh, Glasgow, Aberdeen and Dundee. Among the signatories were Drs D. M. Dunlop (later Sir) and W. D. Small of our College. The others were Professor (Sir) David Campbell (Aberdeen); Professor Geoffrey Fleming and Mr Roy Young, both of Glasgow; and Professors Alexander (Surgery) and Patrick (Medicine) of Dundee. They contended that it was of the utmost importance that steps should be taken to 'increase the prestige of the Scottish Fellowship; to ensure more uniform and higher standard of examination . . . and to create a body which could act on behalf of the consultants in Scotland in negotiations with the Secretary of State'.[32]

An exactly similar letter had been sent to the Royal College of Physicians. Receipt of it is acknowledged in the Council Minutes of 11th June 1946, and it is recorded that the Secretary was instructed to reply that 'the matter was already being considered'. Whether intentionally or not, the nature of the reply was something of an affront having regard to the professional status of the signatories to the letter. Nor is there any evidence that the contents of the letter were at any time conveyed by Council to the College. It is difficult not to link the inactivity of the Council in this matter with the obstructive attitude evident on previous occasions. More precisely the letter had asked for consideration of the possibility of setting up a Royal College of Physicians and Surgeons of Scotland or alternatively two Royal Colleges of Scotland—one of Physicians and the other of Surgeons.

Reverting to the invitation to the College in June 1947, (Sir) Stanley Davidson was called upon to propose a motion. The motion eventually agreed, ran 'That the College having approved that in the interests of Scottish Medicine a National College of Physicians is desirable, requests the President and Council to take the necessary steps in consultation with the Royal Faculty of Physicians and Surgeons of Glasgow, and the leading physicians of Aberdeen and Dundee to set up a joint Committee to investigate the practicability of such a scheme and thereafter to report back to the College before further Action is taken'.[33] Seconding the motion Dr Gilchrist made a plea for the motion to be carried unanimously.

Committee Procedures Criticized

At the next Quarterly Meeting the President on being asked what action had been taken, informed the College that in preparation for an agreed meeting with the Surgical College he had nominated as representatives three Fellows to attend together with himself. His attention was drawn to the absence of (Sir) Stanley Davidson's name from those nominated. At the instigation of Dr McNeil, a man of dour integrity characteristically expressed with tightly pursed lips, Standing Orders were suspended to consider the inclusion of Stanley Davidson among representatives and to enable the President 'to obtain at once the opinion of the Fellows present regarding the composition of the Joint Committee before making his own final decision'. On the motion being put to the vote 28 voted in favour, and 16 against: 12 Fellows abstained from voting. The motion was declared to be lost by the President (Dr D. M. Lyon) as, to be carried, it should have had the support of three-fourths of those voting.[34]

Towards the end of the year (1947) the results of a meeting of the representatives of the three Scottish Medical Corporations were reported to the College. It had been agreed that further information on financial and legal aspects should be obtained and that in due course each Corporation should exchange financial statements. The College was informed that their representatives had since decided to discuss the financial

x

statements with the Edinburgh Surgeons before again meeting the Glasgow Faculty representatives.[35]

FURTHER EFFORTS AT RESUSCITATION FRUSTRATED

In December 1947 a new President (Dr W. D. D. Small) of the College took office. About that time a joint meeting of the representatives of the two Edinburgh Colleges came to the conclusion after consideration of the financial statements that a scheme put forward on behalf of the Glasgow Faculty could not be put into effect. The Faculty was advised by the two Edinburgh Committees of that decision and the hope expressed that negotiations might continue. Discussion in the College of the account given them of their Committee's progress stimulated some highly critical contributions. One Fellow maintained that a lack of sense of urgency on the part of the Committee involved risk of 'the matter dying', and that the Committee would benefit from the addition of more active members. Pursuing the same line, another Fellow made the specific request that a report on the progress of the Committee should be made at the next Quarterly Meeting of the College. Replying to the discussion the President betrayed a sense of irritation. He stated in categoric terms that by the College Laws the appointment of Members to committees was a matter entirely for the President at his discretion; and warned that any attempt to influence the impartiality of the Chair would raise a constitutional problem of the first magnitude. In passing he declared that he had had in his possession for a considerable time the resignation of each member of the Committee for use at any time he might think fit, but he had requested all the members to continue to serve. The President took strong exception to the Committee being constantly harried in the College and declined to give any undertaking other than that a statement of progress would be made as and when there was anything to report.[36] That was in May 1948.

In July progress was reported in so far as proposals agreed by the Committees of the two Edinburgh Colleges were being considered by the Glasgow Faculty. A reference at the Quarterly Meeting in November was limited to a promise of further information after a review of the financial situation.[37] This was forthcoming in the following February in the form of a printed statement issued to Fellows in attendance. The gist of the statement was that a heavy financial obligation would be an inevitable accompaniment of the formation of any National College of Physicians.[38] Later the College of Surgeons confessed to anxiety over a marked decline in the number of examination candidates following the introduction of their Primary Examination; and regarded their financial situation as precluding the setting up of a National College 'at the present time'. Concurrently the Committees of all three Corporations were agreed in their opposition to any proposal that existing Charters should be surrendered because of the risk of privileges being lost.[39] There was a continuous interchange of correspondence between the three Committees but eventually the time arrived when it was realized by all that another meeting was essential in order 'to come to a definite decision as to the practicability of the Scheme'.[40]

Final Joint Meeting of Delegates

Delegates from the three Scottish Corporations met in Glasgow on 17th March 1950. At an interval after the meeting the President of the Glasgow Faculty wrote to the Chairman of the College Sub-Committee, and the following is an excerpt from the letter.

'At the last meeting . . . certain proposals were put forward by the Edinburgh representatives. No joint agreed Minute of that meeting is available but I think I am correct in stating that it was the desire of the Edinburgh representatives that the Faculty Hall, Library and Funds should not be regarded as any part of the new Colleges; that they should become, in effect, the private property of the Fellows of Faculty; and that, if this were agreed to, the Royal Colleges in Edinburgh would have placed before them the advice that negotiations for union should continue. It was felt by the Edinburgh representatives that, until this question was disposed of, there was little use in discussing in any serious manner the question of revision of Charters or of Regulations.

The matter was considered at two Faculty Council Meetings and was referred to the Faculty Meeting on 1st May 1950. A decision was made to refer the matter back to the Council for further negotiations with the opinion that, in terms of the Assumptions in your letter of 6th January 1949 the Faculty Buildings and Library should be maintained in some manner as a Western Branch of the two New Colleges. The following observations may be made on the reasons for this decision:

1. The age and local prestige of the Faculty.
2. The local duties that would require to be carried on.
3. The need for an official centre in the West in view of the number of consultants.

At the same time it was recognised that financial difficulties might arise and indeed other difficulties too, but it was thought that a way out could be found.

At a Council Meeting it was suggested that it might now be advantageous in view of divergent views to seek the advice of some high expert either in Law or affairs. Each Corporation could state to him its desires, difficulties and fears in the hope that he might suggest some arrangement agreeable to all parties. This is merely a suggestion and any views you may put forward can be considered.

> We feel here that the whole trend of events make it more and more desirable that Scottish Medicine and Surgery should soon be able to speak with one voice. The Triple Conjoint in the past and Diploma for the future show that agreement is possible.

> I shall be glad to hear what you now consider to be our next step.'[41]

The above letter was read to the College by the Chairman (Dr D. M. Lyon) of the College of Physicians Sub-Committee of the Joint Committee to consider proposals for a National College. He had been Chairman since the Sub-Committee had been originally nominated by himself in his then capacity of President. Having read the letter the Chairman stated that his Committee felt that further progress was improbable, finance being the main stumbling block, but if progress were to be made it 'might possibly be made by other means or by another Committee'. His Committee therefore reported 'It is with deep regret that the Committee, after prolonged negotiation, have formed the opinion that it is impracticable at present to form a National College of Physicians in Scotland. In these circumstances it is felt that the Committee can no longer serve any useful purpose and should be discharged.' Approval of the Sub-Committee's report was moved by a future President of the College who commented on the desire of the Faculty 'to retain their buildings and Library and to carry on in the same way as they had done in the past'. The motion having been passed the Committee was discharged.[41]

The above Minutes have been reproduced in detail because they reflect the differing outlooks and attitudes of East and West—attitudes which on such information as is available were surely not irreconcilable. An impartial observer must wonder that the last communication from the Glasgow Faculty Committee did not elicit a reply of willingness to co-operate. Certainly a number of Faculty Members were more than taken aback and while they may not have said so, felt affronted.

'. . . never the twain shall meet.' Is this to be the final verdict? It is earnestly to be hoped that such is not the case. A Standing Joint Committee of the three Royal Scottish Corporations was constituted in 1952[42]; an *ex officio* Committee, the representatives of our College are the President, the Vice-President and the Secretary. That the will to co-operate is not entirely lacking was evident at the time when the College required additional clinical facilities to deal with the peak demands of candidates for the Edinburgh Membership Examinations. In 1959 assistance was forthcoming from the Department of Medicine of St Andrews University and the Royal Infirmary, Dundee; and in 1960 arrangements were made whereby clinical examinations were conducted at the Western Infirmary, Stobhill and Yorkhill Hospitals, Glasgow.[43] Similar arrangements continued so long as the need persisted. Much more recently, informal suggestions by the Edinburgh College to the Glasgow College that jointly they might organize a Symposium in Aberdeen won favour. The Joint Standing Committee was not involved; initiative took place at College level and was translated into action without delay by Council. Without indulging in fastidious differentiation of such terms as unification, amalgamation and mergence the evidence points to an unsatisfied wish among many in East and West, and indeed North-east too, for closer, and still closer co-operation of effort.

A great deal rests with the Standing Joint Committee, in the meantime, to keep under constant review ways and means of furthering closer union in the interests of Scottish medicine. The need exists and will remain no matter the increasing closeness of relationships with the London College of Physicians. Disraeli has been credited with saying that London is not so much a City as a Nation. The viewpoint appeals to Government Departments and English Metropolitan Institutions, Guilds and Corporations but is not one favouring the realisation of all that a united Scottish medicine is capable of achieving.

In 1962 the Royal Faculty of Physicians and Surgeons of Glasgow assumed as a new name the Royal College of Physicians and Surgeons of Glasgow. Our Council had confidential advance information of the proposed change and indicated it had no objection. With rigid adherence to democratic protocol Council hastened to emphasize that the decision was that of Council and not the College.[44] No matter, there was a happy culmination with the presentation of an Illuminated Address to the new Royal College by our President (Sir James Cameron).[45]

REFERENCES

(1) KIPLING, R. (1964) The man who was. In his *Life's Handicap*, p. 99. London: Macmillan.

INTER-COLLEGIATE MANOEUVRINGS

(2) CRESWELL, C. H. (1926) *Royal College of Surgeons of Edinburgh. Historical Notes from 1505 to 1905*, p. 119. Edinburgh: Oliver & Boyd.
(3) College Minutes, 28.x.1817.
(4) Ibid., 2.viii.1842.

(5) [BROWN, W.] (1821) *Remarks on the Expediency and Practicability of a Union of the Royal Colleges of Physicians and Surgeons in Edinburgh.* Edinburgh: J. & C. Muirhead.

(6) [DEWAR, H.] (1821) *Observations on the Present Relative Situations of the Royal Colleges of Physicians and Surgeons of Edinburgh.* Edinburgh: Pillans.

(7) CRESWELL, C. H. Op. cit., p. 277.

UNION A DESIRABLE ADJUNCT TO MEDICAL REFORM

(8) College Minutes, 7.viii.1849.

(9) Ibid., 17.v.1848.

(10) Ibid., 26.v.1848.

(11) CRESWELL, C. H. Op. cit., p. 294.

RE-OPENING OF NEGOTIATIONS

(12) Council Minutes, 30.iv.1849.

(13) College Minutes, 17.v.1848.

(14) R.C.P.E. (1857) *General Correspondence,* 6.ii.1857.

(15) College Minutes, 16.iv.1850.

CO-OPERATION REVIVED

(16) Ibid., 24.vi.1859.

(17) Ibid., 12.vii.1859.

(18) Ibid., 26.vii.1859.

(19) Ibid., 19.viii.1859.

(20) Ibid., 30.viii.1859.

TOWARDS A DEFENSIVE ENTENTE CORDIALE

(21) Ibid., 23.xii.1887.

(22) Ibid., 3.i.1888.

(23) Ibid., 9.i.1888.

(24) Ibid., 11.i.1888.

(25) Ibid., 1.v.1888.

SCOTTISH UNIVERSITIES COMMISSION

(26) Ibid., 4.ii.1890.

1946. A NATIONAL COLLEGE

(27) Council Minutes, 13.vi.1905.
(28) College Minutes, 4.vi.1946.
(29) Ibid., 5.xii.1946.
(30) Ibid., 16.vii.1946.
(31) Ibid., 15.iv.1947.

INFORMAL INTER-CITY CONTACTS

(32) Council Minutes, 11.vi.1946.
(33) College Minutes, 10.vi.1947.
(34) Ibid., 15.vii.1947.
(35) Ibid., 4.xi.1947.

FURTHER EFFORTS AT RESUSCITATION FRUSTRATED

(36) Ibid., 4.v.1948.
(37) Ibid., 2.xi.1948.
(38) Ibid., 1.ii.1949.
(39) Ibid., 19.vii.1949.
(40) Ibid., 7.ii.1950.
(41) Ibid., 18.vii.1950.
(42) Ibid., 5.ii.1952.
(43) R.C.P.E. (1959) *Report by the President* [A. R. Gilchrist] . . . *1958–59*, p. 5. Edinburgh: Royal College of Physicians.
(44) Council Minutes, 7.vi.1961.
(45) Ibid., 5.ix.1962.

Chapter XXV

PRECEDENCE: PRIDE OR PREJUDICE?

An two men ride of a horse, one must ride behind.
William Shakespeare (*Much Ado about Nothing*)

Precedent embalms a principle.
Attributed to William Scott, Lord Stowell

'In 1505 the Barber-Surgeons of Edinburgh were incorporated as a Traders-Guild. In 1681 the Royal College of Physicians was established by Royal Charter. Nearly a century later the Guild of Barber-Surgeons, in order to improve their position, and to acquire the same status as the Physicians, applied for and obtained, a Royal Charter as a Royal College of Surgeons. I am advised by eminent Counsel that holders of Charters take order according to the character of the Charters, and that, as a Royal Charter is of higher character than an incorporation as a Trades-Guild, the Royal College of Physicians having held a Charter for a hundred years longer than the other College, was entitled to precedence from the date of said Charter. This precedence has always been accorded . . .

Analogous positions exist in England and Ireland. The Barber-Surgeons of London received a Charter from Edward IV, in 1460 [sic]* but they did not obtain a Charter as a Royal College of Surgeons till 1800. Notwithstanding the greater antiquity of the Guild of Barber-Surgeons, Garter King-at-Arms has decided that the Royal College of Physicians takes precedence over the Royal College of Surgeons. In like manner in Ireland, the Barber-Surgeons of Dublin were incorporated by Queen Elizabeth, a Royal Charter being only granted in 1784. The Royal College of Physicians of Dublin was not incorporated till 1660, [sic]† nevertheless the latter College takes precedence.

I am further advised that in cases not laid down by Tables of Precedence, precedence is fixed by use and wont.'[1]

The above is taken from a letter written by (Sir) John Batty Tuke in January 1898 to the Private Secretary, the Scottish Office, Whitehall.[2] It was written by Tuke following his experience, when as President of the College he attended a ceremony

---

* Charter granted in 1462.
† Charter of Incorporation granted in 1667.

in London for the presentation to the Prince of Wales of loyal addresses on the occasion of the sixtieth anniversary of Queen Victoria's accession.

Some weeks previously the College Secretary, Dr (Sir) Robert Philip, had communicated with the Lord Chamberlain to inform him with diplomatic circumspection that at the ceremony in question 'there seemed to be a departure from accustomed order in giving precedence to the Royal College of Surgeons of Edinburgh over the Royal College of Physicians of Edinburgh', and to enquire with equal courtly caution 'if this departure was of accident or by instruction?' By way of reply Philip was referred to the Secretary of State for the Home Department who was said to be responsible for 'the position of the Societies' and to whom further communications should be addressed. Obediently Philip did as he had been bid only to be told that his letter had been forwarded to the Scottish Office in Whitehall to which all further communications should be sent. Four weeks after sending his first letter to the Lord Chamberlain, Philip received from the Scottish Office a brief but wholly noncommittal reply—'The order in which the several bodies were introduced on the occasion in question does not establish any precedence'.[1]

There was no question of College officials taking petty umbrage, or of the President seeing personal affront where none had been intended. Of this there is ample evidence in action taken by the next President, Sir Thomas Fraser, who a year or two later (1901), on learning of the form of precedence proposed for proclaiming Edward VII's accession to the throne at the Edinburgh Mercat Cross, lodged a strong protest with the Lord Lyon King of Arms 'on my own behalf and on behalf of the Fellows of the Royal College of Physicians'. Concern felt was for the historically acquired pre-eminence of the College, not for the dignity or status of officers or Fellows who are, when all is said and done, but as ships that pass in the night.

The Proclamation was on 25th January 1901. No matter how misguided the civic organizers may have been, early in March the College was in receipt of a gratifying communication from the Office of the Secretary for Scotland to the effect that '... precedence has been established in favour of the Royal College of Physicians'.[1] The date of the communication was of significance—13th March (1901). It provided implied assurance that when in a week's time representatives of the College travelled South to deliver the College's Address of Loyalty, precedence would be in keeping with the wishes of the College.

There must, however, have been something of the terrier in the College Treasurer of the day. He was not yet satisfied. At the Proclamation on 25th January he had an opportunity to speak to the Lord Lyon King of Arms who gave the impression that the offending pattern of precedence had been 'adopted on information supplied by

Officials of the Town Council'. Having wisely first got confirmation of this in writing, the Treasurer (whose duties in these days included those of Secretary) lost no time in seeking an explanation from the Town Clerk. Not surprisingly no satisfaction, and nothing committal was forthcoming from the municipal offices, but our persistent Treasurer did not miss the opportunity 'to point out that in State functions and in general practice the College of Physicians is accorded precedence over the College of Surgeons, and it would be most unfortunate if the Magistrates and Town Council should endeavour to place this College in an exceptional position in functions which take place in Edinburgh under the control of the Civic Authorities'. The Town Clerk cannot be grudged his terse riposte that the Proclamation was not a municipal event! Subsequent correspondence, although not inconsiderable, does not merit quotation. Certainly the College Treasurer gave the impression of rather 'flogging' his contentions, but he himself must have had a sense of accomplishment when to clinch an argument, he enclosed in a letter for the Town Clerk's benefit a copy of the Secretary for Scotland's communication dated 13th March 1901!

In his own way Sir Thomas Fraser apparently continued to press the case of the College in other spheres. A letter dated 9th April (1901) from a University official said 'in view of the decision of the Scottish Office which you have communicated to me I feel that I am bound to give the Royal College of Physicians the precedence over the Royal College of Surgeons, and I shall accordingly call the Physicians first at the Graduation Ceremonial . . . '.[1]

Whatever the expectations the hatchet was not buried. From time to time minor difficulties arose from problems of precedence without creating anything in the nature of a medico-political storm. On 3rd May 1910 the Treasurer reported to Council that on observing the order of marshalling of the Procession at the Accession of King George V the Royal College of Surgeons 'had been given precedence' over our College, he had gone to the Lyon Office only to be told that this had been 'purposely done'. The President was authorized to pursue the matter,[3] in the course of which he had an interview with Sir Thomas Barlow, President of the London College of Physicians[4] with what result is not recorded. Eventually on Council instructions, in May 1911 the Treasurer submitted a Council Report to College imtimating that a recent attempt had been made to reverse the proper order of precedence at State and Ceremonial occasions, and that 'certain proceedings were presently depending in Court'. Apparently despite the Secretary for Scotland's decision in 1901 'the Lyon King of Arms has shewn a disposition to favour the Surgeons . . . '.[5]

Various events had preceded presentation of the Report. A year previously the

Royal College of Surgeons had written to our College expressing satisfaction 'that the Precedence question which arose yesterday at the Proclamation should have passed off in such a friendly manner. At the same time it is the wish of this Council that this question which crops up again and again, should if possible be now settled once and for all.' The letter went on to suggest a joint appeal to arbitration by the two Colleges, mentioning the College of Heralds as one possible arbiter. The College of Physicians replied in a little over five weeks and while making abundantly clear that they saw 'no great advantage' in a discussion, showed readiness to meet. Enclosed with the College reply was a copy of what was becoming an oft-used trump card—a copy of the Secretary for Scotland's letter of 13th March 1901. Correspondence continued in a perfunctory manner and each College consulted Counsel of their own choice. The distinctly opposed views of the Counsels in question cast doubts upon the likely effectiveness of arbitration. Nevertheless the matter was raised again by the College of Surgeons in a letter dated 9th January 1911, in which the desirability of 'a friendly application [to] be made . . . jointly' for a decision was stressed. Otherwise the Surgeons considered they had no option but to present a Petition.[1]

After a meeting of Council and Past Presidents the College of Physicians countered with a reply on 6th February (1911) saying:

> 'We are advised, as it appears your College has been likewise, that precedence depends on the will of the Sovereign. It is therefore the intention of our Council to present to His Majesty a humble Petition praying him to confirm us in the position which we believe we rightly occupy.'[1]

True to their word, the Physicians transmitted a Petition to the King within a matter of days asking that an appropriate directive be issued to the Lord Lyon King of Arms. Not to be outdone, two days later the Surgeons petitioned the Lord Lyon King of Arms for a declaration that they were entitled to precedency. Still not satisfied, the Surgeons then proceeded to petition the King 'craving' him to 'supersede consideration of the petition' of the Royal College of Physicians 'until the Lyon King of Arms had determined the question between the two Colleges'.[1] Were it not that the King is above the Law, the approach certainly had a hint of peaceful picketing about it! In the event, the following Order was issued by the Lord Lyon King of Arms:

> 'Edinburgh 9th March 1911. The Lord Lyon King of Arms, acting on instructions of the Secretary for Scotland, declines jurisdiction in this cause.'

Not prepared to accept the decision, the Surgeons' College appealed to the First Division of the Court of Session. There the Lord President pronounced:

> 'This is either a question of law or it is not. If it is a question of law in the Lyon's Department, then the Lyon is bound to judge of it, and we are over him to put him right if he has gone wrong. If it is not a question of law in that sense none of us have got anything to do with it . . . I think it would be a very heavy onus on those who try to show it that a question of precedence is a question of Law.'

On the 12th of April (1911) the Lord Lyon reversed his previous attitude and decided that he had jurisdiction. Now it was the turn of the College of Physicians to appeal, and in June the Treasurer was able to report to the College that the 'First Division of the Court of Session had . . . unanimously sustained the appeal . . . against the Interlocutor of the Lyon King of Arms, and decided that Lyon King had no jurisdiction to deal with the question of precedence'.[6] The following is taken from the official records of the Court:

> 'Edinburgh, 20th June 1911. The Lords having considered the Appeal, Record and whole proceedings and heard Counsel for the parties, Sustain the Appeal, Recal the Interlocutor of the Lord Lyon King of Arms, dated 12th April, 1911; Find that he has no jurisdiction therefor; Dismiss the Petition and decern.
>
> Sgd. Dunedin J.P.D.'[1]

Complete clarification however had not yet been achieved. During the time that the court case had been proceeding the Secretary for Scotland had asked for the observations of the College of Surgeons on the Petition submitted to the King by the College of Physicians. There later followed a request from the same official for the College of Physicians' observations on those already made by the College of Surgeons in connection with the Petition! The College of Physicians' reply to the Secretary for Scotland had of necessity to follow customary stereotyped lines—until the concluding contention, viz.:

> 'In the King as the Fountain of Honour there resides the exclusive prerogative to deal with questions of precedence, and they [the Petitioners] deny the right of the Lyon King to exercise any jurisdiction in such matters.'[1]

It is difficult indeed to link this fiery declaration with the customarily quiet, dignified deportment of the signatory W. Allan Jamieson.

In September the London Solicitors of the College received the following letter from Sir James Dodds of the Scottish Office:

'Gentlemen.

With reference to previous correspondence, I am directed by the Secretary for Scotland to inform you that the Petition of the Royal College of Physicians of Edinburgh dated the 8th February 1911 has been laid before the King and that His Majesty has not seen fit to comply with the prayer thereof for the issue to the Lyon King of Arms of a Warrant defining the relative precedence of the two Colleges of the Physicians and the Surgeons of Edinburgh,—no sufficient reason having been shown for disturbing the decision intimated by the Secretary for Scotland in 1901, namely that on the occasion of both Colleges appearing to present addresses to the Sovereign, precedence should be accorded to the Royal College of Physicians.'[1]

A classic example of civil service expertise!—it is almost possible to hear the sigh of contented diplomatic achievement as the draughtsman laid down his pen! Fortunately the expertise on this occasion did not cloud the main issue. For the College there was additional satisfaction when a subsequent letter from the Scottish Office intimated that 'His Majesty's Commands . . . have been duly notified to the Lyon King of Arms'.

Understandably the College required the Clerk to compile a complete record of all the circumstances leading up to 'the favourable decision of His Majesty' and 'to ensure that on completion the record is included among Minutes'.[1]

Almost incredibly the subject surfaced again at the time of the Accession of King Edward VIII. Once again the Physicians followed in the wake of the Surgeons in the procession.[7] Verbal remonstrance having proved ineffective a letter of protest was sent to the Lord Lyon King of Arms.[8] There was to be early evidence of a satisfactory outcome. At the proclamation of H.M. King George VI at the Mercat Cross the order of procession as between Physicians and Surgeons was reversed. In the imprecise words of the Clerk to the College 'he had received no complaints'![9] Almost a hundred years had elapsed since as President Dr Pulteney Alison first 'stated to the Lord Provost the propriety of the . . . College . . . being represented' at Royal proclamations.[10]

The whole subject of precedence seems incongruous in the context of late twentieth-century existence. It is difficult to appreciate that the account given relates to events in the late nineteenth and early twentieth centuries, and not wholly to 1681.

The Edinburgh Colleges were not alone in the importance which they, or perhaps more correctly which a few within their ranks, attached to precedence. In 1889 the President of the Royal College of Physicians of London gave it as his opinion that the order of precedence of the Presidents of the two London Royal Colleges and of the General Medical Council required authoritative determination. His reasons were not clearly enunciated. Suffice to say that at different times the subject was raised with the

Garter King of Arms and the Lord President of the Privy Council without apparent result, because indirect reference was again made to the question by the President of the Physicians' College some ten years later.[11] Precedence, however, no matter the mistaken impression it may give in some quarters, retains its place in modern society. It is not a figment of the imagination of medical Corporations.

Fortunately there is a humorous side to it all. The same primeval influence which ordains where and when the new boy at school shall hang his cap or deposit his shoes, determines the grade of desk or carpet allotted to the senior and rising administrator in Whitehall. Nor are local authorities lacking in deference to precedence. Edinburgh knew not a little concern when on the occasion of the marriage of the Prince of Wales in 1863 the Corporation of Dublin was given precedence over the Corporation of Edinburgh at the time of official congratulations being tendered by the Capital Cities at Windsor Castle.[12]

Nor is it wholly irrelevant to mention a fact to which Sir Batty Tuke did not refer in his letter of 1898. Very early in the eighteenth century a Petition was submitted to the 'Right Honourable the Estates of Parliament' on behalf of 'The Lord Provost, Baillies, Town Council of Edinburgh for themselves and their Community, and all the Lieges that may be concerned'. 'The Physicians own Patent is but late in the year 1681', the Petition declared, 'and contains a due reserve in favours of Chirurgion Apothecaries; ... within the Burgh of Edinburgh [they] are generally the best bred, by their service at Home, and Industry and Travels Abroad, for the knowledge of the Nature and Cur of all Diseases, of any sort of People in the Kingdom'.[13]

In 1714 Alexander Pope wrote 'None judge so wrong as these who think amiss'.[14] Unknowingly appropriate and timeous!

REFERENCES

(1) College Minutes, 6.ii.1912.
(2) R.C.P.E. (1898–1900) *Miscellaneous Papers*, no. 391.
(3) Council Minutes, 3.v.1910.
(4) Ibid., 16.i.1911.
(5) College Minutes, 2.v.1911.
(6) Ibid., 27.vi.1911.
(7) Council Minutes, 22.i.1936.
(8) Ibid., 27.i.1936.
(9) Ibid., 30.xii.1936.
(10) College Minutes, 29.vi.1837.

(11) COOKE, A. M. (1972) *A History of the Royal College of Physicians of London*, vol. 3, pp. 897–9. Oxford: Clarendon.

(12) EDINBURGH. City corporation (1929) *Edinburgh, 1329–1929*. [Sexcentenary], pp. 131 f. Edinburgh: Oliver & Boyd.

(13) [ECCLES, W.] (1707) *An historical account of the rights and priviledges of the Royal College of Physicians, and of the Incorporation of Chirurgions in Edinburgh*, p. 55. [Edinburgh: Privately printed.]

(14) POPE, A. The wife of Bath. In *The Rape of the Lock, and Other Poems*, ed. by G. Tillotson (1954) 2nd Edition (rev). London: Methuen.

Chapter XXVI

DISCIPLINARY LAWS:
APPLICATION THROUGH THE CENTURIES

> *... let us remember that the Professions of Law and Medicine have stood with rock-like firmness against all subversive influences. Let us then hold fast to those principles of conduct enunciated by our forefathers, which were their stay and staff throughout the centuries, and pass on undimmed to our successors the torch of knowledge and the ideals bequeathed to us by them.*
>
> Sir Sydney Smith (Promotor's Address: University of Edinburgh, 15th July 1953)

Discipline in a corporate sense is of two kinds—internal and external. The Charter of 1681 took account of both, by conferring on the College powers to enact Laws for their 'own government and welfare' and for the regulation of the practice of Medicine within the City of Edinburgh and Leith, their Suburbs and Liberties (Charter 1681. Appendix A). The very first two Meetings of the College on 7th and 8th December 1681 were devoted to the election of Office-Bearers. On 9th December the time was occupied in drafting Laws for the College. Three was decided upon as the number necessary to constitute a quorum, a decision which has stood the test of time and obtains to this day in so far as the Council is concerned. It was enacted also that any and every new Law before being passed had to be considered at two separate Meetings of the College; and that any and every proposal to abrogate a Law had to be considered at three several meetings of the College before arrival at a decision. This requirement, together with one determined on the same day that proposals being brought before the College shall first have been considered by Council, have also continued in force to the present time.[1]

Nor is it inappropriate to mention again the system of fines to which Fellows were subject for minor offences (Chap. VIII).

PROMISSORY OBLIGATION

The conception of a Promissory Obligation was given birth to on 6th February 1682. There is recorded in the Minute for that day: 'The forme of Declaratione and promeis to be signed by every member of the Colledge Licentiat and Candidat read and to be furder Considered at next meeting'.[2] Actually the subject did not come up for consideration at the next two meetings but on 21st March 1682 it was minuted: 'A paper containing several articles appoynted to be insert in the Register and to be signed by every ffellow of the Colledge voited and approven except the ffyft article which is expunged'.[3] This in effect constituted the draft of the Promissory Obligation to be signed by Fellows on taking their seats. Many years later (1805) loss of the original Obligation was reported to the College who authorized the drafting of a new one.[4] There was little of fundamental significance to differentiate new from old as evidenced by a comparison with the form at present in use and that given by Dr William Eccles in a monograph written in 1707 while he was President of the College.[5] The following is the version given by Dr Eccles:

'To evince to the Reader, That all the Members of the College of Physicians, are bound to defend its Rights and Priviledges, I have adjected the Formula that is subscribed by each Member at his admission, together with their Subscriptions; by which it will appear that they cannot abandon its Defence, without forfeiting any pretence they may have, of being reputed Honest Men and good Christians.

The Promissorie Declaration Subscribed by every Member of the College at his Admission.

I   One of the Fellows of the Royal College of Physicians at Edinburgh do by subscribing these Presents solemnly Declare and sincerely Promise.

1mo. That I shall all my Life according to my power preserve and maintain the Priviledges, Liberty, Jurisdiction and Authority granted to the said College by his Sacred Majesties Patent, for the good and necessary Uses and Ends therein contained.

2do. That I will lay hold on all occasions to promove the Wellfare and Flourishing of the said College, and always give my Vote when it is asked as I think may most conduce thereto.

3to. That I shall as much as I can Advance and Preserve Unity, Amity and Good Order amongst all the Fellows, Candidats and Licentiats thereof, and shall heartily Wish and Endeavour the Prosperity of them all while they continue faithful to the College.

4to. That during my being a Fellow of the College, I shall be always subject to the due Order and Government thereof, according to the foresaid Patent.

5nto. That I shall never divulge any thing that is acted or spoken, in any Meeting of the said College or Council and Court thereof, that I think may tend to the the Prejudice or Defamation of the same, or any Member thereof.

All the foresaid Articles I shall keep, and never wittingly and willingly break any one of them, as I desire to be holden and repute an honest Man and a good Christian. Sic Subscribitur;

Thomas Burnet	Abernethy	Ja. Forrest
Arch. Stevenson	Tho. Spence	Gilb. Rule
An. Balfour	Will. Eccles	Will. Gardyne
Rob. Sibbald	Rob. Hay	J. Riddel
Robert Trotter	Will. Douglas	John Sinclair
Ja. Steuart	Charles Oliphant	Jo. Hay
Will. Stevenson	An. Melvill	Jo. Monro
Jo. Mackgill	Tho. Dalrymple	Jo. Drummond
Will. Wright	J. Robertson	Ja. Lutfutt
J. Leirmont	Da. Dickson	Will. Leirmont
Will. Lauder	George Hepburn	Will. Steuart
Rob. Crawford	Geo. Stirling	Ch. Preston
Matth. Sinclair	Jo. Smellum	Geo. Mackenzie
Pet. Kello	Rob. Carmichael	Fr. Pringle
Alex. Cranstoun	Dav. Mitchel	Da. Cockburn
Ja. Halket	Will. Blackadder	Da. Gregory
Jo. Hutton	Ed. Eizat	Will. Alexander
Arch. Pitcairn	Adam Freer	Ja. Broun
Pat. Haliburtoun	Alex. Dundas	Pat. Sinclair

The new Promissory Obligation was produced at the Quarterly Meeting on 4th February 1806, when it was signed by all present and later laid on the Table 'to be subscribed by such of the Fellows of the College as were not present'.[6]

In his *Abstracts of the Minutes*, Paterson expressed the opinion that it was not possible to say 'whether the terms of the engagement' were 'those originally imposed at the commencement of the College'. At the same time he was certain they had 'undergone only a few verbal alterations since the first edition of the Laws'. He then deals with a subsequent specific change—'the omission of the words "a good Christian"'. In Paterson's opinion the change may not have been made 'by competent authority' and was dated 'at least as far back as 1805'.[7]

SEPARATION OF PHYSICIANS AND SURGEONS

Another declaration of obligation was required of members of the College in 1707 with the object of securing more effectual separation between physicians and surgeons.[8] Recommendation of the new requirement was based on events of over twenty years previously when in 1684 following the Court of Session decision 'Devydeing the calling of Chirurgery and Pharmacy' the College had 'unanimously agried' and registered their agreement by a signed vote.[9] In 1707 differences between the physicians and surgeons had again assumed critical proportions—hence the new and special declaration.[10] The new Law now enacted ordained that it should be signed by all Fellows.[11] Although subsequent references to the Act are sporadic, it can be accepted that admission as a Fellow entailed signing a declaration in conformity with the Act until 1756. In that year the practice was discontinued without, however, any reference to the fact in the Minutes,[12] although in 1750 it had been ordained that Membership of a Corporation of Surgeons or Apothecaries debarred admission to the College as a Fellow.[13] Furthermore in 1763 it was decreed that any Licentiate or Fellow becoming a Member of the Corporation of Surgeons would forfeit his Licence or Fellowship. The month was November: maybe the ghost of Pitcairne was abroad.[14]

EXTERNAL DISCIPLINE

There was one instance in the 1850s of the College being the innocent victim of duplicity of extreme degree. The case concerned a 'Dr' Ryott about whom condemnatory, unsolicited information was sent to the College by a fellow practitioner of the name of Massey, not a Fellow of the College but none the less professedly intent on vindicating its good name. Correspondence between the College and Massey was exchanged over a number of years. The College was too dilatory for Massey who on more than one occasion threatened to resort to 'public exposé in the Medical Journals'. As events turned out Massey's accusation had sound basis. Ryott had claimed in writing to, and when examined by, the College that he was a graduate of Erlangen University. Massey for his part obtained an official letter from the Secretary of the Faculty of that University declaring that Ryott's Diploma had been 'cancelled and a new one refused'. The Secretary's statement terminated: '*He is therefore not a member of the University here.* Wherefore we wish to be relieved from further correspondence with regard to him.' Interestingly this action of the University followed receipt by them of information sent by a practitioner in the same town as Ryott. The College deprived Ryott of its Diploma, but whether he continued to practise in view of his claim to be the possessor of a 'Licence . . . from the Apothecary's Surgeons of England—and also the Diploma in Midwifery—from the Board of the London College', is unknown.[15]

With regard to authority to exercise external discipline the Charter empowered the College to summon before it and fine unlicensed practitioners practising within the jurisdiction of the College; and, in company with a magistrate and chemist, to examine medicines in apothecaries' shops and destroy any of unsatisfactory quality. Moreover, an apothecary had to satisfy the College that he had a competent knowledge of drugs before obtaining the magistrate's authority to open a shop. In addition the College under the terms of the Charter had authority to discipline any Physician, Doctor of Medicine, Licentiate or Fellow who violated any of the Laws of the College while practising within their jurisdiction.

The position of the doctor practising in the country was a special one. In his case a University degree was not obligatory as with those practising Medicine in Edinburgh or the suburbs. Although the College was in no position to enforce their licence in the country, they were ready to grant Licences after examination to the country practitioner. However should such a practitioner contemplate practising within the College's area of jurisdiction he had to be a graduate Doctor, and had to sit a new examination and obtain a new Licence.[16]

At best the supervision exercised by the College over apothecaries' shops was fitful, hesitant and largely ineffective with the result that in the course of time the College ceased to discharge its well intentioned but distasteful inspectorial function. Human nature ensured that personalities disturbed human relationships from time to time, but any hostility cannot have been too long-lived to judge by Cockburn's reminiscence of Dr William Cullen (Chap. XVII).

Adequate indication has already been given in Chapter VIII of the disciplinary exercises conducted by the College in the first hundred years of their existence when dealing with unlicensed practitioners, and with surgeons and druggists who in the opinion of the College were non-conforming. To some extent the College contributed to their own difficulties in dealing with some of the Fellows by their acrobatic vacillations of policy relating to the practice of lithotomy, minor surgery, midwifery and pharmacy (Chap. XIX). This was in the latter half of the eighteenth century. Confusion was worse confounded when in 1764 the College extended the application of their notorious Act of 1754 (Chap. XIX) to all Fellows residing in Great Britain and Ireland. As a result any Fellow practising pharmacy incurred the risk of being struck off the Roll of Fellows.[17] The position with regard to midwifery in the early nineteenth century is clearly evident in a letter dated 6th August 1832 sent by the President (Dr John Macwhirter) to the Clerk (Alexander Boswell). By way of explaining his inability to attend a meeting of Council, the President wrote: 'You must do me the favor to make my apology . . . as being bona fide attending a Lady in Labour which they [the College] will all agree cannot be avoided by me.'[18]

From time to time the College betrayed uncertainty to the point of uneasiness about their position in law when confronted with a disciplinary problem. Ritchie suggested that conflicting interpretations of the law accounted in part for the violent disagreements within the College which led to the suspension of (Sir) Archibald Stevensone, William Eccles, John Robertson, Charles Oliphant, Andrew Melville and John Smelholm—suspensions which were rescinded within a little over four years.[19] There is supporting evidence for this view in the Minutes for 25th September 1695. 'The same day', the Minute ran, 'appoynted Drs. Steivenson, Sibbald and Cranstoune or any two of them with the president to consider the laws and papers referring to the laws and the papers to be delyvered to the president that when they mett they may be written over and put in order and inventar made of them and that every member that hath any papers give them up to the president.'[20] Stevensone did not avail himself of the proferred olive branch.[19]

With the passage of time the College became less concerned with the 'pursuit' of those practising without licence within their juridical domain. For one thing, the number of those who attempted to flout the College's authority decreased notably. Another factor was that in 1829 the College ceased to issue Licences except in so far as they had to be given by the terms of the Charter to all University graduates without examination. A new feature complicated the picture in the nineteenth century. Elsewhere an indication has been given of the reaction south of the border to the increasing number of Scottish Licentiates seeking a livelihood in England (Chap. VII). There were always fingers on the alert to point to misdemeanours committed by the invaders. Moreover the misdemeanours acquired a new medico-political piquancy and the College was faced with the task of dealing with an increased number of disciplinary problems in a variety of circumstances.

THE COLLEGE IS UNEASY

Once again the adequacy of powers possessed by the College came up for review. In its Report submitted in September 1858 the College Committee on Medical Reform (Chap. XIV) gave as one necessary object in any new Charter 'to have the power of suspension and expulsion' of unworthy Members 'vested in the College beyond a doubt'.[21] It may well be that memories of James Gregory were not yet dormant. The new Charter sealed and registered on 31st October 1861, at the same time as authorizing the introduction of a new order of Members, gave power to the College with consent of three-fourths of those present to censure, suspend, or depose any Fellow, Member, or Licentiate of the College who has obtained admission by false pretences or violated any of the Bye-Laws.

POSITION VIS-À-VIS THE G.M.C.

In the years immediately following the passing of the *Medical Act* of 1858 and the granting to the College of a new Charter a somewhat nebulous situation obtained. Of cases coming up for disciplinary consideration by the College, some related to practitioners who had already been struck off the *Medical Register* and some who had not appeared before the General Medical Council. Machinery was set in motion in 1898 to clarify the position. A letter dated 30th November of that year was received by the President of the College from the General Medical Council. The letter stated that consideration had been given to 'the question of penal and disciplinary powers being obtained in order that in the cases of persons whose names had been erased from the Medical Register for a Criminal offence or for professional misconduct . . . these persons should be prevented from the use of any title, diploma or degree so long as the erasure remains in force'.[22]

Enclosed with the letter were copies of two draft clauses intended for amendment of the Medical Acts to deal with the situation. The first clause dealt with proposed conditions governing erasure from the *Medical Register* by the General Medical Council of the names of registered medical practitioners 'convicted in England or Ireland of any felony or misdemeanour, or in Scotland of any crime or offence, or has after due inquiry been judged by the General Medical Council to have been guilty of infamous conduct in a professional respect'. As to the second clause—it dealt with the proposed deprivation of practitioners removed from the Register of all degrees and diplomas conferring a qualification to practice. Apart from a suggested verbal amendment to make provision whereby 'the General Licensing Bodies should be entitled to repone persons who have been deprived of their respective qualifications as granted by the Bodies', the College approved both draft clauses.[22]

In July of the following year (1899) the College received a further letter from the President of the General Medical Council together with new drafts of the two proposed clauses. The amended second clause was of particular significance. It read:

> 'It shall be lawful for each of the Medical Authorities, if and when such Authority thinks fit, summarily and without further enquiry to revoke or cancel the Medical Diplomas or Diploma of such Medical Authority held by any person whose name has been erased from the Medical Register by order of the General Council for any of the causes mentioned in Section 29 of the Medical Act 1858, and subsequently to restore such Medical Diplomas or Diploma to such person without requiring him to pass a qualifying examination.'[23]

The amended draft clauses met with the approval of the College.

LEGAL ADVICE SOUGHT

Apprehension seemingly still prevailed in College circles because in 1910 Council obtained the opinion of the Dean of the Faculty regarding the disciplinary Laws of the College. Among other things they were anxious to know if a determination by the General Medical Council could be considered a conviction by a Law Court. On this particular point they were given a categorical 'No' by way of answer. The Dean's elaboration of his views must have perplexed Council. It was to the effect that 'The General Medical Council is no doubt a very important Body, and is vested with large powers by Act of Parliament. It is however, so far as the College is concerned, a foreign body, and I do not think the College are entitled to accept the decision of the General Medical Council as equivalent to their own decision . . . The General Medical Council cannot . . . be considered for the purposes of these Questions a Court of Law, and the College in my opinion ought not to delegate its duties in matters of discipline to the General Medical Council.' Further advice received by the College was that they must exercise their independent judgment in cases of discipline, and more especially when there was involved 'such a serious and at the same time undefined charge as . . . infamous conduct in a professional sense'.[24] Under the prevailing Bye-Law, the Dean considered that the College was in a position to proceed on the mere production of evidence of the removal of the name from the *Medical Register*.

Present during part of the time at a meeting of Council, the Dean of the Faculty in answer to questions declared that it was obligatory on the College to arrive at decisions only on evidence laid before them; but that if Council were not prepared 'at once to lead evidences', a hearing could be adjourned for a reasonable time to allow of witnesses being summoned. He further advised that an indictment should contain a specific statement of the charge made.[24]

The Dean deserves to be remembered if only because of his innocently audacious description of the General Medical Council as 'a foreign body'!

For some time Council had toyed with the idea of securing a Supplementary Charter with the object of strengthening their disciplinary powers. Notwithstanding the advice given by the Dean of the Faculty, and the opinion of the London solicitors of the College that it was impracticable, Council asked the latter to consult the Lord Advocate 'as to the expediency of promoting a private Bill regarding the matter'.[25] No action eventuated. None the less the possibility of applying for a Supplementary Charter was not abandoned once and for all.

At a Meeting of the College in February 1912, the Treasurer announced that he had been in correspondence with Sir Donald MacAlister, who in turn had been in contact with the Privy Council concerning disciplinary cases of the College. From the correspondence it can be deduced that at some stage the question had been raised as to the desirability, or even necessity, for the College to obtain a Supplementary Charter for dealing with such cases. After consulting the Privy Council, Sir Donald was able to write: 'On the whole, the College has support for the contention that its bylaw is good, and should be acted on, till it is successfully challenged by an aggrieved practitioner in a Court of Law. Then the question of greater powers would take a definite shape.' Even coming from the philosophical highlander Sir Donald, the Council, anxious not to be involved in expensive legal actions, cannot have found conclusive support in his reply. Nor can Sir Donald's postscript, added in confidence, have dispelled doubts. In the course of his consultations Sir Donald had been vouchsafed by a high official the observation: 'Speaking without prejudice it seems to me that the College has been unnecessarily sensitive as to the exercise of the powers it enjoys under the Charter and the Bye Laws incidental thereto'.[26]

Like all great men Sir Donald MacAlister had his detractors who regarded him as aloof. None the less he was greatly respected as Principal and Vice-Chancellor of Glasgow University by students of all faculties. His short stocky figure clad in academic gown, his immaculately trimmed beard, the 'mortar board' and papers under his arm were familiar sights as he made his way on foot from Principal's House to the imposing main entrance of Gilmorehill overlooking industrial Clyde. He seemed to be completely absorbed in his own thoughts. Sir Norman Walker was one of his close friends and great admirers. A few days previous to his visiting the Principal's House on one occasion, a portrait of Sir Donald had been hung in the study—a portrait which has since been described as 'a real work of art—but a pretty grim one'. Asked by Lady MacAlister for his verdict, Sir Norman pondered a while, then turned to his hostess with no hint of malice saying 'The Hanging Judge!' A copy of the portrait now adorns the Council Room of the General Medical Council![27] In 1924 a photographic reproduction of the portrait was given to the College by Sir Norman Walker.[28]

INFAMOUS CONDUCT IN A PROFESSIONAL RESPECT

There was considerable variety in the type of case coming up for review by the College. Advertising and canvassing were invariably dealt with severely, and occurred in different circumstances. In one instance advertising and responsibility for 'quasi-medical publications' resulted in the deprivation of an Indian father and son of their Licences, the son for a considerable time having proclaimed his innocence and attributed his father with complete liability.[29, 30] Claims made in advertisements could be wildly extravagant. An infallible cure for consumption of the lungs as advertised in a notorious weekly journal and as portrayed on cards circulated to patients of other doctors brought about one Licentiate's downfall.[31] An Australian Licentiate inserted an advertisement in the Press, giving his address, headed 'Anglo-Australian Medical Institute' and declaring 'Hundreds treated successfully every year by mail'.[32] On the same continent and in the same year yet another Licentiate linked his name and qualification with an announcement that consultations were free.[32] A few years before the New South Wales Branch of the British Medical Association drew the attention of the College to 'the unbecoming and unprofessional advertisement' being inserted in more than one public newspaper by a Licentiate.[33]

In another instance it was a home Branch of the British Medical Association which brought facts to the notice of the College. According to the Association's letter a Licentiate of the College 'carries on business as Grocer and General Store keeper in the town in which he practises' and 'has been seen behind the counter of the shop selling goods'. The specific question was asked as to his entitlement to pursue his multiple calling but all the Council could write by way of reply was 'whilst it was not common for Licentiates to keep open shop, there was no law against it'.[34] Our practitioner-cum-grocer was not an Edinburgh citizen, nor did he function at the right time—otherwise he would have provided a unique subject for Kay's *Portraits*! On another occasion a Defence Society wrote to inform the College that a Licentiate, struck off the *Medical Register* fourteen years previously, at which time his qualifications were removed, was again using his qualifications and practising. Prosecution was suggested but the College advised that this would be better undertaken by the General Medical Council.[35]

There were the isolated instances of agents being employed to canvas[36] but canvassing in an unusually flagrant form figured in another case. Persuasive, suggestive advertisements adorned every window of the defendant's house frontage. Counsel was employed by both him and the College and after deliberation the College decided upon a motion of censure in preference to suspension.[37, 38] A pronouncement of severe censure in lieu of a severe sentence was agreed upon on another occasion when transport and postal disorganization at the time of a national strike put a Licentiate at great disadvantage when defending an indictment of advertising.[39]

Overprescribing is a sin customarily linked with the wrath of Executive Committees in the National Health Service. Nevertheless the College had a bizarre case to deal with before Executive Committees were in existence. It concerned a Licentiate in the Transvaal. He had prescribed intoxicating liquors 'for divers coloured persons' and to the extent of issuing 971 such prescriptions in a period of less than six months. His sin was the more heinous in that by the law of the land coloured persons were debarred from purchasing or obtaining intoxicating liquors.[40] Other offences providing the substance of indicting motions were drunkenness and disorderliness, felony in the form of procuring illegal abortion or miscarriage, adulterous association with a patient, false certification, and giving false evidence in the Courts. Within recent times excessive alcohol consumption has come to be associated with a greater proportion of driving offences and the incidence of drug offences has increased. False certification was indulged in, in various circumstances. A Licentiate acting as a Medical Referee in Burma gave a certificate in respect of a patient whom he had never examined.[41] Another in India issued medical certificates without having seen the patient[42] and a third was convicted by the Indian Law Courts of giving false evidence.[43] In this last case considerable difficulty was experienced by the College in obtaining an address to which notice of a motion for expulsion could be sent. There was also an isolated instance of intent to mislead a Life Assurance Company.[44] One of those expelled for attempting illegal abortions, of which one proved fatal, was a woman Licentiate.[45] A Licentiate of Dominion extraction was another who was expelled by the College and struck off the *Medical Register*, having been convicted in English assizes of raping a person to whom he had previously administered a drug 'with intent to stupefy' her.[46]

DEFAULTING MEMBERS

Three situations involved Members. The first involved not disciplinary action, but acceptance by the Member of the application of existing College Bye-Laws. Having joined a partnership in which dispensing was carried out, he wrote offering to resign his Membership. The College decreed that he should return his Diploma for such time as he continued to dispense.[47] The situation in which the second Member found himself was very different. Practising in a South Coast resort he 'whilst attending professionally . . . and in conjunction with' a 'nurse companion . . . improperly used undue influence upon' his patient 'to make and execute a transfer to himself of £1,000 National War Loan Stock, and to make and execute a Will . . .' of which he was appointed one of two executors and under which he and the nurse companion were to be 'equal divisees and legatees of the residuary estate . . . .'. Suspension of this Licentiate by the College followed suspension from the Medical Register by the General Medical Council.[48]

The third Member was expelled for indecent publications and unprofessional advertising.[49]

A form of unprofessional conduct which came in for severe censure was association in one way or another with unqualified persons. Thus one Licentiate allowed an unqualified individual to exhibit his name in the Licentiate's surgery and to attend and prescribe for patients. The Council of the College employed Counsel and witnesses including parents and officers in the employ of an English City Education Department, all of whom testified that certificates as to the inability of pupils to attend school had been signed by the unqualified person.[50]

A case with a perhaps fortuitously sad ending was that of a Licentiate in England who admitted to acting as cover to an unqualified 'venereal practitioner'. A member of Council visited the establishment of the unqualified person and found it 'most unprofessional'. Prosecution would appear to have been inevitable. While it was under discussion by Council, the Licentiate died.

THE CASE OF MR OR DR AXHAM

Of cases dealt with by the College arising from assistance given to an unqualified person or persons, the one which received greatest publicity was without question that associated with a Licentiate of the name of Axham and (Sir) Herbert Barker. A motion for expulsion in respect of Frederick William Axham was placed before the College by Council on 6th February 1912. Axham, it was stated, had 'acted in an unbecoming or unprofessional manner in as much as he . . . knowingly and wilfully on various occasions assisted one Herbert Atkinson Barker, an unregistered person practising in a department of surgery, in carrying on such practice, by administering anaesthetics on his behalf to persons coming to him for treatment'. The General Medical Council had previously removed Axham's name from the Medical Register on 24 May 1911[51] but the public outcry to which this gave rise did not dissuade the College from taking action. Council of the College had first resolved to proceed with the case in December of that year.[52] In April of the following year the Clerk received a communication from Mr Axham intimating his intention to be represented by Counsel. The President, Treasurer, Secretary and Clerk were of the opinion that the College should also employ Counsel, but on approaching Counsel were advised that it was 'hardly necessary that the College should be put to the expense' involved. It was decided to accept the advice[53] but the Council Minutes of 11th June 1912 record that 'subsequent events convinced the President and Clerk that Counsel should be retained'.[54]

The circumstances in which Axham's participation was brought into the limelight were unfortunate. (Sir) Herbert Barker was taken to court for damages by a man whom he had examined under gas anaesthesia. He had been approached concerning knee-joint trouble previously suspected of being tuberculous by qualified specialists. Subsequently the man in question had his leg amputated and based his claim on the examination by Barker having in fact been an operation, meaning thereby manipulation, which had reactivated dormant infection. The trial was conducted in the presence of such illustrious legal experts as Sir Edward Carson and Sir Edward Clarke and before that most picturesque of High Court Judges, Mr Justice Darling. Apart from the problems arising from conflicting evidence, the legal arguments were largely concerned with differentiating an 'examination' from an 'operation' in terms of manipulation. Barker lost his case but damages were small.[55]

Axham had given the anaesthetic. He was summoned to appear before the General Medical Council, the complainants being the Medical Defence Union. The verdict of the General Medical Council was that he had been guilty of 'infamous conduct'. His name was erased from the *Medical Register*.[56]

Having been notified of the action taken and intentions of the College Council, Axham pointed out in a letter to the Secretary that '. . . although I had been associated with Mr. H. A. Barker in the interest of the public for several years no exception was taken to this by the Council until the action Thomas v. Barker last February'. 'Mr. Barker', Axham continued, 'was blamed for an act he never committed . . . to my mind, the loss of the leg was due, *not* to his negligence but to orthodox omission.' A significant feature of the case was the fact that four surgeons, one of the highest eminence, gave evidence for the 'Bonesetter'. Admitting to awareness that the law prohibited 'the association of a qualified with an unqualified man' Axham went on to maintain that 'the Act was passed for the protection of the public from charlatanry and *not* to debar them from deriving benefit from valuable methods of treatment because of the discovery of such methods by laymen'.[57]

Mr Axham appeared before the College on 7th May 1912. Additional to (Sir) Byrom Bramwell in the chair, sixty-three Fellows were present. A King's Counsel attended on behalf of the College, and an Advocate and Lawyer on behalf of Mr Axham. King's Counsel read the letter referred to above from Mr Axham to the Secretary of the College and, according to the Minutes, Mr Axham's Counsel 'read extracts from various periodicals, but he did not tender any evidence, or raise any technical plea'. Through the Chairman, Sir Thomas Fraser of the College asked Mr Axham's representatives if Mr Axham intended to continue to administer anaesthesia for unqualified persons. By way of reply Sir Thomas was told that Mr Axham 'had no intention of desisting'.

Thereupon the motion was carried that Mr Axham 'be suspended *sine die* and deprived until the said suspension is removed or remitted of all the rights and privileges, which as a Licentiate he does or may enjoy'.

The decision arrived at by the College was communicated to the General Medical Council.[57]

When in 1917, an offer by Barker to treat soldiers was declined there was a renewed popular clamour for him to be accorded some form of recognition. Previously in 1912 the *Times* had pointed out that Barker's successful 'cures' included a number of patients to whom qualified doctors had failed to afford relief. An approach was made to the Archbishop of Canterbury in 1920 to exercise his erstwhile traditional prerogative of bestowing a degree of Doctorate of Medicine (Chap. XI) on Barker. Action along these lines was not taken, but had the suggestion been implemented it would not have carried with it the right to be included in the *Medical Register* of the General Medical Council. Barker was knighted in 1922.[58]

Mr Axham's case came up for reconsideration by the College in January 1926. On the 19th day of that month, with Dr George Robertson, President, in the Chair, Sir Robert Philip moved on behalf of Council a resolution that '. . . it is now resolved by the College (on proof submitted that the said Frederick William Axham has abstained for the last five years from the practices which led to his suspension and will not resume them) that the said suspension be removed as from this date'. The motion was seconded by Dr William Russell. Several Fellows spoke for and against the motion which was eventually carried by 39 votes to 6.

Thereafter the question arose in discussion as to whether the complete motion should be supplied to the Medical Press only, and intimation to 'the ordinary Press' be limited to a statement of the fact that Mr Axham's suspension had been removed and his Licence restored. Following a vote the College resolved that 'the full motion should be supplied to all the Press'.[59]

TWO DELICATE SITUATIONS

A situation with unusual features arose in 1909 when a doctor who was a Licentiate of the College and also a Fellow of the Glasgow Faculty 'accepted office as Consulting Physician and Surgeon' to an Institute which in the opinion of the Council of the

College conducted 'its operations in an unprofessional manner'. It was resolved by Council that the Secretary 'should write to the Visitor of the Faculty in Glasgow calling his attention to the fact that one of their Fellows held office in this Institution' and that 'the College might feel it necessary to take Disciplinary action . . . unless the Glasgow Faculty resolved to do so'.[60] No motion was presented by Council to the College, but a Council Minute a number of months later noted that it was agreed that no action should be taken.[61]

A curious position arose in 1855 when a Fellow whose name was removed in 1839 from the Roll of Attendance at his own request because of his departure for Canada, on reappearing in Edinburgh asked for his position to be regularized. There were potential legal complications because in the interval between having his name removed and leaving the country the Fellow had attended and taken an active part in sederunts. He had in fact exercised the privileges of an attending Fellow without having been reponed on the roll. The situation was amicably, if from the Fellow's point of view expensively, settled. He resumed his seat unchallenged having undertaken to pay what were regarded as outstanding contributions for 11 or 12 years.[62]

A no less awkward predicament arose on another occasion when a petitioner for the Fellowship from the north unintentionally adopted an unusual method of approach. In the confusion he was mistaken for a namesake outside Scotland. Things were righted at the next Quarterly Meeting.[62]

GET THEE BEHIND ME SATAN

There were times when even the Council themselves had to be on the alert not to commit an unthinking indiscretion. In the early part of the present century the Highland Railway embarked on an ambitious hotel project at Strathpeffer. The then ultra-modern facilities of the new hotel included 'Baths and Wells'. It was to comment—comment not advise—on these that the College was invited to send a deputation. Significantly the deputation was to visit on the opening day of the hotel. In its wisdom the Council did not inform the College at the time and, with puritan austerity worthy of a kirk session, replied to the invitation that they could not consider the proposal.[63]

PROCEDURE

The procedure followed by the College in dealing with disciplinary cases is not designed nor applied with ruthless intent to secure what may be termed a 'conviction'.

For all cases the mode of procedure is laid down in the Laws of the College, and is adhered to strictly and with impartiality. A copy of any motion of indictment, implying liability to censure, suspension or expulsion, is sent with minimal delay under registered cover to the accused. Anyone in receipt of such a copy is given the opportunity to appear before the College and plead personally or by a representative at the meeting at which the motion will eventually be determined.

In the first place a motion which is considered by Council to be necessary is prepared by them and then laid together with their opinion before the College. Decision to entertain or reject the motion is dependent on the voting of Fellows. An instance of rejection of a motion by Council occurred in 1925. 'The infamous conduct in a professional respect' ascribed to a Licentiate consisted of the issue to eleven patients of 'misleading and improper National Health Insurance Certificates'. The motion having been moved and seconded, a senior Fellow in the words of the Minutes 'made a statement against proceeding with the motion and several other Fellows also spoke. On a vote the motion was defeated.'[64] Rejection on another occasion was equally conclusive but again for reasons not precisely explained in the records. It was moved on behalf of Council that a Licentiate had knowingly enabled a woman not certified under the Midwives Act 'to practise as if she were certified'. It was suggested that the woman had attended seventeen cases and that in most of them the Licentiate had signed Maternity Benefit Certificates and Notifications of Birth. After reading a letter from the Secretary of the General Medical Council and a Print of the General Medical Council Minutes, the College Secretary moved a motion for prosecution on behalf of the Council of the College. Sir Norman Walker seconded. The College Minute concluded tersely: 'Dr. William Russell, the representative of the College on the General Medical Council made a Statement with reference to the case and asked the Fellows to vote against entertaining the Motion. On a vote being taken the motion was lost.'[65]

A Motion which has been accepted is brought up for determination at another meeting of the College within two months. For the Motion to be carried at this second meeting a majority of not less than three-fourths of the Fellows present is required. Again subject to there being a three-fourths majority in favour, Fellows may modify a Motion for expulsion to one for suspension or censure; and a Motion for suspension to one of censure. There are a number of recorded instances of Fellows exercising their right to modify in this way.[66] Likewise the College has on occasion taken advantage of the authority it possesses to repone.[67]

The College is not unmindful of the personal tragedy experienced by those whom they feel in duty bound to discipline as required by their Laws drafted specifically for the protection of the public. In a proportion of the more serious cases, letters sent in reply to a notice of disciplinary Motion have been written from prison. Some betray the abject despair of having been already struck off the Register and others again the dread of a future with neither employment nor resources. Few over the years expressed bitterness even when pleading innocence.

REFERENCES

(1) R.C.P.E. (1925) *Historical Sketch and Laws of the Royal College of Physicians of Edinburgh*, pp. 112–13. Edinburgh: Royal College of Physicians.
(2) College Minutes, 6.ii.1682.
(3) Ibid., 21.iii.1682.
(4) Ibid., 5.xi.1805.
(5) [ECCLES, W.] (1707) *An historical account of the rights and priviledges of the Royal College of Physicians and of the Incorporation of Chirurgions in Edinburgh*, pp. 35–6. [Edinburgh: Privately printed.]
(6) College Minutes, 4.ii.1806.
(7) R.C.P.E. [c. 1850] *Abstracts of the Minutes, AD 1682–1731*. By George Paterson, p. 114. (Ms.)
(8) College Minutes, 6.v.1707.
(9) Ibid., 19.xii.1684.
(10) Ibid., 13.iii.1707.
(11) Ibid., 6.v.1707.
(12) R.C.P.E. (1925) *Historical Sketch and Laws*, p. 114. Edinburgh: Royal College of Physicians.
(13) College Minutes, 6.xi.1750.
(14) Ibid., 1.xi.1763.
(15) R.C.P.E. (1853–6) *General Correspondence*, 14.x.1853; 18.x.1853; 23.i.1854; 15.iv.1854; 19.iv.1854; 1.v.1854; 18.iv.1856; 29.iv.1856.
(16) RITCHIE, R. P. (1899) *The Early Days of the Royall Colledge of Physitians, Edinburgh*, p. 93. Edinburgh: G. P. Johnston.
(17) College Minutes, 1.v.1764.
(18) R.C.P.E. (1832) *General Correspondence*, 6.viii.1832.
(19) RITCHIE, R. P. Op. cit., p. 176.
(20) College Minutes, 25.ix.1695.
(21) Ibid., 21.ix.1858.
(22) Ibid., 20.xii.1898.
(23) Ibid., 18.vii.1899.
(24) Council Minutes, 8.vi.1810.
(25) Ibid., 20.xii.1910.
(26) College Minutes, 6.ii.1912.
(27) OAKLEY, C. A. (1971) A College Courant causerie. *The College Courant*, **23**, 47, 29.
(28) Council Minutes, 30.vi.1924.
(29) College Minutes, 27.xi.1862.

(30) Ibid., 3.xi.1868.
(31) Ibid., 4.v.1926.
(32) Ibid., 19.xii.1900.
(33) Ibid., 1.v.1900.
(34) Council Minutes, 31.x.1911.
(35) Ibid., 5.xi.1912.
(36) College Minutes, 5.vii.1932.
(37) Ibid., 6.ii.1934.
(38) Ibid., 1.v.1934.
(39) Ibid., 8.vi.1926.
(40) Ibid., 1.xii.1927.
(41) Ibid., 5.xi.1935.
(42) Ibid., 8.vi.1926.
(43) Ibid., 17.vii.1923.
(44) Ibid., 5.ii.1889.
(45) Ibid., 1.xi.1932.
(46) Ibid., 3.xi.1925.
(47) Council Minutes, 25.iv.1911.
(48) College Minutes, 3.ii.1920.
(49) Ibid., 15.ii.1887.
(50) Ibid., 19.vii.1910.
(51) Ibid., 6.ii.1912.
(52) Council Minutes, 5.xii.1911.
(53) Ibid., 30.iv.1912.
(54) Ibid., 11.vi.1912.
(55) Thomas v. Barker (1911) *Lancet*, **1**, 604.
(56) Supplement (1911) *British Medical Journal*, **1**, 389.
(57) College Minutes, 7.v.1912.
(58) DICTIONARY OF NATIONAL BIOGRAPHY, 1941–50 (1959), pp. 59–60. London: Oxford University Press.
(59) College Minutes, 19.i.1926.
(60) Council Minutes, 26.x.1909.
(61) Ibid., 25.i.1910.
(62) College Minutes, 6.xi.1855.
(63) Council Minutes, 25.iv.1911.
(64) College Minutes, 21.vii.1925.
(65) Ibid., 5.ii.1924.
(66) Ibid., 5.viii.1884.
(67) Ibid., 3.viii.1875.

Y

Chapter XXVII

IN TIMES OF WAR AND BETWEEN WARS

A feature of the early Minutes of the College is the virtual complete absence of mention of current affairs. In the Preface to Duncan's *Memorials of the Glasgow Faculty* the statement appears '. . . the Minute Books are concerned only with the doings of the calling as a corporate body'.[1] This is equally true of the records of the Edinburgh College of Physicians. Reading them it is only the dates of sederunts that serve to remind that concurrently there were taking place Jacobite uprisings, illicit meetings of Covenanters, Napoleonic Wars on the Continent and historic events of national importance in the Crimea, India or South Africa. Not until the advent of the two World Wars is there evidence in the Minutes of the direct impact of hostilities on College affairs and College Fellows. This is to be attributed to the evolution of total war with its involvement of a civilian population organized only slightly less than the fighting services.

COVENANTERS' DEFIANCE

The accession of Charles II to the throne in 1660 was soon followed by legislation designed to nullify the *Solemn League and Covenant* of 1643 by replacing Presbyterianism with Episcopacy. Patronage was restored; ministers unwilling to submit to the authority of bishop or patron were deprived of their pastorates; and attendance by parishioners at 'religious meetings not allowed by law' was proscribed as an act of sedition. Such was the resentment and religious loyalty of Presbyterians that numerous scattered areas of partly organized resistance developed. 'Illegal' religious meetings were held in many places and the Government employed troops to overawe the natives and collect fines. It has been said that 'in every respect the troops acted as if in an enemy's country'.[2] Lives were lost in battle and others terminated at the instance of the Law.

One martyr was William Hervie of whom William Harvey, F.R.C.P. (q.v. under Indian Medical Service) was a direct descendant.[3] The inscription on the martyr's tombstone reads:

HEIR. LYES. WILLI
AM. HERVI. WHO
SWFERED. AT
THE. CROS. OF
LANERK. THE
2 OF. MARCH
1682 AGE 38
FOR HIS ADHERENC
TO THE WORD OF
GOD AND SCOTLANDS
COVENANTED WORK
OF REFORMATION.

Historically it is of interest that the date of Hervie's hanging took place within a few months of the foundation of our College. His 'crimes' consisted of being present at a 'rebellion' and at the publication of a 'treasonable declaration'.[4]

THE JACOBITE RISINGS

But 'tis not my sufferings this wretched—forlorn
My brave gallant friends! tis your ruin I mourn;
Your deeds proved so loyal in hot bloody trial—
Alas! can I make you no sweeter return.

The Chevaliers Lament

Information concerning the involvement of medical men in the Jacobite Risings is scant and not always reliable. This applies particularly to the events of 1715. Not unnaturally discretion compelled anonymity on occasions. A dearth of historical facts is contributed to in so far as the College is concerned, by the lack of any list of Licentiates of the period. There was of course no Medical Register at the time. Moreover there was not always reliable discrimination between practitioners of physic on the one hand and surgeons, surgeon–apprentices and barber–surgeons on the other. Nor can the presence of an occasional 'quack' be ruled out. What is known, however, is that four 'students of physic' belonging to the Edinburgh Company of Volunteers and serving with the Hanoverian forces, were captured at Falkirk, imprisoned in Doune Castle and made a successful escape using their bedclothes to improvise rope ladders.[5] Two of these students later qualified in medicine: William MacGhie who in due course became a physician on the staff of Guy's Hospital and Robert Douglas who joined the Royal Navy as a surgeon.[6] Of the remaining two, one was the son of the parish minister of St Cuthbert's Church, Edinburgh and the other became an author whose play is reputed to have given rise to the comment—'An' whaurs yer Wullie Shakespeare noo?' Historians tell of yet another medical student, a native of the West Indies, who joined Cope's army at Prestonpans and 'who fought well in the battles but was terribly wounded'.[7-9] Of doctors with the Jacobite forces the greatest number came from Angus, and after Angus from Edinburgh.

Considering more particularly the allegiances of individual Fellows of the College, there was no attempt at concealment on the part of Archibald Pitcairne. Nor is his devotion to the Jacobite cause a matter for surprise. To quote Ritchie: 'He was descended from Andrew Pitcairne, who was born after his father had been slain at Flodden Field, and where also his seven sons sacrificed their lives for Scotland and their King. Could the attachment of the Pitcairne family to the House of Stewart be more strongly shown?'[10] The allegiance was transmitted to Archibald Pitcairne's own son who, falling into the hands of the Royalists, was imprisoned in the Tower of London. He was eventually released and pardoned following an appeal to Sir Robert Walpole by Dr Richard Mead, a former pupil of the older Pitcairne at Leyden. Mead, a Fellow of the College, is credited with saying to Walpole: 'If I have been able to save your or any other man's life, I owe the power to this young man's father.'[11]

Archibald Pitcairne died on 23rd October 1713. An ardent Jacobite to the end he dedicated his collected writings thus: 'To God and his Prince, this work is humbly dedicated by Archibald Pitcairne, June 20th, 1713'. He left also a Jeroboam of claret to be opened at the Restoration of the House of Stewart. It was consumed as a memorial gesture on the 148th anniversary of his birth at the restoration of his tombstone.[12]

Another who had connections, albeit remote, with the Jacobites was a grandson of Dr Robert Trotter who was President during the time of strife between the Sibbald and Stevensone-cum-Pitcairne factions in the College Council (Chap. XIX). The grandson was a surgeon in Nithsdale. Because in 1746 he concealed and protected a wounded Jacobite officer in the course of his everyday duties he nearly lost his life at the hands of the Hanoverians. A grandson of the Nithsdale practitioner, also a doctor, was the author of *Derwent Water, or the adherent of King James*.[13] According to

Ritchie, Dr Matthew Brisbane, whose name appeared on the original Charter (Chap. III) could claim that among his ancestors one was killed at Flodden in 1513 and another at the battle of Pinkie in 1547 but otherwise the family does not appear to have been involved in the Risings.[14]

Nor should the name of another Fellow, Charles Congalton, be forgotten. He was a friend of John Gregory and Alexander Carlyle. The latter knew Congalton in Leyden, visited Amsterdam with him and recorded how he was 'one of the best young men I have ever known, having been bred a Jacobite and having many friends and relations in the Rebellion, did not like to keep company with those who were warm friends of the Government'.[15]

Sir Stuart Threipland

If political leanings be put aside, none would begrudge Sir Stuart Threipland of Fingask being given pride of place among Fellows of this period. His father was an ardent supporter of the House of Stewart and had taken an active part in the Rising of 1715. Stuart Threipland was born in the family home at a time when it was occupied by Hanoverian troops and his father was in hiding—or as it was picturesquely described in those days, 'lurking'. Fearful with good reason for the fate of her newly born baby Lady Threipland chose the symbolic name of Stuart for her son. The year was 1716.

When Prince Charles landed at Borrodale and later raised his standard at Glenfinnan, Threipland lost no time in joining him having been recommended by the Old Chevalier as one deserving confidence and not over solicitous for himself.[16] He had already become an alumnus of the University of Edinburgh (M.D. 1742); been admitted a Fellow of the Edinburgh College of Physicians (1744); and commenced practice in Edinburgh. Having assumed the office of medical adviser, Threipland accompanied the Prince on the march south to Derby and was with him at Culloden and during the fugitive wanderings which immediately followed that defeat. They separated, Threipland 'lurking' in the Badenoch country where in company with Dr Archibald Cameron he went to ground in a cave. There he attended Cameron of Lochiel who had grave wounds affecting both ankles. Lochiel having made partial but considerable progress, Threipland departed for Edinburgh disguised as a presbyterian probationer[17] before changing his disguise to that of a 'printer's devil', and escaping to France where he rejoined Prince Charles. While in France his father died and he succeeded to the baronetcy.

With the declaration of an amnesty under the *Act of Indemnity 1747* Threipland was able to return to Edinburgh and there established himself as a notably successful physician. This was recognized by the College when in 1766 they elected him their President. Seven years later he was able to acquire the forfeited estate of his father to which he eventually retired and where he died. His loyalty to Jacobite ideals never wavered. None of those who sharing them, had been less fortunate, came to him in vain for assistance in time of need. Nor over a glass of port was a discreetly disguised toast to the Prince ever omitted.

With justifiable pride and a leavening of Highland fervour Dr Whittet, a Fellow of our College, wrote:

> 'Sir Stuart Threipland of Fingask Perthshire (1716–1805) was born a Jacobite. He was christened one. He was nurtured as one. He died as one—the last one of his generation. He was a devout man, devoted to God and to man—one man—Prince Charles Edward Stuart.'[16]

At the time of his death at the age of 89 years Threipland was the senior Fellow of the College. He had outlived all the Jacobite leaders.

His eighteenth-century medicine chest, which was with him at Culloden, is one of the College's proud possessions. It contains some 160 phials and boxes of pills, powders and tinctures. The chest may originally have belonged to Prince Charles. Before being gifted to the College by Dr John Smith it had been successively the property of Sir Stuart Threipland, Mr Alexander ('Lang Sandy') Wood and Dr George Wood, son of Alexander Wood.

Sir John Pringle

Whereas Sir Stuart Threipland came from the Perthshire Highlands, his counterpart in the Hanoverian forces, Sir John Pringle, was a borderer with origins in Stitchel, Roxburghshire. A student of medicine at the Universities of Edinburgh and Leyden, he graduated M.D. at the latter in 1730 and was admitted a Fellow of the College in 1735. He had a distinguished career on the Continent as physician to the Earl of Stair and later as Physician General to the forces under the Duke of Cumberland with whom he was present at Dettingen.

In 1745 Pringle accompanied Cumberland in his campaign to suppress the Jacobite Rising. According to his own account his main preoccupation was the prevention and treatment of medical conditions until after Culloden when he assumed charge for care of the wounded.[18] Howell declared that 'Pringle's hand can be seen' in all the precautions taken to keep hospitals and jails clean in an endeavour to counter the typhus, influenza and other epidemics with which the Hanoverian forces were plagued after their victory at Culloden.[19] According to Selwyn, he was far ahead of his time in speculating on the use of 'systematic antiseptics'.[20] It is to Pringle's credit that he steadfastly deplored concerted efforts to decry Prince Charles' courage after the Battle of Culloden and maintained that such efforts were motivated by political and not historical considerations. On retiring from practice in London, Pringle returned to Edinburgh only to find not warmth of welcome but 'the wafting smoke from the burning indignation still keenly felt in the Highlands and beyond concerning Cumberland's cold cruelties'.[21] One of his last acts before retracing steps to London was to present to the College the ten manuscript volumes now in the Library (Chap. VI) dealing with military medicine as distinct from military surgery. Pringle's most enduring claim to remembrance is that his suggestion in 1743 that military hospitals should be immune from attack was adopted by the Earl of Stair, commander of the British forces, and his French opposite number the Duc de Noailles. This was an entirely new concept in warfare which in due course provided a basis for the Geneva Convention.

Jupiter Carlyle of Inveresk, an erstwhile pupil of Pringle's, had a grandstand view of the Battle of Prestonpans on which he drew to enliven his *Autobiography*.[22]

In life Pringle's publications on septic and antiseptic substances earned him the Copley medal of the Royal Society of which he was later elected President. It fell to him as President to present the Copley medal to Captain Cook in recognition of the latter's arrangements for preserving the health of his crew. David Hume, philosopher and historian, was one of his patients. To Johnson, Pringle was anathema—his third pet aversion according to Boswell, the others being 'Whiggism' and 'Presbyterianism'.

Gordon-Taylor mentioned a 'Dr James Clerk, of Edinburgh' as among Hanoverian adherents but vouchsafed no further information.[23] If it be accepted that he was a physician as distinct from surgeon and that the spelling of the surname is correct, the doctor concerned *might* be John Clerk who was admitted to the Fellowship in 1714 and elected President of the College in 1740—an office he held for four years. There is no other 'Clerk' in the List of Fellows for the first century of the College's history.

One about whom there can be no question, and who in later years was to be admitted as a Fellow (1756), was Alexander Monro *primus* of firmly rooted Hanoverian convictions. He assisted his father, John Monro, in attending the wounded after the Battle of Sheriffmuir in 1715.[24] It was Monro *primus* who later with Drummond ensured the sustained momentum necessary for realization of the Edinburgh Infirmary project (Chap. XX). The Battle of Prestonpans, in which Cope's men were routed, took place rather less than four years after the Infirmary had opened its doors. Casting aside any political prejudices Monro proceeded straightway to the battlefield and there not only attended to the wounded but also removed many of them to the wards of the Infirmary regardless of whether the unfortunate victims were Jacobite or Hanoverian.[25-27] In addition about 280 wounded were, at the instance of Fellows or future Fellows of the Edinburgh College of Surgeons, George Lauder, John Rattray and Alexander Wood, admitted into the Charity Workhouse in Edinburgh.[28] Movement of the wounded was probably greatly facilitated by use of 'amateur ambulances, coaches, and chaises' which Prince Charles took with him when he left the Scottish capital.[7] In the case of the Infirmary, conditions simulating a military hospital of the period persisted for a considerable time and when Prince Charles left the city to march south, Jacobites among the hospital wounded found to their dismay that they were no longer free men but prisoners.

It is not out of place to recall the contrast between the humanity shewn towards the wounded lying on the field of Prestonpans and the odious brutality meted out to the maimed and stricken strewn over Culloden Moor. According to Whittet, a Thanksgiving Service marked Cumberland's return to London; Cumberland was created Baron Culloden by his father George II; and 'See the Conquering Hero Comes' was Handel's specially commissioned tribute to the returned victor.[29] If this be true—human dignity and human compassion have never been more foully or more abysmally degraded.

Dr Archibald Cameron

No reference to medical participants would be complete without mention of the legendary Dr Archibald Cameron (1705–53), brother of Lochiel. Whether he was a Licentiate of the College is unknown. Indeed it is unlikely, but he certainly established a remote connection with the College by studying anatomy under Monro *primus* and physic under Dr Sinclair in Edinburgh, preparatory to completing his medical studies in Paris.[30] Sent by his brother to meet the Prince and dissuade him from launching on his enterprise, Cameron was ineffective, joined the Jacobite forces and prophetically declared he would be 'the last to quit'. Wounded at Falkirk and Culloden, he escaped to the wilds of Badenoch and later sailed for France with Prince Charles. In 1753 he returned to Scotland, for what exact purpose is uncertain. Suffice it to say he was betrayed, captured and sentenced to be hanged, drawn and quartered. Neither the pathetic pleadings of his wife nor the intercession of Monro *primus*, a staunch Hanoverian but none the less personally aware of the condemned man's worth, prevented the sentence being carried out publicly at Tyburn. Cameron was at one and the same time the last 'rebel' to be sentenced in this way, and as he himself had foretold 'the last to quit'.[31–33]

James Grainger (?1721–66), born at Duns became a Licentiate of the College in 1758 having obtained the Edinburgh University degree of Doctor of Medicine five years previously. After attending University classes he was apprenticed to the Edinburgh Surgeon, Mr Lauder, before entering the Army, in which having been at Falkirk and possibly Culloden, he saw service on the Continent. Leaving the Army in 1748 he endeavoured with limited success to embark on a literary career and although an intimate of Johnson, who praised his 'Ode on Solitude'[34] and of Boswell, he came in for trenchant criticism from Smollett. Grainger died in the West Indies where he had combined medical practice with commercial activities and the successful wooing of the Governor's daughter.[35]

Then there was one William Balfour of Aberdour who took part in the Prince's march to Derby.[36] Admittedly his practice was surgical rather than medical in the narrow sense but his appearance in Robert Louis Stevenson's *Kidnapped* and *Catriona* is excused for latitude on this occasion, more especially as nothing is known of the medical qualifications of the original Balfour. Was there nostalgic significance in the fact that the novelist's mother was a Balfour? Furthermore it was to a Balfour—Dr George Balfour, a President of our College—that the first intimation of Stevenson's death was sent by cable from Samoa.[37]

The Royal Infirmary, Edinburgh

The question of accommodating soldiers in the Infirmary first came up for consideration before 'the '45' when the hospital decided on acceptance of the King's Scots' Invalid Fund. In 1744 the Commander-in-Chief of Forces in Scotland submitted a proposal for a ward to be reserved for sick and wounded in the garrison. Under the arrangements the regimental surgeon was to be in charge and, the hospital physicians—all Fellows of the College at the time—were to have the privilege of visiting patients with their pupils. For many years after the '45 Rising soldiers continued to receive treatment at the Infirmary in accordance with the terms of the Invalid Fund.

Later in the century after the 1763 Treaty of Paris at the end of the Seven Years

War, with the aftermath of 'the '45' still lingering on, many men were discharged from the Army. They included large numbers of sick who wending their way home applied to the Infirmary for admission. Although under no legal obligation the Infirmary invariably complied with such requests from ex-military and naval personnel.[25, 38]

Francis Home was one of those who served in the War of the Austrian Succession and it is on record that while in Flanders he attended Boerhaave's lectures at Leyden.[39] Another future Fellow, who like Home was a Surgeon of Dragoons at this time, was Adam Austin.[40] By the end of the eighteenth century concern over Jacobites had given place to fears of a French invasion, and in 1794 Monro *secundus* became a member of the Committee of Defence of Midlothian.[41]

THE NAPOLEONIC WARS

Of physicians as distinct from surgeons, two with College connections had strangely contrasting links with the Napoleonic Wars. They were Drs David Maclagan and John Moir. Both were destined to become Presidents of our College.

Mention is made elsewhere of Maclagan's service on the island of Walcheren (q.v.). In all he served three years under Wellington in the Peninsular War being awarded the peninsular medal with six clasps. Before returning to Edinburgh in 1816 he was responsible for the hospital arrangements of the Portuguese Army.[42]

The circumstances in connection with Moir were very different. He was born in Verdun where his father, a naval surgeon, and mother were imprisoned after capture by the French. The family returned to Edinburgh in 1814, where John Moir lived to the age of 91 years.[43]

AFTER THE CRIMEAN WAR

Special permission was given to a Fellow at the Quarterly Meeting of the College in May 1864 to raise the question of maladministration of the Army Medical Department. He referred to the dissatisfaction prevalent in the profession and read a recent advertisement over the name of the Director General for Acting-Assistant Surgeons for Temporary Service. Pay was to be at the rate of 'ten shillings a day and allowances equal to those of a Staff-Assistant-Surgeon'. College remitted to Council to consider the present conditions in the Medical Service of the Army.[44]

An outspoken historical lecture to the Royal United Service Institution in 1884 on Army Medical Organization referred to conditions prevailing in the Crimea. 'There was no attempt at ambulance organization. The battalion surgeons of the regiments under fire, aided by the bandsmen, carried away, or tried to carry away, the battalion wounded. There were no trained regimental bearers, no bearer-companies, no field hospitals, no ambulances, no hospital corps, no equipped hospital ships, and behind all was the chaos of Scutari with its "dreary corridors of pain".'[45] There were buried 'before Sebastopol, and at Scutari, not less than 22,000 British soldiers who died of disease, not of wounds, and most of it preventible'.[46] Other less gruesome facts can be gleaned from a short biographical article on the Edinburgh surgeon Patrick Heron Watson. It is interesting that returning to Koolalee in May 1855 after an illness, Watson saw some signs of improvement and to his pronounced dissatisfaction 'only medical work came his way'.[47]

At the Quarterly Meeting of the College in August 1864 it was reported that Council had sent a Memorial dated 12th May 1864 on the subject to Lord Palmerston, First Lord of the Treasury. Certainly the Memorialists did not 'pull their punches'. Having given 'the very unsatisfactory condition of the Army Medical Department' and the increasing aggravation of 'the evils' as reasons for the Memorial the signatories presented a series of baldly stated, historically illuminating facts. Of these the first deserves reproduction.

> 'Previous to 1854 Public attention had not been specially directed to the Medical Department of the Army and though the Officers of that Department considered that they laboured under various hardships, a sufficient supply of Medical Men for the wants of the Service could always be obtained. On the outbreak of the Crimean War it was soon discovered that there was a great deficiency of Medical Officers; and this deficiency was subsequently the cause of a great amount of suffering amongst the Troops. As it was found impossible to obtain a sufficient supply of regular Assistant Surgeons passed according to the requirements of the Army Medical Board, a number of Civilians were engaged as Acting Assistant Surgeons, to perform duties of Commissioned Assistant Surgeons. Notwithstanding, the Medical Department of the Army, confessedly broke down in consequence, not, of the inefficiency of the Officers, but of the smallness of their number.'[48]

The Memorial then proceeded to enumerate subsequent improvements which had stimulated recruitment of eligible medical officers: increased pay and award of rank relative to Combatant Officers. These and other concessions it was argued had not been properly implemented. It was maintained that insult had been added to injury by the issue of an Order in 1862 requiring Staff and Regimental Surgeons to include in their Annual Report information as to the character, sobriety, conduct and temper of their Assistant Surgeons. According to the Memorialists the indecisive attitude of the Army to these and other problems led to many resignations and to a notable lowering of standards of candidates sitting the competitive examinations.

In incisive terms the Memorial stated the case for accelerated promotion; recognition of the right to leave of absence, and to a period of home service as distinct from foreign service; the abolition of confidential Reports of an inquisitorial character and of the requirement that Medical Officers should 'superintend the branding of Deserters'.[48]

After the receipt of the Memorial had been acknowledged, a copy was sent to each Member of both Houses of Parliament. Apart from being advised on behalf of the Secretary of State for War that the Memorial had been referred to him by Viscount Palmerston, the College received no communication on the subject.

The question of relative rank came up again some years later. An Army Warrant having been issued depriving members of the Medical Staff of the Army of relative rank, the College Council lost no time in registering their protest. In doing so they referred to the large number of Fellows, Members and Licentiates of the College who were Medical Officers 'of the Army' and to 'the essential importance' of relative rank to medical officers responsible for the maintenance of discipline when whole hospital establishments were under their command. The unsolicited letter of protest to the Secretary of State for War concluded by representing that 'it would be in the highest degree impolitic to lessen the inducements to competent medical men to enter the Army . . .'.[49]

Presumably the protest of 1887 was ineffective because three years later the College felt the situation called for yet another Memorial, on this occasion addressed to a new Secretary for War. This latest protest contained one new constructive recommendation. The suggestion was advanced that Medical Staff might be 'granted rank as in the Royal Engineers, such rank being effective, as was recommended by Lord Camperdown's Committee "in all respects and for all purposes except that of military command, which last shall appertain to Medical Officers only in hospitals and when on duty with Officers and men of the Medical Staff Corps or attached to it for duty" '.

The motion approving the Memorial and requiring it to be forwarded after signature by the President (Thomas Grainger Stewart) was successfully moved by Dr Young and seconded by Sir Douglas Maclagan.[50]

In this connection it is interesting to note that in January 1898, when president elect of the British Medical Association, Grainger Stewart led a powerful deputation to wait on Lord Landsdowne. Some five months later the creation of the Royal Army Medical Corps with the granting of substantive rank and military titles was declared by Royal Warrant.[51]

Trouble rarely comes singly. Within three years yet another cause for concern presented itself, but on this occasion the College took part in a joint protest agreed by the three Scottish Medical Corporations. A decision by the War Department to restrict the selection of Medical and Surgical Examiners for the competitive examinations for admission to the Army Medical Service solely to past and present examiners of the London Colleges of Physicians and Surgeons set the fuse alight. The Joint Memorial of the Scottish Corporations maintained that if there were to be any limitation of any kind the Army Medical Board as a Public Department should be adequately representative of the Examiners of the different Medical Authorities of the United Kingdom. It pointed out that an inevitable result of the proposed policy would be to attract students from the Scottish to the London Medical Schools with consequent aggravation of the 'cramming' system as the only means of securing success in a competitive examination for which the Examiners are selected from a single centre.

At this stage, nothing daunted, the Scottish lion became proudly rampant! Your 'Director-General', the protest proclaimed, 'holds, as his only qualification, a Scottish Diploma'. Relentlessly it continued—'4 out of 10 Surgeons—Major-Generals hold Scottish Diplomas; as do also 22 out of 73—Surgeon-Colonels; 15 out of 37 Surgeons—Lieutenant-Colonels; and 100 out of 225 Surgeon Majors'. Who could have blamed the anglicized Director General had he indulged in an explosive counterblast?!

The Memorialists concluded with 'if this method of selection should be given effect to, the Medical Corporations of Scotland must naturally feel it as a slight upon the competency of their Examiners . . . and . . . they trust the matter only requires to be brought before the notice of the War Department to be rectified'. It was not without significance that the mover of the successful motion for concurrence with the other Corporations and for transmission of the Memorial to the Secretary for War, was Dr (Sir) Batty Tuke.[52]

A somewhat colourless reply was received within a month. In a way beloved of writers of official communications when opportunity presents, it began with reference to the 'Memorial without date'! What followed may be described as a soft but not wholly committal answer to turn away wrath. It maintained that there was no intention to confer a monopoly on any Medical Corporation; the recently constituted Examining Board differed from its predecessors in that its Members were 'appointed for a limited time'; and that although the latest Members had been selected from the Royal Colleges in London it was 'quite open to the Secretary of State to replace some of them, as vacancies occur, by Members from the Examining bodies in

Scotland and Ireland'. An assurance was given that due weight would be given to the Memorial 'when the time for a further selection arrives'.[53]

In retrospect it is impossible to judge whether a case really existed for the original Memorial. Was it a case of hypersensitivity on the part of the Scots, seeing slight where none was intended, or was it in reality yet another instance of a central department oblivious of the just claims of Scottish medicine?

Account has to be taken of the fact that not all medical degrees of the Scottish Universities enjoyed an altogether savoury reputation in the south. John Hunter sought to impress this on William Cullen (Chap. XI). It is not without interest that the Army Medical Board recorded that 'it is well known that from many of the Scotch Universities a degree may be sent for by the stage coach on paying eleven pounds'.[54] This was in 1796, only three years after the death of Hunter while holding the appointment of Surgeon General.

A determined effort was made in 1796 to improve the standards of medicine in the Army by Sir Lucas Pepys, a distinguished London physician who had been appointed (1794) Physician General and who while holding the appointment was elected President of the London Royal College of Physicians. He adopted the arbitrary policy of limiting promotion *qua* physicians to officers who were graduates of Oxford or Cambridge and who possessed in addition a Diploma of the London College. An inevitable outcome was that graduates of Scottish Universities and diplomates of the Scottish Medical Corporations, together with most regular Army medical officers, were debarred from promotion; and those appointed physicians were almost exclusively individuals recruited from civilian life.[54]

The irrational rigidity with which Pepys' policy could be applied was instanced by the experience of Dr William Wright, a Fellow of the Edinburgh College of Physicians. Wright applied for the post of physician to an expeditionary force bound for the West Indies. A native of Crieff, his previous experience had consisted of a spell in the Naval Medical Service, followed by seventeen years with the Army mainly in the West Indies, and a period of private practice in Jamaica. Wright's application was rejected unless he became a Fellow of the Royal College of Physicians of London. He indicated his readiness to sit the necessary examinations but before this could be arranged the expeditionary force set sail. Exercising his recognized prerogative the Commander of the expedition took it upon himself to appoint Wright physician, contrary to the recommendations of the Medical Board.[54]

In the course of time, Pepys' rules concerning the commissioning of physicians underwent modification. An Oxford or Cambridge degree, and a diploma of the

London College of Physicians remained desirable but were no longer obligatory after 1806. Graduates from other licensing bodies were eligible subject to their satisfying an examination board consisting of the Physician General and two Army physicians.[55, 56]

June 1815 saw the appointment as Director General of (Sir) James McGrigor who, born in Cromdale, Morayshire, took an M.A. degree at Marischal College, Aberdeen before studying medicine in Edinburgh prior to graduating M.D. at Marischal College in 1804. He was elected a Fellow of the Royal College of Physicians, Edinburgh three years later. McGrigor saw active service as a regimental surgeon at Walcheren, in the West Indies, India and Egypt, before joining the staff of Wellington's Army in the Peninsular War. These services and later those as Director General won for him the highest praise from Wellington.[57] Under McGrigor's guidance 'knowledge and ability rather than seniority and patronage' favoured promotion; and first encouragement was given to the creation of certain specialists. He attained his objective as evidenced in his *Autobiography* in which he wrote: 'In the ranks of the medical officers of the Army men are to be found upon a level at least with those in the Colleges of Physicians and Surgeons of London, Edinburgh and Dublin'.[58, 59] Other forms of progress accomplished during McGrigor's term of office as Director General were the initiation of systematized reports and returns from all military stations, the founding of the Anatomical and Pathological Museum of the Royal Army Medical Corps and the establishment of two army benevolent societies.[60]

THE BOER WAR AND AFTER

Young Subaltern: *I do not know how to address you. I do not know whether you should be called major, surgeon-major, mister or doctor. Which is right?*
Surgeon-Major: *On parade you will address me as Sir. Off parade you will not speak to me at all.*

Fotheringham

Victoria Cross Awards

A Licentiate who earned great distinction in the Boer War for the profession and himself was William Baptie, a graduate of Glasgow University, later to become Lieutenant-General Sir William Baptie. He was actively involved in operations directed towards the relief of Ladysmith and the remainder of the South African campaign. His courage in attending to the wounded under fire and his part in the rescue of Lord Roberts' son at Colenso won him the Victoria Cross. Appointed Director of Medical Services in India in 1914 he was the subject of criticism for the defective medical arrangements of the Mesopotamian Expeditionary Force, for which his responsibility was largely nominal. Exonerated by the Commission of Enquiry which followed he was retained as D.M.S. at the War Office.[61, 62]

Henry Edward Manning Douglas, holder of the Scottish Triple Qualification, won the Victoria Cross at Magersfontein. He saw service with the Greeks in the 1913 Balkan War and was in France from 1914 to 1918. Promoted later as Major-General and appointed D.D.M.S. Scottish Command he eventually became D.D.M.S. Southern Command, India.[61]

Prior to the South African War and in an entirely different sphere of operations (Sir) Owen Edward Pennefather Lloyd who had taken the Triple Qualification was awarded the Victoria Cross for gallantry at Sima, Burma in 1893. Retiring as Surgeon-General in 1913 he rejoined in August 1914 serving as D.M.S. Southern Command. From 1922 to 1924 he was a Colonel Commandant R.A.M.C.[61]

Royal Army Medical Corps

At the beginning of the twentieth century the Secretary of State for War was known to be considering the creation of an Advisory Board in connection with the Royal Army Medical Corps. In December 1901 the College was advised by the President (Sir Thos. Fraser) that Council had prepared a Statement for the Secretary for War drawing his attention to the need for adequate Scottish representation on the Board. To press the need more effectively it was proposed that a deputation consisting of representatives of the College and of the other Scottish Medical Corporations, and the Scottish University Members of Parliament should wait on the Secretary of War.[63]

The Statement was duly sent on the 23rd of January (1902). Remarkably, it received a reply within ten days—a reply which was undisguisedly evasive and almost facetious in its reference to Scottish graduates already on the staff of the War Office and on the Board. The details were given to the College by the President who at the same time spoke of a letter he had received from Sir John Batty Tuke, M.P. stating that he had informed the Secretary of State for War that he felt free to bring the subject up in the House of Commons when the Supplementary Estimates came up for consideration.[64]

Territorial Service

With the creation of the Territorial Army after the South African War, a need existed for the organization of a Medical Service for the Territorial Forces. In this connection the D.A.G.M.S. in 1907 suggested the appointment of a local committee to nominate medical officers for the Hospital and Sanitary Services. The President (Dr Charles Underhill) and Vice-President were nominated by the College as their representatives, the University and College of Surgeons also having two representatives each.[65]

1914–1918

THE WAR TO END WARS

When the last round has volleyed, and the boys
Troop through the homeland to the trumpet's blare,
Each back to comfort, love and peaceful ploys,
Shall I be there?

*   *   *   *   *

Victorious, mine effort is not lost;
Vanquished, I ventured all a man could dare;
Enough that when they reckon up the cost,
I paid my share.
T. F. Craig, M.B.Ed. (died of wounds 1918)

Fellows who were members of the Territorial Army and in the Naval Reserve had already been called up for service when war was declared. The majority were attached initially to the 2nd Scottish General Hospital[66] established at Craigleith under the clinical direction of Drs Edwin Bramwell, W. T. Ritchie and Edwin Matthew. From Craigleith the Hospital later moved to Mesopotamia. First reference to the outbreak of hostilities in the Minutes of the College was on 13th August 1914. On that day the President (Dr J. G. Brown) announced that a request had been received from the Chairman of the Territorial Force Association for assistance in the examination of recruits for an Edinburgh battalion which the Lord Provost had offered to raise for the new army. Fellows volunteering to undertake the work handed their names in to the Secretary at the end of the meeting.[67] Because the War Office were unable to accept the Lord Provost's offer, arrangements were subsequently cancelled.[68]

The Scottish Medical Service Emergency Committee

About this time the Chairman of the Scottish Committee of the British Medical Association called a conference of members of the medical profession at which the College was represented. Primarily the conference was called to review the situation which had arisen consequent upon the withdrawal from civilian practice of about 300 medical men. An immediate outcome of the meeting was the formation of a Scottish Medical Service Emergency Committee on 12th August 1914. The Committee consisted of 15 medical men: 7 *ex officio* members, of whom three represented the Royal Scottish Medical Corporations; 4 who were Deans of the University medical faculties; and 8 elected members. (Sir) Norman Walker was Convener and Mr T. H. Graham, Librarian of the College, the Secretary. The headquarters of the Committee were at the Edinburgh College of Physicians.[69]

Ostensibly established with the object of safeguarding civilian practice, the Committee acquired greatly extended functions in the course of time, and came to be accepted by the War Office as their representative authority for medical recruitment in Scotland. Work in the civil sphere consisted in the main of filling vacated general practices and protecting the home interests of practitioners on service. Efforts to organise and co-ordinate measures to recruit medical officers for the Army ran into difficulties with the advent of Lord Derby's Scheme, when practitioners were subject to independent canvassing by Local Recruiting Committees. Eventually the Central Medical War Committee and the Emergency Committee were asked by the Director General of Recruiting, with the approval of the War Office, to undertake all arrangements for procuring medical personnel for the Army, and the Emergency Committee compiled a Medical War Register for Scotland.[70]

With the coming into force of the Military Service Act 1916, involving compulsory service for those aged 18 to 40 years, the Scottish Medical Service Emergency Committee had added to it a Legal Assessor, and became the Central Professional Committee for Scotland with Dr (Sir) Norman Walker as Chairman and with responsibility for dealing with claims for exemption by practitioners.[71] Increasing demands by the Army resulted in burdens being shared disproportionately in some areas. With the object of promoting equality of sacrifice the Emergency Committee recommended a comprehensive scheme of professional mobilization whereby until six months after the cessation of hostilities all doctors of both sexes would be subject to Government direction. A caveat was entered to the effect that the complete organization of the medical profession should be the responsibility of a Medical Committee appointed by the Government.[72]

When the recommendation was reported to the College of Physicians, they resolved unanimously but only after considerable discussion:

> 'That this College, having considered the Resolution . . . endorses the policy of the Resolution, on the understanding that the organization referred to shall be in the hands of a Medical Committee appointed . . . for the purpose, and that this College and the other Scottish Medical Corporations are adequately represented on the Committee.'[73]

The Royal College of Surgeons of Edinburgh was unanimous in passing a similar resolution.[74]

On 6th February 1917 the President of our College (Sir Robert Philip) was able to announce at a Quarterly Meeting that the formation of a Medical Committee to be appointed by the Government along the lines suggested by the Colleges had been approved by the Director General of Medical Service.[75]

The end of the year (1916) saw the creation of a new Government Department—the Ministry of National Service with a medical section concerned mainly with the medical examination by Boards of men called up under the Military Service Act. Dr (Sir) Norman Walker was appointed Commissioner of Medical Services of Scotland while retaining the Convenership of the Emergency Committee. Co-operation between this Committee and the Ministry of National Service became increasingly close. In 1918, under new regulations, special tribunals were created for dealing with applications for granting, renewal or review of certificates of exemption. The Scottish Medical Emergency Services Committee was constituted the Medical Tribunal for Scotland and Dr (Sir) Norman Walker again named Chairman. In the course of its activities the Committee re-edited and elaborated their War Register, practitioners being grouped according to grades.[76]

The Committee was dissolved on the last day of 1919, having concluded its labours by undertaking supervisory work in connection with demobilization. As a final gesture the Committee deposited the accumulated statistics and other material which it had acquired during the time of its existence in the College Library.[77]

Casualties and Distinctions

From time to time as the War progressed, it was the President's privilege to inform the College of distinctions won by those associated with the College. To select one occasion at random—the College heard of the award of the Victoria Cross to Commander P. O. Ritchie, R.N., the son of a former President; the Military Cross while serving in the Flying Corps to the son of another former President, Dr Playfair; the Croix de Guerre (and later Distinguished Service Order) to Dr G. H. R. Gibson, son of a deceased former Councillor; and the Distinguished Service Medal for conspicuous bravery in extinguishing a magazine fire on the old cruiser H.M.S. *Kent* to Mr Leighton, Senior College Officer.[77a]

With the announcement of distinctions it was the sad duty of the President on these occasions to inform the College of those among Fellows and the sons of Fellows who had lost their lives on active service. At the same meeting as the distinctions just mentioned were announced, the College learnt of five deaths. Four were the sons of Fellows. One of these, the son of the Clerk of the College, was a Midshipman on H.M.S. *Monmouth*, an old cruiser in Admiral Cradock's ill-fated Squadron at the Battle of Coronel. The fifth loss related to Dr Melville Dunlop who at the time he left for France was a Member of the College Council. He is selected for mention because of a letter he wrote only fourteen months before his death to the President, his friend Dr Freeland Barbour. In this day and age it is rare to come across sentiments so rich in appreciation and praise and so entirely lacking in destructive criticism, as those in Dr Dunlop's letter. When read to them the College was greatly moved by it. In vivid but restrained terms it recalled the experiences known to the fathers of many of us today. Moreover it is of lasting historical value. The following are extracts:

'Well we have been encamped here "somewhere in France" for about five weeks now, and have had many and varied interesting experiences. We are all under canvas about two miles from the sea with a long range of hilly country behind us, so we are in healthy quarters.

The district for some miles around here is one huge medical camp making provision for something like 30,000 beds, so the authorities are evidently contemplating some big necessity arising. There are hospital units from India, Canada, Australia, America and other places besides many British and French. Some are under canvas, some in huts, while others are housed in large hotels and clubs, in gorgeous casinos and others again in Écoles Militaires or in convents etc. I am simply filled with wonder and amazement at the organization and the forethought of the medical arrangements. There may have been bungling in other departments, but there has been no hitch, so far as I can see, in the medical arrangements.

The equipment of our hospitals in the matter of theatres, bacteriological and X-Ray departments etc. etc. would do credit to any high class hospital at home. The transport arrangements are also beyond all praise. The hospital ships and trains, and the hundreds of motor ambulances that we see daily are fitted with every comfort and luxury that kindly forethought could devise. Yesterday a Red X train carrying about 300 sick and wounded, was evacuated in less than a couple of hours which seemed to me a marvellous performance. It is pitiful to see the train loads of our brave lads arriving daily badly mutilated and many in sore straits from the trenches, but it is at least comforting to know that every provision is made for their care and treatment. That must at least be some consolation to their friends at home. Poor fellows: it makes my heart often sore to see their sufferings but their pluck and endurance makes one proud to think that our old country is still capable of producing men of such unflinching courage. Our hospital I think "takes the cake" for magnificence, as we are housed in the huge Marquees used by the Viceroy at the Delhi Durbar and gifted to us by Indian Princes. Besides being airier and more spacious than the others, they are decorated inside with oriental gorgeousness. I am in medical charge of the hospital, and besides having wards of my own, am medical consultant to the whole hospital and responsible for every medical case. Alexis Thomson acts in a similar capacity to the surgical side. We have a medical staff of 34 . . . our C.O. is a first class man, and we all hit it off excellently, and are fortunate in having a very high class set of men in our unit, several of them being from Edinburgh. It is surprising the number of Edinburgh men one meets here, old friends, residents and students all doing their "little bit". . .

Alexis and I have asked to be sent to the Front to inspect the field hospitals and clearing stations and thus increase our experience . . .'.[78]

There are two others whose experiences on active service need mention if only because they relate to future Presidents—Doctor W. Alister Alexander and Sir Stanley Davidson. Dr Alexander's war-time travels took him to Malta, and later to the North-West Frontier before being brought back to France in the spring of 1918 at the time of the last major German Offensive. In Malta, very conscious of his youth, Alexander accompanied on ward rounds such awe-inspiring consultants as Dr George Gulland of Edinburgh, Sir James Purves Stewart, the neurologist, and Dr (Sir) Archibald Garrod whose name was already linked with his conception of inborn errors of metabolism. Not without relish Alexander tells of how in those days angina was referred to as 'status anginosis' and fibrillation as 'delirium cordis'. On his return from the East the Union-Castle troopship in which he was sailing was torpedoed 'six hours out of Alex', sinking within an hour. 'Sucked under', Alexander attributed his survival to the life jacket he was wearing. In the light of events twenty-three years later in Malayan waters, it was strange to hear from him of Japanese destroyers taking part in rescue operations.

(Sir) Stanley Davidson was the other President who as it happened succeeded Alister Alexander. A second-year medical student at Cambridge, Davidson enlisted as a combatant in August 1914. From his home in Huntly, what more natural than that he should enlist in the Gordon Highlanders, an association which has always been a source of undisguised pride to him? Less easily understood is how little attention was paid by those in authority to the fact that previously the eager young recruit had had a kidney excised.

Possessed of an enviable reputation for discipline and efficiency, the Territorial Battalion in which Davidson enlisted was posted to France and joined a Brigade of Guards in November 1914. This was six months prior to the arrival of the 51st Highland Division to which his Battalion was eventually attached. Within three months of enlistment and at the age of twenty Davidson was promoted to the rank of captain and found himself in charge of 120 men in the front line trenches in Belgium.

Memories of the early days of war in 1914 and 1915 were to prove indelible; and none more so than those of the first twenty-four hours. In the dead of night Davidson's Company clad in kilts, with shoes, not boots, as footwear, struggled through snow and freezing mud up the long communication trenches to reach the water-logged front line. As dawn broke the enemy trenches could be seen no more than 150 yards distant. 'No man's land' was strewn with the dead, many dreadfully maimed and others impaled on the barbed wire defences. Nor was the ugliness of the scene confined to that which could be observed. Everywhere there was evidence of putrefaction emanating from the remains of the unburied. Rodents and body-lice abounded.

German snipers were a constant menace and their victims regularly numbered one or more daily. With the advent of spring and conditions favouring a modicum of mobility the Battalion was involved in attacks and counter-attacks. In one attack the casualties exceeded 600 in number. Davidson's batman—an Aberdeenshire lad—was killed at his side. Those who know Sir Stanley will sense the depth of his reaction in these words of his—'When, later on leave, I called on my batman's parents I was horrified to learn that the boy had barely reached the age of 17'.

What Sir Stanley describes as 'probably the most tragic incident remembered' was encountering the victims of the first enemy chlorine-gas attack on the Canadian Division 'which was next to the Gordon Highlanders'. On the morning following the attack Davidson was under orders to bring up reinforcements from Hazebrouck Junction. His own words best describe his findings: 'Gas casualties lay on stretchers the length of the long railway platform awaiting transport to Base Hospital. Every man was suffering from a chemical broncho-pneumonia with pink coloured froth flowing from their mouths and nostrils. Sixty years have elapsed since I witnessed this ghastly sight, but it will remain with me as long as I live.' And again—'This experience together with those in the trenches, on the battlefield and later in hospital dispelled once and forever conceptions of any glory in war and of ideological heroics'.

As to Davidson himself, he was twice wounded. On the second occasion at Festubert he was particularly gravely injured by an exploding hand grenade. This occurred in the course of a German counter-attack which followed capture by the Gordons of the second-line enemy trenches. After lying for twenty-four hours in the open and having been given up by others as killed, he ultimately found himself in the Gas Gangrene Ward of the Boulogne Base Hospital from which he was, after many months, transferred to a London hospital. His recollections of Boulogne are of the grievous disfigurement and high mortality among his fellow patients; the dreadful odour arising from the black gangrenous flesh of those around; and of indescribably agonizing pain personally experienced on the occasion of each twice daily dressing of his literally huge wound. It remained for the late Sir James Purves-Stewart to recognize that pain rather than sepsis constituted the main threat to survival and to prescribe a deep lanoline-saturated dressing which straightway rendered the pain tolerable.

From London Davidson was sent to a convalescent camp at Ballymena in Northern Ireland; and by 1917 was able to resume his medical studies in Edinburgh, and to develop his interests in medical research. Sir Stanley is deeply conscious of the extent to which his war experiences brought about a great change, known to many others, in his outlook on life. Something approaching an obsession with shooting, fishing and ball games (in all of which he was outstandingly proficient) was supplanted by a determination to devote his energies to improve the lot of those who survived World War I. To hear Sir Stanley is to be conscious of profound conviction and resolute resolve.

His determination has been translated into medical teaching and research. As our College well knows, the beneficiaries have been medicine in general, academic medicine and 'those who survived the First World War'. This same attitude of determination enabled Sir Stanley to overcome in part the handicap of his severely damaged shoulder so that after three years of continuous training he was able to resume golf and shooting.

As the records bear testimony, our College has on many occasions been at the receiving end of the determination and industry so characteristic of Sir Stanley 'in times of war and between wars'.[78a]

President's Advisory Committee

As the War continued, the College became involved in a number of medical questions of national importance. The attention of College was focussed on this by a statement made by the President (Dr Freeland Barbour) towards the end of 1916, in which he raised the possibility of having an Advisory Committee appointed to deal with medical problems arising as a result of conditions of war. Such a Committee, he said, would have the support of Council. A Committee consisting of the Secretary, the Treasurer and six other Fellows was appointed forthwith and suggestions were invited from Fellows as to subjects calling for consideration and action. One problem which had already been considered was that of venereal disease and the College Laboratory facilities had been put at the disposal of the local authority. Another problem concerned disabled servicemen. Prior to the formation of the Advisory Committee, the Council of the College in conjunction with the Councils of the other two Scottish Corporations had sent a joint letter to the Government offering their fullest co-operation in any satisfactory scheme devised for the help of the disabled.[79] The offer was accepted.

At a time when the campaign in France was at one of its most critical phases the President's Committee was responsible for a Report on a subject not directly concerned with the prosecution of the War. The Report dealt with proposals to institute a Ministry of Health, a subject dealt with in Chapter XXVIII.

Disabled Servicemen

Within three months the President's Advisory Committee submitted a Report on the treatment of the disabled. Those who had been disabled and were already discharged were considered separately from those who might be disabled in the future. The first part of the Report urged the need for the provision of arrangements for 'continuance of proper treatment' whereby prospects of a return to civil employment would be improved and the liability to permanent unfitness reduced. For this to be made possible it was argued that co-operation was essential between the War Pensions Department and Local and other Authorities concerned with Public Health, Tuberculosis etc. and the administration of homes; that a Central Medical Authority linked with Local Medical Agencies and in close touch with the Central Pensions Authority, should co-ordinate measures for the selection and distribution of the various groups of patients; and that adherence to recommended treatment should be a condition attached to the continuance of pensions and the granting of supplementary allowances.

With regard to the second part of the Report, it was considered that any man disabled should be retained in the Service during such time as he showed evidence of improvement under treatment. This view did not exclude treatment in civil hospitals and convalescent homes, or of the receipt of special forms of treatment 'while actually living at home'.

The Report was adopted unanimously by the College.[80]

In this connection, while the War was still in progress, a Fellow (Dr H. E. Russell) was instrumental in organizing 'Curative Workshops' for wounded servicemen in Australia.[81]

Hospital and Laboratory Services

In virtue of their civil appointments Fellows were involved as individuals in the inevitable adjustments imposed on hospitals by the exigencies of war. The Royal Infirmary was responsible for the treatment of large numbers of servicemen[82] including men of the British Expeditionary Force, and sailors of the Royal Navy after the Battles of Doggerbank and Jutland. A request to the College to arrange staffing of the medical side of Bangour and Seafield Hospitals was met, the nucleus of staff at Bangour being supplied by the Second Scottish General Hospital at Craigleith (now the Western General Hospital), Edinburgh.[83]

Mention of hospitals would be incomplete without reference to the City Fever Hospital. There under the inspiring leadership of Dr Claude B. Ker, an eminent Fellow, outbreaks involving civilians and servicemen were taken in their stride. They included diphtheria, measles, scarlatina, classic 'spotted fever' and mumps from H.M.S. *Indefatigable* and other battle cruisers lying in the Forth. In 1918 there was the constant stream of admissions as influenza swept the city—patients stricken with terrifying suddenness, livid blue as within hours they struggled desperately for breath, many moribund and some already beyond aid by the time they arrived at the hospital gates. Fatalities included not a few members of the nursing staff. 'Claude B', as Dr Ker was affectionately known, died in 1925, but the remarks of the President (Dr Gulland) at the time deserve quotation. They were:

> 'We all know that he was a keen soldier, and took the greatest interest in military studies, especially in the career of Napoleon, and probably the greatest regret of his life was that he could not be spared for foreign service in the War.'[84]

No contribution to the war effort by the College was of greater significance than that of the College Laboratory. Details are given in Chapter V.

Nor did the College lag in periodically voting sums of money to deserving activities. Those which benefited included the Prince of Wales National Relief

Fund,[85] the Belgian Relief Fund,[86] the Scottish Medical Service Emergency Committee[87, 88] and the Belgian Doctors Fund.[88, 89] In 1917 the Trustees were authorized by the College to borrow from the Bank in order to subscribe £15,000 to the War Loan.[90]

Armistice Thanksgiving Service

A Thanksgiving Service was held in St Giles Cathedral on 21st November 1918. Their Majesties King George V and Queen Mary were present; and the College was represented by the President (Dr William Russell) and three other Members of Council.[91]

Generous Recognition

At the Quarterly Meeting in May 1922, the President (Sir Robert Philip) introduced Lieutenant-Colonel Sir Joseph Fayrer, Bart., C.B.E., M.D. who, on behalf of the Officers of the Second General Hospital, Craigleith, presented to the College a silver bowl 'to commemorate the services of Fellows of this College during the War'.[92]

1932–1939

AFTERMATH AND PRELUDE

Immigrant Refugee Doctors

As a prelude to the outbreak of war in 1939 the great influx of refugee doctors from the Continent presented Licensing Bodies in this country with a perplexing problem. Some disagreement arose between the Scottish and English Conjoint Boards as to the standards to be demanded of these doctors arriving with the object of entering into active practice.

At a meeting held in the London College of Physicians in February 1932 and attended by representatives of the Licensing Bodies but not of the Universities, it was pointed out that of 160 German doctors anxious to obtain a British qualification 120 aimed at obtaining the Licence of the Scottish Conjoint Board. It was suggested that the preference was attributable in part at least to the fact that the Scottish Board Regulations did not require examination in anatomy and physiology, and permitted of entry to the Final Examination after only one year's clinical work. A second meeting took place in January 1934, with Lord Dawson of Penn in the Chair. In the interval between the meetings the Presidents of the two London Colleges had discussed the situation with the Home Secretary, who while agreeing as to the seriousness of the problem stressed the necessity for the proper administration of the Law as regards aliens. He considered that it rested with the Licensing authorities to come into line in the matter of agreeing minimum qualifying tests and periods of study with a view to protecting the interests of the profession and the public.

From the Chair at the second meeting Lord Dawson referred to 'the mass invasion' with which the profession was faced; and indicated that the Dominions had suggested they might have to break off reciprocal relations with regard to practice, as they were not prepared automatically to accept on their Registers those with British qualifications obtained under less stringent requirements than in their own countries. There was agreement at the meeting that there should be a tightening up of regulations but the Scottish Board representatives were adamant that undertakings already given in respect of foreign practitioners should be honoured. These same representatives were equally resistant to a proposal that foreign medical graduates should be required to pass a Preliminary Examination in English, and to pass the examinations in Anatomy and Physiology prior to completing three years' clinical studies as a preliminary to admission to the Final Examination. A compromise was arrived at whereby entry to the Final Examination was subject to the foreign medical graduate '. . . having satisfied the Licensing Corporation of his knowledge of Anatomy and Physiology' and having completed three years' clinical work.

Alterations considered necessary by the English Conjoint Board were made in their regulations and insisted on foreign candidates, even if qualified in the United Kingdom, having completed three years' clinical work. Previously those who possessed Scottish qualifications were entitled to enter the Final Examination of the English Board without further formality. Relaxation of the English Conjoint Board regulations followed in 1938 when the compulsory period of clinical study was reduced to two years. In that year 600 applications for admission to the medical profession in the United Kingdom were received from Austrian doctors, and in 1939 a comparable number of applications was received from Czechoslovakia.[93]

Volunteer Reserves

Meanwhile, as individuals many Fellows and Members of our College were quietly devoting much of their spare time in equipping themselves to take an active part in the struggle that lay ahead. A considerable number held commissions in the Territorial Army, or the Volunteer Reserves of the Royal Navy or Royal Air Force.

1939–1946

TOTAL WAR

Comparison of the Records of the College during the Second World War with those of the First is salutary. In striking manner it demonstrates the repercussions of total war involving almost the entire civilian population in central direction, with 'direction' the operative word. With the organization on an all-embracing national scale of the first-aid post, ambulance and hospital services within the ambit of the Emergency Medical Services, no occasion arose in 1939 or thereafter for anything in the nature of the Scottish Medical Service Emergency Committee of 1914. Without in any way underestimating the immeasurable contribution to the war effort of doctors and nurses in the fighting services, it can be said that in some respects the burden on those remaining in civilian practice approximated more closely to that known to colleagues in the Royal Navy, Army and Royal Air Force than in the War of 1914–18. The extent to which this varied from region to region was related to the degree of involvement in enemy air attacks and in mass evacuation of the civilian population. An incidental outcome which was to produce long-term beneficial results, was closer co-operation between those engaged in private and voluntary hospital practice with members of the profession employed by local authorities.

Especially critical problems followed the evacuation from Dunkirk. Temporarily at least, a large part of the Emergency Medical Services from being potential Casualty Clearing Centres for anticipated air-raid casualties adapted themselves to the functions of Base Hospitals. Meanwhile far-flung campaigns in the vast theatre of global warfare were being pursued on land and sea and in the air. The very immensity of the scale of events greatly limited any corporate contribution of the College, except in so far as countless Licentiates, Members and Fellows made their individual contributions to the innumerable campaigns on every continent, and to the Emergency Medical Services in the United Kingdom. Far from being an apologia, these comments are intended as a factual explanation of the contrast between 1939–46 and 1914–18.

Throughout the war years the College was deeply involved in plans for the situation which would arise after the cessation of hostilities. In this the pace of events was largely determined by Governmental exploratory measures concerned with the future of the Medical Teaching Schools and the possibilities of a National Health Service. A consequence was that anticipatory consideration of Specialist Training and Postgraduate Education became necessary. In all these matters the College was unremittingly at pains to protect the future interests of those absent on active service. Foremost in repeatedly emphasizing the importance of this was (Sir) Derrick Dunlop.[94] Duties undertaken by the College, which in the light of the prevailing circumstances may be termed incidental, were the appointment of a Committee in 1945 to report preparatory to participating in the revision of the British Pharmacopoeia,[95] and the submission by request to the Department of Health of their views on the Control of Radio-Active Substances.[96] During these years Polish doctors in Edinburgh were given Library facilities by the College.[97]

During the period November 1939 to December 1946 the customary Annual and Quarterly Meetings were held without interruption. In that period there were about seventeen Extraordinary Meetings of which eight were concerned in the main with receiving annual reports from the College representatives on the Board of Management of the Edinburgh Royal Infirmary. Reasons for summoning Fellows to Extraordinary Meetings included consideration of Post-War Hospital Problems and the Goodenough Report in 1942; the Goodenough Report again in 1943 and 1945; and the proposed National Health Service in 1944 and 1946. Review of the Membership Regulations, the Future of the College, and the question of a Royal College of Physicians of Scotland came up for discussion at Extraordinary Meetings in 1946. Deliberations by the College on these various subjects are dealt with elsewhere.

Three other Extraordinary Meetings deserve mention: one in 1940 at which the College decided to subscribe to the 'City of Edinburgh Fighter Aircraft Fund'[98]; a second in the following year at which it was resolved to revert temporarily to a five-year curriculum for the purposes of the Triple Qualification; and a third in 1944 to deal with a disciplinary case with wartime implications. The re-institution of the five-year curriculum aimed at increasing the output of qualified men, 'a need for which had been emphasised both by America and Australia'; and resulted in the College requirement being similar to that of the University of Edinburgh which among other teaching bodies had not implemented the recommendation made by the General Medical Council in 1938 for the extension of curricula to six years.[99] As to the disciplinary case, this related to a certificate and letter recommending that a soldier on foreign service should be stationed 'near at home' because his wife was in 'rather a pitiful state of nerves mostly due to air raids . . . [and] not . . . capable of looking after his children'. The patient had not been examined for at least five month before issue of the certificate. There was additional evidence of unprofessional conduct in the fact that the Licentiate involved had attended another patient under the influence of drink and had been 'incapable of properly carrying out his professional duties'. A motion was agreed to suspend. A sad feature was that while serving in the R.A.M.C. in the previous War the doctor in question had been awarded the Military Cross.[100]

Traditionally at Quarterly Meetings the first duty of the President is to refer to Fellows who have died during the preceding Quarter. The custom was continued uninterruptedly during the years under discussion. A poignant feature of these occasions was the frequency with which those who had 'passed on' were noted for their distinguished and gallant service in World War I. To mention by name would have no purpose. They all had in common, service to medicine and allegiance to the College.

In passing it is of interest that one senior Fellow who died at the age of 75 years was the son of the meteorologist whose name is linked with 'Buchan's Cold Spells'.[101] An even more romantic and slightly older Fellow to die was the Maharaja of Gondal. Having successfully passed the examination he became a Member in 1892 and was elevated to the Fellowship in 1895. In addition to obtaining the degrees of M.B. and M.D. at the University of Edinburgh, he was awarded the Honorary Degree of LL.D. of that University and the Honorary Degree of D.C.L. by the University of Oxford. To quote the President of the College (Doctor Fergus Hewat): 'He risked loss of caste by crossing the sea to study Medicine in Edinburgh. . . . It is within the memory of senior Fellows that this distinguished Indian student drove in his carriage to his classes where he had a specially reserved seat for himself and got his secretary to carry out his dissections for him in the Anatomy rooms. He was an intimate friend of the late Dr. Argyll Robertson.' As a Prince he was progressive and philanthropic and abolished taxes in his State. He published his M.D. Thesis *Short History of Aryan Medical Science*, dedicating it to one of his former teachers—the late Sir William Turner.[102]

Another senior Fellow whose death was noted and who had a remarkable career was Dr James Crauford Dunlop. Starting as a paediatrician he developed an interest in research and statistics; delivered several papers before the Faculty of Actuaries of which he was elected an Honorary Fellow; became Director of Statistics in a War Office Department during World War I and was eventually appointed Registrar-General for Scotland.[102] A feature of Dunlop's contribution to College activities was his invariable insistence on the exercise of meticulous care at sederunts in the preliminary consideration of disciplinary cases.

Serving Fellows

On 6th November 1945, the President (Dr Fergus Hewat) welcomed back Fellows who had been absent on active service and expressed the hope that he would soon be extending a similar welcome to those not yet returned home. He mentioned that of Fellows on the Roll of Attendance, 36 had been in the armed services of whom seven had attained the rank of Brigadier.[103]

Today the Roll of Fellows and Members includes the names of many whose war service preceded enrolment. They with their seniors in the College had had experiences which inevitably conditioned their subsequent professional outlook. Unbeknown to them at the time they were forging a link which in later years was to add further meaning to the intangible conception of Fellowship.

For present purposes the achievements of individuals are of less importance than the collective experiences of the many. Generally names will not be mentioned. To do so might quite unintentionally suggest invidious comparison and cause distress by unwitting omission. As to experiences only the most superficial of indications can be given. In 1939 as in 1914, Fellows and Members in the Territorial Army were called up prior to the actual outbreak of hostilities. A number commenced duties at the 2nd (Scottish) General Hospital based at Peebles. A Fellow (J. S. Fulton) was in command and a future President of the College, Ian G. Hill, second in command. The hospital moved on to Palestine (now Israel) in due course. Fulton had seen service in World War I. Mobilized as a student from the O.T.C. to the Field Artillery he served in France and Italy before being sent home to complete his medical course. From Palestine he was posted successively to Greece, Tobruk, Burma as D.D.M.S. (Ops.). When the experiences of most members of the College are reviewed it would seem that one or more of their number must have played a part in virtually all the operations undertaken by the British Armies.

Several aspects impress, particularly on reading available records: firstly, the number who were involved in a whole series of campaigns in different parts of the world, including France, Holland, Germany, Norway, Crete, Africa—North and West, Italy, India, Burma, Singapore, Palestine, the Sudan and Eritrea; secondly, the number for whom active service was no new experience as they had served in World War I; and thirdly, the number of 'old campaigners' from the Dominions of Canada, Australia and New Zealand volunteering for the second time. To illustrate the last group, the case of Sir Samuel Burston, D.S.O. may be cited. A Melbourne graduate (1910) he served in Gallipoli and France in World War I, took his Membership in 1933 and was elected a Fellow in 1937. In World War II he served in the Middle

East and with the rank of Major General later directed the medical services in New Guinea, the East Indies and Burma. He was immensely proud of his association with our College.[104]

Perhaps the highest concentration at any one time of Fellows as O.C.s/Medical Divisions or as Medical Specialists was in the Middle East with its base at Cairo, where a Fellow and future President (W. D. D. Small) was Consultant Physician Middle East Forces. Specialists with College associations on the staff of the Middle East Force, G.H.Q. included, in addition to general physicians, cardiologists, neurologists and a venereologist.

One Fellow,* now the Vice-Chancellor of an English University, after seeing action with a Light Field Ambulance with an Armoured Division at Alamein joined the Blood Transfusion Unit in Cairo. He later commanded the unit. After bringing it home in 1944 he was posted to Tactical Headquarters 21st Army Group as Personal Physician to the then General Montgomery. He remained with the general during his active period of the European Campaign and witnessed acceptance by Montgomery of the German surrender at Lüneburg Heath.[104a]

Tobruk presented its own especial challenges. The A.D.M.S. there (John Fulton), a Fellow of the College, had previously commanded the 23rd (Scottish) General Hospital and in 1942 was followed by John Matheson, now Director of Post-Graduate Medical Studies in Edinburgh after retiral with the rank of Major-General.

When Medical Specialist to the 62nd General Hospital, Melville Arnott was involved in a partial sea-borne relief operation of the beleaguered Tobruk garrison about half way through the siege. Put ashore by the Navy in the dark of night the troops scrambled up a cliff and found comparative safety, conditions which were not vouchsafed to relief parties attempting a similar operation a few days later. The siege was eventually raised after heavy fighting and the Medical Specialist on board the first hospital ship to arrive was H. L. Wallace. Arnott's own words best described the sequel. 'John Fulton and I were the first two to go aboard. Harry greeted us warmly keeping well up-wind of us. He rapidly escorted us to the bathrooms where we had our first bath for several months.'[104b]

At different times a number of Fellows and future Fellows were posted to India and Burma. After a spell in Palestine and a period as Consulting Physician, Southern Command, India (Sir) J. D. S. Cameron went to G.H.Q. Delhi as Consultant Physician All-India. In territorial terms the area for which he was responsible was immense and rivalled only by that of another future President of our College (Sir) Ian G. Hill who became Consultant Physician to the Allied Land Forces, South East

* Dr R. B. Hunter

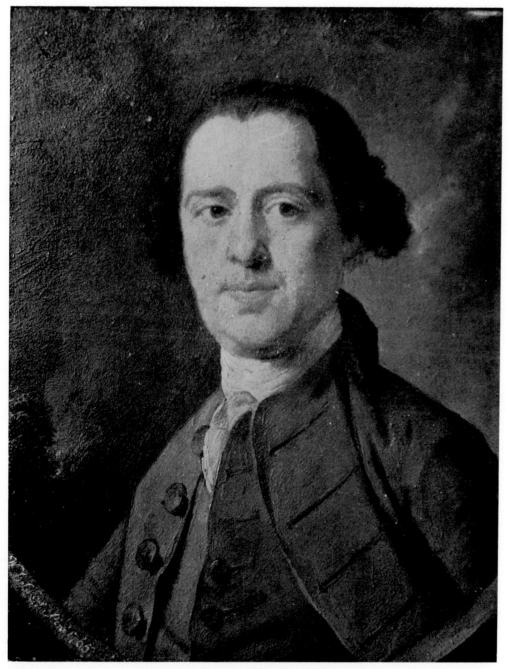

PLATE 38 Sir Stuart Threipland (1716–1805)
Reproduced by Tom Scott from a photograph in the College from the original by Delacour

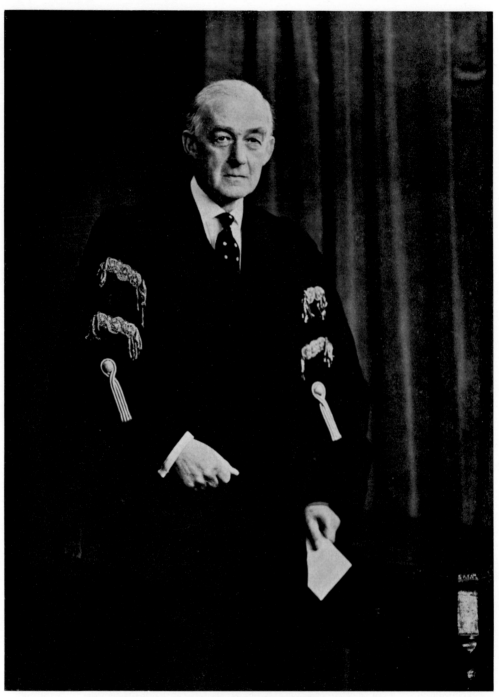

PLATE 39   Dr W. A. Alexander, President 1951–1953
Reproduced by Tom Scott from a photograph in the College

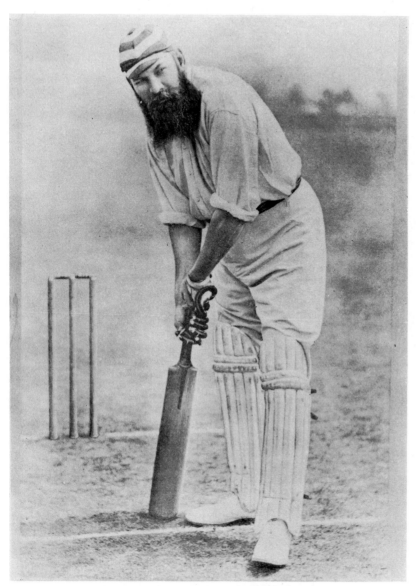

PLATE 40   W. G. Grace, L.R.C.P.E. (1879)
By courtesy of the Marylebone Cricket Club

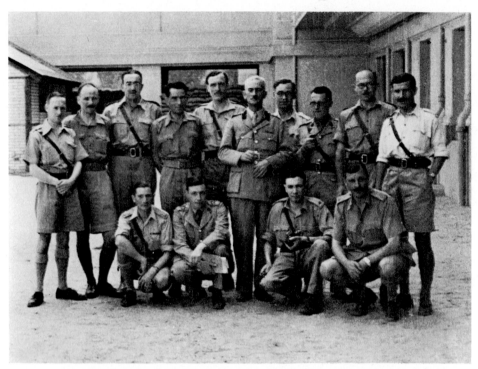

PLATE 41   Cairo: Medical Specialists' Conference, May 1942. Left to right, back row: I. G. W. Hill,
W. M. Arnott, I. Kaplan, J. J. M. Jacobs, J. Mackay-Dick, W. D. D. Small, K. Morris, E. Bulmer,
L. Lamb, J. H. Croom. Front row: A. G. Henderson, J. P. McGibbon, C. E. Van Rooyen, A. Bruce.
By courtesy of I. G. W. Hill

Asia. Previously Sir Ian had been Consultant Physician to the XIVth Army in Burma where his opposite number as Consulting Surgeon was (Sir) John Bruce. Flown to Burma after the fall of Mandalay, Hill encountered General Slim who, quick to note the shoulder flash of the XIVth Army which had been replaced by that of ALFSEA, dubbed Hill a 'deserter'![(104c)]

Ronald Girdwood was another who went from India to Burma where he was assigned responsibility for research into the anaemia which was proving itself to be a crippling scourge among Indian troops fighting in the jungle. Girdwood's work has been described as 'a major contribution to the war effort in the Burma campaign'. Direction of the Malaria Prevention Services in the same campaign was effectively carried out by A. G. Adamson.[(104c)]

There were of course those who took part in the Normandy Beach landings. But they were not the first. The night before the main assault on the beaches an Airborne Division parachuted into Normandy. Among them a young medical officer, now a senior Fellow, was dropped some twenty-five miles beyond the intended British line. He had to rely for forty-eight hours on his ingenuity to escape capture; and on his penetrating rendering of Scottish songs to secure safe entry to the British position. Subsequently this same medical officer was involved in the Ardenne Bulge emergency, and in parachuting over the Rhine as a preliminary to the advance on the Baltic.*[(105)]

The experiences of another future Fellow about this time were no less hair-raising. He was attached to a Marine Commando involved in the capture of the small key port of En-Bessine. Having swum a mile or so ashore after his landing craft had struck a mine, he attended to casualties while 'lurking' Jacobite fashion, knowing the enemy to be in front and to the rear. As the Marines closed in they were exposed to the additional hazard of fire from a flak vessel in the harbour below, and from flame throwers in the hills above. Later this same Commando was given the even tougher assignment of capturing Walcheren Island which, still in enemy hands, prevented effective allied use of the recently captured port of Antwerp. Gilbertian experiences were not lacking. The youthful captain of almost thirty years ago remembers his bewilderment and ignorance of the Geneva Convention when in the heat of battle he had consigned to his care an uninjured captured enemy naval doctor; and his incredulity on another occasion when he learnt that his rucksack, lost many months previously when swimming ashore, had come into the possession of an unknown Field Ambulance Medical Officer, now a Fellow of the College.[(106)] More than 130 years previously a future President (David Maclagan) had seen active service on the Island of Walcheren as medical officer attached to the 91st Regiment.[(107)]

* R. M. Marquis.

z

Not everyone was so fortunate: there were those who were captured. Of these, two M.O.s in the 51st Highland Division were made prisoners at St Valery and only released at the end of the War.[108, 109] Another of today's Fellows experienced the hardships of captivity in Siam and of the notorious 'Burma Road'. Even in this worst of environments there were modest Burns Suppers and improvised St Andrew's Day celebrations—'free to all' including Dutch allies—and occasions for subtle vocal rendering of 'Nipp off, Nippon'.[110] By way of contrast, another future Fellow and Office Bearer, who escaped after capture in North Africa, was able to commence his medical studies while interned in Switzerland.[111]

To turn to other campaigns, Melville Arnott was one who experienced a peripatetic existence. A mutual friend's account best describes events. Posted to Shanghai he (Arnott) then went to Hong Kong. Shanghai fell. From Hong Kong he was sent to Singapore. Hong Kong fell. Next he went to the Middle East. Singapore fell. In the MEF he was in Tobruk, and then in Jerusalem. Tobruk fell. A rumour went round that everyone in Jerusalem packed their bags when they learnt that 'Evacuation Arnott' was coming there. Later Arnott held the post of Officer i/c Medical Division in the 23rd (Scottish) General Hospital where he organized courses of outstanding value for the further education of serving doctors.[104c]

The experiences in North Africa of yet another Fellow were very different. Disembarking at Basra his Division moved to the transit camp at Shaiba where he came across Alastair Bruce who was Officer i/c Medical Division of a base hospital. From Shaiba cattle trucks served as transport to Kirkuk for Divisional training. Thereafter the Division set out for Tunisia via Jordan, Palestine, Egypt, Libya and Tripolitania and went into action at Enfidaville. After a further period of training the Division took part in the landing at Salerno. The building previously earmarked as an Advanced Dressing Station proved to be a Collective Farm; and before the arrival of casualties, unattended cows had to be milked and the stalls cleaned. 'The milk went into a large cauldron together with hens and rabbits on the farm and bully beef from rations to make a magnificent stew.'

In due course the troops advanced northwards and were involved in the crossing of the Garigliano river and the assault of Monte Cassino. The culmination came when they were sent as reinforcements to Anzio. During a subsequent rest period in Egypt the Fellow (R. M. Johnstone) went for a period to the Staff College at Haifa and there, in his own words, his 'acquaintance with the Old Testament helped greatly in solving the tactical problems being studied'. On two occasions—at Enfidaville and at Salerno—Johnstone had to take over the duties of acting C.O. after his Commanding Officer had been killed in action.[111a]

The experiences of those associated with the 7th General Hospital, Crete were in many respects unique. On his way to the island one Fellow★ was hove to for a lengthy period in the Mediterranean, the ship's engines having broken down. An aerial torpedo attack only narrowly missed the motionless target. New arrivals to the island were entranced by the beauty of the mountains, the colours of the rampant wild flowers, the olive groves and the vineyards. The hospital itself was attractively sited, but was handicapped by the total absence of nurses and by having only one source of water. Normal routine was carried out despite exposure of the hospital camp during air-raids in the vicinity to the fire of enemy machine guns and shrapnel from anti-aircraft defences. A visit was paid by General Freyberg V.C.; several hundred patients were evacuated by hospital ship; a number of aircraft were seen to be brought down and on one occasion those in the hospital had a grandstand view of a naval action at night.

The hospital was suddenly faced with a critical situation on the morning of 20th May (1941). In the words of an eye-witness: 'Planes appeared immediately overhead in large numbers—seemingly in hundreds—and of all sorts including gliders; and started to bomb and machine gun the hospital from a very low height. . . . Some of the tents went up in smoke and . . . parachutists landed and proceeded to round up some patients and orderlies whom they marched away.' After an interval New Zealand troops arrived and ordered the removal of the hospital camp to caves in the coastal cliffs. Patients numbering not less than 500 were distributed among five caves, of which one was reserved for dysentery cases. Cave existence continued for five or six days—'lying doggo all day and bringing up rations after dark'.[111b] A vivid if modest account of the work carried out in the 'cave hospital' has been recorded by Debenham.[111c]

In the caves, the progress of fighting on the island could only be guessed by the nearness or otherwise of the sound of gunfire. However on 25th May, orders were received to evacuate the caves and move towards the south coast. Those too ill to be moved were left behind with two medical officers and 30 orderlies. The remainder set out in two parties on a trek across the island. Roads were tortuous, mainly hilly, often precipitous and throughout indescribably rough. Movement was more or less restricted to hours of darkness. Progress was hampered by civilian refugees from bombed villages heading for the mountains, and by the number of walking wounded and vehicles causing congestion. Water was scarce. The footwear of many was soleless.

At long last at 3 a.m. on 30th May the beach appointed for evacuation was reached. The shadowy outline of destroyers lying offshore could just be made out in the dark.

★ W. L. Lamb.

Those from the 7th General Hospital after their trek of more than four days were 'only files from the boat' (ferrying troops to the destroyers) when they were told 'no more to-night'. The destroyers stole away silently into the darkness of the night. As the Fellow of the College who was there laconically recorded—'And that was that'.

There followed a day of uncertainty spent under improvised cover in a badly blitzed village but at 2.30 a.m. (31st May) a hail from the shore was the preliminary to embarkation on a destroyer of the Royal Australian Navy (H.M.A.S. *Napier*). With little delay she sped in company with another destroyer for Alexandria. Relaxed and sleeping in a cabin put at his disposal by a Ship's Officer the Fellow was roused by 'a shattering and deafening noise from the destroyer's A.A. guns firing just above the cabin at nine Stuka dive-bombers'. Violent evasive action saved the vessel from direct hits but not from damage. Frames and shell plates were buckled and propulsion impaired, compelling reduction in speed, but British aeroplanes appeared on the scene and escorted her safely to Alexandria. So ended one individual's experience of Crete.[111b] But there was an ironic outcome of evacuation for the Lieutenant-Colonel. As a mutual friend, and *not* the Fellow himself, wryly remarked—'His reward, reversion to his former rank of major: his job had gone with the invasion'.[104c]

And how did those on foreign service react? As one physician, who from Norway went to Crete and thence to the Middle East before landing in Normandy, wrote: 'I saw a lot of the World and had at the time plenty of opportunity to practise good medicine and learn something about tropical diseases'. Even if everyone was not so appreciative, there are none who would not agree with his: 'I saw the British Tommy at his best and was very proud to be of some small use to him'. Continuing in a way reminiscent of Melville Dunlop Senior in 1915, the writer goes on: 'I was also proud of British Medicine as a whole; for the organisation and standards in the Middle East were very high and the Edinburgh Medical and Our College played no small part in this'.

As to the other armed services—true to its reputation, the silence of the Navy made it more difficult to obtain information from those serving in it. Many R.A.M.C. officers en route to new postings had experience of the hazards of warfare at sea—mines, submarine attacks and aerial bombardment. They were on occasion the victims of the most circuitous of voyages, and at least one medical officer returning home on leave from Cairo spent four months at sea.[111b] In their pre-College days several present-day Fellows served on destroyers hunting U-Boat packs or escorting convoys on the Murmansk or North Atlantic routes. Another Surgeon-Lieutenant was attached to large landing ships in the Far East. One of these young doctors was a son of the Commodore of the Cunard Steamship Company in command for a period of the 'trooper' *Queen Mary*. These doctors were all volunteers 'for the duration'. Reginald Seggar, who was appointed College Officer after 23½ years in the Royal Navy, was recalled to the colours and won a mention in dispatches for his skill and devotion to duty in charge of a Bomb and Mine Disposal Unit.[111d]

In a different category was a Surgeon-Lieutenant Commander R.N., whose wartime service certainly did not lack incident. On board H.M.S. *Royal Oak* when she was sunk at anchor in Scapa Flow by a succession of torpedoes on target, he was thrown into the sea as the battleship turned turtle. Surfacing, there yawned above him the stern and propellers of the rapidly sinking vessel—a vision, with its warning of the possibility of being sucked under, known to many of those who were torpedoed while serving in the Royal Navy and Mercantile Marine. Swimming in sea laden with oil he in time secured a handhold on the freeboard of an upturned boat. The night was coal black. There was no glimmer of light to suggest the coming of rescue craft—whereupon the dozen or so survivors hanging precariously to their upturned boat, broke into song. Their choice: 'Daisy, Daisy, give me your answer do'. *Daisy* was the name of the drifter attached as tender to *Royal Oak*.[112]

For the Surgeon-Commander there lay ahead a period of service in H.M.S. *Prince of Wales*, then the last word in British capital ships. During her commission over some ten months she was visited by H.M. King George VI; carried Mr Winston Churchill to the meeting with President Roosevelt and the signing of the Atlantic Charter; and acted as escort to a vital Malta convoy. Only a few weeks after acceptance trials *Prince of Wales*, in company with H.M.S. *Hood* sighted the enemy cruiser *Prince Eugene* and pocket-battleship *Bismarck*. A converging course was set and *Prince of Wales* followed *Hood* closely astern and a slight degree to starboard. *Hood* was the proud unmodernized 1924 product of Clydebank and in many respects was as impressive as the earlier graceful vessels of the *Queen Elizabeth* class. Straddled, she was then hit amidships by a plunging shell, caught fire, exploded and sank. Of her crew of about 1200 men only three survived. Herself damaged by enemy fire, *Prince of Wales* had to alter helm to avoid the wreckage of the *Hood*.

In due course there came the sudden silent departure for Singapore. Within ten days of arrival there, *Prince of Wales* in company with H.M.S. *Repulse* and four escorting destroyers but no air escort, set sail. Both capital vessels were lost as a result of massive concentrated low and high level air attacks by the Japanese. From his action station on the bridge signal-deck of *Prince of Wales*, the surgeon who had survived the loss of *Royal Oak* was witness to the holocaust which developed in Malayan waters. In many respects his experiences beggar description—seeing

Repulse, a half to a mile distant astern and to starboard, mauled, savaged, rendered helpless and eventually keeling over prior to sinking; and knowing the ominous sickening upward lurch of the *Prince of Wales* as torpedo after torpedo tore into her hull. Casualties were dressed and given morphia: those unable to look after themselves were carried and placed inside Carley floats, and many were taken off by a destroyer manoeuvred alongside the quarter-deck.

Before *Prince of Wales*, listing heavily, finally slipped beneath the waves, hundreds of sailors waited in amazingly relaxed fashion on the fo'c'sle. As the Surgeon-Commander awaited his turn to go overboard he heard a nearby sailor encourage a shipmate with: 'Come on chum, all these explosions'll have frightened the blinkin' sharks away'.

Once again, the surgeon survived. By an extraordinary coincidence he was rescued by H.M.S. *Electra*, the same destroyer which on 25th May 1941 had 'picked up' the sole survivors of the *Hood*. He survived to become Director General of the Medical Services of the Royal Navy.

If the Navy was silent, the Royal Air Force was elusive when approached. To the uninitiated the reaction of a medical of Squadron Leader rank may provide the explanation. Having referred to certain gruesome incidents, he said: ' "Penguins" lived more or less normal lives in pleasant R.A.F. buildings whilst the fighting went on miles away in the sky—giving my war service an air of unreality'. Others again, attached to fighter stations subjected to frequent, selective air attack, knew conditions experienced by Medical Officers in the A.R.P. services of 'blitzed' cities.

In far Bangalore, a Flight-Lieutenant, into whose ken the College had scarcely entered, had occasion to obtain consultant advice from Delhi, some fifteen hundred miles distant. The clinical problem was jaundice; the suspected diagnosis, yellow fever contracted in West Africa en route for India; the consultant's diagnosis, epidemic jaundice. On boarding his plane to return, the consultant (Brigadier J. D. S. Cameron) commented 'My longest domiciliary visit ever!'[113]

How many members of the College were engaged in hospital and civil defence duties is unknown. Certainly they were many, and of them large numbers combined their duties in civil defence and evacuee services with their work in hospital and general practice. Those serving overseas were not unmindful of this. Not a few remarked upon 'the immense strain imposed on the older and senior men left at home to carry on, many of whom knew harder times than those abroad'.

Inevitably in so far as the College is concerned, mention of the war service of members relates almost solely to those with temporary commissions, or commissions in the Territorial Army or the Volunteer Reserves of the Navy and Air Force. This does not imply disregard of the considerable contribution of Fellows with commissions in the regular army. Major-General Sir Alexander Biggam, an Honorary Fellow of the College, was well known for his distinguished military career in France, India, Egypt and elsewhere and for the success which afterwards attended his period as Director of Study at the Edinburgh Post-Graduate Board for Medicine. During World War II he was appointed Professor of Tropical Medicine and Consulting Physician to the Army.

Some idea of the peregrinations and variety of experiences of a regular army medical officer 'during and between wars' can be gleaned from what is virtually an autobiographical article which appeared in the Glasgow Journal *Surgo* in 1960.[114] The writer of the article, a Fellow of the College, would attach greatest importance to his first encounter with bubonic plague among Indian troops serving in the Middle East, to problems encountered in dealing with leptospirosis in Malaysia, and to measures developed to secure the return to a full life and even active service of Gurkha soldiers with proven active pulmonary tuberculosis. The last mentioned was the subject of a leading article and annotation in the *Lancet*.[115, 116]

After World War II the Fellow in question had other experiences of an almost unique kind. He was responsible for the medical care of a number of highest ranking military prisoners and was required to give advice as to their fitness to stand trial.[116a]

THE INDIAN MEDICAL SERVICE

Scots medical men played a notable part in the creation and development of the Indian Medical Service and in the service of the East India Company. The list of those who contributed contains the names of doctors from all the Scottish Universities and a number who were Licentiates of the Royal College of Surgeons of Edinburgh. Unfortunately for the period in question there are no reliable records of Licentiates of the Royal College of Physicians of Edinburgh and sight may well have been lost of many who were associated in one way or another with the Physicians' College. Nevertheless, within comparatively recent years certain Fellows earned considerable distinction in the Indian Medical Service and some of their number on retirement gave both direct and signal service to the College. Their names merit special recording.

There was Sir Robert Charles MacWatt who having seen active service on the North-West Frontier eventually became Director-General of the Indian Medical Service, and who at one time was adviser to General Maharajah Sir Ganga Singh, ruler of the State of Bikanir.[117] Edward David Wilson Greig served on Commissions appointed to investigate the epidemicity of such conditions as plague, cholera and dysentery.[118] Then there was the distinguished trio of I.M.S. Lieutenant-Colonels who on retiral home, co-operated in contributing to the continued success of the College Laboratory (Chap. V), A. G. McKendrick as Superintendent, W. F. Harvey as Pathologist and W. G. Liston as Bacteriologist. The previous records of these three men had been distinguished. After serving in the Somaliland Expedition of 1904, McKendrick became Director of the Pasteur Institute at Kasauli. Rabies was one of his subjects of research, and in the course of time he was appointed Statistician for Rabies on behalf of the League of Nations.[119] Associated in his earlier days with Almroth Wright and Karl Pearson, Harvey became the Director of the Central Research Institute in India, at Kasauli.[120] Pearson's son has paid tribute to Harvey's lack of bias and to his balanced judgment when dealing simultaneously with two such controversial figures as Wright and Pearson.[121] To this day there is in the possession of Harvey's family a signed portrait of Garibaldi. A legacy to Harvey, the portrait had originally been dedicated to a great aunt (Miss Jessie White) who had married an Italian Count—Count Mario—and had provided the frontispiece illustration to a publication of the Countess's posthumous papers.[122, 123]

Plague and malaria were among Liston's main interests and he established, as had been suspected earlier, that plague was essentially a disease of rats, almost always carried by rat-fleas from rat to rat and from rat to man. He served on the India Plague Commission, and on return home was appointed Consulting Physician to the Colonial Office.[124] Notwithstanding the recognition accorded Liston's work during his life-time, the greatest tribute was the posthumous presentation in 1971 of the Karl F. Meyer award by the American Veterinary Epidemiology Society.[125]

Well known to the profession in Edinburgh in his capacity as Superintendent of the Royal Infirmary, Colonel Alexander Dron Stewart had a distinguished World War I record, serving in Egypt, Gallipoli and Iraq and being mentioned in dispatches. Before leaving India he was Professor of Hygiene in the Calcutta School of Tropical Medicine and Hygiene and the First Director of the All-India Institute of Hygiene and Public Health.[126]

The Indian Medical Service was finally dissolved in August 1947 and on 15th July 1969 Sir Robert Hay, K.C.I.E., M.B., Ch.B., D.P.H., who was the last Director General of the Service, was elected an Honorary Fellow of the College. At the same time the Honorary Fellowship was conferred on another erstwhile distinguished physician in India—Sir George Reid McRobert, C.I.E., M.D., F.R.C.P.Lond.

Although perhaps not all so well known to many of the Fellows, there are other distinguished Members of the Indian Medical Service with College links whose names should be mentioned. There was Dr Maung Shwe Zan, a graduate of the University of Edinburgh. Having successfully led his patients and hospital staff out of Burma at the time of the retreat in World War II, he returned to give similar help to others in need. Ultimately he became Professor of Medicine at the University of Rangoon.[127] On retiral from the I.M.S., Lt.-Col. R. V. Morrison was appointed to the Chair of Pathology and later of Medicine at the same University.[128] Lt.-Col. J. H. Barrett was another who became Professor at Rangoon University—in his case—of Anatomy. He entered the I.M.S. after serving in France and took part in campaigns in Burma, Rangoon and Mandalay.[129] The career of Brigadier D. M. Fraser was as varied as it was distinguished. He served as a combatant in World War I and then after graduating in Medicine joined the I.M.S. Following active service on the North-Western Frontier, Fraser returned to civilian employment as a radiologist. In World War II he was created D.D.M.S. with the rank of Brigadier in the 44th Indian Army Division. Later he became the first Director of Health Services in Delhi Province but returned to this country where he secured an appointment as Consultant Radiologist in Liverpool, and continued research on filariasis.[130]

It is convenient at this stage to mention a few Fellows of the College from India and Pakistan who although not in the I.M.S. made a notable success of their professional careers. There were two doctors of the name of Rao of whom one (D.L.N.M.) obtained a Chair in the All-India Institute of Mental Health, Bangalore,[131] and the other (K.K.V.), having studied under Sir Robert Philip, became Professor of Tuberculosis at the Madras and Stanley Medical College.[132] Others who attained professorial status were Drs Premankur De, at the National Medical College, Calcutta; A. M. Kassim at the Dow Medical College, Karachi; P. N. Bardhan and O. P. Malhotra at the Armed Forces Medical College, Poona; and Amir Chand at Lahore Medical College. Professor Kassim was a Fellow of the American College of Chest Physicians, and of the College of Physicians and Surgeons of Pakistan. At the time of his death it was written of him that 'His greatest pride was that he had trained some of the young men of Pakistan, who, in recent years, have become Members of the Royal College of Physicians of Edinburgh. British medicine has lost one of her potentially great Ambassadors in Asia and the world at large.'[133] After retirement, Professor Bardhan became Director of the Central Leprosy Training and Research Institute; Lt.-Col. Malhotra (Indian Army Medical Corps) was personal physician to Prime Minister Nehru; and Major-General Amir Chand became Chairman of the Indian Council of Medical Research Review Committee, and President of the All-India Medical Association.[134]

In 1966 Colonel Mohy Din, a Member of the College, paid a visit to the College when in Edinburgh in his capacity as personal physician to President Ayub of Pakistan.[135] The following year Dr V. T. H. Gunaratne, F.R.C.P.Ed. was elected President of the Twentieth World Health Assembly.[136]

PEACE-TIME COMMUNITY ACTIVITIES

From the earliest days of the College, Fellows have had interests outside their professional activities. The Original Fellows were no exception. Thus Pitcairne is remembered in history as poet as well as physician. Robert Sibbald was outstanding in the multiplicity of his interests which have been recalled by Smout in a way deserving quotation. 'Sibbald', Smout wrote, 'began the first Scottish investigations into archaeology, and into the natural history of fish, birds, plants and whales, founding the botanical gardens at Edinburgh as a herbarium about 1667, and being commemorated to-day in the names of Sibbald's rorqual, the blue whale, the largest of all animals, and of *Sibbaldia procumbens*, one of the smallest and rarest British alpine flowers. He also carried Timothy Pont's geographical work a stage further by initiating the first surveys of the coasts, carried out by John Adair, and by collecting the first detailed topographical descriptions of different Scottish regions later published in Macfarlane's *Geographical Collections* and the inspiration and the model for Sir John Sinclair's eighteenth-century *Statistical Account of Scotland*. It was from his wide curiosity that there developed the first living traditions of study in many natural sciences.'[137]

Wrongly, medical corporations have from time to time been described as being exclusive, and their individual Fellows as tending to be aloof. Certainly in so far as the Edinburgh College of Physicians is concerned, and more especially in so far as more modern times are concerned, this is not difficult to refute. The part played by Fellows and Members in two World Wars has been touched upon, but only touched upon. There is the other side of the picture: participation between wars in the social life and activities of the community. Again no more than a superficial indication can be given, but sufficient to give an idea of the variety of interests enjoyed extra-murally as it were by individuals constituting the College corporate.

Royal Physicians in Scotland

Royal physicians of the sixteenth century were customarily designated 'mediciners', but the seventeenth century saw the appointment of a Principal (or First) Physician and a varying number of Physicians-in-Ordinary. After 1714 there was only one Physician-in-Ordinary and he was sometimes referred to as the Second Physician. Appointments of Physicians-in-Ordinary ceased after 1847. The office of First Physician lapsed in 1844 on the death of the holder, Dr John Abercrombie.

The first to be appointed Principal Mediciner was John Craig, the Scottish physician taken to England by James VI in 1603 (Chap. I): and the second was (Sir) Archibald Stevensone who took up office on 12th November 1681, less than three weeks before the College was granted its Charter of Erection. With two exceptions subsequent Principal Physicians were all Fellows of the Royal College of Physicians of Edinburgh—Sir Thomas Burnet, Doctors Thomas Dalrymple, Andrew Sinclair, Robert Whytt (recorded as Whyte, but with date of death corresponding to Robert Whytt), John Gregory, William Cullen, Joseph Black, James Gregory, Andrew Duncan, sen. and John Abercrombie.

In the list of Ordinary Physicians, the first name of interest from the College point of view is that of Dr Alexander Ramsay who headed the list of signatories appended to new proposals for a College of Physicians, following the death of Dr George Sibbald (Chap. II). Ramsay is known to have held office from about 1631 until his death in 1650. During the years 1660–74 a similar appointment was held by Sir Robert Cunningham (an ancestor of the President of the College from 1756 to 1763). There were fifteen Ordinary Physicians during the inclusive period 1672–1853 and all were Fellows of the College, two of whom were to become First Physician. The complete list consisted of (Sir) Thomas Burnet, (Sir) David Hay, (Sir) Archibald Stevensone, (Sir) Andrew Balfour, (Sir) Robert Sibbald, Thomas Dalrymple, (Sir) Edward Eizat, George Mackenzie, William Douglas, Alexander Dundas, James Lidderdale, Francis Home, James Home, Andrew Combe and John Scott.[138] George Mackenzie was the physician associated with Heriot's Hospital (Chap. XX) and his ardent political leanings may explain why his appointment by Queen Anne in 1714 was not renewed by King George I.

At the present time appointments as Physicians to the Royal Household in Scotland are made on the recommendation of the Lord Chamberlain after consultation with the Scottish Home and Health Department.

The Royal Company of Archers

Membership of the Royal Company of Archers is to be regarded as an activity on a plane of its own. The author was corrected in no uncertain fashion when he suggested it might be included among current select sporting or social activities! He was sternly reminded of the ancient origins of the bodyguard with its technically para-military background. Not a few Fellows have been members of the Royal Company of Archers for Scotland and one of Raeburn's masterpieces depicts a President of the College, Dr Nathaniel Spens, wearing the uniform of the Company in which he was an Adjutant-General.

Sporting Activities

There have been and are anglers, climbers and yachtsmen innumerable. Sir Byrom Bramwell was an enthusiastic angler. It is possible that he acquired this from William Stewart, author of the *Practical Angler*, with whom as a student he once shared rooms. What is certain is that his enthusiasm led to his two professorial sons taking up the art.[139] While the tales of fishermen do not always bear scrutiny, it is on record that Dr J. P. Leckie created history in his day when he sailed round Great Britain in an engineless yacht,[140] and there are few who have not heard of the climbing feats in mature age of Sir Robert Christison[141] or of Dr Andrew Duncan's annual pilgrimages, continued until he was over eighty years of age, to the top of Arthur's Seat. Duncan had many other extraordinary interests. Elsewhere an indication has been given of his part in the founding of the Royal Edinburgh Asylum and the Royal Public Dispensary. In addition, he was largely instrumental in obtaining Charters for the Royal Medical Society and the Royal Caledonian Horticultural Society: and in founding a Gymnastic Club. Apparently too Duncan had time for golf because it is on record that when aged fifty years he and his five-year-old son were soundly trounced by septuagenarian Alexander Wood and his grandson aged seven.[142] It was Duncan's custom to befriend promising young men, one of whom was (Sir) Henry Raeburn the artist: and Duncan's tombstone has around it small memorial stones erected to the memory of some of his students.

Within recent times, at least two golfing Fellows, J. L. Cowan and J. Lawson were Members of the Royal and Ancient Club.[143, 144] Both had distinguished war service records; Dr Cowan was a Justice of the Peace and Dr Lawson in addition to being a Member of the University Court of St Andrews was a Member of the Scottish Hospitals Endowment Research Trust. A man of great versatility and charm, an A.R.C.M. and L.R.A.M., Dr J. B. McDougall played for Scotland at Rugby both before and after World War I during which he commanded Number 30 General Hospital at Calais, and after which he became Director of the British Legion Village in

Kent. An authority on tuberculosis, he acted as adviser to U.N.R.R.A. and the World Health Organization, and as Secretary to the Joint Tuberculosis Council.[145] Harking further back in time, one of the Licentiates of 1879 was none other than the famous cricketer, Dr W. G. Grace.[146] Nor is it out of place to mention the prowess of Professor Alexander Kennedy as an amateur boxer. His other activities included professional broadcasting and playwriting for the radio medium: and among his research subjects was the psychology of parachute training.[147]

Exploration: Philately

Dr J. H. H. Pirie's claim to mention is unique. Following graduation he went to the Antarctic as a medical scientist with the Mawson Expedition, and after serving in East Africa with the R.A.M.C. in World War I, joined the South African Institute for Medical Research of which he eventually became Acting Director. Plague was one of his particular studies. A philatelist of note, he possessed a well-known collection of stamps.[148] Another Fellow with philatelic interests was Dr J. C. Webster who became Professor of Gynaecology and Obstetrics at Rush Medical College, Chicago. When a research student in Edinburgh he sold a collection of stamps for £5, to learn later to his mortification that a number of stamps in the collection were each worth £100.[149]

Botany

Botany has been a major hobby with some Fellows. Dr C. H. Fox was a Member of both the Botanical Society and the Society of Antiquaries of Scotland[150]: and Dr R. Brooks Popham was another recognized botanist who for a number of years was Surgeon to the Mission to Deep Sea Fishermen.[151] A native of Ceylon (Sri Lanka) Dr Andrew W. E. Soysa was an expert in the cultivation of orchids of which several varieties are named after his wife and himself.[152] In command of the Medical Division of a Military Hospital in Ceylon during World War II, Dr Soysa did not disguise his pride in being connected with the R.A.M.C., and he and Dr J. D. S. Cameron knew immense mutual pleasure when the former acted as host to Dr Cameron who was touring the Commonwealth.[153]

Astronomy seems to have found little favour but Dr Ernest Watt was Vice-President of the Edinburgh Astronomical Society.[154] Dr James Burnet was another with unusual interests. He was a Fellow of the British Esperanto Association, and of the Institute of Linguists.[155]

Music and Education

Dr John Orr, a busy General Practitioner, was Chairman of the Directors of the Edinburgh Concert Society. Such was his impact on the Society that on his death, as a tribute to his memory, the Scottish Orchestra played the 'Nimrod' variation from Elgar's 'Enigma' *Variations*. In the College he was industriously involved in the affairs of the School of Medicine for sixty years and his interest in medical education took him to the U.S.A., Canada and India.[156] Another who travelled far in the interests of medical education was Sir Norman Walker, successor to Sir Donald MacAlister as President of the General Medical Council. He paid two official visits to India and two less formal visits to the U.S.A. in this connection.[157]

The Mission Fields

Others found their interests in very different fields not entirely divorced from their professional activities. Dr Ella Pringle, the first lady to be elected a Fellow, was a well-known missionary in Manchuria. Born in 1880, she obtained the Membership in 1925 and became a Fellow four years later.[158] An even more widely known medical missionary was Dr George Keppie Paterson who was associated for more than fifty years with the Edinburgh Medical Mission and Cowgate Dispensary. He visited Damascus on no fewer than eight occasions in order to report to his Directors on the progress of missionary work in Palestine.[159]

Religious principles exercised a notably profound effect on the professional careers of two other Fellows. Dr G. R. E. G. Mackay served with the Argyll and Sutherland Highlanders in World War I being awarded the Military Cross with bar and the Italian Bronze Medal. In 1938 he gave up his practice in Edinburgh in order to devote his energies to Moral Rearmament.[160] The case of Father Joseph Whitaker was rather different. The son of a celebrated teacher of anatomy, he was awarded the Military Cross for gallantry while serving with the Royal Field Artillery in 1914. On his return from Flanders he took the Triple Qualification and M.B., B.S.London. A Roman Catholic, he took Holy Orders, and in the course of time was appointed in succession as Chaplain to Liverpool and Glasgow Universities before undertaking pastoral work in the Orkneys and Shetlands.[161]

The professional career in earlier years of Dr David Daniel Davis was equally unusual. A Welshman, he intended to go in for the ministry but on matriculation at Glasgow University combined studies in the Arts with others leading to a medical degree. After graduating M.D. in 1801 he practised medicine in the north of England and for some years gave service also as a nonconformist minister. In 1804 Davis was appointed physician to Sheffield General Infirmary but moved nine years later to London where he developed his special interests in midwifery and was in the course of time selected for the post of physician-accoucheur for the birth of the future Queen Victoria. Although present at the birth Davis did not take an active part in the delivery. It has been said that his 'recognition (1836) of the transmissible nature of puerperal fever' predated the classic descriptions of Oliver Wendell Holmes (1843) and Semmelweis (1846).

Davis was admitted to the Fellowship of our College shortly before he moved to London, by which time he had given up the ministry and taken out a patent for a not wholly successful propulsive mechanism for canal barges. His third son (Edward Davis) was a gifted sculptor and a bust by him of his father is on view at the University College Hospital Medical School, London, where Daniel Davis was Professor in Midwifery.[162, 163]

Scholarship

'A scholar physician' was the enviable description applied to Dr Adam Patrick, who was Professor of Medicine at the University of St Andrews, and President of the Scottish Society of the History of Medicine.[164] Drs J. D. Comrie and Douglas Guthrie come into the same category in virtue of their major writings on the history of Scottish Medicine. Dr H. Graham Langwill, a Fellow and nephew of the Scottish historian Henry Gray Graham, wrote among other papers, a monograph on stammering with which he had been afflicted and which was cured by Dr John Wyllie, the author of an early classic on aphasia.[165]

Civic Honours and Activities

A striking number of the Fellows of the College have taken an active part in civic affairs. Chronologically Monro *secundus* has legitimate claim to pride of place. He was appointed under one of the earliest Burgh Police Statutes in Scotland to be a Commissioner with responsibilities in connection with the 'cleansing, lighting and watching the South Side of . . . Edinburgh'.[166] At a later date Dr Alexander Wood also held office as a Police Commissioner. On one occasion his duties involved leading a contingent of special constables up the Mound through volleys of stones hurled at them by a hostile crowd as the constables made their way to the Meadows to suppress a seditious meeting.[167] This same Alexander Wood after retirement from active medicine became interested in the establishment of the Edinburgh Tramway Company of which he became chairman.

Sir James Alexander Russell was Lord Provost of Edinburgh for the period 1891–94[168] and Dr G. F. Barbour Simpson, grand-nephew of Sir J. Y. Simpson, was a Member of Edinburgh Town Council for twelve years.[169] Across the water in Fife, Dr A. L. S. Tuke, youngest son of a former President, Sir Batty Tuke, M.P., was a Free Burgess of the Royal Burgh of Dunfermline and a Deputy Lieutenant of the County of Fife. A general practitioner in Dunfermline for sixty years he held a unique position among fellow practitioners and the community at large.[170] An Orcadian by birth and contemporary of Sir Batty Tuke, Sir Thomas Clouston was made a Freeman of the town of Kirkwall in recognition of his life-long interest in the affairs of his native islands.[171] Two others who were appointed Deputy Lieutenants were Dr E. Bulmer for Warwickshire[172] and Dr J. Kinnear for the City of Dundee.[173] Dr P. M. Tolmie of Nairn having retired from practice became in succession Town Councillor, Dean of Guild, Baillie and Provost[174]; and in Wales, Dr D. R. Lewis, a Governor of the National Library of Wales, was appointed a High Sheriff of the County of Brecknock.[175]

Reverting to the early days of the College particular interest attaches to Dr John Boswell, President in the years 1770–2 and previously Treasurer on two occasions. In 1748 he was made 'burges and freeman of the Burgh of Musselburgh' in recognition of 'the singular regard' in which he was held: and Boswell's Court on the south side of Castle Hill in the Royal Mile, Edinburgh is named after him.[176] John Boswell was the last British student to be promoted M.D. by Boerhaave at the University of Leyden. A son (Robert) and grandson (Alexander) were successive Clerks to the College and a nephew, James Boswell, was biographer of Samuel Johnson.[177]

In quite another sphere Dr G. S. Brock[178] and Dr W. Hughes[179] held appointments to British Embassies, the former at Rome, and the latter at Tokyo where he was Professor of Medicine in the Japanese Medical School. Two Fellows of the College were appointed Honorary Physician to the Governor General of New Zealand. The first of these, Dr J. R. Boyd, was a Founder Member of the Royal Australasian College of Physicians and a prize was established by his colleagues in his name in recognition of his services in peace and war.[180] The second, another Founder

Member of the Australasian College, who was Director of Medical Services of the New Zealand Army and Air Force in 1940, was Sir Fred Bowerbank.[181]

In a racy autobiography Bowerbank described how studying for the Edinburgh Membership was more difficult for the older candidate than for the young. However he was successful at his first attempt, although losing a stone in weight in the process! He recalled the value to him in general practice of experience gained in the Cowgate Dispensary, and of how when visiting one district 'a woman opened the door and in we went to find ourselves in a large lofty room with 3 or 4 shakedowns on the floor, a table, some chairs and little else. There was a hugh fireplace and above it was the coat of arms of the once aristocratic owners . . .'.[182] Nor had Bowerbank forgotten his Edinburgh venereologist's dictum in the days of mercury and potassium iodide— 'One night with Venus means two years with Mercury'.[183] Referring to the primitive instruments upon which the Edinburgh Biochemical Laboratory was dependent and contrasting them with the facilities available in the wealthy Rockefeller Foundation he made the comment: 'I may be prejudiced, but this lack of finance seemed to stimulate the real research student'.[184] Those whom Bowerbank met and had discussions with when he re-visited Edinburgh included Drs W. T. Ritchie, Rae Gilchrist, C. P. Stewart and (Sir) Derrick Dunlop.[185, 186]

It would be presumptuous and incautious to make selective reference to Fellows and Members who have achieved great professional distinction during the last twenty or thirty years. That is a task for whomsoever is responsible in the future for continuing the History of the College. The College however has been associated with certain events in medical progress, varying in significance but meriting brief mention as events rather than as achievements of individuals.

Service on National Committees

To mention by name the many Fellows who have served on important National Advisory Committees is quite impracticable. Indeed the same can be said of the not inconsiderable number of Fellows appointed Chairmen of such Committees during the last thirty years or so. Suffice to say that in the course of their activities these Fellows have contributed to national policy in such varied fields as the use and dangers of drugs, cancer, radio-active isotope services, health services for the Highlands and Islands and the training of health visitors. In 1969 a Past President was appointed Chairman of the Scottish Council for Postgraduate Medical Education— being the first to be so appointed. He was succeeded by another past President.

An unusual appointment accepted by yet another past President on the invitation of the Lord Provost was the Chairmanship of the Medical Committee for the Commonwealth Games in Edinburgh in 1970. There were nine sub-committees which between them dealt with such subjects as Tropical Medicine, Orthopaedics, sexing entrants for women's events and testing for 'pep-drugs'.

Research

Of Dr William M. Court Brown it can be said without reservation that despite his untimely death at the age of fifty he acquired an international reputation as a result of his work on cytogenetics. The M.R.C. Research Unit in Edinburgh for the study of the Clinical Effects of Radiation of which he was Director made many discoveries concerning chromosomal abnormalities. Court Brown was given an Honorary Professorship by the University of Edinburgh.[187]

While working under Professor Sharpey-Schäfer, Dr (later Professor) P. T. Herring described the granules in the neurohypophysis which have come to be known as the 'Herring Bodies'.[188]

Administration

In the field of administration considerable credit was due to Dr A. M. Fraser who, in his capacity as Medical Officer of Health of the County and Borough of Inverness, contributed greatly to the establishment of consultant medical and obstetric services and the creation of a satisfactory Highlands and Islands Medical Fund. Fraser's efforts were effective in inducing general practitioners to continue practising in remote areas.[189] The posts of Chief Medical Officer of a number of Government Departments have been held by Fellows of the College. They include Sir Cuthbert G. Magee at the Ministry of Pensions[190] and Sir James M. McIntosh,[191] Sir Andrew Davidson,[192] Sir Kenneth Cowan and Sir John Brotherston, all of the Department of Health for Scotland (or later equivalent); and, Dr J. M. Rogan at the National Coal Board. McIntosh left to occupy in succession the post of Professor of Public Health at Glasgow University and a similar post at the London School of Hygiene and Tropical Medicine. Davidson was a Member of the Willink Committee. Sir Francis R. Fraser, son of Sir Thomas Fraser, became Director General of the Emergency Medical Services during World War II in succession to Sir John Hebb who, previously transferred to the Ministry of Health from the Ministry of Pensions, had already laid the foundations. During World War I Sir Francis was Consulting Physician to the British Army on the Rhine; and after World War II became Director of the British Post-Graduate Federation.[193] He was succeeded as Director at the (Royal) Medical Post-Graduate School at Hammersmith by another distinguished émigré of our College, Sir John McMichael whose name is associated with outstanding cardiological research.

Overseas Dr J. F. Campbell Halsam after distinguished military service in World War I and after three years as C.M.O. Barbados was appointed D.M.S. for Northern Rhodesia. He was largely responsible for the development of the Rhodesian Health Service and on retirement in 1947 was Chairman of the Silicosis Medical Bureau and of the African Affairs Board.[194]

Medical Exploration

In the clinico-administrative field of venereology a very considerable contribution was made by Dr L. W. Harrison. He served throughout the South African and 1914–18 Wars, being awarded the D.S.O. in the latter when he became adviser in venereal disease in Western Europe. Subsequently he was for a number of years adviser on his specialty to the Ministry of Health, and in the course of his work was given the Freeman Snow award of the American Society of Hygiene.[195] He was responsible in 1938 for a Report entitled *Anti-venereal measures in certain Scandinavian countries and Holland.*

Dr Alexander Brown's accomplishments as clinician, administrator and pioneer will long be remembered by Asians as well as Europeans, and by the laity as well as the medical profession. After being associated in Edinburgh with Sir Derrick Dunlop he joined the R.A.M.C. in 1946 and saw service in Sierra Leone. The war over, he again went out to Africa. With companions his purpose was to create a new University at Ibadan and this he achieved within ten years by which time a new medical school and teaching hospital were effectively functioning. Thereafter Professor Brown devoted much of his time and energy to the development of a rural health centre where students could be taught community health and where it was possible to carry out epidemiological research.[196] Brilliant as a student, Brown's life work will long be remembered for its vision and its compassion.

An interesting side-light was the bringing of the first insulin to Great Britain by Dr George C. Lambie. He was an outstanding instructor of junior students in clinical medicine; served in Mesopotamia, India and France winning the Military Cross in World War I; and eventually emigrated to Australia to become Professor of Medicine at the University of Sydney. One of the first to benefit from Lambie's importation of insulin was Sir Norman Walker.[197] Dr F. E. Reynolds had an unusually colourful career. Having studied in Wasserman's Laboratory he later joined the Plague Commission, with duties taking him as far afield as Siberia and China. His inborn love of horses led to the friendliest of relations with the Russian Cavalry. After being in charge of a hospital in the Middle East he became Professor of Pathology in Cairo.[198]

Mention of Cairo immediately brings to mind the work there of (Sir) Sydney A. Smith as Professor of Forensic Medicine. A pioneer in firearm identification he later occupied the Chair of Forensic Medicine at Edinburgh University becoming Dean of the Medical Faculty.[199] It is a measure of the esteem in which he was held that the students elected him to be their Rector. Greatly to his credit he gave the full weight of his support to the creation in 1941 of a war-time Polish School of Medicine in Edinburgh. During the time of its existence the School produced more than 225 doctors.[200] His popularity was rivalled by a much younger Fellow (Sir) James D. S. Cameron who retired four years before the customary age from his position as senior consultant physician to the Edinburgh Royal Infirmary and the Scottish Borders Group of Hospitals, in order to become adviser on medical education to the Government of East Pakistan. His accomplishments in Pakistan were monumental and in a short period of time he was Professor and first Director of the Institute of Post-Graduate Medicine at Dacca which was largely of his own creation. Among his many achievements as President on behalf of the College were the Founding of the St Andrew's Day Symposium and the inauguration of Conferences of Presidents of the Royal Colleges of Physicians. He was a Member of the Merit Award Committee and Consultant to W.H.O. on Medical Education in Baghdad and Alexandria.[201]

Sir Stanley Davidson is another Past President to whom the College is immensely indebted in numerous ways. No President has had the welfare of Scottish Medicine and with it that of the College more near to his heart than Sir Stanley. Should, as many if not most Fellows hope, the Royal Colleges of Edinburgh and Glasgow in the future mutually agree to unification, amalgamation or whatever form of close alliance may be considered proper in the interests of Scottish Medicine the staunch, courageous, persistent efforts of Sir Stanley in the 1940s will prove not to have been in vain. The rôle of Sir Stanley will then be seen to have been on a par with that of Dr Purves (Chap. II) and Dr George Sibbald (Chap. II) in relation to Sir Robert Sibbald's culminating success in obtaining our College's first Charter (Chap. III).

Already very considerable, in virtue of his eminence as a clinician and medical writer, of the professional posts he held in the Universities of Aberdeen and Edinburgh, and of his great generosity, Sir Stanley Davidson's stature within the history of the College will with time most certainly acquire even greater significance. The enrolment of Sir Stanley as an Honorary Fellow in 1972 was a timely tribute of admiration and affection.

The purpose of this section has been to give a brief inkling, and only an inkling is possible, of the many and varied interests of those associated with the College over the years. To revert momentarily from the internationally eminent to the less obviously distinguished is in no sense to pass from the sublime to the mundane. Our College is an ancient corporate body. The Fellows, Members, Licentiates and Officers as they come and go each and all contribute in their own individual way to the approaching three hundred years old heritage. In this context there are four others whose activities and interests must be recorded. One was a biochemist: two were Fellows of the College: and the fourth a Librarian.

Eminence Despite Prolonged Ill-health

James Walker Dawson (1870–1927) acquired eminence in virtue of his character as a man, his skill as a micro-pathologist and his integrity as a research worker. Illness which first caused serious concern in his schooldays compelled him to abandon medical studies four years after commencement. Dawson resumed his studies some twelve years later having in the interval been to America, India and New Zealand; and having laboured as lumberjack and shepherd in the last named country. Returned to Edinburgh he resumed his medical studies in 1903. Charles McNeil understandingly described what eventuated—'The only field open to him (Dawson) was the laboratory, and there he went not from inclination but necessity. In this sheltered corner he remained for twenty-three years, sorely hampered ... by continual ill-health and with occasional attacks of serious illness, but sustained ... by his indomitable spirit.'[202]

In 1908 Dawson was awarded a gold medal for his M.D. thesis on *Inflammation and repair, and the evolution of an abscess*: and, in 1916, his thesis *The histology of disseminated sclerosis* for the degree of D.Sc. was published in the *Transactions of the Royal Society of Edinburgh*.[203] In addition to less ambitious contributions to the literature Dawson published five major monographs. All were recognized as being outstanding and authoritative and the last entitled *The melanomata* appearing in 1925 was described as 'a classic work of reference'.[204]

Dawson's meticulously performed research embodying unrestrained self-criticism supported by exquisitely informative illustrations and convincing mode of expression brought fame. Appreciation by surgeons no less than physicians was evident in his election as a Fellow of the Royal College of Surgeons of Edinburgh. Earlier in his career he had been awarded the Syme Surgical Fellowship. For reasons of health, offers of appointments at home and abroad had perforce to be declined. He was however an assistant pathologist to the Edinburgh Royal Infirmary for a limited period, and at the time of his death was pathologist to the Longmore Hospital for Incurables. During World War I he acted as Lecturer in the University. Essentially however Dr Dawson's major work was conducted in the Research Laboratory of our College. He was elevated to the Fellowship in 1924. Sadly, a deterioration in his physical condition prevented him from delivering in the spring of 1927 the Morison Lecture which the College had invited him to give and for which he had undertaken much preparatory work. His choice of subject had been *Some fundamental conceptions in the pathology of the nervous system.*

To quote McNeil again, James Dawson left 'an example and an inspiration'.[205] His widow is an eminent pathologist in her own right and herself worked in the College Laboratory. She was made an Honorary Fellow of our College in 1969. During her husband's lifetime Dr Edith Kate Dawson, M.B.E. was responsible for a number of drawings in his publications.

Brilliance in the Face of Adversity

William Ogilvy Kermack (1898–1970) was the scientist—an M.A. and D.Sc. of Aberdeen, an Honorary LL.D. of St Andrews and a Fellow of the Royal Society, the Royal Society of Edinburgh and of the Royal Institute of Chemistry. A native of Kirriemuir, the birthplace of Sir James Barrie and the distinguished surgeon Sir David Wilkie, Kermack was appointed in charge of the Chemical Department of our College's Research Laboratory in 1921. Three years later, when only 26 years of age, he met with a laboratory accident which resulted in permanent, total loss of sight. No longer able to take an active part in practical work, he kept abreast of the literature with the aid of friends and continued to design experiments which were carried out by his co-workers. Kermack's brilliant work despite handicap earned for him the Freeland Barbour Prize of our College and the Makdougall Brisbane Prize of the Royal Society of Edinburgh. In 1949 he was appointed to the newly created McLeod-Smith Chair of Biological Chemistry at the University of Aberdeen where he continued his research despite the demands of teaching and administration. In the words of one obituary appreciation—'By any yardstick, his achievements were outstanding, but for one handicapped by blindness they were almost unbelievable'.[206]

Student Health

The other Fellow was Dr R. E. Verney. A South African by birth and a general practitioner by choice, he developed a deep affection for Edinburgh, and the University and College of Physicians within its boundaries. From this there grew an intense interest in Student Health which led to his being appointed the University Medical Officer for Student Health. A pioneer in the field he made an outstanding success of his task and his success in turn attracted large benefactions for use in furthering the interests of the Student Health Service.[207]

Prolonged and Varied Service

The Librarian was Thomas Harkness Graham. To him the College was indebted for no fewer than forty-two years of unstinted arduous service, and during World War I the Scottish Medical Service Emergency Committee (q.v.) was fortunate to have him as their Secretary. Deservedly Mr Graham had conferred upon him the O.B.E. in 1919. He was also Registrar for the Scottish Branch of the General Medical Council.[208] His memory is still revered by older Fellows, and his work as Librarian remains a subject for admiration by the several who have since succeeded him in office in the persons of Mr L. Jolley, Mr G. R. Pendrill and Miss J. P. S. Ferguson.

In 1915 Graham at his own request was granted release from his duties as Librarian in order to apply for a commission in H.M. Forces. To his great regret he was not accepted on account of his eyesight.

George Home, Graham's assistant, was wounded by shrapnel at the Dardanelles, but returned to his regiment on Gallipoli after a spell in hospital at Malta. While in hospital he was visited by (Colonel) G. Lovell Gulland who at the time was in medical charge of the Malta Hospital.

By way of postscript it may be added that an Honorary Member of the College named John Stewart Muir who practised in the Scottish Borders was credited with having been in attendance at the birth of 3344 babies.[209] Whether the Honorary Membership is to be regarded as a case of *ad* or *propter hoc* is uncertain! Be that as it may, Muir's accomplishment recalls Rorie's tribute to another:

To this cauld warld in fifty year
She'd fosh near auchteen hunner.
Losh keep's! When a' thing's said an' dune,
The cratur' was a won'er![211]

REFERENCES

(1) DUNCAN, A. (1876) *Memorials of the Faculty of Physicians and Surgeons of Glasgow, 1599–1850.* Preface, p. vi. Glasgow: Maclehose.

(2) THOMSON, J. H. (1875) *The Martyr Graves of Scotland.* First series, p. 12. Edinburgh: Johnstone, Hunter & Co.

(3) HARVEY, W. R. (1974) Personal communication.

(4) THOMSON, J. H. (1877) Op. cit. Second series, pp. 163–5.

THE JACOBITE RISINGS

(5) HOWELL, H. A. L. (1914) The story of the army surgeon and the care of the sick and wounded in the British army, from 1715 to 1748. *Journal of the Royal Army Medical Corps,* **22,** 463 f.

(6) MACNAUGHTON, W. A. (1932) The medical heroes of the 'Forty-five. *Caledonian Medical Journal,* **15,** 113 and 119.

(7) HOWELL, H. A. L. Op. cit., p. 464.

(8) MACNAUGHTON, W. A. Op. cit., p. 124.

(9) CARLYLE, A. (1910) *Autobiography of Dr. Alexander Carlyle of Inveresk, 1722–1805,* p. 145. Edinburgh: Foulis.

(10) RITCHIE, R. P. (1899) *The Early Days of the Royall Colledge of Physitians, Edinburgh,* p. 160. Edinburgh: G. P. Johnston.

(11) Ibid., p. 184.

(12) Ibid., p. 186.

(13) Ibid., p. 152.

(14) Ibid., p. 148.

(15) CARLYLE, A. (1973) *Autobiography of Dr. Alexander Carlyle. Anecdotes and characters of the times.* [1st Edition reprinted.] Ed. by J. Kinsley, pp. 86 and 91. London: Oxford University Press.

(16) WHITTET, M. M. (1914) Medical resources of the Forty-five. *Transactions of the Gaelic Society of Inverness,* **44,** 8.

(17) FORBES, R. (1895) *The Lyon in Mourning,* vol. I, p. 348. Edinburgh: Scottish History Society. (Scottish History Society, vol. XX.)

(18) PRINGLE, J. (1752) *Observations on the Diseases of the Army in Camp and Garrison,* pp. 48–64, passim. London: A. Millar & D. Wilson.

(19) HOWELL, H. A. O. Op. cit., p. 468.

(20) SELWYN, S. (1965) Sir John Pringle (1707–1782): hospital reformer; moral philosopher; and pioneer of antiseptics. In *Scottish Society of the History of Medicine. Report of Proceedings.* Session 1964–5, p. 16. Edinburgh: [Scottish Society of the History of Medicine].

(21) WHITTET, M. M. Op. cit., p. 14.

(22) CARLYLE, A. (1910) Autobiography . . . 1722–1805, pp. 143 f. Edinburgh: Foulis.

(23) GORDON-TAYLOR, G. (1945) The medical and surgical aspects of 'the 'Forty-five'. (The Vicary lecture.) *British Journal of Surgery*, **33**, 129, 7.

(24) WRIGHT-ST. CLAIR, R. E. (1964) *Doctors Monro; a medical saga*, p. 52. London: Wellcome Historical Medical Library.

(25) TURNER, A. L. (1937) *Story of a Great Hospital; the Royal Infirmary of Edinburgh, 1729–1929*, pp. 94–5. Edinburgh: Oliver & Boyd.

(26) MACNAUGHTON, W. A. Op. cit., p. 122.

(27) WHITTET, M. M. Op. cit., p. 12.

(28) GORDON-TAYLOR, G. Op. cit., p. 8.

(29) WHITTET, M. M. Op. cit., p. 27.

(30) MACNAUGHTON, W. A. Op. cit., p. 64.

(31) Ibid., p. 66.

(32) WHITTET, M. M. Op. cit., p. 15.

(33) AMULREE, B. W. S. MACKENZIE, Baron (1971) Dr. Archibald Cameron. *Medical History*, **15**, 230–40.

(34) HOWELL, H. A. Op. cit., p. 470.

(35) MACNAUGHTON, W. A. Op. cit., p. 114.

(36) Ibid., p. 61.

(37) DAVIDSON, C. H. (1973) Personal communication.

(38) TURNER, A. L. Op. cit., p. 96.

(39) COMRIE, J. D. (1932) *History of Scottish Medicine*, 2nd Edition, vol. I, p. 317. London: Baillière, Tindall & Cox.

(40) CARLYLE, A. (1973) Op. cit., p. 102.

(41) INGLIS, J. A. (1911) *The Monros of Auchinbowie*, p. 106. Edinburgh: Constable.

THE NAPOLEONIC WARS

(42) THIN, R. (1927) *College Portraits*, p. 91. Edinburgh: Oliver & Boyd.

(43) Ibid., pp. 93–5.

AFTER THE CRIMEAN WAR

(44) College Minutes, 3.v.1864.

(45) EVATT, G. J. H. (1914) Army medical organization in war, with suggestions as to militia and volunteer aid. *Journal of the Royal Army Medical Corps*, **22**, 91.

(46) FOTHERINGHAM, J. T. (1914) Some historical notes on the British medical services. *Journal of the Royal Army Medical Corps*, **22**, 527.

(47) WATSON, W. N. B. (1966) An Edinburgh surgeon of the Crimean war—Patrick Heron Watson (1832–1907). *Medical History*, **10**, 173.

(48) College Minutes, 2.viii.1864.

(49) Ibid., 2.viii.1887.

(50) Ibid., 3.vi.1890.
(51) CANTLIE, Sir N. (1974) *A History of the Army Medical Department*, vol. II, pp. 357–8. Edinburgh: Churchill Livingstone.
(52) College Minutes, 18.vii.1893.
(53) Ibid., 7.xi.1893.
(54) CANTLIE, Sir N. Op. cit., vol. I, p. 181.
(55) MacLELLAN, A. (1974) Personal communication.
(56) Ibid., p. 201.
(57) COMRIE, J. D. Op. cit., vol. II, pp. 747–8.
(58) CANTLIE, Sir N. Op. cit., vol. I, p. 431.
(59) McGRIGOR, Sir J. (1861) *The Autobiography and Services of Sir James McGrigor, Bart.*, p. 97. London: Longman, Green, Longman & Roberts.
(60) CANTLIE, Sir N. Op. cit., vol. I, p. 452.

THE BOER WAR AND AFTER

(61) [MORTON, L. T.] (1956) Centenary of the Victoria Cross; the awards to medical men. *British Medical Journal*, **I**, 227.
(62) College Minutes, 2.xi.1920.
(63) Ibid., 17.xii.1901.
(64) Ibid., 4.ii.1902.
(65) Council Minutes, 5.xi.1907.

1914–1918

(66) R.C.P.E. (1925) *Historical Sketch and Laws*, p. 109. Edinburgh: Royal College of Physicians.
(67) College Minutes, 13.viii.1914.
(68) Ibid., 21.viii.1914.
(69) CURRIE, J. R. (1922) *The Mustering of Medical Service in Scotland, 1914–1919*, pp. 5–6. Edinburgh: Scottish Medical Service Emergency Committee.
(70) Ibid., pp. 50–2.
(71) Ibid., p. 85.
(72) Ibid., pp. 94 f.
(73) College Minutes, 21.xii.1916.
(74) CURRIE, J. R. Op. cit., p. 96.
(75) College Minutes, 6.ii.1917.
(76) CURRIE, J. R. Op. cit., p. 140.
(77) R.C.P.E. (1925) *Historical Sketch and Laws*, p. 110. Edinburgh: Royal College of Physicians.
(77a) College Minutes, 4.v.1915.
(78) Ibid., 20.vii.1915.
(78a) DAVIDSON, Sir S. (1971–5) Personal communications.
(79) Ibid., 7.xi.1916.
(80) Ibid., 6.ii.1917.

(81) Ibid., 5.ii.1952.
(82) TURNER, A. L. Op. cit., p. 321.
(83) College Minutes, 30.xi.1916.
(84) Ibid., 5.v.1925.
(85) Ibid., 13.viii.1914.
(86) Ibid., 3.xi.1914.
(87) Ibid., 2.xi.1915.
(88) Ibid., 5.ii.1918.
(89) Ibid., 5.xi.1918.
(90) Ibid., 6.ii.1917.
(91) Ibid., 5.xii.1918.
(92) Ibid., 2.v.1922.

1932–1939

(93) COOKE, A. M. (1972) *A History of the Royal College of Physicians of London*, vol. III, pp. 1069 f. Oxford: Clarendon.

1939–1946

(94) College Minutes, 18.vii.1944.
(95) Ibid., 1.v.1945.
(96) Ibid., 5.ii.1946.
(97) Council Minutes, 29.x.1940.
(98) College Minutes, 16.vii.1940.
(99) Ibid., 22.v.1941.
(100) Ibid., 20.vii.1943.
(101) Ibid., 1.ii.1944.
(102) Ibid., 2.v.1944.
(103) Ibid., 6.xi.1945.
(104) R.C.P.E. (1960) *Report by the President* [*A. R. Gilchrist*] . . . *1959–60*, p. 4. Edinburgh: Royal College of Physicians.
(104a) HUNTER, R. B. (1975) Personal communication.
(104b) ARNOTT, Sir Melville (1975) Personal communication.
(104c) HILL, Sir I. G. W. (1975) Personal communication.
(105) MARQUIS, R. M. (1972) Personal communication.
(106) FORFAR, J. O. (1972) Personal communication.
(107) THIN, R. Op. cit., p. 91.
(108) College Minutes, 15.vii.1947.
(109) WALKER, E. R. C. (1972) Personal communication.
(110) MACARTHUR, P. (1972) Personal communication.
(111) KEAY, A. J. (1972) Personal communication.
(111a) JOHNSTONE, R. M. (1975) Personal communication.

(111b) LAMB, W. L. (1975) Personal communication.

(111c) DEBENHAM, R. K. (1942) R.A.M.C. hospital in Crete. *Journal of the Royal Army Medical Corps*, **78**, 183–5.

(111d) College Minutes, 5.v.1959.

(112) CALDWELL, E. D. (1972) Personal communication.

(113) DOUGLAS, D. M. (1973) Personal communication.

(114) MACKAY-DICK, J. (1960) A medical officer in the Royal Army Medical Corps looks back. *Surgo*, **36**, 3, 24.

(115) Leader (1958) Tuberculosis among the Gurkhas. *Lancet*, **2**, 1053.

(116) Annotation (1960) Resection for pulmonary tuberculosis in the army. *Lancet*, **2**, 639.

(116a) MACKAY-DICK, J. (1975) Personal communication.

THE INDIAN MEDICAL SERVICE

(117) College Minutes, 1.v.1945.

(118) Ibid., 2.v.1950.

(119) Ibid., 20.vii.1943.

(120) Ibid., 2.xi.1948.

(121) PEARSON, E. S. (1938) *Karl Pearson; an appreciation of some aspects of his life and work*, p. 73. Cambridge: University Press.

(122) HARVEY, R. W. (1974) Personal communication.

(123) MARIO, J. W. (1909) *The Birth of Modern Italy*. London: J. Fisher Unwin.

(124) College Minutes, 7.xi.1950.

(125) LISTON, W. G. Posthumous presentation of the 1971 Karl F. Meyer award. Lieutenant-Colonel W. G. Liston. *Journal of the Royal Army Medical Corps*, **119**, 49–56.

(126) College Minutes, 4.xi.1969.

(127) Ibid., 3.v.1966.

(128) Ibid., 5.ii. 1963.

(129) Ibid., 4.xi.1969.

(130) Ibid., 6.ii.1968.

(131) Ibid., 5.ii.1963

(132) Ibid., 26.vii.1960.

(133) Ibid., 3.xi.1964.

(134) Ibid., 3.xi.1970.

(135) Council Minutes, 15.xi.1966.

(136) College Minutes, 7.xi.1967.

PEACE-TIME COMMUNITY ACTIVITIES

(137) SMOUT, T. C. (1972) *A History of the Scottish people, 1560–1830*. Rev. Edition, p. 174. London: Collins/Fontana.

(138) Murray, A. L., comp. [1966] *Lists of Royal Physicians in Scotland, 1568–1853.* Comp. by A. L. Murray, Scottish Record Office. (Typescript.)

(139) Bramwell, J. Crighton (1973) Personal communication.

(140) College Minutes, 6.v.1952.

(141) Christison, Sir R. (1886) *The Life of Sir Robert Christison, Bart.*, vol. II, p. 371. Edinburgh: Blackwood.

(142) Pottinger, G. (1972) *Muirfield and the Honourable Company*, p. 114. Edinburgh: Scottish Academic Press.

(143) College Minutes, 21.vii.1970.

(144) Ibid., 1.xi.1966.

(145) Ibid., 7.xi.1967.

(146) Ibid., 2.xi.1915.

(147) Ibid., 26.vii.1960.

(148) Ibid., 26.vii.1966.

(149) Ibid., 2.v.1950.

(150) Ibid., 1.ii.1916.

(151) Ibid., 1.v.1951.

(152) Ibid., 4.v.1965.

(153) Cameron, J. D. S. (1968) Personal communication.

(154) College Minutes, 6.v.1947.

(155) Ibid., 4.ii.1958.

(156) Ibid., 7.ii.1950.

(157) Ibid., 2.ii.1943.

(158) Ibid., 16.vii.1963.

(159) Ibid., 21.vii.1942.

(160) Ibid., 1.ii.1966.

(161) Ibid., 2.ii.1965.

(162) Jones, G. R. B. (1972) David Daniel Davis, M.D., F.R.C.P. (1777–1841). *The Carmarthenshire Antiquary*, **8**, 91–100.

(163) Jones, G. R. B. (1973) David Daniel Davis, physician and his son, Edward Davis, sculptor—a supplementary note. *The Carmarthenshire Antiquary*, **9**, 119–30.

(164) College Minutes, 3.xi.1970.

(165) Ibid., 5.xi.1946.

(166) Inglis, J. A. Op. cit., p. 103.

(167) Brown, T. (1886) *Alexander Wood, M.D., F.R.C.P.E.; A sketch of his life and work*, p. 141. Edinburgh: Macniven & Wallace.

(168) College Minutes, 5.ii.1918.

(169) Ibid., 6.v.1958.

(170) Ibid., 20.vii.1948.

(171) Thin, R. Op. cit., p. 44.

(172) College Minutes, 25.vii.1967.

(173) Ibid., 17.vii.1962.

(174) Ibid., 4.v.1965.

(175) Ibid., 5.xi.1957.

(176) SKINNER, R. T. (1947) *The Royal Mile*, p. 9. Edinburgh: Oliver & Boyd.

(177) College Mss. *Boswell family papers*. [c. 1750].

(178) College Minutes, 3.v.1949.

(179) Ibid., 4.xi.1958.

(180) Ibid., 3.v.1960.

(181) Ibid., 1.xi.1960.

(182) BOWERBANK, Sir F. (1958) *A Doctor's Story*, p. 31. Wellington, New Zealand: Tombs.

(183) Ibid., p. 33.

(184) Ibid., p. 179.

(185) Ibid., p. 176.

(186) Ibid., p. 206.

(187) College Minutes, 4.ii.1969.

(188) Ibid., 6.ii.1968.

(189) Ibid., 7.xi.1961.

(190) Ibid., 5.xi.1963.

(191) Ibid., 26.vii.1966.

(192) Ibid., 1.v.1962.

(193) Ibid., 3.xi.1964.

(194) Ibid., 1.xi.1955.

(195) Ibid., 28.vii.1964.

(196) Ibid., 6.v.1969.

(197) Ibid., 7.xi.1961.

(198) Ibid., 2.v.1967.

(199) Ibid., 22.vii.1969.

(200) TOMASZEWSKI, W., ed. (1968) *The University of Edinburgh and Poland*, p. 50. Edinburgh: W. Tomaszewski.

(201) College Minutes, 6.v.1969.

(202) [McNEIL, C.] (1927) Obituary. James Walker Dawson, M.D., D.Sc., F.R.C.P.E., F.R.C.S.E. *Edinburgh Medical Journal*, **34**, 480.

(203) DAWSON, J. W. (1916) The histology of disseminated sclerosis. *Transactions of the Royal Society of Edinburgh*, **50**, 517–740.

(204) Obituary. James Walker Dawson (1927) *Lancet*, **2**, 90.

(205) [McNEIL, C.] Op. cit., p. 481.

(206) ROYAL SOCIETY OF EDINBURGH (1972) *Yearbook, 1971–72*. (Session 1969–71), p. 57. Edinburgh: Royal Society of Edinburgh.

(207) College Minutes, 3.ii.1970.

(208) Ibid., 6.xi.1962.

(208a) Ibid., 2.xi.1915.

(209) Ibid., 7.ii.1939.

(210) RORIE, D. (1920) *The Auld Doctor and Other Poems and Songs in Scots*. London: Constable.

Chapter XXVIII

TOWARDS A NATIONAL HEALTH SERVICE

So often do the spirits of great events
stride on before the events,
And in to-day already walks to-morrow.

Samuel Coleridge

The genesis of the as yet imperfect National Health Service is to be found in the beginning of the present century. A resurgence of the nation's social conscience gave an impetus and new momentum to social legislation. For the purpose of this history certain enactments call for particular consideration. They are the National Insurance Act of 1911, the National Health Service Acts of 1946 for England and Wales, and of 1947 for Scotland. In their peri-natal days these Acts all stirred up mighty furores but their supposedly demoniacal features have almost assumed benignity with the passing of years. Now they can be seen in truer perspective.

Concern over the physical welfare of the nation was stimulated by the recorded findings of school teachers who even before the introduction of compulsory education in 1880 found many pupils incapable of benefiting from instruction because of their physically debilitated state. This was followed in the course of time by grave disquiet over the poor physique of army recruits at the time of the Boer War.[1] In quick succession the Midwives Act was passed with the creation of the Central Midwives Board in 1902; a Royal Commission on Physical Training (in Scotland) was appointed in 1903; and an Inter-departmental Committee on Physical Deterioration formed in 1904. Provision of school meals in certain circumstances was legalized in 1906 and with the passing of the Scottish Education Act the School Medical Service was launched in 1906.[2] A new Workmen's Compensation Act was placed on the Statute Book in 1906 and the first Old Age Pensions Act in 1908. About this time (1905) the Poor Law and Relief of Distress was the subject of investigation by a specially appointed Royal Commission, which recommended the transfer of the administration of the Poor Law and Poor Law Institutions from the Poor Law Boards to County and County Burgh Authorities.

Progress towards social emancipation led to the passing of the National Insurance Act in 1911 'to provide for . . . insurance against Unemployment and for purposes incidental thereto'.[3] Far from being steam rollered through Parliament, the Bill was introduced and passed with a speed more in keeping with the 'Jet Age'. On all sides feathers flew, skulls were cracked and deep-seated enmities created. Distrust was bred. In his ruthless, not far short of fanatical determination, the main protagonist ignored cabinet colleagues, side-stepped Government Departments other than the Treasury, and remained oblivious of the existence of negotiating bodies representative of the medical profession.[4, 5] The appellation 'Lloyd George' soon acquired, and long retained a double significance—appreciative or 'snide' according to circumstances. Such was the antipathy aroused among many of the profession that, when some thirty-five years or so later the possibility of a National Health Service became a live issue, they, although now mature and senior, were prejudiced from the start with revived memories of 1911. Their grievance was not against the Insurance Scheme which in its day had justified itself, but against the political manoeuvring, the unscrupulous manipulation and contemptuous handling to which the profession as a whole had been submitted. The suave accounts in some Public Health text books pay scant regard to the emotional and professional turmoil known to general practitioners and their families when the Insurance Act was introduced.

In the first decade of the century many family doctors ran family clubs for their poorer patients and employed a collector who, debarred from canvassing, was paid on a commission basis. There were also numerous Approved Friendly Societies which made arrangements with individual family doctors to provide services to their members for an annual membership fee as small as 2/6d. Elsewhere it was not uncommon for a young doctor to 'put up his plate' in a poor industrial district and provide surgery and dispensary services at the rate of 6d. per visit. When, having at long last discharged his debts with income derived from his 'Sixpenny practice', the doctor often but not always moved to a more salubrious and lucrative area in the same city or elsewhere.

Underlying all was the fear of ill health and of inability to pay for treatment if needed. The National Insurance Act was intended as a first major step towards the abolition of these fears. Subject to restrictions of age and income, it provided a means of insurance against ill health for a large part, but not all of the working population. Weekly contributions were paid by insured workers and their employers, and a new National Health Insurance Commission with Sir Robert Morant as Chairman, was

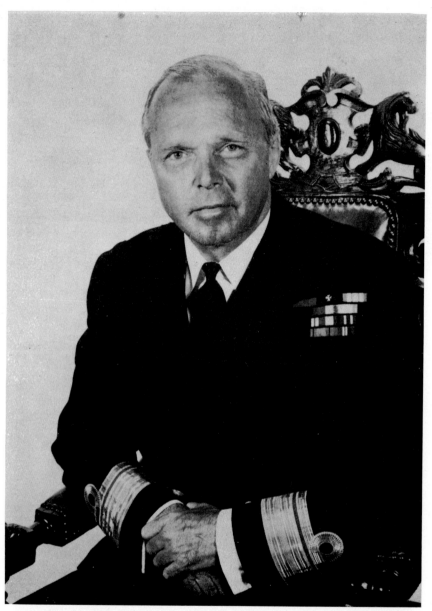

PLATE 42 Surgeon Vice-Admiral Sir Dick Caldwell, Medical Director General of the Royal Navy,
1966–1969
Photograph by Devon Commercial Photos Ltd., Plymouth

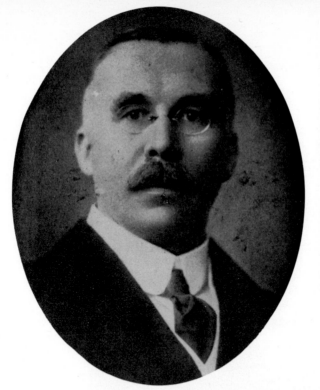

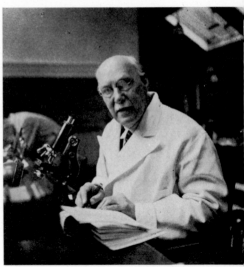

PLATE 43c   Lieutenant-Colonel W. F. Harvey
(1873–1948)
By courtesy of Miss B. Harvey

PLATE 43a   Lieutenant-Colonel W. G. Liston (1873–1950)
By courtesy of the Director, the Haffkine Institute, Bombay

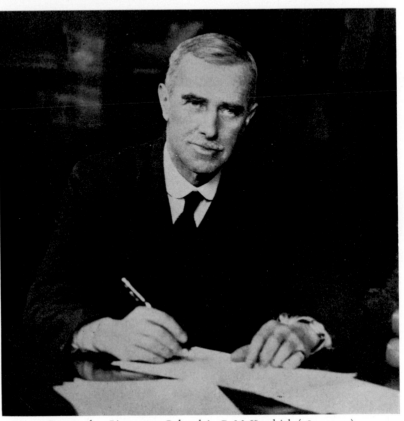

PLATE 43b   Lieutenant-Colonel A. G. McKendrick (1873–1943)
By courtesy of Mrs Joyce Matthew

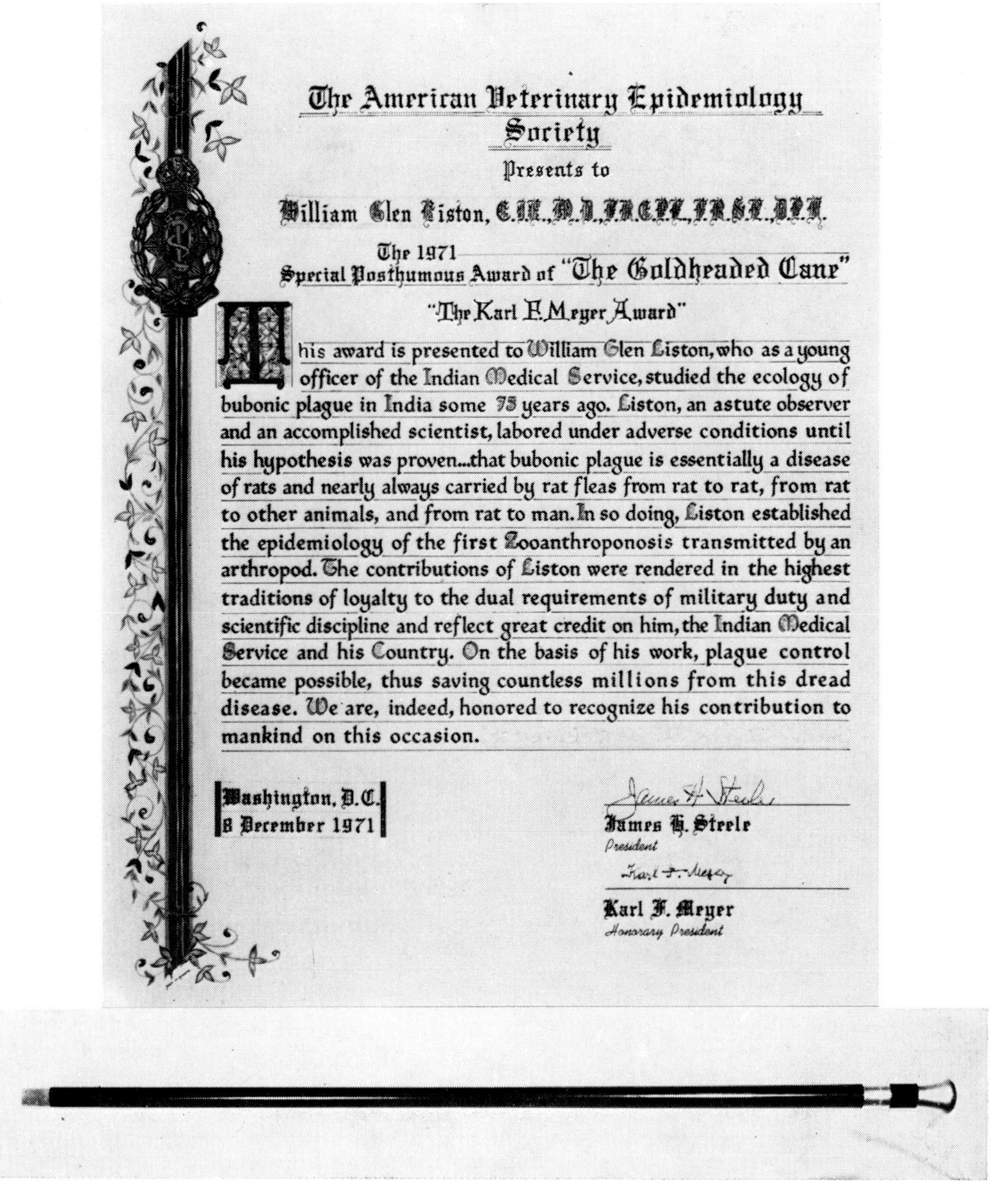

The American Veterinary Epidemiology
Society

Presents to

William Glen Liston, C.IE. M.D. F.R.C.P.E. F.R.S.E. D.P.H.

The 1971
Special Posthumous Award of "The Goldheaded Cane"

"The Karl F. Meyer Award"

His award is presented to William Glen Liston, who as a young officer of the Indian Medical Service, studied the ecology of bubonic plague in India some 75 years ago. Liston, an astute observer and an accomplished scientist, labored under adverse conditions until his hypothesis was proven...that bubonic plague is essentially a disease of rats and nearly always carried by rat fleas from rat to rat, from rat to other animals, and from rat to man. In so doing, Liston established the epidemiology of the first Zooanthroponosis transmitted by an arthropod. The contributions of Liston were rendered in the highest traditions of loyalty to the dual requirements of military duty and scientific discipline and reflect great credit on him, the Indian Medical Service and his Country. On the basis of his work, plague control became possible, thus saving countless millions from this dread disease. We are, indeed, honored to recognize his contribution to mankind on this occasion.

Washington, D.C.
8 December 1971

James H. Steele
President

Karl F. Meyer
Honorary President

PLATE 44   W. G. Liston: Posthumous award of 'The Goldheaded Cane' by the American
Veterinary Epidemiology Society, 8th December 1971
By courtesy of the Editor of the *Journal of the R.A.M.C.* (1973) 119

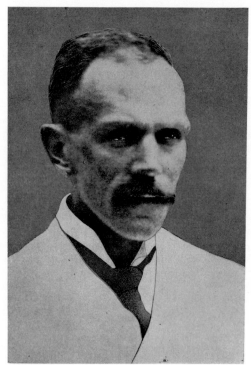

PLATE 45   Dr J. W. Dawson (1870–1927)
By courtesy of Dr Edith K. Dawson

entrusted with central administration. Morant was an eminent Civil Servant with a redoubtable reputation in Whitehall circles. Local administration was made the responsibility of Local Insurance Committees with medical service subcommittees. Decision as to the capitation fee to be awarded doctors on the panels rested with the Commissioners.

Although intended 'to provide . . . against loss of health and for the prevention and care of sickness' the Act did not make provision for the dependants of insured persons, or for specialist treatment other than maternity benefit and a sanatorium benefit for phthisical patients. Under a special section of the Act arrangements for the setting aside of one penny per insured person for medical research were authorized: the estimated total sum involved amounting to approximately £57,000 per annum.[6] This sum contributed towards the establishment of a National Institution for Medical Research and the creation of the Medical Research Committee. Attached at first to the Insurance Commission, the Research Committee was reconstituted in 1920 as a special committee of the Privy Council and renamed the Medical Research Council.

Ironically some of the basic ideas in the National Health Scheme were acquired in Germany by the man who not many years later was to contemplate the hanging of the Kaiser!

THE NATIONAL INSURANCE ACT, 1911

Suspension of Standing Orders was moved by Dr William Russell at an Extraordinary Meeting on 19th December 1911 to enable the College to request 'Council to consider the National Insurance Act, and to consult with the other Royal Colleges in connection therewith'. The motion was carried in its entirety. Later another motion was successfully passed to the effect that the Council was instructed to report to the College as soon as possible 'and before committing their College, the result of the Conference with the Councils of the other Colleges'.[7]

At an Extraordinary Meeting of the College three days later the President (Sir) Byrom Bramwell in the Chair, reviewed the provisions of the National Insurance Act and of action taken by Council.[8] In the interval since the previous meeting there had been a meeting of the Councils of the three Scottish Medical Corporations at which complete agreement had been reached in drawing up a Joint Manifesto for consideration by their respective Colleges. Adoption of the Manifesto having been proposed and seconded, Sir Thomas Fraser recommended that no matter its unanimous adoption it should 'be gone over paragraph by paragraph'. This course was

2A

agreed to and several constructive amendments were made in the discussion which followed. The College then instructed Council to remit the amended Manifesto to the two other Corporations for any further adjustments, after which the Manifesto was to be forwarded on behalf of the three Corporations to every practitioner in Scotland, the four Scottish Universities and to the Insurance Commissioners. Council were not required by the Edinburgh College to refer back any further 'minor and verbal alterations'.

The Manifesto commenced with the all important statement that 'The National Insurance Bill has now become law': and lost no time in declaring that 'The six cardinal points again and again insisted upon by the profession as a minimum, have not all been incorporated in the Act'. In the circumstances the three Corporations considered it incumbent on them 'to advise the profession in Scotland as to what . . . should be done'. At pains to assure the B.M.A. in Scotland of their desire to assist, the Corporations emphasized their cordial sympathy with the Profession. In more practical terms they advised that since under the Act, Scotland was to have an Executive of her own, separate Commissioners and a Separate Fund, it was essential that the Medical Profession in Scotland should have 'a strong and thoroughly representative Central Medical Council . . . endowed with full advisory and administrative powers, with a paid secretary and an office in Scotland'. Such a Council, it was suggested, might consist of the Scottish Committee of the B.M.A.; a representative from each Insurance Area; and representatives from the Scottish Corporations and the four Scottish Universities. Coupled with an offer to co-operate was another to contribute to costs.

The Manifesto ended on a note of crescendo. 'The Scottish Corporations', it declared, 'are of opinion that the Members of the medical profession in Scotland should refrain from undertaking any medical work under the Insurance Act until Regulations have been framed by the Scottish Insurance Commission which are entirely in accordance with the six fundamental requirements of the profession and that the Scottish Insurance Commission should forthwith be informed of this.' Brave and strongly expressed words indeed, followed as they were by an exhortation on 'the paramount importance of loyal co-operation and of determined and unflinching adherence to the six cardinal points'. Additional to the President, sixty-seven Fellows signed the Roll on this occasion.[8] Some six weeks later the President reported that the Scottish Corporations had decided to form a General Medical Insurance Council with as previously suggested an office and paid secretary, a share of the expenses involved to be borne by the College.[9]

A special meeting of the College was called on the first day of February (1912) to consider a letter of invitation from the Insurance Commissioners. The invitation was to take part in a conference of representatives of the medical profession to discuss important questions of procedure, the Commissioners having already had a conference with 'representatives of prospective insured persons'. To this second conference the College was invited to send two representatives, a similar invitation having been extended to 'the General Medical Council, the M.B.A. and other medical bodies'. A major purpose of the meeting was to discuss the selection of medical members of the Advisory Committee who were to advise the Commissioners on the drawing up of Regulations. The invitation had been sent by the Assistant Secretary of the Health Insurance Joint Committee: and the meeting was to be held at the Home Office, Whitehall but notification of postponement was received by telegram twenty-four hours before the appointed day.[9]

There is no further recorded mention of College concern over the Insurance Act for a further ten months when an Extraordinary Meeting was called to consider a Report from Council on the relation of the College to the Scottish Medical Insurance Council. The Report sought the views of the College. Fifty-eight Fellows were in attendance. After summarizing the history of the Scottish Medical Insurance Council, Dr William Russell read a Manifesto which he moved should be sent to the profession in Scotland on behalf jointly of the two Edinburgh Royal Colleges. The declared intent of the Manifesto was to assist the profession in their efforts to secure alteration of certain undesirable features of the Insurance Act. Exception was once again taken to the way in which 'cardinal principles' had been ignored—only on this occasion the number was given as seven and not six as previously. It was pointed out that in all matters in all Areas, control was vested in the Local Committee which was 'composed . . . of not less than three-fifths of representatives of insured persons': and that the Local Medical Committee had no executive rights. The intended Memorial maintained that only an Amending Act would establish medical provisions on a satisfactory basis in the face of the consolidated power wielded by the Local Insurance Committee under the terms of the Act then in force. 'In the view of the Colleges', it was stated, 'the Act will perpetuate and extend some of the worst features of club practice; and if 'members of the profession in Scotland are satisfied . . . and are prepared to accept service under Local Insurance Committees on the terms indicated, the Royal Colleges, while not attempting to dissuade them, cannot be parties to any agreement derogatory to the status of the profession.'

The proposed Manifesto met with a mixed reception. The 'Previous Question' was moved and lost, as was a motion for delay. Eventually Dr Russell's motion was passed *nemine contradicente*, but at the instigation of several Fellows the Manifesto was read through in detail, and a number of modifications of wording suggested of which the Council undertook to take account.[10]

Research Fund

On 6th May 1913 Sir Robert Philip on behalf of Council proposed the following motion, which after being seconded by Dr James Ritchie *Secundus*, was agreed to unanimously:

> 'That it be remitted to the Council of the College to approach the Chancellor of the Exchequer with an expression of the view that the money available for research under the National Insurance Act amounting to £57,000 per annum should be expended in the development of original investigation in recognised laboratories throughout the United Kingdom.'[11]

With little delay a Memorial was presented to Mr Lloyd George, the then Chancellor of the Exchequer. By way of introduction the Memorialists expressed their appreciation of the wisdom of the provision whereby under the National Insurance Act money provided by Parliament was to be devoted to research: and drew attention to their favoured position 'to judge of the best means of stimulating and fostering original investigation' as a result of experience derived over many years from administration of 'their extensive Research Laboratory'. After consideration of all the circumstances the view was advanced that available moneys should be utilized for the endowment of research workers in the numerous well-equipped laboratories throughout the United Kingdom as had been suggested in the Final Report of the Departmental Committee on Tuberculosis. While not ignoring the attractions of co-ordinated effort the Memorial embodied the firm opinion that 'to establish at once a new Institute of Research implies grave oversight of the very complete facilities already existing . . .'. A plea was advanced that any scheme in connection with research should be kept as fluid as possible, and subject to centralization only to the extent required by direction of the main lines of work and by apportionment of moneys to workers in approved laboratories.[12]

Sir Arthur Newsholme later described the investigations made possible by the allocation of National Health insurance funds for research as 'one of the most satisfactory bye-products of national insurance'. At the same time he commented upon the unsuitability of the Treasury requirement in the days of the Local Government Board whereby grants had to be completely expended within the financial year. The requirement was incompatible with the exigencies of scientific work.[13]

THE NATIONAL TREND PERSISTS

*A recent statement . . . that scientific advice should be 'on tap and not on top' is profoundly
foolish. The relation of the secretary to the expert should be that of 'primus inter pares'.*
Sir Arthur Newsholme

Proposal to Institute a Ministry of Health

Mention is made in Chapter XXVII of the creation in 1916 of a Special Committee
to advise the President (Dr Freeland Barbour) on problems arising as a result of war
conditions. Although the subject could not be said to be directly related to the war
effort, this Committee had referred to it proposals which were due for presentation to
Parliament for the institution of a Ministry of Health.[14]

The Report of the Special Committee was medical as distinct from political in
character, and was in the nature of a Statement for submission to Council and ultimate transmission to the College. It commenced by drawing attention to the disadvantages arising from a multiplicity of Government Departments having sectional
interests in a variety of aspects of the health of the Community. 'A fundamental
weakness', it was maintained, lay 'in the fact that in none of the Departments concerned is the control vested in a Minister appointed primarily to deal with Health
problems.' Essential interest in Health questions was considered to be 'obscured' and
effective machinery for dealing with the complex problems of National Health,
lacking. In categorical terms the Statement declared a need for 'the creation of a
Ministry which shall concern itself with Health matters pure and simple, and to
whose jurisdiction shall be transferred from other Departments the operations of all
existing enactments in so far as they deal with Health'. Attention was drawn to
omissions 'in the purview of the Acts'. It was recommended that any new Ministry
should consist of the Minister and a Board of Health, with the Minister as Chairman
and members representative of administrative officials, laymen with experience of
health problems, and medical men with knowledge of public health service, general
practice, special clinical departments including industrial medicine, medical research
and medical statistics.

The Statement was approved on the motion of Dr Lorrain Smith with Sir Robert
Philip seconding. After discussion the draft Statement was remitted to Council for
certain amendments prior to being sent to among others, the Government.[14] In the
covering letter sent with the Statement in final form mention was made that 'the
prevailing opinion of the College is that the establishment of a Ministry of Health

ought to be postponed until after the War'. There is nothing in the College Minutes or correspondence to suggest that consideration of the subject by the College followed a request for their views. Available evidence points to the College having taken the initiative.[15]

At the first Quarterly Meeting in 1919 the formation of a Scottish Ministry of Health Committee was announced and the College on being invited to participate nominated two representatives in the persons of Sir Robert Philip and Dr A. H. Freeland Barbour.[16] A decision was arrived at by the College about this time to prepare a second Statement. On this occasion Council had more obvious regard to national interests. It expressed satisfaction that provisions relating to Scotland had been removed from the Ministry of Health Bill, 1919 and that a separate Health Ministry for Scotland was contemplated. A plea was submitted for control of health measures applicable to Scotland being vested ultimately 'in one official, specially appointed and responsible for this office only—who should be a Member of Parliament'. A larger medical membership than that proposed in the Bill was urged: and emphasis was attached to the importance of Consultative Councils as 'effective bodies initiating as well as qualifying proposals', with ready access to the Minister.

After considerable discussion and agreement as to minor amendments the College decided unanimously that the Statement should be sent to 'all Members of Parliament and Departmental officials, including the Secretary for Scotland'. A motion that the Statement should be sent simultaneously to the Press was lost.[17]

A Board of Health for Scotland, the precursor of today's Scottish Home and Health Department, was created in 1919, the Ministry of Health having been established in the same year.

Scottish Board of Health

Social progress was far from being wholly arrested by World War I. The Scottish Board of Health had responsibilities which embraced housing, local government and the requirements of the Poor Law. Previously the Highland and Islands (Medical Service) Grant Act of 1913 had been placed on the Statute Book and virtually created a state-subsidized scheme to meet the peculiar needs, beyond the scope of the National Insurance Scheme, of the Highlands and Islands. Two other major enactments were the Maternity and Child Welfare Act of 1918 and the Nurses Registration (Scotland) Act of 1919. In the interval between the two world wars progress was continued as a result of a comprehensive series of enactments designed to provide assistance for necessitous families; and families faced with unemployment, sickness and temporary incapacity of the mother on account of pregnancy.

Consultative Council on Medical and Allied Services (Scotland)

Following on the creation of the Scottish Board of Health, a Consultative Council on Medical and Allied Services was established under the chairmanship of Sir Donald MacAlister. The purpose of the Council was 'To consider and make recommendations as to the systematised provision of such forms of medical and allied services as should in the opinion of the Council, be available for the community'. In their interim Report issued in 1920 the Consultative Council maintained that 'public provision should be made for a complete medical service for the whole population of the National Insurance grade'. The Report gave a comprehensive outline of requirements covering domiciliary, hospital and convalescent care. It stated in unequivocal terms:

> 'We regard it as of primary importance that the organisation of the health service of the nation should be based upon the family as the normal unit, and on the family doctor as the normal medical attendant and guardian. It is not for disease or diseases in the abstract that provision has to be made; but for persons liable to or suffering from disease.'[18]

Department of Health for Scotland: Local Government Act

In 1928 the Scottish Board of Health was re-designated the Department of Health for Scotland with as ministerial head the Secretary of State for Scotland. With the passing in 1929 of the Scottish Local Government Act a conversion of Poor Law Institutions into General Hospitals was initiated by certain local authorities. Of these authorities the City Councils of Edinburgh, Glasgow, Dundee and Aberdeen were the most important having regard to their new responsibilities in connection with the administration of converted hospitals.

Cathcart Report

Some years after the creation of the Department of Health a Committee on Scottish Health Services was appointed. In response to a request from the Committee, the

College submitted a lengthy Memorandum fully warranted by the challengingly comprehensive remit—'as to the lines along which . . . National Health Policy should be directed so as to secure the best possible results from all the agencies concerned with the health of the people'.[19]

In its Introduction the College Memorandum made brief mention of notable advances in the past, and of diseases which continued to provide a challenge despite improved social and economic conditions. Passing reference was made to the continuing need for after-care of victims of the Great War, and to the pervading effects of stress and anxieties associated with everyday existence.

Proceeding to considerations of general policy the Memorandum touched on heredity and environment in relation to disease prevention, the significance of eugenic studies, the long-established virtue of antenatal clinics, the work of Health Visitors, and School Inspections. In a way reminiscent of Christison's appraisal of Abercrombie and others the College of 1934 attached the utmost importance to the contribution of the family doctor. He it was maintained 'must remain the pivot of all schemes which concern the national health'. Expansion of his responsibilities was foreseen. Additional to dealing with illness it was regarded as 'a matter of supreme moment' that he should 'superintend and advise as to the health of the family'. To assist and encourage him it was considered that he should have a comprehensive laboratory service at his disposal.

The College favoured extension of the National Health Insurance Scheme to dependants; the provision of a consultative service for National Health Insurance patients; and the payment individually, on an insurance or contributory basis, or by the Local Authority for maintenance and treatment of patients in general hospitals. An unquestioned need for co-ordination of the work of Voluntary and Local Authority Hospitals was voiced: and a case presented for 'Paying Blocks'. Emphasis was attached to limiting the use of Out-patient Departments to consultative purposes (or emergencies): and to discourage patients from consulting directly with the specialist of their choice. In the event of hospitals receiving fees from patients, payment should, it was thought, be made to members of staff. Hospital Paying Blocks were deemed to be better suited than Nursing Homes for the needs of many patients. Small voluntary hospitals of 50–100 beds staffed by practitioners and visited by consultants from teaching hospitals should in the opinion of the College be 'continued and extended'. The arrangements in them had been found to work 'admirably'.

Replying to wide-ranging specific questions on Medical Teaching the Memorandum was unavoidably superficial. In many instances the answers betrayed the views strongly adhered to by unnamed but well-known teachers of the time! Many subjects were dealt with and it is of interest that there was ready recognition of the importance of Nutrition as a subject; and that it was recommended that medical students should be given a short course of instruction in Dentistry with particular reference to prevention.

Prospects of clinical material in Municipal Hospitals being made available for the teaching of medical students were warmly welcomed.[20]

The Departmental Committee on Scottish Health Services issued a Report in 1936 of which it was said 'in its breadth and detail and statesmanship [it] became at once a classic in the literature of Scottish medical, school and administrative history'.[21] Commonly associated with the name of the second chairman, Professor E. P. Cathcart, the Report emphasized how the vital statistics of Scotland were 'disquietingly less favourable than those of England and Wales'[22] and that 'the first essential . . . is to integrate the separate services into a national health policy'.[23] Co-operation between voluntary and statutory hospitals and the public authorities was advocated together with the creation of Regional Advisory Hospital Committees. Vital importance was attached to education for health.[24]

The imminence of hostilities seriously limited effective application of the majority of recommendations. In the years immediately preceding the outbreak of War, statistical studies pointed to the persistence of disabling chronic conditions, the comparative youth of many chronically handicapped and the need of family doctors for improved facilities for diagnosis and treatment.

Emergency Medical Services

The year 1938 witnessed the beginnings of the Emergency Medical Services which were designed to deal with anticipated air raid casualties in the cities and industrial areas, casualties which as events turned out were at no time on a scale approaching that forecast. In so far as hospitals were concerned, the services provided for interrelated casualty clearing and base hospitals of which the rôles were subject to adjustment as the pattern of air attack unfolded. Other factors influencing policy were the changed circumstances immediately following Dunkirk, and the requirements of civilian evacuees. *Pari passu* with the Emergency Hospital Service, organized Hospital Laboratory, Public Health Laboratory and Blood Transfusion Services were developed.

B.M.A.: Medical Planning Commission

Post-war policy came up for consideration while hostilities were still at their height. With the active co-operation of the Royal Colleges and Corporations, the British Medical Association in 1940 established a Medical Planning Commission 'To study war-time developments and their effects on the country's medical services both present and future'. A Draft Interim Report representing the integrated findings of twelve committees was produced by May 1942.[25] The Report accepted the need for a regionally based unified hospital system and recognized the crucial importance of the family doctor in any medical service. A whole-time salaried service was not generally favoured, and preference was expressed for a national medical service along the lines of the National Health Insurance Scheme. An end to the buying and selling of practices was foreseen. A Government Department with a Central Medical Advisory Committee, or an independent corporate Body responsible through a Minister to Parliament were suggested as alternatives for central administration. Originally intended for submission to the Government, the Report never got beyond the interim stage, but did nevertheless exercise considerable influence on future discussions.

Beveridge Report

While the Medical Planning Commission was still sitting the Government appointed an Inter-Departmental Committee under the chairmanship of Sir William Beveridge 'To undertake with special reference to the inter-relation of the schemes, a survey of the existing national schemes of social insurance and allied services, including workmen's compensation, and to make recommendations'. The Committee was appointed in June 1941. Their Report was submitted in November 1942, and gave a clear impression of the limited scope of medical provisions among social services. Social security was given as the objective and Want, Disease, Ignorance, Squalor and Idleness as obstacles to be removed. It was maintained unreservedly that Comprehensive Health and Rehabilitation Services were fundamental to any comprehensive national social policy while at the same time recognizing the importance of such services in securing a reduction in legitimate claims for high benefits in disability. More specifically it was declared that 'a comprehensive national health service will ensure that for every citizen there is available whatever medical treatment he requires, in whatever form he requires it, domiciliary or institutional, general, specialist or consultant, and will ensure also the provision of dental, ophthalmic and surgical appliances, nursing and midwifery, and rehabilitation after accidents'. Considered in relation to the paramount claims of Social Security, the challenge to a fully effective Health Service was seen as the provision of 'full preventive and curative treatment of every kind to every citizen without exceptions, without remuneration limit and without an economic barrier at any point to delay recourse to it'.[26]

Comprehensive Medical Service: Principle accepted by Government

It rested with Sir John Anderson (later Lord Waverley) in his capacity as Lord President of the Council to inform the House of Commons on 16th February 1943 of the Government's reaction to the Beveridge Report.[27] In the course of a massive statement on the Government's social programme, he declared acceptance in principle of Beveridge's three basic assumptions—Children's Allowances: a policy of Maintenance of Employment: and a comprehensive medical service. Sir John Anderson was educated at George Watson's Boys' College and was an alumnus of the University of Edinburgh. When Anderson was transferred from the Colonial Office to the embryonic National Insurance Committee the Secretary of State minuted: 'Mr. Lloyd George and Sir R. Morant have done well for themselves, an ill-service to the Colonial Office, and, I hope, good to Mr. Anderson, whose admirable services I gratefully acknowledge'.[28]

The last to lay claim to it himself, Anderson was the most distinguished British Civil Servant of his period. If only for their historic importance, the following words from his speech to the House of Commons require to be recorded:

> 'The object is to secure, through a public, organised and regulated service, that every man, woman and child who wants it can obtain, easily and readily, the whole range of medical advice and attention . . . The idea of the new service must be one of the co-operation of public authorities, voluntary hospitals, and other voluntary agencies, and the profession, towards one common end . . . Experience justifies us putting this ultimate responsibility in any area on to the well-tried local government machinery, working very often over large areas . . . and certainly working in . . . collaboration with voluntary agencies . . . The well-being and integrity of the medical profession . . . must be amply and properly safeguarded.'[29, 27]

Hetherington Committee

Meanwhile the Secretary of State for Scotland had in 1942 appointed a Committee on Post-war Hospital Problems in Scotland with Sir Hector Hetherington as chairman. It was intended that the Committee should submit recommendations to implement 'a policy aimed at the post-war development of a comprehensive and co-ordinated hospital service . . . on a regional basis'. Reporting in August 1943 the Committee assumed that the dual system of voluntary and local authority would persist and that the larger local authorities would be expected to maintain a comprehensive regional Hospital Service. An advisory Regional Council, representative of all the interests involved, was recommended for each of five regional hospital areas. Complicated financial proposals were submitted about which the Chairman had doubts and he personally considered a case existed for a State Grant to Voluntary Hospitals in recognition of the threat to their solvency from social and economic causes not of local origin.[30]

White Paper: a Sequel

Following Sir John Anderson's statement in the House of Commons and with a minimum of delay, exploratory discussions were started. Initially they were largely confidential. Partaking were a number of organized groups which included one nominated by the British Medical Association and the Royal Colleges; a second representative of the voluntary hospitals; and a third representative of the large local authorities. In due course (February 1944) the Government published a White Paper entitled *A National Health Service* which in a plan submitted for discussion proposed that:

(i) A Minister with a Central Health Service Council and a Central Medical Board should be vested with central responsibility.

(ii) The Councils of Counties and County Burghs would undertake the organisation of the Service, and the administration of the hospitals—administration of the latter to be, where local circumstances indicated a need, by Joint Boards with major authorities as constituent members. Local Health Service Councils were to advise those responsible for administration.

(iii) While retaining their administrative autonomy voluntary hospitals were to be invited to take part, in accordance with the terms of contracts to be agreed, in the plans of those administering hospital areas.

(iv) Group Practices were advocated as cardinal features of any future General Practitioner Service, but not to the exclusion of individual practice. There was to be no interference with the professional freedom of the doctor or the freedom of choice of doctor by the patient.[31]

B.M.A. Reaction

Within six months of its issue, the B.M.A. published the results of a Questionnaire on the White Paper distributed to all doctors in Great Britain.[32] Replies, representing

48 per cent of those to whom the questionnaire had been sent, revealed majorities in favour of Joint Hospital Boards, and Health Centres; and notably significant majorities against control of the Medical Service by Local Authorities, and against representation of the Local Authorities by Joint Hospital Boards possessed of Health Advisory Councils. In the ensuing months confidential negotiations took place dealing more particularly with the possibility of creating Regional Councils exercising authority over areas not necessarily determined by local authority boundaries; and of professional guidance in planning the service being given greater scope, having the potential contribution of universities with medical schools particularly in mind.

A New Government: a Second White Paper

A change in Government took place in July 1945, and private meetings between the new Ministers and the Negotiating Committee followed. A second White Paper was published simultaneously with the presentation to the House of Commons in March 1946 of a Bill applicable to England and Wales.[33] It was not until the English Bill became law that a Bill for Scotland was introduced. Reverting to the first White Paper, the English Bill embodied new administrative proposals. Of these the most important was transfer of all hospitals to the State; the delegation of administrative responsibility for hospitals to Regional Boards; and the vestment of local hospital administration in Hospital Management Committees. As to the General Practitioner Service, administration was to become the responsibility of local Executive Councils. While the Councils of Counties and County Boroughs were to retain environmental health services in extended form, their hospitals were to be transferred to the Regional Hospital Boards. Allowing that the General Practitioner Service should not be subject to control by local authorities, the Minister of Health, in a statement to the House, insisted that the sale and purchase of practices would have to come to an end; and gave the gradual redistribution of doctors as a need requiring priority consideration.

Remuneration of Doctors

Inevitably questions of professional remuneration loomed large. Two Inter-Departmental Committees were appointed, both with Sir Will Spens as chairman—the first in February 1945 to consider the case of general practitioners, and the second in May 1947 to review that of consultants and specialists. The findings of both Committees were accepted by the Government. Proposals in respect of family doctors related to net incomes after deduction of allowable professional expenses and on the assumption that provision for illness, premature decease and retirement was the private concern of the individual doctor. For consultants and specialists the appropriate Committee suggested for trainees, graded salaries based on periods of training: for specialists, basic salaries rising to a maximum by annual increments: and for specialists aged more than forty years, special awards for those selected by a national committee on the score of outstanding merit. The awards were to be in three grades and to consist of additions to salary, and the percentage of specialists eligible for each grade of award was stated.

Smouldering Suspicions

The English Bill became law on 6th November 1946. Although the general principles underlying a National Health Service were accepted by a great majority of the doctors, there persisted in the profession a genuinely grave disquiet at the possible loss of professional freedom, and an undisguised apprehension that the introduction of a salaried service would only be a matter of time. A large section of the profession was averse to accepting assurances on these particular points. Considered impartially the attitude was understandable. Those concerned with the drafting of Statutory Rules and Orders can be almost obsessionally influenced by the need to close loopholes and forestall possible evasions. In the words of a Leading Article in the *British Medical Journal*, 'Parliamentary drafting is a fine art and to the uninitiated phrases with simple intent can sound quite sinister, and harmless sounding phrases disguise startling implications'.[34] Historically the tendency can be traced to the earliest seventeenth-century (1603) Poor Law enactments: more concerned to protect the community than to ease the lot of the necessitous. Understandably, a defensive suspicion is bred in the minds of those who are subject to control by enactments and who are conscious of the often remote and frequently incomplete appreciation by legislators and those who advise them. It is small wonder that, when as does happen, central and local authorities fail to achieve mutual accommodation, a profession dependent upon individualism for much of its strength should be wary about being traduced by political oratory—and more especially by political oratory embellished by lilting Welsh wizardry. To witness Lloyd George and Nye Bevan captivate their audiences were experiences not to be forgotten, but they were experiences calling for reflection in an unemotional atmosphere before coming to conclusions.

In the same month that the National Health Service Act was placed on the Statute Book the British Medical Association conducted a Plebiscite which sought guidancee from its Members as to whether negotiations should be entered into with the Minister on the regulations authorized by the new Act. Voting was 18,972 in favour of and 23,110 against negotiations[35] : and of family doctors, 64 per cent were opposed to negotiation. In the circumstances the Council of the B.M.A. had no option but to inform the Minister that they had no mandate to negotiate.

Mutual Hostility Persists

The Plebiscite had been taken in November 1946. An impasse had been reached. Negotiations were not resumed until February of the following year. Relationships between the negotiating parties deteriorated and, on 8th January 1948 a special representative meeting of the B.M.A. passed a unanimous resolution recommending unqualified rejection of the Act by all practitioners. The date requires emphasis—8th January—exactly six months before 'the appointed day' when the requirements of the Act were to be implemented. Yet another Plebiscite was arranged by the B.M.A. and on 18th February (1948) it was announced that 40,814 doctors had recorded disapproval and 4735 approval of the National Health Act in its form at that time.[36] The probability, if not certainty, is that the voting reflected a deep-rooted antipathy to anything savouring of a whole-time state medical service. An assurance was soon forthcoming that a whole-time service would not be introduced by invoking the statutory powers in the form of regulations. Further reiterated assurances were given that there would be no interference or curtailment of a doctor's existing freedom of writing and speech.

Final and Third Plebiscite

After clarification of certain points the B.M.A. embarked on a third Plebiscite, general practitioners being asked for a 'Yes' or 'No' reply to acceptance in the light of modifications now proposed by the Government. The B.M.A. made it plain at the time that they would advise co-operation if 13,000, or less, general practitioners voted otherwise. In the event the number voting against co-operation fell short of the stipulated figure by more than 3400.[37] Subject to certain reservations the decision was arrived at by the B.M.A. on 28th May 1948 to recommend the profession to take part in the National Health Service.[38]

The National Health Service (Scotland) Act, 1947

Introduced in December 1946 the Scottish Bill received the Royal Assent in May 1947. The purpose of the Act was 'to provide for the establishment of a comprehensive health service for Scotland, and for purposes connected therewith'. There was much in common between the Scottish and the English (and Welsh) Acts more especially in the matter of conditions of service applicable to the medical profession. Central administration of the Scottish Act was made the responsibility of the Secretary of State for Scotland acting through the Department of Health: five Hospital Regions were designated each with their supervisory Regional Hospital Boards; and the administration of Hospital Groups was to be undertaken by Boards of Management. In direct contrast with arrangements south of the border, Teaching Hospitals were to be administered by Boards of Management responsible to the Regional Hospital Boards.

Provision was made for University representation on the Boards of Management of Teaching Hospitals, and University influence was further enhanced by representation on Medical Education Committees of which there was to be one in each Region. Inverness served as an administrative centre for the Region embracing the Highlands and Islands of the north and north-west: Edinburgh, Glasgow, Aberdeen and Dundee were with their Universities regarded as the centres for the other four regions. Large burghs, counties or groups of counties as defined under the Local Government (Scotland) Act of 1929 constituted Local Health Authorities for the purposes of the Scottish Health Service. By the terms of the new Act of 1947 the development of health centres rested with the Secretary of State with powers to delegate to Local Health Authorities: and all hospital endowments after initial transfer to newly created Boards of Management, were subject to distribution according to the decisions of a Hospital Endowments Commission.[39]

THE NATIONAL HEALTH SERVICES ACTS

ENGLAND & WALES 1946: SCOTLAND 1947

. . . I never could get accustomed to the annoyances caused me by the obstructive tactics of much of the Civil Service, not the faults of individuals but rather of the machine.

Sir Wilson Jameson

The first significant reference in the College Minutes to developments in connection with a national service was dated 21st July 1942. On that day the President (Dr

Charles McNeil) referred to the Draft Interim Report of the Medical Planning Commission (q.v.) a copy of which had been received by Council for their considered opinion. Fellows were invited by the President to submit their views in writing.[40] Discussing representation of the Scottish Medical Corporations the President informed the College in April of the following year that, while they were not represented on the Advisory Committee, they were represented on a United Kingdom Committee and a Scottish Representative Committee established to keep Government policy under review.[41] The College was informed that there was reason to think that policy favoured the creation of a Central Medical Appointments Board, and the use of major local authority machinery to establish Local Health Authorities. Significantly reference was made to the Hetherington, Beveridge and Goodenough Reports. With regard to the threatened closure of the Extra-Academical School contained in the Goodenough Report, an appeal was made by one senior Fellow 'that neither sentimental nor historical considerations' should have overmuch importance attached to them and that 'harmony with the University in the general interest of medical education' should be maintained.[41]

White Paper: Mixed Reception by College

In May 1944 the College were advised that the Council had considered the Government White Paper, having been informed ten months previously by their representative Dr McNeil on the Medical Planning Commission that the most he was at liberty to convey was that of administrative proposals contemplated by the Government, a number had met with considerable opposition.[42] Now in 1944 developments had reached the stage of the College being invited to enter into free discussion about the White Paper. Before it was decided to call an Extraordinary Meeting, apprehension was expressed by those present lest the profession became part of the Civil Service, and about the future of the voluntary hospitals. A Fellow with particular interests in general practice declared that, as depicted in the White Paper the Health Service was quite inadequate, and that its development should follow and not precede the creation of a new social service for the prevention of disease.[43]

An Extraordinary Meeting was called in a month's time. Opening the discussion, Dr McNeil reminded Fellows that the B.M.A. Planning Commission had advocated extension of the basis of Medical Insurance, a complete service for everyone with retention of freedom of choice of doctor, and agreement that administrative arrangements should have first consideration. The White Paper was described as a Government compromise; and the proposed Medical Advisory Committees as machinery designed to preserve a balance between the medical administrator and practising doctor. One view expressed concern that the Scottish Medical Advisory Committee had been appointed without reference to the Scottish Medical Corporations, but did not win general support. Some doubts were felt as to the ability of voluntary hospitals to make their proper contribution in the face of rising costs: and a Fellow with predominantly administrative interests urged a realistic view with acceptance of the White Paper 'lest worse befall'. The position of the numerous Fellows on active service was not forgotten and the College was reminded that they would wish to make their views known before decisions were made. Eventually after a fairly wide-ranging but not impressively constructive discussion the course was adopted of remitting the White Paper to Council for joint consideration with the other medical Corporations. A Committee was thereupon appointed by Council[44] which following discussions with the other Corporations,[45] drafted a Memorandum which after amendment was sent by Council to the Secretary of State for Scotland.[46]

College Memorandum on First White Paper

While agreeing with the general principles of the Scheme, the College Memorandum on the proposed National Health Service urged that administrative machinery should be kept as simple as possible: development should be gradual; and that legislative measures should be deferred until the return home of men and women on active service.

The Memorandum confirmed acceptance of the view that the hospital services in Scotland should be based upon five Regions and at the same time strongly recommended that these same regions should provide the foundations for comprehensive unified health services to meet all the needs of the people. Disagreement was expressed with the intention rigidly to retain local government boundaries as probably being contrary to efficiency of the health services in certain circumstances. With undisguised emphasis it was declared that 'the central responsibility must lie with the Secretary of State for Scotland, acting through the Department of Health': and that regardless of the arguments advanced in the White Paper for the continuance of medical services in various Government Departments these services should be transferred to the Department of Health. As to representation, the College urged that 50 per cent of the part-time members of the Central Medical Board should be nominated by the profession: and that a number of those on the Central Health Council should be nominated by medical organizations.

With regard to local administration the College were 'firmly of opinion that all local services should be more closely integrated' and, with the furtherance of this objective in mind suggested that all medical services should be within the control of a single administrative body—the Regional Health Board. This Board should, the Memorandum suggested, assume the 'responsibilities at present assigned to the Joint Hospital Boards' and 'would administer all clinics and domiciliary services . . . of the region'. Local advisory bodies, it was maintained, 'should not contain more than a nominal number of local authority representatives'. Trial of Health Centres in densely populated areas was considered desirable.

Dispersed throughout the Memorandum was evidence of certain anxieties. Thus to the College the proposed scheme seemed 'to deal with a Sickness Service rather than with a Health Service' and it was considered that 'more should be made of the essentials of health and preventive medicine, namely, housing, good nutrition, sanitary services and education of the public along lines of disease prevention'. The College viewed proposals to *direct* young graduates 'with alarm', as a measure raising issues of grave importance extending beyond purely professional considerations. Fears were expressed that voluntary hospitals would find themselves in difficult financial situations, and the need was foreseen of teaching hospitals being assured adequate material for teaching requirements.

Commenting on the absence in the White Paper of details for providing a consultant service, the College Memorandum stated that the College had already approved standards of training, and had already recommended the maintenance of a specialist–consultants register by the General Medical Council. Appointments, it was considered, should be made 'by the Board of Management of the hospital concerned on advice from the Regional Hospital Council and the staff of the Hospital'. Other points dealt with were the conditions of service of junior hospital appointees and part-time consultants. The final comment was:

> 'The College is strongly in favour of freedom for the medical profession in matters of scientific investigation and publication.'[47]

The Memorandum is of historical interest in a number of respects. Its subject matter was, at the time, unique. The presentation of the material was outstanding in its clarity of expression, economy of words, and the courageous incisiveness with which carefully considered convictions were conveyed. Nor should it escape notice that in 1944 as in 1681, Fellows were acutely aware of the contributions they had to make to community medicine. Events since 1944 have in many ways confirmed the foresight of Fellows in 1681.

Uneasy Forebodings

Four months after transmission of the College Memorandum Dr McNeil reported on such progress as had been made by the Negotiating Committee on the White Paper. His account could not be described as entirely encouraging from the College standpoint. He warned that while considerable progress had been made with general practitioner services, a great deal remained outstanding in so far as Hospital and Special Services were concerned. In similar vein he told of failure to postpone or phase legislation with a view to hospital requirements being given priority over extension of benefits to dependants; and of the dogged unwillingness of the Minister to concede in the matter of the intended Local Administrative Structure. In conclusion Dr McNeil made mention of a forthcoming second White Paper (q.v.) which contemplated an increase in the powers to be granted to Regional Bodies and the establishment of the General Practitioner Service on lines resembling those of the existing National Health Insurance Scheme.[48]

Request from Negotiating Committee

. . . the great thing to remember about these committee people who come in and pretend to run our shows for us is that we generally outlive them and, fortunately, from time to time they change.

Sir Wilson Jameson

The next development was a request by the Negotiating Committee for the views of the College on two confidential documents containing tentative modifications of the White Paper aiming at the abandonment of control of young doctors: the prohibition of the sale of practices: and changes in the administrative structure. Without delay the predictable Extraordinary Meeting was arranged.[49] This took place in June 1945. The meeting was of particular significance in that there was first early evidence of the possibility at least of proposals for Scotland differing in some respects from those for England and Wales. It was pointed out that Regional Councils were contemplated for Scotland, each to consist of representatives of Voluntary and Local Authority Hospitals in equal numbers, and to have the guidance of an essentially medical advisory body. There was no mention of medical representation of hospital areas. By way of contrast, contemplated provisions for England were, according to McNeil, to take the form of composite authorities each consisting of local Boards, voluntary hospitals, and selected medical individuals to plan for a Region and Constituent Areas. Discussion concluded with the College resolving that Local Clinics, including Maternity and Child Welfare Services should be brought into closer relationship with hospital services and that arrangements for Scotland should be the same as those for England.[50]

By the time of the Quarterly Meeting in May 1946 the National Health Service Bill for England and Wales was before Parliament. A statement of some length was made by Dr McNeil (now an ex-President) in his continuing capacity of College representative and he asked for the observations of Fellows on specific points. Four College resolutions on this occasion require quotation. Of these the first was to the effect that the College 'accepts the administrative arrangements in the National Health Service Bill regarding Hospitals as likely to provide a better distribution and co-ordination of work among existing hospitals and an orderly development of new hospitals'. Voting was 27 in favour and 1 against the motion.

The second motion for which 17 voted 'for' and 11 'against' was 'new proposals in the Bill replacing existing purchase and sale of private practices are likely to provide a better distribution of general practice among the whole people'.

Of the remaining two motions, both were seconded and accepted *nemine contradicente*. They were:

> 'The maximum of professional freedom compatible with efficiency, discipline and order, should be enjoyed by all practitioners, general or specialist', and
> 'The College is opposed to and regrets the disintegration of the Maternity Services treatment in the Bill, and still more the absence of provision for linking together the personal services dealing with children.'

It requires no stretch of imagination to attribute part at least of the last motion to the vocational perspicacity of a former paediatric President.

The Scottish Bill: a 'Watching Committee'

As already mentioned, this Bill was brought before Parliament in December 1946. At the Quarterly Meeting of the College in the previous month the President (Dr

Murray Lyon) drew the attention of Fellows to the fact that 'no request for help had been received from the authorities in connection with the National Health Service Bill for Scotland'. He gave it as his opinion that a Committee should be appointed 'whose duty it would be to watch the progress and study the Bill for Scotland, and to draw attention to all points of interest and questions which might affect the College'. A Committee was duly nominated and consisted of Drs Charles McNeil (Chairman), W. D. D. Small, C.B.E., Thomas Ferguson, D. K. Henderson, James G. M. Hamilton, J. L. Cowan, A. W. Stewart, C.I.E., and W. S. Clark.[52]

This 'Watching' Committee reported in three months' time. The Negotiating Committee in London was faced with the decision whether or not to continue negotiations with the Government (q.v.). Speaking for the Committee, McNeil said the Bill gave the medical profession a share in the responsibility for administration and formation of policy but there was without doubt still reason for anxiety. None the less he considered an opportunity was being offered for general improvement of the medical services, and that the profession was sufficiently well organized to be able to protect its own interests. Once again the Fellow with an administrative background who in October had urged acceptance of the White Paper 'lest worse befall' spoke up, and on this occasion to the effect that the 'time for negotiations was past' and the College should now help the Secretary of State to frame the necessary Regulations 'to make the best possible of . . . a very bad job'. There was no indication as to whether 'badness' of the job was in any way attributable to political bias, legislative ineptitude or professional obduracy! Be that as it may the College authorized its representative to indicate that it was the view of the College that negotiations should continue.[53]

London: Points at Issue

Negotiations did continue, if in creaking fashion and sultry atmosphere. Less than six months before the appointed day for England and Wales a letter of enquiry was received by the College from the Negotiating Committee. The College representative (Dr McNeil) enumerated the persisting differences between the Minister and the Profession. They were the method of entry by appointment; the restriction of entry by the operation of Medical Practices Committees; payment by basic salary and capitation fee; the excessive powers to be assumed by the Minister; uncertainties concerning compensation in the case of partnerships; and the position with regard to dismissal from the Service. Discussion was conditioned by fears of ministerial monopolistic control of consultants and competition among them; of a whole-time service; and of the insidious introduction of political issues. (Sir) Stanley Davidson with characteristic forthrightness urged that any thought of fighting the purchase of practices on a patient–doctor relationship should be discarded straightway. Depending on the outlook of the individual the outcome of the meeting was sagacious, or timorous. A reply to the Negotiating Committee was postponed until the result of the second Plebiscite only very recently decided upon by the B.M.A.[54]

Six days after announcement of the results of this Plebiscite (November 1946— q.v.) an Extraordinary Meeting of the College was called to consider among other aspects of the situation the past and future negotiations of the Negotiating Committee. Discussion was wide and views expressed varied. Prospects of a basic salary invoked severest criticism. Amendment of the Act was proposed which prompted (Sir) Andrew Davidson of the Department of Health to point out the impossibility of any such course of action in advance of the introduction of the Principal Act. Dr McNeil with his accumulated intimate knowledge of proceedings called on the College to assist the Negotiating Committee and the B.M.A. by approving the attitude adopted by the latter in its efforts to safeguard professional standards. A somewhat nebulous suggestion that some form of positive action should be taken to break the deadlock did not win the sympathy of the Vice-President who considered it would place 'too great a burden on the . . . College'. It was however left to Council to draft a Statement for consideration by the Fellows.[55]

This Statement was drawn up and circulated among Fellows before another Extraordinary Meeting in March. Once again in accordance with expectations discussion was considerable, and McNeil urged that the General Practitioners should be given weighty support as a means of maintaining the bargaining power of the B.M.A. and the Negotiating Committee. Numerous amendments to the draft Statement of Council were proposed but all defeated. The final outcome was that a Resolution based on Council's Statement was sent to the Prime Minister and the Press; and a copy of the Resolution was enclosed in a letter to the Negotiating Committee by way of a reply to their request of some weeks previously.

Resolution sent to the Prime Minister

The Resolution sent to the Prime Minister embodied four sections. Of these the first consisted of a reflective Preamble reminiscent of Memorials submitted in the distant past, except in so far as it was less verbose. The following were the three other sections:

'2. The College shares the desire of the entire community for a National Health Service which will afford to the people the highest standard of medical service attainable. It views with disappointment and disquiet the failure of the negotiating parties to reach agreement.

3. The College is of opinion that the overwhelming vote of every section of the medical profession disapproving of the National Health Service Act 1946 in its present form can only be explained by fear that professional freedom is gravely endangered. The essential fear centres round the power of the Minister to alter by order or regulation the fundamental terms of service of the medical profession.

4. The College urges in the national interest that negotiations should be resumed and that the matters in dispute be re-examined and adjusted so that the profession will feel able to co-operate with confidence in the development of the comprehensive service desired by all.'[56]

Final Advice to the Negotiating Committee

Of equal importance as a historical milestone was the letter from the College which accompanied the Copy of the Resolution sent to the Negotiating Committee. 'The view of the College on the Minister's reply', it began, 'will be expressed by its representative Dr. Charles McNeil, as he may think opportune. Meantime . . . the College considers certain concessions may have to be made by both sides . . . The Minister might be pressed to include in an amending Act certain safeguards to maintain the policy which he has indicated to be that of the Government—for example a clause which would forbid the introduction of a whole-time salaried service without further Act of Parliament. Were this done, the questions of basic salary and of the right to buy and sell practices would become of less importance and might leave room for concession. "Negative direction" and right of appeal are other matters which should be further discussed.'

> 'The Committee should concentrate its efforts on securing the limitation of the powers of government by Ministerial regulation whereby fundamental matters of principle may be determined without full parliamentary debate, and on freedom to practise, to write, and to speak without interference or dictation.'[56]

On 28th May 1948 the profession was recommended to take part in the National Health Service Scheme and on 5th July of the same year the Scheme came into operation throughout the United Kingdom. At a Quarterly Meeting in July, Dr Charles McNeil resigned from his post as Negotiator and Observer on behalf of our College, duties which in one way or another he had undertaken from the time he was first elected President in 1940.[57] In many ways his activities in connection with the

National Health Service resembled those in the nineteenth century of Dr Alexander Wood (Chap. XII) on behalf of the College in connection with Medical Reform. Both men were ardent Collegiates: where Wood was relentlessly determined, McNeil was quietly pertinacious: both men rendered the College exceptional service each in his own way—and the calculated steadying influence of McNeil's hand on the helm will become increasingly recognized with time.

REFERENCES

(1) CRAIG, W. S. (1946) *Child and Adolescent Life in Health and Disease: a Study in Social Pædiatrics*, pp. 136–7. Edinburgh: E. & S. Livingstone.

(2) ROSS, J. S. (1952) *The National Health Service in Great Britain*, p. 37. London: Oxford University Press.

(3) Ibid., p. 41.

(4) BRAITHWAITE, W. J. (1957) *Lloyd George's Ambulance Wagon. Being the memoirs of William J. Braithwaite, 1911–1912.* London: Methuen.

(5) CONYBEARE, Sir J. (1957) The crisis of 1911–13: Lloyd George and the doctors. *Lancet*, **1**, 1032.

(6) 1 & 2 Geo. 5, c. 55 (1911).

THE NATIONAL INSURANCE ACT, 1911

(7) College Minutes, 19.xii.1911.

(8) Ibid., 22.xii.1911.

(9) Ibid., 1.ii.1912.

(10) Ibid., 12.xii.1912.

(11) Ibid., 6.v.1913.

(12) Ibid., 23.vi.1913.

(13) NEWSHOLME, Sir A. (1936) *The Last Thirty Years in Public Health*, p. 120. London: Allen & Unwin.

THE NATIONAL TREND PERSISTS

(14) College Minutes, 6.xii.1917.

(15) Ibid., 18.xii.1917.

(16) Ibid., 4.ii.1919.

(17) Ibid., 11.iii.1919.

(18) SCOTLAND. BOARD OF HEALTH (1920) *Consultative Council on Medical and Allied Services. Interim report.* (Chairman: Sir Donald MacAlister.) Edinburgh H.M.S.O.

(19) College Minutes, 6.xi.1934.

(20) R.C.P.E. (1934) *Memorandum on Scottish health services . . . to the Committee on Scottish health services.* Edinburgh: [Privately printed].

(21) ROSS, J. R. Op. cit., p. 69.

(22) SCOTLAND. DEPARTMENT OF HEALTH (1936) *Committee on Scottish Health Services. Report,* p. 83. (Chairman: E. P. Cathcart.) Edinburgh: H.M.S.O.

(23) Ibid., p. 87.

(24) Ibid., p. 248.

(25) MEDICAL PLANNING COMMISSION (1942) *Draft Interim Report.* London: B.M.A. House.

(26) INTERDEPARTMENTAL COMMITTEE ON SOCIAL INSURANCE AND ALLIED SERVICES (1942) *Report by Sir William Beveridge.* London: H.M.S.O.

(27) *Hansard,* 386, H.C. Deb., 5s, 16th Feb., 1943, 1655 f.

(28) WHEELER-BENNETT, J. W. (1962) *John Anderson, Viscount Waverley,* p. 25. London: Macmillan.

(29) ROSS, J. S. Op. cit., pp. 83–4.

(30) SCOTLAND. DEPARTMENT OF HEALTH (1943) *Committee on Post-war Hospital Problems in Scotland. Report.* (Chairman: Sir Hector Hetherington.) Edinburgh: H.M.S.O.

(31) MINISTRY OF HEALTH *and* DEPARTMENT OF HEALTH FOR SCOTLAND (1944) *A National Health Service* [White paper]. London: H.M.S.O.

(32) ROSS, J. S. Op. cit., p. 88.

(33) MINISTRY OF HEALTH (1946) *National Health Service Bill: summary of the proposed new service* [White paper]. London: H.M.S.O.

(34) Leader (1972) Next step in Scotland. *British Medical Journal,* **1,** 462.

(35) ROSS, J. S. Op. cit., p. 123.

(36) Ibid., p. 125.

(37) Ibid., p. 126.

(38) BRITISH MEDICAL ASSOCIATION (1948) Special Representative Meeting. *British Medical Journal* (Supplement), **1,** 147–55.

(39) 10 & 11 Geo. 6, c. 27 (1946–7).

THE NATIONAL HEALTH SERVICES ACTS

(40) College Minutes, 21.vii.1942.

(41) Ibid., 22.iv.1943.

(42) Ibid., 20.vii.1943.

(43) Ibid., 2.v.1944.

(44) Ibid., 6.vi.1944.

(45) Ibid., 18.vii.1944.

(46) Ibid., 6.x.1944.

(47) R.C.P.E. (1944) *Memorandum by the Royal College of Physicians of Edinburgh on the proposed National Health Service.* Edinburgh: [Privately printed].

(48) College Minutes, 6.ii.1945.

(49) Ibid., 1.v.1945.

(50) Ibid., 4.vi.1945.

(51) Ibid., 7.v.1946.

(52) Ibid., 5.xi.1946.

(53) Ibid., 4.ii.1947.

(54) Ibid., 22.i.1948.

(55) Ibid., 24.ii.1948.

(56) Ibid., 15.iii.1948.

(57) Ibid., 20.vii.1948.

Chapter XXIX

COMMUNITY HEALTH AND WELFARE:
SOME OTHER COLLEGE ACTIVITIES

Welfare is a whole, built up from many interconnected elements. It includes elements physical, intellectual, emotional and spiritual, family relationships as well; and social— since the welfare of the individual depends on that of the society in which he lives, as its welfare depends upon him.

Lord Samuel (Romanes Lecture, 1947)

With events moving irreversibly over the years towards a National Health Service as an integral part of overall social legislation, the College was inevitably involved in developments with a direct or indirect bearing on the medical profession. These developments dealt with a wide variety of subjects related to medico-social problems.

VENEREAL DISEASES

In March 1899 Council submitted to College a Report on a Memorial received from 'a meeting of ladies with reference to a proposed inquiry regarding venereal diseases'. After approving the Report the College resolved to petition Parliament for the appointment of a Royal Commission on Venereal Diseases.[1]

THE HEALTH OF SCHOOL CHILDREN

On 8th March 1904 the College had submitted to it by the President (Sir Thomas Clouston) a Report of a Sub-Committee of the Royal College of Physicians, Royal College of Surgeons of Edinburgh and of the Faculty of Physicians and Surgeons of Glasgow on 'Health Conditions of School Children of Scotland'.

The Report opened with the statement that accurate data would be of considerable value in 'determining the question which is at present disturbing the public mind viz:—Whether degeneracy of the race is taking place'. Responsibility for ascertaining the position was considered to rest with the State, with practical contributions from such Bodies as the Medical Corporations. Initiation of an Enquiry was given as an understandable sequel to the Royal Commission on Physical Training in Scotland,[2] and a large section of the public was described as looking to 'our profession for light and guidance'. A case was presented for voluntary effort on the part of the Medical Corporations with the co-operation of local authorities, which would involve the former in only limited expenditure and which through the influence of public opinion might persuade the Government to appoint a Royal Commission.

The scheme of examination of children suggested by the Committee for a progressive series of ages, embraced height, weight, chest measurements; muscular power, nutrition and general development; diseases and malformations; malfunctions of organs of special senses; mental development; and the condition of teeth. Examinations satisfying the highest attainable scientific standards of accuracy were regarded as *sine qua non*.

Specific points for urgent attention were given as ascertainment of the readiness or otherwise of local authorities to co-operate in the areas contemplated—Edinburgh, Leith, Glasgow and Govan, and the availability of limited funds from College sources. The College approved the proposed investigation 'on the understanding that the College may contribute towards the expense of such Inquiry'.[3]

There was an interlude at this stage. At the Quarterly Meeting in May Dr Clouston moved the suspension of Standing Orders, the reason being that the Education (Scotland) Bill was before Parliament and contained no clauses for medical and hygiene measures; the Bill might reach the committee stage at any time and Sir John Batty Tuke, M.P. had given notice of an amendment to make good the deficiencies, and College support would strengthen his hand. A motion was passed calling on Council to endeavour to secure the insertion in the Education (Scotland) Bill of clauses making it incumbent on School Boards to provide medical inspection, for the supervision of school hygiene and for suitable physical education.[4]

A Minute of 7th February 1905 referred again to the plan to be undertaken jointly by the College and the Glasgow Faculty into the 'Health Conditions of School Children of Scotland'. To further the proposed enquiry the College voted a sum of £250 with the reservation that any action by the Joint Committee of the two Medical Corporations should be postponed 'until it is seen whether provision for such an inquiry is introduced into the new Education Bill for Scotland during the ensuing session of Parliament'. The motion was proposed on behalf of the Council, and seconded by Scotland's pioneer physician in the health and diseases of children, Dr John Thomson.[5]

Details of the Bill became known within a few months and the Council considered it appropriate to send to the Secretary of State for Scotland what can only be described as an appreciative Memorial. Referring to 'the effects of Educational methods on the health of school children dealt with in the Education (Scotland) Bill now before Parliament' the Memorial stated that the College shared public concern 'as to the physical and mental effects of our increasing urban life'; and felt that 'those evil effects might be largely counteracted by better conditions during school life'. Unqualified approval was given to proposals in the Bill 'for the Medical Inspection of Schools, and for the making of Physical Education a part of school training' and it was urged that 'the Education Department should have specific powers over the Local Bodies to render' the proposals effective. It was made abundantly clear that implied in the recommendation was authority on the part of the Medical Inspector 'to examine into the health of the school children, and their capacity for Education, Mental and Physical, and also into the School Hygiene'. Almost certainly this comprehensive appraisal of the Bill owed much to John Thomson's broad conception of Child Life and Health. Approval contained in the Memorial extended to the special provisions contemplated for certain handicapped children, and for the Sanitary Inspection of Schools. Finally the Memorialists concluded with an expression of conviction that 'Physical Education on a scientific basis is needed in many of our City Schools . . .'. The Memorial had the unanimous support of the College.[6]

While on the subject of the health of the school child it is not out of place to mention a letter received in June 1914 from the Chairman of the Edinburgh School Board. It asked if the College 'had any means of putting a stop to what is not only a scandal but a danger to the health and the morals of the public'. The 'scandal' referred to was 'the sandwich men . . . carrying bills . . . on which are advertised the businesses of a "Dr." Temple and a "Dr." Massey'. With disarming delicacy the writer allowed that 'the meaning of these is sufficiently obvious'. Nothing daunted the College Council referred the problem to the Procurator Fiscal with a request that he prosecute. The President (Dr Graham Brown) and Clerk even went the length of meeting the Fiscal. But twentieth-century administrative procedure was already in vogue. The Fiscal disclaimed responsibility and recommended that the General Medical Council should be asked to prosecute, a recommendation which the Clerk to the Council of the College was instructed to implement.[7]

Eventually the College decided to prosecute[8] and Temple and Massey were fined with the option of imprisonment.[9]

MIDWIVES

THE MIDWIVES (SCOTLAND) ACT, 1914

Having considered the Midwives (Scotland) Bill, Council recommended its approval to the College.[10] At one time certain reservations had been held concerning representation of the College on the Central Board for Scotland but as explained by Dr Freeland Barbour these had been accepted as relatively insignificant in the light of the importance of the major principles involved.[11] The motion for approval was successfully proposed by Dr Haig Ferguson and seconded by Dr J. W. Ballantyne[12] —both distinguished obstetricians with wide socio-medical interests. Dr Ferguson's name was for long associated with the care of the unmarried mother and her child, and that of Dr Ballantyne with pioneer work in the field of antenatal care and the study of fetal morbidity.

The Petition subsequently sent to Parliament was emphatic in declaring that the College 'highly approve' the Midwives Bill which they were convinced would if passed into law 'secure the better training of midwives in Scotland, and thus conduce to a diminished childbed and infantile mortality'. Historically, the interest of the Petition is in the obvious desire of the preamble to forestall any challenge of the College's claim to pronounce judgment on matters obstetric or neonatal. The College's Charter was quoted as evidencing that their establishment had '*inter alia* consolidated the medical profession and encouraged and advanced medical learning and science'; and that they were authorized to make Bye-Laws and Regulations for promoting the science of and ordering of the practice of the science of medicine.[13]

NURSES

NURSING SERVICES IN SCOTLAND: STATEMENT BY THE COLLEGE (MAY 1938)

This Statement was submitted in response to an approach by a Scottish Departmental Committee on Nursing; and was prepared by a College Committee consisting of Drs J. D. Comrie (Vice-President), R. B. Campbell, C. McNeil, D. M. Lyon, T. Y. Finlay and T. D. Inch.[14] College evidence was submitted according as it related to (*a*) Recruitment and Conditions of Entry or (*b*) Terms and Conditions of

Service. With regard to the first of these recruitment was considered to be too haphazard, interchangeability between different branches for the purposes of training was recommended and the desirability of a superannuation scheme stressed. As to the age at entry the College favoured girls of 17–18 starting to work in hospitals for children or in the children's wards of fever hospitals, it being accepted that these girls could at the age of 19 years be drafted to general hospitals. At the same time it was recommended that the position of 'untrained nurses or home-helps' should receive consideration.

A series of suggestions concerning conditions of service were incorporated in the Statement. Ninety-six hours' duty per fortnight was given as the optimum to be aimed at. Administrative adjustments by senior staff and the employment of more nurses were suggested as possible means of offsetting the uncertainties associated with off-duty periods and the undesirable deduction of time for lectures from those periods. An adequacy of ward-maids was regarded as necessary to reduce the amount of purely domestic work undertaken by nurses. Hostels for nurses were advanced as a possible solution in dealing with unsatisfactory service of meals and the lack of adequate opportunities for recreation. A system of inspection of the conditions under which nurses lived and worked was advocated.

In the opinion of the College, training for a period of three years in a general hospital was adequate for a girl commencing at the age of 19 years and possessed of a suitable preliminary education. Without ruling out the possibility of more male nurses being employed, it was considered at the time of the Statement that the supply of such nurses was 'sufficient and suitable'.[15]

MATERNITY AND CHILD WELFARE

The preparation of a Maternity and Child Welfare Bill was pursued in the years 1916–18 while the nation was facing a succession of grave military crises. In March 1917 the President of the College (Sir Robert Philip) suggested the calling of a meeting in the College to discuss the Edinburgh Civic Welfare Scheme. His intention was to invite the attendance, in addition to Fellows, of local members of the profession and representatives of the civic authorities. Doctors John Thomson, J. W. Ballantyne and Lorrain Smith were entrusted to draw up a preparatory Report.[16]

A comparatively early result was the receipt of a letter from the Edinburgh and Leith Division of the B.M.A. which urged that any proposed Welfare Scheme should be limited to the poor, make provision for illegitimate infants and ensure adequate

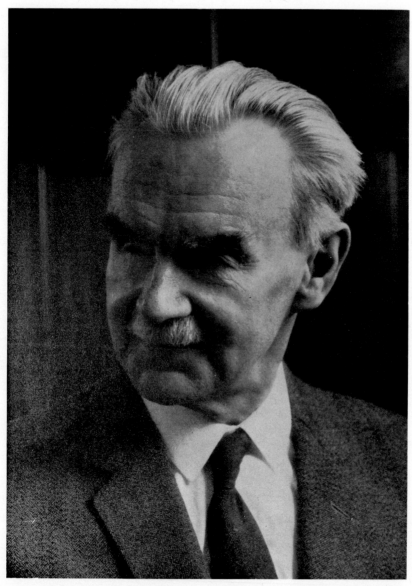

PLATE 46   Professor W. O. Kermack (1898–1970)
Photograph by Studio Morgan, Aberdeen

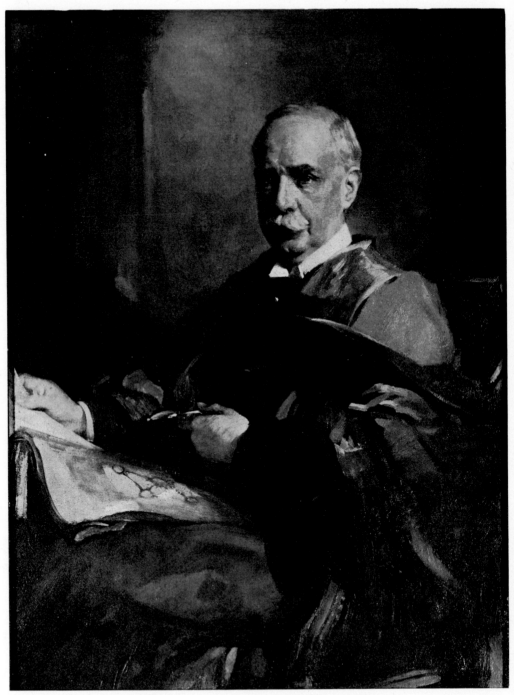

PLATE 47   Sir Robert W. Philip (1857–1939)
Reproduced from portrait in the College by Sir James Guthrie, R.S.A.; photograph by Tom Scott

remuneration of doctors. A point particularly stressed in the letter was the necessity for the administrative departments to obtain advice from a 'duly recognised . . . Committee of clinicians', and this was heartily endorsed in the reply sent by the College. In due course a College Committee was formed which consisted of the President and the Secretary (a paediatrician—Dr Dingwall Fordyce) together with those who had been responsible for the preparatory Report, and the full co-operation of the Royal College of Surgeons and the British Medical Association was secured.[17] A conference eventuated and, in accordance with a resolution passed, the Town Clerk of Edinburgh was advised of the formation of a Joint Committee representative of the two Edinburgh Colleges and the British Medical Association to assist the Public Health Authorities.[18]

MILK SUPPLIES

On 21st July 1914 a Committee was appointed 'to consider the question of the Milk Supply of the City'.[19] There is no evidence that any report was produced or that the City Public Health Committee or Medical Office of Health received any communication from the College.[20] The outbreak of war on 4th August may well explain this. At the time in question doubts were being entertained in some quarters about the freedom from tuberculosis infection of milk coming from surrounding rural areas.

MENTAL DEFICIENCY

SCOTTISH LUNACY AND MENTAL DEFICIENCY LAWS: COLLEGE STATEMENT (JULY 1938)

In the Statement submitted by request of a Departmental Committee on the Scottish Lunacy and Mental Deficiency Laws the College expressed the view that emendation and consolidation of the law relating to mental diseases was highly desirable. Essentially the Statement dealt with questions raised under a series of headings determined by the Departmental Committee in the terms of reference. These questions dealt with certification, detention and supervision in relation to unsoundness of mind in a variety of situations.

A case does not exist for detailing the answers given to the various questions but it

2B

was noteworthy that the College was opposed to continuation of the practice involving 'the sub-division of mental defectives into idiots, imbeciles, feeble-minded persons and moral defectives'; and it considered that Local Authorities should have power to accommodate mental defectives irrespective of age in separate blocks in existing mental hospitals and that, where necessary, the Public Health Authorities should have made available to them provision for the care of mentally defective children under the age of five.

The College Statement took the opportunity of urging the abolition of dual control of rate-aided hospitals by the Public Health and Public Assistance Authorities, and of ventilating the need for legal provisions to protect medical officers from 'frivolous or vexatious actions at law in connection with their duties under the lunacy acts'. Finally the point was made that the connotations 'person of unsound mind', 'rate-aided person' and 'mental hospital' should be substituted in the laws and documents for 'lunatic', 'pauper' and 'asylum' respectively.[21]

THE INDUSTRIAL POPULATION

A year prior to the outbreak of World War II the College, at the request of a Royal Commission, submitted a Statement on the Geographical Distribution of the Industrial Population. When making their request the Commissioners drew the particular attention of the College to the disadvantages in the past to health of life in large industrial towns; the improvement in conditions of health in such towns during the preceding 50–75 years; and to a comparison of conditions of health in those towns with those in rural areas. Two specific questions were asked: does or does not the balance of advantage still rest in favour of the country; and if so, to what extent?

In their Statement the College drew attention to the handicaps imposed by the vagueness of the 'notion of health conditions involved', the lack of direct observations on the actual physical condition of individuals, and the necessity of depending on relevant statistics from official sources. To arrive at their conclusions the College first studied General Death Rates, Infant Mortality Rates, National Health Insurance Sickness Rates, and data obtained from the Medical Inspection of School Children. From their findings they were satisfied that a marked improvement in health conditions, reflected in almost all aspects of bodily health, had taken place in both country and town during the preceding 100 years. If anything the extent of improvement had been greater in the towns, but the Report went out of its way to emphasize that this in no way applied to infant mortality which in towns was 'peculiarly backward' and still 'substantially behind the country'. It was considered that this discrepancy, which was most evident in limited regions of cities, was due to features incidental to urbanization and not to urbanization *per se*; and that it would probably disappear with 'slum clearance and overcrowding schemes'.

Turning to 'future probable trends' the Report stressed the need to discriminate between 'industrialisation' and 'urbanisation'. How refreshing it is not to come across even mention of that modern monstrosity 'conurbation'! General conclusions arrived at were that in part public health had suffered disastrously from urbanisation particularly when associated with industrialisation; that poverty, malnutrition and hygiene rather than population concentration had been major contributory factors; and that objection on health grounds did not constitute valid reasons for deprecating well-planned urban areas. Finally the opportunity of the Report was taken to urge that 'an effort should be made periodically to estimate' the health of the people.[22]

The Report is an admirable one. Preparation of it and the appendices and tables must have entailed an immense expenditure of time and effort. Members of the Committee responsible were Drs A. Goodall (President) (Chairman), J. D. Comrie (Vice-President), E. Bramwell, W. T. Ritchie, C. McNeil, A. F. Hewat, A. G. McKendrick (Lt.-Col.), J. D. Gilruth, W. T. Benson, E. Watt, T. D. Inch, associated with Mr W. J. Stuart (President, Royal College of Surgeons of Edinburgh), Dr G. A. Brown (Royal Faculty of Physicians and Surgeons of Glasgow) and Dr P. L. McKinlay (Department of Health, Scotland).[14]

WORKMEN'S COMPENSATION

Another Report prepared in the pre-war months was one for the Royal Commission on Workmen's Compensation. The request was described as urgent and the College lost no time in appointing a Committee.[23] Dr Alexander Goodall (President) was Chairman, the other members being Drs J. D. Comrie (Vice-President), J. Orr, C. M. Pearson, A. L. S. Tuke, T. Ferguson, J. K. Slater, T. D. Inch, W. R. Russell, S. A. Smith, J. M. Dewar and D. J. A. Kerr (Secretary). Disadvantages of the system in force at the time which had come to the notice of the College were described. They included:

    (i) lack of wages or sick benefit, and prolonged delay of compensation during the investigation of circumstances giving rise to sickness or industrial disease;

    (ii) the possibility of claiming a lump sum encouraging exaggeration of symptoms;

(iii) delay in arranging compensation prejudicing recovery;

(iv) bias on the part of medical men in favour of a client, whether employee or employer;

(v) accident-prone workmen, and

(vi) increased duration of disability favoured by the existing system.

Among remedies suggested were:

(i) Entitlement to Sick Benefit as soon as declared unfit.

(ii) Greater care in the appointment of medical referees having knowledge of conditions under which men work.

(iii) Conclusive decisions should not rest with *one* medical referee: the possibility of a medical board or medical tribunal of appeal should be considered.

(iv) Wastage would be lessened were workmen submitted to a medical examination at the beginning of their career and possibly also again at the age of 50 years, and

(v) Consolidation of the National Insurance, Workmen's Compensation and Unemployment Insurance Acts and their administration on a National Basis to eliminate 'most of the existing difficulties, such as definition of an accident, delay in payment of persons unfit through injury, and antagonism between employer and employee . . .'.[24]

SCOTTISH HOUSING

In February 1943 a letter was received by the College on behalf of the Sub-Committee on Housing Design of the Scottish Housing Advisory Committee asking that the College should submit evidence.[25] The Committee appointed with Dr W. G. Clark as Chairman to deal with the matter, considered the Remit to be too narrow and in preparing their evidence deliberately aimed at expressing their 'views on every medical aspect of housing'. Previous housing programmes had, in the opinion of the Committee, made inadequate provision 'for the artisan population' and they considered that provision of this kind should have priority over slum clearance. Having advised this they focussed attention on the vital importance of education without which 'all housing plans might be brought to nought'.[26]

THE FUTURE OF HOSPITALS

Early in 1942, acutely aware of the extent of discussions in progress concerning the development and organization of hospitals on a Regional basis, the College on its own initiative resolved to ascertain the views of the Edinburgh Royal College of

Surgeons and the Glasgow Royal Faculty as to establishing a Joint Enquiry. A College Committee was then appointed.[27] It was about this time that the Hetherington Committee (Chap. XXVIII) had commenced its labours. Within three months the College was invited by the Department of Health for Scotland to submit evidence and another Committee was appointed for the purpose.[28]

The Memorandum prepared by this Committee as a preliminary to giving oral evidence was discussed by the College who agreed that a central body was best suited to correlation and control of voluntary, local authority and Emergency Medical Service hospitals. Colonel Stewart, Medical Superintendent of the Edinburgh Royal Infirmary advised the Committee to elaborate their proposals and instanced the need for further elucidation on the composition of Medical Advisory Committees.[29]

As central authority plans began to take shape the College was again approached by the Department of Health. On this occasion the views of the College were sought on the Areas of Regional Hospital Boards which were contemplated by the Department. Replying the College Council suggested that Dumfries, Kirkcudbright and Wigtown should be transferred from the Western to the South-Eastern Region. This, it was argued, would serve to equalise the amount of clinical material available to Edinburgh and Glasgow with medical schools of approximately the same size.[30]

PROPOSED SPECIALIST POLYCLINIC

The Act of 1947 gave powers to the Secretary of State to develop Health Centres (Chap. XXVIII). A proposal three years previously represented an endeavour to anticipate events. It was brought to the notice of the College in a letter from the Department of Health for Scotland and emanated from the Court of the University of Edinburgh. At an earlier date an informal conference had taken place between representatives of the Department of Health, the South-Eastern Area Committee of the British Hospital Association, the Corporation of Edinburgh and the University to discuss the proposal. Approach to the College by the Department had been prompted by the divergence of views expressed at the conference.

The contemplated project was for the establishment of a Specialist Polyclinic which it was envisaged would undertake the admission to hospitals from a defined area, of patients after examination; or, in the case of patients acutely ill through the agency of the Polyclinic's Assignment Department. It was claimed for the proposed scheme that it would facilitate the centralization of records and the accumulation of morbidity statistics at the same time as having attractions 'from a purely medical point of view'. Among other objectives were the provision of a consultant service by appointment, the separation of the problems of diagnosis from those of treatment, a statistical survey of certain types of morbidity, and the training of students and post-graduates. The diagnostic approach would, it was suggested, consist of a general physical examination and 'such simple laboratory tests as are commonly included in the term "clinical pathology" '. At the conclusion of this general examination the patient would be 'seen by a consultant'.[31] Studied in retrospect, the proposals showed only limited evidence of regard for essentially human considerations and bore the hallmark of ruthless theoretical administrative efficiency combined with a pre-dominantly surgical outlook.

To study the proposals and the accompanying plans the College appointed a comprehensively representative Committee, membership of which included in addition to general physicians, a cardiologist, a dermatologist, an ear, nose and throat specialist, an obstetrician and the medical superintendent of the Royal Infirmary. Their unanimous conclusion was that, although many improvements might be effected in the Infirmary Out-Patients Department, the Polyclinic merited examina-tion only if more detailed information was made available.[32]

The proposals did not materialize.

MEDICAL PROFESSION: CONDITIONS AND CIRCUMSTANCES OF SERVICE

REMUNERATION OF THE MEDICAL PRACTITIONER

At the Quarterly Meeting in May 1945 a letter from the Department of Health was read asking 'as to the proper range of income for General Practitioners etc.'. A small Committee which included the Secretary of the Scottish Branch of the B.M.A. was appointed.[33] The Minutes of the Extraordinary Meeting at which the Committee's Memorandum was submitted and approved were admirably discreet. The only information vouchsafed was that the Memorandum 'answered fully the two ques-tions put . . . by the Inter-Departmental Committee' and was forwarded to the Ministry of Health.[34]

SPECIALISTS AND CONSULTANTS

The College was a constituent member of the Joint Committee on Specialized Status consisting of representatives of the three Scottish Corporations and Scottish representatives of the Royal College of Obstetricians and Gynaecologists.[35] As Chairman of the Joint Committee, Dr Charles McNeil explained to the College at a Quarterly Meeting that the Committee's remit covered all aspects of consultant and specialist training, practice and status, it being accepted that supervision for control of education and training would be provided by the General Medical Council. A Report submitted by the Committee was approved and copies sent to the English Joint Committee and the Department of Health for Scotland.[36, 37]

In mid-1945 the Government sought information as to the number of specialists who would probably be available for the contemplated National Health Service Scheme. The same information had been asked for by the Department of Health for Scotland and in order to provide it, a meeting was arranged at St Andrew's House. There an estimate of the number of specialists in various categories was produced to a Group Committee but only after an undertaking had been given that the name of no individual was to be disclosed until the date for Public Registration. The Edinburgh Group Committee consisted of one representative each from the two Edinburgh Royal Colleges, the Royal College of Obstetricians and Gynaecologists, the University, Public Health Specialists and the British Medical Association. Names submitted included service specialists.[38]

By 1948 considerable developments had taken place and the President (Dr W. D. P. Small) was able to inform the College that they would have an official contribution to make to the panel for selection of specialists under the National Health Service; and, that names of Fellows were being put forward. Furthermore he indicated that two additional considerations were under review. Firstly, whether Merit Awards as suggested by the Spens Committee should be made on a Scottish or a British basis; and secondly, whether the Royal Colleges or the British Medical Association should represent the consultants in negotiations with the Government.[39] Later in the year the B.M.A. set up Regional Consultant Bodies with one Central Committee for the entire body of consultants. A Scottish Committee was appointed by the B.M.A. but was not subject to its control. (Sir) J. D. S. Cameron was the Edinburgh College of Physicians' representative on the B.M.A. Exploratory Committee and it was he who explained a Memorandum produced by that Committee and who, at the same time as recommending approval, urged harmony among all the Corporations.

A conference had been held on 28th July 1948 in London at which it was agreed that the Joint Committee must speak with one voice for consultants; and that there should be two Joint Secretaries, one appointed by the Colleges and Corporations, and the other by the B.M.A. The agreed composition of the Joint Committee was: the Royal College of Physicians, London and the Royal College of Surgeons of

England—three representatives each; the Royal College of Obstetricians and Gynae-cologists—two; the two Royal Colleges of Edinburgh and the Royal Glasgow Faculty—one each; and the B.M.A.—six.[40]

Within a few months the President informed the College that it had been sug-gested to the London Joint Committee that a special subcommittee should be appointed to deal with Scottish affairs and that it should consist of two representatives of each of the Royal Scottish Corporations, one of the Royal College of Obstetricians and Gynaecologists, and four of the Central Consultants and Specialists (Scotland) Committee set up under the aegis of the B.M.A. Scottish Branch. It was intended that the Scottish Committee should be a separate committee, co-operating closely with the Main Committee. To facilitate this it was proposed that Scottish representatives on the London Committee should be *ex officio* members of the Scottish Committee.[41]

Further developments were reported to the College at an Extraordinary Meeting in June 1949 by (Sir) James Cameron. The purpose of the meeting was to consider revised terms of service for consultants. It was explained that the proposed terms were incorporated in a recently published Memorandum[42] and as amended they partially met the views of the Joint Committee. Cameron considered that the terms should be accepted as the best obtainable despite the inclusion of provision for a permanent contract. He was influenced by his conviction that the Ministry of Health had reached the limit of concession. The College thereupon resolved that the revised terms of service should be approved and instructed their representatives on the Joint Committee 'to support the recommendation that consultants be advised to accept permanent contracts'.[42]

At this time, a Fellow resident in England wrote to the College about his expense allowances under the new régime. In retrospect and in parenthesis his experience had an element of whimsical pathos, with which many would sympathize. On submit-ting his claims the Fellow in question was abruptly informed by the Inspector of Taxes that he was now a Civil Servant and his expense allowances would be dealt with accordingly.[42] Such were the implications of lost caste! Or was it a case of 'the wages of sin'?!

RELATION OF GENERAL PRACTITIONERS TO CONSULTANT SERVICES

Following an indication by the Secretary of State for Scotland that he was considering the relationship between general practitioners and the Hospital Service, the Scottish Health Services Council appointed a special subcommittee. This in turn sought an expression of opinion by the College, and the President (Sir David Henderson) nominated a Committee consisting of consultants and general practitioners to draw up a Memorandum.[43] Those on the Committee were Drs L. S. P. Davidson, D. N. Nicholson, J. Halliday Croom, J. L. Cowan, R. E. Verney, H. P. Tait, W. F. T. Haultain, N. Macmichael and J. Laurie with Dr W. A. Alexander (Vice-President) as Chairman. When the Committee reported verbally, Fellows in attendance were asked to submit any comments they might wish to make within two weeks. While of the opinion that no effort should be spared in integrating and co-ordinating the work of the family doctor with the hospital services, the Committee emphasized that the general practitioner had little time 'to increase his contacts and widen his horizon and hopes'.

Answering specific questions put by the Joint Subcommittee of the Scottish Health Services Council, the College Committee expressed the view in so far as laboratories were concerned that large cities were in general satisfactorily served and that the needs of the rest of the country were met by regional services. Facilities for blood examination were said to need improvement urgently, and it was suggested that greater availability of laboratory assistance would enable practitioners effectively to treat more patients. As to the employment of general practitioners in hospital, the Committee considered they could assist in the out-patients department of the larger hospitals and in 'some institutions, even in the cities which could be staffed with advantage by general practitioners with consultant advice as required'. It was not thought that practitioners should have responsibility for the care of in-patients 'in large and intermediate general hospitals'. On the other hand, every encouragement should, it was stated, be given to continuation of the practice whereby in Cottage hospitals the family doctor retained responsibility for his own patients. In the matter of fostering closer and more constant contact of practitioners with consultants, the College Committee was fully alive to the difficulties of the family doctor whose needs and interests they thought 'might be more widely recognised'. At the same time tribute was paid to the practice in some hospitals of welcoming the family doctor on ward rounds and at staff clinical meetings, and to the B.M.A. branches and well-established medical societies organizing clinical meetings, lectures and discussions. Such difficulties as existed were described as being 'not so much of opportunity as of time'.[44]

REFERENCES

VENEREAL DISEASES

(1) College Minutes, 7.iii.1899.

THE HEALTH OF SCHOOL CHILDREN

(2) ROYAL COMMISSION ON PHYSICAL TRAINING (Scotland) (1903) *Report.* 2 vols. (Chairman: Lord Mansfield.) Edinburgh: H.M.S.O.
(3) College Minutes, 8.iii.1904.
(4) Ibid., 3.v.1904.
(5) Ibid., 7.ii.1905.
(6) Ibid., 20.vi.1905.
(7) Ibid., 21.vii.1914.
(8) Ibid., 3.xi.1914.
(9) Ibid., 2.ii.1915.

MIDWIVES

(10) Ibid., 5.v.1914.
(11) Ibid., 3.v.1898.
(12) Ibid., 20.v.1914.
(13) Ibid., 21.vii.1914.

NURSES

(14) Ibid., 3.v.1938.
(15) R.C.P.E. (1938) *Departmental committee on nursing services in Scotland. Statement by the Royal College of Physicians of Edinburgh.* Edinburgh: Privately printed.

MATERNITY AND CHILD WELFARE

(16) Council Minutes, 26.iii.1917.
(17) Ibid., 10.vii.1917.
(18) Ibid., 30.x.1917.

MILK SUPPLIES

(19) Ibid., 21.vii.1914.
(20) TAIT, H. P. (1973) Personal communication.

MENTAL DEFICIENCY

(21) College Minutes, 19.vii.1938.

THE INDUSTRIAL POPULATION

(22) Ibid., 1.xi.1938.

WORKMEN'S COMPENSATION

(23) Ibid., 2.v.1939.
(24) Ibid., 18.vii.1939.

SCOTTISH HOUSING

(25) Ibid., 2.ii.1943.
(26) Ibid., 4.v.1943.

THE FUTURE OF HOSPITALS

(27) Ibid., 3.ii.1942.
(28) Ibid., 5.v.1942.
(29) Ibid., 2.vii.1942.
(30) Council Minutes, 13.v.1947.

PROPOSED SPECIALIST POLYCLINIC

(31) College Minutes, 6.x.1944.
(32) Ibid., 7.xi.1944.

MEDICAL PROFESSION

(33) Ibid., 1.v.1945.
(34) Ibid., 4.vi.1945.
(35) Ibid., 4.v.1943.
(36) Ibid., 2.xi.1943.
(37) Ibid., 1.ii.1944.
(38) Ibid., 1.v.1945.
(39) Ibid., 20.vii.1948.
(40) Ibid., 2.xi.1948.
(41) Ibid., 1.ii.1949.
(42) Ibid., 21.vi.1949.
(43) Ibid., 18.vii.1950.
(44) Ibid., 7.xi.1950.

Chapter XXX

1950 AND AFTER: ADJUSTMENTS IMPOSED BY CHANGING CIRCUMSTANCES

. . . medicine, professedly founded on observation, is as sensitive to outside influences, political, religious, philosophical, imaginative as is the barometer to the changes of atmospheric density.

Oliver Wendell Holmes

OUTSIDE INFLUENCES

For the College, the situation which obtained after World War II compelled major readjustments and a reappraisal of the function of the College more particularly in the spheres of Medical Education, Medical Research and Hospital Services. A position had to be faced in which the College no longer exerted an influence on undergraduate medical training through the agency of an Extra-mural Medical School, and in which, bereft of a Laboratory, its potential in the promotion of research was considerably curtailed. With the advent of the National Health Service another new situation arose in so far as the experience of the College was available in an essentially advisory capacity. An accompaniment of the vast expansion of legislation involved in the phase by phase evolution of the Welfare State was the creation of a host of Select Committees and Departmental Committees. The trend was accentuated by the circumstances of war and by the eventual establishment of a National Health Service. In consequence, direct official contact between the Government and College as known in the nineteenth century had well nigh disappeared. Likewise, save in the most exceptional circumstances, representations on the part of the College which in earlier times would have been submitted as Suppliant Memorials or Petitions, now take the form of Memoranda and Reports not to the Heads of Government but to the appropriate Government Department or Departments. *Pari passu* the occasions on which the Government or Government Departments make a direct approach to the

College for advice or comment have lessened. This is largely explained by the multiplication within recent decades of professional and administrative organizations concerned in depth with highly specialized interests. In years past, advice was sought from the College by central and local authorities on public health, epidemiological, nutritional, housing and other community problems, for studying which there are now recognized, firmly established separate professional Bodies, expert but by no means infallible. Nevertheless, during the period 1953 to 1968 the College submitted some twenty reports to various professional and government sponsored organizations.

Research Potentialities

The existence of separate organizations, however, does not and has not precluded the College from partaking in and actually initiating research enquiries. An illustrative case was the comparatively recent issue of the Report on *The Care of the Elderly in Scotland*.[1] Requiring financial backing beyond the resources of the College, and necessitating access to sophistically equipped laboratories which the College does not possess, clinical and biological research on a significant scale is not possible. However, certain of the bequests for research which the College administers are available for the financing, in part or whole, of fact-finding surveys by expert working parties. Policy in this connection is now under constant review and may be expected to assume more definite shape at an early date. No matter the changes taking place in research participation by the College as a corporate body, it can be accepted as a *sine qua non* that Fellows will, in their individual capacity, continue as in the past to make major contributions to advances in the many medical disciplines.

Examinees en masse

In the years following World War II the College was faced with an entirely unprecedented problem: the situation arising from a rapid progressive increase in the number of candidates for the Membership Examination. The increase acquired momentum in almost alarming degree: the figures (Table 1) speak for themselves.

TABLE I

Year	Total No. of Candidates in 12-month Period	Year		Total No. of Candidates in 12-month Period
1925	37	1960		1262
1935	52	1961		1323
1939	110	1962		1373
1946	119	1963		1559
1948	349	1964		1413
1955	539	1965		1418
1956	604	1966	Pt. I	1024
			Pt. II	728
1957	781	1967	Pt. I	722
			Pt. II	1092
1958	887	1968	Pt. I	657 (old regns.) +150 (new)
1959	1031		Pt. II	815

From the figures it will be seen that while a slight increase in the number of candidates was evident in 1939, the tidal wave of demand, and such it was, first appeared after the cessation of hostilities.

More than one factor explained the situation. Service medical officers lost no time in taking the examination on demobilization. The trend was further aggravated by the requirement attached to many of the new National Health Service posts that candidates should possess a higher diploma. Similar influences were operating overseas which accounted in part for the number of candidates who came from abroad. The repercussions were cumulative.

The College owed an immense debt to Dr Alister Alexander for the wisdom of his counselling in these difficult circumstances. Elected President in 1951 he endeared himself to Fellows of all ages. His affection for the College is profound. He brought to the Meetings of Council and College the same quiet, gracious understanding which characterized his attitude at the bedside and in the out-patient clinic. Where principle was involved he could be relied upon to be resolutely obdurate, but expression of his obduracy was invariably tempered by transparently sincere modesty. Having accepted a challenge he gave of his all, as borne out by his services to the College as President, Councillor and Honorary Librarian. Those who know him cannot fail to recognize the quality of goodness in him—a quality he has always applied for the better advancement of the College.

Before long, accommodation to meet examination needs presented a problem. In the course of time resort had to be made to the use of University rooms for the written examinations[2] and the co-operation of no fewer than thirteen hospitals in Edinburgh, five in Glasgow and two in Dundee. Peel Hospital, Galashiels was enlisted for the supplementary requirements of the clinical examinations.[3] Seen in correct perspective these problems were essentially a challenge to the administration. Another administrative situation needing diplomatic negotiation was the almost exorbitant demands by the examinations on the time of physicians in the employ of the National Health Service. Gratifyingly, agreement was reached with the Department of Health for Scotland and the Ministry of Health that examinations for higher qualifications were an essential part of National Health Service duty in that they were concerned with the provision of suitably qualified persons for training and future work in the Hospital Service.[4]

Standards of Examination

Of infinitely greater moment, however, was the growing concern felt by the College about the standard of a very large proportion of the examination entrants. Indirectly, the status of the College Membership was at stake, not because of the standards of the examination which never relaxed their exacting demands, but because of the inadequate preparation and experience of many of the candidates from overseas. The best indication of this is the year-by-year pass-rate (Table 2).

TABLE 2

Year	Approximate Percentage Pass	Year	Approximate Percentage Pass
1950	28	1957	19
1951	25	1958	19
1952	28	1959	20
1953	25	1960	15
1954	29	1961	17
1955	25	1962	15
1956	20	1963	16

The variations in the pass-rate did not reflect adherence to an imposed low percentage pass, but the low standard of many candidates. Any candidate who satisfied the examiners was recommended for Membership regardless of what the pass-rate proved to be.

The Membership Candidate who Fails

Always jealously concerned for the reputation of the College Membership Examination for fairness, the Council in 1971 endorsed a recommendation of the College Advisory Committee on Examinations that a Counselling Service should be available for failed candidates.[5] Almost twenty-five years previously the subject had been raised by Sir Stanley Davidson in a letter to Council.[6]

Dr Henry Matthew was the main instigator of the development and he, together with the Registrar or another member of the Committee, explained to candidates invited to attend for interview the nature of their unpreparedness. There has been an excellent response to invitations to attend.

Underlying the counselling procedure there is undisguised humanitarian understanding which has been a feature over the decades of the Edinburgh Membership Examination. There can be few, if any, who in their professional careers have sat the examination and later in life acted as examiners, who have not been aware of the fairness, consideration, courtesy and unhurried tempo of the examination in all its phases. Candidates—successful and unsuccessful—have on numerous occasions expressed appreciation of just those aspects of the examination, a fact in which the College takes legitimate pride.[7]

A Warning Amber-light

In 1966 an event took place which might well, although it did not—have entailed serious administrative and other difficulties. A patient sustained injury as a result of over-vigorous clinical examination by a candidate.[8] At a later date, after consultation with an Insurance Company, an Indemnity Insurance was taken out as a safeguard for the future.[9, 10]

The Membership an Index of Potentiality

There was evidence of the need for concern in the previous examination records of candidates. Thus in 1963, of 244 successful examinees 83 had appeared for the first time, 57 for the second, 104 for a third and subsequent attempts. Two candidates passed on the occasion of their eleventh appearance,[4] but their experience could not compare with that of a candidate who succeeded in July 1962 at his sixteenth attempt.[11] The general experience of the College in this connection was not unique: the London and Glasgow Colleges were equally perturbed and inevitably the subject from being a topic of conversation became a matter for joint consultation by all the Medical Colleges. These Colleges agreed in their evaluation of the Membership as an index of potentiality on the part of the holder 'to become a specialist or consultant after further training'. This viewpoint was not always appreciated abroad by a proportion of Members who on their return assumed consultant responsibilities without further training.[12] The Edinburgh Membership was particularly prone to abuse in this way, because the profession of a chosen specialty in a subsidiary part of the examination was interpreted by some successful candidates lacking in discrimination as proof of acquired specialist status. Some of the criticism by sister Colleges of the Edinburgh Membership Examination on this score ignored the proven educational value of having to aquire knowledge in depth of a selected specialty.

'Multiple Diplomatosis'

Another anxiety shared by the three Colleges was the increasing tendency among candidates for hospital posts to secure the Membership of more than one College in the hope thereby of improving their prospects.[13] This outlook was not wholly lacking in historical substance. It was not unknown for a new incumbent of a senior academic post to be told shortly after appointment that the University concerned was embarrassed by teaching hospital representations that the appointee although a Fellow of one College was neither a Fellow nor Member of another specified Royal College. This situation obtained until the advent of the N.H.S.

In 1968 the Todd Report (Royal Commission § 92) stated baldly: 'Some English regional hospital boards have declared that qualifications of the English and Scottish Colleges are equally acceptable, but in practice a candidate with an English higher diploma is likely to be preferred in England, though the converse does not hold. As a result Scottish graduates (they constitute at present about a quarter of the British total and many of them must leave Scotland to secure hospital appointments) often find that they must spend time and money seeking the qualification of an English as well as of a Scottish College.'[14] Nevertheless in this connection the conditions applicable to the appointment of physicians to the Edinburgh Royal Infirmary prior to the N.H.S. cannot be ignored (Chap. XX).

Today eager prospective candidates for hospital posts can be forgiven if they are fearful about discrimination along these lines. They are the victims of perpetuated beliefs based on largely discontinued practices.

An indirect outcome of the phenomenal increase in the number of candidates for the Membership Examination of the College was an altogether notable growth in the list of Members of whom the majority were resident outside the British Isles. To quote from the President's Report for the year 1959–60: 'In round numbers, there are now close on 2000 Members, approximately 1300 of whom reside abroad, as against 700 living in the United Kingdom'.[3] The distribution of Fellows and

Members within the Commonwealth at that time is shewn in Table 3. Twelve years later the distribution in those countries is shewn in Table 4.

TABLE 3

Country	No. of Fellows	No. of Members
Sri Lanka (Ceylon)	2	62
Pakistan	3	54
India	30	496
Australia	8	101
South Africa	15	183
New Zealand	11	75
Canada	14	44
United Kingdom	364	732

TABLE 4

Country	No. of Fellows	No. of Members
Sri Lanka (Ceylon)	19	98
*Pakistan	36	121
Bangladesh	6	32
India	137	781
Australia	41	182
*South Africa	45	157
New Zealand	31	66
Canada	47	73
United Kingdom	555	851

(* No longer Member of Commonwealth in 1972.)

The Objectives of Postgraduate Training

Closely allied to the problems of examination were those of Postgraduate Medical Education. The evolution and activities of the Edinburgh Post-Graduate Board for Medicine are described later in this chapter. In considerable measure the courses organized by the Board were designed to meet the needs of graduates from abroad. Although never officially presented as useful preparation for the Membership Examination, they were regarded as such by most of those enrolling for them. Over the years, in addition to activities under the auspices of the Board, strictly College provisions for the postgraduate have taken the form of Lectures, Symposia and

Scientific Publications. These have been directed towards the provision of continuing education for Members and Fellows as distinct from pre-examination preparation for Membership aspirants. Of particular importance and encouragement is the initiative shewn by Collegiate Members in organizing College educational activities.

In 1969 a new Standing Committee of the College was established with a name so lengthy and so circumlocutory as almost to suggest despair at the outset! It was the Standing Committee on Specialist Standards, Vocational Registration and Post-graduate Medical Education, which straightway sponsored no fewer than 19 Specialty Committees, subsequently reduced to seventeen.[15] In the course of time the parent Committee came to be known as the Standing Committee on Education and Specialist Standards. Each Specialty Committee submitted recommendations for the training suited to preparation for their separate disciplines. The Standing Committee consists of Fellows and Collegiate Members who at the time of writing include representatives from Glasgow, Aberdeen, Dundee and Perth. At a later date, with the full approval of the Edinburgh College of Physicians, the Royal Colleges co-operated with the Association of Professorial Heads of Departments in Medicine and Paediatrics and with the Universities and certain Specialist Associations to form the Joint Committee on Higher Medical Training.

A certain change in emphasis has taken place with greater attention being paid to 'in-service training' as recommended by the Royal Commission on Medical Education. A Scottish Council for Postgraduate Medical Education was first established in 1970. Among this Council's Regional Committees is the South-East Regional Committee for Postgraduate Medical Education. There is a representative of the College on the Scottish Council and another on the Regional Committee.

Raising the Sights: Widening the Horizon
The arrival from almost all the world's continents of graduates for training and to sit examinations compelled an adjustment of outlook on the part of the College. From being essentially inward looking it has become dominantly outward looking. Relationships with sister Colleges in the United Kingdom have acquired a more meaningful friendliness, and contacts with medical interests overseas have increased in frequency—sometimes the result of intercollegiate arrangements, and sometimes due to the travels of Fellows under the aegis of W.H.O. or the British Council. The pace of events has been conditioned at home, albeit unobtrusively, by the arrival of the Welfare State and National Health Service; and abroad, by changes which have occurred within the spheres of Empire and Commonwealth. There is other evidence that the College has been alerted within itself in the encouragement being given to

Members to take an active part in the counsels and the activities of the College—a policy urged so forcibly and so persistently over the years by Sir Derrick Dunlop.

THE FUTURE OF THE COLLEGE: THE CROOM REPORT

The College entered the second half of the twentieth century with its Fellows and Members dispersed as never before. At a time when medicine had undergone changes probably unprecedented both in scale and pace the College was under the necessity of reviewing its relationships with other bodies, functions in the fields of research, position and influence as an advisory body, and its responsibilities in the furtherance of postgraduate education and training. At the same time the need was recognized for a critical study of the administrative structure of the College, the place and activities within the structure of Members and Fellows, and the desiderata for an improved Membership Examination. To consider these and other problems the President in office in 1968 (Dr Christopher Clayson) appointed a Committee 'to consider the rôle of the College in the light of the Report of the Royal Commission on Medical Education and to make recommendations'. The Committee without sacrifice of efficiency or thoroughness, produced an admirable report with remarkable expedition in October 1969. Entitled *Report of College Committee to Consider the Future of the College*,[16] the report is customarily referred to as the *Croom Report*.

In previous years, at the risk of incurring unpopularity, Dr Charles McNeil and Sir James Cameron had drawn attention to the need for the College to look to its laurels and to have thought for the problems looming ahead.[17, 18] The Croom Report served to present the problems in stark reality and made a number of far reaching constructive suggestions. Accepting the views of the Royal Commission concerning the responsibilities of professional bodies in relation to professional training and examinations, the Report recommended the establishment of the Standing College Committee already mentioned—the Committee on Specialist Standards, Vocational Registration and Postgraduate Medical Education, and the setting-up of Specialty Committees by the parent Standing Committee (q.v.). While commending planned appointments for a three-year period of general professional training, the Croom Committee took strong exception to the Commission's proposals for assessment of general professional training. The Commission condemned assessment based on a 'single major "pass or fail" examination' and advanced the view that trainees should be assessed on 'a progressive basis throughout the three-year period' involving reports by 'supervisors and the chiefs of units' in which trainees had been working.[19] It was maintained by the Croom Committee that the assessor should be the appropriate College, that examination for Membership of the College should be 'the principal mechanism of assessment' and that progress reports should be regarded as a form of 'secondary mechanism of assessment'. As to the accreditation of training posts, the Report assumed that the College contribution would operate within the framework of the proposed Scottish Council for Postgraduate Medical Education. At the same time as agreeing that the establishment of specialist standards and the acceptance of vocational registration were necessary corollaries to specialist training, the Committee advocated registration by the General Medical Council on presentation of a certificate from the appropriate College.

Other points in connection with postgraduate training to which the College Committee attached particular importance were the creation of regional postgraduate committees and local postgraduate centres; continued College activities within the ambit of the Edinburgh Post-Graduate Board for Medicine and the Scottish Post-graduate Medical Association; further development of College Scientific Meetings and publications; and formal liaison among all professional bodies involved in postgraduate education.

For the particular requirements of overseas doctors the provision of in-service hospital training was regarded as fundamental; and it was recommended that overseas graduates should be sponsored from their country of origin, be accepted for approved posts before coming to the United Kingdom, and be subject to continuous counselling from the time of arrival.

Detailed consideration was given by the Croom Report to the future of the Membership Examination. Continued trial for a limited period of the Common Part I Examination (q.v.) was recommended together with an increase in the interval between success in the Part I Examination and completion of three attempts at the Part II Examination; and proposals for reciprocity of Membership between the three Colleges were described as meriting all support, with a common Part II Examination as ultimate objective.

Specific reference was made to the Royal Commission's desire that 'the satisfactory completion of general professional training should be marked by the trainee's acceptance into the main grade of membership of the appropriate college . . .'.[20] Because of the obvious implications to the detriment of the College Membership the suggestion was summarily rejected. As one means of securing active participation of Members in College activities and affairs the Committee recommended the creation of a category of Collegiate Members with privileges additional to those of other

Members (p. 777); and the formation of a Collegiate Members' Committee with authority to elect annually two of their number to become additional members of the College Council. The system of election to the Fellowship, the administrative structure of the College, and the question of public relations were given as subjects deserving critical review. Little time was lost in implementing many of the recommendations of the Report which was approved by the College at an Extraordinary Meeting attended by the President and 58 Fellows on 15th October 1969.[21]

POSTGRADUATE EDUCATION

. . . the graduate . . . whether he determines to enter one of the Services, to devote himself to Public Health administration, to adopt a scientific career, or to engage in general practice or one of the many specialties . . . will soon find that, if he is to be efficient, he must keep in touch with modern progress and remain a student throughout his professional life.

Edwin Bramwell

If every symposiast were a Dr. Samuel Johnson, perhaps . . . discussions at a symposium might strike more fire and distil less mutual admiration. Symposia, like hard liquor, should be taken in reasonable measure at appropriate intervals.

Sir F. M. R. Walshe

The College has had a keen interest in medical education from its earliest days. This is borne out by the Laws and Regulations which reflect efforts on the part of the College to promote and ensure professional proficiency on the part of Licentiates, Members and Fellows. There is further evidence in the active encouragement given the University of Edinburgh to establish a Faculty of Medicine in the early eighteenth century. The contrasting conceptions of under- and post-graduate training took shape in the late nineteenth century, assuming clear definition in the present century. Both forms of education were accepted as a College responsibility. A direct result of post-World War II developments in the spheres of medical administration and politics has been an inevitable concentration of College interests in medical education on the training of the postgraduate. This training embraces vocational preparation, refresher courses and instruction of those concerned to acquire intermediate qualifications.

Lectures, Symposia and Publications
Influence on measures for postgraduate education is exerted in a variety of ways by the College. These include Lectures and Symposia with the College Hall as venue and

the publication of scientific papers. The Symposia and almost all the Lectures are scientific in character and at different times deal with the various disciplines within the field of medicine. At least two Symposia are held every year, the first having been arranged at the instigation of Sir James Cameron to take place on the occasion of the inaugural St Andrew's Day Festival in 1961. Traditionally a Symposium now constitutes an integral part of the annual St Andrew's Day Festival. Indeed it can be said to be gaining a rightfully dominating place in the Festival proceedings in so far as present policy is to combine Lectures with Symposia, thus extending free discussion to the Lectures. To an increasing extent those participating in the Symposia have included eminent members of the profession of international repute. This has for many years been characteristic of those chosen to deliver the Endowed Lectures, and lists relating to the past contain the names of recognized authorities from many countries. A decision to initiate a College Publication Series was decided by Council in 1953 and finally implemented by College in 1954.[22, 23] Many of the Lectures and a proportion of the Symposia have been published and the demand for the scientific publications has in a number of instances been very considerable. A list of recent publications of the College is given at the end of the section and includes publications of Symposia (q.v.).

Symposia hold out great possibilities as a means of furthering the College's influence. This was well demonstrated by arranging one at what may be called a thriving College outpost at Stockton-on-Tees. The date—a historical one—was 13th October 1972, and the subject *Recent Advances*. Yet another development of considerable importance is the active participation in educational activities of Collegiate Members, who in 1971 organized with great success their first Symposium, with as subject *Medicine and the Mass Media*.[24] This took place in the College Hall.

Many regard Symposia as relatively recent innovations. But are they? Are they not rather revivals of the Dissertations so highly valued by Robert Sibbald some 300 years ago?

Membership of Committees

Postgraduate education promoted in the form of Lectures, Symposia and Publications constitutes an organized corporate contribution on the part of the College. Numerous other contributions are made jointly with other bodies. To understand these an elementary knowledge of a somewhat confusing administrative background is necessary.

In practice what bodies are interested in the promotion of postgraduate medical education? They are many and it goes without saying that they include the Scottish

Royal Colleges and University Medical Schools. To these must be added the Scottish Home and Health Department, the Scottish Council for Postgraduate Medical Education, the Regional Hospital Boards, the British Medical Association and the Royal College of General Practitioners. A direct consequence of the number of interested parties has been the formation of a series of Joint Committees, the activities of which are at times liable to suffer from inadequate liaison.

Mention has been made of the Standing College Committee on Specialist Standards, Vocational Registration and Postgraduate Medical Education. Within the College itself, the value of the Committee's work is greatly enhanced by the wide geographical representation characterizing membership (q.v.).

No formal machinery exists for the specific purpose of discussion of postgraduate medical education between the Edinburgh and Glasgow Colleges. There are, however, the regular meetings of the Standing Joint Committee of the Scottish Royal Colleges at which the subject can always be raised. Representatives on the Committee are for the Edinburgh Physicians—their President, Vice-President and Secretary; the Edinburgh Surgeons—their President, one Vice-President and Secretary; and for the Glasgow College—their President, Visitor and Secretary. In addition the Chairman and Secretary of the Scottish Branch of the Royal College of Obstetricians and Gynaecologists attend.

In the realm of hospital practice 'in-service training' has prior claim on postgraduate educational activities. For administrative purposes there is the Scottish Council for Postgraduate Medical Education with Regional Committees of which the South-Eastern Regional Committee for Postgraduate Medical Education is the one with which the College is directly concerned. The College has one representative on the Scottish Council and one on the South-Eastern Regional Committee. Discussions or negotiations with the Hospital Services may be conducted by the College through these representatives directly, or through its representatives on the Edinburgh Post-Graduate Board for Medicine. This last named Board is in outstanding measure the most potent body for the successful promotion of postgraduate education more especially in an age of rapid clinical and scientific progress. Moreover the Board has all the advantages of long-established close alliance between the Edinburgh Colleges and the University. The history is one of mutual pooling of resources to favour maximum effectiveness.

At the present time the Board has an independent Chairman with the Royal College of Physicians, the Royal College of Surgeons and the University of Edinburgh each having three representatives. Within comparatively recent years provision has been made for the co-option of one general practitioner, one representative of the

Regional Hospital Board and one other from the South-Eastern Regional Committee for Postgraduate Medical Education. Co-option along these lines has materially facilitated arrangements for developing in-service training; and has offset such handicaps as may have arisen from the Board being 'a Committee to advise the University Court' which in turn could not accept, by the terms of the constitution, advice from any body other than the Faculty of Medicine.

The Board was a member of the Scottish Postgraduate Medical Association which was founded in 1963 and consisted of the three Royal Colleges and the four Universities in Scotland.[25] Previously Dr Rae Gilchrist had represented the College at a meeting at Dundee to consider the formation of the Association. Happily the train of events was very different from that of the exploratory meeting in Dundee two centuries before! (Chap. II.). On this occasion it was decorous and devoid of cloak and dagger tactics. In accordance with correct procedure, as a first step an Executive Committee was appointed with the object of approaching the University Vice-Chancellors and of securing integration of the activities of those interested.[26] The Association did not accomplish anything of great note and has ceased to function.

PUBLICATIONS OF THE ROYAL COLLEGE OF PHYSICIANS OF EDINBURGH

1. RITCHIE, J. (1953) *History of the Laboratory of the Royal College of Physicians of Edinburgh.*
2. PATRICK, A. (1955) *The Enteric Fevers, 1800–1920.*
3. MACKINTOSH, J. M. (1955) *Research in General Practice.*
4. KENNEDY, Sir D. K. (1955) *Society and Criminal Conduct.*
5. SMITH, J. (1955) *The Aetiology of Epidemic Infantile Gastro-enteritis.*
6. WATTS, C. A. H. (1956) *Neuroses in General Practice.*
7. WITTS, L. J. (1956) *Anaemia and the Alimentary Tract.*
8. SMIRK, F. H. (1956) *The Treatment of High Blood Pressure.*
9. ANDERSON, W. F. (1957) *The Care of the Elderly in General Practice.*
10. RUSSELL, W. R. (1957) *The Physiology of Learning.*
11. GARROD, L. P. (1959) *Chemotherapy of Infections of the Urinary Tract.*
12. SELLORS, T. H. (1960) *The Contribution of Surgery to Clinical Cardiology.*
13. COWAN, Sir K. (1960) *The Climate of Health.*
14. DAVIDSON, Sir S. (1960) *Anaemia and Operations on the Gastro-intestinal Tract.*
15. CRUICKSHANK, R. (1961) *Measurements in Medicine.*
16. STOKER, M. (1962) *Tumour Viruses.*
17. GRAY, J. D. A. (1963) *Antibiotics in Medicine.*
18. R.C.P.E. (1963) *The Care of the Elderly in Scotland.* (Report of a College Committee.)
19. MILLAR, W. M. (1963) *Models and Methods in Psychiatric Research.*

20. BURCHELL, H. B. (1964) *Lesions of the Aortic Root.*

21. NABARRO, J. D. N. (1964) *Corticosteroid Therapy—uses and abuses.*

22. CHRISTIE, R. V. (1964) *Respiratory Failure.*

23. BEATTIE, C. P. (1964) *Toxoplasmosis.*

24. SPINK, W. W. (1967) *The Dilemma of Bacterial Shock: with special reference to endotoxin shock.*

25. FLOREY, Sir H. (1967) *The Responsibilities of Medicine in the Modern World.*

26. DACIE, J. V. (1967) *The Hereditary Haemolytic Anaemias.*

27. R.C.P.E. (1970) *The Care of the Elderly in Scotland: A follow-up report.*

28. RUSSELL, H. (1971) *J. W. Ballantyne: M.D., F.R.C.P.Edin., F.R.S.E. 1861–1923.*

29. EASTWOOD, M. & SMITH, I. D. (1973) *Medicine and the Mass Media: answering press questions.*

PUBLICATIONS OF SYMPOSIA HELD AT THE ROYAL COLLEGE OF PHYSICIANS OF EDINBURGH

1. *Some Aspects of Renal Disease.* (1965)
2. *The Study of Normal and Disordered Functions of the Small Intestine.* (1962)
3. *Genetics in Medicine.* (1962)
4. *Chronic Respiratory Disorders.* (1963)
5. *Polyarthritis.* (1964)
6. *Disorders of the Blood.* (1965)
7. *Disorders of the Heart and Circulation.* (1966)
8. *Thyroid Disease and Calcium Metabolism.* (1967)
9. *Some Aspects of Neurology.* Ed. by R. F. Robertson. (1968)
10. *Hazards of Therapy.* Ed. by R. F. Robertson. (1969)
11. *Intensive Therapy.* Ed. by R. F. Robertson. (1970)
12. *Developments in Postgraduate Medical Education.* Ed. by R. F. Robertson and J. I. Hall. (1971)
13. *Liver Disease.* Ed. by R. F. Robertson and J. I. Hall. (1972)
14. *Anorexia Nervosa and Obesity.* Ed. by R. F. Robertson and A. T. Proudfoot. (1973)
15. *Preventive Medicine.* Ed. by A. T. Proudfoot. (1973)
16. *Advances in Laboratory Medicine.* Ed. by A. T. Proudfoot. (1973)

THE EDINBURGH POST-GRADUATE BOARD FOR MEDICINE

The quotation on page 758 is taken from the Foreword to the first volume of Edinburgh Post-graduate Lectures in Medicine. The writer was Dr Edwin Bramwell, than whom nobody did more to make the Edinburgh Postgraduate Medical Courses a resounding success. In his foreword he traces the evolution of these courses.

Early in his career, Bramwell was an extra-mural lecturer and associated with his father, Sir Byrom Bramwell, in providing a course in systematic medicine. During World War I, after being called up, he served on a Committee appointed to advise the War Office on shell-shock, and when made physician to the Royal Infirmary in 1919 developed courses of lecture-demonstrations which although voluntary won great favour among postgraduate and undergraduate students. His skill and courtesy as a clinician, and his writings won him a host of admirers. Bramwell married the eldest daughter of the distinguished anatomist Professor J. D. Cunningham, two of whose sons achieved great distinction in World War I—Admiral of the Fleet, Viscount Cunningham of Hyndhope as Commander in Chief Mediterranean, and Sir Alan Cunningham as G.O.C. in Chief, 8th Imperial Army in the Middle East.

As to Sir Byrom Bramwell, Sir Robert Philip referred to his return to Edinburgh as 'the curious perversion of circulation—which does not often occur—which brought an Englishman north of Tweed'.[27] Sir Byrom acquired international fame. Osler was one of his personal friends and admirers.[28] An altogether outstanding teacher, Byrom Bramwell's clinical demonstrations in the 'Infirmary Duck Pond' became and remain a byword. As a Fellow of over forty years' standing, Councillor and President, he was held in the highest esteem in our College, which knew great gratification when its Hall was chosen as venue for the presentation of his portrait. In actual fact two portraits were presented—one for retention by Sir Byrom and one to hang on the walls of the College. Sir Robert Philip, the President of the College, took the chair at a meeting attended by some two hundred people. Subscriptions towards the portraits had come from friends and former pupils of Sir Byrom dispersed throughout the Old and New Worlds and the Far East.[27] In 1933 Edwin Bramwell was elected to the Presidential Chair vacated by his father twenty-one years previously, and in 1960 his brother Professor Crichton Bramwell had the Honorary Fellowship of the College bestowed upon him.

Serious consideration was first given to organized postgraduate teaching in Edinburgh in 1905. By happy coincidence the Governing Board of the School of Medicine of the Royal Colleges and the Medical Faculty of the University simultaneously came to the conclusion that a need existed for the inauguration of organised postgraduate teaching. Independent Committees were formed by both these bodies. From these there evolved a Joint Executive Committee which derived immense benefit from the intimate friendship shared by Dr George Gibson and Professor J. D. Cunningham respective Chairmen of the College and University Committees. The Joint Committee consisted of Drs George Gibson, J. W. Ballantyne and Logan

Turner representing the Colleges' School of Medicine; and Professors Cunningham, John Chiene and Harvey Littlejohn the University. Professor Cunningham was Chairman and Dr Edwin Bramwell, Secretary. Dr H. Rainy was co-opted to represent the independent lecturers. In later years the duties of Honorary Secretary were undertaken in succession by Dr J. D. Comrie, Professor R. W. Johnstone, Drs W. D. Small, Douglas J. A. Kerr and J. K. Slater of whom the last-named made a particularly noteworthy contribution during a period of office extending over no less than eleven years. The Committee reserved the right to invite lecturers and, at the same time as insisting that there should be no interference with undergraduate training, decided that private postgraduate courses might if approved by them be advertised in the annual Syllabus.

Beginning in 1906 with a course for general practitioners, postgraduate vocational teaching underwent progressive extension. This applied to both the number and scope of courses. By 1913 subjects dealt with, in addition to those intended specifically for general practitioners, included surgery, internal medicine, diseases of children, diseases of the ear, nose and throat and urology. After World War I an elaborate Syllabus was drawn up providing intensive courses for no less than nineteen subjects. These were not uniformly successful and policy reverted to that in force in the pre-war days with the addition of extra courses on such selected subjects as appeared desirable from time to time. In 1938, at the behest of the Department of Health for Scotland, the Joint Committee arranged experimental courses for panel practitioners with immediately gratifying results. Earlier, tentative trial had been given to a limited number of graduate clinical demonstrations during term time at the Royal Infirmary and Royal Hospital for Sick Children.

Encouraged by the success to date, a further step was taken in the autumn of 1937 of instituting an eight weeks' course in Internal Medicine during the academic term. Thirty-two graduates enrolled and four were attached for ward work under each of the eight Physicians in the Royal Infirmary. The various departments in medicine combined to provide in addition integrated teaching sessions, demonstrations and opportunities to take case records over the eight weeks period of the course. From the experience gained the Joint Committee were satisfied that the course, although provided during the academic term, had not interfered with undergraduate training or imposed an unfair burden on the teaching staff.[29] Postgraduate teaching activities ceased, following the outbreak of World War II.

Dr Rae Gilchrist well remembers the enthusiasm with which the project had been launched under the stimulating leadership of Dr Edwin Bramwell. The enrolled graduates together with members of the postgraduate teaching staff were invited to breakfast in the Students' Union prior to the first instructional session at 9.30 a.m. A more promising initiation could not be imagined. It met with the enduring success which it deserved.[30] Doubtless Dr Bramwell knew that he was resuscitating a persuasive custom of the College which centuries before preferred a breakfast to a dinner for its annual celebrations!

Early in 1944, while hostilities were still in progress, Dr Edwin Bramwell as Chairman of the College Committee on Postgraduate Teaching urged upon the Council the need for a new Watching Committee 'which would be ready to discuss at once any proposals made by the Government or otherwise'. To meet what he regarded as an urgent situation Dr Bramwell recommended the immediate appointment of 'three representatives each from the College, the [Royal] College of Surgeons and the University'. Council shared his view as to the urgency of the need. At the same time as informing the College of the position the President (Dr Fergus Hewat) advised Dr Bramwell as to Fellows whom he had nominated.[31]

By the time of the next Quarterly Meeting the College was told that a Joint Committee had been formed and had already had several sessions; and that a letter had been received from the University dealing with preparations for a postgraduate course to be held when hostilities ceased.[32] The subject came up for further consideration at the next two Quarterly Meetings. At the first, the Joint Committee's Report was received and generally approved by the College and (Sir) Derrick Dunlop took the opportunity to suggest that if touch was to be maintained with younger doctors there should be an adequate number of junior Fellows on any future Joint Board.[33] On the occasion of the next meeting the President (Dr Fergus Hewat) explained that although the College had conducted a successful postgraduate course 'for 40 or 50 years', reconstitution of the Committee was necessary if the proposed Edinburgh Post-Graduate Board for Medicine was to be eligible for Government grants. Unanimous approval was given by the College to the new Constitution[34] and subsequently the Laws were amended to meet the situation.[35]

Some years later, on the invitation of the President (Sir Stanley Davidson), the Senior Representative of the College (Dr Rae Gilchrist) gave a review of developments. He began with a summary of attendances during the immediate post-war period. The average attendances at the twice yearly surgical courses had been 180; and at the thrice yearly course in Internal Medicine, 80 to 90. When account was taken of Refresher Courses for General Practitioners approximately 700 to 800 postgraduates were working in the Postgraduate School in each of the three post-war years.

By 1951 the numbers had declined considerably and totalled only 300 for the whole year. This Dr Gilchrist attributed to there having been fewer graduates in need of instruction, and only two courses in Internal Medicine during the twelve months in question, and to a marked fall in applications for the Surgical Course following the institution of the Primary Fellowship Examination. In conclusion the College was urged to recognize the contribution made by the University which had guaranteed the working expenses in addition to giving help in other ways.[36] Previously, when agreement had been reached that control of postgraduate medical education should be vested in the University of Edinburgh with the primary object of qualifying for participation in Exchequer Grants, it was decided that the arrangements should become effective on 1st October 1953, with Sir Alexander Biggam continuing to officiate as Director.[37] Further details were given to the College at the February Quarterly Meeting in 1954 when the President (Sir Stanley Davidson) announced that the Board was to be known as 'The Post-Graduate Board for Medicine' with a chairman to be appointed by the University Court after consultation with the Royal Colleges. There was a clear understanding that members of the Board were to function as individuals and not as representatives of any office they might hold, and that while the Board would submit annual reports to the University Court, the College would receive a copy.[38]

When the Annual Report for 1954 was presented to the College reference was made to it being the fiftieth year of postgraduate work in the Medical School. In that year 580 graduates enrolled—'a quarter from India or the Orient, a quarter from Great Britain and the remainder from the Dominions or the Commonwealth'.[39] Co-operation between the Colleges and the University paid handsome dividends; the numbers attending continued to rise,[40] the courses in Internal Medicine and the Refresher Courses for General Practitioners maintaining their popularity. Provision was made also for Dental Practitioners.

The College at its Quarterly Meeting in May 1957 received a Report on Postgraduate Education produced by a Committee of the Court of Edinburgh University. In the course of their deliberations the Committee had consulted Sir Stanley Davidson, (Sir) Derrick Dunlop and Dr Rae Gilchrist representing the College; and Sir Alexander Biggam and Mr James Graham, F.R.C.S.E., representing the Edinburgh Post-Graduate Board for Medicine. A major point made in the Report was an urgent need for the development of instruction in the pre-clinical or basic sciences, development to promote an outlook of application to clinical circumstances, and to have the advantage of integration with clinical facilities in hospital wards. It was recognized that improvement along these lines would involve additional appointments and accommodation. A clear elucidation of the position was given by (Sir) Ian

Hill who maintained that while 'Post-graduate Education was a function of the Royal Colleges and the University . . . it was for the University to take a dominant share in the teaching of the basic sciences'. Approval of the Report by the College was *nemine contradicente*.[41]

In 1960 the College was informed that Sir Derrick Dunlop had been appointed independent Chairman of the Edinburgh Post-Graduate Board for Medicine following the retirement of Sir Alexander Biggam.[42]

The Pfizer Foundation Donation

In February 1961 the College were informed that three lecturers had been appointed by the University whose time would be devoted entirely to the instruction of postgraduates, but that accommodation continued to present a problem.[43] A year later almost to the day, the College learnt of a generous donation by the Pfizer Company for the erection of a Foundation for postgraduate teaching; the Foundation to include provisions for a lecture theatre, library and refectory. The Post-Graduate Board's good fortune could not have been more timely, coming as it did during what was described as 'a record year' and with the courses in Internal Medicine 'booked up' for two years in advance.[44]

Applications by postgraduates, and support from Trusts continued to grow in the ensuing year. In 1962, 825 postgraduates attended from thirty-six different countries and bookings for the course in Internal Medicine were complete for four years ahead. The need for further clinical facilities remained, and part solution was greatly aided by funds made available by the Nuffield Provincial Hospital Trust for courses organized for General Practitioners in South-East Scotland. An attractive feature of the resultant arrangements was the proximity of the meeting places to the areas from which the postgraduates were drawn. To promote effectiveness the Post-Graduate Board appointed Regional Directors.

Dr Archibald Davidson Bequest

At the Quarterly Meeting at which they were given these facts, Fellows were advised also that the building of a Postgraduate Medical School might well prove possible as a result of funds made available by the Lister Memorial Trust, and as a result of a bequest of a former holder of the Triple Qualification of the Scottish Colleges, Dr Archibald Davidson of Australia. The building, it was stated, would probably be erected on a site near and owned by the Royal College of Surgeons, and would be furnished, equipped and maintained by the University.[45]

There could not have been a more opportune windfall. In 1962 the College had approved in principle that the Lister Memorial Funds should be used to erect a Lister Memorial Post-graduate Medical School.[46] It became apparent however that liquid assets from the Lister Memorial Funds fell short of the sum required for the erection of a new building. As it happened Dr Archibald Davidson had directed that his bequest should be used in such manner as the governing body of the School of Medicine should determine, in order to provide, erect and equip new buildings for the School of Medicine. In the circumstances, and with the agreement of the Governing Board, the College approved in principle that 'the Lister Memorial Funds be conjoined with the Archibald Davidson Bequest for the erection of a Lister Memorial Post-Graduate Medical School'.[47]

There was an encouraging response to the Nuffield sponsored scheme in the South-East of Scotland, and the Post-Graduate Board were successful in securing an increased number of clinical attachments including some at Newcastle.[48] In due course it became necessary to limit enrolments to students who had had previous hospital experience.[49]

About this time greater attention was being paid to the widespread growth and distribution of demands for postgraduate education and the College was reminded of the need for integration of the Post-Graduate Board's activities with those of the Regional Hospital Board and possibly also those of the (Royal) College of General Practitioners. There had already been recognition in a Report on the University Structure (Chap. XXXII) of the desirability of closer association between the academic interests of Fellows and Members in training for teaching and research, and the vocational interests of the Post-Graduate Board in training for intermediate qualifications and in providing refresher courses.[50] Little time elapsed before the Regional Hospital Board made arrangements for the instruction of general practitioners at peripheral hospitals.[51]

Another aspect of postgraduate education was the subject of special study at a Conference in London sponsored by the six Royal Colleges in Great Britain, the expenses of which were borne by the London College of Physicians. The subject concerned was the training of specialists. Reporting to our College after the Conference the President—(Sir) Ian Hill—drew particular attention to the relevant sections in the Draft Regulations on Medical Education issued by the General Medical Council.[52]

Discussion of future policy within the College was greatly influenced by the contents of a Report of a Council Committee on Post-Graduate Medical Training submitted to Council in September 1967.[53] This Report allowed that there had been criticism, both of the educational activities of the Board as a whole and of the

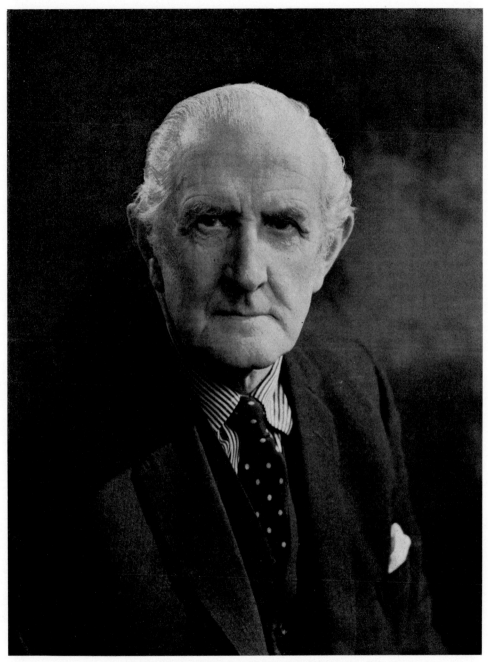

PLATE 48   Sir Derrick M. Dunlop, Chairman of the Appeal Committee
Photograph by E. R. Yerbury & Son, Edinburgh

contribution of the College to those activities. Endeavouring to assess the grounds for criticism, the Committee considered that in point of fact the Board merited unreserved credit in virtue of the proven success of their 'personal programmes' such as clinical attachments and assessment of unsponsored Commonwealth students; occasional specialist courses; constantly over-subscribed refresher courses for general practitioners; and in particular the courses designated 'intermediate' leading to higher qualifications and legitimately claiming to be second to none available in the United Kingdom. Acceptance of deficiencies by the Committee was frank. Their candour was to their credit. They freely allowed that educational programmes for pre-registration house officers were virtually non-existent in contrast to the position in London; that 'intermediate' courses catered in the main for overseas graduates and were unsuited to senior house officers and registrars in need of facilities suitably integrated with their daily commitments; and that provisions in Edinburgh for 'advanced' level studies could not compare with those available at Post-graduate Institutes in London. Furthermore it was noted that Edinburgh had made no concerted effort to provide basic training for potential general practitioners.

In the matter of postgraduate activities of the College in its own right, the Committee accepted that the lectures, symposia, publications and Library facilities of the College might be construed as constituting only a limited contribution, but with ample justification focussed attention on the altogether outstanding part played as individuals by Fellows and Members of the College in postgraduate instruction. Wisely, and showing practical realism, the Committee advised the Council concerning the need to consider whether further postgraduate activities on the part of the College should be along independent lines or channelled through the Board which it was 'clearly bound to support'. Among constructive recommendations advanced by the Committee one was to the effect that 'intermediate education' for hospital staffs offered a field for new development, organized on specialist section bases comparable to those of the Royal Society of Medicine.[53]

In 1968 the Edinburgh Post-Graduate Board gave trial to a modification of the Spring Course. This was extended from 13 to 18 weeks. It was composed of a number of short courses in certain specialties in such a way that the whole course of Internal Medicine was covered without preventing attendance by those who wished for personal reasons to confine their studies to a special subject.[54]

The Lister Institute was opened on 11th November 1967,[55] the Pfizer Foundation building having been opened by H.R.H. the Duke of Edinburgh on 2nd July 1965. Complementary to one another the two buildings made a major contribution to solution of accommodation difficulties. Administratively there then arose need for an

2C

adjustment to meet the situation following involvement of the National Health Service in postgraduate education and the coming into existence of a Regional Post-graduate Committee. Provision was made for representatives of the Service and the Regional Committee in a revised constitution of the Post-Graduate Board. The revised constitution was circulated among Fellows together with a Memorandum of the Dean of the University Faculty of Medicine, and an interpretation of the constitution as agreed between the President (Dr Christopher Clayson) of the College and the Dean of the Faculty at the time.[56] As evidenced by the Annual Report of the Board in 1970, an element of uncertainty about the future of the Board persisted as a result of a continuing fall in the numbers applying for courses. Among possible contributory factors were a tendency for the traditional lecture system to fall out of favour, and the presence of a competitive element in measures developing for 'in-teaching'.[57]

Reference to the Post-Graduate Board for Medicine would be incomplete were acknowledgment not made of the invaluable services as Directors of Sir Alexander Biggam, an Honorary Fellow of the College, and his successor, Professor E. C. Mekie, a surgeon and Fellow of both Edinburgh Colleges.

THE MEMBERSHIP AND THE MEMBERSHIP EXAMINATION

Examinations are formidable even to the best prepared, for the greatest fool may ask more than the wisest man can answer.

Charles C. Colton (1780–1832)

Council Committee Appointed

Having regard to the difficulties being experienced in administering the examination (q.v.) it came as no great surprise to Fellows when, at the February Quarterly Meeting in 1963, the President announced that Council were of opinion that changes should be made in the Membership Examination and that a Committee with Dr J. D. S. Cameron as Convener had been appointed to advise Council.[58] There was evidence that concern extended beyond Edinburgh in the fact that the subject came up for serious discussion at a later date in Glasgow at a meeting of the Presidents of all Colleges of Physicians in Great Britain and Ireland.[59] In both Edinburgh and Glasgow considerable disquiet was felt by Fellows concerning the effects of the examinations on the care of patients. Encroachment on the time of physicians was another source of worry. To some extent the problems were aggravated by the holding of examinations simultaneously in both cities, and a motion was passed by the College by a majority of 36 to 6 inviting Council to review the situation with their opposite numbers in Glasgow.[60]

The Committee appointed to review the Membership Examination reported in May 1965. They were emphatic that there were too many unsuitable, ill-prepared candidates and that the interests of patients required that screening procedures should be operated to limit the number of candidates sitting Part II of the Examination. As to Part I, the Committee after considering other possibilities and mindful of the interests of patients, were of the opinion that the fairest screening procedure would be a written paper consisting of a large number of questions each requiring only a literally brief answer. Other recommendations were that, whenever practicable, four instead of two examiners should be allotted to each candidate in the clinical examination; and that in order to eliminate the 'chronic examinee' a restriction should be imposed on the number of times a candidate could take the Part I Examination in order to become eligible to sit Part II.

Reciprocity: Early Soundings

Although strictly speaking not in their remit, Sir James Cameron gave it as the unanimous desire of the Committee that the possibilities of reciprocity should be discussed 'with assiduity'. Referring to consideration of the subject on more than one occasion by the Standing Joint Committee of the Scottish Colleges, Sir Ian Hill expressed the somewhat equivocal view that the College should not suggest reciprocity but should rather 'welcome proposals to that end'. The Committee's Report was approved by the College.[61]

Scottish Colleges Approach the London College

A few months later reciprocity came up for discussion at a meeting of the Standing Joint Committee of the Scottish Colleges. It transpired that only recently the Glasgow College had published new Regulations for their examination and they had only just come into force. Understandably the Glasgow representatives asked that a year or two should be allowed to elapse before further discussion of changes involving 'reciprocity and amalgamation of facilities for the examinations'.[62] Nevertheless, tentative exploratory talks continued. At a meeting in January 1967 of the same Standing Committee it was suggested that representatives of the Edinburgh and Glasgow Colleges should again meet to discuss the subject. Those representing Edinburgh were the Committee appointed to review the Membership Examination. They were able to report some months later that two fruitful meetings had been held with their Glasgow opposite numbers, at the second of which the question of reciprocity with the London College of Physicians arose in so far as the Part I Examination was concerned. Arrangements had already been made for a meeting in London.[63]

Part I Common Examination Agreed by the Three Colleges

The Quarterly Meeting of the College in July 1967 was the occasion for a resolution which was to set in train a momentous series of decisions in the years to follow. Approval was given to a motion on behalf of Council 'That the College empower the President and Council to continue exploratory discussions with representatives of the Royal College of Physicians of London and the Royal College of Physicians and Surgeons of Glasgow regarding the establishment of a common Part I for the Membership Examination'. Previous to the motion being put, it had been reported that the Council Committee to review the Membership Examination were unanimous in condemning the Part I as an ineffective means of screening candidates, and in considering a multiple choice paper as the best alternative in all the circumstances.[64] At the next Quarterly Meeting the College were informed of proposals, after discussion between the three Colleges of Physicians, to form a Joint Examining Board to set questions in accordance with multiple choice practice; a Membership Committee to receive applications and to determine where the examination should be held; and a Finance Committee.[65]

Further details were given in May 1968. The Joint Examination Board for the Part I Examination was to consist of 12 members—6 representatives of the London College, and 3 of each of the two Scottish Colleges. Drs Henry Matthew, K. G. Lowe and R. F. Robertson represented our College. It was further announced that a separate panel was going to be appointed 'to take in turn (with colleagues from other Royal Colleges) to sit the Common Part I examination at a date in advance of the candidates in order to discard any questions which appeared to be doubtful or ambiguous'.[66] October 1968 saw the introduction for the first time of the Common Part I Examination and Multiple Choice Paper. An early result was a dramatic fall in the number sitting the Examination through the College. While no single causative factor could be identified, possible contributory causes were the higher pass-rate in London where the Part I Examination started in 1961, and the contrasting complicated nature of the Edinburgh Examination.[67]

A point of some practical importance is that other Colleges expressed a wish to make use of the facilities provided for the M.R.C.P.(U.K.). In May 1970 the College recommended approval to an application of the Royal College of Physicians of Ireland. The resolution took account of the fact that the London and Glasgow Colleges had passed similar resolutions, and of conditions suggested as necessary by the Joint Negotiating Committee of the Edinburgh, Glasgow and London Colleges.[67] Among the conditions was one that a pass in the Multiple Choice Question paper through the Irish College would lead to the M.R.C.P. Ireland only, but would not entitle a candidate to enter for Part II of the M.R.C.P.(U.K.). Some months later a letter sent to the President of the College of Physicians of Ceylon and signed by the three Presidents of the United Kingdom Royal Colleges of Physicians indicated the terms and conditions under which a Part I Examination for the Membership could be held in Ceylon, prior to successful candidates taking Part II of the Examination at the College of their choice in the United Kingdom.[68] The Proposals in this connection were discussed further on the occasion of a visit to Sri Lanka by the Vice-President (Dr Halliday Croom) of our College; and the arrangements are now in operation.[69] Other centres for Part I examinations have been established in Egypt, Ghana, Iran, Malaysia, Sudan, West Indies and Ethiopia.[70, 71] Furthermore it has been arranged that British service officers can sit the Part I Examination in Singapore.[72]

Part II Reciprocity: Cautious Approach

Meanwhile approach to the problem of reciprocity in connection with Part II was being considered by the Council Committee. Immediate action was discouraged until the recently published Todd Report and the pending findings of the Croom Committee had been studied.[73] In November 1968 the President (Dr Christopher Clayson) referred to a meeting in London of the Joint Committee of the Royal Colleges of Physicians to consider the Membership Examination. Written assurance had been received that the College would be kept advised concerning progress. According to the Minutes the meeting 'had arisen out of the 450th Anniversary Celebration of the Sister College in London'.[74] Therein there may well be a pointer and good augury for our own celebrations in 1981! At the first Quarterly Meeting in 1969 the President proposed that the College should have a strictly informal discussion on the Membership Examination in the light of opinions expressed at the two most recent meetings of the Joint Committee of the Scottish Royal Colleges. Discussion was concerned with the possibility of reciprocal Memberships and the financial problems which might arise.[75]

Thereafter events proceeded apace. A Joint Committee was appointed by the three Royal Colleges to study the implications of reciprocity of the Membership Examination. In April 1969 an Extraordinary Meeting of the Edinburgh College was held at which another session of informal discussion took place. The President outlined the Joint Committee's views, stated that the objects of the exercise had already been approved by the College, described a common Part II examination as providing an effective way of preventing 'multiple diplomatosis', but concluded by saying that such a common examination was 'perhaps undesirable at present'. Considerable discussion followed, many of the 64 Fellows in attendance contributing. There was general but not unanimous agreement that reciprocity in principle was desirable. At the same time it was made clear that to be acceptable a Common Part II Examination would have to maintain the College method of examination more especially in so far as retention of selected subjects was concerned. Sight was not lost of the possible effects of the proposals on the income of the College.[76]

Implementation of a Common Part II Examination remained in abeyance despite agreement among the three Colleges as to the desirability of reciprocity. Delay was attributable to persisting differences. Nevertheless, the President felt able to explain to the College at their 1969 July Quarterly Meeting that reciprocity would involve the award of the Diploma for M.R.C.P.(U.K.) in lieu of the Diploma of individual Colleges; successful candidates would be elected as Members by all three Colleges without any modification in prevailing arrangements enabling eminent men to be elected as Members under the Laws of each College. A motion for approval of Draft Regulations submitted to the College was carried unanimously.[77]

M.R.C.P.(U.K.): *Reciprocity*

In anticipation of the ultimate achievement of complete reciprocity based on a common examination the M.R.C.P.(U.K.) was introduced in October 1969 while each College adhered to its own form of examination. Implied in this joint acceptance of the new Diploma was acknowledgment by each College of the equality shared by the three Memberships. By way of consolidating this new found community of outlook the Presidents of the three Colleges agreed to impose a limit on the number of attempts which any candidate could make in an endeavour to pass the Part II Examination.

Shortly after the introduction of the M.R.C.P.(U.K.) an Advisory Committee on Examinations was appointed by the Council of the College to keep the College Examination under review. One of the first observations made by the Committee concerned a pronounced fall in the number of candidates entering the Part II Examination through the Edinburgh College. This they attributed to candidates being deterred to some extent by the greater complexity of the examination as compared with those of the London and Glasgow Colleges, although other factors were almost certainly operating. Other attractions being equal the English Metropolis has a certain historical mesmeric influence in a host of spheres including that of medicine. Another factor which impressed the Committee, whether favourably or otherwise, was the implication contained in the Report of the Todd Commission that candidates sitting the Membership would be expected to do so at a notably earlier stage than hitherto. Without doubt the policy advocated paid little regard to the time required to acquire the skill and knowledge necessary to pass the examination in selected subjects incorporated in the Edinburgh Membership Examination. There were, and still are many, including experienced teachers and examiners, who regret a change of attitude contributed to in some measure at least by administrative expediency.

Nevertheless, with the long-term object of complete reciprocity in mind, the Advisory Committee of the College Council had no option but to conduct a comprehensive review of the content of the Part II Examination of the College with particular reference to Selected Subjects. Early in January 1970 the London College published a report based on a review of their own examination. On the instructions of Council the Edinburgh Advisory Committee studied the London Report with meticulous care. Council was advised by the Committee that the most recent recommendations possessed the ingredients of an examination of greater objective merit than either the Edinburgh or London Examinations in operation at the time. The Committee, with a magnanimity which was both accommodating and realistic, went further and recommended that taking the overall situation into account the College should contemplate, with minimal delay, planning a Common Part II Examination along the lines of the London College Report. The recommendation had the approval of the College at its Quarterly Meeting in May 1970.[67]

M.R.C.P.(U.K.): Reciprocity and Common Examination

An early outcome was regular meetings of the Joint Committee of the three Royal Colleges. It soon became apparent that each College would require to appoint a group of examiners to supervise the collection of examination material. For this purpose the Edinburgh College formed what was termed a 'Part II Question Group' in June 1970, and this was followed in five months' time by the establishment of a Common Part II Planning Committee, on which there were representatives of the Question Groups of each of the three Colleges. The Planning Committee is responsible for recommending the detailed format of the examination and the scoring system to be employed. The first Common Part II Examination came into operation in October 1972.

Part II Examination: the Former Edinburgh and New Common Forms Compared

Of first importance are the conditions governing the number of times a candidate may sit the Part I Examination as a preliminary to proceeding to Part II. It is now laid down that four attempts only are permitted, although in exceptional circumstances each College may allow a further two attempts. In no circumstances can a candidate sit on more than six occasions. As to the Common Part II Examination, six attempts are allowed but with two important provisos. Not more than two of the attempts can be made through the agency of any one College, and all attempts to pass Part II must be completed within three years of success in the Part I Examination. A candidate who has failed six times to pass Part II is debarred, once and for all, from sitting again either Part I or Part II of the Examination.

Two major changes were made in the Part II Examination. The former essay type examination in Applied Basic Sciences, Medicine and Therapeutics was replaced in its entirety by a written section composed of three parts. These subsections were as follows:

> 1. Case histories. The candidate is required to answer questions on three of five histories offered to him. Of the five histories at least one deals with a paediatric patient.
> 2. Interpretation of data. The candidate is required to identify abnormalities and answer specific clinically orientated questions (e.g. X-rays, electrocardiograms, laboratory data etc.).
> 3. Interpretation of slides. The candidate is required to identify abnormalities and answer specific questions relating to the abnormalities in 20 slides projected on a screen.

The overall purpose of the new form of question was to minimize 'examiner variability', while at the same time providing a more comprehensive field of examination. In the particular case of the subsection dealing with case histories, the aim was to test a candidate's ability in clinical interpretation and deduction.

The second major change was that with the one exception of Paediatrics no provision was made for a candidate to offer a Selected Subject. Any candidate who chose to be tested in Paediatrics in the oral and clinical examinations was still required to sit the same written examination as other candidates. Under the modified Regulations introduced in September 1970, the Part II Examination remained unchanged except for candidates choosing to be examined solely in the Medicine of Childhood. Candidates in Paediatrics could either take the examination under the old system and offer Child Life and Health as a Selected Subject, or take the examination in the Medicine of Childhood. This examination consisted of a Clinical Paper in the General Medicine of Childhood and another in Neonatal Paediatrics, and an oral session dealing with both General Medicine of Childhood and Paediatrics.[78]

Recognition of the special position of paediatrics within the overall discipline of medicine was tantamount to acceptance of the pioneer work of the Edinburgh Medical School in promoting understanding of Child Life and Health. In this the Edinburgh College of Physicians had contributed a notable supporting rôle. It was significant that encouragement was forthcoming from the Croom Committee for a request from the Academic Board of the British Paediatric Association, for Medicine of Childhood as an alternative subject to General Medicine.[79]

In the light of experience further changes in the Examination for the M.R.C.P. (U.K.) were introduced in August 1972. They related to the Oral and Clinical Sections of the Common Part II Examination. Under the new Regulations (1972) candidates can opt to be tested in either General Medicine or Paediatrics in these sections, but no provision is any longer made for candidates in Paediatrics to take an Examination in the Medicine of Childhood. In the written section *all* candidates are, as previously, offered five cases of which at least one will be paediatric, and are required to answer questions on three of the five cases.

Minor differences apart, the procedure at clinical examinations remains basically unchanged. Oral examinations are conducted by two examiners of whom one may be a specialist. The policy of exchanging examiners with the Colleges of Glasgow and London continues but with the number of examiners involved increased.

THE COLLEGIATE MEMBERSHIP

Following on the creation of the M.R.C.P.(U.K.) the three Colleges agreed that each might establish a category of Members called 'Collegiate Members', with the object of encouraging them to take part in the activities of Members of the College of their choice. The Edinburgh College Laws were altered accordingly to enable Collegiate Members, whether M.R.C.P.(Edin.) or M.R.C.P.(U.K.) to have a closer association with the College than that enjoyed by ordinary Members.[80] Concern that Members should be brought into the corporate life of the College was of long-standing. It had been the subject of discussion by Council in 1953.[81]

A Reception was arranged for Collegiate Members on 12th October 1970. At the Reception the names were announced of those elected to the Collegiate Members' Committee as a result of a postal vote. The elected Members were drawn from Edinburgh, Glasgow, Aberdeen, Perth, Dundee and Stracathro and at the first meeting Dr M. A. Eastwood of Edinburgh was elected Chairman. This first meeting was attended by the Secretary (Dr Alex. Keay) and the Treasurer (Dr William Mac-leod) of the College. The former outlined to the Committee the administrative procedures of the College, and the latter made it known that the College had placed a sum of £600 at the disposal of the Collegiate Members' Committee for the ensuing year.

The Council of the College and the Collegiate Members held a joint meeting on 29th April 1971, at which the latter presented, among other proposals, the following:

1. the existing privileges of ordinary Members should remain unchanged;
2. the fostering of additional privileges for Collegiate Members;
3. full participation by Members in all College and Council Committees;
4. development within the College of a social and academic life for Collegiate Members;
5. active participation in postgraduate medical education by the College;
6. preparedness on the part of the College to show interest and offer expertise in the ethical and moral issues presenting to the profession;
7. more extensive publicising of the excellent library facilities, and
8. the organisation by Collegiate Members of lectures of general interest, followed by some form of social gathering.

To quote from the First Annual Report of the Collegiate Members' Committee signed by their Chairman: 'These proposals were discussed, and with only one reservation, namely Membership of the Fellowship Committee, the proposals were warmly received by the Council'.[82] Following the discussion the Council acted as host at an informal dinner.

The maiden voyage of the Collegiate Members' Committee was as auspicious as its launching. Within approximately eight months of election the Committee organized what proved to be a highly successful Symposium with *The Wind of Change* as subject and without suggestion of threatening revolution or anarchy! Another equally interesting and successful Symposium followed in October 1971. On this occasion the subject was *Medicine and the Mass Media* and speakers were drawn from the National and Scientific Press, the Universities—including the Open University—the National Health Service and the House of Commons opposition back bench. The imaginative programme met with the response it deserved.

HONORARY MEMBERSHIP

When in 1916 the College wished to honour three Royal Army Medical Corps Officers for outstanding service in the typhus-stricken camp at Wittenberg by including their names on the Roll of Members, it transpired that by their Laws the College could only elect these officers to the ordinary Membership 'without examination and without fee'.[83] A new Law was passed in 1918 under which on the nomination by Council and subject to approval by a majority of seven-eighths of the Fellows voting at an Extraordinary Meeting called for the purpose, the Honorary Membership can be offered to men of distinction.[84]

THE FELLOWSHIP

In the course of informal discussion of the Report on the Future of the College, the Croom Committee responsible for preparation of the Report gave it as their firm, unanimous conviction that the Fellowship was and must be retained as what they termed *'an additional honour'*.[85] This is the view to which the College continues to adhere. While Collegiate Members enjoy certain privileges, advancement of a Member to the Fellowship is in no way dependent upon, or conditioned by his being a Collegiate Member.[80] During the discussion already mentioned, consideration was given to the possibility of a Member suitable for elevation being overlooked, but there was no general agreement as to a feasible solution. Of Fellows speaking, most were not merely opposed but strongly opposed to a suggestion that candidates for admission to Membership should be asked to submit a Curriculum Vitae which would be revised every three years.[85] Altogether the suggestion was too reminiscent of dubious, if not unsavoury machinery in connection with merit awards in the National Health Service. Another suggestion which found favour with several was that Regional Committees of Fellows might be vested with the responsibility of recommending to the College Fellowship Committee, Members for advancement.[85] The subject is not lacking in pitfalls, but this suggestion has attractions and in Yorkshire and Wessex, if not elsewhere, there already exist informal regional associations capable of co-operating with the Fellowship Committee.

A need for a Roll of Fellows similar to Munk's *Roll* of the London College of Physicians has been recognized but still remains to be met.[81]

HONORARY FELLOWSHIP

Policy with regard to the admission of Honorary Fellows has altered radically since the early days of the College. The custom of electing distinguished laymen as well as eminent members of the medical profession lapsed with the admission of Dr Matthew Baillie in 1809. Previously in 1773 the number of Honorary Fellows had been restricted to ten.[86] By Laws enacted in 1909 the Honorary Fellowship can be offered to individuals of high distinction who have been nominated by Council and whose nomination has been approved at an Extraordinary Meeting of the College by a majority of nine-tenths of the Fellows voting. The first Honorary Fellow to be elected under the new law and the first to be elected for 110 years was H.R.H. Edward, Prince of Wales.[87] Appendix L gives the names of those subsequently elected in the last fifty years or so. The complete list includes Honorary Fellows elected during the period 1696–1809 during which time Diplomas of Membership were not granted by the College, despite the fact that they are frequently referred to in the literature as Honorary Members.

COMMUNICATIONS

Mountains divide us, and the waste of the seas . . .
Canadian Boat Song

Awakening of the College to the need for maintaining the closest possible ties with Members and Fellows scattered far and wide over the continents has been slow. One, if not the most precious, asset of the College is its conception and practice of Fellowship. The closest of friendships exist among those working as 'mates', 'brothers' or 'comrades' at the bench, in the workshop or in the office; and among doctors engaged in clinical, research or academic pursuits. But no matter how deep and sincere the relations may be, they lack an undefinable, intangible something that is the spirit of Fellowship known to the Royal College of Physicians of Edinburgh— interpreting Fellowship in its widest and not narrow or titular sense. The like does not exist in all Universities no matter how loyal the student bodies and academic staffs. Nor, it is suggested, do all if any of the other medical corporations know quite the same intensity of unspoken Fellowship shared by young and old, junior and senior, within the walls of the Edinburgh College. 'Within the walls of the Edinburgh College'—those words are crucial. The College has ever been ready to evince this Fellowship to the exile calling *en passant*, the prodigal son returned in retirement or the visiting stranger no matter how young or old, how eminent or unknown, and no matter his country of origin. But in the case of a stranger or forgotten exile the initiative has to be taken by him. Too little thought has been given until recent years by the College to sharing its unique awareness of true Fellowship with those among its number who are far removed from Edinburgh.

That which applies to the Member or Fellow domiciled in the Highlands, south of Tweed, in Wales and across the Irish Sea applies also, if in a different way, to those in Canada, Australasia and the Far East. The impression is confirmed by letters from distant lands—distant despite modern air transport. It is not without significance that the letter of one correspondent opened with the quotation which heads this section. At the same time as betraying true sentiment the quotation was intended to convey the silent regret of a Fellow conscious of the remoteness of ties with our—with *his* College. If truth must be told the College while aspiring to nation-wide influence has been inclined to take for granted the unique Fellowship it enjoys within the environs of Edinburgh and to be blind to the desire of Members and Fellows else-where to share that Fellowship as fully as possible and practicable.

One small step taken to remedy the situation was a decision by the College Council in 1953 that each year the President should circulate to all Fellows a report on College affairs during the preceding twelve months.[88] With the appearance for the first time of the College quarterly publication entitled *Chronicle* the President's Report no longer appears independently but as a routine integrated part of the quarterly issue. The risk is that the contribution may in the course of time assume too rigidly the form of a Report and tend to lose the sense of being a personal message. Sir Hector Hetherington when Principal and Vice-Chancellor of Glasgow University established the immense value of an annual personal letter to all members of the General Council, informative in the extreme although couched in the most informal terms. His letters stimulated as they galvanized. They were invariably the subject of admiring discus-sion at Glasgow Graduate gatherings throughout the United Kingdom. Hethering-ton was vividly alive to the impact of outward-thinking. There is growing realiza-tion that our College should with minimum delay adopt a less inward looking atti-tude in its approach and initiatives if its conception of Fellowship is to be shared by all who are entitled to it and by all who would welcome it.

REFERENCES

OUTSIDE INFLUENCES

(1) R.C.P.E. (1963) *The Care of the Elderly in Scotland.* Edinburgh: Royal College of Physicians.
(2) R.C.P.E. (1959) *Report by the President* [A. R. Gilchrist] ... *1958–59.* Edinburgh: Royal College of Physicians.

(3) R.C.P.E. (1960) *Report by the President* [A. R. Gilchrist] . . . *1959–60*. Edinburgh: Royal College of Physicians.

(4) R.C.P.E. (1963) *Report by the President* [J. D. S. Cameron] . . . *1962–63*. Edinburgh: Royal College of Physicians.

(5) Council Minutes, 24.viii.1971.

(6) Ibid., 31.x.1944.

(7) MATTHEW, H. J. S. (1972) Personal communication.

(8) Council Minutes, 23.iv.1963.

(9) Ibid., 1.vii.1963.

(10) Ibid., 19.xi.1963.

(11) Ibid., 5.ix.1962.

(12) R.C.P.E. (1966) *Report by the President* [I. G. W. Hill] . . . *1963–65*. Edinburgh: Royal College of Physicians.

(13) R.C.P.E. (1969) *Report by the President* [C. W. Clayson] . . . *1967–68*. Edinburgh: Royal College of Physicians.

(14) ROYAL COMMISSION ON MEDICAL EDUCATION 1965–68. (1968) *Report*. (Chairman: Lord Todd.) § 92. London: H.M.S.O.

(15) R.C.P.E. (1969) *Report of the Standing College Committee on specialist standards, vocational registration and postgraduate medical education*. (Typescript.)

THE FUTURE OF THE COLLEGE

(16) R.C.P.E. (1969) *Report of College Committee to Consider the Future of the College*. (Convener: Dr J. Halliday Croom.) Edinburgh: Royal College of Physicians.

(17) College Minutes, 5.xii.1946.

(18) Ibid., 4.vi.1946.

(19) ROYAL COMMISSION ON MEDICAL EDUCATION 1965–68. Op. cit. § 93 & 94.

(20) Ibid., § 98.

(21) College Minutes, 15.x.1969.

POSTGRADUATE EDUCATION

(22) Council Minutes, 31.iii.1953.

(23) College Minutes, 4.v.1954.

(24) Ibid., 4.xi.1971.

(25) Ibid., 7.v.1963.

(26) Ibid., 2.v.1961.

(27) R.C.P.E. (1923) *Presentation of Portrait to Dr. Byrom Bramwell. Report of proceedings at the Royal College of Physicians, Edinburgh. Saturday, 19th May, 1923*. [Edinburgh: Privately printed.]

(28) CUSHING, H. (1925) *The Life of Sir William Osler*, vol. I, pp. 517 & 527. Oxford: Clarendon Press.

(29) EDINBURGH POST-GRADUATE LECTURES IN MEDICINE (1940) *Foreword*, by Edwin Bramwell. Vol. I, pp. IX–XVI. Edinburgh: Oliver & Boyd for the Honyman Gillespie Trust.

(30) GILCHRIST, A. R. (1972) Personal communication.
(31) College Minutes, 1.ii.1944.
(32) Ibid., 2.v.1944.
(33) Ibid., 18.vii.1944.
(34) Ibid., 1.v.1945.
(35) Ibid., 15.vii.1947.
(36) Ibid., 5.ii.1952.
(37) Ibid., 21.vii.1953.
(38) Ibid., 2.ii.1954.
(39) Ibid., 1.ii.1955.
(40) Ibid., 5.ii.1957.
(41) Ibid., 7.v.1957.
(42) Ibid., 2.ii.1960.
(43) Ibid., 7.ii.1961.
(44) Ibid., 6.ii.1962.
(45) Ibid., 5.ii.1963.
(46) Ibid., 17.iv.1962.
(47) Ibid., 7.v.1963.
(48) Ibid., 4.ii.1964.
(49) Ibid., 2.ii.1965.
(50) Ibid., 1.ii.1966.
(51) Ibid., 7.ii.1967.
(52) Ibid., 1.xi.1966.
(53) R.C.P.E. (1967) *Report of Council Committee on Post-Graduate Medical Training.* (Typescript.)
(54) College Minutes, 4.ii.1969.
(55) Ibid., 6.ii.1968.
(56) Ibid., 4.xi.1969.
(57) Ibid., 3.ii.1970.

THE MEMBERSHIP AND THE MEMBERSHIP EXAMINATION

(58) Ibid., 5.ii.1963.
(59) Ibid., 7.v.1963.
(60) Ibid., 3.xi.1964.
(61) Ibid., 4.v.1965.
(62) Ibid., 26.vii.1966.
(63) Ibid., 2.v.1967.
(64) Ibid., 25.vii.1967.
(65) Ibid., 7.xi.1967.
(66) Ibid., 7.v.1968.
(67) Ibid., 5.v.1970.
(68) Ibid., 21.vii.1970.

(69) Ibid., 3.xi.1970.

(70) CROFTON, J. W. (1974) President's Report. *Chronicle*, **4**, 2, 3.

(71) FLEMING, P. R., MATTHEWS, M. B. *et al.* (1974) Evolution of an examination: M.R.C.P.(U.K.). *British Medical Journal*, **2**, 99.

(72) MACLEOD, H. M. (1972) Personal communication.

(73) College Minutes, 23.vii.1968.

(74) Ibid., 5.xi.1968.

(75) Ibid., 4.ii.1969.

(76) Ibid., 16.iv.1969.

(77) Ibid., 22.vii.1969.

(78) Ibid., 22.ix.1970.

(79) Ibid., 4.ii.1969.

THE COLLEGIATE MEMBERSHIP

(80) R.C.P.E. (1970) *Report by the President* [C. W. Clayson] ... *1968–69*. Edinburgh: Royal College of Physicians.

(81) Council Minutes, 31.iii.1953.

(82) R.C.P.E. (1971) *The First Annual Report of the Collegiate Members' Committee, 1970-1971*. [Edinburgh: Royal College of Physicians.]

HONORARY MEMBERSHIP

(83) College Minutes, 2.v.1916.

(84) Ibid., 5.ii.1918.

THE FELLOWSHIP

(85) Ibid., 6.v.1969.

HONORARY FELLOWSHIP

(86) Ibid., 3.xi.1773.

(87) Ibid., 3.vi.1919.

COMMUNICATIONS

(88) Council Minutes, 17.ii.1953.

Chapter XXXI

1950 AND AFTER: COLLEGE ADVISORY
REPORTS, COMMUNITY PROBLEMS

Medicine is a profession for social service and it developed organisation in response to social need.

Charles H. Mayo

DISABLEMENT

Tis not enough to help the feeble up,
But to support him after.

William Shakespeare (*Timon of Athens*)

The two Reports which follow should be considered in historical perspective. They deal with disablement under modern conditions. War injuries and those arising from road accidents have focussed attention on disablement in the present century. Industrial employment has added to the toll, but it is salutary to remember that this applied not only to the present century but to the nineteenth century from the earliest days of the industrial revolution when frequently women and children as well as men were the victims of disablement—temporary and permanent.

Committee of Inquiry into Questions affecting Disabled Persons
Evidence submitted by the College, 1954[1]

A College Committee with Dr W. A. Alexander as Convener was appointed in July 1953 to give evidence.[2] 'The responsibility for continued care until patients are re-established in the community rests firmly with the medical profession.' This declaration appeared in the opening statement and continued to dominate the theme of the evidence submitted. No attempt was made to conceal the partial failure of the profession to realize fully their responsibilities in this sphere, and to co-operate to the full with agencies empowered by Act of Parliament to further efforts on behalf of the disabled. Attention was focussed on the detrimental effects of prolonged periods of inactivity after the termination of active medical treatment involving growing fears of unemployment and financial disaster.

Exception was taken to the conception embodied in the Beveridge Report[3] differentiating 'medical' and 'post-medical' treatment in measures for rehabilitation. It was noted that 'this fundamental error' was perpetuated in the Tomlinson Report[4] which ultimately led to administrative responsibility for the rehabilitation of disabled persons being vested in the Ministry of Labour in accordance with the requirements of the *Disabled Persons (Employment) Act 1944*.[5]

Reference was then made to certain studies which had been made in the preceding decade in Scotland.[6, 7] The combined findings of these studies revealed the extent to which social and environmental circumstances conditioned the success or otherwise of resettlement, and warranted the conclusion that some of the shortcomings of the system in operation at the time were attributable to ineffective follow-up and failure to concentrate on groups offering prospects of the best results 'in relation to efforts expended on their behalf'. A special enquiry into the problems of disabled youth in Glasgow attached importance to improved basic living conditions, the availability of intensive medical and surgical treatment, the provision of necessary medical and surgical appliances, the 'mitigation of . . . gross educational lack', satisfactory settlement before 'the young person begins to drift', and training courses for disabled young people.[8] Other West of Scotland investigations dealt with the contrasting difficulties of skilled and unskilled workers in obtaining employment suited to their disability.

In their evidence the College drew particular attention to the success which had attended the joint efforts of a Consultant in Social Medicine, a Medical Officer in Charge of Physical Medicine and a Senior Almoner at a Resettlement Clinic established in the Western Infirmary, Glasgow. Appraising the achievements of this Clinic, the College in their evidence suggested 'that action taken at the time of discharge from hospital by a group representing all interests involved is productive of results as good as, if not superior to, those attained by the existing official machinery alone'.

Continuing, the College evidence commented briefly on some aspects of the administration of official measures for the industrial rehabilitation and resettlement of disabled persons. Tribute was paid to the well-intentioned efforts of Disablement Resettlement Officers but, it was suggested that their knowledge should not be limited to available vacancies and should extend to the stresses and strains entailed in the nature of the employment involved. Moreover it was stated to be common knowledge that the official register of disabled persons included a number not in real need of help in obtaining or holding employment, whom the Ministry felt unable to differentiate from others in real need of assistance. Placement, the College maintained, could not be regarded as assurance of successful resettlement and the need was for a systematic follow-up more comprehensive than that dependent solely on postal communications. Credit was given to industrial rehabilitation units for their skill in re-assessment but, it was pointed out that a need existed for a readjustment providing for more consideration of complex medical problems involving psychological disturbance. As the number of disabled requiring sheltered employment far exceeded the places available, it was recommended that every effort should be made to ensure that priority was given to those in undoubted need of sheltered employment. A case was advanced for exploring the possibility of providing suitable work for those who were home-bound.

By way of summary the College evidence made a series of additional specific constructive suggestions. These included:

'The development of an efficient rehabilitation scheme within the Health Service, with appropriate facilities for both in-patients and out-patients; and the inclusion in facilities of regional residential rehabilitation centres, and 'day-to-day' rehabilitation centres serving concentrated populations with provisions for physiotherapy, a gymnasium and an occupational therapy department. Close co-operation between family doctors, the hospital service, rehabilitation centres and Ministry of Labour officials was urged. Pursuing prospects of increasing integration and extending it to central supervision, the College instanced the Royal Danish Invalidity Court as meriting emulation. Some members of that Court were medical and others were representative of the two sides of industry. Alternatively it was suggested that a Joint Board representative of the Ministry of Labour and the Central Health Departments might be established.

Of disabled persons those most likely to show a maximum response were given as young persons, and those 'fresh from medical treatment' and in need of suitable work. Vocational training courses in increased numbers geared to a reasonable prospect of suitable employment were described as essential. Finally the College raised the question as to whether rehabilitation and resettlement should not be more effectively linked with the 'general "after-care" responsibilities . . . laid upon local authorities' under the *National Health Service Acts of 1946 and 1947*.'[9, 10]

Departmental Committee of the Ministry of National Insurance to Review the Present Provisions of the National Health (Industrial Injuries) Act

Memorandum of Evidence submitted by the College, 1954[11]

A Committee with Dr W. A. Alexander as Convener was appointed by the College in November 1953.[12] In retrospect the evidence sought from the College Committee is of special interest in that it illustrates the difficulties confronting a medical committee where no clear-cut line of demarcation separates medical from administrative considerations. It is not unknown for a medical statement taken out of context to be misrepresented or applied in an unwarranted general way at a later date. Allowing that it may be entirely in error, the impression gained from the College evidence is that their representatives trod warily lest they might expose themselves to misinterpretation in this way.

A major observation made by the College at the outset of their evidence was that they were impressed by the advantages which would accrue were payment of sickness and industrial injuries benefit on the same scale. Were this to obtain, it was pointed out that general practitioners would be relieved of the difficult and often odious task of deciding whether an injury or an illness was or was not due to employment, and that it would obviate the discontent, bitterness and frustration known to many workers who felt that they should be paid industrial benefits when in receipt of sickness benefit only. It was also argued that a change along the lines suggested would serve to remove the anomalies of the Act, and to bring to an end the 'practice of certain Trades Union officials putting pressure on general practitioners to sign certificates for those of their patients who are contesting an award for partial disablement'. Before presenting their evidence on this particular point the College had appointed a general practitioner member of the College Committee to investigate the problem and to let them have the benefit of the views of his colleagues in general practice and of himself. Having expressed their opinion the College allowed that they realized the Government 'might not be able to accept the principle of equal payments because of financial and/or political considerations', and that being so had decided to examine certain provisions of the *Industrial Diseases Act* in detail.

The College devoted a considerable amount of time to consideration of the industrial dermatoses which they declared accounted for more lost working time than all other conditions 'put together', and which when the question of cause and effect arose presented particular difficulty because of the numerous causes unrelated to occupation. In the circumstances the College sought the advice of a consultant dermatologist with wide experience in the working of the *Industrial Injuries Act*, who did not miss the opportunity to point out that there was no dermatologist serving on the Departmental Committee. The Dermatological Report submitted to the College and conveyed in substance to the Departmental Committee, instanced situations in which dermatologists frequently classified a genuine industrial disease as 'injury by accident' because of the incompleteness of the official list of Prescribed Diseases; recommended the differentiation of dermatoses essentially occupational in character from those exacerbated by a man's work; and considered that earlier reference of cases to a dermatologist would be in the interest of all concerned, including the Exchequer.

It was in their attempts to answer questions contained in a Memorandum of the Departmental Committee that the College showed greater hesitancy, which at times was the reaction to questions of uncertain meaning or intent. To reproduce all the questions and answers would be pointless for present purposes. If only because of the long-term sagacity of the answer given to it, one question in the Departmental Memorandum deserves mention. It was—'Is there any middle way, wider than the present system but short of giving cover for all diseases arising out of work in insurable employment, which would be practicable without producing anomalies?' To this the College replied—'This is the most important question asked . . . The College does not approve of giving general cover for all diseases arising out of work in insurable employment, but suggests that the gradual addition of carefully selected hazards to the list of prescribed diseases over a period of years would perhaps be more acceptable to the Ministry of National Insurance and to the industrial workers. The *Industrial Injuries Act* is a comparatively new form of health benefit brought to the notice of the workers and it is felt that it would be wrong to attempt any drastic alteration in its form at the present time. As medical knowledge and business interest in the problems of occupational health increases some of the present-day hazards will no doubt be eradicated. On the other hand new unexpected hazards will arise from new industrial processes as these are developed and these hazards will, in the course of time, merit consideration by the authorities.'[11]

REHABILITATION

Scottish Health Services Council Report on Medical Rehabilitation: the Pattern of the Future
Comments of a College Committee, October 1972[13]

In October 1972, a College Committee under the Chairmanship of Professor A. Mair gave its comments on a *Report on Medical Rehabilitation* issued by the Scottish

Health Service Council.[14] The Committee had obviously considered the Report with considerable care and in great detail. Their comments were essentially practical, wide-ranging and made no pretence to 'pull punches'. The absence of facts to substantiate some of the firm opinions expressed was noted, as was the generality of recommendations relating to consultant staff. Whole-hearted approval was given to contemplation of a comprehensive approach to research but attention was focussed on the importance of securing evidence as to need before embarking on extensive new departments and the appointment of new staff in large numbers. As to finance, emphasis was attached to the importance, in marshalling support for the Health Council's recommendations, of obtaining and providing evidence on the cost-effectiveness of an efficient medical rehabilitation service.

The College Committee was not convinced that the appointment of large numbers of consultants was the answer to many of the problems confronting the service; and drew attention to the importance of the consultant as a co-ordinator for the purposes of rehabilitation service, teaching and research within such disciplines as Paediatrics, Psychiatry, Neurology, Surgery and Geriatrics. Short-term planning was urged in the first place with the object of strengthening the resources of existing departments. Appointments of consultants, it was considered, should be limited in number and restricted to teaching hospitals in Scotland. Desirably, it was stated, the new appointments should be made jointly by the National Health Service and the Universities, and should recognize the needs of research and teaching.

In the opinion of the College Committee, the Health Council Services' recommendations for a new specialty of medical rehabilitation were to a certain extent lacking in 'realism and practicality'. The main grounds for criticism were that the Report failed—to quote the rasping terminology of the Committee!—'to eliminate replication' of certain services. Unreserved support was given to proposals for the better dissemination of information, and the simultaneous preservation of 'the identity of voluntary organisations'.

Teaching came in for special comment by the Committee. They were emphatic about their reservations concerning inclusion of Rehabilitation as a separate subject in the undergraduate curriculum. 'This discipline', they argued, 'seems much more suited to the postgraduate phase of a doctor's education and training, and to his "continuing education", than to the undergraduate curriculum. The recommendation for undergraduate teaching in rehabilitation we regard therefore as more of a criticism of existing arrangements for postgraduate education and training than as a practicable solution to a rather pressing problem. In the meantime however, and until more effective arrangements can be made, clinical undergraduate teaching should include as far as possible some instruction on rehabilitation services.'[13] This however should not be regarded as a substitute for a more vigorous approach to the need for training in the postgraduate phase of the doctor's career.

DRUG ADDICTION

> *Thou hast the keys of Paradise, oh, just subtle, and mighty opium.*
> Thomas De Quincey

> *Calamy, laudamy, poultices, pills,*
> *They are the stuff for bodily ills.*
> *Thingummybobs of a different kind*
> *Are the stuff for disorderliness of the mind.*
> *When with distresses your psyche is wracked,*
> *Relax. Think of nothing at all. Abreact.*
> James Bridie

The date of the College Report referred to below affords evidence that the question of drug addiction has been a matter of concern for some considerable time.

Drug Addiction: Report of Committee appointed by the Council, 1959[15]

The College was informed at the February Quarterly Meeting 1959 that an invitation had been received from the Minister of Health and Secretary of State to give advice to the Interdepartmental Committee on Drug Addiction.[16] A Committee was accordingly appointed with Dr T. A. Munro as Convener and Dr A. G. MacGregor as Secretary. A feature of the Committee was that membership included Fellows closely concerned with the legal aspects of addiction, the statutory restrictions and regulations in force, and with the care and treatment of addicts in hospital; and that they had the benefit of advice from the Physician-Superintendents of the Royal Edinburgh Hospital for Mental Disorders and the Crichton Royal Hospital, Dumfries.

(Sir) Derrick Dunlop was a member of the Ministry of Health Committee on the joint nomination of the College and of the Royal College of Physicians of London.

The terms of remit require mention in some detail. They were 'to consider whether any revised advice should also cover other drugs liable to produce addiction or to be habit forming; to consider whether there is a medical need to provide special, including institutional, treatment outside the resources already available, for persons addicted to drugs; and to make recommendations, including any proposals for administrative measures that seem expedient . . .'.[16]

Regulations Adequate

The Committee's Report took the form of answers to a series of questions submitted to them. On the particular question of increased addiction to Dangerous Drugs the Committee had no information to suggest that there was such an increase, and from evidence derived from police reports in Edinburgh concluded that there was no rise in the amount of excessive prescribing of narcotic drugs 'as would cause the circumstances to be reported to the police'. Taking these observations into account, and from a study of admissions to the Royal Edinburgh and Crichton Royal Hospitals on account of drug addiction during the years 1950–8 inclusive, the Committee concluded that there was 'no evidence of any increase in addiction to opiates and synthetic opium substitutes'; and that 'the unauthorised obtaining of D.D.A. drugs is not a problem, that illicit drug traffic appears to be non-existent in Scotland, and that, providing the existing regulations under the D.D.A. are properly enforced, an adequate amount of control' was being exercised.

Professional Personnel at Risk

Of 77 addicts in the two Mental Hospitals already mentioned 58 were 'professional' addicts but the Committee did not consider that the figures reflected any particular trend. Morphine addiction was considered to be probably less common than prior to 1939 but there was reason, it was stated, to think that addiction to pethidine among doctors and nurses had increased. The College had no doubts as to the need for more stringent controls to prevent the accumulation of excessive quantities of dangerous drugs by the 'professional' addict. Full implementation was urged of the recommendations embodied in *Report on the Control of Dangerous Drugs and Poisons in Hospital* published by the Central Health Service Council in 1958.[17]

Sources of Information

The College Committee was opposed to the institution of compulsory notification and for the registration of addicts as being likely to militate against successful treatment, and inappropriate for patients receiving increasing doses of drugs during the terminal stages of fatal illness.

Forms for Prescribing

In the opinion of the College distinctive forms for prescribing potentially addictive drugs would have no advantage but several disadvantages, and might well alarm patients for whom such drugs were prescribed for legitimate reasons.

The Elderly Morphine Addict

Corroboration of the opinion of the Rolleston Committee[18] was forthcoming in that the College Committee was satisfied concerning the validity of the concept of a stabilized addict, and that some cases would be stabilized on a greatly reduced dose and could lead a normal life. There was agreement among the members that in many cases there was 'no good purpose . . . in attempting to "cure" an elderly morphine addict'.

Institutional Treatment Essential

Institutional treatment was described by the Report as essential for complete and certain drug withdrawal and as requiring highly skilled nursing. The institution, it was stated, need not necessarily be a mental hospital. Support and supervision given as out-patient treatment were considered essential sequellae to institutional in-patient care; but the Committee regarded treatment during drug-withdrawal of the potential "pre-addict" to be within the competence of the general practitioner.

Compulsory Institutional Treatment

The Committee were of the opinion that existing powers were adequate and that the national problem of addiction to D.D.A. drugs was not sufficient to warrant compulsory powers. The *Criminal Justice Act*,[19] it was argued, gave sufficient control were the Law broken and in practice the doctor could often bring about admission for treatment by withholding the prescription for the addictive drug.

Extent of Success in Treatment

Drawing on their own experience the Committee were satisfied concerning the effectiveness of institutional treatment in securing drug withdrawal but were well aware that a large proportion of addicts 'subsequently relapse after varying periods of time'. Nevertheless the re-admission rate for drug addicts was found to be less than for alcohol addiction.

Instruction in the Use and Abuse of Dangerous Drugs

Instruction of students and practitioners was considered to be adequate by the Committee, but the implementation of the D.D.A. regulations variable.

Interim Embargo on New Analgesics
A suggestion that all new analgesics likely to prove addictive should be reserved by law from general prescriptions until adequately investigated was ruled out as 'quite impracticable'. General use for some time was regarded as fundamental to assessment of addictive properties.

Use of Sedatives, Hypnotics, Central Nervous Stimulants and Tranquillisers
In this connection the Committee had been asked to specify drugs giving 'cause for alarm'.

Barbiturates, the Committee were satisfied, were used excessively, and to a considerable extent because of lack of precision in diagnosis. Dependence upon barbiturates was recognized as not uncommon among chronic neurotics, but the Report made the point that there was a subtle difference between dependency upon, and addiction to, drugs. Barbiturates were described as one of the commonest of drugs giving rise to skin eruptions. An observation of particular practical significance was the belief of the Committee that some of the increased morbidity associated with barbiturates was attributable to excessive use of these hypnotics when patients were in hospital. A special study of this aspect of the problem was carried out which led the Committee to conclude that 'in respect of the use of barbiturates, more attention should be paid in hospitals to the selective and discriminating use of barbiturate sedation, particularly during the week before the patient's discharge home'.

Carbromal, named as an addictive drug which was available without prescription, was rapidly acquiring increasing popularity as a hypnotic and was a common secondary drug in cases of alcoholism. The Committee went so far as to say that Carbromal as an important drug of addiction was 'probably more important in this respect than any of the barbiturates'.

Excessive use of amphetamine was said to be increasing despite the withdrawal of 'Benzedrine' inhalers.

According to the Report, habituation to tranquillisers was 'fairly common' and morbidity from their use increasing. Summarizing their views the Committee considered that it was undesirable, in principle, that powerful and potentially dangerous drugs (e.g. chlorpromazine or meprobromate) should be available for distribution to the public without control. Many such drugs were known to be injurious to health without necessarily being classified as poisons, and the Report maintained that a prescription should be a prerequisite for their sale. Moreover the Committee was of the opinion that in addition to sedatives, hypnotics, central nervous stimulants and tranquillisers—'sex hormones, anti-histamine preparations, anti-spasmodics, diuretics etc., should likewise be available only on prescription'.

It was further suggested by the Committee that consideration of the general principle of control should have regard to the desirability of diminishing 'the extent of self-medication'. In furtherance of this it was suggested as possibly appropriate that the above preparations might be included under Part II of the *Therapeutic Substances Act (1956)*.[20]

Drugs acting on C.N.S.: Clinical Trials

Dealing with the final question posed by the Interdepartmental Committee, the College Committee was emphatic that it would be unreasonable to limit the use of all new drugs acting on the central nervous system until adequate clinical trials had been completed; and that initial clinical trials should continue to remain the responsibility of the sponsoring pharmaceutical manufacturing house.

Addiction to alcohol was described as a subject calling for a full review and enquiry into the social and medical problems involved.

The Report of the Committee appointed by Council was approved by the College at the Quarterly Meeting in May 1959.[21]

NATIONAL STATISTICS

. . . there is a definite task before us—to determine from observation, the sources of Health, and the direct causes of death in the two sexes at different ages and under the different conditions.

William Farr

Ensuring the accuracy of statistics touching on personal and domestic matters is notoriously difficult. Periodic review of the legislative background is important if socio-medical studies are to be provided with reliable information even in an age of computer analyses.

Registration of Births, Deaths and Marriages, 1962

Not for the first time the College in 1962 adopted a strong line in seeking to remedy the deficiencies in the methods of Registration of Births, Deaths and Marriages. Over 120 years had passed since the College gave their unstinted support to recommendations advanced by the British Association for better registration in Scotland (Chap. IX). Furthermore in 1875 the College in reply to an enquiry from the Lord Advocate concerning the Registration of Still-Births left him in no doubt that their views were unchanged from those contained in their Memorial of 1858.[22]

The Committee appointed by the Council of the College in 1962, with Dr Henry Matthew as Convener and Dr J. O. Forfar as Secretary,[23] published a report in June 1962[24] which was outstanding for its incisive brevity, convincing lucidity and practical recommendations.

In the introduction attention was drawn to the tendency at times to certify with a view to satisfying the Law rather than to provide information of medical value; and the failure of many doctors to appreciate the crucial importance of statistics available to medical research workers and socio-medical planners being reliable. Published investigations were quoted purporting to demonstrate the inaccuracy of death certification by comparing clinical diagnosis with pathological findings.

Death Certificate

Human fallibility apart, the Committee considered that inaccuracies in the completion of death and still-birth certificates were contributed to by the form of the certificates themselves and of the instructions accompanying them. Selection by the Registrar-General of the *International Classification of Causes of Death* was considered to be unsuited to the modern pattern of disease; and the measures employed to discourage use of indefinite and undesirable terms and impose diagnostic precision were seen as involving a very real risk of distortion and falsification of the Registrar-General's statistics. Although permissible in Law, certification of the cause of death based on inspection of the body after death was condemned. Exception was taken to the confusion arising from the designations of Primary and Secondary Diseases; and to the absence of mention on the certificate of a post-mortem having been performed. Furthermore it was felt that the issue of death certificates to informants who in turn register the death may on occasions encourage modification of the certified diagnosis with the object of sparing the feelings of relatives.

Still-birth Certificate

Criticism of the still-birth certificate resembled that of the death certificate in many respects. In addition it was pointed out that the *International Classification of Causes of Still-Birth* as adopted by the Registrar-General for Scotland (1958) contained terms no longer widely accepted; and that an unquestionable need existed for information containing maternal age and parity for the purposes of medical research.

Birth Certificate
As the full birth certificate is normally issued, it was suggested that production of the shortened form could under certain circumstances 'raise the implication of illegitimacy'.

Specific Recommendations

The following were among specific recommendations made in the Report:

Death Certificate
The Death Certificate for Scotland should conform to the Medical Certificate of Cause of Death as used in England in so far as the respective legal systems of the two countries will permit. The book of certificates should contain instructions similar to those in the English book modified to give effect to the other recommendations made in the Report.

Adoption of the form of the English Death Certificate involving abandonment of the terms Primary and Secondary and adherence to the system approved by the World Health Organization viz. a *Direct* cause of death followed by *Antecedent* causes followed by *Other Significant Conditions*.

Expansion and modernisation of the 'International Classification of Causes of Death as adopted by the Registrar-General for Scotland (1958)' included in the books of death certificates, to provide a more comprehensive and appropriate classification.

Omission of the list of 'Terms which are Indefinite or Undesirable for purposes of Medical Certification' and replacement by the suggested new expanded International Classification of Causes of Death as adopted by the Registrar-General for Scotland.

A certifying doctor should have the right in exceptional circumstances to go outside the official list of causes of death and in rare instances to certify causes of death as unknown. It should be pointed out in the instructions however that diagnoses outside the official list will involve correspondence with the Registrar-General.

An indication in the new instructions regarding death certificates that 'Specific Disease' would always be understood to mean Syphilis.

Improvement of the 'Examples of Method of Using the Form of Medical Certificates of Death': e.g. a neonatal death should be included.

An indication in the Scottish Death Certificate as in the English Death Certificate whether a post-mortem examination has been or will be carried out. When it has been notified on the certificate that a post-mortem examination has been or is to be made the Registrar-General should, not earlier than one month after the date of certification, send the certifying doctor a further form requiring him to give information regarding the final post-mortem diagnosis.

Certification of death should not be made by a doctor on mere inspection of a body after death. Where the patient was not under medical attendance within a reasonable time of death and no certificate can be issued by a doctor, Procurators Fiscal in discharging their obligation for arranging for the issue of a death certificate should, in the interests of accurate certification as well as of justice, make more frequent use of post-mortem examinations. Such examinations should be carried out by those who have had a full training in pathology and have at their disposal facilities for full pathological examination.

Adoption in Scotland of the procedure employed in England whereby the certifying doctor posts the death certificate to the Registrar without transmitting it to the relatives of the deceased.

Still-birth Certificate

The Scottish Certificate of Still-birth should conform to the Certificate of Still-birth as used in England (Form 34) with the deletion on the reverse side of the 'Note to Informant' but with the attachment to the certificate of a 'Notice to Informant', similar in form and in purport to that attached to the English Death Certificate. The books of certificates should be accompanied by instructions similar to those contained in the books of English Certificates of Still-birth.

As with the Death Certificate the terms 'Primary' and 'Secondary' should be replaced by 'Direct', 'Antecedent' and 'Other Significant Conditions'. It should be made clear in respect of 'Cause of Death' (Direct Cause, Antecedent Cause or Other Significant Conditions) whether the cause was in the mother or the foetus.

A more comprehensive and up-to-date *International Classification of Causes of Still-birth* as adopted by the Registrar-General for Scotland (1958), should be provided.

The list of 'Terms which are Indefinite or Undesirable for purposes of Certification' should be omitted.

As with the English Certificate of Still-birth, 'Examples of the Method of Using the Form of Certificate of Still-birth' should be given.

The certificate should indicate whether a post-mortem examination has been or will be carried out. Where a post-mortem examination has been carried out the procedure followed should correspond to that recommended for death certificates.

Provision should be made in the Still-birth Certificate for recording maternal age and parity.

The same procedure for posting direct to the Registrar should be adopted for the Still-birth Certificate as recommended for the Death Certificate.

Birth Certificate

The abbreviated Birth Certificate should be the one normally issued, the full certificate being issued only on request.

Other General Recommendations

Measures put forward as likely to improve accuracy in certification were arrangements for medical students to be addressed at an appropriate stage in their curriculum by a member of the Registrar-General's Department, and the issue to all doctors of an explanatory leaflet which might be included in the *Prescriber's Journal* issued by the Department of Health for Scotland. Exception was taken to some of the legal phraseology embodied in the Death and Still-birth Certificates, and the emphasis attached to the mandatory basis of the certificates. It was considered that considerable benefit to research would result were the Annual Report of the Registrar-General to differentiate where possible between statistics based on post-mortem examination and those based on clinical diagnoses.

A plea was submitted for uniformity in Scotland and England in the time within which Birth Certificates, Death Certificates and Still-birth Certificates should be delivered to the Registrar. Seven days for the Death Certificate and 21 days each for the Birth Certificate and Still-birth Certificate were considered appropriate. It was pointed out that access to original records held by the Registrar-General or to tabulations not normally published by him, is only obtainable on payment of a fee and subject to the agreement of the Registrar-General. Bona fide medical investigators should, it was contended, have ready access without payment to birth, death, still-birth and marriage certificates and to the additional information given by the informant to the Registrar under the Population (Statistics) Act 1960.[25] Further it was considered that under similar conditions access to categories of disease should be facilitated.

The Report concluded with the dogmatic assertion that amendment of the *Births, Deaths and Marriages (Scotland) Acts 1854–1938* was regarded as a matter of urgent necessity.

Historically, acceptance of current English procedure in a number of respects by the College Report of 1962 is of interest. It represented a reversal of attitude to that shown in 1854 when English proposals were regarded as too complicated (Chap. IX).

In due course the form of death certification was modified by the Registrar-General following receipt of the various reports asked for by him. What precise influence the College Report had is a matter for conjecture. The fact remains however that the eventual alterations were very much along the lines recommended by the College. In particular it was required that notification of death must indicate that a post-mortem was being held when such was the case.

FETAL AND CHILD LIFE

The best gifts . . . are from those who have nothing but themselves to give.
Neil Munro

The expectant wee things, toddlin' stacher through
To meet their Dad, wi' flichterin noise an' glee.
His wee bit ingle, blinkin bonnilie,
His clean hearthstane, his thrifty wifie's smile
The lisping infant prattling on his knee
Does a' his weary kiaugh and care beguile.
Robert Burns (*Cotter's Saturday Night*)

ABORTION

Macduff was from his mother's womb
Untimely ripp'd.

William Shakespeare (*Macbeth*)

Sir, it would astonish you to know what improvements we have made of late years in all
branches of obstetrical knowledge, but particularly in that one single point of the safe and
expeditious extraction of the foetus . . .

Laurence Sterne (*Tristram Shandy*)

So farewell hope, and with hope farewell fear,
Farewell remorse: all good to me is lost:
Evil be thou my good.

John Milton (*Paradise Lost*)

Towards the end of 1965, when invited to give evidence to a B.M.A. Subcommittee
to review legislation on abortion, the College felt unable to do so as a Corporate
Body.[26]

Memorandum submitted by the College to the Committee on the Working of the Abortion
Act 1967, 1971[27]

A Committee consisting of Dr R. M. Marquis (Convener) Drs J. Smith, W. D.
Boyd and D. Baird (Secretary) was appointed by Council to consider the subject.[28]
The Committee's Memorandum welcomed the opportunity to submit comments
while at the same time recognizing that College members were less directly involved
in the working of the Act than other branches of the medical profession. After reviewing the general and local situation the following Conclusions and Recommendations
were submitted for consideration:

(i) The provision of a comprehensive family planning service and free contra-
ceptive advice within the Health Service; and the inclusion of free contraception in
services available at obstetrical centres where abortions are performed.

(ii) Modification and improvement of gynaecological facilities, including the
provision of special facilities for minor gynaecological surgery on an out-patient
basis. This recommendation took account of the fact that the Abortion Act[29] had
led to a redistribution of work within the Health Service, the redistribution being
characterised by increased gynaecological demands as distinct from an increase in
total load.

It was considered that out-patient services catering for the termination of early pregnancies should be provided within hospitals possessed of facilities for resuscitation and in-patient care to deal with complications should they arise. Strong preference was expressed for the performance of abortions within the gynaecological services rather than in Abortion Clinics.

(iii) The public and the medical profession required to have impressed upon them the urgency of early diagnosis, the need for speedy diagnostic procedures and prompt referral for gynaecological opinion.

(iv) The prevailing system of notification was described as unsatisfactory and notification confined to the statutory elements was recommended.

(v) Conscientious objection to abortion must be respected but should not be allowed to hinder the development of facilities for the early assessment of unwanted pregnancies and their efficient termination in the presence of indications.

(vi) More research on the practical implications of abortions was urged, in view of medical decisions on the termination of pregnancy having to be arrived at without full knowledge of the long-term physical and psychological effects of abortion.

In the opinion of the Memorialists differences between regions in Scotland in the interpretation by doctors of criteria for abortion were diminishing; the system of approval of private nursing homes in Scotland had been found satisfactory; and no difficulty had been encountered over the ability of staff to contract out of abortion procedure on conscientious grounds.

The Memorandum was approved by the College on 21st December 1971.[30]

ASSESSMENT

Do you know who made you?
'Nobody as I knows on', said the child . . . 'I 'spect I grow'd'.

Harriet B. Stowe (*Uncle Tom's Cabin*)

Children you are very little,
And your Bones are very brittle;
If you would grow great and stately,
You must try to walk sedately.

R. L. Stevenson

Comments submitted to the Secretary of State on the Report of the Study Group on the Assessment of Children, April 1971[31]

The Comments were submitted in response to a request from the Secretary of State for opinions on the recommendations contained in the Study Group Report, the practicability of implementing the recommendations, and the priorities to be observed in developing assessment services. The College Committee consisted of Drs A. J. Keay, J. Syme and H. J. Walton. Forceful agreement was expressed in the Comments with the Report's acceptance of the need 'for a more formal system of inter-disciplinary assessment to procure the most effective use of treatment facilities', and for 'review and re-assessment of children once they are in care'. Rightly the College emphasized the particular importance of interdisciplinary assessment of children coming before the Panel hearings. A point thought to merit 'serious criticism' was the way in which the Report considered assessment in isolation and 'not in conjunction with the provision of continuing responsibility for treatment and care'. Children in need of expert assessment and who may not be in the care of the Social Work Department should, it was recommended, be referred to the 'ordinary hospital (paediatric and psychiatric) and school psychological services'. At the same time it was stressed that inefficiency might result where large numbers of children were involved, more especially if staff undertaking assessment did not have a continuing responsibility and if facilities for implementing recommendations did not exist.

To whom are assessment teams to be responsible? The Comments posed this direct question and stated unreservedly that doctors should 'continue to see their responsibility as to the child and his parents (or substitute parents), and not primarily to the Social Work Departments'. Great importance was attached to sustained closest possible contact between Social Work Departments on the one hand and the Health Services on the other; and to effective use of Health Visitors, with their intimate knowledge of, and experience in, the support of problem families. Social Work Departments were seen as being well placed to assist in educational measures by facilitating the attendance of doctors at assessment centres, and the interchange between doctors and social workers at both graduate and undergraduate levels.

A plea was submitted by the College Committee for the avoidance of standardization in the development of homes for residential care. As to children in care, attention was drawn to the need for the essential safeguard of review and re-assessment being implemented in such a way that it does not interfere with the ordinary provisions of specialist care from hospitals and school psychological services. It was considered that substitute parents should not be denied direct access to these services.

In general the College Committee considered the Study Group's recommendations to be an ideal solution incapable of immediate total realization; and agreed with the concept of Pilot Assessment Projects as a first step in development.

Approval to the Committee's Comments, subject to the inclusion of reference to psychiatrists, was given by College on 13th April 1971.[32]

ADOPTION

And he who gives a child a home
Builds palaces in Kingdom come.

John Masefield

Report of a Council Committee of the College on a Working Paper containing Provisional Proposals of the Departmental Committee on the Adoption of Children, February 1971[33]

The Committee appointed by Council consisted of the Vice-President, Dr J. G. M. Hamilton (Convener) and Drs J. O. Forfar, M. D. W. Low and A. J. Keay.

The Committee was in general agreement with the greater part of the Report and made particular reference to its agreement:

(a) that the welfare of the child should be the paramount consideration in adoption proceedings;
(b) with the concept of financial aid for adoptive parents of children with medical problems which cause extra expense, and
(c) that the appointment of a guardian *ad litem* should be left to the discretion of the court.

A number of other essentially constructive observations of major significance were made by the College Committee. Thus:

(a) While agreeing that registration of Adoption Agencies should be central and according to agreed national standards, it was recommended that renewal of registration should be the responsibility of local authorities and, in Scotland, in collaboration with and with the advice of, the Social Service Group, Scotland. In the opinion of the Committee, Social Services legislation and practice were more advanced in Scotland than in England and Wales, and "the best features in the Scottish scene should be incorporated in the agreed national standards." The appointment of a National Consultative Group or Panel to advise on the standard of resources to be required for registration of Adoption Agencies was recommended for consideration. Such a Panel would continue to advise on policy, and an independent Medical Group, it was suggested, could advise on medical aspects of adoption and the medical resources available to agencies.

(b) Adoptive parents in the case of a defective or handicapped child offered for adoption should have the opportunity of discussing the implications with a consulting paediatrician or other expert. Of no less importance, it was recommended that all significant medical information essential for the child's future welfare be conveyed to the family doctor of the adoptive parents—and that necessary regulations directed to this end should be made.

(c) Allowing that a mother shortly after childbirth is often not in a position to give a final irrevocable decision with regard to adoption of her infant, the view was expressed that 'where there has been good agency work with the mother before delivery . . . an early decision by the mother can be appropriate and thus allow of early placement'.

(d) The College was emphatic about not being satisfied that under the present law and in agency practice, the importance of the medical aspects of adoption (including mental health) was sufficiently recognised.

(e) Ascertainment of certain medical facts in regard to applicants should not be the responsibility of the guardian *ad litem*, and such medical evidence should be obtained from a medical source.

(f) When a comprehensive medical report is to be submitted to a Court, the Court should be advised by suitably qualified and experienced medical practitioners.

(g) Desirably all medical forms used in adoption medical practice should be made statutory.

In conclusion the College recommended that the National Health Service should ensure that accommodation and other facilities for medical adoption examinations are available. Such provision was not, it was stated, always made.

The Report was approved on 23rd February 1971.[34]

THE AGED

> *Grow old along with me!*
> *The best is yet to be,*
> *The last of life, for which the*
> *   first was made.*
>
> Robert Browning

> *There is more danger of the individual rusting out, than wearing out.*
> Sir Humphrey D. Rolleston

The Care of the Elderly in Scotland
Report by a Committee of the College, 1963[35]

The time was in Scotland's history when old age and poverty were virtually synonymous. This still applies in part but not in general. Aspects which do persist are the physical, mental and emotional handicaps to which the elderly are liable and to which loneliness contributes so much. Viewed in this light, the College Report of 1963 took its rightful place in a long line of historical pronouncements by the College, going back to the occasion in 1840 when the College asked that the Poor Law Commissioners should extend their activities to Scotland. Indeed it can be maintained with justification that interest of the College in the aged commenced with the establishment of their Dispensary in 1682. The situation and the problems have changed, but the fundamental humanitarian approach has remained.

The Committee, of which the Convener was Dr Christopher Clayson and the Secretary Dr James Williamson, was appointed by the President (Sir) J. D. S. Cameron, on 7th November 1961, 'to consider the arrangements for the care of the elderly in Scotland and to make recommendations'.[36] Their Report was, and indeed is, of outstanding importance and vividly illustrates the intense interest in community aspects of medicine which has been a feature of the activities of the College from the time of the original Charter. The Report was noteworthy also for its comprehensiveness in terms of both depth and breadth, its judicious criticisms and far-seeing recommendations, and for its clarity of exposition. Where it occurred, repetition was deliberate and for a purpose. Without being in any way emotional the Report conveyed a sense of immediate urgency about problems which if not dealt with could result in a social catastrophe. Furthermore it is to be noted that initiative came entirely from within the College itself. This Report was not a response to enquiries from central departments.

For their purpose the Committee adopted the definition that the elderly comprised men and women of 65 years of age and over; and it interpreted the challenge in the terms of reference, as the need to assess the size of the existing problem, to give detailed consideration to existing facilities and their inadequacies, and to state what in its view would be a suitable geriatric service in Scotland. The Committee's approach was based on a critical analysis of already available information, and information obtainable without undue delay from a variety of sources including Local Authorities and Regional Hospital Boards.

Objectives
Early in their Report the Committee defined the aims of their proposals for the care of the elderly as:

> '(a) to sustain them in independence, comfort and contentment in their own homes, and when independence begins to wane, to support them by all necessary means for as long as possible;

(b) to offer alternative residential accommodation to those who by reason of age, infirmity, lack of a proper home, or other circumstances are in need of care and attention; and

(c) to provide hospital accommodation for those who by reason of physical or mental ill health are in need of skilled medical or nursing attention or both.'[35]

Before detailing the aims of geriatric care, the Report pointed out that subject to possible modifications resulting from changes in the birth rate, the proportion of elderly persons in the population will probably continue to increase to an approximate figure of 13 per cent by 1980; the increase will be even more pronounced in women than in men, and single and widowed elderly women will present special problems; and that the proportion of old people living alone is probably 20 per cent of the total number of aged. As the number of old people in the population was expected to rise by 30·5 per cent from 545,000 in 1961 to 711,000 in 1981, the Committee believed that frailty and sickness in the elderly 'will be an increasing challenge to both our preventive and therapeutic services'.

Against this background the Report proceeded to consideration of the contribution to care of the elderly by the general practitioner, local authorities, the hospital service, voluntary bodies and the National Assistance Board. Mention was made of the particular problem of terminal care, and by way of conclusion the Report gave a succinct summary of conclusions and recommendations.

The General Practitioner

Tribute was paid to the amount of work undertaken for the elderly by general practitioners whose difficulties were fully appreciated. These difficulties were considered to be aggravated by the total inadequacy in the case of the elderly relying on 'the self-reporting of illness which appears to be reasonably satisfactory in younger age groups'. Allowing that there was no simple remedy for the problem the Committee gave as one possible important line of action, the reduction in size of 'the maximum permitted list for general practitioners without loss of income'. Other suggestions were that practitioners should have the assistance of health visitors with the object of favouring earlier detection of disabilities in old people; and that the appropriate authorities should be encouraged to offer general practitioners part-time posts in geriatric long-term, assessment and rehabilitation units. These were seen as measures which would incidentally enable practitioners to appreciate modern methods which they could apply to elderly patients in their own practices.

Local Authorities

Reference was made in more than one section of the Report to difficulties in the way of establishing the best care of the old arising from division of function. These were encountered in the statutory allocation of responsibilities to Regional Hospital Boards and Local Authorities in the National Health Service; and the historically explained policy adopted by local authorities of separating health and welfare functions. In these and similar potentially conflicting situations the importance of integration could not, in the opinion of the Committee, be over-emphasized 'since the needs of old persons change frequently and rapidly'. Comments on local authority services took into account replies received from 50 out of the 55 Scottish local authorities to a detailed schedule of enquiry. Replies were not received from Glasgow, Aberdeen, Clydebank and the counties of Ross and Cromarty and Dunbarton.

Housing
The scope of special provisions for old people was found to vary widely but most local authorities provided special housing in small apartment houses within general housing schemes thus retaining the elderly within the general community. Referring to the hostel accommodation provided by some authorities the Report expressed a desire for 'much more imaginative attempts . . . by providing more houses and hostels with shared facilities (dining, laundry, entertainment rooms, central heating etc.) and in particular with resident wardens'. The recommendation aimed at enabling more old people to remain in the general community.

Institutional Care
Provisions under this heading came in for severe criticism. Centrally recommended policy was (under Part III of the 1947 *National Assistance Act*)[37] to concentrate welfare homes provision 'on the frail'. Information given to the Committee indicated that in two cities, 82 per cent and 72 per cent of welfare beds were in former poor law accommodation. In large Burghs the average was 69 per cent and in County Council areas 41·2 per cent. Care in these circumstances clearly pointed to the fundamental need for increased staff, structural alterations and lifts. Recurring national financial crises had resulted in the perpetuation of wholly unsatisfactory conditions. Promises made by Governments since July 1948 to discard old poor law institutions and to reduce the size of homes to less than 50 beds had not been implemented. In the opinion of the Committee 'every effort and priority should be given to providing

more purpose-built accommodation'. 'Frail Ambulant Homes' as developed by a few authorities were regarded as having a temporary expedient value only. The following quotation from the Report provides a cogent summary of the Committee's reactions:

> 'We . . . feel bound to report that the provision of welfare accommodation for the frail is seriously below the required level and that many local authorities seemed to have failed to comply with this part of the recommendations contained in S.H.M. 58/51. It is for such frail old persons that the dividing line between the spheres of hospital and local authorities is most ill-defined, and it seems to us that in some areas old people in this "frail ambulant" category are apt to be consigned to a sort of "no man's land".'

Voluntary homes were described as fulfilling a great service to the community but surprisingly, in general, high voluntary bed ratios were not a feature of areas with low welfare bed ratios. It was in the opinion of the Committee essential for local authorities to undertake energetic programmes to replace the old unsuitable homes and to provide new places for the increasing numbers of old people. Estimates, it was maintained, should be prepared forthwith and ultimate implementation of plans should be achieved within ten years.

Hostels for the mentally disturbed old person as required under the *Mental Health (Scotland) Act, 1960*[38] constituted another unsatisfactory aspect of institutional provisions which should be corrected in the opinion of the Committee. It was presumed that such persons were being looked after unsatisfactorily at home or wrongly occupying welfare or hospital beds.

Consultative Health Centres

Basing their views on the success which had attended consultative health centres for old people pioneered by two Local Authorities, the Committee recommended that more of these clinics should be established by Local Authorities in consultation with Regional Hospital Boards and Executive Councils as a method of preventing disability in old people. These centres were seen as foci favouring team work, bridging the gap between local authority and hospital doctors, and facilitating effective continued charge of patients by the general practitioner originally referring them.

Domiciliary Care

Considerable attention was given in the Report to the contribution of health visitors and district nurses to care of the elderly. This was seen as constituting a problem of clamant urgency. It was ascertained that three, and only three, of the 50 authorities who replied to the College questionnaire employed health visitors on whole-time geriatric work; and the impression gained was that in general the proportion of health visitors' time devoted to old people was surprisingly low. In Edinburgh a survey had shown that whereas 38 per cent of old people would have benefited from health visitor services, only $2\frac{1}{2}$ per cent received them. In contra-distinction to health visitors, most district nurses were found to be spending the greater part of their time in caring for the elderly. Unhesitatingly the Report declared that district nurses were certainly not devoting too large a proportion of their time on old people and that 'the health visitor spends far too little of her time on this section of the community'. Two observations came in for selected comment. Secondment of health visitors to general practitioners was favoured, and at the same time as accepting the possible importance of geographical factors, it was recommended that extended trial should be given to combining the duties of health visitors and district nurses.

Among doctors and patients who have had opportunities to study the work of health visitors and district nurses from a variety of viewpoints there are undoubtedly many who would heartily approve of these recommendations of the Committee. Quest for administrative tidiness or even economy should not deprive elderly people in their own homes of the vital benefits to them which prompted these particular suggestions of the Committee.

Tribute was paid in the Report to the established importance in hospital practice of social workers, who should, it was urged, be employed in services concerned with the maintenance of old people in the general community. All grades of social workers as defined in the *Younghusband Report*[39] were considered to be needed, together with programmes of training for 'middle grade' workers to meet a known discrepancy between supply and demand. The possibility of employing welfare assistants to assist health visitors and trained social workers, and of the employment of enrolled nurses to assist the district nurse in the domiciliary care of old people was raised.

The Committee had no doubts about the fundamental importance of home helps but were alive to the difficulties in the way of organizing an ideal service. Immediate consideration was urged for the development of a special corps of home helps for the elderly. Available information showed that in all areas a high proportion of home helps' time is devoted to the care of the elderly, the trend being most in evidence in rural districts. Exception was taken to certain restrictions imposed on the use of home helps. The restrictions in question were disallowing home help assistance if a daughter was living in the area; the imposition of a fixed time limit; and the absence of provision for weekend help.

Still considering domiciliary care, the Report focussed attention on the maintenance of sound nutrition, adequate arrangements for chiropody, the fundamental necessity for comprehensive provisions for physiotherapy, and the desirability of assistance in doing laundry. With regard to nutrition the value of mobile meals services and of dining and lunch clubs was stressed. Day centres were suggested as another means of providing comparable services. Greater importance was attached to the real need among the whole population than to an increase in the number of meals provided to those already in receipt; and an assurance was sought that services catered for by the school meals service would maintain standards during school holidays. The number of old people in need of chiropody was said to be considerably in excess of the number known to family doctors. Physiotherapy under close supervision by the family doctor was described as essential for the preservation of independence or partial independence. The Committee was satisfied that confusion existed as to which authority was responsible for providing domiciliary therapy, and that immediate elimination of this confusion was fundamental to the establishment of an adequate service. Expansion of arrangements to enable old people or their relatives to have occasional holidays was considered necessary.

A scheme of registration of old people was recommended in the Report, which maintained that only a complete register would be successful. Two possible mechanisms were put forward—one dependent upon the Ministry of Pensions notifying medical officers of health when people reached pensionable age; and the other relying on the extraction of the list of names from the indices of the Executive Councils. The Committee did not share the view that registration and subsequent visitation by local authority officers would be resented by many old people as an intrusion on their privacy. Together with registration, arrangements whereby old people could summon help were described as needing careful thought.

Administration

Finally on the subject of local authority contributions to the care of the aged the Committee expressed agreement with the recommendations of the *Guillebaud Committee*[40]; considered that there should be one head of the local health and welfare service, and that an assessment of priorities for admission to institutional care was essentially a medical matter; and recommended that the health and welfare services under a local authority should be amalgamated under the medical officer of health. The Committee were convinced that health visitors and district nurses were in inadequate supply, and that research studies were required.

The Hospital Service

The Number and Siting of Geriatric Beds

Satisfied that the need for hospital beds would continue to increase, the Committee estimated that by 1975 approximately 11,000 beds would be required. Approximately 20 per cent of the recommended accommodation for old people administered by hospital boards should, it was advised, be allocated to assessment and rehabilitation, and 80 per cent to long-stay units, which 'would in general be smaller than 100 beds except in large urban communities where economy may be served by having larger units'.

In the opinion of the Committee all the Scottish Universities should request the Scottish Home and Health Department to provide geriatric assessment units in teaching hospitals. Were the request granted, they foresaw enhanced opportunities for instruction of medical and nursing students and medical postgraduates; more readily available geriatric advice for medical colleagues; and more expeditious transfer of geriatric patients from general and special wards.

The College Report was prepared before publication of the findings of the Committee appointed by the Secretary of State to review the medical staffing structure of hospitals. It considered that two consultants with supporting staff would be required for a population of 200,000, and that an increase in the senior registrar establishment was urgently needed. Suggestions were advanced concerning the training of geriatric physicians and the teaching of geriatrics.

Out-patient Facilities

The Report freely allowed that there were strong arguments in favour of geriatric out-patient clinics. It considered that these clinics favour unhurried attention, permit of preliminary medico-social assessment additional to clinical diagnosis, facilitate early decision as to the desirability of domiciliary, welfare home or hospital care and permit of priorities for admission being determined. Further a geriatric out-patient clinic was considered well suited for follow-up requirements. Surprise was expressed at the scarcity of developments along these lines.

As to day-hospitals, the Committee, almost ecstatically, declared their value to be enormous, but found that they were little utilized. In these units, it was pointed out, general care can be carried out; self-respect and morale boosted; physiotherapy, occupational therapy and chiropody administered; and suitable meals provided.

The Mentally Sick Old Person

Difficulties confronted the Committee when considering this aspect of their remit. The incidence of mental disorders in old age was, and indeed is, unknown. While some of these old people were admitted to hospital, others found their way to geriatric units, nursing homes, voluntary old people's homes and welfare institutions. A further complication was the conflicting advice given to the Committee by experts on the subject.

In the circumstances and having regard to the resources which existed, the Report recommended as a general line of approach to the admission of elderly patients to hospital, that:

(a) in straightforward physical illness the patient should go to the assessment unit of a geriatric department,
(b) in straightforward mental illness the patient should go to a mental hospital,
(c) where any doubt exists the patient should be admitted to a geriatric assessment unit in the first instance, and
(d) at all stages, and despite separation of their units by physical distance, the geriatric consultant and the psychiatrist must have a close and continuing association so that a patient's misplacement in a wrong hospital can be speedily corrected.

Liaison

Improved co-operation between general practitioners, local authorities and the hospital service was stated by the Committee to be essential if geriatric care was to attain desired standards. Possibilities suggested were giving the Medical Officer of Health an honorary appointment with the Regional Hospital Board; increasing employment of general practitioners appointed for the purpose of taking part in the care of old people in welfare homes and hospital; and more extended trial of reciprocal medical appointments between local and hospital authorities.

The Report paid tribute to the outstanding contribution of voluntary organizations and urged that more local authorities should take advantage of their powers under the *National Assistance Act*[37] to give financial assistance to Old Peoples' Welfare Committees. Great importance was attached to regular visiting of the elderly by voluntary workers, and retirement counselling and education for leisure were named as subjects needing greater attention.

The Financial Circumstances of the Elderly

The Committee commented on 'the fine work' done by officers of the National Assistance Board. Despite this, however, a number of old people who qualified for assistance did not obtain it, either from lack of knowledge or mistaken pride. A flat increase of retirement pensions with regular reviews and related to the cost of living was recommended in the Report as the most effective way of meeting the problem of undeclared need. Strong exception was taken to the levying of prescription charges if only because at times they discouraged the elderly from seeking necessary medical advice, and because many old age pensioners did not exercise their right to reclaim from the National Assistance Board. Another 'strong recommendation' of the Committee was that wider use should be made of National Assistance Board powers to meet part of the charges for old people in approved private lodgings. Arrangements for the use of suitable selected private lodgings were described as often desirable in the interests of the old person and the general economy.

The College is entitled to modest satisfaction in the fact that as long ago as 1852 it memorialized the Treasury, or more precisely the Lords of the Treasury, on the inadequacy of what they termed medical grants under poor relief (Chap. IX).

Throughout, the outlook of the Report of 1963 was influenced by:

1. The urgency of the situation, and
2. the fact that the real need is considerably in excess of the actual demand for care.

The Report was approved by the College in July 1963.[41]

The Care of the Elderly in Scotland: A Follow-Up Report, 1970[42]

As the title indicated, this was a follow-up Report consisting of records of the proceedings of a Conference organized by the College and held in the Queen Street Hall in October 1969. Progress since the issue of the previous Report was reviewed and reappraisal of future needs considered by a number of experts. The Conference took the form of three sessions at each of which there were three major contributors followed by general discussion. Speakers were representative of the interests of general practitioners, nurses, consultants, academics, local authorities, hospital and central government departments. They included members of University Departments of Geriatrics, Social Medicine and Mental Health.

At the opening session of the Conference the first paper was given by Dr James Williamson who had acted as Secretary to the Committee producing the Report of 1963. He took as his title that of the 1963 Report and gave his personal impressions of progress achieved and lacking in the interval between 1962 and 1969. For the purposes of his comparison Dr Williamson had obtained the assistance of the same hospital boards and local authorities who had provided information for the earlier official Report of the College. Even allowing that seven years was a short period for much to be accomplished, Williamson's findings gave no reason for waxing wildly enthusiastic. Certainly considerable progress had been made in providing hospital and welfare beds but the progress was unevenly distributed and pockets of great need persisted. Perhaps most disconcerting, remembering the emphasis attached to retention of the elderly in their own homes, was that 'provision of community support in the form of domiciliary services' showed little change. In the matter of 'specialist' health visitors so strongly urged by the College, Edinburgh employed one, Aberdeen two and Glasgow 33 'engaged solely in visiting old people'. In country areas where the problems of old age were as acute and as varied as in the cities, four out of a total of 360 health visitors had 'specialist' duties with the elderly. Findings with regard to medical staffing were paradoxical to say the least in the light of views previously expressed by the College. Williamson found that 'medical staffing in the geriatric service has increased greatly' but that 'the greatest effort has gone into expanding in-patient care, while out-patient and day-patient facilities have expanded relatively little'. Virtually no significant progress had taken place in developing consultative health centres; and the College recommendation that more general practitioners should be employed in assessment and rehabilitation units had met with little response. A review of transport facilities was given as necessary to popularize out-patient and day-patient services which were in less favour in Scotland than south of the border. In housing of the elderly, counties had the best if moderate record of advance—'otherwise changes are meagre'.

Almost inevitably Dr Williamson gave vent to the plaintive cry heard so often, in so many places, and in so many circumstances—'although there is much talk of integration of the health services, the administrative pattern remains the same as 21 years ago'. Some facets of the administrative pattern might with justification be said to have their origins in the sixteen hundreds! Understandably Dr Williamson saw a break in the clouds with the recent institution of a Chair of Geriatric Medicine by the University of Glasgow.

The next paper on demographic and social aspects was given by Professor S. L. Morrison. He referred to the continuing increase in the proportion of old people in the Scottish population, and the inevitable effect on what he termed 'the economic load on the bread winners'. This he followed with a warning to which all with specialist interests in any scientific discipline the country over might with advantage give serious attention. 'If planning is to be realistic, expectations about the scale of increased resources . . . must be kept within reasonable bounds. However, there is ample scope for the better use of present resources.' As one form of possible adjustment he instanced 'some reallocation of services from the young to the old' and in his concluding remarks argued that 'the cultural lag exemplified by their [local authorities and the Health Service] concentration on child health and welfare must be corrected'. Without in any way belittling the urgency of the needs of the aged, a policy developed along such lines would be in danger of ignoring the immeasurable preventive value of services organized for child life and health—a preventive value analogous to that so ardently advocated as essential to geriatric services. Furthermore the attitude recommended would seem to ignore how much preventive domiciliary geriatric and paediatric care have in common. Such is the considered reaction of a paediatric septuagenarian.

'Planning for the Elderly' was the subject of the next paper by Miss G. Sumner who gave as the fundamental requisite for planning, 'better information concerning needs'. She argued it was essential to arrive at an estimate of total needs to ensure perspective; arrive at rational decisions concerning priorities; determine the right remedies; and make reasonable attempts at forecasting future needs.

Outlining the psychiatrists' viewpoint, Professor W. M. Millar allowed that the number of elderly persons requiring psychiatric treatment or care was not known, and quoted evidence suggesting that a large overlap existed between patients in mental hospitals and geriatric wards in regard to both mental and physical illness. He referred to the difficulties experienced in mental hospitals related to overcrowding, the unsuitability and age of many hospitals, and the staff shortage, all with an important bearing on the crucial problem of morale. Although an urgent case existed for new and reconstructed buildings and the recruitment of appropriate staff, Professor Millar suggested that 'our limited resources might best be directed away from the institutions and into appropriate facilities in the community'. His concluding comment was to the effect that the main bulk of comprehensive psychiatric care and treatment could be transferred to the community services.

Dr A. G. Donald made a contribution as refreshing as it was realistic. It was based on his experience of a general practice consisting of 10,000 patients attended by five partners with the supporting services of one full-time and one part-time health visitor, one full-time State Registered Nurse and one full-time State Enrolled Nurse.

He gave evidence in support of his view that the elderly know how to, and do 'initiate for themselves medical attention'. In prevailing circumstances Dr Donald saw the factor of time as a major impediment to the general practitioner improving his service for the elderly. Doctors in his practice had seen 75 per cent of elderly patients living alone during the previous three months, and 60 per cent of those not living alone during the same period. He extolled the value of the nurse and health visitor in the performance of their key rôles, and regarded their attachment on a full-time basis as of fundamental importance. Added benefit would he thought result from attachment of a social worker. Dr Donald was entirely in favour of the general practitioner treating his own elderly patients in the hospital environment but stressed that for this to be a practicable proposition in terms of available time, administrative adjustments would have to be made by the central authorities. He credited the home help service with having 'revolutionised the maintenance of the elderly in their homes' and with probably being the most vital single provision; and in paying tribute to the voluntary services, singled out for special mention Lamb's House, a pioneer Day Centre attended by no less than 2000 elderly persons. Praise was forthcoming for the Geriatric Consultative Service which provided among other features assessment of an elderly person at home within twenty-four hours of receipt of a telephone call.

The nurses' point of view was presented in a notably practical way by Miss M. A. Brayton, a Regional Nursing Officer with considerable paediatric experience. After reviewing prevailing problems Miss Brayton made certain suggestions for furtherance of the aims of the College Report (1963). These included measures to encourage the return to service of retired married nurses; extension of the home help service to cover weekends; the employment of a nurse in the locality to assist in 'supervised housing'; recognition of the fact that in so far as equipment was concerned 'what is standard for acute medical and surgical wards is not necessarily right for a geriatric ward'; and eventual insistence on a nurse having had previous experience of the care of the elderly in home or hospital.

The Medical Officer of Health for Edinburgh (Dr J. L. Gilloran) outlined steps taken by his Authority in catering for the needs of the elderly, at the same time explaining such administrative difficulties as those arising from development of warden-type housing units encroaching upon the overall housing allocation, and the question of prior demands on the services of a limited number of health visitors. There was, he suggested, a case for greater deployment of social workers to deal with the problems of the elderly, and he stated that lack of home helps in the necessary number had rendered impossible extension of the service provided to include domestic work as recommended by the College. Because the need of many elderly people is a 'willing pair of hands . . . rather than social work', Dr Gilloran suggested that 'fit older people themselves' might be employed as home helps, with adequate remuneration and without their pensions being affected.

Putting the Regional Board point of view Dr C. Bainbridge (a Senior Administrative Medical Officer) declared that in the interests of future planning, geriatricians should 'be honest and truthful in their returns of how many beds are really used for assessment purposes and how many for long-term cases'. He was pessimistic about the prospects of 'many more new units . . . in the near future'; questioned the College recommendations concerning the size of long-stay units but supported those advocating the inclusion of a geriatric assessment unit in teaching hospitals; and drew attention to the drain on the overall supply of trained nurses which would result were the College recommendation to employ more health visitors translated into action. In an indirect way Dr Bainbridge was discouraging rather than encouraging about day-hospitals. In his summary dealing with central administration, a Deputy Chief Medical Officer of the Scottish Home and Health Department expressed appreciation of the initiative shewn by the College. The general views he expressed concerning aims in future development of the care of the elderly were not at variance with those of previous speakers, and it was encouraging that support was given by him for greater attention to be devoted in academic spheres to the problems of old age in medical education and research.

The two Reports on Care of the Aged were successful in stimulating Regional Hospital Boards to review their geriatric services. Some improvement in amenities and in the number of beds available followed in due course. Of equal importance was an increased awareness of the need for the closest co-operation between Hospital Boards and Local Authorities. There was a simultaneous recognition of a need for new consultant appointments, and a wider acceptance as a top priority of sheltered housing for the elderly in Scotland. Both College Reports received widespread notice throughout the British Isles, and abroad.

MONOPOLIES

The Monopolies Commission
Report of a Subcommittee of the College Council, 1971[43]

The Monopolies Commission presented their Report to Parliament in October 1970. It was entitled *A Report on the general effect on the public interest of certain restrictive practices so far as they prevail in relation to the supply of professional services.*[44] Comments from the College were invited by the Secretary of State, the Department of Trade and Industry and by the General Medical Council. Previously a Statement had been submitted to the Commission following receipt of a questionnaire dealing with functions of the College, the Fellowship and the Membership, the control of fees charged by Fellows and Members, and discipline as exercised by the College.

A Subcommittee of the Council appointed to consider the Commission's Report stressed the importance of a Report being produced by the General Medical Council embodying the views of all the medical professional bodies concerned. Attention was drawn also to the fact that although a letter to the President of the College (Dr Halliday Croom) from the Secretary of State for Trade and Industry adopted the attitude that 'Transactions for the Supply of Professional Services are business transactions', the Report of the Commission referred to characteristics of the professions which belied the Secretary of State's dogmatic assertion.

Restrictions on Entry

Other comments by the College Committee were confined to seven 'practices' specified by the Commission. The prevention of unregistered practitioners from practising in the National Health Service, signing death certificates and prescribing dangerous drugs was described as 'entirely in the public interest'. Insistence on a recognized training course and on passing a series of carefully controlled tests in order to be registered was described in like fashion.

The College expressed the view that it was 'entirely reasonable' that there should be a minimum age limit in medicine and agreed that the sex of applicants was irrelevant. However, referring to the findings of the Royal Commission on Medical Education that wastage of women qualifying in medicine is much larger than that of men, the College considered that the informal limitation whereby the percentage of women students was in the neighbourhood of 20 to 25 per cent was reasonable. At the same time the hope was expressed that in the future women would be encouraged to combine full-time duties with their domestic and other commitments. As to the particular question of nationality the College pointed out that in accordance with academic tradition this did not involve restricted entry, but that a general feeling prevailed that medical students from developing countries should receive their professional education in their own countries. In practice a limit was imposed on undergraduate students from abroad but few medical schools restricted the number of postgraduate students. It was submitted that the required evidence for registration of employment in the form of a pre-registration house appointment served as a reasonable criterion of competence. With regard to election to a Membership or Fellowship after a suitable professional examination, the procedure was described as a reasonable safeguard of the public interest and safety. The fact that the Royal Colleges include among their functions the maintenance of specialist standards was considered to reinforce the contention.

Discussing other possible restrictive practices, the College did not consider that points raised concerning fees were relevant to the medical profession; and gave it as their opinion that 'as far as the medical profession is concerned there appears to be no reason why a doctor should not engage in some other profession such as accountancy, or indeed in some commercial enterprise unrelated to medicine'. They did agree however that it would be inappropriate for a doctor in clinical practice to engage in the business of pharmacy or, while in clinical practice, to be engaged in the pharmaceutical industry. Considering isolated districts in particular, the Memorandum considered it was in the interests of the service that practitioners might dispense medicines and that visiting ophthalmologists might engage in practice in the premises of the local optician. The same view was expressed about the collaboration taking place in group practices with physiotherapists and chiropodists.

Advertising

The College expressed complete agreement with the view that freedom to advertise would involve readier resort by patients to incompetent service, and opposed more widespread publicity in the various public media. It was pointed out that in the event of specialist registration being introduced, lists of specialists in the various disciplines would probably be made available to the public.

The Memorandum concluded by noting the Commission's recommendations that particular professions should be referred by the Department of Employment and Productivity to the Commission for examination. Comment was made on the obscurity of the Commission's Report in so far as the medical profession was concerned, and readiness expressed to provide any further enquiring body with evidence.

ALCOHOL

Fifteen men on the dead man's chest—
Yo-ho-ho and a bottle of rum!
Drink and the devil had done for the rest—
Yo-ho-ho and a bottle of rum!

R. L. Stevenson

Evidence to the Standing Medical Advisory Subcommittee on Alcoholism, 1963

The Committee appointed by the College in 1959 to report on drug addiction (q.v.) did not include alcohol in their studies. They considered that addiction to alcohol required to be studied from a number of angles. One approach was dealt with in the Report below. There can be no gainsaying that the scale of consumption of alcohol in Scotland has always been and continues to constitute a national problem. Whatever the position at the present time, the doctor was not immune from the dangers in the nineteenth century. Describing his experiences as a general practitioner in East Lothian, Samuel Smiles told of kindness among farmers always willing to entertain him with a 'glass of whisky toddy' while he was attending their households. 'This', said Smiles, 'is one of the perils of the profession.'[45]

There was no hesitancy in the attitude of the College to the problem of the habitual drunkard in 1890 (Chap. XXI). They were fully alive to both the social and medical challenges involved. In 1963 the College was approached for its views and these were given in the form of Evidence by the Council submitted to the *Standing Medical Advisory Committee Subcommittee on Alcoholism*. Records of the evidence appear in the College Guard Book.

The Council considered that arrangements for the treatment of alcoholics were inadequate if lacking a specialist medical team or unit, or supervisory facilities for in-patients in other than mental hospitals. No exception was taken to the emergency treatment of acute complications in the acute medical wards of general hospitals, but strong exception was taken to any policy involving the stigma of admission to a mental hospital for subsequent convalescent treatment. Specialized units under the overall charge of a consultant physician assisted by a consultant staff and junior medical staff were described as necessary. In their evidence Council considered these specialized units should cater for emergency cases, in-patients and out-patients, and persons referred by family doctors, and should assist in dealing with the inadequacy of existing after-care and rehabilitation services. Other improvements recommended were group meetings, day hospital facilities and sheltered workshop employment but without segregation of alcoholics as a class.

A special plea was submitted for greater liaison among organizations interested in the protective care of alcoholics in Edinburgh, and for better appreciation of the temptations inseparable from certain specified types of employment. It was considered there was no evidence of 'an increase in the direct physical complications of alcoholism' but that alcoholism was contributed to by physical disease. With calculated insistence the evidence concluded that effective care of alcoholics 'must include, in addition to adequate medical facilities, the enlisting of full co-operation by employers, labour exchange managers, social welfare workers and even, at times, by the courts'.[46]

Scottish Licensing Law

Report by the College to the Committee on Scottish Licensing Law, 1971[47]

In April 1971, at the instigation of the Secretary of State for Scotland a Departmental Committee on Scottish Licensing Law was appointed with Dr Christopher Clayson, a past President of our College, as Chairman. Following a request from the Departmental Committee for the views of the College and for answers to listed specific questions, Council appointed a Committee with Dr H. J. Walton as Convener and Dr A. T. Proudfoot as Secretary.

Unsuccessful in a search of the world medical literature for clear evidence of the effects of changes in licensing laws on health, the Committee aimed at providing what they termed background medical information. They found that available historical evidence pointed to a reduction in gross public drinking following the introduction of licensing measures in Britain. Licensing controls were seen as intended in part to protect public health in that, while allowing citizens to drink, they controlled the availability of drink to those who misuse it. Figures were given showing that among premises licensed to sell intoxicating liquor the number of registered clubs, licensed restaurants and residential premises was proportionately small in Scotland as compared with England and Wales, and Northern Ireland. The Committee regarded the relationship between 'drunkenness statistics' and 'alcoholism prevalence' as undetermined, despite an increase in the incidence of drunkenness offences being generally accepted as an indication of an increase in the prevalence of alcoholism.

Provided they are interpreted with reserve, the number of drunken driving offences was however accepted as an indication of the incidence of abnormal drinking, and the Report accepted that available evidence supported the view that alcoholic legislation had influenced the occurrence of road traffic accidents. A study of data based on the screening for alcohol of patients admitted to a Regional Poisoning Centre gave scientific confirmation of the high proportion of suicides in which alcohol is involved, but did not establish any relationship between ingestion of alcohol and consumption during licensing hours. No figures were available on the proportion of divorces granted for cruelty prior to the *Divorce Reform Act (1969)*,[48] in which drunkenness was mentioned as a cause.

The Committee referred to the position with regard to all admissions to mental hospitals on account of alcoholism. Admission rates were stated to have risen yearly since 1960, a similar steep rise having characterized also first admissions, 'the Scottish rate being seven times higher for men and five times higher for women than the England and Wales rates'. Even when cautiously interpreted the trends in drunkenness and cirrhosis death rates were accepted as providing supporting evidence for the view that alcoholism had been increasing between 1950 and 1970. A categorical statement was included to the effect that young people were becoming addicted to alcohol in increasing numbers and that alcoholism was presenting at an increasingly early age.

The Committee in their Report drew special attention to two persisting complications. Many doctors, it was maintained, recognized only the 'loss-of-control' type of alcoholism and were liable to be ignorant of the type described as 'inveterate' drinker. As to the incidence of alcoholism in relation to social class, the liability of information and figures being misleading was mentioned; and one possible explanation advanced was that the more socially advantaged patients sought treatment more readily, but some on the other hand descended to levels associated with the socially and economically least fortunate. A Report of the Department of Customs was quoted showing that expenditure on alcohol by manual workers, the professional classes and administrative classes represented 4.9, 3.3 and 3.3 per cent respectively of total household spending.

As to education, it was pointed out that the need to keep the public informed would acquire even greater importance were drinking provisions made more liberal. The question was raised as to whether as a measure for the protection of youth, advice on the subject should be included in school education programmes.

The summarized conclusions of the Committee favoured continuation of some external control, and opposed on health grounds extensive relaxation of the licensing laws. Increasing the number of licensed restaurants in Scotland and the social and recreational facilities in public houses were suggested as possible ways to dispel the conception of 'drinking shops'. Finally, the Committee advocated 'strongly' that the consequences of any change in the licensing laws should be carefully studied. There should, it was urged, be monitoring of offences against those associated with drinking; injuries to self and associates; the pattern of admission to hospital for diseases associated with alcohol; and the pattern of admission for acute intoxication. To this end a case was presented for the creation of a research unit in Scotland; and for the collection of data before as well as after any alteration in the licensing laws. In this way it was maintained a rational basis could be established for future changes.

Report of the Departmental Committee on Scottish Licensing Law (Clayson Report)[49]

The Clayson Report was published in **August 1973**. It is at present receiving the consideration of the Scottish Office. Suffice it to say at this stage, the recommendations contained in the Report were in a number of respects liberalizing while at the same time intended to discourage the less attractive aspects of Scottish drinking. Retention of 18 years as the minimum age for public drinking was strongly advocated.

SMOKING

> *A branch of the sin of drunkenness, which is the root of all sins.*
> James VI of Scotland (James I of England) in *A Counterblast to Tobacco*

With increasing frequency of recent years there has been recurrent mention in symposia arranged by the College of the dangers inherent in the smoking habit. References to the subject in College Minutes are few and far between. The first reference of significance appeared in 1959 following receipt of a letter from the City Medical Officer of Health who was promoting an anti-smoking campaign. 'Canny' is the only description applicable to the College attitude at that time! A representative who it was agreed might be sent was under specific instructions as to what he should say if approached by the Press. He was to state that 'the College was sympathetic to any campaign designed to promote better health or to prevent disease in the community, but that the College was not in a position to support without reservation a specific anti-smoking campaign on the premises of which there was still some divergence of medical opinion'.[50] Such modern equivocation must surely have caused James VI to writhe in his grave!

Colloquium held at the College: 20th January 1972[51]
With time, caution if not cast to the winds, certainly became less evident. The College became a corporate member of ASH (Action on Smoking and Health Ltd.) and subsequently decided to hold a Colloquium which was attended by representatives of many branches of hospital staffs. As a prime objective the Colloquium aimed at recommending a uniform hospital policy on smoking.

Participants included nurses, physicians, surgeons, hospital secretaries, members of

Hospital Boards, a Medical Officer of Health, the Director of the Scottish Health Education Unit and members of the Scottish Home and Health Department. Discussion was wide ranging and separate sub-groups discussed the problem from the standpoint of (*a*) patients, relatives and visitors, (*b*) hospital staff, (*c*) availability of cigarettes in hospitals, and (*d*) health education.

After considerable debate it was recommended that:

1. Non-smoking areas should include medical and related specialities, surgical, obstetric and gynaecological wards, out-patient departments, laboratories, areas where patients undergo treatment or investigations, lecture rooms, libraries, canteens and staff dining rooms.

2. Smoking areas might include certain wards where a ban would be inhuman, e.g. some geriatric and psychiatric wards, and in those wards looking after terminal and long-stay patients: but should be limited to certain restricted areas and to certain times.

3. Subject to future reconsideration cigarettes should be available though not on display at hospital shops and on trolleys.

4. Hospital profits from cigarette sales should be returned to an appropriate anti-smoking campaign fund.

5. Hospital staff should not smoke in front of patients and teaching staff should be encouraged not to smoke in the presence of students.

6. Hospital smoking policy and the underlying reasons should be already set out for staff, patients and visitors on notice boards and in booklets.

7. The hazards of cigarette smoking should be dealt with in lectures on preventive medicine in training courses for future hospital staff.

8. Each Hospital Board of Management should establish a working party comprising all types of staff to assess the hospital's position as far as smoking is concerned and to continue to review this in the light of new developments.

One devotee of the briar noted with disguised relief the absence in the meantime of reference to pipe smoking. In the words of Kipling, will the eventual decree be—'. . . knock out your pipes an' follow me.'?![52]

After careful preparation a Report of the Colloquium proceedings was forwarded to the Scottish Home and Health Department, Scottish Regional Hospital Boards and the various Boards of Management within the South East Region, Scotland.

REFERENCES

DISABLEMENT

(1) R.C.P.E. (1954) *Committee of inquiry into questions affecting disabled persons. Evidence submitted by the Royal College of Physicians of Edinburgh.* (Typescript.)

(2) College Minutes, 21.vii.1953.

(3) INTERDEPARTMENTAL COMMITTEE ON SOCIAL INSURANCE AND ALLIED SERVICES (1942) *Report* by Sir William Beveridge. London: H.M.S.O.

(4) INTERDEPARTMENTAL COMMITTEE ON THE REHABILITATION AND RESETTLEMENT OF DISABLED PERSONS (1943) *Report.* (Chairman: G. Tomlinson.) London: H.M.S.O.

(5) 7 and 8 George 6, c. 10 (1944).

(6) DEPARTMENT OF HEALTH FOR SCOTLAND (1943) *Health and Industrial Efficiency: Scottish experiments in social medicine.* London: H.M.S.O.

(7) FERGUSON, T. & MACPHAIL, A. N. (1953) A Scottish study of persons registered as disabled under the Disabled Persons (Employment) Act, 1944. *Glasgow Medical Journal,* **34,** 343–53.

(8) MEDICAL RESEARCH COUNCIL (1952) *Employment Problems of Disabled Youth in Glasgow,* by T. Ferguson, A. N. MacPhail and M. I. McVean. (M.R.C. memorandum, no. 28.) London: H.M.S.O.

(9) 9 and 10 George 6, c. 81 (1946).

(10) 10 and 11 George 6, c. 27 (1947).

(11) R.C.P.E. [1954] *Memorandum on the submission of evidence . . . to the Departmental Committee of the Ministry of National Insurance . . . to review the present provisions of the Industrial Diseases Act.* (Typescript.)

(12) College Minutes, 3.xi.1953.

REHABILITATION

(13) R.C.P.E. *Scottish Health Services Council report on medical rehabilitation: the pattern of the future. Comments of a College committee. October 1972.* (Typescript.)

(14) SCOTTISH HEALTH SERVICES COUNCIL. Standing medical advisory committee (1972) *Medical Rehabilitation: the pattern for the future: report of a subcommittee.* Edinburgh: H.M.S.O.

DRUG ADDICTION

(15) R.C.P.E. (1959) *Report of Committee on Drug Addiction Appointed by Council.* Edinburgh: Royal College of Physicians.

(16) College Minutes, 3.ii.1959.

(17) CENTRAL HEALTH SERVICES COUNCIL (1958) *Joint Sub-committee On the Control of Dangerous Drugs and Poisons in Hospital. Report.* London: H.M.S.O.

(18) MINISTRY OF HEALTH (1926) *Departmental Committee on Morphine and Heroin Addiction; report.* London: H.M.S.O.

(19) 4 and 5 Eliz. 2, c. 34 (1956).

(20) 4 and 5 Eliz. 2, c. 25 (1956).

(21) College Minutes, 5.v.1959.

NATIONAL STATISTICS

(22) Council Minutes, 10.ii.1875.

(23) Ibid., 23.i.1962.

(24) R.C.P.E. (1962) *Report of Committee . . . on the Registration of Births, Deaths and Marriages* (Scotland) *Acts 1854–1938 for submission to the Registrar-General for Scotland.* (Typescript.)

(25) 8 and 9 Eliz. 2, c. 32 (1960).

FETAL AND CHILD LIFE

(26) Council Minutes, 29.xii.1965.

(27) R.C.P.E. [1971] *Memorandum for submission to the Committee on the working of the Abortion Act.* (Typescript.)

(28) Council Minutes, 14.ix.1971.

(29) Eliz. 2, c. 87 (1967).

(30) Council Minutes, 21.xii.1971.

(31) R.C.P.E. [1971] *Comments on Report of the Study Group on the assessment of children.* (Typescript.)

(32) Council Minutes, 13.iv.1971.

(33) R.C.P.E. [1971] *Report of Council Committee . . . on the Working Papers containing the provisional proposals of the Departmental Committee on the 'Adoption of children'.* (Typescript.)

(34) Council Minutes, 23.ii.1971.

THE AGED

(35) R.C.P.E. (1963) *The Care of the Elderly in Scotland.* Edinburgh: Royal College of Physicians. (Publication no. 22.)

(36) College Minutes, 7.xi.1961.

(37) 11 and 12 George 6, c. 29 (1947).

(38) 8 and 9 Eliz. 2, c. 61 (1960).

(39) MINISTRY OF HEALTH AND DEPARTMENT OF HEALTH FOR SCOTLAND (1959) *Working Party on Social Workers in the Local Authority Health and Welfare Service. Report.* (Chairman: Eileen L. Younghusband.) London: H.M.S.O.

(40) MINISTRY OF HEALTH AND SCOTTISH OFFICE (1956) *Report of the Committee of Enquiry into the Cost of the National Health Service.* (Chairman: C. W. Guillebaud.) London: H.M.S.O.

(41) College Minutes, 16.vii.1963.

(42) R.C.P.E. (1970) *The Care of the Elderly in Scotland: a follow-up report.* Edinburgh: Royal College of Physicians. (Publication no. 37.)

MONOPOLIES

(43) R.C.P.E. (1971) *The Monopolies Commission. Report of a sub-committee of the Council.* (Typescript.)

(44) MONOPOLIES COMMISSION (1970) *Report on the General Effect on the Public Interest of Certain Restrictive Practices so far as They Prevail in Relation to the Supply of Professional Services.* London: H.M.S.O.

ALCOHOL

(45) SMILES, S. (1905) *Autobiography*, ed. by T. Mackay, p. 49. London: Murray.

(46) R.C.P.E. (1963) *Evidence submitted by the Council . . . to the standing medical advisory committee sub-committee on alcoholism.* (Typescript.)

(47) R.C.P.E. (1971) *Report . . . on Scottish licensing law to be submitted to the Committee on Scottish Licensing Law.* (Typescript.)

(48) Eliz. 2, c. 55 (1969).

(49) DEPARTMENTAL COMMITTEE ON SCOTTISH LICENSING LAW (1973) *Report* (Chairman: Dr Christopher Clayson). London: H.M.S.O.

SMOKING

(50) Council Minutes, 20.i.1959.

(51) Colloquium on smoking in hospitals, Royal College of Physicians, Edinburgh, 1972 (1972) *Smoking in hospitals. Report.* (Typescript.)

(52) KIPLING, R. Follow me 'ome. In *Rudyard Kipling's verse* [n.d.] Inclusive Edition. 1885–1918, p. 507. London: Hodder & Stoughton.

Chapter XXXII

1950 AND AFTER: COLLEGE ADVISORY REPORTS, MEDICAL EDUCATION AND REGISTRATION

I believe that emphasis on security is overdone and that we should revert to leadership with authority, but without security. I believe that as in the days of Harvey an important part of medical education should be discussion, disputation and debate.

R. V. Christie

I've been at their lectures on health an' High Jean
Gude kens that I niver was wearier!
Use your ain commonsense when ye're treatin your wean
An ye'll find there's naethin superior.

D. Rorie

The hardest conviction to get into the mind of a beginner is that the education upon which he is engaged is not a college course, not a medical course, but a life course, for which the work of a few years under teachers is but a preparation.

Sir William Osler

The College has been deeply interested in medical education from the time of its Charter as evidenced in the Chapters describing the Leyden Inheritance (Chap. XVII) and the early relations with the Town's College and Civic Authorities (Chap. XVIII). Interest was maintained in later years in the form of the Extra-mural School of Medicine (Chap. XVI), the College Laboratory (Chap. V), and sustained participation in the activities of the School of Medicine for Postgraduate Education. With the advent of the National Health Service in 1948 and the appointment in 1965 of a Royal Commission on Medical Education entirely new problems arose. These were reflected in the College Reports which follow. Close collaboration with the University of Edinburgh continued.

MEDICAL EDUCATION

Report on Teaching Facilities and Students' Amenities in Scottish Hospitals, July 1957[1]

Despite its temperate phraseology and despite its unemotional presentation there is no disguising that this Report was a cry of despair—or rather *cri de coeur*. It was produced at the instance of the President (Sir Stanley Davidson) and with the approval of the Council by ten Fellows of the College, all clinical teachers—three each in Edinburgh and Glasgow and two each in Aberdeen and Dundee. The Fellows were Drs (Sir) Stanley Davidson, A. R. Gilchrist, J. Innes, J. Craig, H. W. Fullerton, J. L. Henderson, (Sir) Ian Hill, T. Anderson, L. J. Davis and E. J. Wayne. Awareness of a growing intense concern among clinical teachers at the persistently anachronistic standards of teaching facilities and students' amenities prompted the appointment of the Committee. It was the hope of the College that the views expressed in the Report might be of value to both the Regional Hospital Boards and Universities.

The Historical Background

Teaching hospitals in Scotland were built between 50 and 100 years before the time of the Report and any reconstruction or rebuilding of them between the two world wars was minimal in amount. Subsequent to the War of 1939–46 the national economy compelled restrictions of the severest kind on expenditure incurred in modernizing old and building new hospitals. In North America, Norway, Sweden and Switzerland the late 1920s saw new hospital construction gain momentum. There the hospital facilities for care of the patient, teaching and research were of standards which showed up those of our Scottish hospitals in sad relief.

Historically, co-operation between the Universities and the great voluntary hospitals provided a basis for medical teaching from the beginning. A new feature was introduced with the passing of the *Local Government (Scotland) Act, 1929* which transferred administrative responsibility of the Poor Law hospitals in the four principal Scottish cities to the municipal authorities. In the course of time, encouraged by the co-operative attitude of these authorities, the Universities began to use the municipal hospitals for clinical teaching. Originally 'purpose-built' to meet the needs of the poor and chronic sick, the local authority hospitals were not entirely suited to teaching requirements and were seriously deficient in essentials of equipment. With increased usage of local authority facilities the position developed wherein at least one-third of all hospital beds were used for teaching.

By the time the *National Health Service (Scotland) Act* was placed on the Statute Book the majority of the erstwhile Poor Law hospitals taken over by the local authorities showed evidence of the benefits of association with teaching activities. In accordance with the terms of that Act all the teaching hospitals, those which had been voluntary and those which had been municipal, were placed under the Regional Hospital Boards. Had Teaching Hospital Boards after the English pattern been created, Regional Hospital Boards would have been deprived of large numbers of beds essential for the care of patients for whom they were legally responsible. Opinions were not unanimous as to whether the system in England was to be preferred. Suffice it to say there were not a few clinicians in the South who with good reason came to envy Scotland its wholly regional hospital administrative framework.

All these facts were outlined in the Introduction to the College Report together with a summary of the relative position of the Regional Hospital Boards and those responsible for medical education under the terms of the National Health Service Act. It was explained that the Scottish Universities had the right of nomination to Boards of Management of teaching hospitals; that, acting through the Regional Hospital Board the Secretary of State for Scotland was responsible for the provision of reasonable facilities for clinical teaching and research in hospitals; and that each Scottish Region embodying a medical school was required by statute to establish a Medical Education Committee. The purpose of the Committee was to advise the Regional Hospital Board on the administration of the hospital service in so far as it related to facilities for clinical teaching and research.

Procedure Adopted by College Committee

The College Committee collected data for clinical teaching in the main Scottish hospitals and compared data with similar data from teaching hospitals elsewhere in Great Britain, Scandinavia and North America. The facilities available for clinical research and postgraduate education were not studied. A standard *proforma* was used and in the case of the four Scottish teaching centres the returns were analyzed by local subcommittees, who distinguished between major teaching hospitals in which the students spent a considerable amount of time, and hospitals visited by students for short periods of instruction.

General Recommendations

Provision for Students

The Committee based their recommendations on an estimate that junior students should spend two hours and senior students at least three hours each morning in the main general teaching hospitals; and with advancing seniority most afternoons in special hospitals or out-patient clinics. Amenities considered essential included adequate cloakroom and lavatory accommodation for both sexes; appropriate accommodation for reading and studying including a common room and 'silent room' available day and night for both resident and non-resident students; simple meals served under aesthetic and hygienic conditions; and residential accommodation reserved for the sole use of Final Year students, with single bedrooms and a sitting room. Approximation of charges for board and lodging to those payable by students in hostels or private lodgings was considered essential.

Provision for Teaching Staff

Teaching staff was defined as including the complete range of members from Consultant to House Officer. For them it was considered each unit should have a suite of rooms consisting of a combined office-cum-consulting room; a secretary–typists' room with provision for the storing of records; and a common-room to be used for study, reading, staff meetings and tutorials to students in small numbers.

Provision for Postgraduate Students and Teaching Staff

Where separate provisions were not made, more especially where postgraduates regularly attended in large numbers, it was recommended that facilities suggested for undergraduate students (q.v.) should be correspondingly expanded.

Lecture Theatres

These were given special and detailed attention in the Report. A large theatre seating not less than 200 persons was given as an essential requisite for the medical division, and another for the surgical division of every major teaching hospital. To deal with unavoidable conflicting demands one or more subsidiary theatres with seating accommodation for 50 to 75 persons was recommended, it being understood that these theatres would be available also for the teaching of technicians, physiotherapists, radiographers etc.

Great importance was attached to the details of construction and equipment of lecture theatres. Air conditioning and lighting easily controlled by the lecturer;

projection apparatus for lantern slides of different sizes and both silent and sound films; and epidiascopes suited to illustrations, graphs and X-ray films were regarded as essential. It was further recommended that in one theatre each seat should be wired to allow for the instalment of a didactophone apparatus. Attention was drawn to the need for a waiting and dressing room adjoining the patients' entrance to a theatre; and for each clinical unit to have a small teaching room fitted out as a side-room, in which small groups of students could have demonstrated to them patients 'wheeled' directly from the ward.

Out-patient Department for Teaching Purposes

The mere mention of teaching instruction in an out-patient department conjures up visions of inflexible but fallible appointment lists, patients irate and others forgiving, anxious but helpful nursing staff, conciliatory social workers, bemused students, and the ominous ticking of the clock overhead. Doubtless some or all of the members of the College Committee had recollections of similar sessions. Certainly they went to great lengths to underline the increasing importance being attached to medical instruction given in out-patient departments. They suggested that the following facilities were necessary for an out-patient department to contribute to maximum teaching efficiency:

(a) A sufficient number of consulting rooms additional to those required for day-to-day routine demands;

(b) a number of small rooms close to the consulting rooms where students can discuss with patients or relatives in private;

(c) within the out-patient precincts technician(s) capable of carrying out side-room techniques; and a laboratory of a size where a student can undertake side-room investigations;

(d) a suitably equipped room in which various simple clinical investigations can be carried out, with students in attendance to receive instruction and assist;

(e) one or more X-ray screening rooms in the out-patient department, and

(f) a lecture theatre with undressing cubicles, rest room and suitable projection apparatus.

Out-patient departments operating 'on at least some days of the week' from 9 a.m. to 9 p.m. would, it was considered by the College, be advantageous to both patient and student.

Administrative Aspects of Medical Education

The concluding section (other than the Summary) of the College Report was of considerable significance. In essence it consisted of criticism not of the Medical

Education Committees but of their inability, in the face of frustrating circumstances outside their control, to secure implementation of their unanimously agreed recommendations for improving teaching facilities. There was no question of antagonism between Universities and Regional Hospital Boards. Frustration arose directly from inadequacy of funds and the absence of any authoritative statement as to whether the University or the Regional Hospital Board was primarily responsible for expenditure incurred in providing within hospitals, building and equipment for the teaching of medical students. As the College Report explained, 'it was not until June 1957 that the Universities were notified of the administrative arrangements agreed between the Treasury, the University Grants Committee and the Health Department for financing the facilities required for teaching and research in hospitals'.

In the opinion of those drafting the College Report the Medical Education Committees required improved status in order to become more effective. This, it was suggested, could be secured were Hospital Boards and University to give early advance notice to the Medical Education Committees about developments touching on medical education and related facilities. Furthermore it was argued that the promotion of medical education would derive overall benefit on a national basis were the Department of Health for Scotland to take the initiative, and make available to the Medical Education Committees in all regions, plans designed in any one region for hospital projects concerned with improvement of facilities for teaching and research. Initiative along these lines, it was maintained, would promote constructive criticism, favour standardization of plans and foster a close association among the Regional Hospital Boards and Universities of Scotland.

After approval by the College the Report was communicated to the Medical Press[2]; and at a later date the President (Sir Stanley Davidson) was able to report to the College that the Minister of State for Scotland had received a College Deputation at St Andrew's House where a lengthy and helpful discussion of the Report took place.[3]

Evidence submitted to the Committee appointed by the University of Edinburgh 'to examine the structure of the University and to report on the changes, if any, in constitution, organisation, or procedure desirable to ensure the proper discharge of the University's functions', 1962[4]

Council appointed an Advisory Committee consisting of Drs (Sir) Ian Hill (Convener), J. G. M. Hamilton, T. Anderson, R. H. Girdwood, E. B. French (Secretary) and J. S. Robson.

2E

The fact that Fellows of the College had taken an active part in determining the pattern of undergraduate and postgraduate teaching since clinical instruction began in the Edinburgh School inevitably resulted in the College's evidence being concerned mainly with medical teaching during the clinical years. The first point made by the College was that of those on the University Committee who might be expected to represent the interests of the Faculty of Medicine not one was a clinician or holder of a Regional Hospital Board contract. This, the College considered, called for review if only because in practice the principal Edinburgh hospitals constituted a vital part of the University structure. Further cause for concern was seen in the possible loss of a measure of freedom by the governing bodies of the Universities as dependence upon Treasury Grants underwent inevitable increase.

The University and Regional Hospital Board
In the judgment of the College the Faculty of Medicine was in a particularly vulnerable position as compared with other Faculties. One special reason was that contrary to the established framework in England, one authority (the Regional Hospital Board) was responsible for the administration of both teaching and non-teaching hospitals within its area. In effect this exposed the teaching of medicine in undue measure to the vagaries of Government policy and the inelasticity of Treasury control; and experience of the National Health Service during the fifteen years prior to evidence being submitted warranted the view that teaching and research had received less consideration than was their due. Moreover that situation had evolved despite there being specific mention in the *National Health Service (Scotland) Act* to the provision of facilities for teaching and research. In their evidence, however, the College allowed that, in general, staffing of teaching institutions had been more generous than in non-teaching hospitals, although the extent of generosity bore no direct relation to the load of patient care, teaching and investigative demands.

Should additional money for research be forthcoming under Regional Board auspices, the College considered that the University should be assured of freedom to prosecute research which might 'not seem immediately practical to the Regional Board' and for which 'access to patients and hospital laboratories' would be required by members of university staffs. It was pointed out that a situation might even arise in which the Hospital Board would be called upon to accept responsibility for applying a form of routine investigation which had originated as a research procedure. Although liaison between Board and University was already satisfactory, it was urged that it would have to be even closer and be extended to cover problems of staffing, finance and provision of research.

To assist in promoting this, three suggestions were submitted, viz:

(a) University members of Regional Hospital Boards should be empowered to report back to Faculty, and to advise the Board of items of common interest arising in Faculty;

(b) there should be regular meetings of the Standing Committee of the University and Regional Hospital Board, and

(c) the Medical Education Committees should be rendered more effective, especially as machinery for liaison in relation to teaching.

Academic Committees

Then followed a series of recommendations concerning statutory Academic Committees. The University Court should, it was suggested, include the Chairman of the Regional Hospital Board and the Dean of the Faculty of Medicine; and the representation of non-professorial members of the Faculty should be increased. Because of the growing complexity of the Deanship it was felt that consideration should be given to making the post a full-time one. As to the Faculty itself it was thought that its representation would be secured were non-professorial members elected as representatives of specified groups of interests, and there were at least two of these members on the clinical teaching staff. Furthermore the view was advanced that elected members of Faculty who raised business on behalf of their groups should be permitted to report back. Suggestions advanced to improve the influence of the Board of Studies in Medicine were that the Board, consisting of well over 300 members, should be subdivided into subcommittees representative of all the special interests; and that an Executive Committee should be formed of one member from each subcommittee.

Professorships

Reversion to the policy of having two complementary Chairs in Medicine was favoured by the College. Underlying the recommendation was the object of lightening the load of administration, and enabling the research-inclined appointee to cope with the increasing complexity of scientific medicine, while at the same time making provision for a clinical Chair of which the occupant would be concerned primarily with applying up-to-date scientific knowledge to the diagnosis and treatment of disease. Personal Chairs were approved, it being felt that there was a case for establishing a small number of 'floating Chairs' in Edinburgh. At the same time the College recognized the difficulties in the way of implementing such a policy. Financial and legal requirements made for slow progress in promoting the necessary Ordinance in Parliament, in a way contrasting unfavourably with English procedure. This fact prompted the College to assert that 'there is need to re-examine this whole question with a view to permitting more freedom to the University to manage its own affairs in its own way'.

Lectureships and Research Workers

Considerable disquiet was expressed by the College over the difficulty of correlating the number of training posts with the probable number of consultant vacancies. Co-existence of University and Regional Board gradings aggravated the situation. Anxiety arose from the fact that an excess of training posts might result from the existence of University lecturers with honorary Regional Board attachments; and from the fact that preferential advance of those holding University trainee posts might develop in virtue of the additional advantageous opportunities for research associated with the University posts.

The College Report was not hesitant in its recommendations. In the light of prevailing requirements it considered that the autonomy of the University in 'the creation of or in appointments' to these posts should cease. Instead of the University making an appointment and then asking the Board to grant honorary clinical status to the appointee, the College urged that appointments and grading should be discussed and agreed by the University and Hospital Board before advertisement. It was further recommended that the appointing Committees should be subject to the statutory rules governing appointments under the National Health Service.

Clinical Teaching

Logically the Report proceeded from consideration of the position of individuals to that of their functions as clinical teachers. In a sense a plea was made for the more wholehearted admission of the part-time consultant into 'the body of the Kirk'. At the same time as endorsing the policy of whole-time professorial appointments, the College drew attention to the continuing need for part-time clinical teachers who, it was urged, should have numerically improved representation on the Faculty of Medicine. 'These Consultants appointed to the teaching hospitals by Regional Boards', the Report continued, 'enjoy autonomy in their clinical responsibility. We believe that they must continue to enjoy a similar autonomy in their clinical teaching.' In how many places and how often have similar views been heard expressed with less responsibility and less dignity!

Because of the disparity between the number of students and the number of clinical teachers in some units, the suggestion was advanced that 'for teaching purposes only' junior staff might be seconded from the more generously staffed units. Reading between the lines, the implication is that University units would undertake the secondment and by doing so facilitate the instruction of students in small groups. The impact of the increasing specialization and growing complexity of modern medicine on the type and extent of clinical material available for teaching were considered. Allowing that solution of the problem called for compromise, the College gave it as its opinion that 'suitable special units should be incorporated whenever possible within larger general units', but that the number of specialized beds should constitute no more than a relatively small, fixed proportion of the total number of beds in the unit.

Among general topics dealt with in the Report were the desirability of all teachers having access to courses of instruction on modern developments in teaching methods and expertise; and the unquestionable necessity for students, postgraduates and staff to have reasonable and readily available library facilities.

Postgraduate Education

Most of the points dealt with in the Report had a bearing on postgraduate as well as undergraduate education and understandably the former did not receive lengthy consideration. Details, given elsewhere (Chap. XXII), were mentioned concerning the scope of instruction organized by the Post-Graduate Board, the influence of the College through Fellows in their capacity as clinical teachers, and the standard of knowledge and achievement insisted upon for election to the Membership. About one quarter of the total number of postgraduate students in any one year were said to attempt the examination of the College, many of whom returned to teaching posts in their own countries. At the time the Report was submitted to the University Committee the conditions under which many postgraduates worked and lived were described as deplorable. This the College considered more than sufficient reason for the position being righted whereby the University should receive the financial support accorded to institutions in other parts of Britain. The large contribution made by Edinburgh to postgraduate training in medicine fully warranted the view. The Report of the College of Physicians to the University Committee concluded: 'We feel that pressure should be brought to bear on the University Grants Committee to distribute their funds for postgraduate education more equitably'.

The Report met with the unanimous approval of the College when presented at an Extraordinary Meeting, and was the subject of special congratulations from Sir Stanley Davidson, (Sir) Derrick Dunlop and Dr Rae Gilchrist. Forty-two Fellows were present.[5]

Memorandum of Evidence on Medical Education: Submitted to the Royal Commission on Medical Education, July 1966[6]

The Report was prepared by a College Committee nominated by the President (Sir Ian Hill) with Dr Rae Gilchrist as Convener, and took into account the views of those Fellows of the College in the United Kingdom who had made written submissions in response to an invitation from the Committee.

At the same time as briefly reviewing the cumulative success of the Edinburgh Medical School in undergraduate education the introductory section of the Report underlined the debt of Scottish medicine to Dutch influence. It declared that at Leyden the 'atmosphere was vital and the spirit adventurous', an influence even greater than that exerted by the courses in the basic sciences and the teaching organized there. Reviewing the development of postgraduate education in Edinburgh, the Report foresaw a considerable expansion in the functions of the Post-Graduate Board for Medicine with as one outcome increasing participation in the provision of educational facilities in the spheres of both hospital and general practice within the National Health Service. While in Edinburgh there was co-operation between the two Royal Colleges and the University, it was pointed out that in Glasgow there was fruitful collaboration between the Royal College and the University; postgraduate instruction was given in both Dundee and Aberdeen; and that each school had its own particular pattern of postgraduate education. The introduction of the Report drew attention to the independence of the Royal Colleges in terms of financial status and opinion on medical affairs, and to the part played by their nominated members on the Joint Consultants Committee responsible for, among other conditions, those relating to undergraduate and postgraduate teaching. It was maintained that the Royal Colleges were ideally equipped to maintain their rôle in the development of medical education in Scotland and might well serve as 'the focal point of co-ordinated activity among the Scottish Universities, the National Health Service and the Colleges themselves'.[7]

The introduction was followed by separate sections dealing with undergraduate education, postgraduate education and medical manpower. That on undergraduate education dealt firstly with the intense competition for places in medical schools, and an increasing tendency towards specialization commencing at school with the growing emphasis attached to science and allied subjects. Some anxiety was expressed at the lessening importance being attached to a more liberal school curriculum prior to entry to a medical school; and consideration was given to the not inconsiderable risk of an immature choice of career being contributed to by direct entry into the second year medical course of pupils suitably qualified in science subjects. To meet the situation the College were of the opinion that pupils with adequate scientific qualities should continue to enter directly into the second year, while those who have devoted more time to the humanities at school should be given increased opportunities to pursue the necessary scientific subjects at the University. Means were advised whereby schools and school teachers could be made better acquainted with the requirements for preparation and entry into a medical school. Boldly in an age of pedagogic and pupil militancy the Report almost went so far as to teach the teacher. To facilitate assimilation into university life, it was argued, pupils 'in their final year at school (if not before)' should acquire the art of learning for themselves and 'Schoolroom teaching should be punctuated extensively with "free periods" designed to stimulate the pupils' independence of thought and learning'.[8] As a member of the teaching profession remarked, only the deference due to 300 years protected the College from ripostes concerning grandmother and the sucking of eggs!

Selection of Applicants

Selection procedures for places in a university were recognized as constituting a thorny problem. Academic achievement was given as the most reliable criterion for the recognition of future successful examinees but as having no proven value in detecting applicants who will be the best doctors in all fields or any one particular field. Urgency was attached by the Report to the need for prospective studies to consider ways and means for discriminating between the potentially able examinee and the potentially good doctor.[9] Surprisingly to some readers at least, personal interviews were credited with minimal value which, if justified, would seem to imply an element of deficiency on the part of medical staff and others involved.

Undergraduate Training

Passing from the school to University, the College Report did not spare criticism of the undergraduate curriculum which it maintained suffered from lack of departmental and interdepartmental adaptability to outside influences, and from being conditioned by the fact that at one time 50 per cent of medical graduates were destined for general practice. In the opinion of the College 'the purpose of undergraduate medical education is to provide the student with some understanding of the normal structure and function of the human body and of the way it is disturbed by disease and modified by therapy'; and the enlightened teacher no less than the apprehensive student would wholeheartedly agree that successful undergraduate instruction does not require 'burdening the mind with the vast body of detailed knowledge which is needed in the practice of any branch of medicine'. Undergraduate education, it was urged, must attain its objectives by sustaining curiosity, encouraging active participation in studies, increasing powers of observation, and developing the capacity to obtain and assess evidence and to make judgments. Expressed another way, the student should 'be taught less and educated more'.[10]

In the opinion of the College, the conditions necessary to attain these objectives did not exist. To remedy the situation the College recommended reduction of the curriculum to a period of five years for ordinary students and six years for honours (B.Sc.) students.[11] Of the five years it was considered that three should be allotted to preclinical studies and two only to clinical work. With shortening of the undergraduate clinical curriculum it was envisaged that attention should be focussed on an integrated approach to the patient on a physical and psychological level; and that coincidentally the instruction in the surgical subspecialties and kindred subjects should be limited to general considerations and an elementary introduction to diagnostic methods.[12] Fundamentally the recommendations implied modification of the undergraduate training by reduced emphasis on vocational content and transfer of a considerable amount of that content to postgraduate instruction.

Clinical Material and Clinical Instruction

Discussing the effect of increasing specialization on the character of clinical material available for undergraduate teaching, the Report considered that the tendency was less evident in Scottish than in London teaching hospitals. Nevertheless the Report accepted that the evolution of special units within teaching hospitals was both necessary and desirable, and that the interests of undergraduate teaching would be safeguarded were there greater collaboration between teaching and other hospitals, and were more extensive use made of district hospitals and out-patient departments.[13] Attention was drawn to the fact that contrary to the position in England and Wales, Regional Hospital Boards in Scotland had by the *National Health Service (Scotland) Act* a statutory responsibility for medical education. The committee framework was responsibly criticized as having functioned unsatisfactorily, and recommendations were made for improvement of the situation.[14]

Principles of Examination

A short but incisive paragraph of the Report was critical of prevailing methods of examination on the grounds that they perpetuated objectionable features of the undergraduate course, including in particular the demand for excessive factual information.[15]

Postgraduate Education

Postgraduate education was considered under four headings—the Pre-registration period, the Intermediate period, Advanced Training and Continuing Education. Two consecutive years in hospital practice prior to registration were advocated by the Report, the first to be spent in junior general medicine and general surgery house officer appointments, and the second in similar further house appointments in those subjects or in a series of specialist units including obstetrics. It was felt that appointments in the first postgraduate year should if possible be 'within the region associated with the graduate's University'. Without saying so directly, the Report rather implied that circumstances might necessitate taking posts in the second year outside that region. It did not mention the advantages that can accrue from seeing methods employed in another region. However there was no concealing the College's concern that all these resident house posts, whether in a teaching or peripheral hospital should be subject to adequate consultant supervision, associated with suitable clinical work, both qualitatively and quantitatively; and provide duties dominantly practical in nature and with 'patient care in hospital as the most important component'. Great importance was attached to achieving these essential requirements and to the greatest care being exercised in the recognition of posts as suited to pre-registration graduates.[16] Throughout there was an appreciation of the need of those in training to be given a share of controlled responsibility—an appreciation closely resembling that expressed by Glasgow's Lord Rector 'Jimmy' Reid when discussing the justification for wider participation generally by students in administration.[17] No one can question the need of many house officers to be given greater responsibility and less 'paper work' under the personal supervision of their 'chiefs'.

Intermediate Training

Turning to intermediate training for registered doctors intending to enter general or hospital practice, academic or laboratory work the Report was satisfied that this could be procured as senior house officer, registrar (or University equivalent) or unpaid clinical assistant, or from organized courses of instruction. Rightly, attention was drawn to the disadvantageous position in which registrars found themselves when the centres in which they were working lacked undergraduate or postgraduate facilities. To quote—'While these doctors are of value to the Health Service, their full potential is not realised'. In the opinion of the College these and similar discreditable situations would eventually cease to arise were senior house officers and registrars linked to a Postgraduate Centre; advice to registrars on their careers routinely given by a Director of Studies at the Postgraduate Centre; and were the graduates undergoing further training assured of time, opportunity and study leave to use the facilities of Postgraduate Centres.[18]

Consideration was given to the special problem of graduates from medical schools overseas. The need for an initial period of assessment rarely in excess of one month was stressed; and attention was focussed on the need of many of these graduates for further practice and training involving continued supervision by the Director of the Postgraduate Centre until their work was of a standard acceptable for employment.[19]

Advanced Training

The Report described Advanced Training as training normally following the intermediate period after a higher qualification has been obtained. Customarily the individual held a senior registrar post or University equivalent. In the opinion of the College the practice of regarding senior registrars as supernumerary to service establishment was to be condemned, and in the later years of their appointment they should have opportunities to undertake locum consultant work. Furthermore it was maintained that secondment should be extended to include all teaching hospitals and that opportunities to work abroad should be encouraged with a guarantee of reappointment on return. Satisfaction was expressed with the administrative arrangements, dependent on geographically widely based committees, for the supervision of training in the South Eastern Region of Scotland.[20]

Finally in the matter of Advanced Training, the Report described hospital clinical conferences as playing a vital part and urged that attendance at them should have high priority in a consultant's routine, the attendance of general practitioners should be encouraged, and 'the staff of smaller hospitals should not be left in isolation'. It was recommended by the College that, with the co-operation of the hospital administration and Boards of Management, arrangements should be made for joint activities to meet the needs of the smaller hospitals and areas removed from the main teaching centres.[21]

'Research interests, committee work or other commitments are too often allowed to take precedence over teaching duties.' This was another significant pronouncement in the College Report and one which would find favour with a not inconsiderable section of older members of the profession on both sides of the border. Most certainly in more than one medical school, house officers are aware of the position and are justifiably resentful of its impact on the guidance and instruction they receive, whether in the form of precept or example. Few if any Fellows or Members of the College would disagree with another declaration in the Report, viz.:

> 'Teaching incentives are still required in the hospital service. In our opinion teaching ability should carry greater weight in determining advancement at all stages of the hospital doctor's career.'

This statement was amplified as follows:

> 'Universities, Regional Hospital Boards, Hospital Boards of Management and their Appointments Committees should be alive to their obligations to promote and encourage teaching of the highest standard in the areas under their supervision. By so doing the whole Health Service stands only to gain.'[22]

The admonition, for such it was, could at one time have been extended with justification to some of the Teaching Hospital Boards in the south.

Continuing Education for General Practitioners

Concerning general practitioners the College gave unqualified support to proposals that postgraduate training should extend over five years. Appointments in paediatrics, obstetrics or psychological medicine were described as 'particularly desirable' in the second pre-registration year. Two years as assistants in approved practices were recommended, with a possible return thereafter to a nearby hospital for clinical attachment on a part-time basis. Refresher Courses were described as already generally accepted as a regular necessity, and the employment of suitably qualified general practitioners in the hospital as meriting trial. The possible activities of general practitioners engaged in this way were envisaged as the day-to-day care of patients presenting less obscure problems.[23] Attention was drawn to the necessity for arrangements to retrain married women doctors returning to active professional work after some years of absence.[24] Funds which had been allocated by the Nuffield Provincial Hospitals Trust for the appointment of postgraduate advisers were described as having given rise to 'an organisation of immense educational significance' in furthering continuing education and as deserving every encouragement from Regional Hospital Boards and local Postgraduate Boards.[25]

Administration and Finance

The College considered that a case existed for a thorough review of existing arrangements. Arguments were advanced for the creation of the equivalent of a clearing house for postgraduate students who would be suitably distributed without interfering with the policies or activities of area postgraduate boards. In the particular case of Edinburgh, it was stated, lack of funds had limited developments necessary for advanced training designed for selected individuals attached to specialized clinical units and departments. The Report advocated the establishment in Scotland of an organization to plan and develop postgraduate education, the organization to be based on the existing Scottish Postgraduate Medical Association, with direct financial support from the University Grants Committee and the National Health Service.[26]

Medical Manpower

This was the subject of special consideration in the College Report. It is necessary to remember the year of the Report was 1966. Factors given as contributing to the shortage of medical manpower in Great Britain included the increase in population, a more exacting consumer demand, the increasing complexity of techniques employed in patient care, a growing realization of the need for expanded facilities for research and continuing education, and the emigration of doctors. Particular attention was drawn to the reduction which had taken place in the previous 15 to 20 years in the number of graduates from Scottish schools registering with the General Medical Council. The College arrived at the conclusion that an increase in the number of doctors graduating from medical schools was necessary. While unable to give an estimate of the desirable increase, they drew attention to the danger that any considerable addition to the number of places would involve a scarcity of applicants for other disciplines and a fall in the standard of students accepted for medicine. In the opinion of the College an increase in the output of doctors should be secured by expanding existing medical schools. Such a policy, it was pointed out, would obviate the need to provide the expensive pre-clinical departments necessarily required for any new medical schools. It was considered that full use of all clinical facilities in the Medical Schools of Edinburgh, Glasgow, Aberdeen and Dundee, and greater use of smaller hospitals could increase the annual output of graduates from the Scottish medical schools from 400 at the time of the Report, to 550 or 600. The newer Universities, it was suggested, might assist in providing accommodation in the basic sciences for an increase of medical students on that scale. Moreover the Report was satisfied that, were clinical resources utilized on the proposed comprehensive basis, individual teaching units would not be embarrassed by an excess of undergraduates. With circumstances as described, the College was emphatic in its view that a new medical school in Scotland was not, and would not be necessary 'in the foreseeable future'.[27]

Coupled with the problem of adequate recruitment there were those of the conservation of existing resources of medical undergraduates and the most effective deployment of doctors. Considering these the Report repeated its desire for improved methods for the selection of students; adjustments in the curriculum as a whole to permit of a longer and more functionally practical pre-registration period; and the elimination of the inefficient use of expensively trained doctors. Particular attention was focussed on the waste of skill of general practitioners entailed in dealing with 'a burden of trivialities making up a considerable portion of their day's work'. With good reason the College expressed undisguised concern about the inefficient use of junior hospital staff. They declared: 'Many housemen are overworked. Much of their time is occupied in duties devoid of educational value.' At the time under consideration these strictures were more than justified.

Reverting to the conditions of work expected of general practitioners the statement is made that many were 'no longer willing to accept the rôle in which they are cast'. By way of partial remedy of the situation, group practices of varying types were seen as offering the best prospects favouring as they might the most economical use of 'supporting workers such as nurses, social workers, secretaries and public health employees'. The recommendations which followed had as common denominator a closer association between general practice and the hospital service. Indeed the Report went so far as to urge serious consideration of a medical framework with the hospital as core, and highly organized group practices in support along the lines described by Biörck in Sweden. Then in somewhat pensive visionary mood the College said: 'We pause to wonder, therefore, if general practice as we have known it in the past has a place in the future. We envisage highly trained practitioners taking their places in medical centres attached to hospitals and in time becoming what are called today "general physicians".'[28]

That the College should commit such a statement to writing was highly significant. Without doubt much has taken and will take place along the lines foreseen by the College. Not all of even the most fervidly loyal Fellows and Members would accept what was foreseen as wholly desirable. Certain questions should be left to the readers of the Report to answer for themselves. To what extent if any may this particular paragraph of the Report have been conditioned overmuch by a purely hospital consultant approach? In a number of respects the views expressed were in line with the thoughts of some civil servants and members of the medical profession (not of our College) more administratively than clinically active. Can it be therefore that the Report attached overmuch importance to 'administrative tidiness', the bogey in so many ways of so many national organizations? Thirdly, did the conception of general practice in the future as postulated in the Report take adequate account of what the discriminating patient wants and pays for as tax-payer? Throughout the social spectrum there is much disillusionment at the erosion of the primary importance of the home in the services as they are now being provided by general practitioners and hospital in- and out-patient services. How many younger consultants have had practical experience of seeing patients in a remote shepherd's cottage, in a highland croft, or in the home of a long-distance lorry driver or mass-production worker? Personal relationship between patient and doctor is a subject dear to the heart of many patients no matter how much it has been denigrated at times on the public media. Its unquestionable diminution is regretted by many who have known it. Should the hospital outlook develop to the increasing exclusion of fundamental consideration of the patient *in his home*, paediatrics and geriatrics will be the first to suffer. Other disciplines will follow suit, and with them teaching. Finally, is any one tidy administrative paper scheme capable of catering humanely for the contrasting problems in health and disease of urban *and* rural areas? There is ample evidence all around to aid the reader to arrive at a factually based opinion.

Women Doctors

Still on the subject of effective recruitment and employment of doctors, the Report recognized that many women graduates were not fully employed, a fact largely accounted for by domestic responsibilities. Factors needing attention to encourage full-time professional activities by women doctors were given as opportunities for retraining, modification of the income-tax law relating to a wife's earnings, and greater adaptability on the part of employing authorities particularly in the matter of part-time occupation.[29]

The Medical Needs of Developing Countries

Permanent emigration of doctors from the United Kingdom could not be contemplated as an answer to the tremendous medical needs of the developing countries in the opinion of those responsible for the Report. The view was largely influenced by the manpower position at home. Agreement was expressed with the greater part of the findings of the Commonwealth Medical Conference in Edinburgh in 1965 (q.v.). Support was given to expanded postgraduate training in Great Britain for doctors from abroad; secondment of medical teachers from regional as well as teaching hospitals in this country; and schemes for special post-registration training for young British doctors undertaking to work for a period in an underdeveloped country and guaranteed an appointment on their return to Great Britain.[30]

In the concluding general discussion, family practice was regarded as a specialty in its own right, training for which requires study over a wide field. The point was made that the best teaching from the most experienced cannot be maintained continuously throughout the year despite the economic attractions of limiting long vacations now that practically all students are supported by public funds.[31] Considering the teaching duties undertaken by clinicians, the College Report, at the same time as submitting a plea for more standardization of clinical methods far short of uniformity, readily allowed that the student in 'building his own pattern' was well able to determine for himself that which he regarded as most desirable in the contrasting approaches, methods, emphasis and deportment of his teachers.[32] The unquestionable scarcity of clinicians specifically trained for teaching was underlined, and the positive recommendation made that registrars aiming at a career in the hospital service would profit from formal training in this connection. This strongly worded and realistic recommendation reflected the insistent importance attached by the Report to ascribing much greater value to teaching ability when considering the advancement of doctors in the hospital service.[33]

Quotation, albeit at some length, from the last two paragraphs serves to crystallize the general tenor of the Report. Having again emphasized the vital importance of two years of pre-registration it stressed the need for subsequent supplementary education during which

'the outlook of the young doctor should be broadened, his experience, confidence and judgement greatly enhanced. With this background his personal inclinations and aptitudes should provide him with a lead to his future career. He may then choose to train for the hospital service as a consultant, for academic medicine as an investigator and teacher, for general practice as a family doctor, or for public service as an administrator.'[34]

'It is at this point of divergence that education in depth must begin in the subject of his chosen field . . . It remains to provide every facility to promote and maintain the professional standards of the doctor, both consultant and general practitioner, throughout their subsequent careers.'[35]

Not a few administrative schemes have fallen short of their target because obsession with structure has led to disregard of human and personal considerations. By way of contrast, where in the past the development of educational programmes has been tardy, the explanation has not been lack of foresight or enthusiasm on the part of teachers, but failure of the administrators to provide the facilities. There is ample evidence to substantiate the wisdom underlying the recommendations submitted by the College.

An Extraordinary Meeting called to consider the Report was attended by 49 Fellows, with the President (Sir Ian Hill) in the Chair. Written comments had been submitted by a number of those unable to attend and extracts were read from letters from Sir Stanley Davidson, Dr D. C. M. Walker, Sir John McMichael and Dr G. M. Wilson among others. A notably serious and 'most informative discussion' followed 'in which there took part *inter alia* the Deans of the Faculties of Medicine in the Universities of St. Andrews and Edinburgh and nine other Fellows'.

The motion of approval of the Report which was eventually passed required that consideration should be given 'to the remarks and suggestions voiced during the debate when drawing up the final report to be submitted to the Royal Commission'.[36]

Response to St Andrew's House Enquiry

A sequel to the above events took place two years later following publication of the Todd Report. A letter dated 15th July 1968 from the Scottish Home and Health Department had a list of questions enclosed, answers to which were sought from the College. With wise and timely circumspection the College supplied comments, not answers, and made clear that the comments were of an interim nature. Two months previously the College had appointed a Committee to consider the *Report of the Royal Commission on Medical Education* and was already in a position to give a considered reply. The Chairman was Dr Christopher Clayson and a feature of the Committee was the absence of hitherto active, highly respected senior Fellows and the inclusion of prominent but younger Fellows certain to be deeply involved in future developments in the years ahead.

In broad terms the College comments agreed with the Commission's recommendations for postgraduate training; and made a particular point of the fact that posts for general professional training should be a College responsibility, and that subsequent approval would incorporate assessment of hospital standards, the maintenance of a register of posts, regular inspection of the hospitals and correlation of training posts with the performance of trainees. As to further professional training, the Commission's proposals for junior specialists were considered to differ little from arrangements already in existence in Scotland for senior registrars; and those for Continued Education and Training met with the College's approval, particularly in so far as increasingly active participation of Postgraduate Medical Centres was contemplated.

Attention was drawn by the College to problems with which integrated training programmes might have to contend. The purpose was not to discourage, but to give the Scottish Department of Home and Health the benefit of the experience of certain Fellows in the College. These Fellows had had experience of relatively small-scale regional schemes for the allocation of pre-registration house officer posts and the rotation of senior registrars.

In their reply the College made it clear that they did not entirely agree with the Commission's suggestions for assessment in the case of the hospital doctor. The College gave it as their opinion that a trainee's professional training having been completed, his assessment should be carried out by 'the appropriate College', and that examination for Membership of the College should constitute the principal mechanism of assessment. Progress reports during general professional training should, it was maintained, be regarded as available as a secondary mechanism of assessment in the case of doubtful candidates. Astutely the College elaborated their views by declaring that 'whilst the main assessment, namely the examination for Membership, is a matter for the Colleges alone, continuing assessment might, in view of the work involved, require the establishment of an assessment committee in which the Colleges, the Universities and the Regional Hospital Boards might have to be represented'.

When it came to the question of the interrelationship of vocational registration and postgraduate qualifications, the College with truly Edwardian grace exposed the uncertainty which had prevailed in the minds of the Commissioners when determining a doctor's readiness for vocational registration. 'We believe', continued the College commentary, 'that a national committee for specialist training and vocational registration will have to be set up consisting of representatives from the Royal Colleges, the Universities and certain specialist organisations . . . to advise the General Medical Council.' At the same time it was made emphatically clear that scrutiny of individuals' applications for registration should be the responsibility of individual Colleges and not of any national committee.

Wisely the comments continued in this increasingly assertive tone. Dealing with the Membership of the College they stressed that it was normally regarded as 'an essential pre-requisite for vocational training and vocational registration *qua physician*', but allowed that at the commencement of the proposed scheme specially experienced doctors would be entitled to registration although not in possession of a Membership Diploma.

And of the Fellowship of the College? The College wrote by way of comment— *The Fellowship of the College is an entirely different matter and is not related to vocational registration.* The terse declaration left no room for dubiety: the attitude of the College could not have been more effectively indicated.

Likewise in the matters of career structure in the hospital service and manpower problems, the College were disinclined to make comments in advance of the conclusion of consultations proceeding at the time elsewhere. Suggestions made for arrangements for overseas doctors did not differ from those previously submitted to the Royal Commission by the College[37] (q.v.).

The Scottish Royal Colleges and the Evaluation of Trainee Paediatricians, 1968[38]

If I had my time again . . . and were planning a course as physician . . . I would undoubtedly choose to be a paediatrician.

Hugh Barber

It is natural to consider this Report after that of the Edinburgh College's Report to the Royal Commission on Medical Education. Deliberately the Report on Trainee Paediatricians was delayed until the views of the Royal Commission were known in April 1968. The Report was the result of a request by the Academic Board of the British Paediatric Association to whom it was submitted by Dr James Farquhar of our College in an individual capacity, after discussion with the Presidents of the Royal Colleges of Physicians of Edinburgh and Glasgow and with the Council of the former. Discussions were especially concerned with 'the present state, and possible future pattern' of the examinations for the Memberships of the two Colleges.

At the time of the discussions both Colleges held Part I examinations and refused permission to reattempt the Part II examination in the case of persistently unsuccessful candidates. The Part II examinations were similar in so far as they consisted of papers, and clinical and oral examinations, but differed in that Paediatrics constituted one of five sections in the Glasgow papers and orals from which candidates were required to select one, whereas in the Edinburgh examination Child Health was one of 32 approved subjects of special interest available for choice by candidates. In Glasgow the clinical examination was in general medicine; in Edinburgh written, clinical and oral examinations were conducted both in general medicine and the selected subject. Available Edinburgh figures indicated that 1 in 2 or 3 passed the selected subject but that failure in General Medicine 'reduced the paediatric pass-rate to 1 in 5 or 1 in 10 or less. The final pass list almost always included candidates whose *failure* in Child Health was compensated by double the number of surplus marks in General Medicine, whereas no reverse compensation was ever allowed', and by way of contrast 'candidates in any section, other than Child Health', were 'almost immune from examination on the general medicine of infants and young children'.

Possible developments of the examination system were mentioned in the Report and for present purposes it is sufficient to point out that, while there was no questioning the fundamental necessity of retaining an effective test of general medicine within the examination, the Presidents of both Colleges favoured the view that paediatrics was 'perfectly appropriate' general medicine for the requirements of Part II. Not without good reason, the President (Dr Christopher Clayson) and Council of the College were gratified to learn that of British Paediatric Association members the proportion who were Members of the Edinburgh College had increased from 1 in 6 of those admitted to the Association before 1960 to 1 in 2 since 1960. This did not however dissuade the President and Council of the College from understanding the desire among paediatricians for major adaptation of the examination to meet paediatric needs.

It has to be appreciated that the Report was not prepared on behalf of the College, but on behalf of the British Paediatric Association by one of their Scottish representatives who was a Fellow of our College. Nevertheless, the Report served to reveal the College's attitude in the matter of paediatrics and it is for that reason that detailed reference has been made to selected sections. Furthermore, the Report virtually prefaced a major step taken by the College in 1970.

In that year at an Extraordinary Meeting in September new Regulations for the Part II Examination in Paediatrics for the Membership were unanimously approved. Under the new Regulations, candidates in paediatrics were given a choice of examination. Either they could take the examination in accordance with former Regulations and offer Child Life and Health as a selected subject, or they could take the examination in 'The Medicine of Childhood'. The last named new examination contained the same components as the examination in adult general medicine. The prescribed form of examination consisted of two written papers—one in the General Medicine of Childhood and the other in Neonatal Paediatrics. There were in addition a clinical examination on the General Medicine of Childhood and a second on Neonatal Paediatrics, followed by an oral examination covering the whole field of the Medicine of Childhood. There was only one oral examination. The new Regulations were not applicable to the Common Part II Examination for the Membership (U.K.).[39]

J. A. Froude declared that 'the first duty of a historian is to be on his guard against his own sympathies'. The warning is one to be heeded with even greater stringency by the amateur historian, who however cannot forbear on this occasion from expressing the conviction that the new Regulations represented an advance as outstanding as it was enlightened. Nor could conception have been more appropriate, occurring as it did in a medical environment which had long since discarded the discordant term Paediatrics in favour of Child Life and Health.

REGISTRATION BY THE G.M.C.

The Pre-Registration Year
Report of College Council Committee, 1972[40]

A Conference on the Pre-Registration Year was held under the auspices of the General Medical Council in 1972. The Conference was attended by Dr J. G. M. Hamilton in his capacity as College Representative on the G.M.C. Prior to his attendance the College Council considered the Report prepared by their specially appointed Committee, with Dr A. J. Keay as Convener and Dr J. Syme as Secretary.

The Committee was emphatic that the educational value of the pre-registration year suffered from the lack of continuing assessment by the medical school of the posts themselves and of the progress of occupants. While in favour of retention of the pre-registration year, it was considered that its educational value would be improved by having a better relationship to the undergraduate curriculum. With this object in view it was recommended that the final undergraduate and the pre-registration years should be restructured as a single two-year entity. This period would, it was assumed, be preceded by provisional registration, count towards general professional training, and be followed by full registration. It was recommended that a first examination primarily on theoretical knowledge should be sat on completion of the penultimate undergraduate year, and a second consisting essentially of a formal assessment of clinical ability at the end of the two years. Accepting that frequent assessment of the suitability of pre-registration posts was essential the Committee favoured external assessment.

Registration of Overseas Medical Graduates
Report of Council Committee, 1972[41]

The Council of the College appointed a Committee (with Dr J. Williamson as Convener and Dr N. C. Allan as Secretary) on being invited by the General Medical Council to comment upon an interim report by their Special Committee.

The College Committee of Council allowed that formal evidence was lacking but were agreed that, in some ways, existing arrangements were unsatisfactory especially in certain parts of England and particularly in connection with certain specialties. Selected points commented upon by the Committee were the five-fold increase of medical schools in the Indian sub-continent since 1946, instances of difficulty in patient-care arising from inadequate knowledge of the English language, and, the problems presented by highly qualified and experienced overseas doctors from medical schools in countries without reciprocal arrangements.

Suggestions advanced by the Committee were:

1. A review by the General Medical Council of arrangements with medical schools in countries covered by reciprocal agreements, and the termination of recognition of schools not subject to continuing assessment.

2. An examination to assess basic professional competence of overseas doctors from medical schools in countries not the subject of reciprocal agreements, and a test of competence in the English language to precede or be included in the examination. Success in the examination would qualify for temporary registration.

3. 'Attachment posts' should be restricted to hospital departments approved for the purpose by the G.M.C. and possessed of adequate facilities and staffing for supervision and assessment. Success in the examination (q.v.) followed by satisfactory performance during attachment would qualify for temporary registration involving, if necessary, a period in a recognised pre-registration post.

4. Review of the legislation to enable overseas graduates who have satisfactorily completed the period of temporary registration to become eligible for full registration.

5. Special facilities for full registration of highly qualified, experienced and reputable overseas doctors without examination or assessment-by-attachment. A panel of experts in each specialty might be set up by the Royal Colleges to assess individuals.

REFERENCES

(1) R.C.P.E. (1957) *Report on Teaching Facilities and Students' Amenities in Scottish Hospitals.* Edinburgh: Royal College of Physicians.

(2) College Minutes, 23.vii.1957.

(3) Ibid., 5.xi.1957.

(4) R.C.P.E. (1962) *Evidence submitted . . . to the Committee appointed by the University of Edinburgh 'to examine the structure of the University and to report on the changes, if any, in constitution, organisation, or procedure desirable to ensure the proper discharge of the University's functions'.* (Typescript.)

(5) College Minutes, 17.iv.1962.

(6) R.C.P.E. (1966) *Memorandum of Evidence on Medical Education . . . to the Royal Commission on Medical Education.* Edinburgh: Royal College of Physicians.

(7) Ibid., paras. 1–6.

(8) Ibid., paras. 8–10.

(9) Ibid., para. 12.

(10) Ibid., paras. 14–15.

(11) Ibid., para. 16.

(12) Ibid., paras. 18–19.

(13) Ibid., para. 23.

(14) Ibid., para. 25.

(15) Ibid., para. 21.

(16) Ibid., para 27.

(17) REID, J. (1972) *BBC broadcast,* 25.v.1972.

(18) R.C.P.E. (1966) *Memorandum of Evidence on Medical Education.* Para. 29. Edinburgh: Royal College of Physicians.

(19) Ibid., para. 30.

(20) Ibid., para. 31.

(21) Ibid., para. 33.

(22) Ibid., para. 35.

(23) Ibid., paras. 36–8.

(24) Ibid., para. 40.

(25) Ibid., para. 39.

(26) Ibid., para. 41.

(27) Ibid., paras. 42–4.

(28) Ibid., paras. 45–6.

(29) Ibid., para. 47.

(30) Ibid., para. 48.

(31) Ibid., paras. 51–2.

(32) Ibid., para. 55.

(33) Ibid., para. 57.

(34) Ibid., para. 59.

(35) Ibid., para. 60.

(36) College Minutes, 21.vi.1966.

(37) Council Minutes, 23.vii.1968.

(38) FARQUHAR, J. W. (1968) *The Scottish Royal Colleges and the evaluation of trainee paediatricians; a report to the Academic Board of the British Paediatric Association.* (Typescript.)

(39) College Minutes, 22.ix.1970.

(40) R.C.P.E. (1972) *The pre-registration year. Report by a Council committee.* (Typescript.)

(41) R.C.P.E. (1972) *Registration of overseas medical graduates by the General Medical Council. Report by a committee of the Council . . .* (Typescript.)

Chapter XXXIII

1950 AND AFTER: COLLEGE ADVISORY REPORTS, THE NATIONAL HEALTH SERVICE

FINANCIAL CONSIDERATIONS

Removed from kind Arbuthnot's aid,
Who knows his art, but not the trade
Preferring his regard for me
Before his credit, or his fee.

Jonathan Swift

And yet he was but esy of dispence;
He kept that he wan in pestilence.
For gold in physik is a cordial,
Therefor he loved gold in special.

Chaucer

There were few if any aspects of the National Health Service in which Fellows were not involved directly or indirectly from its commencement. Indeed many were involved in the preliminary planning. It was inevitable therefore that the advice of the College was sought from time to time by Government Departments and Hospital Authorities. As will be seen from the College Reports which follow, the subjects raised were related to problems of medical establishments in hospital, the provision of their pharmaceutical and scientific services, the organization of regional laboratory services, and the cost of the National Health Service.

In addition to the contributions of these Reports, the views of the College were made known on many other subjects by a considerable number of Fellows who were members of national, regional and hospital committees.

COMMITTEE OF ENQUIRY INTO THE COST OF THE NATIONAL HEALTH
SERVICE:
MEMORANDUM FROM THE COLLEGE, 1954[1]

The Memorandum began by expressing the view that as a social experiment the
National Health Service had already achieved a considerable measure of success. In
the main the Memorandum was concerned to discuss means whereby efficiency of
the Service might be improved in the light of experience gained during the previous
five years. The views expressed related particularly to the National Health Service in
Scotland.

Organization and Administration
Reference was made to the doubtful wisdom of the Cathcart Committee's[2] conclusion that it was essential for the general practitioner and other medical services to
be brought under one administration. As events turned out many of the difficulties
in all areas had been foreseen. The creation of liaison committees had not resulted in
the necessary degree of co-operation between the administrative bodies. Indeed the
College went so far as to say that 'the one effective co-ordinating factor has been the
central Department'. High tribute was paid to the self-effacing way in which by their
unostentatious influence officers of the central department enabled 'the Service to
work as well as it has'.

Two factors militated against success: strictly limited resources and the absence of
any regional or local body with authority to determine priorities in the overall
interests of the Service. Competition between interests developed. Perspective was
at a discount. If only because of inherited deficiencies in hospital and specialist
provision, the College considered it was probably inevitable that in the early days of
the Service a disproportionate emphasis was given to hospital requirements. Lack of
adequate safeguard against such over-emphasis was given as an important weakness in
the existing administration.

The Memorandum favoured a feasibility study intended to consider the creation of
all-purpose authorities charged with planning and administering all services which
at the time were the responsibility of Regional Hospital Boards, Local Authorities
and Executive Councils. Population and geographical considerations would condition
the areas over which the suggested overall authorities would exercise jurisdiction. It
was the opinion of the College that Scotland 'might be covered by 8–10 authorities
in place of the 5 present Regional Hospital Boards, 25 Local Executive Councils and

55 Local Authority Health Committees'. For effect to be given to any such suggestion it was realized that time and legislation would be required. The recommendation was made, however, that there need be no delay in considering rationalization in the form of pooling of administrative staff and equipment of Hospital Boards and Executive Councils.

Hospital Administration

The Memorandum unequivocally favoured the prevailing system of Regional Board or alternatively the hospital committees of the suggested all-purpose authority (q.v.). Adherence to the Scottish policy of employing administrative Medical Superintendents was unhesitatingly urged in the interests alike of efficiency and economy.

Hospital Finance

Criticism was levelled at the closely centralized system of finance and accounting making for inflexibility of the Service which by its very nature was dependent upon adaptability for efficiency, and at the encouragement given to 'over-budgeting'. Inseparable from the system was a need for the closest scrutiny and control of the budgets at all administrative levels, which contributed to cumulative frustration and a sense of deprivation of responsibility throughout the hospital service.

The College, using the proven success of university finance as an analogy, recommended that careful consideration should be given to the adoption of a block grant system. A further major point made was that the running costs of many hospitals were being inflated by inefficiency, attributable to lack of capital funds with which to rebuild, re-equip and modernize out-dated buildings neglected during periods of war.

Doubtless the Memorialists were mindful of an element of disgruntlement in the neighbourhood of Edinburgh. Hospital Endowment Funds were governed by the *National Health (Scotland) Act, 1947*.[3] In the course of time special legislation in connection with the Endowment Commission enabled Scottish hospitals to retain a portion of their endowments. Distribution of funds becoming available in this way was the responsibility of Regional Boards. The Hospital Endowments Commission with Sir Sydney Smith as Chairman submitted a Report to the Secretary of State for Scotland in 1955.[4] The impression gained ground that allocation to the Royal Infirmary (Edinburgh) was penalized by the necessary priority conferred on the modernization of other hospitals in the area in process of being upgraded.

Charges in the National Health Service

Continuation of token charges on prescriptions and the charges for spectacles and dentures were favoured as a means of discouraging frivolous and extravagant use of the Service and of encouraging a sense of ownership. At the same time as expressing a wish to see their expansion the College considered home-help services should continue to be subject to charges. The Memorandum made clear that payments should be subject to exemption or modification in the case of children, war pensioners, those in receipt of grants under the National Assistance Act, and those in receipt of old age or widows' pensions. Arrangements imposed on Hospital Management Boards concerning charges in respect of private beds were criticized as having contributed to a loss of revenue in certain specified circumstances. Hospital Boards, it was considered, should have authority to charge according to their discretion.

Drug Bill

Expenditure on drugs was, according to the Memorandum, 'seriously prejudicing many urgent developments in the National Health Service'. It was of the order of £46½ millions in 1953–4, exclusive of the cost of drugs administered to patients in hospital. The 'profound appeal' of proprietary preparations was seen as posing a serious problem. 'If', the College stated, 'there is a real desire to economise in this connection, then the way in which economies may be effected is the way of proscription rather than that of the qualified right of prescription.' A further statement in the Memorandum was to the effect that to limit prescribed drugs to official preparations in the British Pharmacopoeia, the British Pharmaceutical Codex and the National Formulary 'would not be to the detriment of a single patient'. None the less the College were well aware that they were treading difficult, as distinct from dangerous ground. Rigorous curtailment of the right to prescribe proprietary remedies was recognized as certain to have serious repercussions on the large pharmaceutical firms which had contributed so much to the advancement of therapeutics. The College did not venture further than to suggest that 'steps should at any rate be taken to supply information to the profession of comparative costs of drugs and to encourage the recent tendency among manufacturers to indicate the cost of their preparations in their advertisements'.[1]

Subsequent events have justified the College's caution. Increasing knowledge of the bioavailability of drugs no longer warrants the assumption that generically named drugs are invariably therapeutically similar to their branded equivalents. Enlarging on this, Sir Derrick Dunlop explained how absorption of an active therapeutic agent can be subject to the influences of a variety of 'compounding factors' all having a bearing on 'the therapeutic efficacy of the dosage form'. The procedure adopted in preparation and the effectiveness of successive controls are of especial significance.

A further although unrelated point to note is that, among Fellows of the College, there are some who feel that the emphasis on the cost of drugs is sometimes excessive, when considered in conjunction with hospital expenditure incurred in connection with bed-occupancy and laundry work. Even so, there remains reason to be reminded of James Gregory's warning—'None but those who are in the secret have any notion how much easier it is to *prescribe* than to *think*: and of course how much oftener the former is done than the latter . . .'.[6] Nor would Gregory have taken exception to a recent American statement that while 'formerly the pharmacist made what the physician prescribed; now the physician prescribes what the industry makes'.[7]

The Aged and Infirm

'The College believes that the care of the aged . . . needs to be tackled in a bolder and more imaginative way if the already considerable volume of distress and extravagance is to be mitigated.' Such was the opinion of the College. While not questioning the decline in standards of social responsibility they were satisfied that the major contributory factors were inadequate housing and overcrowding, the employment of women and the increasing proportion of elderly persons in the population. It was considered that an urgent need existed for an expansion of hostels and old folks' home facilities with assured services of physiotherapists and occupational therapists. Such provisions would, it was maintained, shorten the prolonged occupation of acute beds by the convalescent aged without detriment to the infirm patient. Further easement of the situation would, it was argued, follow expanded services of home nurses, domestic helps and 'meals on wheels' by enabling more elderly people to be efficiently treated at home.

In conclusion the Memorandum submitted a plea for greater financial and other encouragement of the public health and preventive medicine facets of the National Health Service. Withal the College shared the general concern about the cost of the Service but saw 'little prospect of any spectacular reduction without serious sacrifice of quality'.

REMUNERATION OF GENERAL PRACTITIONERS

A Memorandum[8] was prepared by the College in response to a letter dated 13th March 1945 from the Inter-Departmental Committee on Remuneration of Medical

Practitioners. The Memorandum dealt with Recruitment and Remuneration. With regard to recruitment to a publicly organized medical service, it was maintained that coupled with an adequate salary there should be an effective superannuation scheme; while accepting that a publicly organized service might require a measure of supervision, practitioners should retain the maximum possible freedom 'to do in his own way what he considers best for his patients'; and clerical work expected of the practitioner should be kept down to a minimum. Provision of locums was advanced as necessary to enable practitioners to have regular study leave and to enable whole-time members in the Service to take a reasonable annual holiday.

Urging a remuneration appropriate to the demands made on the profession the Memorandum listed such important considerations as the long expensive training, the grave responsibilities inseparable from the practice of medicine, the inevitably irregular hours of duty and the unavoidably high expenses incurred by practitioners. Limitation of the number of patients for whom a practitioner should be held responsible was given as a fundamental necessity in any attempt to encourage a higher standard of practice. Conditions of service and remuneration should, it was stated, be the same for both men and women, and the possibility of an additional annual payment in respect of approved registrable higher qualifications was raised.

Rather more than ten years later the subject of Remuneration again came up for consideration after a Meeting between representatives of the General Medical Services Committee and the Joint Consultants Committee. Discussion took place at a Quarterly Meeting of the College in February 1956, a Report of the joint meeting of the two Committees having been previously circulated. The Chairman of the Joint Consultants Committee had asked for the views of the College. There was fairly general agreement among Fellows that, after making full allowance for the position of junior members of the profession and taking into account the restriction of wages urged by the Government, the time was inappropriate for seeking increased remuneration. Some few of those present doubted the justification for an increase regardless of other considerations. Eventually it was resolved:

> '. . . no claim for a general increase in medical remuneration based upon "the betterment factor" should be made at the present time, but . . . if and when an appropriate time should arrive . . . the method of joint action . . . is acceptable'.[9]

The 'joint action' envisaged was a joint claim on behalf of general practitioners and hospital medical staff.

ROYAL COMMISSION ON REMUNERATION OF DOCTORS & DENTISTS:
MEMORANDUM OF EVIDENCE SUBMITTED BY THE COLLEGE. OCTOBER
1957[10]

In effect the Memorandum constituted the College's response to a request on the part
of the Royal Commission for the views of the College on twenty-one defined topics.
The College Committee felt competent to provide information on fifteen of the
topics raised. Before dealing with these topics, the Memorandum opened with three
brief Sections—Introductory, The Present Situation and The Future. Two significant
sentences appeared early in the Introductory section. Firstly—'Remuneration must
not be the main preoccupation of the medical graduate or of the bodies that represent
him, but the doctor should not have to worry constantly about financial difficulties'.
The principle involved was in reality applicable to any breadwinner. Not so the
second statement, one pregnant with significant forewarning—'He [the doctor] must
remain an individual with a personal relationship to the patient rather than become a
civil servant'.

Accepting that an understandable decline in the standard of living of doctors had
accompanied the development of the Welfare State, the Memorandum declared that
recruitment to the profession of persons of the right type would suffer serious handicap were remuneration not commensurate with the long training, intellectual
talents and service to the community expected. A reminder was inserted of the Spens
Committees' recommendations that the standard of living enjoyed by the Profession
in 1939 should be maintained. The College Committee was of the opinion that
implementation of the Spens recommendations[11, 12] was dependent on the 'most
vigorous steps to reduce taxation and counter inflation', in the absence of which the
Profession would have no option but to seek 'just and practicable' increases in
remuneration.

Discussing the general situation prevailing at the time the Memorandum was
produced, several important points were made. One was to the effect that uncertainties about professional prospects and economic standing in the community fostered
reluctance among parents, including those with medical qualifications, to encourage
their children to embark on a medical career. At the same time it was allowed that not
all parents shared this pessimism. In so far as grants to medical undergraduates were
concerned, the justice of assessing need and determining amount on the basis of the
gross income of the parent was questioned. In support of their contention the
Memorialists instanced how a doctor might be unable to educate his children at a

university whilst 'his working-class patient' might be 'able to obtain the means to do so'. Among newly qualified medical graduates the house officer was described as having 'little cause for complaint about . . . his security'. Today, not everyone would subscribe to the view expressed that 'there can be no doubt, even in his own mind, that he [the house officer] is a trainee', or that he is always alive to being financially better off than his counterparts were in the days before the National Health Service. On the other hand the Memorandum appreciated the apprehensions of hospital officers derived from the experience of able senior registrars who had been unable to obtain consultant posts.

Prospects for an aspirant to general practice were not described as wholly encouraging. The main problem in general practice was given as 'how to become a principal'. Attention was drawn to the notably small number of assistantships in Scotland in relation to the annual number of Scottish graduates as strongly suggestive of the considerable extent to which Scottish graduates sought employment 'in other spheres or even in other countries'. Factual evidence was given to show that success in becoming established as a principal in general practice carried no assurance of an adequate income.

Genuinely sympathetic understanding was shewn for the position in which registrars were liable to find themselves. In pre-National Health Service days a registrar who failed to achieve consultant status was able to enter general practice in which his experience and contact with hospitals stood him in good stead. As the Memorandum pointed out, with the greater rigidity which followed the transition of 1948, progress along normal channels was 'difficult enough', but 'to change direction in midstream' was 'even less easy'. The argument was advanced that the standard of work in the National Health Service would benefit were it made easier for registrars to work part-time in general practice while attached to a hospital. To deal with the position of the 'time expired' senior registrar undertaking consultant duties while awaiting a retiral or death vacancy, the suggestion was made that the post of senior registrar should be made a permanent one, re-designated Senior Assistant Physician/Surgeon and recognized as a normal stepping-stone to consultant status.

As to consultants, the College Committee stated that there was 'ample evidence to show that many consultants are acutely anxious about the present situation and about the future'.

The section of the Memorandum dealing with 'The Future' was notable for its emphatic expression of opinion. Unhesitatingly it maintained that it was 'essential that the machinery for adjusting remuneration and terms of service should be drastically overhauled' if smooth and equitable resolution of controversies between the profession and the State was to be achieved in the future. A small permanent Committee had been previously recommended by the Priestley Commission to keep the salaries of senior civil servants under review.[13] In the opinion of the College a similar neutral body would 'serve the interests of the medical profession, the Government and the public'.

As to the specific questions put by the Royal Commission and the answers given to them in the College Memorandum—no purpose would be served by giving these in detail. In the course of replying however the College placed on record a number of other important impressions of which condensed mention is essential.

The Committee responsible for the Memorandum considered a possibility existed that Medicine as a career was declining in popularity but, basing their opinions on impressions only, did not think that there had been any recognizable decline in the quality of applicants for medical training or of newly qualified doctors. Emigration was not regarded as an important reason for wastage in the early years after qualification. None the less, coming from so influential a body as the College, it would be unwise to ignore their view in 1957 that: 'We fear a deterioration in the quality of those seeking a career in the medical profession . . . The factors are many and complex, but they include:

1. Competition from Science and Business . . .
2. The politically involved state of Medicine . . . and consequent uncertainty about the future.'

Incidental mention was made of an insufficient desire among well-trained men to enter in the first instance the specialties of Radiology, Dermatology and Psychiatry; and, of greater importance, concern was expressed about the growing schism between hospital doctors and family practitioners. Exception was taken to the practice of giving newly appointed part-time consultants such a small number of sessions that their income was quite inadequate, particularly in areas where private work was negligible. In diplomatic terms, the practice was tentatively traced to London and 'possibly other medical centres' where it was believed physicians with large consultant practices established prior to the inception of the National Health Service, were not desirous of more than three or four weekly sessions.

Another point coming in for severe stricture by the College Committee was the diversity of procedures adopted by those dealing with income-tax allowances—a diversity which discriminated particularly severely against whole-time medical members of the National Health Service and of University staffs with similar clinical responsibilities. Approval was given to the merit award system as a valuable incentive.

With the development of the Nuffield and other provident schemes it was envisaged that a certain demand would continue for private consultant advice. That being so, it was pointed out that with the closure of nursing-homes mainly due to domestic staff difficulties, there was a need for the provision of private beds in hospitals. Although there was adequate provision in this respect in many regions, there were no fee-paying *medical* beds in hospitals in the South-Eastern Region of Scotland. There were however amenity beds in the Simpson Memorial Maternity Pavilion, and a few private beds in the Infirmary neurosurgical unit of which Mr Norman Dott was in charge.[14]

Agreement by the College to co-operate with the Royal Commission was first given in May 1957 when a Committee was appointed with the President (Sir Stanley Davidson) as Chairman, Dr J. K. Slater as Convener, and Dr R. H. Girdwood as Secretary. Other members were Drs W. I. Card, J. Halliday Croom, A. Rae Gilchrist, I. W. B. Grant and J. H. Wright.[15] The Committee reported back six months later, and it is of interest that a Fellow in general practice expressed warm approval of the proposal that registrars might act as part-time general practitioners. On the instructions of the College the Report was circulated to the Royal Commission, the British Medical Association, the Joint Consultants Committee (U.K.) and the Scottish Central Consultants Committee.[16] Early in 1958 the College was invited to give evidence before the Royal Commission.[17] At a later date the President (Dr Rae Gilchrist) reported having attended and having received a sympathetic hearing. He had submitted a personal supplementary statement to the Commission as there was occasion after the Meeting for some slight modification of the original Memorandum.[18] Two years later the President (Dr Rae Gilchrist), in moving the approval of the Government's proposals pointed out that they showed realistic appreciation of the position of junior members of the profession, and that they made provision for the establishment of a reviewing body.[19]

MEDICAL STAFFING

O' a' the jobs that sweat the sark
Gie me a kintra doctor's wark,
Ye ca' awa' frae dawn till dark,
Whate'er the weather be, O!

D. Rorie

The essential unit of medical practice is the occasion when, in the intimacy of the consulting room or sick room, a person who is ill . . . seeks the advice of a doctor whom he trusts. This is a consultation and all else in the practice of medicine derives from it.

Sir James Spence

LEGAL LIABILITY OF THE DOCTOR IN THE NATIONAL HEALTH SERVICE

A printed document with the above as title,[20] carefully supplemented with 'Not for publication' and issued in 1955 by the Central Consultants and Specialists Committee (Scotland) brought the subject of altered relationships between members of the profession and the hospital authorities to a head as far as the College was concerned.

More than a year previously at a Quarterly Meeting the College had approved a motion to the effect that:

'The Consultants' and Specialists' Joint Committee (Scotland) be requested to discuss with the Department of Health for Scotland:

    1. the need to preserve the present position in Scots Law in respect of the professional acts of doctors, and

    2. the steps which require to be taken to this end,

    3. to suggest to the Scottish Joint Committee that Membership of one of the Medical Defence and Protection Societies should be a condition of employment in the Hospital Service.'[21]

At a Quarterly Meeting on 26th July 1955, the Secretary (Dr Henry Matthew) moved on behalf of the Council that the paper in question should be considered by the College. Seconded by the Treasurer (Dr J. Alastair Bruce) the motion was carried unanimously. On the invitation of the President (Sir Stanley Davidson), Dr J. G. M. Hamilton proposed a motion which had been considered by Council and referred *simpliciter* to the College. Speaking to the motion Dr Hamilton spoke of the change in relationship arising from court decisions in recent legal actions. Dr W. A. Alexander seconded the motion and other speakers referred to the possible infringement of professional freedom and to the large number of practitioners who had already declared their wish for action to be taken. A fear in the light of recent judgments was that to safeguard public funds hospital authorities might seek to determine clinical procedures. With this there was anxiety over the confidentiality of medical records which when required for legal purposes were to be transmitted only by the hospital authority's solicitor.

The motion under discussion was passed by 26 votes for and 6 against, and read as follows:

2F

'That the Royal College of Physicians of Edinburgh, believing it to be in the public interest and in the interest of the progress of Medicine that doctors should be solely responsible at law for their clinical actions, urges the Scottish Joint Consultants Committee and the United Kingdom Joint Consultants Committee to approach the Government with a view to promoting the legislation necessary to re-establish in law the former relationship between hospital doctors and the management of the hospitals in which they work.'[22]

Some years later the President (Dr Rae Gilchrist) informed the College that a draft Circular on the prevention of untoward incidents due to the conduct of members of hospital staff had been prepared by the Ministry of Health. Contained in the Circular was a suggestion to set up a Medical Ethical Committee to consider incidents arising from professional incompetence or misconduct. The Joint Consultants Committee was described as viewing the suggestion with considerable misgivings and it was stated that they had postponed arriving at any decision until further legal evidence was forthcoming from the Medical Defence Unions.[23]

NUMBER OF MEDICAL PRACTITIONERS AND MEDICAL STUDENTS, 1955

To meet a request of the Ministry of Health a Committee was appointed by the College to estimate on a long-term basis the number of medical practitioners qualifying and the number of medical students required to meet commitments. The Committee encountered so many unpredictable factors that it concluded a satisfactory estimate was impracticable, and the College thereupon advised the Ministry of Health of their opinion that they could give 'no valid estimate'.[24] Subsequent events and more especially the outcome of the Willink Report,[25] pointed to the wisdom of the College's attitude. Considered from the point of view of the medical profession the recommendations contained in that Report and the Government policy to which it gave rise were not far short of disastrous.

The attitude of the College must not be misinterpreted. Concern over the inadequacy of medical personnel in relation to population and rural needs had for more than a century been uppermost in College deliberations. This concern prompted the publication by the College in 1852 of the *Statement on the situation in the Highlands and Islands of Scotland* (Chap. IX). The theme will be found constantly reiterated in later reports submitted by the College in connection with the National Health Service.

MEMORANDUM OF EVIDENCE TO BE SUBMITTED TO THE JOINT WORKING PARTY OF THE MINISTRY OF HEALTH, DEPARTMENT OF HEALTH FOR SCOTLAND AND THE JOINT CONSULTANTS COMMITTEE ON THE MEDICAL STAFFING STRUCTURE IN THE HOSPITAL SERVICE. 1959[26]

An Extraordinary Meeting was called in November 1952 to consider 'the Proposals of the Department of Health in regard to the structure of Hospital Medical Staffing in Scotland', with a view to the opinion of the College being conveyed to the Joint Committee of Consultants and Specialists (Scotland). Discussion was considerable and largely revolved round the difficulty of reconciling the training of consultants with the staffing of hospitals. A body of opinion favoured a consultant grade between senior registrar and full consultant. Eventually the Department of Health's proposals received general approval by 24 votes to 23.[27]

At a Quarterly Meeting six years later the President (Dr Rae Gilchrist) announced that a Committee had been appointed to prepare evidence for a Joint Working Party which would receive written and oral evidence on the medical staffing structure in the Hospital Service and which would visit hospitals in different parts of the country.[28] The Committee were required to base their findings 'in the light of experience of the hospital service since 1948'. They numbered eight and were comprehensively representative consisting of two full-time members of university staff and honorary consultant physicians to teaching hospitals; three part-time consultant physicians in teaching hospitals; one part-time consultant in a non-teaching hospital; one full-time consultant in a teaching hospital and another in a peripheral non-teaching hospital. Nineteen Fellows responded to the Committee's invitation to submit memoranda. Study by the Committee was confined to the broader aspects of hospital medical staffing, and did not deal with all the specialties.

Consultants
Considering the responsibilities of the consultant the Report drew attention to the time given to committees, conferences and examinations and to the particular need for provision of 'consultant cover'. That every consultant should 'by right have a definite number of beds as his own responsibility' was given as 'an essential feature . . . in the best interest of patient and consultant alike'. At the same time it was recommended that the senior consultant in any unit should be the consultant-in-charge for the purposes of administration and organization. Unable to lay down a fixed number of beds for medical units, the Committee suggested a range between 40 and 70 irrespec-

tive of whether a hospital was a teaching or a non-teaching hospital. Peripheral hospitals were found to be understaffed as regards consultants and it was categorically stated that a defect of the hospital service was the employment in non-teaching hospitals of consultants working in isolation. Redistribution of consultant staff was described as a means of securing more efficient and economical use of staff and of encouraging closer liaison between teaching and non-teaching hospitals. Importance was attached to abolishing anomalies in consultant staffing in comparable units and to ensuring that no consultant had less than seven sessions.

Registrar Grades

Discussing registrar grades the Committee recognized the validity of reasons given for embittering frustration among those having a fixed and non-renewable term of office, with at best limited prospects of early advancement to consultant rank while at the same time becoming increasingly unsuited to entering general practice. Appointments as senior registrar should, it was considered, carry with them security of tenure and 'a fair chance of becoming a consultant' and in general should be limited to teaching hospitals. The Committee did not conceal the fact that it had come to be tacitly accepted in both teaching and non-teaching hospitals that the registrar grade existed primarily for staffing duties, thereby implying that a post as registrar was no longer regarded as a step capable of leading to eventual consultant status.

The Committee favoured the abolition of the entire registrar structure as a training framework; the integration with security of tenure of the equivalent of senior registrar in the 'working hospital staff'; and replacement of the title of senior registrar by that of assistant physician. Implementation would, it was recognized, necessitate appointments being made by an Advisory Committee. Information available to them convinced the Committee that non-teaching hospitals tended to be understaffed in all grades, with as one outcome that senior registrars were assuming responsibilities appropriate to consultants. While discouraging the appointment of senior registrars to non-teaching hospitals, the Committee was opposed to the two-tier system of consultants and house officers in these hospitals, and considered that a strong case existed for the introduction of intermediate medical staff in the persons of registrars.

To overcome the disparity between the prospects of teaching and non-teaching hospitals the Committee recommended 'most strongly' a system of interchange of registrars between the two types of hospital. It considered also that a case existed for part-time appointments in the senior registrar and registrar grades, and for financial easement for the registrar to move into general practice. Senior hospital medical officer posts should, it was recommended, be abolished whenever possible.

Integration of Hospital and General Practice

The Committee came out in favour of closer integration of the hospital and general practitioner services which it argued might well be favoured were registrars enabled to work part-time in general practice and were part-time hospital appointments made available to general practitioners. At the time the Memorandum was drawn up there was good reason to accept that extra hospital experience and higher qualifications frequently proved a handicap to those anxious to enter general practice. This finding prompted the Committee to urge a more positive approach: 'A determined effort should be made on the one hand to encourage young doctors to widen their hospital experience, and on the other to persuade principals to welcome them . . . into general practice'. Considerable space was devoted in the Memorandum to the closer integration of hospital and general practice. Two sections in particular deserve mention as revealing visionary foresight unwittingly admixtured with the traditional outlook of the College more than a century previously.

> 'General practitioners working part-time in hospital should not be debarred from promotion in the normal framework of the hospital service, even to consultant level, so long as they can satisfy Appointment Advisory Committees of their qualifications, skill and experience.
> 'It has been argued that as most general practitioners are now in direct competition one with another for N.H.S. patients, they would not be acceptable as hospital doctors looking after one another's patients. We believe that . . . this difficulty could be overcome.'

The Committee were of the opinion that the employment of general practitioners on the staff of hospitals would raise the standards of general practice. Unfortunately no mention was made of the inevitable benefit to hospitals with whole-time medical staff which would be derived from the domiciliary outlook of the family doctor. On more than one occasion Sir James Spence was known to urge that teachers of medicine should seek the views of family doctors before deciding upon what to teach. Changes wrought by the National Health Service have in no way altered the soundness of Spence's dictum.[29]

House Officers

The difficulties in the way of filling house officer posts were elaborated and the particularly precarious position of special units emphasized. An increase in the number of senior house officer posts was advocated, but any suggestion of their use to subsidize trainees attending courses for higher qualifications was deprecated. Attention was drawn to the potential value of senior house officer posts in providing continuous locum cover in a hospital, account being taken of the too often ignored fact that 'provision of locum H.O.'s. must be made'.

The concluding section underlined the benefits to efficient use of medical staff which would follow increased secretarial and technical assistance.

The Report was approved *nemine contradicente*[30] and at a later date the College accepted an invitation to offer oral evidence which was given by the President, Dr Halliday Croom and Dr Card.[31] In November 1961 the College was informed that in a pending review of hospital medical establishments investigations were to be carried out on a regional basis in England and Wales and on a national basis in Scotland. It was the purpose of the Department of Health for Scotland to appoint six assessors who would visit each Scottish Region, meet the four Scottish members of the Platt Working Committee and later meet representatives of each Regional Hospital Board.[32]

It is not possible to assess the precise influence exerted by College Reports on those designing and executing plans embodied in the National Health Service. Intended as a *Health* Service it is not out of place to consider what in broad terms the Service has achieved in the first quarter century of its existence. The subject was touched on by Professor Stuart Morrison in his Sydney Watson Smith Lecture on *The Future of Preventive Medicine* delivered before the College in December 1972.[33] He described the measurable results of the Service as disappointing despite soaring costs, and referred to the steady increase in 'sickness absence'. Evidence was given suggesting that while all social classes made full use of 'curative services', the extent to which modern medicine modified the cause of chronic and degenerative disease was open to question. This Dr Morrison attributed in large part to the restrictive conception of preventive medicine as incorporated in the National Health Service; but saw prospects of improvement in the reorganization of the Service contemplated for 1974. Reorganization, with tripartite control a thing of the past, was seen as opening the doors to clinicians and preventive medicine specialists jointly *organizing* screening, treatment, rehabilitation and after care services.

With regard to integration of the hospital and general practitioner services the Scottish Home and Health Department issued a Report entitled *General Practitioners in the Hospital Service* in 1973.[34] The Report urged greater participation in hospital work by general practitioners and called on the Royal Colleges to consider how encouragement could be given to the early establishment of general practitioner hospital units.

TECHNICAL SERVICES

Where she [Medicine] nam'd the disease she now separates the bacillus;
Sets the atoms of offence, those blind and sickly bloodeaters,
'Neath lens and daylight, forcing their foul propagations,
Which had ever prosper'd in dark impunity unguest,
Now to behave in sight . . .

Robert Bridges

As Physic advances farther and farther every day and develops new axioms, it will require
fresh assistance from Mathematic.

Sir Francis Bacon

When you cannot measure it, when you cannot express it in numbers,—you have scarcely,
in your thoughts, advanced to the stage of Science . . .

Lord Kelvin

LABORATORY SERVICES IN SCOTLAND: REPORT BY SPECIAL COMMITTEE, 1957[35]

The College was invited by the Department of Health for Scotland to give advice on the present organization of laboratory services. A special Committee was formed to review the position. In presenting their Report the Committee reviewed the administrative framework existing at the time and then submitted a number of suggestions.

Central Responsibility
Responsibility for providing hospital and specialist services including laboratory services was vested in the Secretary of State for Scotland under the terms of the *National Health Service (Scotland) Act*. By the same Act he was empowered to provide or arrange for the provision of a bacteriological service for the control of the spread of infectious diseases. The duty of providing these services was delegated by the Secretary to the Regional Hospital Boards who in turn delegated some functions to Hospital Boards of Management. In practice Boards of Management undertook the staffing, equipping and management of the laboratory among other hospital services; and the Regional Hospital Board remained immediately responsible for the provision, organization, and planning of the laboratory among other services in their area.

A Scottish National Joint Committee for Laboratory Services was created in 1948, with one representative from each Regional Hospital Board and one from each of the Scottish Universities under a Chairman appointed by the Secretary of State. The Committee's terms of reference were 'To advise and assist the Regional Hospital Boards in Scotland in the development of the laboratory services provided as part of the National Health Service, with special regard to the need for inter-regional planning and co-ordination'.[35]

The Pattern of Services

Available laboratory services in Scotland were in the main provided in association with the hospitals but, in Edinburgh and Dundee there were contractual arrangements with University Departments and in Glasgow the Corporation Public Health Laboratory undertook a considerable amount of bacteriological work for the Regional Hospital Board. A Regional Hospital Board laboratory was developed as an integrated service intended to serve all interests in the Health Service including those of general practitioners and local health authorities. Each Regional Board had a Laboratory Services Sub-Committee.

The two University Departments participating in the regional laboratory services were said to be subject to undesirable pressure owing to the superimposition of large-scale routine work on teaching and research activities.

The Committee's Suggestions

The review required by the College Committee's remit was of 'the *organisation* adopted in Scotland for the provision of laboratory services'.

Separation of public health work from the main stem of laboratory medicine was not favoured by the Committee who considered that the principle of an integrated laboratory service for all purposes should be retained. Laboratory provision in each region should, it was recommended, be organized around one or more parent laboratory with associated district laboratories on the periphery. As to committees, it was considered that a National Laboratory Service Committee should be appointed to advise the Secretary of State, and that in each region a Laboratory Service Committee should be formed to advise the Regional Hospital Board on the needs of the region and of the means for satisfying them. The recommendations in respect of these Committees emphasized in detail the need for comprehensive representation. Fully informed of the difficulties being faced by the University Departments, the College Committee came to the conclusion that 'While this state of affairs is doubtless due to lack of resources in personnel and accommodation to meet the expanding requirements of the National Health Service . . . the University Departments should continue to participate actively in day-to-day work to the extent necessary to maintain their efficiency as teaching and research units'.

The Report was approved by the College *nemine contradicente.*[36]

HOSPITAL SCIENTIFIC AND TECHNICAL SERVICES: COLLEGE MEMORANDUM ON THE ZUCKERMAN REPORT[37]

A Committee was appointed by Council on 24th October 1967[38] to consider the Zuckerman Report.[39] The members consisted of Dr R. H. Girdwood (Professor of Therapeutics, University of Edinburgh), Dr E. Samuel (Consultant Radiologist, Royal Infirmary, Edinburgh) and Dr L. G. Whitby (Professor of Clinical Chemistry, University of Edinburgh).

Of necessity the Memorandum verged on the technical. It was none the less an admirable example of '*multum in parvo*'. In their preamble the College Committee emphasized that there were many medically qualified graduates who were well orientated scientifically, and deprecated excessive attention being focussed on the difference between medical and science graduates. Furthermore it was pointed out that in Scotland the considerable reliance by hospitals on the Universities resulted in a close interrelationship between the National Health Service and Universities.

Adequacy of Services in Hospitals
To a varying extent the services were described in the Report as 'inadequate in scale, personnel and organisation'. A contrast was drawn between the rapidly increasing work loads, amounting to as much as 100 per cent each five years in the case of biochemistry laboratories, with the financial level of $2\frac{1}{2}$ per cent per annum determined by the Government for the growth rate of the National Health Service. A need was foreseen for a limit to be applied to the way in which consumer demand was exercised, and for the establishment of a correct relationship between that demand and the use of scientific and allied services. Educational adjustments favouring the informed use of new developments were called for, and problems of organization resulting from acceptance of previous research activities as constituting routine services were stressed. The rate of development of new techniques was given as reason for organization being flexible in character in order to deal with necessary adjustments in terms of technical procedures and scientific personnel. Operational research was advanced as a possible method of anticipating changing emphases. The Report attached special importance to changes in the hours of work in departments,

involving the operation of a shift system to ensure economic use of automatic equipment, and to deal with the increasing demands of immediate access to a wide range of supporting investigations required by modern patient care. Competition between the N.H.S., University and Medical Research Council laboratories specially qualified to provide scientific and technical services in short supply, was cited as a possible cause of disharmony. Reference was made to experience with automatic equipment and 'work-simplified measures' and the view advanced that it was 'very possible that departments of medical automation, working like factories to a clearly defined schedule, will be needed in the near future'.[37] Warnings were uttered concerning the inevitably high capital expenditure involved, and the importance of accountancy allowing for greater productivity without comparable additions to staff when evaluating increased running costs on consumable items. Finally in this connection, a plea was made for improvement in the pharmaceutical and hospital engineering services and in the promotion of satisfactory career structures.

Staff Organization in relation to Physical Factors

Accommodation for scientific and technical services added to previously existing hospitals was described as frequently 'far from ideal', but capable of improvement in the event of the hospital rebuilding programme being implemented. Where rebuilding was not contemplated the Committee were convinced problems would persist for many years and recommended that in all hospitals the accommodation provided for these particular services 'should at least conform to the standards laid down by the Factories Acts'. Discussing location they gave as factors needing consideration the need for patient and equipment to be in juxtaposition, the speed with which the answer to a question is required, and the fact that specimens may deteriorate if transported some distance. Decisions, it was accepted, would necessarily vary from hospital to hospital, and from discipline to discipline, but it was recognized that while centralization might be the best policy for computer and high capacity automatic equipment a need would remain for smaller laboratories to meet out-patient and certain other local needs. Special mention was made of problems inseparable from peripheral hospitals remotely situated as in the Highlands and Islands of Scotland.

Classification, Recruitment, Training and Further Education

Considering classification of the services, the Memorandum suggested a grouping of the services into the following subdivisions: Laboratory Medicine; Clinical Investigative Areas (e.g. Clinical Physiology, Anaesthetics, Electroencephalography); Ionizing Radiations (e.g. Radiotherapy, Radiodiagnosis, Radioactive Isotopes);

Locomotion and Rehabilitation (e.g. Orthopaedics, Physiotherapy, Prosthetics, Artificial Limb Departments); Hospital Supply (e.g. Pharmacy, Electronic Apparatus, Dietetics); and, Statistics and Computers.

The Committee were unable to draw up a *general* career structure.

Among other points made in this section of the Memorandum were the discouragement of interchange of staff between N.H.S. and University or M.R.C. appointments by differing salary scales and difficulties related to superannuation. Mention was made of the better financial inducements in industry for graduates. Moreover, it was said that 'possibly graduate scientists . . . should have salary scales that are equivalent to those of medical graduates doing similar work'. Replacement of 'apprenticeship-and-day-release' by block tuition was given as deserving consideration.

Scope and Organization

In the opinion of the Committee there was a case for both national and regional organization—the former to exercise the maximum measure of devolution. Recruitment and the scale of staff appointments were seen as subjects calling for settlement on a national basis but a regional basis was advocated for the organization of laboratory services, with a few exceptions. Reference laboratories and those functioning in a consultative capacity were among the exceptions. Sight was not lost of the possibility that if carried to excess centralization could result in those running the service being isolated from their clinical colleagues. Dealing with the possible extension of service, the Memorandum laid down as a basic principle that whenever practicable, people should be kept out of hospital and with this end in view practitioners should be encouraged to adopt ways calculated to make the best use of diagnostic services available to them.

Relationship between Clinicians and Members of Staff

The Memorandum urged the integration of clinical and non-clinical staff; considered that non-medical graduates in hospital laboratories should be given an honorary consultant contract, and raised the question as to whether they might not be made eligible for merit awards; and suggested the possible advisability of reviewing the legal implications of increased dependence of patient management on scientific and technical services in so far as members of staff of those services were concerned. One paragraph of this section of the Memorandum requires to be quoted in full, if only because it touches upon the fundamental concept of patient care by the physician as it has evolved over the centuries. It read as follows:

'The individual doctor must always be responsible ultimately for the care of the patient whatever support he invokes at any time to provide the best possible investigative facilities and opportunity for cure or relief of disease. We may perhaps be relinquishing this concept to some degree and replacing it by management of the patient and his illness by a unit, a specialty group employing several disciplines, or perhaps a division. It is doubtful whether this will ultimately be acceptable to the patient unless it still permits him to identify the Consultant who is personally responsible for his care and welfare.'[37]

Scientific and Technical Staff—Pooled or Exclusive?

A possible conflict of interest was seen by the Committee. For the staff, recruitment to a 'pool' favoured a better career structure and better opportunities for interchange of experience and ideas. From the point of view of a specialist team engaged on research, considerable advantage was derived from having the exclusive use of a small group of scientific and technical staff. The Report presented the 'pros and cons' for both attitudes and was opposed to any rigid policy whereby the two systems of employing staff were mutually exclusive. None the less it favoured the attachment of staff to a central department as benefiting the career prospects of the scientist and favouring maximum utilization of expensive scientific equipment. An important proviso incorporated in the recommendation was that there should be no undermining of the confidence of clinical departments in the availability of staff and equipment when required.

The Memorandum was presented to and approved by the Council of the College on 27th December 1967,[40] being later forwarded to the Ministry of Health.

Subsequently Professors Girdwood, Whitby and Samuel of the College were invited to appear before the Zuckerman Committee to discuss points arising out of the College Memorandum. One outcome of the Zuckerman Report was the setting up in Scotland of the Scottish Health Services Scientific Council on which the Royal College of Physicians of Edinburgh is represented. The first representative of the College was the President in office, Dr J. Halliday Croom.

FUTURE OF THE SCIENTIFIC SERVICES: REPORT OF A WORKING PARTY OF
THE SCOTTISH HEALTH SERVICES SCIENTIFIC COUNCIL[41]
COMMENTS OF COLLEGE COUNCIL, FEBRUARY 1972

The Working Party consisted of five individuals including Dr Halliday Croom who was Chairman.

Commencing with a concise review of scientific services in the existing organization, the Report went on to deal with services contemplated in the Reorganized Health Service and outlined in the White Paper (*Reorganisation of the Scottish Health Service*); and to consider foreseeable problems arising as a result of the major administrative adjustments. Conclusions incorporated in the Report included the necessity for organization to meet the needs of patient care, public health and epidemiology; Health Boards being responsible for the management of scientific services in their own areas; effective national planning combined with local management, with a national committee to advise on policy and planning; and for local co-ordinating arrangements between adjacent Boards or groups of Boards.

On 29th February 1972, the Scottish Home and Health Department was informed that the Council of the College approved of the Report and the proposals. At the same time it was emphasized that the Council were concerned lest development of services might lead to diminishing concern with service to patients, and attached the greatest importance to close daily contact with clinical staff.[42]

In an age in danger of being dominated by administrators and architects it is reassuring to note how often in its Reports on many subjects the College had occasion to utter reminders of the need for prior consideration of the patient in planning.

BLOOD TRANSFUSION SERVICE: DEPARTMENTAL DISCUSSION PAPER

REPORT BY COUNCIL OF COLLEGE, JUNE 1972

Review of the Blood Transfusion Service in the course of the proposed reorganization of the Scottish Health Service was the subject of a document described as a 'discussion paper' and sent by the Scottish Home and Health Department to the College for comment.[43]

Proposals submitted in the document for the reorganization of the Blood Transfusion Service contemplated among other changes the appointment of a National Medical Director and a full-time Secretary and Treasurer with supporting staff. It was visualized that the National Medical Director would be of consultant grade, have an honorary appointment with a Regional Hospital Board, and be responsible for co-ordinating the activities of the five Regional Centres together with those of the Protein Fractionation Centre being established in Edinburgh. The officers and staff referred to were all to be employees of the Scottish National Blood Transfusion Association.

In their Report of 2nd June 1972, the College expressed agreement with the proposals. The College were more cautious in their view about a suggestion in the 'discussion paper' that the Blood Transfusion Service might 'be embraced within' what was termed a 'Common Services Agency'. With a view to sustaining voluntary aspects of the Service the discussion paper suggested that a national committee with regional representation might prove useful. Mindful of experience in other medico-administrative spheres, the College took the opportunity to stress the need to preserve the voluntary principle linking donor and Transfusion Service; and to enter a caution against the development of a too formal and rigid administrative structure.[44]

WORKING PARTY ON THE HOSPITAL PHARMACEUTICAL SERVICE: MEMORANDUM OF EVIDENCE GIVEN BY THE COLLEGE TO THE MINISTRY OF HEALTH ON THE REPORT, 1970[45]

A Working Party 'to advise on the efficient and economical organization of the hospital pharmaceutical service' with particular reference to organization units, the best use of pharmacists and supporting staff, and a suitable career structure for staff was appointed by the Minister of Health and Secretary of State for Scotland in April 1968. The Report of the Working Party which obtained evidence from the College was published in February 1970.[46] A letter was received by the President (Dr Christopher Clayson) from the Department of Health and Social Security enclosing advanced cyclostyled copies of the Working Party's Report, comments on which were desired by the Secretary of State.

A Committee was thereupon appointed by Council of the College, consisting of Dr R. H. Girdwood and Dr J. Laurie, who obtained evidence from the Group Chief Pharmacist, Royal Infirmary, Edinburgh (Mr J. A. Myers) and the Chief Pharmacist, Dumfries and Galloway Royal Infirmary (Mr D. Macfarlane).

While accepting the four broad headings of the Working Party's Report based on the original terms of reference from the two central departments, the College Committee stated that additional factors which had acquired increasing importance required consideration: these were the manufacture of sterile infusion fluids; sterile water and haemodialysis solutions etc.; pharmaceutical research in teaching hospitals; and the maintenance of appropriate records. Subsequent events have certainly confirmed the wisdom of the proposed additions.

The Desirable Unit of Organization

The Committee were emphatic that 'the number of beds . . . is no criterion'. In support of their contention they contrasted the differing demands of advanced surgical techniques and certain specialized medical units, with geriatric and mental hospital wards. Mention was made of the growing requirements of large out-patient departments incorporating major diagnostic and research units. Lack of pharmacists due to low salary scales was given as a major factor preventing efficient organization. To a large extent, the Report maintained, the organization was dependent upon the part-time services of retired pharmacists and housewives.

Existing hospital groups were described as wasteful of qualified staff and equipment. A city area with a population of 300,000 to 500,000 was regarded as a suitable basis for organization, with as centre the major teaching hospital or major district general hospital. At the centre, it was envisaged there would be manufacturing laboratories capable of meeting the needs of hospitals, large and small, of sterile solutions over a wide range; equipment for supplying the smaller hospitals with haemodialysis solutions etc.; a pre-packing unit; a quality control laboratory; adequate storage and office facilities to cope with area requirements. It was recommended that co-ordination should be the responsibility of an Area Principal Pharmacist attached to an area hospital (e.g. Edinburgh Royal Infirmary, Aberdeen Royal Infirmary etc.). Glasgow in virtue of its large concentrated population, and the Highlands and Islands with their sparsely distributed population were cited as situations calling for special adjustments. Emphasis was attached to reliable efficient transport arrangements.

Integrated Regional Pharmaceutical Services to be developed by Regional Pharmacists and based on Area Pharmacists were advocated as a means of securing economic redeployment of pharmacists and pharmaceutical work. It was considered that while the appointment of Area Pharmacists should rest with Regional Hospital Boards, Regional Pharmacists should be appointed by the Secretary of State for Scotland, and that an Area Pharmacist should have direct access to the Board of Management of the main hospital where his headquarters would be located.

Continuation as a forum for the interchange of ideas of the existing two Regional Pharmaceutical Advisory Committees in Glasgow and Edinburgh was recommended.

Retail Chemists
In the opinion of the Committee 'the services of the local pharmacist in general practice in a small rural village forty or more miles from the nearest hospital pharmaceutical department could be utilised where it is not economic or practicable to provide a service from the hospital pharmaceutical department'.[45] Another example of private enterprise, no matter on how minute a scale, coming to the rescue of a national organization!

National Co-ordination

In so far as Scotland was concerned the Report considered that a goodly measure of national co-ordination had been effected with 'the purchasing of drugs, dressings and disposables etc., through the Scottish Hospital Pharmacists' Advisory Committee, at the Home and Health Department'. The scheme was described as 'well run' and in what followed there was a veiled and indirect hint that Scotland's experience might be of value to 'other regions of the United Kingdom'. How colourlessly unromantic 'other regions of the United Kingdom' reads when compared with the old-time unashamed references to the Kingdom of Scotland and the Kingdom of England!

Effective Employment of Pharmacists

A detailed list of duties and responsibilities was given in the Report according to whether they should be undertaken by a pharmacist-in-charge personally; by a pharmacist personally; directed and controlled but not supervised by a pharmacist; and supervised by a pharmacist. It was accepted that variations were inevitable in hospitals of different type and size, and were determined by the calibre of supporting staff. The importance of technical and clerical staff and of porters being well trained was stressed.

Further Training for Pharmacists

On this subject the Committee was undisguisedly dogmatic. They drew attention to the need for postgraduate courses in pharmacy of which none were provided in Scotland, and for the institution in Scotland of an M.Sc. degree which suitable pharmacists might be encouraged to take. Present and prospective Chief Pharmacists in the larger hospitals should, it was argued, be sent by Boards of Management to 'high level residential courses' at a carefully selected administrative college, or be encouraged to study for an academic diploma or the professional examinations of a reputable institute concerned with public administration. Refresher courses in pharmacology and therapeutics and meetings of pharmacists on a national basis were described as essential in the light of the rapid evolution of pharmacy and its applications.

Supporting Staff

'To talk of the best use of supporting staff in Scottish Hospital Pharmacies is premature' stated the Report and went on to produce factual supporting evidence. In 1965 the basic grade for pharmacists in the United Kingdom contained 52 per cent part-time pharmacists; 73 per cent were women of whom many were expected to marry and leave the service, 60 per cent being aged less than 31 years. High wastage of staff was further contributed to by the much better financial prospects in industry and business. Competition for advertised posts was minimal. In the quoted words of a Group Chief Pharmacist: 'The present staffing situation in hospital pharmacy is chaotic . . . Standards of work have not been increased in many hospitals and often the standards have fallen in a National Health Service which was intended to raise standards and provide better patient care . . . Responsible Heads of Schools of Pharmacy . . . can no longer honestly recommend pharmacy as a career.' With fullest justification he further described the situation as verging on the desperate and one 'little appreciated by doctors and nurses working in hospitals'.

The Committee had no doubts that an urgent need existed for better financial rewards for increased skills both in relation to pharmacists and supporting staff, and the Report embodied suggestions for career structures for these two groups.

Research

Facilities for research, liaison with the local pharmacy and/or medical school, and joint university hospital pharmaceutical appointments at senior levels were advocated; and mention was made of the fact that the Chief Pharmacist of the Edinburgh Royal Infirmary was an honorary senior lecturer in the University Department of Therapeutics.

After the Working Party's publication of their Report in February 1970, the President (Dr Christopher Clayson) received a request in mid-March (1970) on behalf of the Joint Consultants Committee for observations on the Noel Hall Report as the Working Party publication had come to be known. Understandably in drafting their reply Council were advised by Dr Girdwood.[48] The reply was extremely concise and indicated general agreement with the Report. At the same time the opportunity was taken to underline the crucial importance of rapid agreement and implementation of suitable salary scales if technical and supporting staff were to be recruited and retained in adequate numbers. Renewed attention was drawn to the importance of records being standardized on a national basis.

From the point of view of the College, a gratifying feature of the Working Party Report was that the Memorandum of Evidence submitted by the College was one of the few to be quoted. It may be claimed with justification that the College views were an important factor in influencing the decision ultimately arrived at to organize the Hospital Pharmaceutical Service in Area Units supplying 4000–6000 beds. Furthermore Regional Pharmacists were appointed in Edinburgh, Glasgow, Aberdeen, Dundee and Inverness with as one major responsibility the assistance of Regional

Boards in preparing schemes for the reorganization of the pharmaceutical services. Area pharmacists have also been appointed.

THE PHARMACOPOEIA

. . . the greatest therapeutic gift is the gift of Charity and that should be a permanent and not a changing fashion in therapeutics.

Sir Derrick Dunlop

Ah! the paradise that awaits us in 1984! . . . For every ill a pill. Tranquillizers to overcome angst, pep pills to wake us up, life pills to ensure blissful sterility.

Malcolm Muggeridge

REPORT OF COLLEGE COMMITTEE ON THE REVISION OF THE BRITISH PHARMACOPOEIA, 1958[48]

In accordance with custom since disappearance of the *Edinburgh Pharmacopoeia* and the institution of the *British Pharmacopoeia* last century (Chap. XXV) the College was asked for its opinion concerning proposed changes to be embodied in a new edition of the latter.

The College appointed a Committee to consider the scope of the next edition of the *British Pharmacopoeia* and more especially a list of drugs which the British Pharmacopoeia Commission had under consideration for retention in, deletion from, or addition to the Pharmacopoeia. Membership of the College Committee numbered three—(Sir) Derrick Dunlop, and Drs A. G. Cruickshank and A. G. Macgregor.[49] Their Report was notably succinct and incisive, dealing as it did with classified and unclassified drugs and groups of drugs. For one reader at least the Report provided moral rearmament in goodly measure when he read of a drug concerning the value of which one of the three wise men was 'convinced', while his two collaborators 'were more impressed by its toxicity'. Agreement to disagree artfully expressed!

The College Committee found themselves in 'very general agreement' with the provisional tentative suggestions of the Commission, but foresaw the day when the inclusion of '*all* good new drugs in the Pharmacopoeia' might prove impossible because of the number involved.

REORGANIZATION

In any organisation there is need to ensure that information passes both from the centre to the perimeter and from the perimeter to the centre.

Sir Edward Appleton

Initiative must be preserved in spite of organisation.

Bertrand Russell

WHITE PAPER ON REORGANIZATION OF THE SCOTTISH HEALTH SERVICES

A White Paper was presented to Parliament by the Secretary of State for Scotland in July 1971.[50] It represented the Government's proposals for a reform of the administrative structure of the National Health Service in Scotland in advance of the changes in local government expected to be completed in 1975. The White Paper attached considerable importance to the establishment of a strong professional consultative structure as a means of ensuring an effective partnership between those responsible for the management of, and the professional individuals providing, the health services.

Arrangements for reorganization aimed at the creation in Scotland of fourteen Health Boards which would be responsible for the health services in their respective areas. Implied in this was the unification under each Health Board of the hospital service, family practitioner service and local authority health services. Furthermore it was intended that a single-tier structure should replace the existing two-tier form of Regional Boards and Boards of Management, and that strong professional committees with statutory recognition would advise a Health Board on current and long-term problems. It was proposed that the new Health Boards should be represented on a central Scottish Health Service Planning Council, establishment of which would synchronize with the creation *de novo*, of a Common Services Agency. This Agency, the White Paper stated, 'would provide a wide range of services for the Planning Council, the health boards and the Department'. The probable activities of the Agency were outlined in terms which were somewhat superficial and vague, but sufficient to betray the ambitious alternate objective that it would develop into 'a new type of National Health Service body of central importance to the efficient day-to-day running and long-term planning of the service . . .'. Flexibility was to be the key-note of the external and internal activities of the Agency—a most obvious and necessary administrative defensive interpolation while so much remained to be defined.

Close co-operation with local authorities was underlined as essential. Legislation in precise terms was not considered necessary for the fostering of such relations. Human nature being what it is, will the challenge of reorganization serve to bring to an end inter-departmental rivalries, suspicions between local and central authorities, and distrust between experienced clinicians and administrators superabundantly confident in their growing power? Noteworthy was the White Paper's intended allocation of responsibility for medical and dental examination within the School Health Service to the Health Boards with the caveat that 'education authorities will have a strong and continuing interest'. The child guidance and speech services in schools were to remain the responsibility of the education authority.

It was intended that doctors, nurses and other professional people should be employed by, or in contract with Health Boards instead of Hospital Boards, Executive Councils or Local Authorities; and that the services of Health Boards would be centrally financed, and so fall into line with the existing hospital and family practitioner services.

As to endowments, those given before November 1946 having been transferred to the Scottish Hospitals Trust under the *Hospital Endowments (Scotland) Act, 1971*,[51] the income due would be paid to Health Boards; and those given after 1946 would be vested in Health Boards for use so far as possible for the objects specified by the donors.

Mention was made in the White Paper of the possibility of establishing a Health Commissioner to handle complaints about the health service.

The Council of the College considered the White Paper and forwarded their observations to the Scottish Home and Health Department after their meeting in September 1971.[52] While in general agreement with the recommendations of the Government, Council made comments on certain specific points.

Referring to the appointment by the Secretary of State of certain members of Health Boards after consultation with the Universities concerned, Council of the College considered that further information was desirable about the total number of members who might be appointed after consultation with the University in areas with Medical Schools. While supporting the statutory recognition proposed for professional committees, Council drew attention to the desirability of, in addition, 'statutory provision for consultation of such committees in matters which affect patient care'. The need for the administrative and professional staff of Health Boards to be of 'high quality' was emphasized, and the principle underlying the concept of a 'Health Commissioner' was accepted.

Council, it would seem, were in some doubt about the Common Services Agency as forecast in the White Paper. There was, it was felt, a need for information concerning the availability of Agency Staff at local level, and, to avoid remoteness from those concerned with local planning on the part of a centralized body. Particular concern was expressed over the proposed division of certain services between the Medical and Social Services (q.v.). Welcoming the inclusion of the School Health Service among Health Board responsibilities, Council advocated a similar arrangement for the Child Guidance Service. It then proceeded to conclude with a strongly worded caution, deserving of quotation at length:

> 'The provision of a comprehensive service to the Community on the lines suggested [in relation to local authority responsibilities in social work and environmental services] . . . is entirely dependent on the effective provision of services under the *Social Work (Scotland) Act*. The Council wish to express their disquiet concerning the provision of such services and consider that further investigation and clarification of the division between the responsibilities of the Medical and Social Services is required.'

Almost certainly there was uppermost in the minds of Council the situation with regard to the care of children and the aged.

In the months following the publication of the White Paper the College were in receipt of a series of communications, designated 'consultation papers', from the Scottish Home and Health Department. These documents dealt with a variety of problems subsidiary to the overall plan of reorganization. Their very number serves as an indication of the extent of College involvement in the reorganization of the Scottish Health Services. Thus, subjects on which in 1972 alone their comments were invited by the Scottish Home and Health Department included the administrative structure of Health Boards; Common Services Agency; Administration of the Ambulance Service; Management at District Level; Transfer and Appointment of Staff; Computers and Computing; and Proposed Health Board Areas. No purpose would be served by detailing the comments of Council, but a certain few selected observations need to be mentioned. Thus in the matter of the administrative structure of Health Boards, the College 'stressed the principle that medical opinion should not be expressed by a medical administrator' and that the Chairman of an Area Medical Committee should have the right to membership, with voting rights, of the Executive Group.

DOCTORS

The Report of a Joint Working Party (*Doctors in an Integrated Health Service*)[53] appointed by the Secretary of State for Scotland was submitted to the College for comments. Membership of the Working Party numbered twenty-six and included the following Fellows of the College—(Sir) John Brotherston (Chairman), Drs T. Anderson, J. Crooks, A. R. Currie, A. S. Duncan, A. K. M. Macrae, J. G. M. Hamilton and D. M. Pendreigh (Joint Secretary); and the following Members of the College—Drs K. M. Parry, F. D. Beddard and S. J. Hadfield (Observer). Dr P. A. P. Mackenzie in the Working Party was a Licentiate of the College.

The Report dealt separately with the contributions of General Practice, the Specialist Services, Community Medicine and Medical Organization and concluded with a chapter on the 'Need for Change: Conclusions and Prerequisites'. It was considered by the Council of the College which gave their views in a short document in October 1971.[54]

Council expressed general agreement with the Working Party's findings but felt that certain sections of the Report called for special comment. Agreeing whole-heartedly that the important part played by general practitioners needed to be strengthened, Council drew attention to their need for adequate facilities for investigation and treatment in Health Centres or Hospitals. These facilities were described as fundamental to professional satisfaction, and Council were of the opinion that the Report did not appear to give 'adequate weight . . . to the special demands of the breadth of general practice'. Support was given to 'a trial of the reintroduction of general practitioners into the hospital team' which it was considered could best be achieved by 'the progressive introduction into general practice of suitably trained young graduates . . . able to continue an involvement in one of a limited number of specialties in which they had received some training . . .'. Import-ance was attached to continuing education for general practitioners and approval given to the view expressed in the Report that 'organisational changes must be reinforced by changes in medical education and in the attitude of medical educators'. The scarcely euphonious phraseology consisted of a quotation from the original Working Party Report.

A closer integration between specialist practice and the rest of the Health Service was regarded as essential by the Working Party. Towards this end they considered that specialists must become increasingly involved in the work of health centres. The College Council had doubts about the immediate practicability of such a develop-ment. Their doubts centred on the availability of existing specialist staff to provide a service which although eminently desirable would inevitably prove time consuming.

Certain sections of the chapter on Community Medicine in the Report elaborated on the place of statistical analyses aided by modern systems of information storage. While in no way decrying the accurate evaluation of statistical data, Council submitted an earnest plea that central provision of facilities for this purpose should not lead to underestimation of requirements at hospital level, and would need to ensure the accurate recording of basic medical data. At the same time Council drew attention to the importance of greater financial allocation at hospital level if improvement of existing record systems was to be secured.

Council's concluding comments indicated agreement with the divisional system already in operation in some hospitals; and expressed unqualified approval of 'the central professional advisory body' postulated in the Report to provide professional advice at national level on planning and development, the promotion of research and the best deployment of resources.[54]

NURSES AND NURSING

The nurse's tongue is privileged to talk.
Old English Proverb

Inevitably, with the impetus given to reorganization of the National Health Service, the future of nurses and nursing came up for special consideration. Two Departmental Reports were issued in the year 1972. Of these the first was the Report of a Working Group appointed by the Scottish Home and Health Department[55]; and the second, the *Report of the Committee on Nursing* (Briggs) appointed by the Secretary of State for Social Services.[56]

Written evidence was submitted to the Briggs Committee by the College, and both Reports were referred by the Scottish Home and Health Department to the College for consideration.

Nurses in an Integrated Health Service
Report of a Working Group appointed by the Scottish Home and Health Department

The terms of reference of the Group were to consider the organization of the nursing work in the National Health Service in Scotland in the context of the proposed reorganization of the administrative structure of the Service. The Group consisted of fifteen nurses. Additional members were co-opted to serve on Subgroups which gave special consideration to problems of organization related to nursing service in child health, mental health, geriatrics and midwifery.

Among major recommendations in the Report were greater attention to specialization in nursing; recognition of the importance of nursing research; and acceptance of the team concept as a means of fostering co-operation between members of the different professions involved in health care. Education was given as the key to success in bringing together the hospital and community services. To this end it was recommended that initial training should equip nurses to work at basic level in both hospital and community; and that at post-basic level there might be a multi-disciplinary approach to clinical specialization and research.

Report of the Committee on Nursing (Briggs Report)

By its terms of reference the Committee was required to review the rôle of the nurse and the midwife in the hospital and in the community, and the education and training for that rôle. Oral and written evidence was submitted by the College to the Nursing Committee.

Written Evidence submitted by the College

Council appointed a Subcommittee which consisted of Drs W. A. Murray (Convener), J. Williamson (Member of Council and Secretary to the Committee), A. W. Wright (Member of Council) and J. W. Affleck.[57] Their Report, after acceptance by Council, was submitted to the Committee on Nursing.[58]

In the opening paragraphs emphasis was attached to the fundamental aims shared by nurses and doctors; and to the recognized fact that in the past the vocational urge possessed by nurses had militated against the recognition of a nurse's entitlement to proper status and opportunities for advancement. There followed a summary of what the Committee considered to be the nurses' duties. These were given as the provision of physical care and psychological support of the patient; participation under medical guidance in therapeutic and diagnostic procedures; to have an educational rôle in relation to the patient, and persons other than patients, including members of other professions; and to contribute to management and planning within the Health Service. At the same time a caveat was entered concerning excessively ruthless interpretation of a policy to free nurses from 'non-nursing duties'. Specific circumstances were given in which the special skill and understanding of the trained nurse were essential for the effective discharge of certain duties which might 'superficially' be assessed as 'non-nursing'.

Discussing the existing and future demand for nurses, considerable attention was given to the repercussions of increased specialization in medicine. Intensive care units were described as 'taking nurses away from other activities' and the view advanced that there was a strong case for non-nursing duties to be 'devolved on to other staff' and for enrolled nurses, if given suitable training, to play an important part in these units. Care of the elderly was seen as one of the greatest increasing problems facing the hospital service, and it was recommended that training of all nurses should include a period in a geriatric assessment unit, and that geriatric units should have close associations with district general hospitals and teaching hospitals.

The statement was made that 'the welcome renaissance in general practice has led to a belated recognition of the fact that the family doctor can cope adequately with a very large part of community health problems'. True although this is, it might have been amplified by reference to those aspects of what is now ponderously called community medicine which were so unostentatiously and so ably performed by family doctors of previous generations. There are alive today many elderly individuals who spontaneously testify to this. However the Report realistically commented on the new and varied demands on nursing establishment being made by the general practitioner and organized community services, which with development will ease the burden on hospitals and family doctors. In the opinion of the Committee community duties were particularly suited to married women resuming nursing activities, and provided opportunities for an important contribution by enrolled nurses. Nurses working in the field of psychiatry came in for special comments. They were not, it was maintained, to be regarded any longer as having a purely custodial rôle, but were to be valued as members of a multi-disciplinary team concerned with social therapy and rehabilitation. Furthermore psychiatric nurses were, it was noted, involved in educational programmes designed to explain their function and practice to other nursing groups, social service students and medical students.

Medicine is peculiarly susceptible to changes in emphases determined by fashion. This Report was noteworthy in a number of respects but not least for the fact that it was prepared by a Committee lacking paediatric representation and that from beginning to end contained no mention of infant or child. None is more indebted to, or understanding of the nurses' contribution than the children's physician. Hospital and community paediatrics have been subject to evolutionary progress in recent decades no less than adult medicine. Nurses together with their medical colleagues have of necessity to make adjustments of a nature not dealt with in the Report. In the interests of the infant, reorganization of paediatric nursing must not be determined by remote academics or professionals-become-administrators with only distant contact with the practical realities of current nursing care. The view is based upon both administrative and clinical experience.

Wisely or unwisely the Council Committee exercised considerable restraint when dealing with the training of nurses. It did however express certain views on general aspects of the subject. A very broad training with emphasis on the basic care of the sick patient was advocated for all nurses. It was considered that a year of general nursing practice should be required of any nurse after registration or enrolment before she specialized should she so wish. For nurses so inclined, specialist vocational schemes were regarded as essential.

With regard to the functions and practice of tutor nurses the College Committee did not disguise its doubts although the impression given is that diplomacy alone prevented stronger expression of their views. Their implied criticism was summed up in their opinion that 'it is anomalous that a young nurse can forsake clinical nursing forever in her twenties, train as a tutor and thereafter have generations of student and pupil nurses entrusted to her care, and yet never again do any practical nursing'. It might well have been added that many Ward Sisters of long experience regret the extent to which theoretical as distinct from practical considerations often dominate the instruction given. Throughout, the remarks on the training of nurses dwelt understandably on the analogy with 'modern thinking on doctor training'. In actual fact, the analogy could be extended to the training given to apprentices and students in heavy industry.

Doubts were expressed in the College Report about the career structure recommended by the Salmon Committee. In particular, there was apprehension over the proposals implying that a good, competent nurse possessed of a strong sense of vocation and by instinct clinically orientated, would after reaching a specified grade (Grade 7) have to resign herself to being divorced from ministering directly to the sick should she be offered further advancement. The College Report suggested that the salary scale for Grade 7 should be 'considerably extended upwards . . . so that the best individuals in this grade might be attracted to remain therein and be able to attain near-parity with their colleagues who chose administration as their field'.[59]

To some, administrative posts represent the peak of professional achievement, to others, the loss of professional soul and idealism. Rothschild stated 'the acquisition of administrative experience at a fairly early age is also necessary to enable scientists to make their proper contribution in policy-making posts at headquarters'.[60] To the ambitious young nurse and young doctor, the early deceptive lure of administration is attended with not inconsiderable risk.

The 'Briggs' Report
Of mammoth proportions the Report concluded with a Summary of what were described as 'main recommendations', of which there were seventy-five. For present

purposes, reference to only a selected few of these is necessary. A Central Nursing and Midwifery Council with three distinct Education Boards for England, Scotland and Wales and with, in addition, a statutory Standing Midwifery Committee was recommended. This Council was to be responsible for professional standards, education and discipline in nursing and midwifery in Great Britain, and the central government departments in London, Edinburgh and Cardiff were to be ultimately responsible for nursing and midwifery education. It was contemplated that the age of entry to the nursing/midwifery profession should be reduced to seventeen years by 1973; there should be one basic course of eighteen months leading to a statutory qualification, the Certificate in Nursing Practice; and that a further eighteen months' course for those holding the Certificate in Nursing Practice should be established leading to a second statutory qualification of Registration. Implied in this last recommendation was that unlike the existing Register, the new Register would not have separate parts. For students with the ability and desire to 'train further' it was suggested that courses leading to Registration could include, or be followed by, instruction leading to a non-statutory Higher Certificate in a particular branch of nursing/midwifery.

With regard to personnel, increased male recruitment, special attention to the recruitment of more A-level entrants, and the encouragement of nurses/midwives whose careers have been interrupted to return to the profession, were all advocated. Dealing with conditions of work, numerous aspects were considered including night shifts, on-call systems, personnel departments, travel schemes and secondment for academic studies. In the matter of organization and career structures improved liaison between hospital and community services was urged forcibly, and suggestions advanced for adjustments in ward organization. The emergence of a 'new caring profession' for the mentally handicapped was foreseen.

Comments of Council Committee of the College on the two Reports, November 1972

Both the above Reports were referred by the Scottish Home and Health Department for the comments of the College. Council accepted the comments of their Committee on each occasion.[61]

Comments on the Report of the Working Group: 'Nurses in an Integrated Health Service'

The Council Committee were in general agreement with the Report but would have preferred more enthusiasm for experimentation and pilot schemes for nurses to work in both hospital and community. They suggested also that wholly effective representation of nurses at decision-making level might be hampered by the hierarchical nursing structure. A caution was entered lest the undeniable need for well-planned programmes of research should contribute to 'research becoming an end in itself and of research achievement acquiring too much emphasis in securing advancement to higher posts in nursing'.[62]

Comments on the Report of the Committee on Nursing (Briggs Report)

The Council Committee was impressed as much by the amount of information in, as by the length of the Report, with which they were in general agreement. They did however allow of one major source of disquiet. The reason for concern was uncertainty as to the prospects of advancement for Ward Sisters and they reiterated the views they had already expressed when submitting evidence (q.v.). Their concern and lack of conviction by the Briggs Report on this particular point were undisguised.

As to the proposed new Central Council, the College without betraying apprehension, expressed the hope that the best features of the existing Scottish General Nursing Council would be preserved. While giving a general welcome to the educational recommendations, the College was doubtful whether provision of a basic course for all entrants to training regardless of their educational qualifications was a realistic proposal. Recommendations concerning manpower and conditions of work were accepted without reservation. Referring to the 'new caring profession' for the mentally handicapped, the College expressed the view that 'for the foreseeable future considerable numbers of mentally handicapped patients of all ages with multiple physical and mental disabilities will pose irresistible calls upon the nursing profession'.[63]

Can 'caring profession' be accepted as a happy form of nomenclature? It seems to convey a sense of apology for nursing activities in the past. Or does it reflect current obsession for a change of connotation for change's sake? To this day there are rural 'rodent officers' who much prefer their former designation of 'rat catcher' as more truly indicative of their skill!

SOCIAL WORKERS

Employment in the Health Service

A Document with the above as subject[64] was received for comment from the Scottish Home and Health Department, and replied to in June 1972. The Document, which was not for publication, was produced by the Social Work Sub-Committee of the Working Party on Relationships with Local Authorities. Certainly in so far as the National Health Service was concerned it contemplated what might fairly be termed a revolutionary change with inevitable repercussions on the medical services provided by hospitals.

After defining the social worker's function the Document gave as its fundamental objective 'to meet the needs of patients and their families for social work services in the most effective way possible'. To this end it was recommended that a patient and his family should receive continuity of care 'before, during and after his illness . . . from the same social worker'; the social worker in a health service setting should have direct access to the community services, and the local authority social work department should have direct access to the skill and experience of social workers in hospitals and health centres; and that the social worker should be trained to be and accepted as an essential member of the professional team in a hospital or health centre.

In the opinion of the Working Party all social workers should be employed by local authorities whether working in hospitals or in local authority posts, and eventually decision as to which social workers would serve in hospitals would rest with the local authority. The whole tenor of the Document was crystallized in its first recommendation to the effect that 'when the reorganization of the health service takes effect, full responsibility for the provision of social work services in hospitals and other health establishments should be placed on local authorities, with a consequential adjustment in Rate Support Grant'. Among other recommendations was one that a Working Party should be appointed as soon as possible to draw up general guidance on the social work staffing requirements of the health service.

In the first instance the Document was referred by the College Council to Dr J. Williamson for comments. His opening comment was delightfully puckish: 'Paper is written in 1st person plural. It would have been useful to know who "we" are'.

He pointed out also that the theory underlying the *Social Work (Scotland) Act* was that social workers were 'generic', having a general knowledge and general ability in practice, whereas prior to the Act there were such specially trained and experienced employees as Children's Officers, Mental Health Officers and Probation Officers.[65]

With these and other comments from Dr Williamson to help them Council replied to St Andrew's House in terms as important as they were emphatic. Because of their importance a lengthy quotation from the reply is justified.

'The Council feel that the Social Work (Scotland) Act of 1969[66] produced a complete separation of social work from the Health Service resulting in the formation of a larger, more centralised and more bureaucratic organisation. This Act, they feel, gave the new social work departments many more responsibilities than they could adequately discharge. The Council felt that the doctrine of the "generic" social worker had had adverse effects. Some members of Council from their experience were not content with the present liaison between their hospital medical social worker and social work departments. Others felt that the present Social Work Act was proving to be much less effective than it might be. Three years of experience of the present system had left profound dissatisfaction with its working. The proposal to take the hospital social worker into the social work departments might well mean that social work for hospitals would deteriorate and that close team work as in psychiatry, paediatrics and geriatrics would be much more difficult to secure.

There was general satisfaction with the quality of the social worker at present in hospital and the Council felt that hospital social work should not be taken over by an organisation which had already given rise to grave misgivings concerning its ability to discharge its responsibilities under the Social Work (Scotland) Act.'[67]

Report of the Working Group on the Training Needs of Staff in Day Centres, 1972

A copy of the above was received by the College from the Social Work Services Group, Edinburgh. The Group consisted of social workers, psychologists and educationists and obtained evidence from thirty-six sources of which none was medical. Recommendations made by the Group included training courses for day-centre staff; generic training to provide basic knowledge for work in any type of centre; and a Central Training Council.[68]

In their comments sent to the Social Work Services Group the Council of the College took full account of views expressed by Dr J. Williamson. The general theme of the Group Report met with agreement but attention was drawn to the desirability of medically qualified people including a doctor with psychiatric training being in the Working Group. This suggestion was reinforced by mention of the fact that most persons attending day centres did so basically on account of physical or mental disability. At the same time a firm recommendation was made that the Training Council proposed by the Group should include a doctor with special experience in the problems of the disabled, and a psychiatrist.[69]

RESEARCH

Research that holds no hope of potential benefit to the patient may be research, but it is not medical research.

Henry Miller

. . . a research committee can do one useful thing and one only. It can find the workers best fitted to attack a particular problem, bring them together, give them the facilities they need, and leave them to get on with the work. It can review progress from time to time and make adjustments: but if it tries to do more, it will do harm.

W. W. C. Topley

A Framework for Government Research and Development, 1971

This publication consisted of two main sections: the first a Report commissioned by the Government on *The Organisation and Management of Government Research and Development* by Lord Rothschild, Head of the Central Policy Review Staff[60] : and the second the Report of a Working Group of the Council for Scientific Policy on *The Future of the Research Council System.*[70]

Certain background facts to Government Research need explanation at the outset. The Department of Education and Science supports basic research at the Universities through the agency of the University Grants Committee; and at the institutes and units of 'subordinate' Research Councils through the Council for Scientific Policy. The functions of the Council for Scientific Policy are purely advisory and its advice is tendered to the Secretary of State for Education and Science to whom the Research Councils have direct access. There are five Research Councils including the Medical Research Council which are 'subordinate' to the Council for Scientific Policy only in respect of the allocation of funds. An appreciable portion of the work of the Medical Research Council is in the field of applied science.

One thing the two Reports had in common was an overwhelming attachment to abrasive abbreviations. The end results were better suited to digestion by a computer than by more humbly orientated physicians. Lord Rothschild's Report was based on the principle that applied Research and Development with a practical application as objective must be done on a customer–contractor basis. 'The customer says what he wants; the contractor does it (if he can); and the customer pays.' With almost indecent haste and, one might say, with political myopia the Government in an introductory memorandum to the Report verged on the eulogistic in the matter of the 'customer/contractor' principle. Rothschild was critical of the Medical Research Council background in so far as the Council were autonomous in respect of their programmes, and that their applied research activities had 'no customer to commission and approve it'. Curtly he summed up the situation: 'This is wrong'. His argument was that no matter how distinguished, intelligent and practical scientists may be, 'they cannot be so well qualified to decide what the needs of the nation are and their priorities, as those responsible for ensuring that those needs are met'.[71]

No one would question the generalization. The fact remains, however, there have been occasions in times of grave crises when the administrator has been relieved to see the scientist assume responsibility. And as Rudyard Kipling almost 50 years ago reminded the Royal Society of Medicine, there are other aspects deserving consideration by the pragmatist and scientist alike!

> 'Isn't it likely that the multitude and significance of the revelations heaped upon us within the past few years have made men in self-defence specialise more and more narrowly? Haven't we been driven headlong to abandon our conceptions of life, motion and matter? And isn't it human that in that upheaval men may have carried off each his own cherished prepossession . . . ? . . . Suppose, then, at some future time when the bacteriologist and the physicist are for the moment at a standstill, wouldn't it be interesting if they took their problem to the astronomer, and—in modern scientific language, of course—put to him Nicholas Culpepper's curious question: "What was the aspect of the heavens when such-and-such phenomena were observed?" '[72]

The section contributed by the Working Group (with Sir Frederick Dainton as Chairman) of the Council for Scientific Policy was concerned essentially with the conception underlying Research Council structure. While allowing that the structure had certain disadvantages the Group considered that its retention was essential and were firmly opposed to any suggestion that each Research Council should be administered by an executive department. A proposal of almost Juggernaut proportions was however advanced. The Group advocated the replacement of the Council for Scientific Policy by a Board of the Research Councils which was to be responsible to the Secretary for Education and Science for ensuring that Research Councils were meeting the requirements of executive departments for scientific support. Membership of the Board would include among others the Scientific Heads of Research Councils, the President of the Royal Society, a University Vice-Chancellor, and representatives from the University Grants Committee and other Government departments.

The Green Paper Considered

The subject of the Green Paper on Organization and Management of Government Research and Development was considered by Dr J. A. Strong and Dr M. A. Eastwood who reported their opinions to the Joint Committee of the Scottish Royal Colleges.[73] Subsequently a joint letter was sent on behalf of these Colleges to the Chief Scientific Officer in Whitehall.

Despite having extracted one extension from the central authority, the Joint Committee remonstrated tactfully that 'the time available for the discussion of matters of the importance of those contained in the Green Paper is still inadequate'. The Committee stated they were 'on the whole' satisfied with the way in which Research Councils, and the Medical Research Council in particular, discharged their responsibilities. Of special significance was the opinion given that 'the separation of basic from applied research, which is implicit in the Rothschild Report, cannot be sustained in medical research where the interface between these two fields of research is complex'. Approval was given to the promotion of research on a customer-contractor relationship 'provided that such funds are not subtracted from the budget of the Medical Research Council'. It was pointed out that adoption of a customer-contractor relationship would necessitate the introduction of safeguards as to rights of publication of research.[74]

As events turned out, the Council of the Edinburgh College of Physicians felt constrained to submit supplementary points which were concerned primarily with medical and related research. These additional comments provided the substance of a letter signed by the President (Dr Halliday Croom) on 11th February 1972 and sent to the Chief Scientific Officer on behalf of himself and Council.[75]

The letter was refreshingly pungent. Diplomatic phraseology in no way detracted from the conviction compelling expression of Council's views. Because of the extent to which the doubts expressed were shared by members of the profession within and outside the College, there is adequate reason for quoting sections of the letter.

Concern was expressed that changes made in the organization of Government Research 'should not involve sacrificing any of the desirable and indeed often admirable features of the organisation and support of medical research in the United Kingdom at this time'. Appreciation of past activities of the Medical Research Council in the organization and support of medical research was unstinted. Importance was attached to the fact that it was extremely unlikely that other bodies responsible for spending government funds on medical research would 'have access to better advice and information than that available to the Medical Research Council'. While decrying any suggestion that there should be anything in the nature of a

2G

potential monopoly of government support, Council declared it to be 'important that nothing should be done, for example by reducing the proportion of direct support for medical research provided through the M.R.C., to reduce the contribution that this organisation makes to knowledge and understanding in medicine'.

Reduction of support given to the M.R.C. might well, it was argued, lead to deterioration in the training given to young medical scientists and clinical investigators in establishments administered by the M.R.C. and in University and Hospital departments. The Council of the College reinforced their argument with the statement that 'much of the credit for the extension and for the improvement in the standard of clinical research in the National Health Service must be attributed to the support provided, directly or indirectly, by the [Medical Research] Council . . .'. This function within the ambit of the National Health Service 'must', it was insisted, 'be provided for now and in the future as a deliberate act of policy, rather than be allowed to happen incidentally, or worse, to languish . . .'.

In the matter of 'tardiness' in implementing the findings of research the College declared that 'this has not usually been the result of delay on the part of the research organisations, but rather on the part of those to whom the task of administering changes naturally falls'. The question was raised in rather tentative fashion as to whether the Health Departments concerned should not be made more clearly responsible for developing the results of medical research.

In conclusion, the letter drew attention to the benefits derived from the work of the Advisory Committee on Medical Research in Scotland. Subject to proper safeguards, research projects supported by the pharmaceutical industry were regarded as suited to promotion.

The Use of Fetuses and Fetal Material for Research
Report of Advisory Group: Comments of College: October 1972

In May 1970 the Secretary of State for Social Services and the Secretaries of State for Scotland and Wales appointed an Advisory Group to consider the ethical, medical, social and legal implications of using fetuses and fetal material for research. Sir John Peel, K.C.V.O. was Chairman and Dr Christopher Clayson, President of our College at the time, was one of the eleven Members of the Group which issued their Report in 1972.[76] The Report, having given concise summaries of the medical and legal backgrounds to the subject, dealt with the implications of research, the future control of research and terminated with a 'Recommended Code of Practice'. Evidence was obtained by the Advisory Group from a number of organizations and individuals representative of, among others, religious denominations, medical including obstetric and paediatric interests, midwives, nurses, patients and those engaged in research. Other evidence was obtained from the Society for the Protection of Unborn Children.

A request for comments on the Report was received by the College from the Scottish Home and Health Department in August 1972. Comments were sought on the recommendations and in particular on the Recommended Code of Practice embodied in the Report, which was considered by the President and Council. A communication sent to St Andrew's House on 4th October (1972) expressed 'approval of the Report as a valuable document'. The Council were especially impressed by the importance attached in the Report to ensuring a continuing supply of fetal material for services and research purposes; and by the clarity of the Recommended Code of Practice.

To many research is an emotive subject. It is appropriate to remember the words of Lord Samuel in his address on Science and Philosophy to the British Association in 1948: ' "The troubles of the world have come from science having advanced faster than morals: yes", he said, "but the remedy is not to hold up science; it is to speed up morals".'[77]

NATIONAL HEALTH SERVICE: PRIVATE PATIENTS

A letter dated 23rd June 1971 was received by the College from the Clerk to the Employment and Social Services Sub-Committee of the House of Commons Expenditure Committee. The purpose of the communication was to ask 'whether the College would wish to submit' a written memorandum 'on the provision of N.H.S. facilities for private patients'. Thereupon the Council of the College appointed a Committee to study the subject.[78] Members of the Committee were Drs A. W. Wright (Convener), J. C. Gould (Secretary), J. G. Macleod and H. J. S. Matthew, and their Report was presented to and agreed by Council in September 1971.

The Report stated categorically that the aim of the National Health Service must be to provide the highest possible standard of care for all patients and that arrangements for private patients within the Service must in no way interfere with this objective. Advantages to private patients, which formed the basis of objections to the provision of facilities for them, were given as choice of consultant and time of hospitalization; the waiving of certain hospital regulations such as restricted visiting hours; and additional amenities such as telephone and television. Nevertheless the Council considered that proposals for the inclusion of private in-patients and out-patients within the Service could be implemented without creating any differences in the standard of medical care. It was pointed out that failure to achieve this would have an adverse effect on the morale of hospital staff.

To some extent, the Report maintained, objections to private practice were contributed to by deficiencies in accommodation and staffing within the National Health Service. Deficiencies in these respects could result in long waiting lists, and the private patient could avail himself of an opportunity to avoid 'such bottle necks so that he may be said "to jump the queue" '. It was frankly allowed that criticism was most valid where priority in treatment was obtained by the private patient because the ordinary National Health Service facilities being unable to cope with prevailing overall demands. The Report emphasized the importance of private patients not being enabled to jump the queue when there are waiting lists, and gave as the only satisfactory solution to the problem the provision of adequate facilities for all medical requirements in terms of the number of beds and consultants. Provision of a larger number of single multi-purpose rooms, flexible in use and available for all patients, was suggested as a way of offsetting drawbacks resulting from the inter-mingling of private and non-paying patients. Medical indications would determine use of such rooms, which would be available for private patients if their medical condition warranted it, or if the rooms were not required for other patients.

Considering Scotland as a whole, the Committee recommended an increase of private beds in hospitals to at least 2 per cent of beds for acute cases as already obtained for England and Wales. A case was also advanced for the development of out-patient facilities for private patients. With not a little ill-disguised ingenuity it was said: 'The provision of adequate private in-patient and out-patient facilities in hospital allows part-time consultants, who presently require to see their private patients elsewhere than in hospital, to become more "geographically whole time". Working in one area such as the hospital would allow part-time consultants to make more efficient use of their sessional time' and so increase their availability for the benefit of N.H.S. patients. Towards the end of 1969, there were in all Scotland 395 part-time consultants inclusive of surgeons, obstetricians and anaesthetists.

Passing reference was made to the levying of charges in respect of drugs and medical supplies ordered for the private patient, and for the laboratory and diagnostic tests carried out on him. Exception was taken to the practice. In the wider fields of finance a policy was advocated whereby funds other than Treasury funds might be utilized for new buildings and equipment programmes, and as contributions to running costs. Possible sources suggested were the Provident Associations, Charitable Trusts and local benefactors. Commenting upon the disadvantage to hospitals and Boards of Management of payments by private patients being diverted directly to the Treasury, the opinion was expressed by the Committee that at least a proportion of these monies should go directly to the hospital managements.

Three other observations made in the Report deserve mention. Firstly, exception was taken to the frequent denial that there was a sizeable demand for private beds, largely based on low bed occupancy. Figures in this connection were regarded as meaningless in view of their scattered nature and the poor amenity offered in relation to the charges levied. Secondly, medical graduates, in the opinion of Council, left this country and the N.H.S. 'for improved medical facilities elsewhere rather than for income derived from medical practice'. Thirdly, there was a gain in prestige through influential patients, both from home and abroad, being attracted to have their medical attention in British hospitals. To attract these patients the quality of treatment and nature of the amenities offered were instanced as important.[79]

Such was the Committee Report on a subject which none would gainsay is somewhat delicate in this day and age. Reading between the obviously carefully chosen lines the impression—which may be entirely erroneous—was gained that the writers were aware of a certain unease. Doubtless they were conscious of being orientated by a primarily consultant outlook. What can be said however is that, in certain fundamental ways, views based on one region or one country for that matter cannot avoid being conditioned by distinctive local, regional or national attitudes. Interpretation by patients of their rights and by the profession of points of etiquette varies widely. Industrialization breeds materialism which in turn encourages elements of at times aggressive insistence in all economic strata of society. Complete appreciation of domiciliary situations does not always come easily to the hospital-bound doctor.

The House of Commons Expenditure Committee issued its Report in March 1972, and in April 1973 the Government published a White Paper entitled *Private Practice in National Health Service Hospitals*.[80] It was the declared policy of the Government 'to continue to make facilities available in N.H.S. hospitals for the treatment of private patients to the extent that this can be done without detriment to N.H.S. patients'. In the opinion of the House of Commons Committee abuses were not widespread or of any magnitude but the White Paper accepted the recommendation that control procedures in hospital should be more strictly observed.

REFERENCES

FINANCIAL CONSIDERATIONS

(1) R.C.P.E. (1954) *Committee of enquiry into the cost of the National Health Service. Memorandum.* (Typescript.)

(2) DEPARTMENT OF HEALTH FOR SCOTLAND. Committee on Scottish Health Services (1936) *Report.* (Chairman: E. P. Cathcart.) Edinburgh: H.M.S.O.

(3) 10 and 11 George 6, c. 27 (1947).

(4) DEPARTMENT OF HEALTH FOR SCOTLAND. Hospital endowments commission (1955) *Hospital Endowments: report.* Edinburgh: H.M.S.O.

(5) DUNLOP, Sir D. (1971) *Good Practices in the Manufacture and Quality Control of Drugs.* Basle: Pharma Information. (Address at the International Federation of Pharmaceutical Manufacturers Associations' Symposium, Geneva, September 20–23, 1971.)

(6) GREGORY, J. (1800) *Memorial to the Managers of the Royal Infirmary*, p. 96. Edinburgh: Murray & Cochrane.

(7) DOWLING, H. F. (1970). *Medicines for Man*, p. 31. New York: Knopf.

(8) R.C.P.E. (1945) *Memorandum . . . on Remuneration of Medical Practitioners.* Edinburgh: Royal College of Physicians.

(9) College Minutes, 7.ii.1956.

(10) R.C.P.E. (1957) *Memorandum of Evidence to be Submitted to the Royal Commission on Remuneration of Doctors and Dentists.* Edinburgh: Royal College of Physicians.

(11) MINISTRY OF HEALTH AND DEPARTMENT OF HEALTH FOR SCOTLAND (1948) *Inter-departmental Committee on the Remuneration of Consultants and Specialists.* (Chairman: Sir Will Spens.) London: H.M.S.O.

(12) MINISTRY OF HEALTH AND DEPARTMENT OF HEALTH FOR SCOTLAND (1946) *Inter-departmental Committee on the Remuneration of General Practitioners.* (Chairman: Sir Will Spens.) London: H.M.S.O.

(13) ROYAL COMMISSION ON THE CIVIL SERVICE 1953–55 (1955) *Report.* (Chairman: Sir R. E. Priestley.) London: H.M.S.O.

(14) DOTT, N. (1972) Personal communication.

(15) College Minutes, 7.v.1957.

(16) Ibid., 5.xi.1957.

(17) Ibid., 4.ii.1958.

(18) Ibid., 6.v.1958.

(19) Ibid., 3.v.1960.

MEDICAL STAFFING

(20) CENTRAL CONSULTANTS AND SPECIALISTS COMMITTEE (SCOTLAND) (1955) *Legal Liability of the Doctor in the National Health Service.* [Edinburgh: Privately printed.]

(21) College Minutes, 4.v.1954.

(22) Ibid., 26.vii.1955.

(23) Ibid., 3.xi.1959.

(24) Ibid., 24.vii.1956.

(25) MINISTRY OF HEALTH AND DEPARTMENT OF HEALTH FOR SCOTLAND (1957) *Committee to Consider the Future Numbers of Medical Practitioners and the Appropriate Intake of Medical Students.* (Chairman: Sir Henry Willink.) London: H.M.S.O.

(26) R.C.P.E. (1959) *Memorandum of evidence . . . to the Joint Working Party of the Ministry of Health, Department of Health for Scotland and the Joint Consultants Committee on the medical staffing structure in the hospital service.* (Typescript.)

(27) College Minutes, 4.xi.1952.

(28) Ibid., 4.xi.1958.

(29) SPENCE, Sir JAS. *et al.* (1954) *A Thousand Families in Newcastle upon Tyne*, p. 178. London: Oxford University Press.

(30) College Minutes, 28.vii.1959.

(31) Ibid., 3.xi.1959.

(32) Ibid., 7.xi.1961.

(33) MORRISON, S. L. (1973) The future of preventive medicine. In *Symposium on Preventive Medicine, Edinburgh, 1972*, ed. by A. T. Proudfoot, pp. 90–102. Edinburgh: Royal College of Physicians. (Publication no. 43.)

(34) JOINT WORKING PARTY ON THE INTEGRATION OF MEDICAL WORK. Sub-group on general practitioners in the hospital service (1973) *Report.* Edinburgh: H.M.S.O.

TECHNICAL SERVICES

(35) R.C.P.E. [1957] *Laboratory services in Scotland. Report by special committee.* (Typescript.)

(36) College Minutes, 5.ii.1957.

(37) R.C.P.E. (1967) *Memorandum on Hospital, Scientific and Technical Services, prepared by the . . . sub-committee.* (Convener: Dr R. H. Girdwood.) (Typescript.)

(38) Council Minutes, 24.x.1967.

(39) *Hospital Scientific and Technical Services:* report of the Committee (1968) (Chairman: Sir S. Zuckerman.) London: H.M.S.O.

(40) Council Minutes, 27.xii.1967.

(41) SCOTTISH HEALTH SERVICES SCIENTIFIC COUNCIL (1972) *The future of the scientific services. Report of a working party.* (Typescript.)

(42) Council Minutes, 23.ii.1972.

(43) SCOTTISH HOME AND HEALTH DEPARTMENT (1972) *Reorganisation of the Scottish Health Service: blood transfusion service. A discussion paper.* (Typescript.)

(44) Council Minutes, 31.v.1972.

(45) R.C.P.E. [1970] *Memorandum of evidence to the Ministry of Health on the report of the working party on the hospital pharmaceutical service.* (Typescript.)

(46) WORKING PARTY ON THE HOSPITAL PHARMACEUTICAL SERVICE (1970) *Report.* (Chairman: Sir Noel Hall.) London: H.M.S.O.
(47) Council Minutes, 14.iv.1970.

THE PHARMACOPOEIA

(48) R.C.P.E. [1959] *Report of the Committee on the revision of the British Pharmacopoeia 1958.* (Typescript.)
(49) Council Minutes, 1.vii.1959.

REORGANIZATION

(50) SCOTTISH HOME AND HEALTH DEPARTMENT (1971) *Reorganisation of the Scottish Health Services.* Edinburgh: H.M.S.O.
(51) Eliz. 2, c. 8 (1971).
(52) Council Minutes, 10.ix.1971, 23.ix.1971.

DOCTORS

(53) SCOTTISH HOME AND HEALTH DEPARTMENT (1971) *Doctors in an Integrated Health Service.* Report of a joint working party. Edinburgh: H.M.S.O.
(54) R.C.P.E. [1971] *Doctors in an integrated health service.* [Comments by Council.] (Typescript.)

NURSES AND NURSING

(55) NURSES IN AN INTEGRATED HEALTH SERVICE (1972) *Report of a Working Group Appointed by the Scottish Home and Health Department.* Edinburgh: H.M.S.O.
(56) COMMITTEE ON NURSING (1972) *Report of the Committee on Nursing.* (Chairman: Asa Briggs.) London: H.M.S.O.
(57) Council Minutes, 29.vii.1970.
(58) Ibid., 27.i.1971.
(59) R.C.P.E. [1971] *Report prepared by the . . . sub-committee . . . for submission to the Committee on Nursing.* (Typescript.)
(60) ROTHSCHILD, N. M. V., 3rd Baron (1971) Organisation and management of government research and development. In *Framework for Government Research and Development,* p. 16. London: H.M.S.O.
(61) Council Minutes, 25.i.1973.
(62) R.C.P.E. (1972) *Opinions of Committee of Council . . . on the Report 'Nurses in an integrated health service.'* (*Powell Committee.*) (Typescript.)
(63) R.C.P.E. (1972) *Opinion of Committee of Council . . . on the Report of the Committee on Nursing.* (*Briggs Report.*) (Typescript.)

SOCIAL WORKERS

(64) SCOTTISH HOME AND HEALTH DEPARTMENT. Working party on relationships with local authorities. Social work sub-committee [1972] *Employment of social workers in the Health Services.* (Typescript.)

(65) WILLIAMSON, J. [1972] *Comment on 'Report of working party on relationships with local authorities. Social work sub-committee. Employment of social workers in the health services.'* (Typescript.)

(66) Eliz. 2, c. 49 (1969).

(67) R.C.P.E. (1972) *Letter to Scottish Home and Health Department,* 2.vi.1972.

(68) SCOTTISH OFFICE. Social work services group (1972) *Report of the working group on the training needs of staff in day centres.* (Typescript.)

(69) R.C.P.E. (1972) *Letter to Social Work Services Group,* 11.x.1972.

RESEARCH

(70) COUNCIL FOR SCIENTIFIC POLICY (1971) The future of the research council system. Report of a C.S.P. working group. In *A Framework for Government Research and Development.* London: H.M.S.O.

(71) ROTHSCHILD, N. M. V., 3rd Baron. Op. cit., pp. 3–4.

(72) KIPLING, R. (1928) The story of Nicholas Culpepper: astrologer-physician. *Lancet,* **ii,** 1061.

(73) Council Minutes, 23.ii.1972.

(74) STANDING JOINT COMMITTEE OF THE SCOTTISH ROYAL COLLEGES (1972) *Letter to the Chief Scientific Adviser.*

(75) R.C.P.E. (1972) *Letter to the Chief Scientific Officer,* 11.ii.1972.

(76) SCOTTISH HOME AND HEALTH DEPARTMENT (1972) *The Use of Fetuses and Fetal Material for Research:* report of the Advisory Group (Chairman: Sir John Peel). London: H.M.S.O.

(77) SAMUEL, H., Viscount Samuel (1949) *Creative Man and Other Addresses,* p. 63. London: Cresset Press.

NATIONAL HEALTH SERVICE: PRIVATE PATIENTS

(78) Council Minutes, 13.vii.1971.

(79) R.C.P.E. [1971] *Provision of National Health Service facilities for private patients. Report by a Committee of the Council.* (Typescript.)

(80) DEPARTMENT OF HEALTH AND SOCIAL SECURITY (1973) *Private Practice in National Health Service Hospitals,* para. 40. London: H.M.S.O.

Chapter XXXIV

THE COLLEGE TODAY

In common language we speak of a generation as something possessed of a kind of exact unity, with all its parts and members one and homogeneous. Yet plainly it is not this. It is a whole, but a whole in a state of constant flux. Its factors and elements are eternally shifting. It is not one but many generations.

John Morley (*On compromise*)

THE CONSTITUTION: SALIENT FEATURES

The right of election is the very essence of the constitution.

Junius

For forms of government let fools contest;
Whate'er is best administered is best.

Alexander Pope

At the time of the erection of the College on the 29th November 1681 there were twenty-one Fellows listed in the Original Patent (Chap. III). Today (1974) there are 1729 names on the Roll of Fellows and 2490 names on the Roll of Members. Collegiate Members are included in the Roll of Members.

Responsibility for the management of College business is vested in the Fellows of the College who in the discharge of their duties administer the property and affairs of the College, enact its Laws, elect Fellows and Members and grant Licences and Diplomas. Fellows of the College elect their President, Vice-President and Council. In the words of Chapter I, Section 3 of the Laws 'a Meeting of the College shall be constituted by a Meeting of the Fellows'.

ANNUAL MEETING OF THE COLLEGE

The Annual Meeting of the College is held on St Andrew's Day should it fall on a Thursday, otherwise on the first Thursday after St Andrew's Day. At the Annual Meeting there are elected for the ensuing year the President, Vice-President, Council, four Fellows to be members of the Library Committee, two Fellows to be members of the Fellowship Committee and the members of other Standing Committees. Fellows who have not signed the Promissory Obligation and who, not being exempt, have not paid their annual subscription are not entitled to attend the Annual Meeting. On the other hand, a Fellow who has satisfied these conditions and who is unable to attend the Annual Meeting can vote by post for the election of the Council. By applying to the Secretary of the College he can obtain a voting paper with voting instructions and a College envelope in which to return his recorded votes. Only Fellows may attend an Annual Meeting, of whom twenty-five constitute a quorum.

ADMINISTRATIVE FRAMEWORK AND PERSONNEL

The Council

The Council consists of the President, the Vice-President and five Fellows. Fundamentally the Council is concerned with the general administration of College business and property, subject always to the Regulations and Laws of the College as they have from time to time been determined by the Fellows and subject to 'such instructions as may be given from time to time by the Fellows in Meeting assembled'.[1] This involves the consideration of business to be brought before Fellows at their next meeting, advising the Secretary in the preparation of billets for meetings, arranging such parts of the Examination for the Membership as come within the Council's jurisdiction and arranging the Examinations for the Licence of the College. It is required of the Council that at the Quarterly Meeting of the College in July, they submit for approval the Regulations for the Membership, and the Regulations and Plans for the Examination for the Licence of the College and for Diplomas in Special Subjects in Medicine. In addition the Regulations dealing with the annual subscription payable by Fellows have to be submitted at this same meeting. Should any question of censure, suspension or expulsion of a Fellow, Member, Licentiate or other Diplomate arise it is the responsibility of the Council to prepare an appropriate motion and arrange for the case to be considered at a meeting of the College.

Three members of Council constitute a quorum and it is within the competence of Council to appoint Committees to advise them, and membership of Council Committees need not be confined to members of the Council.

Council Minutes are preserved from 1844.

Committees

Standing Committees are elected annually and, with the exception of the Library and Fellowship Committees, membership by election is not necessarily limited to Fellows of the College. With the single exception of the Fellowship Committee each Standing Committee includes in its membership a co-opted Collegiate Member nominated annually by the Collegiate Members' Committee and enjoying the status of an elected member. Standing Committees include the Fellowship and the Library Committees, and the Committee on Specialist Standards, Vocational Registration and Postgraduate Medical Education. *Council Committees*, as for example the Laws Committee and the Advisory Committee on Examinations, are appointed by the Council. Membership is not necessarily limited to Councillors. Other *College Committees* are appointed and discharged by the President and are required to submit quarterly reports until discharged. Their membership is not confined to Fellows of the College. The Croom Committee on the Future of the College (Chap. XXX) is a recent example of a College Committee.[2] With regard to expenditure special provisions are made in the case of the Library Committee, but otherwise Council approval is necessary before any expense can be incurred by a Committee. A Collegiate Members' Committee is elected annually, consisting of nine members who are resident in the United Kingdom.

The President

Any Fellow may propose one of the Fellows as President at the Annual Meeting. On the motion being seconded, the nominee is elected President unless more than one Fellow is proposed and seconded in which event voting is carried out by card, votes being counted by Scrutineers nominated by the President still in office. In the event of a tie between two candidates, the senior on the Roll is elected, and if there are more than two nominations any Fellow receiving more than three-fourths of the votes is elected President, otherwise a further card vote is taken on the two names which have received the greatest number of votes.

A poignant College Minute recorded in December 1912 that 'owing to the state of his health' Dr George Gibson was unable to allow his name to be proposed as President.[3] He died within weeks leaving behind him memories of 'all that was best and highest in medicine'.[4]

An unusual situation arose at the Quarterly Meeting in August 1773. The Vice-President (Dr Boswell) was in the Chair. A letter was read from the President (Dr Drummond) resigning his office as he had gone to live in Bristol. Accepting the resignation, College decided 'it was not incumbent on the Society to continue the Propreses in the chair as President'. Dr Boswell thereupon retired. Dr James Baird was then elected propreses and this was followed by the election of Dr William Cullen as President, who forthwith 'made choice of Dr. Boswell as propreses'. Seventeen members including Dr Cullen were present at the sederunt.[5] An interesting feature was that Cullen was not, and had not previously been, a member of Council. Poole in his personal notes written about fifty years later expressed the view that the President should in accordance with the Laws at the time have been elected by the Council and not by the College at large.[6]

Three Presidents died while holding office. The first was Dr James Forrest in 1722. There is no mention of his passing in the Minutes but Dr William Eccles 'acted as Praeses till next Election day'.[7, 8] In 1766, Dr Robert Whytt died in similar circumstances. No difficulties of procedure arose in connection with the election of a successor. Dr Whytt 'haveing at Last Election Continued Doctor Porterfield Propreses . . . the College' continued 'him President till next General Election in December'.[9] The Minutes gave no inkling of the professional distinction of the recently departed President. A hundred and forty-two years were to pass before a similar situation arose. Dr Underhill died while holding presidential office in 1908. Council recommended that the College should elect a successor to hold office until the Annual Election Meeting and that any vacancy which might arise in Council as a result should not be filled. The Vice-President (Dr John Playfair) was 'unanimously elected President', the necessary motion being moved by Sir Thomas Fraser who referred to 'the course adopted . . . in May 1776 [sic] when a vacancy had occurred by death' but made no mention of the circumstances which had followed the resignation of Dr Drummond in 1773.[10]

Laws of the College at present in force (1972) determine that if the President (or any member of Council) shall die or resign during his period of office, the Fellows present at any Ordinary Meeting or at an Extraordinary Meeting called for the purpose may elect a President (or member of the Council) in place of the deceased, and that any Fellow so elected shall serve for the remainder of the period of office for which the deceased was elected.

Today formalities are reduced to a minimum when a newly elected President assumes office. Election having been determined by the College, the outgoing President transfers the Robes of Office to his successor. Confident that there will be no resurgence of Stevensones and Trotters, past and present Presidents do not jointly sign an inventory of College documents as in bygone days. The following illustrates the practice followed in the early years.

'Inventarie of what was delivered by Dr. Wm. Eccles late Pres^t of the R.C. Phy^s in Ed^r to Dr. M. Sinclair, after his election as Pres^t—Decr 1708.

1. 'Im: The principall Patent, with the Great Seal appended dated at Whitehall 29 Novr 1681'
2. 'Ratification thereof in Parl^t dated 16 June 1685. These two in a black box'
3. 'The Act and Decreet. The Lords of Session, in favours of the said College, against George Stirling, Chirur^n., Apothe:^{e}, dated 25 March 1685, Marked N.1'
4. 'Act and Decreet, the Lords of Session, in favours of the said Coll. agt. the said Geo. Stirling, dated 19 Feby 1686, marked No. 2.'
5. 'Decreet pronounced by the Pres. & Censors of the said Coll: agt. the said Geo. Stirling, dated 18 Decr. 1685. Marked 3.'
6. 'Act of the Privie Councill, discharging the passing of the Chirurgions' Signature, dated 19 Jany. 1682, marked No. 6.'
7. 'Act of the P.C. ordaining the Coll. of Phys^s to visit the Apothecaries Shops, and examine themself^s dated 21 Nov: 1684. Marked N.4. This is ratified with the Patent.'
8. 'Act of the Lords of Session ordaining letters of Horning to be direct agt. George Stirling, dated 30 March 1686. Marked N.5.'
9. 'Another Act of the Privie Councill requiring the College of Phys^s. to visit the Apoth^s. shops, dated 8th Jany 1685, marked N.7.'
10. 'Warrant for a grant in favour of the said College authorizing them to examine graduates of Medicine in our own Universities befor their being allowed to practise Medicine in Ed^r, dated 19 Nov: 1686 Marked N.8.'
11. 'Act of the Privie Councill exeeming the Members of the said Coll. from attending the King's host, dated 12 Nov. 1688, marked No. 9'
12. 'Warrant to the Lyon anent the armes of the College, dated 25 Novr 1682. N.10'
13. 'Commission. The said Coll. to Dr. Dickson to agree with the Chirur^s. dated 9 Feby. 1695. Marked N. 11'
14. 'Dr. Dickson's agreem^t: with them, dated 11 July 1695, marked N. 12'
15. 'Dr. Trotter then Pres^t. has approbation thereof, marked N. 13. All those papers are in bundle A.'
16. 'Bundle B containing doubles of papers in which the College is concerned, being 19 in number. This bundle wants one.'

17. 'Bundle C containing papers relating to James Nisbet's process, being in number twelve.'
18. 'Bundle D containing doubles of papers in which the College is concern'd, being in number thirty three.'
19. 'The Seal of the College cut in copper with this inscription round it "Sigillum etc., etc.".'
20. 'The reverse of the said Seal likeways cut in copper with this motto "prudentia vigilantia".'
21. 'Bundle E. containing papers relating to the process intended by the Coll: agt. George Stirling, being in number eight.'

'Edin. 1 Feby. 1709. The above papers were delivered by Dr. Eccles to Dr. Matt: Sinclair, present Prest in witness whereof they have both signed this prests day and year forsaid

(signed) Matt: St. Clair. P.
Will: Eccles'

'Edin. 20 Decr 1716. Then received the above mentioned papers (except one amissing in Bundle B.) from Dr. Sinclair late Prest: in witness whereof I have signed this prest. day and year forsd.

(signed) Will: Stewart
Matt: Sinclair

Ther was likewise delivered by the said Dr. Sinclair the rights of the Lands disponed by Sir James McKenzie to the Colledge.

As also Rights of the Lands purchased from Baillie Jeffrey etc. . . .'[11]

In their day two Presidents had the altogether unusual experience of holding similar office in the Royal College of Surgeons of Edinburgh. To add to the uniqueness of the experience the two concerned were father and son. David Maclagan was President of the Surgeons in 1826 and of the Physicians in 1856, and his son Andrew Douglas Maclagan, President of the Surgeons' College in 1859 and of our College in 1884. A brother of Douglas Maclagan was Archbishop of York.[12]

Membership of Council

Nominations for election as *Councillors* require to be submitted to the Secretary at least five weeks before the Annual Meeting. Any two Fellows can nominate one or any number of Fellows not exceeding six. A Councillor can hold office for five successive years if elected annually, after which he can be re-elected if he has been out of office as Councillor for one year. If only six Fellows have been nominated, those six are automatically declared by the President to be Councillors for the ensuing year. In the event of nominations exceeding six, decision is arrived at by the use of voting papers to which are added the closed envelopes containing the papers of

Fellows who have voted by post. The four Scrutineers count the votes. Should nominations prior to the meeting be less than six, further nominations are invited after those originally proposed have been declared Councillors. A card vote in respect of new nominations is carried out if they exceed the required number.[13]

It is intended that Council shall include three co-opted members—two Collegiate Members and one representative of the Faculty of Community Medicine. Pending necessary adjustments of the Royal Charter these representatives attend as observers.

Election of Councillors is followed by that of the *Vice-President* from among the newly elected Council. A card vote is employed, each Fellow writing the name of the Councillor whom he would wish to be Vice-President. Any Councillor receiving three-fourths of the votes is automatically elected, otherwise a second card vote is conducted in connection with the two names which received the greatest number of votes on the previous occasion. Seniority determines final choice in the event of a tie.[14]

In the absence of the President, his duties devolve upon the Vice-President.

The first Vice-President was Sir Robert Sibbald, being nominated by the President.[15] Initial attempts to modify the right of the President in this connection were unsuccessful.[16, 17] In 1695 a Regulation was passed determining that the oldest Censor or failing him the oldest Councillor in Town should act as Vice-President[18] but the old practice was reverted to within four months and persisted with for many years.[19]

Committee Membership

At the Annual Meeting there remain to be elected four Fellows for the Library Committee and two for the Fellowship Committee. One or more Fellows can be nominated by any two Fellows for each of these Committees, election being by card vote if necessary. Any two Fellows may also make one or more nominations for other Standing Committees—these being elected annually and with membership not confined to Fellows.

The Treasurer

Abstracts of the Treasurer's Accounts appeared for the first time in the Minutes for 1696. This followed the compulsory vacation of his office as Treasurer by Dr Oliphant.

The practice was then established of appointing a Committee to report on the accounts of a retiring Treasurer soon after the election of his successor. This was followed in the course of time by the appointment of the Committee every year or other year. The accounts were kept in Money Scots until 1723 when a change was made to Money Sterling—£8:6s:8d. Sterling being equivalent to £100 Scots. Funds passing through the Treasurer's hands usually included Bonds for Fees payable by Fellows on entering the College with the result that recorded balances of accounts were apt to be misleading. During the period 1696 to 1736 there was an annual balance in hand on eighteen occasions, the amount varying from £736. 11. 4 Scots in 1713 to £1. 9½ Sterling in 1730. Deficiencies, euphemistically referred to as 'Due Treasurer', occurred on four occasions amounting to as much as £928. 1. 4 Scots in 1723.[20]

Today election of the Treasurer is by Council within seven days of the Annual Meeting. The same applies to the Secretary, Registrar and Honorary Librarian and all must be Fellows of the College.

The Treasurer is accountable for the College Funds and has to ensure that the balanced College Accounts are presented, duly audited, at the May Quarterly Meeting. Titles and securities other than those in the custody of the Bank are in his care. Subject to an overriding figure of £400 the Treasurer can expend money on essential repairs to buildings; and his many duties, subject to control by Council, include those of manager of the College Hall, supervision of the College Officers and domestic staff, and the organization of the ceremonial and social activities of the College.

On his retirement the Treasurer's books and vouchers must by the Laws be examined by a special Council Committee.[21] In 1961 it was resolved that the Committee should consist of the President.[22]

The College accounts are audited by a Chartered Accountant appointed by the Council.

The Secretary

From 1709 to 1772 the office of Secretary and Librarian was conjoined.

As in the case of the Treasurer, the Secretary's duties today are multifarious. In addition to taking charge of all general correspondence and administrative supervision of clerical staff, he is responsible for summoning meetings, ensuring the efficient recording of Minutes and when instructed, submitting to College Meetings the Opinions of Council on matters previously considered by them.[23]

Early in their existence the College had borne in on them the imperative necessity of reliable recording. In 1707, the following Minute was made: 'The Colledge takeing into their Consideratione the manifold prejudices they have sustained by wryteing the minuts of their sederunts on loose shedules and not Ingrosseing them in the minut book, whereby the Colledge Registers have been rendered . . . Imperfect, severall years minuts haveing been [sic] Intirelie lost . . . ordain' the Scroll Minute of each Meeting to be engrossed in the Book before the next Meeting, and the Minute Book after comparison with the Schedule to be 'subscrybed by the President in presence of the Colledge'.[24]

Without question the new Minute was intended to prevent a repetition of the loss of records revealed at the time of 'The Ryot' (Chap. XIX). At that time Dr Trotter maintained 'that the Books and Papers were keeped up by Doctor Stevinson for eight Moneths, and that when delivered, he found all the Laws and Acts for the space of four years, taken out of the lesser Register, and that many Acts and Minuts are still un-delivered'. Stevensone's defence in his 'Information' was that this 'last Misrepresentation anent Abstracting the Registers, is a very heavy Charge, but he is so Wise in his Wrath, as only to Libel it at random, because he is Conscious he cannot fix it on any particular person. The Truth is, the first three years after the Erection, Hugh Stevinson was Clerk, and the Register for the most part lay in his House, and what was done in the Colledge, was Minuted in Papers a-part, which were to be inserted in the Registers, if the Clerk neglected this, it was none of Doctor Stevinsons fault, for the Clerk continued after Doctor Stevinson was off, all Doctor Sibbalds time, who got the Books, Seals, and Papers from the said Hugh Stevinson, and what was delivered by Doctor Sibbald to Balfour, and by him to Doctor Stevinson, was re-delivered and brought in entire to the Colledge, and if any Papers be Abstracted or amissing, Doctor Stevinson and his Party, will heartily concur for finding them out.'[25]

The fact remains however that the original papers were never found. To attempt to apportion blame at this late stage would be pointless.

Paterson drew attention to an absence of Minutes for the periods 5.xii.1700–16.v.1701, and 4.xii.1701–16.xi.1702; and suggested that there may have been no meetings or that difficulty had been experienced in getting attendances necessary for a quorum.

Loss of Minutes was even more serious than appeared on the surface because, previous to printing of the Laws in 1789 the practice had been adopted of periodically copying out 'Resolutions sembling Laws' into a separate book which was subject to occasional revision.[26]

Dr Boswell, during the time he was Treasurer, was granted permission to take delivery of the Minute Book with a view to making 'excerpts relative to the History of the College'. There is no record of a History having materialized.[27]

The Registrar

The duties of the Registrar may if thought desirable be combined with those of the Secretary. They include responsibility for all correspondence in connection with qualifications granted by the College after examination, and making the necessary arrangements for candidates to attend such examinations.

An almost intolerable responsibility was imposed on administrative officers and staff with the massive increase of candidates for the Membership Examination in the 1950s and 1960s. The Secretary bore the brunt of the new burden as the duties of Registrar had been combined with that of Secretary for as long as can be remembered. In seeking to ease the situation the Council decided to appoint a Registrar who, with duties as already defined in the Laws, would be responsible for all examinations and would attend Council Meetings as required. To date the office has been a preserve of the Macleods—William of that ilk having been appointed in 1960 and Hugh in 1968.[28, 29]

The Bursar

A final decision to appoint a College Bursar was arrived at in September 1972.[30] In addition to supervision of administrative and office staff his duties include assistance to the Treasurer in the inspection and maintenance of the College fabric and buildings and in organizing entertainments; to the Secretary in dealing with correspondence, maintaining the Roll of Diplomates, and preparing Diplomas; and to the Registrar in organising the Examinations Office. The Bursar attends meetings of College and Council and where appropriate meetings of Committees.

The Librarians

The *Honorary Librarian* acts as Convener of the Library Committee; exercises general control of the Library; supervises the Librarian and Library Staff; and presents the annual Library Committee Report at the November Quarterly Meeting of the College. He is elected by the College.

Among the duties of the *Librarian* are the cataloguing of all new acquisitions in the form of books and periodicals, and attendance at all Library Committee meetings at which he minutes proceedings. A definition of duties gives no indication of the bulk of work entailed, when account is taken of the time involved in obtaining references, exchanges and translations, aiding lines of research being studied by Fellows and Members, and periodically preparing exhibitions of selected books in the Library.

The Auditor

The Auditor is a Chartered Accountant who in addition to auditing the Accounts of the College prepares an annual abstract of the accounts for circulation to Fellows and submission at the May Quarterly Meeting.

The Clerk

Paterson considered that the Clerk had always been a member of the legal profession.[31] This may have been true of the first fifty years, but apparently was not the case in the mid-nineteenth century to judge by the irate words of an exasperated Honorary Secretary—Dr Alexander Wood. 'Can you tell me', he asked, 'of what profitable use a Clerk is . . . ? While he was a law agent, there might be some apology for the office. Now there is none.'[32] But generalizations are dangerous. There was a time when the office of the Clerk was certainly no sinecure. It is on record that in 1724 a Mr Riddell after twenty-six years' duty as Clerk, gave in an account of his services 'since his entry. And therupon the Colledge ordered' him to be paid 'five guineas In full of his said accompt Which he accepted of though his accompt Extended to much more, And then the Colledge gave him thanks for his good services'.

Nor was that the end of matters: Mr Riddell permitted himself to be re-engaged, perhaps because henceforth the Clerk was 'to have a Croun for his paynes' whenever any of the Fellows attended at the University to examine for Medical Degrees.[33]

Mr Riddell had been preceded in office by Hugh Stevenson (1682–4), Alexander Home (1693–5) and R. Trotter, W.S. (1695–7), and was followed in 1727 by H. T. Balcanquall, Writer.[31]

Referring to the comparative scarcity of early records Jolley attributed it in part to the Clerks having been lawyers, who treated College papers passing through their hands in the same way as papers belonging to other clients. Clerks held office until their decease and the probability is that College papers were never handed over to newly appointed successors.[34]

At the present time the appointee is required to be a solicitor in practice in Edinburgh and normally acts as Legal Adviser to the College. His appointment is an annual one, and he attends all the Meetings of the College and the Quarterly Meetings of the Council. The technical proceedings in connection with the election of Councillors including the arrangements dealing with postal voting are his responsibility, as are the preparation and issue of all Diplomas of the College under the direction of the President and Secretary. In the event of the College entertaining a disciplinary motion for censure, suspension or expulsion, it rests with the Clerk to send within three days a copy of the motion to the accused individual.

Other Officers elected by the College are the *Editor of Publications* and the *Editor of the College Chronicle*.

REPRESENTATIVES OF THE COLLEGE

The General Medical Council

Under the terms of the Medical Act 1956 'the choosing of an appointed member [of the G.M.C.] shall be for a term not exceeding five years, and a person may be chosen to be an appointed member who has previously been a member of the General Council'.

Nomination of any one Fellow for election can be submitted by two Fellows, and in the event of no nominations being received by the Secretary any two Fellows at the College Meeting can nominate a Fellow for election as the College Representative on the General Medical Council. Election is by ballot in the event of there being only one nomination, and by card vote if there are two or more nominations.

The Conjoint Committee of Management of the Triple Qualification

A Fellow is elected annually at the Quarterly Meeting in May as one of three representatives of the College and customarily holds office for a period of three years. Any two Fellows can nominate any one Fellow for election, and if no nomination has been received any two Fellows can nominate a Fellow at the College Meeting.

The Edinburgh Post-Graduate Board for Medicine

Annually at the July Quarterly Meeting the College elects a Fellow to serve for a three-year period, with eligibility for reappointment. The position with regard to nomination is the same as that in connection with the Conjoint Committee except that election takes place at the July Quarterly Meeting.

As need arises the Council appoints representatives of the College to act on other medical and charitable boards.

MEETINGS OF THE COLLEGE

Meetings fall into the customary three broad categories: the Annual Meeting already dealt with (q.v.); Quarterly Meetings; and Extraordinary Meetings. Ordinarily only Fellows may attend an Annual Meeting. Collegiate Members may attend Quarterly Meetings. Extraordinary Meetings can be called for Fellows only, or Fellows and Members. Twenty-five constitutes a quorum. The general pattern in force dates back to 1681.

Quarterly Meetings are held on the first Thursday of February, May and November and on the third or fourth Thursday of July each year. Billets are issued not less than four days before each meeting. Informal discussion on any matter of interest may be permitted by the Chair at a Quarterly Meeting but no binding decision can be taken at the meeting on any subject raised in discussion.

Should the President or Council consider it necessary on account of business of a special nature arising, an *Extraordinary Meeting* is called. Furthermore should the President or the Secretary receive a requisition signed by any five Fellows calling for an Extraordinary Meeting and indicating the purpose for which it is sought, it is incumbent upon the President to call the meeting within twenty-one days of receipt of the requisition. Similar conditions apply to the calling of an Extraordinary Meeting of the Fellows and Members to consider business affecting the general interests of the medical profession and the public. At an Extraordinary Meeting no business can be transacted other than that for which the meeting was originally called.

Fellows and Collegiate Members may inspect the Minutes of College Meetings both prior to and after their approval.

Points of Procedure

Business for transaction at any meeting has been previously considered by the Council and is brought before the meeting as a Committee Report, a Motion by Council or a

Motion by a Fellow, duly seconded. In broad terms the practice dates back to 1681. During Sir Robert Sibbald's Presidency a Committee appointed to revise the College Laws commented in relation to an Act of 1681: 'Whereas by the said . . . act for avoiding of confusion and losse of tyme it is provided that befor any thing be considered by the Colledge it shall first be considered by the President and Council, which some have misconstructed as if there were a negative power in the Council, which was never intended', and then adjured the College to consider 'whether or not it is not consistant enough with the same law that things may be only communicated to the President in some cases'.[35]

The Billet summoning a meeting contains notices of any Committee Report, Motion by Council or Motion by a Fellow which is to come up for consideration by the College, and where a Committee Report is involved, it is either circulated with the Billet or made available in the College to Fellows in advance of the meeting. At the meeting amendments are put in writing: it is not competent to move a direct negative to a motion, and a Fellow unwilling that the College should come to a decision on any motion, may move 'the previous question'. A Fellow or Collegiate Member protesting against a decision reached by the Fellows may request that his dissent be recorded in the Minutes.

A motion for the suspension of Standing Orders has to be submitted in writing to the President or Chairman together with a statement of the business proposed to be discussed and of the reasons for urgency. To be carried a motion for suspension requires a three-fourths majority of those voting.

A two-thirds majority of the Fellows voting at two Meetings of the College is essential for the carrying of a motion for the abrogation or alteration of a Law. In the event of an amendment of the original motion being approved at the second Meeting, the amended motion is determined at a third Meeting.

The following are among other situations for which special majorities are prescribed:

Election to Honorary Fellowship	— 9/10
Election to the Fellowship	— 3/4
Election to the Membership	— 3/4
Alienation of Property	— 3/4
Money Votes	— 3/4
Penal Cases	— 3/4

Motions and amendments are determined by a simple majority of the Fellows voting, except where special majorities are required by the Laws. The President has one vote as a Fellow and a casting vote in the event of an equal division, except where voting is in connection with the election of a new President or Vice-President.

It is interesting to compare present requirements with those of Laws enacted on 9th December 1681 on the occasion of the third meeting of the College. On that day it was determined that:

(1) new Laws should be considered at two separate meetings before being enacted,
(2) every proposal to abrogate a Law must be considered at three several meetings before a decision is made, and
(3) every proposal before being laid before the College 'shall be represented to the President and Council, who shall take it into consideration, and report the same at the next Meeting of the College with the sense of the Council thereupon'.[36]

THE COLLEGE LICENCE IN MEDICINE

A candidate seeking admission to examination for the Licence must possess a medical qualification approved by the Council, which must be satisfied that he is of good moral character; or he may obtain the Licence of the College conjointly with those of the Royal College of Surgeons of Edinburgh and of the Royal College of Physicians and Surgeons of Glasgow—The Triple Qualification. Before receiving the Licence, the Applicant is required to sign a Promissory Declaration undertaking 'under pain of forfeiture' of the Diploma, not to advertise or be connected with anyone who is engaged in any discreditable kind of medical work, and to obey the Laws of the College.

At first no regular list was kept of Licentiates who did not proceed to the Fellowship, but the College does have a record of those awarded the Diploma of Licentiateship since 1858.

THE AWARD OF DIPLOMAS IN SPECIAL SUBJECTS

The College grants, after examination by themselves or in conjunction with the Royal College of Surgeons of Edinburgh and the Royal College of Physicians and Surgeons of Glasgow, Diplomas in Psychological Medicine, and may grant Diplomas in other special subjects in medicine as may be considered desirable from time to time.

Those to whom the College has granted Diplomas are known as Diplomates.

MEMBERS OR FELLOWS OF A FACULTY OR JOINT FACULTY

The College may establish a Faculty in the College or may combine with any other body or bodies to establish a Joint Faculty in the College, and can delegate powers separately or jointly with other bodies to members of a Faculty or Joint Faculty. It is decreed that the affairs of each Faculty or Joint Faculty shall be managed and administered by a Board of Faculty, and shall be regulated by Standing Orders approved by the College. The College retains the right to revoke any powers which it has delegated to any Faculty.

Admission to Membership of a Faculty is by examination in all but exceptional cases: admission to Fellowship of a Faculty may or may not be by examination. On admission, Members or Fellows of a Faculty or Joint Faculty are presented with appropriate Diplomas after having signed an undertaking to abide by the Standing Orders of the Faculty and the Laws and Regulations of the Royal College of Physicians of Edinburgh as they apply to Members or Fellows of the Faculty.

On 3rd February 1972 it was resolved that in combination with the Royal College of Physicians and Surgeons of Glasgow and the Royal College of Physicians of London a Joint Faculty of Community Medicine should be established.[37]

In retrospect it should be recorded that when in 1960 consideration was being given in the South to the creation of a Faculty of Pathology or College of Pathology, the Council of our College was emphatic that the Membership Examination should not be modified to suit specialists and that Clinical Medicine should remain an integral part of the examination.[38]

ELECTION AS A MEMBER OF THE COLLEGE

In the early days of the College there was an intermediate grade of 'Candidat' through which Licentiates had to pass before becoming Fellows. Although not named in the Charter the procedure was prescribed in the bye-laws. According to Paterson the aim was to ensure deliberation before admitting to the Fellowship although in most instances admission in practice as Licentiate, Candidate and Fellow took place at one meeting after the three several examinations prescribed for the Licence had been passed. The grade of 'Candidat' was tacitly allowed to disappear after 1710.[39]

The new order of Membership was established in 1861. At a Council meeting over a hundred years later it was determined that election to Membership was not the hallmark of a specialist but indicated suitability to undergo training for specialization.[40]

For election as a Member a person must have held a qualification in Medicine approved by the Council for not less than two years, and must have undergone training of a nature and duration which satisfies the Council. Other than in specified exceptional circumstances the passing of an examination arranged in accordance with College Regulations is a prerequisite to election as a Member. Selection of examiners is a responsibility of Council. It is within the authority of Council to exempt a person from the whole or a part of the prescribed examination who has been proposed by two Fellows, and about whom supporting evidence as to his qualifications and training and as to his having attained professional eminence has been given in writing. Motions for the election of candidates to the Membership are determined at a Quarterly Meeting and the names of those elected are placed on the Roll of Members maintained in the College.

At a Meeting of Council on 12th July 1966 a letter was received from the Secretary of the Board of Medical Examiners of New York State asking for information concerning the standard of examination for the Edinburgh Membership. The enquiry had been prompted by consideration by the Board of possibly exempting those in possession of the M.R.C.P.Ed. from its State Examination, along lines already obtaining in connection with holders of the M.R.C.P.London. Information was sent, as requested.[41] Rather surprisingly the College did not pursue the subject further nor did it receive unsolicited information. However enquiries have established that 'in 1970 the New York State Board of Medical Examiners decided to exempt members holding the M.R.C.P. of Edinburgh in the same manner as those holding London membership'. A prerequisite for any candidate applying for exemption is that he shall have passed the examinations of the Educational Council for Foreign Medical Graduates, and that the State Board are satisfied with his qualifications and professional experience.[42]

Collegiate Members

Since 1970 any Member after election can apply to be designated a Collegiate Member and to have his name placed on the Roll of Collegiate Members after signing 'the Declaration'. Collegiate Members are required to conform to all Laws and Regulations pertaining to Members; are entitled to certain privileges in addition to those of Members including attendance at Quarterly Meetings; and annually have to elect from among their number a Collegiate Members' Committee. The Collegiate Members' Committee represents the view of Members to the Council, and nominates one Collegiate Member for co-option to each Standing Committee of the College other than the Fellowship Committee. An annual report is submitted by the Collegiate Members' Committee at the November Quarterly Meeting of the College.

ELECTION AS A FELLOW OF THE COLLEGE

And there's a hand my trusty fiere,
And gie's a hand o' thine.

Robert Burns

It is a privilege and duty to nominate Members for election to the Fellowship. Nominations are scrutinized by the Fellowship Committee which consists of two Members of Council, and two Fellows who are not Members of Council and who are elected by the College. Asked by the Fellowship Committee in 1956 how soon a Member might be advanced after election as a Member, Council left the Committee entirely free but considered that 'only in exceptional circumstances and in Members of outstanding ability should such recommendation be put forward within one year', and advised two to three years.[43] A statement concerning the merits of each nominee is submitted by the Committee to Council which is responsible for submitting to the College names of Members considered suitable for advancement to the Fellowship. In giving their considered views Council take account of qualifications, professional standing, appointments held and contributions to literature. It is within the power of Council to recommend Medical Graduates or Licentiates of exceptional distinction who are not Members of the College for election to the Fellowship, but in any one year not more than four such Fellows can be elected.

Proposals for advancement to the Fellowship are intimated in the Billet for, and announced at the May Quarterly Meeting; and motions for the election to the Fellowship are proposed and seconded on behalf of the Council at the following Quarterly Meeting in July. The motion for the election of Members to the Fellowship may take the form of a single motion or a series of motions according as the President may think desirable. Aware that there might be deserving Members in the United Kingdom and abroad who had escaped the notice of the Fellowship Committee, the President and Council asked Dr Lindsay Lamb to investigate the position of Members of more than ten years' standing. Dr Lamb conducted two studies: one of Members elected in the United Kingdom and Ireland during the period 1950–9, and a second of Members living abroad elected during the years 1950–5. The studies took the form of letters of enquiry and *pro forma* asking for certain particulars. A paper entitled 'The Member's Route to the Fellowship' based upon his factual findings was prepared for Council by Dr Lamb and later discussed informally by the College at the Quarterly Meeting in February 1971.[44]

On election the names of Fellows are placed on the Roll of Fellows. A newly elected Fellow can take his seat at the next Quarterly Meeting after his election or at any subsequent Quarterly Meeting, but cannot attend the Annual or any Extraordinary Meeting until he has first taken his seat at a Quarterly Meeting. Before taking his seat each Fellow is introduced to the President and Fellows present; has the Promissory Obligation read aloud to him before affixing his name to it in the presence of the Fellows; and has extended to him by the President on behalf of the Fellows, the right hand of Fellowship. Any Fellow resident abroad, who is temporarily in the United Kingdom but unable to attend a Quarterly Meeting, can by arrangement appear before the President and affix his name to the Promissory Obligation after having had it read aloud to him. Thereafter he is entitled to the rights and privileges of Fellows who have taken their seats as mentioned above.

In 1695 a Regulation was passed excusing Fellows who did not reside within the area of the College's jurisdiction from paying the full admission fee. These *Non-Resident Fellows* who represented a considerable body of individuals were not permitted to participate in the privileges of, or to sit and vote in the Meetings of the College. First official use of the term 'Non-Resident Fellow' appeared in a Resolution of 1726 which at the same time as recognizing the preferential fees accorded them, required that Bonds should be given to meet the difference in the event of their coming to reside in Edinburgh.[39]

Subscription rates to the College still take account of a Fellow's place of domicile. Use of the term 'Non-Resident Fellow' has disappeared these many years and as the official lists demonstrate satisfaction is known in linking the names of Fellows and Members with their country of residence. In no sense of the word is the association of distant Fellows and Members with the College a nominal one. This nurture of distant links has been for long the intent of the College as evidenced in a letter from the Honorary Secretary (Dr R. D. Haldane) answering a Fellow's enquiry in 1859. Dr Haldane wrote: 'We are taking steps to procure a new Charter and the almost universally expressed wish has been that the Non-Resident Fellows should be brought into a real Connexion with the College . . .'.[45]

Humility is a desirable attribute. Jolley contributed to it when he wrote about the College archives: 'It is possible to establish the exact date when a man is elected a Fellow. It is not possible to establish the date when he ceases to be a Fellow . . . A Fellow who remained in Edinburgh made no impact on the College when he died.'[46] However correct, a little unintentionally unkind!!

THE HONORARY FELLOWSHIP OF THE COLLEGE

The College can offer its Honorary Fellowship to persons of high distinction, whom the Fellows desire to honour. Nominations are made by the Council and proposals are considered at an Extraordinary Meeting called for the purpose. Honorary Fellows who are medically qualified are entitled to all the privileges of ordinary Fellowship.

During the first twenty-five years of the College's existence the privilege of voting was granted to four non-medicals who were made Honorary Fellows—Lord Polwarth,[47] Mr Scougal,[48] Lord Anstruther[49] and the Earl of Wemyss. [50] In so far as records can be relied on it would seem that prior to 1800 there was only one Honorary Fellow *ex officio*.

INHERITED RESPONSIBILITIES

THE LIBRARY

The Library is the College's richest possession—materially, historically and spiritually. It is in the literal sense of the words a national treasure and as such the College's responsibility for it is immense.

Superintendence of the Library, the purchase of books and the making of recommendations to the Council for the disposal of unwanted books is vested in the Library Committee. This Committee consists of the President, the Vice-President, Treasurer, Secretary, Honorary Librarian, four additional Fellows elected annually and a co-opted Collegiate Member nominated by the Collegiate Members' Committee. Three members form a quorum.

Use of the Library is governed by Regulations drafted by the Library Committee, submitted to Council, and finally approved by the College. The extent to which all classes of readers and borrowers can use the Library is determined by the current

Library Regulations which are displayed in the Reading Rooms. Provision is made under the Regulations for other than Fellows and Members to consult or borrow books, and for the application of graded special penalties in the event of failure to return, loss of or damage to a book or books. Council's approval is required for the loan of manuscripts, and no book can be sent or taken out of the British Isles without the express permission of the President and the Honorary Librarian. The Librarian has authority to refuse to issue on loan any book on the score of its rarity or physical condition.

ALIENATION OF COLLEGE PROPERTY: TRUSTEESHIP

The subject is not lacking unsavoury links with the not very remote past history of the College (Chap. XXIV).

No motion involving the alienation of any part of the property of the College, or the application of it to other than the ordinary purposes of the College, can be determined unless approved by a majority of three-fourths of the Fellows voting at two Meetings of the College (Quarterly or Extraordinary), six days at least intervening. Similar conditions apply to the payment by Council of donations, subscriptions or other payments exceeding £50 for other than ordinary College expenses. In the case of the proposed sum not exceeding £200 Fellows can vote such a sum at any Meeting by a majority of three-fourths of those voting.

The securities for all the sums of money and property constituting part of the College funds and all associated heritable rights are taken in favour of the College in its corporate name, or in favour of the Trustees 'for the time being and their successors in office'.

The Trustees consist of the Treasurer and four Fellows. Three constitute a quorum. Vacancies occurring from whatever cause are filled by Council who advise the College at the next Quarterly Meeting of action taken. It is the duty of theTrustees to manage the investments of the College and to invest all monies (other than those retained by permission in the Bank and by the Treasurer) in the name of the College in its corporate capacity. They have power to lend out and invest the monies belonging to the College in the purchase of real or heritable property, or upon real or heritable security, or upon bonds, mortgages, debentures, debenture stock, deposit receipts, preference, guaranteed, deferred or ordinary stocks, shares or other securities of any Company, Bank, Insurance Company, Corporation, or Public Trust or Board.

FORFEITURE OF FELLOWSHIPS, MEMBERSHIPS, DIPLOMAS AND LICENCES

Chapter IX of the Laws (1974) is entirely devoted to this situation. Happily recourse to application of the Laws in question is a rarity. None the less when circumstances compel, the problems to be dealt with bristle with legal complexities. For this reason alone Chapter IX of the Laws (1972) is given below, verbatim.

'Of Forfeiture of Fellowships, Memberships, Diplomas and Licences

1. Any Fellow, Member, Licentiate or Diplomate who shall have been convicted by the Law Courts of the United Kingdom, of the Republic of Ireland or of any other country, of any felony, misdemeanour, crime or offence, or who shall, after due inquiry, be judged by the Fellows to have been guilty of infamous conduct in any professional respect, or who shall, after due inquiry, be judged by the Fellows to have acted in an unbecoming or unprofessional manner, or who shall, after due inquiry, be judged by the Fellows to have violated this or any bye-law, rule or regulation of the College, may if the Fellows see fit, be censured or be deprived, *sine die* or for such time as the Fellows may determine, of all the rights and privileges which as Fellow, Member, Licentiate or Diplomate he does or may enjoy, or may, if the Fellows see fit, be expelled from the College and deprived of his Fellowship, Membership, Licence or Diploma, and of all the rights and privileges which as Fellow, Member, Licentiate or Diplomate he does or may enjoy.

2. The proceedings for censure, suspension or expulsion shall be the following:— The motion for the censure, suspension or expulsion of the Fellow, Member, Licentiate or Diplomate shall contain a statement of the offence of which the Fellow, Member, Licentiate or Diplomate is accused. This motion shall be prepared by the Council and shall be laid, with the Council's opinion thereon, before a Meeting of the College at which the motion shall be proposed and seconded. A vote of the Fellows shall then be taken as to whether it is expedient to entertain the motion. In the event of its being decided by a majority that the motion shall be entertained, the further proceedings shall be the following:— The motion shall be determined at another Meeting of the College specially summoned for the purpose and held at an interval of not less than two months after the first. The object of this Meeting shall be announced in the Billet which shall be issued at least fifteen days previous to the Meeting. A majority of not less than three-fourths of the Fellows present shall be required to carry the motion. At the determination of a motion for expulsion it shall be competent for the Fellows to modify the same to a motion for suspension or censure, and in like manner at the determination of a motion for suspension it shall be competent for the Fellows to modify the same to a motion for censure, such modifications being carried always by a majority of not less than three-fourths of the Fellows present.

3. Within three days after the Meeting at which the Fellows decided it to be expedient to entertain the motion for censure, suspension or expulsion the Clerk shall transmit a copy of it to the Fellow, Member, Licentiate or Diplomate accused.

It shall be held sufficient evidence of this Law having been fulfilled, if the notice has been posted in a registered envelope bearing the address of the Fellow, Member, Licentiate or Diplomate, as given in the latest issue of the Medical Register. The Clerk shall also, and as soon as possible, inform the accused of the date of the Meeting of the College at which the motion of his censure, suspension or expulsion will be determined, at the same time informing him of the terms of Law 4 of this Chapter.

4. The Fellow, Member, Licentiate or Diplomate accused may appear and plead, either personally or by a representative, at the Meeting at which the motion is to be determined.

5. It shall be in the power of the Council to shorten the period of two months between the proposal and the determining of the motion, should the Fellow, Member, Licentiate or Diplomate accused petition to that effect.'[51]

FINANCIAL POLICY

> . . . *Learning sits*
> *Remote from worldly cares,*
> *And leaves to skilled financiers its*
> *Pecuniary affairs.*
>
> A. D. Godley

> *I do proclaim*
> *One honest man—mistake me not—but one;*
> *No more, I pray—and he's a steward.*
>
> William Shakespeare (*Timon of Athens*)

The Early Background

Poole summarized the position admirably and honestly when he wrote that the financial transactions of the College 'in borrowing, prosecuting for, receiving donations of money disclose a long state of undignified penury, notwithstanding many beneficent deeds almost to ostentation. They had even the will to comfort themselves nobly, while the scantiness of their Funds either perpetually impeded their generosity or chastised them for exercising it.'[52] Moreover, as Paterson stated: 'From 1704 to 1731 we find constant records of debts contracted by the College; and it seems to have been by no means an unusual thing to contract fresh loans in order to pay off sums already borrowed from other parties—so that the College was never really out of debt all the time'.[52] One scarcely credible Council Minute records how in order to pay a debt due to the Bank of Scotland, £50 was borrowed from the Secretary of the Bank![53]

At the time in question two major factors contributed to the financial insecurity. First of these was involvement of the College in the disastrous affairs of the Darien Scheme sponsored by the Company of Scotland trading to Africa and the Indies (Chap. I). Ironically, although understandably, in June 1697, the African Company asked that two or more members of the College should 'visite the droggs that are come home for thyr use'. According to Poole the College acceded to the request, but with what result he does not say.[54] Eventually the College having originally invested £200 Stg. in the venture[55] was fortunate to recover about £120 Stg. when the Company was wound up. The other factor was the proclivity of the College in purchasing properties for which money had to be frequently borrowed.[56] From time to time, to meet recurrent crises recourse was made to various expedients. Thus on one occasion at short notice selected Fellows were called upon to make part payment of outstanding Bonds,[57, 58] and on another occasion an attempt was made to secure immediate and full payment of Bonds by dispensing with the need to pay interest due.[59]

From the outset Bonds played a fundamental rôle in College finances. They were required as a security that individuals obtaining the College Licence would, when called upon, proceed to take the Fellowship. In effect the Bonds were security for payment of the remainder of fees chargeable upon Fellows. The sums due upon Bonds were not necessarily paid immediately on attaining the Fellowship. According to the convenience of the College the Treasurer held them in pledge and called for payment in whole or in instalments. Why this should have been is not stated, but the fact remains that interest was payable on unredeemable bonds after they had become due! On the other hand, a small minority of Licentiates, for reasons unknown, were never called upon to redeem their pledges.[39]

Apparently in 1693 it was recognized that there was a need for a tightening of procedure. The College required that a candidate for the Licence should 'Consigne in the Thesaurers hands The soume of Thrie hundreth merks scots' to be returned if, 'at his Tryall he shall be found unsufficient … and if he be found qualified Then befor he be Licensed he is to give bond to the Thesaurer for ane hundreth merks to be payed whenever he shall be admitted Socius'.[60] But there were other difficulties. A custom, not without attendant risks, had developed of Bonds being given in the name of the Treasurer and not of the College. This was put right by requiring that all Bonds given by Intrants should be 'for the use and behoof of the colledge'.[61] When on a future occasion the procedure was not adhered to, the offending Bond was destroyed and a new one made out correctly.[62]

2H

1950–1974

The Treasurer is responsible for advising Council in so far as day-to-day income and expenditure are concerned. Advice about Investments and Property ownership is the responsibility of the Trustees who have the unremitting assistance as adviser of an expert in Finance (q.v.).

In recent times successive Treasurers have promoted a policy directed towards keeping expenditure within reasonable bounds despite progressively increasing costs; maintaining and improving the fabric and furnishings of the Hall with as one object the safeguarding of the College in the future from a possible combination of unavoidable inordinate expenditure and a worsening of the financial climate; and utilizing any favourable balance as between income and expenditure to increase capital investment. The task of Treasurers has been no easy one. Their problems have been accentuated by both national and Collegiate factors. The barometric state of the money market and the creeping trend towards inflation need no elaboration. In many respects domestic factors were more variable and almost equally unpredictable. A judiciously cautious policy, uninfluenced by either extravagant optimism or morbid pessimism, has contributed greatly to a situation of stability allied to a rational confidence, at a time when international, national and medical affairs have been in a state of constant flux.

Paradoxically a considerable part of the twenty years under consideration was one of prosperity for the College. This was attributable in almost total measure to an unprecedented increase in the number of Fellows and the number of candidates for the Membership Examination. Whereas the number who sat the Examination in 1952 was 396, it rose to a peak of 1559 in 1963 with a subsequent fall to 1024 by 1966. It redounds to the credit of Treasurers during these and subsequent years that they missed no opportunity to reiterate their insistent opinion that this source of income on an altogether unique scale had to be evaluated as a temporary and not a permanent phenomenon. In this they were largely influenced by the fact that the policy of many of the countries overseas from which collectively the majority of candidates were coming, was to establish their own Colleges of Physicians with powers to issue their own diplomas. Subsequent events confirmed the accuracy of the forecast. Again as later predicted, a decline in the number of candidates was accentuated by changes in the form of the Membership Examination. This became evident with the introduction in 1968 of a two-part examination, Part I being common to the three British Royal Colleges of Physicians; and even more dramatically in 1972 when a common Part II Examination was instituted.

Reference has been made to the progressive rise of costs. Naturally their mention conjures up visions of increased expenditure on stationery, wages, heating and lighting. What could escape notice is an 85 per cent increase in the rateable value of the College Buildings. Major expenditure was incurred in redecorating the Entrance Hall, Assembly Hall and New Library for the first time in over forty years. Cleaning of the portraits was undertaken at the same time. There then followed cleaning of the stonework of the building, the provision of long overdue satisfactory amenities in the way of cloakrooms for both sexes and modernization of antiquated kitchen facilities. The antiquity of some fittings was typified when the need arose to exclude light from the large glass windows in the cupola-type roof of the Assembly Hall. Not only were the old blinds in use worn out and ineffective but a team of skilled tradesmen had to be employed to install and later remove them on each occasion the Hall required to be darkened.

Accommodation for administrative and secretarial staff continues to be seriously inadequate. Some relief was provided when No. 8 Queen Street, which had been College property for over one hundred years, was occupied by the College for the first time. Internal structural alterations were involved in providing new office accommodation and the opportunity was taken to effect major changes in the central heating system to enable the total requirements of the College to be catered for by one plant. Wisely having regard to the considerable and, in many instances, inestimable value of some of the College's books and other possessions, a strong room was installed. Most impressive of all was the opening as library reading rooms in 1955 of an Adam Suite which formed part of the original house at No. 8 Queen Street. The suite has been described by authorities as the finest of the Adam period in Edinburgh. Prior to being opened as reading rooms the suite was decorated and furnished in keeping with the period of the original architect. In 1974 the College decided that the Adam Suite should be named after Sir Stanley Davidson.[63]

Further property was purchased in May 1970. This consisted of No. 11 Queen Street. The purchase followed acceptance of the Croom Committee's recommendation to the effect that the College should remain on its present site. One use to which the newly acquired building will be put is the establishment of a modern seminar room which will constitute a memorial to a former highly esteemed member of Council, the late Dr James Laurie. The time of implementation of this decision will be determined by the results of a public appeal launched by the College in 1972 and by the phasing of any new structural programme.

Two subjects appear with understandably unfailing regularity in the Annual Reports of successive Treasurers. The first of these is the Library Endowment Fund, the resources of which are entirely at the disposal of the College in the same way as the General Funds. The Endowment Fund was initiated in 1953, by using the proceeds of the sale of the College Laboratories. The fund has always been regarded as a reserve fund and donations to the College are added to it provided always that such a procedure is not precluded by conditions attached to the donation or legacy. In reality the existence of the Library Endowment Fund is evidence of adaptability to unpredictable impact on College activities and procedures, of changes in the shape of medicine—clinical and educational. The College administers over twenty other Bequests and Funds, to which widely varying conditions are attached sometimes making for great difficulty in utilizing the legacies for the maximum benefit of medicine in general and the College in particular. This is the second subject not infrequently raised in the Reports of Treasurers. It is eminently desirable that any testator making a bequest to the College should allow as much discretionary power as possible to the College.

Reference to the Library is essential if not only because it is at one and the same time the most valuable possession of, and one of the most expensive charges on, the College. Some of the problems facing those in charge of Library affairs have been detailed in Chapter VI. Economies must be effected. To this end agreement has been reached with other medical libraries in the City to terminate the duplicate and sometimes triplicate purchase of what have been termed 'the more esoteric journals'.

INHERITED TRADITION

In the continual remembrance of a glorious past individuals and nations find their noblest inspirations.

Sir William Osler

In everything the old overlaps the new.

G. M. Trevelyan

Tradition, together with such words as patriotism, ideology, nationalism, and democracy are often only hesitantly used in modern times lest their intended meaning be misconstrued. A fear of undertones prevails. But can there be, even in the minds of the most sceptical of Fellows, Members and Licentiates, doubts concerning the significance and meaning of tradition in relation to our almost three-hundred-year-old College?

In having regard to tradition the College is mindful of the strivings and example of those who have gone before. To remain proudly conscious of the past does not imply blind worship of, or for that matter, uncritical deference to our predecessors. We are as aware of their errors as of their accomplishments and we have lessons to learn from them all as the College applies the experience of three centuries in facing the challenge of the future. Tradition is the product of Corporate Fellowship over the years and not a by-product of individual Fellows. Therein are to be found the very beginnings and continuing strength of College Tradition. If great men among Fellows are remembered, it is because their greatness has stood the test of time. There is no need for any apologia. Consider the major religious, national and political ideologies prevailing in our own time, and how one and all embody ancestral figures and customs in their avowed convictions.

Some find the preservation or perpetuation of aspects of traditional ritual irksome, if not unacceptable. To see at a graduation ceremony a senator clad in sports jacket and grey flannel trousers only partially hidden by academic robes was not an elevating experience—more especially as the offender was a northern Scottish graduate and the University an English one. None the less, there can have been few who participated in the spectacularly impressive quincentennial celebrations of the University of Glasgow who were not moved in ways incapable of tangible expression. Some who were critical at the outset soon became vociferously appreciative. A surprising experience was to witness an elderly alumnus of long-standing international fame battling for a place in the auditorium among recent graduates and students. There was no aversion to tradition by the young on that occasion, even although there may have been failure to pay deference to a generation twice removed. When the day of our College's Tercentenary arrives, it behoves the College (as indeed it will the University of Edinburgh in 1984!) that a generation once or twice removed is as meaningfully concerned in celebrations as those still hale and hearty.

Let it not be forgotten that for almost three hundred years the Royal College of Physicians of Edinburgh has played an important part in the civic life of the City of Edinburgh and in the national life of Scotland. This has long been recognized by the medical profession over a wide area and by many of the laity in our own islands. Throughout its existence the College has adjusted itself to changes in the social milieu, and has shared in the vicissitudes of national survival, cultural progress and scientific advances. It would be strange indeed had there not been a simultaneous growth of tradition—a tradition of which if seen in true perspective, the College is entitled to be proud. Nor is the tradition of the College of a purely symbolic nature. It is imbued with a conception of Fellowship never more evident than at the present time. Allied to it is a rarely declared but undisguised affection among Fellows for the

College. As one Fellow wrote to the President after a social occasion: 'The warmth of the welcome and the whole friendly atmosphere made me appreciate the Fellowship as something much more valuable than a mere academic qualification'.[64] Convention does not account for the relative frequency with which generous gifts and munificent bequests to the College have been coupled with expressions of affection and gratitude.

Fellows and Members of the College today and in the years to come, can scarcely claim to be respecting the spirit underlying their Promissory Declarations if they seek to discard Collegiate tradition *in toto*. Present-day procedures may include some which, being inherited, appear irrelevant, inappropriate and unnecessary. What of procedures initiated today? How many of them will be regarded as irrelevant and inappropriate in the future? No matter—their place in the evolution of College Policy and Tradition will deserve to be remembered.

A complete definition of tradition is impossible. Elsewhere in the text there are scattered evidences of it in practice. Certain aspects of College Tradition have a recent, if not immediate significance and are mentioned below. Some are associated with a harmless but whimsical pedantry, pardonable if only because of their historical origins in the dim and distant past.

The Charter

The original Charter granted by Charles II in 1681 is in the possession of the College, framed and housed in the Queen Street Library. Unfortunately the Royal Seal is missing although the mark of its former place of attachment to the bottom of the parchment is easily discernible. Disintegration of the Seal, a not uncommon occurrence, probably explains its absence. The probability, taking the date of the Charter into account, is that the Scottish Great Seal used had been that of 1660, with as legend IVSTITIA ET VERITAS. This particular Seal had on the reverse side: 'The King on horseback to dexter with curling hair, clad in plate armour . . . The horse has no caparisons, only a small saddle cloth. It gallops over hilly country with a view of Edinburgh from the south and the Firth of Forth in the distance.'[65]

The College Seal and Coat of Arms

Incorporated by Royal Charter in 1681, the College took advantage of their rights under the letters patent to design a seal for themselves in the following year. Their next step was to seek what was technically termed a Royal Augmentation of a canton of the Royal Arms of Scotland. This entailed obtaining a Royal Warrant. Application for this was favourably received; and a Warrant issued by King Charles II, and countersigned by the Earl of Moray as Secretary of State, instructed the Lord Lyon King of Arms '. . . to allow and confirm into the said Colledge of Physicians our Coat of Scotland in the Dexter Canton of their Armes; and that as a Mark of our Royal favour to the said Colledge, and as the proper nationall difference'.[66] Two Seals are extant—one inscribed '1682' and the other '1861–1681': both embody the Royal Augmentation.

There is no official record of the Arms to which the newly authorized canton was added and to complicate the position, unsigned and undated manuscript papers in the possession of the College indicate that at some later date further steps were taken to obtain 'Armes'. One document is linked with the name of 'John Campbell Hooke of Bangeston Esquire, Lyon King of Arms'—Lyon for the period 1759–96. Because of the absence of any Royal Augmentation, Barden concluded that the document was in all probability no more than a draft.[67]

Even if only a draft, the document is of particular interest in the light of the 'Armes' eventually granted to the College (q.v.). The proposals for the 'Ensigns Armorial' were:

> 'Or, an Esculapean Club in pale, wreathed about with a dead Serpent distilling drops of Blood, his head in Base, supported by an Imperial Crown, between three Laurel Garlands, one in chief, and two in the flanks, all proper; within the Royal tressure gules. Above the Shield instead of an Helmet, is placed a Physicians Cape, with a Plume of Laurel; and on each side thereof instead of a Mantling, a Physicians Robe, all proper; and on a wreath of their Liveries is set for Crest, A Game Cock in a Crowing posture, trampling on a Serpent which raises itself, aiming a stroke at his breast both proper. And in an Escroll above, this Motto Eia! et magnos dirigit Urbes, and below, Pro Sceptro tuemur. On a Compartment under the Shield, and of which spring Thistles and Poppies surrounding the same, are placed for Supporters, on the Dexter the God Apollo Pythicus, with his Bow in his hand, a Quiver of Arrows at his back, a Radiation round his head, and a dog sitting and looking up to him at his feet; And on the Sinister the Goddess Hygieia, in purple Rayment, fringed with gold, bruising a Serpent below her feet all proper.'[68]

Gruesome indeed!—more so even than Edgar Allan Poe.

The subject evidently came up again in an indirect way in 1830. In July of that year a letter from the Lyon Office addressed to Dr G. A. Borthwick was emphatic: 'There seems to have been no Patent of Arms asked for or obtained from this Office at any period for the College—those for the College of Surgeons are matriculated in the common form'.[69] This did not discourage the Council of our College from inserting the Common Seal into the Laws in 1852.[70]

More than sixty years later, on 4th December 1897 an Extraordinary Meeting of the College remitted to Council '. . . to consider the expediency of obtaining a Grant of Arms'.[71] Doubtless to the surprise of Council, they were advised by an Advocate that the College Arms had never been registered but that the same Arms had been in use by the College 'since shortly after the date of the first Charter (1681) up to the present time'. As a result the Council decided to apply to the Lord Lyon King of Arms for a grant of Arms.[72] At their next meeting Council authorized the Treasurer to proceed with Registration of the College Arms at a cost of approximately £70.[73] In January 1900 the Council studied and approved a drawing of Arms drafted by the Lord Lyon King of Arms.[74]

Matriculation of the Arms was not finally effected until 5th April 1900. The Extracts of the Matriculation contained the following:

> "Whereas Sir John Batty Tuke . . . President of THE ROYAL COLLEGE OF PHYSICIANS OF EDINBURGH and the Council and Fellows . . . have by Petition of date the sixteenth day of March 1898 . . . represented unto US THAT on the twenty-ninth day of November 1681 the Royal College . . . received a Charter of Incorporation under the Great Seal of King Charles II and that a second Charter . . . was granted . . . the sixteenth day of August and sealed . . . the thirty-first day of October 1861: THAT by both these Charters the said College was empowered to use a common seal and that certain heraldic devices have been used on the said seal from a period very shortly after the date of the first mentioned Charter . . . but have never been recorded in the Public Register of All Arms and Bearings in Scotland as the Ensigns Armorial of the College.'[75]

The Matriculation then proceeded to indicate that Ensigns Armorial had been devised, assigned, ratified, confirmed and matriculated. In all the circumstances the College met with more tolerance and understanding from the Lyon Clerk and Keeper of the Records, than the defaulting citizen of today expects from his Income Tax Inspector. Among Edinburgh academic institutions, the 'Honourable College of Chirurgeans' was the first to acquire a coat of arms.[76]

And what of the detailed particulars of the newly acquired Arms of our College? They certainly reflect changes which had taken place since the days of Lyon John Campbell Hooke of Bangeston! Had the image of the College acquired docility, the fire in the bellies of the Lords Lyon lost lustre, or Victorian prudery gained ascendancy?! The following is the description of the Coat of Arms as recorded in the Public Register:

'Argent, issuing from a mount in base an oak tree proper fructed Or, on a canton of the last a lion rampant within a double tressure flory counter Flory Gules being the Royal Coat of Scotland the right to bear which in dexter canton was granted to the College of Physicians at Edinburgh by Royal Warrant under the sign manual of King Charles II of date 25 February 1682 (1681 old style in England) directed to Lyon. Above the Shield is placed a helmet befitting their Degree with a Mantling Vert doubled Argent above which is set for Crest—issuing out of a ducal coronet the figure of Apollo couped at the waist with bow and quiver on his back and holding a lyre in his hands wreathed about the temples with a garland of bay all proper and in an Escrol over the same this Motto NON SINIT ESSE FEROS. And upon a compartment below the Shield are placed for Supporters two savages wreathed about the middle with oak proper the one on the dexter holding in his exterior hand a covered cup Or and that on the sinister a sprig of rue Vert.'[75]

It is thought that the motto is derived from Ovid (Epistulae ex Ponto, II, ix, 47—Adde quod ingenuas didicisse fideliter artes Emollit mores *nec sinit esse feros.*' ('Note too that a faithful study of the liberal arts humanises character and *permits it not to be cruel.*' If this be accepted the motto is a modified quotation of part of a sentence from Ovid. Translated the original part read 'and he is not permitted to be cruel'. By substituting 'non' ('not') for 'nec' ('and not') in the original wording a motto was devised which was independent of anything in the nature of the original extraneous context. Such it is assumed was the reasoning of those who decided upon the form of words for the motto of our College.[77]

The oak tree is a device closely connected with King Charles II and sprigs of oak have been used as Royal badges since his reign, and 'there are very few grants of arms which include the Royal Coat and the bearing of such an "augmentation" must be considered a great privilege'.[78]

As to the Legend of the College Heraldic Seal, Stevenson and Wood described it as SIGILLUM COLLEGIJ REGIJ MEDICORUM EDINBURGI. 1682. At end a thistle head slipped, leaved and inverted. Cabled border. Diam. 2 1/8 in.'[79]

Mention in the Minutes of the College Arms does not occur again until July 1959. Reporting on a consultation with the Lord Lyon, the College Librarian described having been told that 'the correct form for cap badge and buttons is the coronet and Apollo only'. The shield would appear only on the lapels of the uniform. At the time of the interview the Lord Lyon had suggested that 'the College should have its own flag and this would show the Oak tree with the Lion rampant in the top left hand corner'.[80] Within a week Council resolved that the College should have a flag.[81]

Eventually a flag was obtained displaying the Lion rampant, and oak tree with acorns. It is flown at the time of such College functions as Quarterly Meetings,

Symposia and, perhaps ironically for some candidates, at the time of examinations. On Royal occasions and on St Andrew's Day the Saltire flag is invariably 'run up'.

When later in 1961 the Treasurer had occasion to consult the Lord Lyon King of Arms regarding a Medallion for the President, the Lord Lyon recommended that the College Crest in enamel should be worn by the President 'suspended by a green ribbon as green is the colour of the College Livery'.[82] Previously, extreme erudition on the part of the President and Secretary had emboldened them to question the accuracy of the wording on the Crest. Doubts were expressed as to whether Ovid had not been misquoted. With understandable and sagacious agility Council arrived at a compromise agreement and transferred further consideration to the College Laws Committee.[83] The views arrived at have already been given (q.v.).

Censors

Inevitably with the passage of time, some features of early procedure and tradition have disappeared into the limbo of the past. The appointment of selected Fellows as Censors is a case in point. Maitland, writing in the middle of the eighteenth century, gave an account of the background to the duty of the Censors at that time. He described how persons practising 'the Art of Physick, without an immediate Warrant from the . . . President and College' were liable to a 'Penalty of Sixty pounds Scotish, or Five Pounds Sterling for every Month they practise Physick without such Warrant; and every Person continuing to practise after the first Mulct . . . the Fine to be doubled monthly . . . one Moiety of the said pecuniary Mulcts to the Use of the Poor, the other to that of the College'.

Continuing, he explained that

> 'the College is . . . impowered to chuse yearly two of their Members Censors, who, together with the President, may summon before them all unqualified Practitioners of Physick within the Jurisdiction . . . whom they may severally punish by pecuniary Mulcts . . . and as often as the . . . President and College shall think fit to hold a Court for that Purpose, they shall previously acquaint the Lord Provost, or other Magistrates of Edinburgh . . . in order for a Bailiff of the Town's being appointed to sit with them on the Trial of each Offender; for it shall not be lawful for the . . . President and College to fine any Surgeon or Apothecary, Citizens of Edinburgh, without the Consent of the Provost, or one of the Bailiffs of Edinburgh, who is to be present at all judicial Proceedings in such Affairs; and if at any Time the said Provost and Bailiffs should refuse to be present, it shall be represented to the Privy Council, that the College may be inabled to proceed against the . . . Offenders'.[84]

The Censors had also duties involving the inspection and maintenance of standards in druggists shops. It is questionable whether these functions were ever discharged other than perfunctorily and they gradually ceased to be exercised. Likewise the prosecution of unwarranted practitioners fell into abeyance many years before the Medical Act of 1858. A natural consequence was that the new Charter granted to the College after the passing of that Act contained no reference to the appointment of Censors. This however did not deter Council in 1953 from nominating two Fellows 'to act as Censors for a period of two years as from the forthcoming examination'.[85] The resuscitation, if such it could be called, was shortlived.

The following were the Censors in the first few years of the College's history:

>   1681–2. Dr. Balfour and Dr. Livingstone (died whilst in office).
>   1682–4. Sir Andrew Balfour and Sir Robert Sibbald.
>   1684–5. Dr. Learmonth and Dr. Trotter.[86]

Other departures from long-established traditional procedures took place in the present century. In 1904 the sederunt was for the first time ascertained by cards instead of roll call[87], and in 1958 the Roll of Attendance was abolished.[88]

The Fiscal/Procurator Fiscal

This office was finally relinquished at the same time as that of Censor. The first persons appointed were medical men (Archibald Pitcairne 1682; Dr Cranstoun 1684; Dr Spence 1693) but after about 1695 lawyers were appointed.

Mr W. Riddell, appointed Clerk in 1698, undertook the additional duties of Fiscal until 1706 when he was followed by Robt. Stewart (1706–26) and Henry Balcanquall (1726). In 1727 Riddell resigned the Clerkship and was succeeded by Balcanquall who then 'of consent of . . . Wm. Riddell the College choysed him [Balcanquall] for Proc^r Fiscall' (q.v.).[89, 90] Their duties were to institute and conduct prosecutions for irregular practice and infringement of the rights of the College.

Precedence without and within College Precincts

An indication has already been given of the significance attached to precedence by the College on State and other occasions (Chap. XXV). Public functions at which the College is represented by the President and at which the President is preceded by the

College Officer bearing the College Mace include the Medical Graduations of the University of Edinburgh; the 'Battle of Britain' and Royal British Legion annual commemoration services in St Giles Cathedral; the annual Inaugural Church Service in St Giles Cathedral of the Edinburgh Festival; and the annual Church Service on St Andrew's Day at the same High Kirk. The President attends also the Triple Qualification graduations in Edinburgh and Glasgow.

For reasons unknown the College is not, as previously, officially represented at the annual inaugural service in St Giles of the General Assembly of the Church of Scotland. A pew is none the less reserved in St Giles Cathedral for the College on special occasions, being the front pew on the north side of the chancel. For the President a stall is allocated for official occasions below the organ, and his macer sits below him.[91] There are in the possession of the Cathedral a Bible and a Hymnal, both bound in green leather with the crest of the Royal College of Physicians engrossed upon them. Inscribed on the two volumes are 'This Bible [Hymnal] given to St. Giles Cathedral for use in the Stall of the Royal College of Physicians, Edinburgh by Charles McNeil President. All Saints Day 1942.'

At some time, the exact year being unknown, doubts arose as to the processional order of precedence to be observed by individual Fellows taking part in these and comparable occasions. This prompted the Council of the College to issue the following directions:

Royal College of Physicians

ORDER OF PRECEDENCE

As Manager of all Ceremonies in which the College may take part, the Treasurer has felt the want of any definite order on which he may rely. The Council have therefore approved the following Order of Precedence to be observed at Ceremonial Functions, and they trust that the Fellows of the College will co-operate in carrying it into effect:—

The President

———

The Vice-President

———

Past Presidents in the order of their seniority as Presidents

———

The Council in order of seniority on the College Roll

———

The Secretary

———

The Fellows of the College in their order on the Roll of Attendance

———

The Treasurer, as Master of Ceremonies.

When the College attends any functions robed, any Fellows who attend without robes should bring up the rear of the procession.

As far as the President, Vice-President, Members of Council, the Secretary and Treasurer are concerned, the Order of Precedence holds good at all sederunts when they enter the College Hall, the company of Fellows being already assembled. The Registrar follows the Secretary, the Treasurer as dictated by long-established custom bringing up the rear from which position he can best exercise his control as Master of Ceremonies.

Insignia of Office

The Mace referred to above was gifted to the College in 1893 by (Sir) Alexander Russell Simpson towards the end of his period of office as President.[92] Previously in 1831 Dr W. Moncreiff, a Fellow and Librarian of the College had presented a gold-headed cane to the President and Fellows for the use of the President.[93] A second cane was gifted twenty-two years later by Mr Craig, Surgeon, Ratho and had a particular historical value in that it had originally belonged to, and been regularly used by Dr William Cullen.[94] From the time that it came into the possession of the College this second cane has been treasured as one of the insignia of the Vice-President. A third cane, or 'baculum' as it is referred to in the records was presented to the College for the use of the Morison Lecturer.[95] Incorporated in it are the coiled serpent and cock associated with Aesculapian mythology.

There is in the possession of the College another insignia of office consisting of 'a brass mounted mace with ebonised handle'. The Aesculapian serpent and cock are incorporated in the design of the mace. Little if anything is known of the origins of this insignia other than that there is an item in the Treasurer's Accounts for the year ending 1st February 1847—'Peter Muir for Officers Staff £1: 1: —.' [96] It is the custom for the staff to be carried by the Officer who uses it when introducing guests on such occasions as receptions.

'Collegiate Costume'

Through tatter'd clothes small vices do appear;
Robes and furr'd gowns hide all.

William Shakespeare (*King Lear*)

In the case of other Members of Council, College gowns constitute the only insignia of office and are worn at all Ordinary and Extraordinary Meetings of the College. A long time elapsed before a decision was arrived at to have an official gown, and the decision made, it took almost as long to agree on the form the gown should take. First consideration seems to have been given to the needs of the President. In August 1822 the suggestion was made that as 'it had formerly been the custom for the President on particular occasions to wear a gown' the President and Treasurer should make enquiries 'on this subject'. To this the College agreed and gave authority to them to provide a suitable gown.[97] Apparently no immediate action was taken, possibly because of heavy expenditure incurred in other ways. However, the subject was again raised in 1830, but consideration was further delayed[98] for three months when a Committee was appointed 'to consider of a suitable dress to be worn by the President on public occasions, and also of Gowns to be used by the Fellows . . .'.[99] There is no further reference to the matter in the Minutes until 1846 when 'the President exhibited . . . a gown which the Council recommended should be adopted as part of the official costume of the Fellows'. The intention was that the Fellows should provide themselves with gowns and this may account for the College deciding to delay any decision yet again.[100] Discussion was renewed at the next Quarterly Meeting when a motion to accept the recommendations made at the previous meeting was lost by a majority of 16 to 10.[101]

More than twenty years elapsed before prospects of Fellows being suitably robed assumed really tangible form! At a Quarterly Meeting in November 1865 Council recommended to the College 'that a Costume should be adopted' and that the question of choice of costume should be remitted to them [the Council]. College agreed.[102] At long last in May 1867 it was reported that Council had determined that 'the Collegiate Costume should consist of a Black Stuff Gown, a Black Cloth Hood lined with crimson silk and bound with crimson velvet inch wide, and an Academical Cap'. 'A specimen'—a most appropriate description it would seem!—'of the Gown, Hood and Cap' was thereupon laid on the table. There followed a considerable amount of discussion. On behalf of Council it was recommended that 'each

Fellow . . . should procure the costume . . . and . . . wear it on all occasions when the College appears in public and that it be imperative on the Examiners to wear the costume on all Examinations held in the College'. Exception was taken by one Fellow to the stipulation about examinations, and another urged that there should be 'no Special Hood for the Fellowship of the College, but that the Fellows may wear the Hood belonging to their University medical degree'. It was eventually agreed that 'Fellows should be at liberty to wear the distinguishing badge of any degree in Medicine they may possess if they should prefer it to the sample costume submitted'.[103]

That was far from being the end of the matter. The Council had had reason to review their original recommendation concerning a hood! Doubts had arisen as to the legality of adoption of a hood by the College. With graceful naïvety the Council now took the view that 'hoods have generally been regarded as distinctive marks of the profession by the wearers of a University Degree . . . and . . . it would be a mistake to infringe a custom' established 'by habit if not opinion'. In the circumstances the College were asked to reconsider their former resolution and to authorize a change in the recommended Collegiate costume affecting the crimson velvet trimming. The width of the trimming was to be increased from one inch and a half to two inches! A 'Specimen of the Gown' so altered 'was exhibited'. There was considerable discussion among the twenty-seven Fellows present before final agreement was reached, of which details are not given in the Minutes.[104] It is a challenge to the imagination to visualize a company of mature males engrossed in solemn conclave on matters of apparel! Eventually, the gown as altered and without hood came to be recognized as the Collegiate costume. Whether Fellows ever took advantage of their right to wear the hood appropriate to their University medical degree is uncertain. Nor, despite the fact that his robing was the first source of sartorial concern, is there further mention of any particular costume for the President. None the less, as is apparent at all meetings of the College, the President and Vice-President appear in distinctive gowns, appropriately adorned—the President's with gold braiding and the Vice-President's with silver braiding. Since 1962, when the President officially represents the College on public occasions he wears a handsome gold medallion gifted anonymously to the College.[105] The Secretary's and Treasurer's gowns also have distinctive, but less obvious, maroon trimmings.

Over the years there has been recurrent consideration of an 'academic dress' for Licentiates. On more than one occasion consideration has been prompted by specific enquiries on the part of Licentiates themselves, but Council appears to have been habitually reluctant to make any positive recommendation. This reluctance was evident when the question was raised by one Licentiate in 1904[106] while another enquirer received from the Secretary (Sir Robert Philip) a reply to the effect that 'the College has not seen its way in the meantime to sanction a distinctive Costume for the Licentiates'.[107] Again in 1942, no decision was reached after viewing a special gown submitted for consideration.[108]

The Promissory Obligation

The requirement that a Fellow before taking his seat shall sign the Promissory Obligation is of course steeped in tradition extending back to the earliest days of the College. Having been introduced by the Secretary, the President and Fellows, all standing receive the Fellow. The President then reads aloud the Promissory Obligation, whereupon the Fellow having signified his assent to the requirements of the Obligation affixes his name to it. For the purpose of signing he is proferred a pen which was once the property of Sir James Mackenzie. The pen was a gift to the College from an Honorary Fellow, Sir John Parkinson[109] who on another occasion gave the College two letters written by Sir James Mackenzie.[110]

Within comparatively recent times signing of the Promissory Obligation has come under closer scrutiny, largely as a result of the pertinacity of an ultra-efficient College Secretary with a paternal pedagogic background. It was pointed out how difficult overseas Fellows found signing when visiting this country for a short period after election. To meet the situation the Council resolved that Fellows in such circumstances should be allowed to sign the Promissory Obligation at a Meeting of the Council if unable to attend a College Meeting.[111]

Links with Past Personalities

Over the course of years the College has benefited greatly from donations which have preserved links with outstanding College personalities and traditions. To cite only a few examples—manuscript lectures of Matthew St Clair, Charles Alston, William Cullen, John Rutherford, Joseph Black, Francis Home and James Gregory given by Dr James Home in 1845; the original MS. of Dr John Brown's *Rab and his Friends* presented by a number of Fellows in 1906; a collection of medical writings belonging to Sir James Young Simpson, presented by Sir Alexander Simpson[112]; manuscript writings and articles by Dr William Cullen; an autograph letter and pocket medicine case belonging to Sir James Young Simpson gifted by Dr Berry Hart; a desk which had been the property of Dr John Gregory; and the presentation to the College by Dr William Phillips, F.R.C.P.Lond. of Dr Argyll Robertson's Travelling Case of Lenses. The link between Prince Charles Edward Stuart and Sir Stuart Threipland has already been mentioned (Chap. XXVII).

The Chiron Motif

Coming to more recent times, there is the long-established use of green in connection with College publications, stationery and livery. It has been modestly incorporated in the College tie of comparatively recent origin. Is there a College Colour in the traditional sense of the word? There are no records to confirm any such belief but it has been suggested that the green is that of the oak tree incorporated in the College Coat of Arms and associated with King Charles the Second who granted the College its original Charter in 1681. For motif the tie has embodied in it the early Greek physician Chiron, depicted as a centaur in keeping with the accounts of Grecian mythology. Renowned for his pharmaceutical skill rather than his surgical accomplishments, Chiron included among his disciples Achilles, Castor and Aesculapius. According to one legend Chiron, having been accidentally shot by Hercules with a poisoned arrow renounced his immortality in favour of Prometheus and was established by Zeus among the stars in the constellation of Sagittarius. Chiron appears as motif in the mural decoration of the Entrance Hall and main Stairway of the College, and a silver statuette of the Centaur was given to the College by Sir James Cameron when President.[113]

The Membership Examination

Of necessity procedure in connection with the Membership Examination underwent modification to deal with the large number of candidates in the 1950s and subsequently. As recently as the years between the two World Wars candidates at any one sitting rarely exceeded ten or twelve in number. The final part of the examination, the oral, was held in the New Library. There each candidate faced his last examiners who were comfortably ensconced in one of the several recesses with shelves of massive tomes behind, to left and to right of them. The surroundings were impressive and the atmosphere considerate and understanding. With a concluding 'thank you', the examiners eventually directed the candidate to what is now the room reserved for the President. There the small côterie of aspirants awaited their fate. The wait seemed interminable. With every minute that passed, the picture they presented increasingly resembled that of fearful patients in a dentist's waiting room. Only a Bateman could have done justice to it!

Then—the door was opened from without, with the utmost deliberation. Modestly resplendent in his green uniform and with great dignity the College Officer entered; called Dr So-and-So by name; handed him his hat and coat; and as tenderly as his office permitted ushered the named gentleman into the vestibule and thence to the steps leading down to Queen Street. Seven, eight or maybe nine times the solemn ritual was repeated. What followed? Without any candidate's hat or coat but with a hint, but only a hint of a smile, the Officer entered once more and called out not one, but all the names of the few survivors, gathered them up as a hen collects her chickens—and led them into the presence of the President, to be informed of their success!

Today candidates are spared that ordeal but how much more nerve-racking, much more prolonged and how mundane it must be to await the postman's knock for official intimation of the examination result.

Persistent Pickwickianism

To say that tradition dies hard savours of the trite. Nevertheless some aspects of tradition which are slow a-dying have subtle significance and contribute a certain Pickwickian pawkiness to proceedings. It will be remembered that there was a time when lists of Fellows were required to have asterisked the names of those admitted in virtue of being professors (Chap. VIII). At least it was one way of reminding the academics of their good fortune! But the tradition has not yet assumed morbid skeleton form! In February 1969 a Standing College Committee felt it necessary to request the Council's permission to use the title 'Professor' where appropriate in correspondence with other Royal Colleges and Specialist Associations, who were accustomed to using the title. Agreement was granted to the extent that the title might be used in inter-collegiate matters but at the same time the Council resolved 'to maintain the tradition of not using this title within this College'.[114] Even correspondence had been previously subjected to an element of traditional procedure. In 1916 the Treasurer was instructed by Council on how Fellows were to be addressed. Appropriate forms of address were given as 'Dr. . . . F.R.C.P.' for domestic use;

'Sir . . . F.R.C.P.' in the case of a Knight; and 'F.R.C.P.E.' for 'outside domestic use'.[115]

The Resting Places of three Great Physicians

There is however a wholly different aspect to tradition: respect for the memory of those who have long-since passed on. Archibald Pitcairne died on 23rd October 1713, aged 61 years and was buried in the Greyfriars Churchyard, Edinburgh. In 1800, at the instance of the Aesculapian Society of Edinburgh a statement was issued to the effect that Pitcairne's 'tombstone lies flat upon the ground and is almost covered with earth'. Subscriptions were obtained from members of the Society, the two Edinburgh Royal Colleges and other medical men with a view to restoring the monumental tomb. In all there were forty-nine medical subscribers, Dr Andrew Duncan, sen. having been largely responsible for marshalling support. The restoration was completed on the 148th anniversary of Pitcairne's death. On the tombstone was the following inscription:

> 'There lyes Doctor Archibald Pitcairn, who died 26th★ day of October 1713, aged 61; also Elizabeth Pitcairn, his daughter, who died the 18th day of March 1718; Elizabeth Stevenson, his widow, died 5th October 1734; Margaret Pitcairn, his daughter, died August 1777; Janet Pitcairn, Countess of Kellie, his daughter, died 7th June 1776; Lady Ann Erskine, his last surviving grandchild, one of the best of women, died 18th March 1803.
>
> Ecce mathematicum, vatem, medicumque, sophumque, Pitcairnum magnum haec urnula parva tenet. Ergo, vale, lux Scotigenum, princepsque medentium. Musarum columen deliciaeque, vale.'[116]

One hundred and fifty years later, in 1952, the tercentenary year of Pitcairne's birth, the Council of the Royal College of Physicians decided to have his tombstone renovated and the subsequent commemoration included a lecture on the life and work of Pitcairne.[117]

A not wholly dissimilar train of events followed the death of Dr William Cullen. His death took place on 5th February 1790 when within one month of his eightieth birthday. Dr John Brown has left us a colourful picture of Cullen's small estate of Ormiston Hill. The house had a 'magnificent outlook across the Vale of the Almond to the Ochils, and the outlying Grampians from Benlomond to Schiechallion, and across the Firth to Benarty and the Lomonds'.[118]

★ The *Greyfriar's Records* give this as the day of burial *not* of death.

Cullen was buried on 10th February in his home parish of Kirknewton. In the words of his biographer:

> 'No evident memorial or inscription distinguishes this sepulchre from those by which it is surrounded. But in the inner . . . surface of the eastern wall there is inserted a marble slab, which records the name, the death, and the accomplishments of Cullen's eldest son, Robert, the judge . . . By this alone the place is recognised as the tomb of William Cullen.'[119]

On 24th October 1862, at the instance of the College, the Council, Secretary and Treasurer visited the Kirknewton burying ground. According to the President (Dr Craigie) he had previously been there in 1856, 1857 and 1858 and sought the co-operation of the Parish Minister with a view to gaining entrance 'to the place' for the Council. The general findings of the Council were in keeping with those described by Cullen's biographer. They did however obtain information of value from 'an aged inhabitant of the village', who stated that he had been a servant in the family of Lord Cullen [the judge]. According to this informant the remains of Dr Cullen and his son were deposited 'not side by side, but the one above the other' immediately in front of the marble tablet to the memory of Robert Cullen the judge. As to the stonework, the Council found this to be so weathered as to be in a state of considerable disrepair.[120] It was left to Council to 'take what steps might seem requisite'.

After much cogitation and with, it would seem, a certain awareness of embarrassment, it was decided to approach surviving relatives of Dr Cullen with 'some hopes' that they might see 'the propriety of taking some measures, not only to keep the Sepulchre in decent memory of their distinguished ancestor'. Dr Cullen's only surviving son, General William Cullen, died in India before being approached and subsequent correspondence led to negotiations, if such they could be called, with a grand-daughter of Dr Cullen. She, while ready to further measures for effecting repairs gave no indication of a possible contribution to a memorial. In the opinion of Council she left 'the matter altogether in a state of polite obscurity'! This however did not prevent the College from placing 'a sum not exceeding one hundred pounds . . . at the disposal of the Council for providing a suitable Memorial to Dr. Cullen'. Events proved that obscurity on the part of Dr Cullen's grand-daughter had been misinterpreted in part at least, because three months later the President informed the College that one of their number when in London had seen the lady in question and returned the richer by 100 guineas as a contribution to the Memorial fund. In due course, the sepulchre repaired, a modest memorial was erected.[122]

By a strange coincidence, in common with other outstanding men among our predecessors, Sir Robert Sibbald's later days were 'almost unnoted' and until recent times his place of death and burial and indeed the date of his death were matters of considerable doubt. In Jolley's words, 'even Sir Robert Sibbald . . . passes out of its [the College's] records without a trace'.[123] All credit for dispelling doubts on these scores is due to Dr Peel Ritchie who in his Harveian Oration outlined how step by step he arrived at convincing conclusions.[124] These were that Sibbald died in Carruber's Close, Edinburgh on 9th August 1722 aged 82 years, and that he was buried on 12th August 1722 within the burial place of the Phesdo family in Greyfriars Kirkyard, Edinburgh. This last conclusion was based on the finding by Ritchie in the 'Records of Burial in Greyfriars Churchyard' of the following entry:

> 'Sunday, 12th August 1722, Sir Robert Sibbald of Kipps, Doctor of Medicine, aged 82 years, dyed 9th, buried 12th, lyes the foot of the middle Phesdoes ground, hearse, Turff.'

This was confirmed by an entry in the 'Records of Interments in Greyfriars' Burying-ground from 1st April 1717 to August 31 1728' to the effect that:

> 'Sir Robert Sibbald of Kipps, Doctor of Medicine, aged 82 years, died 9 and buried 12 (August) within Phesdoes ground, Middle East End thereof.'[125]

Ritchie's conclusions appear fully warranted despite the fact that there are no monumental or other references to Sibbald.

It is a matter for conjecture why Sir Robert Sibbald was interred in the burial ground of another family. Ritchie suggested that access to his own burial ground was impossible because major structural alterations were known to have been in progress. He postulated also a sympathy between the Phesdo family and Sibbald in their 'Church and Political views'.[126]

Centenaries

No mention of the first centenary of the College appears in the Minutes and this despite the fact that Monro *secundus* was President during the period 1779–82. Monro did in 1781, however, present to the College a copy of his father's (Monro *primus*) works. The absence of any commemorative celebrations may possibly be explained by a variety of circumstances such as involvement in reports to the civic authorities, a certain difficulty in securing payment of overdue subscriptions, and controversies with the architect of the Hall in George Street. Even the Library was proving to be a source of trouble at this time. It was in 1781 that the Library was removed from the Infirmary to George Street.[127] The Catalogue of books was badly in need of revision and Sir Stuart Threipland and Dr Cullen who had been entrusted with 'looking into this matter' were roundly rebuked and required to 'set about and finish the necessary revisal thereof with first conveniency'.[128] How the circuitously polite diction of the day lent itself to telling admonition!

The second centenary of the College being granted its original Charter did not pass unrecognized. Celebrations took place on the occasion of the annual dinner on 8th December 1881. Those who attended included most of the resident Fellows of the College, Representatives of both Houses of Parliament, the Fighting Services, the Magistracy of Edinburgh, the College of Justice and other eminent citizens. Members of the medical profession from Glasgow and other cities and towns in Scotland were also present as guests.[129] The national financial crisis in 1931 compelled partial abandonment of intended celebrations on the occasion of the 250th anniversary.[130]

Reference was made on the occasion of the Service of Commemoration of St Andrew's Day on 3rd December 1961 to the Centenary of the second Royal Charter granted to the College. The Dean of the Thistle, Dr Charles Warr was indisposed but a special message was read from him.

> 'I would like to extend a special greeting to those who are representing the Royal College of Physicians at this Service. On 29th November 1681 King Charles II granted a Charter to the College. In 1861 a second Charter was granted by Queen Victoria.' 'During the past few days', the Dean's message continued, 'the College has been celebrating the Centenary of the second Charter, and included in these celebrations is attendance at this St. Andrew's Day Service in the High Kirk of Edinburgh. As they look back with pride on the history of their College, our congratulations and our gratitude go forth to them. For all that they and their forbears have done to advance the ministry of healing we would offer our heart-felt thanks to God. We pray that the Divine blessing may continue to rest upon the Royal College of Physicians, and that its future may still further enhance the achievements of the past.'[131]

Long-standing Links with Edinburgh Societies

A debt owed to our predecessors is the close and, on suitable occasions, convivial links of many years standing with certain Edinburgh Societies. Moreover the traditional association derives special significance from the fact that Fellows of the College were involved directly or indirectly in the founding of the Societies in question.

The Royal Medical Society dates back to 1737. That was the year when the Society was formally constituted, but the origins can be traced back to 1734 when six students of medicine 'fired by the example of their masters, who had nothing more at heart than the improvement of those who committed themselves to their tuition' began to hold informal meetings when they discussed among themselves papers which they had written.[132] At first the Society met in a tavern but, in 1771, a committee was appointed to consider the erection of premises and the establishment of a library. The Committee consisted of the four Society Presidents together with Drs William Cullen, John Gregory and Andrew Duncan, sen. A subscription list was launched and was headed by Drs Cullen, Monro *secundus*, John Gregory, John Hope, Francis Home and Professor Black. John Morgan was one of those who subscribed. In 1775 the Foundation Stone of the new building was laid by the then President of the Royal College of Physicians, Dr Cullen. The need for a new building arose in 1819 when a Committee was once again appointed, the members including Dr Andrew Duncan, Dr James Gregory and the President of the Royal College of Physicians, Dr James Buchan.[133]

With legitimate pride this pioneer Medical Society which had acquired a Royal Charter in 1778, celebrated its first centenary in 1837. The occasion was marked by more than twenty toasts! Admission was restricted to Members only, with the exception of the Principal of the University (George H. Baird), the President of the Royal College of Physicians (Dr Alison) and the President of the Royal College of Surgeons (Sir George Ballingall). Those on whom the Society conferred Honorary Membership included (Sir) J. Y. Simpson, and three Americans all of whom had been ordinary Members in their student days—John Morgan, Benjamin Rush and William Shippen.[134] It is of interest that Morgan was responsible for starting the first medical society in Philadelphia about 1763–5. This venture was shortlived as an independent entity. When in 1766 it merged with another society to form the American Philosophical Society, Redman and Morgan were members.[135] Dr William Shippen, jun. was president in 1790 of a society in Philadelphia which owed its foundation to students.[136]

The first distinguished man of science not an ordinary member to be elected an Honorary Member of the Society was Dr John Purcell, Professor of Anatomy in Trinity College, Dublin. Dr William Cullen was the second. Sir Byrom Bramwell was the recipient of a unique honour at the hands of the Society. In the words of the historian he was 'in one respect, the most outstanding figure in the history of the Society, for upon him alone was conferred the dignity of Honorary President.'[137] A compliment in reverse was paid in 1902 when, Sir Thomas Fraser being in the chair, Dr Kenneth Downie presented the Society with a photograph of Fellows of the Royal College of Physicians.[138]

In 1969 the Royal Medical Society initiated a scheme which was as magnanimous as it was imaginative, for the production of a descriptive catalogue of the older collections of printed medical books in Edinburgh libraries. Possessing as it does the largest single collection of historical medical works in Edinburgh, the College is considerably involved. Other institutions which are co-operating include the National Library of Scotland, the Royal Botanic Garden, the Royal College of Surgeons, the Royal Observatory, the Royal Society and the University of Edinburgh; and, the Royal Medical Society is itself including its own important collection of older books. The Royal Medical Society was instrumental in engaging a research worker to undertake the cataloguing, and assumed full financial responsibility for a period of three years.[139]

Eighteenth-century Edinburgh was renowned for its numerous social clubs. Primarily medico-social clubs did not exist at first although there was one named 'Doctors of the Faculty Club', the members of which according to Dr Watson Wemyss were 'imaginary physicians'. In the course of time medical clubs with an essentially social objective such as the 'Celsian Club', the 'Galenian Club' and the 'Dissipation Club' appeared on the scene.[140] For the purpose of this history two Societies or Clubs call for special mention. They are the Aesculapian Club and the Edinburgh Harveian Society which continue to thrive to this day. Both owed their origin to a Fellow and one-time President of the College—Dr Andrew Duncan, (sen.), whose name has already been mentioned in connection with the founding of the Royal Public Dispensary and Morningside Hospital.

The Aesculapian Club was founded on 2nd April 1773. Membership was limited from the outset to Fellows of the Royal College of Physicians and the Royal College of Surgeons. At first total membership was fifteen but this was increased later to twenty-two when it was decided that Aesculapians from each of the Edinburgh Royal Colleges should be equal in number. Festivities consisted of supper in the early years, but later assumed the form and proportions appropriate to a Dining Club. For one hundred years smoking was not permitted. The subject was still somewhat contentious after relaxation of the rules in 1882 when cigarettes only were permitted and then only 'after a certain period of the evening'. Evidently 'cigarettes of a mild character' were provided at the club's expense but the policy was changed in 1894 when an increase in the cost of the dinners was accompanied by a ruling that smokers 'must provide their own tobacco'. In 1924 the College agreed to the Aesculapian

Club holding its dinner in the New Library, but at the same time politely required that, for the future, annual applications would be necessary 'as the Council cannot bind their successors'. It may be that the Club was rather taken aback! They did make an application in twelve months' time, but according to their historian, were slow to return to the College for their annual dinner. Dr Andrew Duncan functioned as Honorary Secretary for fifty-four years; and Sir Douglas Maclagan, who designed a badge for the Club, was a member for no less than fifty-seven years.[141]

The Edinburgh Harveian Society was founded on 12th April 1782 to establish 'an Annual Festival in honour of deceased Medical Worthies, particularly of Dr Harvey the discoverer of the Circulation of the blood.'[142] Membership was restricted to Fellows of the two Edinburgh Royal Colleges and limited to about thirty, but in 1832 all Fellows of both Colleges were regarded as eligible 'provided they pass the ordeal of the ballot box'.[143] Later it was extended to medical graduates of Edinburgh University residing in Edinburgh; and among non-local residents, to medical graduates and licentiates in Medicine or Surgery. In its earliest days the Harveian Society had a close affinity with the Aesculapian Club, perhaps as a result of one or two Harveian Orations having been given at the latter prior to 1782. For some years the Harveian Society was known as the 'Circulation Club' and proposals for Membership were submitted at the April meeting of the Aesculapian Club or the March meeting of the Dissipation Club.

A requirement of the Harveian Society's Laws was that the President should deliver a discourse at each April Festival of the Society. Those Presidents who over the years selected Harvey as the subject of their Oration included Drs Andrew Duncan, J. W. Ballantyne, Sir Thomas Fraser and Sir Robert Philip. An Oration of particular interest was delivered in 1778 on the 200th Anniversary of the birth of Harvey—four years before the founding of the Edinburgh Harveian Society. It is on record that the Oration was entitled *De laudibus Gulielmi Harvei Oratio* and that it was delivered in Latin *habita in Aedibus Academiae Medicae prope Aulam Collegii Regii Chirurgorum Edinburgensis* [144] The Orator was the irrepressible Andrew Duncan, sen.

In 1884, the year of Edinburgh University's Tercentenary, the Society held their annual Festival in the College of Physicians when Professor Virchow attended and an apology for absence was received from Louis Pasteur. The presence of distinguished guests was a departure from precedent, but the holding of the Society's Festival in the Royal College of Physicians has become an established custom, business meetings of the Society being held in the Royal College of Surgeons. It can be safely presumed that there was no recurrence of the Society's experience in 1856. On that occasion the Festival took place in a tavern or hotel. With dyspeptic displeasure the Minutes recorded 'disastrous because there was not enough to eat'![(145)]

The Festival is an occasion for tradition and levity. A figure representing Harvey with a heart in his hand stands in front of the Society's President, and a bust of Harvey adorns another table. When the time comes for the ox-heart to be served, the President calls upon the neophytes present to stand up and appointed scrutineers note the way in which the neophytes partake of the heart. Professional eminence does not absolve from lack of expertise. Wit readily wins expiation. Dr Underhill failed to dispose completely of his portion. Required to make amends his retort of 'nothing left but vegetations' secured pardon. Professor Annandale's tactics as a neophyte were otherwise. He demanded three helpings! With what exact purpose has not been stated, but a clergyman is invariably invited to attend the Harveian Festival and in doing so join the ranks of the 'Socii adjuncti'. In 1892 Professor Grainger Stewart had no doubts as to the purpose when, introducing the Reverend James Macgregor, D.D. of St Cuthbert's, he said 'the Society wanted a Chaplain with a heart, and they had found him in Dr. Macgregor'.[(146)]

Edinburgh Pathological Club. Founded in 1886, this Club contrary to the impression conveyed by its name, has always been actively interested in disciplines ranging beyond those of pathology rigidly interpreted. Policy has consistently recognized the importance of cross-fertilization in an era of rapidly increasing specialization. In addition to pathology, general medicine and surgery, gynaecology, anatomy, physiology, ophthalmology and laryngology were represented in the original membership which was restricted to twenty-five. More than half the original members were Fellows of the College.

The prime mover in the establishment of the Club was (Sir) John Batty Tuke. One original law that has stood the test of time is that there is only one office-bearer, the Secretary. It was determined also that the Chair at any meeting should be taken by the third person entering the room; and that Communications should not exceed thirty minutes' duration. Not noted in Guthrie's article is that the time was when 'a bottle of whisky was passed round during deliberations'. Members now number almost 400. There may be some who, in the words of Tom Fleming, think wistfully of 'The years that got away'!

The first Secretary to be elected (1886) was Dr (later Sir) Sims Woodhead who in the following year was appointed the first Superintendent of our College Laboratory. Other Fellows of the College have figured prominently as Secretaries of the Club in subsequent years, and as contributors of papers and to discussions. At different times contributions at meetings have dealt with subjects coming within the spheres of haematology, dermatology, child health, body metabolism and veterinary conditions. During World War I Professor Lorrain Smith demonstrated experiments in connection with Eusol and, in conjunction with Professor J. S. Haldane, tests concerning the efficacy of charcoal-filled masks as a protective measure against the inhalation of chlorine gas.

Proposals for child welfare provisions on a national scale came up for consideration by Parliament in the latter years of the War, and this prompted the Pathological Club to organize a series of meetings dealing with the subject. In the following winter (1917–18), a course of twelve discussions was held on improvement in the education of medical students. At one session the Headmasters of George Watson's Boys' College and Merchiston Castle School and the Headmistress of a girls' school delivered addresses on 'School Education in relation to the Study of Medicine'. Some thirty-seven years later (1955), the challenge of medical education again came up for consideration by the Club when asked by the University for its opinion of the undergraduate curriculum.

In 1900 the 100th meeting of the Edinburgh Pathological Club was followed by a dinner in the College of Physicians.[146a]

Medico-Chirurgical Society of Edinburgh. Foundation of this Society dates back to August 1821. Those responsible were frank in their 'approval of the objects and constitution of the Medico-Chirurgical Society of London'.[146b] Succinctly expressed, the aim of the Society was 'to place medicine on a scientific basis'.[146c] Launching of the project was due mainly to an ophthalmologist, Robert Hamilton.

The first President was Dr Andrew Duncan, sen., and Dr W. P. Alison was one of the first two joint Secretaries. In the words of the surgeon Caird: 'The Society prospered, especially fostered by the College of Physicians, who generously granted it a room in which to meet'.[146b] The accommodation was in the George Street Hall, but in the course of time the Society moved to a series of temporary quarters, one of which was the apartments tenanted for a short period by the College at 119 George Street[146d] (Chap. IV). Referring to the Society's Jubilee Conversazione, Handyside mentioned that: 'The Royal College of Physicians had the courtesy to permit their valuable Collection of Portraits of celebrated Physicians and Surgeons, and many rare and valuable works in Medical Literature, to be exhibited'.[146e]

A reliable if superficial indication of the part played from the outset by Fellows of the College can be obtained from study of the *Transactions* of the Society. Among those who were most prolific with their contributions were Drs John Abercrombie, J. H. Bennett, W. P. Alison, (Sir) Robert Christison, William Cullen, Andrew Duncan, sen., W. T. Gairdner, (Sir) James Y. Simpson and Alexander Wood. Of these Abercrombie was the first to communicate a paper, his subject being *Contributions to the pathology of the heart*. The date was 5th December 1821. Over the years the erudition and number of original communications has been prodigious. Mention of an extremely limited and necessarily selective few will serve to illustrate the wide range of interests of Fellows of the College in earlier years. Thus arsenical poisoning was dealt with by Christison in 1825, vegetable alkaloids by Thomas Fraser in 1868, experiments on electro-biology by Alexander Wood in 1851, prolonged total deprivation of food by Douglas Maclagan in 1835, diphtheria by Begbie in 1862, and the practical significance of the stethoscope by Abercrombie in 1841. Among communications which have proved to acquire a particular historical significance were Bennett's *On leucocythemia* (1850); Argyll Robertson's *Observations of the action of light on the pupil* (1869); Christison's . . . *of the occasional milky appearance of serum* (1828 and 1830) and *On the adulteration of drugs* (1836); Alison's *On quarantine houses in checking the diffusion of cholera* (1832); William Begbie's *On the relation of rheumatism and chorea* (1846); and Alexander Wood's *On a new method of administering medicine, more especially applied to painful local afflictions* (1855). Inevitably there was a host of contributions by an infinite variety of Fellows on different aspects of tuberculosis infection.

The above examples provide evidence of the extent to which, from the early nineteenth century, our College and the Society shared, as would be expected, a common approach to research and practice in the field of clinical medicine. Happily perhaps, today's outlook might question the propriety of such communications as Goodsir's *Report of the lesions discovered in the post-mortem examination of the late Dr. Abercrombie* (1844) and Newbigging's *History of the case of the late Dr. W. P. Alison* (1859).[146f]

Edinburgh Obstetrical Society. The Society was founded in January 1840 largely at the instigation of younger members of the profession who were practising midwifery. In the previous month ten doctors had attended a preliminary exploratory meeting at which letters of support for the project were received from the others. Of the twenty doctors concerned more than half were either Fellows or future Fellows of our College. They included Doctors William Beilby, Peter Fairbairn, Robert Lewins, R. B. Malcolm, John Moir, George Paterson, Alex. Peddie, Charles Ransford, R. Renton, Alexander Wood and A. Ziegler.

At the inaugural meeting Dr Beilby was elected President; Dr Renton one of the two Vice-Presidents; and Drs Paterson and Ransford Secretaries. The first discussion in the Society was introduced by Beilby, and at the same meeting an application for admission was successfully submitted by J. Y. Simpson who gave a communication to the Society two months later. In subsequent years a number of Fellows of the College have been elected President of the Obstetrical Society. They included (Sir) John Halliday Croom, Alexander Keiller, John Moir, (Sir) J. Y. Simpson, A. R. Simpson and C. E. Underhill. At different times the responsibilities of Secretary of the Society were discharged by the following Fellows of the College—Drs J. W. Ballantyne, Freeland Barbour, James Carmichael and Robert Thin, A. Keiller, Peel Ritchie and C. E. Underhill. Dr Oliphant Nicholson was Editor of the Society's *Transactions* for a period of two years; and it is of particular interest that the first volume of the published *Transactions* was edited by Peel Ritchie who was author also of *The Early Days of the Royall Colledge of Physitians of Edinburgh*.[146g] In their day Thatcher and John Brown were Fellows of the Society, as in more recent times were two Presidents of our College—Charles McNeil and Rae Gilchrist.

Current records testify to the effective continuation of links between the Society and our College.

Another active group in which a number of Fellows of the College have played a prominent part is *The Scottish Society of the History of Medicine*. It was founded in Edinburgh in 1949 at the instance of Dr Douglas Guthrie, and support was straightway forthcoming from Glasgow, Aberdeen and other centres not confined to Scotland. Guthrie was the first President, being subsequently elected Honorary President; and Dr H. P. Tait was the first Honorary Secretary, the responsibilities of which office he still continues to discharge (now jointly) with characteristic thoroughness and zeal. Other Fellows who have, among others, actively contributed to the affairs of the Society and its Council include Drs W. A. Alexander, W. D. H. Conacher, A. M. Gillespie, Charles McNeil, John Ritchie, W. D. D. Small, T. R. R. Todd and E. R. C. Walker of Edinburgh; Stanley Alstead and G. D. Forwell of Glasgow; John Craig of Aberdeen; Martin Whittet of Inverness; and J. L. Henderson of Dundee. To these names must be added those of L. J. Jolley, G. R. Pendrill, and Miss J. P. S. Ferguson—successive Librarians of our College. In general an autumn meeting is held in Edinburgh and a winter meeting in Glasgow, the venue on these occasions being one of the Royal Colleges. Summer meetings tend to take the form of pilgrimages to places selected for their historical interest. Meetings are invariably delightful social occasions. Annual reports of the Society are ambitious in the way they provide summaries of relevant events and publications in the English-speaking world, indications of topical domestic interest and brief résumés of papers not published elsewhere.

The Royal Society of Edinburgh. It is not suggested that this Society is to be regarded as a Medical Society. It is a Society of which many of its numerous origins have roots in Edinburgh medicine of the eighteenth century, and which as a scientific society has over the years been concerned in varying degrees with science as applied in medical practice. Furthermore as a Society with early literary associations it has interests in the history of applied science in medicine. For present purposes interest is concerned mainly with the influence exerted by medical men in their dual capacity as Fellows of our College and Members of the Senate of the University of Edinburgh.

Mention has been made (Chap. VIII) of the relatively short lived Medical Society founded in 1731 and of how it was followed by the Philosophical Society. The reason for the demise of the Medical Society is uncertain: it may have been the outcome of declining interest or of a genuine desire to encourage interests not confined to medicine. Whatever the reason Monro *primus* was not averse to the change to judge by his preface to the fifth volume of *Medical Essays* of which the following is an extract:

> 'A Society being formed in this Place for the Improvement of Natural Knowledge, in which all the Branches of Medicine are included; and the Members of the Society being adopted into this new one, the Design of publishing more Volumes of Medical Papers was dropt some Time ago.'[147]

Fellows of the College who were members of the Philosophical Society in 1739 included Charles Alston, John Boswell, John Clerk, Andrew Plummer, William Porterfield, (Sir) John Pringle, Andrew St. Clair, and John Stevenson. Other names which appear on the admission roll for 1782 include Joseph Black, Henry Cullen, William Cullen, Andrew Duncan, James Gregory, James Hamilton, Francis Home, John Hope, James Lind, Alexander Monro *secundus*, Donald Monro, Daniel Rutherford and Charles Stuart. Dr John Clerk, once described as 'the most celebrated physician that has appeared in Scotland since Dr. (Archibald) Pitcairn' and as 'an excellent classical scholar and critic'[148] was Vice-President of the Philosophical Society, and Dr Andrew Plummer, a Fellow of the Royal Society and friend of Boerhaave was Joint Secretary as he had been of the earlier Medical Society. At different times Monro *primus* and Monro *secundus* shared the Secretaryship with David Hume.[149] It was while Plummer was Secretary of the Philosophical Society that an announcement appeared in an Edinburgh magazine that the Society was prepared to undertake the study of minerals their 'nature and uses', on behalf of any interested parties.[150] Plummer's particular interests were, it will be remembered, chemistry and pharmacy and it was he who commended the therapeutic value of the waters of Moffat Spa.[151]

With the mutation of the Society from one to improve medical knowledge to another to improve Arts, Science and particularly Natural Knowledge, the *Medical Essays and Observations* were replaced by *Essays and Observations, Physical and Literary* which however never attained regular publication. Despite the change, medical subjects continued to predominate, and in the first volume of the new publication Dr Alston contributed an article consisting of a vigorous criticism of the Linnaean System of Classification.[152] This article caused Linnaeus temporarily to hesitate to accept the Honorary Fellowship of the Royal Society in later years. As further evidence of the widened interests of the Philosophical Society as compared with its predecessor, William Cullen as Vice-President was constantly subject to pressure by the President, Lord Kames, to embark on a book on agricultural holdings.

Passing mention of the *Select Society* (*1745*), a short-lived esoteric off-shoot of the Philosophical Society, is justifiable if only because two Fellows of the College, Monro *primus* and Sir Alexander Dick were among its members who included Adam Smith and David Hume. Unabashed by the erudition of their fellow members the records indicate that Monro and Dick were exemplary in attendance and uninhibited in debate.[153]

The equanimity of the *Philosophical Society* was disturbed when the *Society of Antiquaries of Scotland* petitioned for a Royal Charter in 1782. One result was that consideration was given by Members of the University, Faculty of Advocates and the Philosophical Society to the creation of a Royal Society of Edinburgh. Dr William Cullen as Vice-President was in the forefront of action taken by the *Philosophical Society*. In a Memorial to the Lord Advocate, Cullen outlined why it was desirable that the *Philosophical Society* should have a Charter, but stated that the Society considered that their own cause would be best served by the creation of a single general Royal Society along lines favoured by the University to cater for the cultivation of 'every branch of science, erudition and taste'.[154, 155] The University Senate of which he was a member provided Cullen with another avenue for expression of his views. His fellow senators included Drs Joseph Black, John Hope and Alexander Monro—all members of the Philosophical Society. A Memorial drawn up by the Senate betrayed undisguised apprehension that injury to the University would follow recognition of the *Society of Antiquaries* as a corporate body. The arguments and negotiations that followed have no bearing on the history of our College except in so far as the *Society of Antiquaries* referred to the loss of the Natural History collections of Sir Robert Sibbald and Sir Andrew Balfour as evidence of the insecurity of the University Museum were it proposed that antiquities should be deposited in it.

The University's petition was for a Royal Charter for a *Royal Society of Edinburgh for the advancement of learning and usefull knowledge.* A Charter was granted in 1783 and depicted the new Royal Society of Edinburgh as a forum for those 'well versed, not only in the Sciences of Mathematics, Physics, Chemistry, Medicine and Natural History, but also in matters that relate to Archaeology, Philology and Literature'. The newly established Royal Society of Edinburgh consisted of two components or 'Classes' as they were termed—a Physical one embracing the 'sciences of Mathematics, Natural Philosophy, Chemistry, Medicine, Natural History and whatever relates to the improvement of Arts and Manufacturers'; and a Literature 'Class' embracing 'Literature, Philology, History, Antiquities and Speculative Philosophy'.[156] Cross-fertilization between the two 'Classes' was not precluded as evidenced by the frequency with which the chair at the Literary Section was taken by the ubiquitous Dr Andrew Duncan, and by the delivery before that same section of a paper on *Theory of the Moods of Verbs* by Dr James Gregory. Among the mainstays of the Scientific or Physical section at various times were Drs William Cullen, Alexander Monro *secundus*, John Hope and Joseph Black.

Monro *secundus* wrote several papers embodying essentially anatomical observations. Another College Fellow and University Professor of the name of Hope—Thomas Charles Hope—made a classic contribution, *An Account of a Mineral from Strontian, and of a Peculiar Species of Earth which it contains,* in which he announced the discovery of strontia. Over the years a number of notable papers dealing with pharmacology and therapeutics written by Dr Alison, Sir Robert Christison, Sir Thomas Fraser and Dr William Rutherford appear in the Society's *Transactions.* In the field of obstetrics, widely interpreted, Dr Matthews Duncan and Sir James Y. Simpson both contributed to the *Transactions*—the former a paper *On the Power exerted in the Function of Parturition*[157] and the latter a description of the *Structure of the Human Umbilical Cord and Placenta.*[158]

Two features characterized the subsequent course of the *Royal Society of Edinburgh.* A decline took place in the activities of the 'Literature Class' and by the beginning of the nineteenth century the number of other than scientific papers was meagre. At the same time, despite the Society developing a predominantly scientific character, Medicine as a scientific discipline did not acquire a significant niche for itself in the affairs of the Society. As Guthrie (1958) commented, 'the strictly medical papers' were few in number.[159] To some extent this may have been due to the competitive

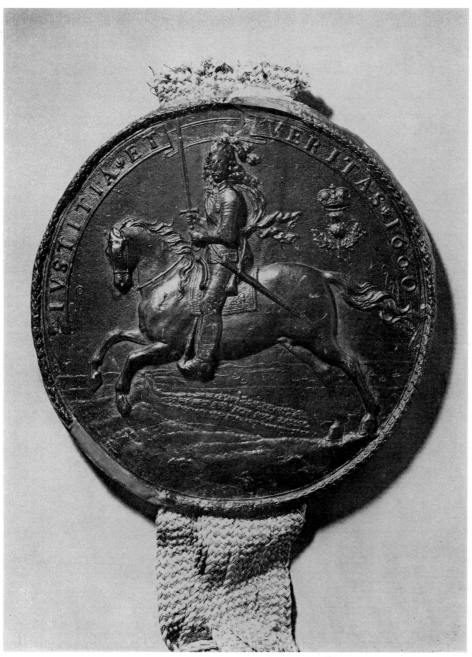

PLATE 49   Great Seal of Scotland: Charles II
By courtesy of the Scottish Record Office; photograph by Tom Scott

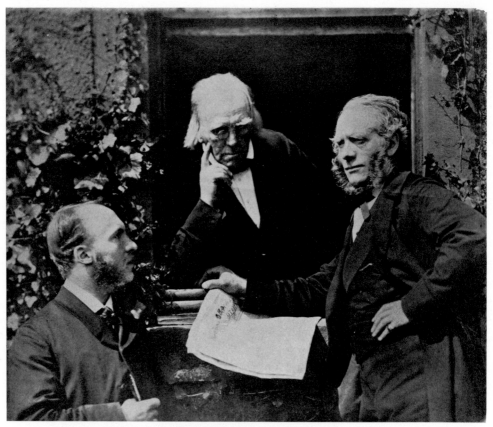

PLATE 50   Three Generations of Maclagans (*c.* 1850)
Reproduced from an original photograph by D. O. Hill; courtesy of Christie's, London

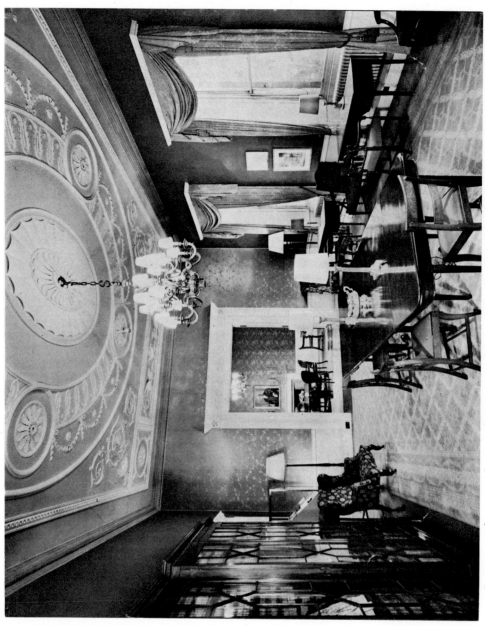

PLATE 51 The Sir Stanley Davidson Rooms (Adam Suite). Sir Stanley's portrait by Raeburn Dobson, R.S.A., can be seen above the fireplace in the Fellow's Room

Photograph by Tom Scott

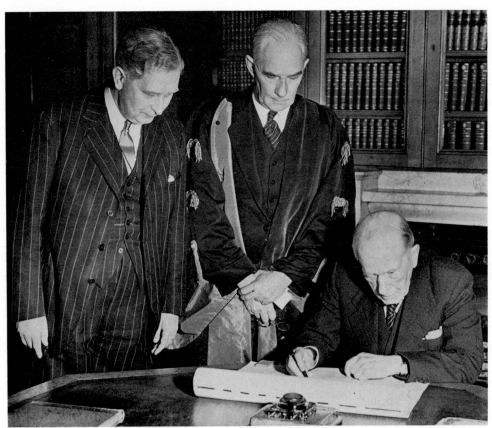

PLATE 52   Honorary Fellows: signing the Roll (Left, Sir Walter Russell Brain, Bt.; centre, Sir Stanley
Davidson, President; right, Sir Robert Muir)
Photograph by the Scotsman Publications Ltd.

publishing attractions of Dr Andrew Duncan's *Medical Commentaries*, *The Edinburgh Medical and Surgical Journal* and the *Transactions of the Edinburgh Medico-Chirurgical Society*. Nor should the attractions of the Royal Medical Society as a forum be forgotten.

Throughout the Royal Society of Edinburgh's existence their Roll has always included individuals who were Fellows of both the Royal Society and the Royal College of Physicians of Edinburgh. It cannot be said however that the influence on, or indeed active participation of Fellows of the College in the affairs of the Society within recent years bears even remote resemblance to the situation obtaining in the days of the Monros, Cullen, Alston and Plummer. Moreover it has to be remembered that the influence of these men probably owed more to their University than to their College associations.

In 1916, the Council on behalf of the College readily concurred with a suggestion of the Royal Society that there should be collaboration in compiling a list of *Scientific Serials in Edinburgh Libraries*. College representatives were appointed to attend a preliminary meeting.[160]

A happy innovation took place in 1972. In February of that year a Symposium with as subject *Blood and Blood Products* was organized jointly by the Royal Society and the Royal College of Physicians of Edinburgh and held in the Hall in Queen Street.

REFERENCES

THE CONSTITUTION

(1) R.C.P.E. (1974) *Laws*, Chapter XI, para. 2, Law 9.
(2) R.C.P.E. (1969) *Report of College Committee to Consider the Future of the College.* (Convener: J. Halliday Croom.) Edinburgh: Royal College of Physicians.
(3) College Minutes, 5.xii.1912.
(4) Ibid., 4.ii.1913.
(5) Ibid., 3.viii.1773.
(6) POOLE, R. [c. 1823] *Miscellaneous Minutes respecting Dr. Cullen*, pp. 12–13. (Ms.)
(7) RITCHIE, R. P. (1899) *The Early Days of the Royall Colledge of Physitians, Edinburgh*, p. 293. Edinburgh: G. P. Johnston.
(8) College Minutes, 1.v.1722.
(9) Ibid., 6.v.1766.
(10) Ibid., 23.vi.1908.

(11) POOLE, R. (1838) *Preparatory Notes for a History of the College*, pp. 261–4. (Ms.)

(12) THIN, R. (1927) *College portraits*, p. 91. Edinburgh: Oliver & Boyd.

(13) R.C.P.E. (1974) *Laws*, Chapter X, Laws 5–9.

(14) Ibid., Chapter X, Law 10.

(15) College Minutes, 21.xii.1693.

(16) Ibid., 3.xii.1694.

(17) Ibid., 17.i.1695.

(18) Ibid., 28.v.1695.

(19) Ibid., 21.ix.1695.

(20) R.C.P.E. [c. 1850] *Abstracts of the Minutes, A.D. 1682–1731*. By George Paterson. Treasurer's accounts. (Ms.)

(21) R.C.P.E. (1974) *Laws*, Chapter XI, para. 4.

(22) Council Minutes, 5.xii.1961.

(23) R.C.P.E. (1974) *Laws*, Chapter XI, para. 7.

(24) College Minutes, 6.v.1707.

(25) R.C.P.E. (1696) *Miscellaneous Papers*, no. 98.

(26) R.C.P.E. [c. 1850] *Abstracts of the Minutes . . . 1682–1731*. By George Paterson. Laws and Minutes. (Ms.)

(27) College Minutes, 2.ii.1762.

(28) Council Minutes, 29.vi.1960.

(29) Ibid., 18.x.1960.

(30) Ibid., 12.ix.1972.

(31) R.C.P.E. [c. 1850] *Abstracts of the Minutes . . . 1682–1731*. By George Paterson Clerk. (Ms.)

(32) R.C.P.E. (1851) *Letter book*, 14.ii.1851.

(33) College Minutes, 5.v.1724.

(34) JOLLEY, L. (1958) The records of the Royal College of Physicians of Edinburgh. *Bibliotheck*, **1**, 3, 20.

(35) POOLE, R. (1838) *Preparatory Notes for a History of the College*, p. 52. (Ms.)

(36) R.C.P.E. (1925) *Historical Sketch and Laws of the Royal College of Physicians of Edinburgh*, p. 113. Edinburgh: Royal College of Physicians.

(37) College Minutes, 3.ii.1972.

(38) Council Minutes, 23.ii.1960.

(39) R.C.P.E. [c. 1850] *Abstracts of the Minutes . . . 1682–1731*. By George Paterson. Fellowship & License (sic). (Ms.)

(40) Council Minutes, 21.iv.1964.

(41) Ibid., 12.vii.1966.

(42) CONE, T. E., jun. (1972) Personal communication.

(43) Council Minutes, 15.v.1956.

(44) College Minutes, 4.ii.1971.

(45) R.C.P.E. (1859) *Letter Book*, 8.ii.1859.

(46) JOLLEY, L. Op. cit., pp. 23–4.

(47) College Minutes, 15.v.1696.

(48) R.C.P.E. (1925) *History and Laws*, p. 22. Edinburgh: Royal College of Physicians.

(49) College Minutes, 6.xi.1699.

(50) Ibid., 13.xii.1705.

(51) R.C.P.E. (1974) *Laws*, Chapter IX.

FINANCIAL POLICY

(52) R.C.P.E. [c. 1850] *Abstracts of the Minutes . . . 1682–1731.* By George Paterson. Financial transactions. (Ms.)

(53) College Minutes, 7.v.1728.

(54) Ibid., 29.vi.1697.

(55) Ibid., 30.iii.1696.

(56) Ibid., 23.ix.1707.

(57) Ibid., 5.ii.1697.

(58) Ibid., 14.x.1698.

(59) Ibid., 31.i.1700.

(60) Council Minutes, 9.xi.1693.

(61) Ibid., 24.ix.1695.

(62) Ibid., 4.iii.1696.

(63) Council Minutes, 23.iii.1973.

INHERITED TRADITION

(64) R.C.P.E. (1959) *Report by the President [A. R. Gilchrist] . . . 1958–59.* Edinburgh: Royal College of Physicians.

(65) STEVENSON, J. H. & WOOD, M. (1940). *Scottish Heraldic Seals.* Vol. 1, Public seals, p. 19. Glasgow: Privately printed by Maclehose.

(66) R.C.P.E. (1681/2) *Miscellaneous Papers*, no. 45, 25.ii.1681/2.

(67) BARDEN, P. J. (1961) Edinburgh's academic heraldry. *University of Edinburgh Gazette*, **30**, 12.

(68) R.C.P.E. [1781] *Miscellaneous Papers*, no. 217.

(69) R.C.P.E. (1830) *General Correspondence*, 29.vii.1830.

(70) Council Minutes, 3.iv.1852.

(71) College Minutes, 4.xii.1897.

(72) Council Minutes, 22.ii.1898.

(73) Ibid., 15.iii.1898.

(74) Ibid., 30.i.1900.

(75) *Register of all Arms and Bearings in Scotland* (1959) Vol. XVI (Folio 1). (Ms.)

(76) Ibid., vol. I.

(77) ROBERTSON, R. F. (1972) Personal communication.

(78) BARDEN, P. J. Op. cit., p. 13.

(79) STEVENSON, J. H. & WOOD, M. Op. cit., p. 168.

(80) Council Minutes, 1.vii.1959.

(81) Ibid., 14.vii.1959.

(82) Ibid., 5.xii.1961.

(83) Ibid., 3.i.1961.

(84) MAITLAND, W. (1753) *The History of Edinburgh, from its Foundation to the Present Time*, p. 376. Edinburgh: Hamilton, Balfour & Neill.

(85) Council Minutes, 20.i.1953.

(86) R.C.P.E. [c. 1850] *Abstracts of the Minutes . . . 1681–1731*. By George Paterson. Censors. (Ms.)

(87) College Minutes, 3.v.1904.

(88) Ibid., 6.v.1958.

(89) R.C.P.E. [c. 1850] *Abstracts of the Minutes . . . 1681–1731*. By George Paterson. Fiscal. (Ms.)

(90) College Minutes, 30.xi.1727.

(91) MACLEOD, W. (1972) Personal communication.

(92) College Minutes, 18.vii.1893.

(93) Ibid., 2.viii.1831.

(94) Ibid., 1.xi.1853.

(95) Ibid., 6.xi.1923.

(96) R.C.P.E. (1846–7) *Treasurer's Account*. (Ms.)

(97) College Minutes, 6.viii.1822.

(98) Ibid., 3.viii.1830.

(99) Ibid., 3.xi.1830.

(100) Ibid., 4.viii.1846.

(101) Ibid., 4.xi.1846.

(102) Ibid., 7.xi.1865.

(103) Ibid., 7.v.1867.

(104) Ibid., 6.viii.1867.

(105) R.C.P.E. (1963) *Report by the President* [*J. D. S. Cameron*] *. . . 1961–62*. Edinburgh: Royal College of Physicians.

(106) Council Minutes, 20.xii.1904.

(107) R.C.P.E. (1904) *Letter book*, 13.x.1904.

(108) Council Minutes, 14.vii.1942.

(109) College Minutes, 23.vii.1957.

(110) Ibid., 26.vii.1966.

(111) Council Minutes, 19.vi.1956.

(112) College Minutes, 4.ii.1913.

(113) Ibid., 17.vii.1962.

(114) Council Minutes, 25.ii.1969.

(115) Ibid., 26.ix.1916.

(116) RITCHIE, R. P. Op. cit., pp. 185–6.

(117) College Minutes, 4.xi.1952.

(118) BROWN, J. (1882) *Horae Subsecivae*. Third series, p. 341. Edinburgh: David Douglas.

(119) THOMSON, J. (1859) *Life of William Cullen, M.D.*, vol. II, p. 661. Edinburgh: Blackwood.

(120) College Minutes, 4.xi.1862.

(121) Ibid., 5.v.1863.

(122) Ibid., 4.viii.1863.

(123) JOLLEY, L. Op. cit., p. 24.

(124) RITCHIE, R. P. Op. cit., pp. 256–64.

(125) Ibid., p. 262.

(126) Ibid., p. 263.

(127) R.C.P.E. (1925) *Historical Sketch and Laws*, p. 82. Edinburgh: Royal College of Physicians.

(128) College Minutes, 6.xi.1781.

(129) Ibid., 7.ii.1882.

(130) Council Minutes, 14.xi.1931.

(131) Ibid., 5.xii.1961.

LINKS WITH EDINBURGH SOCIETIES

(132) FOTHERGILL, J. (1783) *The Works of*. Edited by John Coakley Lettsom. Vol. II, p. 367. London: C. Dilly.

(133) GRAY, J. (1952) *History of the Royal Medical Society 1737–1937*, p. 120. Edinburgh: Edinburgh University Press.

(134) Ibid., p. 48.

(135) PACKARD, F. R. (1900) Medical societies in this country founded prior to the year 1787. *Transactions of the College of Physicians of Philadelphia*. Third series, **22**, 18.

(136) RADBILL, S. X. (1953) The Philadelphia Medical Society, 1789–1868. *Transactions and Studies of the College of Physicians of Philadelphia*. 4th series, **20**, 103.

(137) GRAY, J. Op. cit., p. 256.

(138) Ibid., p. 229.

(139) HARGREAVES, G. D. (1973) Old medical books in Edinburgh libraries: the Royal Medical Society Catalogue project. *Chronicle*, **3**, 1, 3.

(140) WEMYSS, H. L. W. (1933) *A Record of the Edinburgh Harveian Society*, pp. 1–2. Edinburgh: Constable.

(141) [STUART, W. J.] (1949) *History of the Aesculapian Club, 1773–1949*. [Edinburgh, n.p.]

(142) WEMYSS, H. L. W. Op. cit., p. 5.

(143) Ibid., p. 10.

(144) Ibid., p. 26.

(145) Ibid., p. 42.

(146) Ibid., p. 37.

(146a) GUTHRIE, D. (1966) The Edinburgh Pathological Club. *Medical History*, **10**, 87–91.

(146b) CAIRD, F. M. (1922) Valedictory address. *Transactions of the Medico-Chirurgical Society of Edinburgh*, **36**, 4.

(146c) HANDYSIDE, P. D. (1874) Valedictory address. *Edinburgh Medical Journal*, **XIX**, 772.

(146d) Ibid., p. 1104.

(146e) Ibid., p. 1101.

(146f) CRAIG, W. (1884) On the early publications of the Medico-Chirurgical Society of Edinburgh. *Transactions of the Medico-Chirurgical Society of Edinburgh*, **3**, 38–49.

(146g) UNDERHILL, C. E. (1890) Jubilee address: sketch of the history of the Obstetrical Society. *Transactions of the Edinburgh Obstetrical Society*, **15**, 1–23.

(147) [MONRO, A., *primus*] (1742) Preface. In *Medical Essays and Observations*. Revised and published by a society in Edinburgh. Vol. V, part 1, p. iii. Edinburgh: Ruddiman.

(148) ALLARDYCE, A., ed. (1888) *Scotland and Scotsmen in the Eighteenth Century, from the Mss. of John Ramsay, Esq. of Ochtertyre*, vol. 1, p. 234. Edinburgh: Blackwood.

(149) INGLIS, J. A. (1911) *The Monros of Auchinbowie*, p. 102. Edinburgh: Constable.

(150) *The Scots Magazine* (1743) **5**, 385.

(151) COMRIE, J. D. (1932) *History of Scottish Medicine*, 2nd Edition, vol. I, p. 299. London: Baillière, Tindall & Cox.

(152) ALSTON, C. (1754) A dissertation on the sexes of plants. In *Essays and Observations, Physical and Literary*, vol. 1, pp. 205–83. Edinburgh: Hamilton & Balfour.

(153) INGLIS, J. A. Op. cit., p. 72.

(154) CULLEN, W. (1783) Memorial of the Philosophical Society of Edinburgh. *Scots Magazine*, **45**, Appendix, p. 676.

(155) THOMSON, J. Op. cit., p. 219.

(156) History of the Society (1788) *Transactions of the Royal Society of Edinburgh*, **1**, 12.

(157) DUNCAN, J. M. (1867) On a lower limit to the power exerted in the function of parturition. *Transactions of the Royal Society of Edinburgh*, **24**, 639–51.

(158) SIMPSON, J. Y. (1864) On the anatomical type of structure of the human umbilical cord and placenta. *Transactions of the Royal Society of Edinburgh*, **23**, 349–53.

(159) GUTHRIE, D. (1958) Medical and literary contributions to the Transactions of the Royal Society of Edinburgh, 1783 to 1900. In *Yearbook of the Royal Society of Edinburgh*, p. 7. Edinburgh: Royal Society of Edinburgh.

(160) Council Minutes, 4.iv.1916.

Chapter XXXV

FAR FLUNG OVERSEAS LINKS

For a' that and a' that,
It's coming yet, for a' that,
That man to man the warld o'er
Shall brothers be for a' that.

Robert Burns

The preservation of links with Members and Fellows dispersed throughout the world provides the College with a serious challenge. There can be no doubt that the College values existing links and is anxious to see them not only firmly established but also expanded, and there is ample evidence that Members and Fellows abroad welcome any move in this direction.

SOME PROBLEMS

It is necessary to consider the implications in true perspective. A sense of urgency has only come into the picture with the rapid increase in the number of Members and Fellows domiciled overseas in the years following World War II. This in itself warrants criticism of the College in that previously insufficient thought had been given to those among them practising in such great countries as New Zealand, Australia, Canada and South Africa. Indeed it has been said that, by its apparent limited interest in Australasian developments the Edinburgh College lost an opportunity of exercising a helpful influence comparable to that exerted by London in the early days of the Royal Australasian College of Physicians. A Royal College of Physicians and Surgeons has been in existence in Canada for over one hundred years and a College of Physicians, Surgeons and Obstetricians in South Africa for eighteen years. India, Pakistan and Sri Lanka (Ceylon) have each their own College of Physicians and each awards its own diplomas. The trend illustrates the alliance between national sovereignty and medical progress—an alliance which augurs well for the countries concerned.

To a varying extent Edinburgh medicine and with it the Edinburgh College of Physicians has been associated with the early years of medicine in those countries. Academic posts have been, and in a number of instances are, held by Fellows of the College who have inevitably fostered in different degrees the principles of medicine as taught and practised in Edinburgh. Of necessity this influence has declined with the professional authority and independence acquired in these countries. This fact in no way warrants the assumption that the need to maintain virile, meaningful links no longer obtains. On the contrary, the College having accepted the new situation and adjusted its outlook, can perpetuate existing links to the ultimate mutual benefit of its Members and Fellows overseas and of itself.

With time the same trend will almost certainly evolve in countries which for want of a better name are still referred to as developing nations. So many factors, definable and indefinable, are involved that the question of time cannot be foretold with any accuracy. That being so, the necessity for the College to maintain and intensify

TABLE I

No. of Fellows and Members according to Geographical Distribution, 1972.

Geographical Location	No.		Total
	Members	Fellows	
Asia	136	24	160
Australia	182	41	223
Bangladesh	32	6	38
Canada	73	47	120
Sri Lanka (Ceylon)	98	19	117
East Africa	68	17	85
Egypt	63	12	75
India	775	138	913
Malaysia	38	9	47
Singapore	30	20	50
New Zealand	66	31	97
Pacific: Fiji, Solomons	1	1	2
Pakistan	118	36	154
South Africa	157	55	212
South America	—	9	9
U.S.A.	45	39	84
West Africa	40	19	59
West Indies	39	9	48
Total	1961	532	2493

measures for continuing contact with its Fellows and Members in those countries is the greater. The College is indeed fortunate in the enthusiasm shewn by a number of Fellows in fostering under a variety of auspices this form of professional entente.

Before outlining the ways in which overseas links have been maintained within recent years it is not out of place to indicate the practical difficulties in the way of complete success. First and foremost among these is the problem of numbers allied to wide dispersal. This is well illustrated by the record for 1972 (Table 1).

To complete the picture, in Table 2 are the corresponding figures for the Home Islands—using the term Home Islands as a means of editorial expediency and with no intent to disturb nationalistic susceptibilities.

TABLE 2

Country	No.		Total
	Members	Fellows	
Scotland	254	500	754
England	543	380	923
Wales	31	21	52
Northern Ireland	23	18	41
Eire	13	1	14
Total	864	920	1784

In Europe there were 3 Fellows in Malta, 2 in the Channel Islands, and 1 each in Gibraltar, Cyprus, Switzerland, Denmark and France. Of Members there were 3 in Malta, 2 in the Channel Islands, and 1 each in Cyprus, Norway and Belgium.

To quote Dr James Farquhar, one of our much-travelled Fellows,

> 'the countries . . . are as remote from each other as they can be in space, race, religion, language and politics. A less likely combination would be difficult to imagine, and yet there may be a message in it. East, West, Black, White, Arab, Jew, Hindu, Moslem, Catholic, Protestant, Marxist and Capitalist, we share a common bond—the Royal College of Physicians of Edinburgh.'[1]

Another aspect requires mention, no matter although essentially material in nature—the question of expense. Air travel is taken for granted. In reality it alone has made frequent and effective global contact possible. It involves considerable expenditure and on a scale which may well prove beyond the capacity of some of those who in virtue of their collegiate office might be expected to travel hither and thither, at any and all seasons. This was recognized by the College when Council considered the purposes to which the Verona Gow Bequest might best be used. Council arrived at the decision that the income from the Bequest should be used to advance medical research by financing visits by senior Fellows of the College to Commonwealth Countries. The wisdom of the decision has been more than justified by the accomplishments of senior Fellows who were assisted from this source. (Sir) James Cameron, (Sir) Ian Hill, and Drs Christopher Clayson and John Halliday Croom were among the first to receive the award.

Coupled with the financial aspect there require to be considered the extent to which travelling abroad can impinge on Area Health Board and academic teaching commitments. There are patients in need of care and students requiring to be taught. This is not mentioned in any critical spirit, but the fact remains that in some medical schools comments by patients and remarks by junior staff and students at the prolonged absence of 'chiefs' are occurring with increased frequency. The reaction is healthy and merits consideration. Allowance should be made for it by those intent on expanding travelling commitments.

VISITORS FROM OVERSEAS

In the course of any one year numerous visitors from overseas come to the College—some to take advantage of the Library facilities, others to participate in symposia and others again to see the College about which they have heard from their fellow-countrymen. Every now and again there are Members who, having been advanced to the Fellowship, take the opportunity of a visit to this country to sign the Promissory Obligation, and others not associated with the College who arrive with notes of recommendation and introduction from their senior colleagues abroad. Mention has been made of organised visits such as those of doctors from the United States of America, Holland, Denmark and Russia. There was further evidence of the international significance of College activities in notable visits by Her Excellency Mrs Pandit when High Commissioner for India (1960), Dr Thomas M. Greenaway, the President of the Royal Australasian College of Physicians (1961), Sir Robert Menzies, K.T. when Prime Minister of Australia (1963), and by Dr Rudolph Kampmeier, President of the American College of Physicians (1968).

REPRESENTATION ON OFFICIAL OCCASIONS

In 1957, Sir Edward Appleton attended the Centenary Celebrations of the Academy of Medicine of Cincinnati as representative of the University of Edinburgh, and took the opportunity to convey the greetings of the Royal College of Physicians of Edinburgh. In the same year the College was represented at the 41st South African Medical Congress by Mr Norman Dott, LL.D., F.R.C.S. Two years later the President of the College (Dr A. Rae Gilchrist) was present at the Annual Meeting of the Royal Australasian College of Physicians. It was the first occasion on which a President of our College had paid a visit to the sister Australasian College during his term of office.[2] Sir Ian Hill emulated Dr Gilchrist's example, and attended the annual meeting of the Australasian College by invitation in 1966.[3] In the previous year Sir Ian represented the College at the opening of the new Faculty of Medicine in the University of Malaya at Kuala Lumpur.[4] Dr Christopher Clayson and Dr John Halliday Croom, while holding presidential office, each in turn attended the annual meeting of the Australasian College (in 1969 and 1971 respectively), and the former was present in an official capacity at the Annual Convocation at Boston, Massachusetts of the American College of Physicians in 1968. The Boston Convocation consisted of a joint meeting between the American College and the Royal College of Physicians of London in recognition of the 450th Anniversary of the latter.[5] Previously in 1966 Dr Clayson had, as one of the first of his official duties as President, attended the Centenary Celebrations in Ottawa of the Royal College of Physicians and Surgeons of Canada, and took the opportunity of being present at the Annual Convocation of the Canadian College.[6] The Colombo Medical School celebrated its Centenary in 1970 and on this occasion the Edinburgh College was represented by the Vice-President (Dr Halliday Croom). Dr R. H. Girdwood represented the College in 1972 at the Second International Medical Congress at Bulawayo. Previously in 1967 he had attended a meeting of the Pakistan Medical Association in Karachi where he was entertained by Fellows and Members.[7] Invitations were received also for the College to be represented at the induction of the President of the University of Illinois (1965), and at the installation of the Vice-Chancellor of Lagos University (1968).

These many duties discharged abroad by Officials of the College in no way reflect the amount of travelling undertaken by them. Considering our Presidents—Dr Gilchrist visited both New Zealand and Australia; Sir Ian Hill's various itineraries embraced in addition to Australasia, Malaya, Singapore, India, Burma, Ceylon, East and North Africa and Khartoum; Dr Clayson included Singapore and Malaysia on his return from Australia; and Dr Halliday Croom, Canada, Australasia, Hong Kong and Singapore.

Representation of our College at two other notable anniversary celebrations must be mentioned. They both took place in London and are referred to here as a matter of convenience, and with no intent to suggest that the Tweed is to Scotland what the English Channel was to England in pre-Common Market days. The celebrations were those of the 450th Anniversaries of the Royal College of Physicians of London in 1968 and of the Worshipful Society of Apothecaries in 1967. On both occasions the Edinburgh College was represented by their President, Dr Christopher Clayson.[5]

Among Presidents, mention of Sir J. D. S. Cameron has been left to the last deliberately. The reasons are two-fold. In the first place his contributions to the fostering of overseas links were in many respects unique in conception and in realization. Secondly, his periods in far away countries took place in the main after demitting Presidential Office. An indication has been given of Sir James's pioneer work in bringing together the Presidents of the Colleges of Physicians in the Commonwealth and Associated Republics (Chap. XXXVI). No matter the bewildering changes being undergone by the Commonwealth, none can gainsay that Sir James's accomplishments have sown seeds which will continue to bear fruit in the sphere of world medicine. As the end of his third year of Presidency approached, Sir James was invited by the Council of the College to undertake under the terms of the Verona Gow Bequest a visit to Pakistan, India, Burma and Ceylon 'to make contact with Fellows and Members . . . Medical Schools and Hospitals'; to consider training received by medical graduates there, and to lecture.[8] In his Report for 1962–3, written only a short time before leaving for the East, Cameron said '. . . a strenuous tour has to be faced. The knowledge that it is College work, that it is a service to a loyal and grateful group of Fellows and Members of our College will give ample recompense for the energy and effort expended.'[9]

Active as Councillors of the College have been it must be remembered that a considerable number of other Fellows have travelled overseas, many of them on numerous occasions. For present purposes the difficulty is that their visits abroad have been sponsored by a wide variety of organizations which include the British Council, the Inter-University Council for Higher Education Overseas, the South African Medical Association, and the World Health Organization.

Some indication of the ramifications of Edinburgh Medicine in developing countries was given in a survey of the involvement of the Medical Faculty of the University in Overseas Aid. Members of staff in the employ of the University in 1970 had during the previous ten to eleven years visited no fewer than fifty countries dispersed over Arabia, Tropical Africa, Asia, the Pacific, Indian Ocean, South America and the Caribbean. University clinical medical departments were associated with the greatest number of visits which varied in length from one or two weeks to over twelve months. Participating doctors lived, worked and discussed medical education and practice with overseas colleagues. In virtue of their close contacts and their ultimate knowledge of socio-environmental factors these doctors were in a position to exercise a particularly powerful and personal influence. A number of those involved in these essentially University projects were Fellows or Members of our College.[10]

Regardless of the aegis under which visits are paid, travelling Fellows have innumerable opportunities of meeting other Fellows and Members in their native or adopted countries. As will be appreciated from the foregoing table there are few countries in the world in which a meeting with collegiate colleagues cannot be anticipated.

COLLEGE INFLUENCE AND STATUS OVERSEAS

An impression shared by Fellows who have travelled abroad is the warmth of the welcome received by all wherever they have gone. Successive Presidents and other Fellows travelling in a variety of capacities have told of this and how 'our own Fellows and Members rally round with private parties and indulge in chats about "home" and mutual friends'.

There is however no escaping the fact that ties in relation to different countries have undergone changes in different ways and in different degrees. Thus, in countries possessed of their own Colleges, interest in our College is understandably on the wane, certainly in so far as the Membership and Fellowship are concerned. That is not to say that genuine sentimental friendship has not stood the test of time. It certainly has, but a new generation of *Dominion* doctors is arising whose natural inclination is to aspire to Fellowship of their own College. More than one correspondent from New Zealand at the same time as expressing regret, referred to the apparent lack of active interest until comparatively recent times of the Edinburgh College in its Fellows and Members in the Antipodes. Nor can the adjustments in international political relations be discounted as of no significance. Australians, New Zealanders and Canadians, aware of their immense contributions in two world wars, have been bewildered, chagrined and at times hurt by the implications of the European

Common Market. Memories of the Anzacs at Gallipoli and the Canadians at Dieppe still live. And rightly so.

Historically it is of interest that Sir James Young Simpson's only sister emigrated with her husband to Tasmania. Later she went to Victoria to which a brother of Simpson also emigrated.[11] A comparable connection exists between New Zealand and our College. After graduating in medicine at Edinburgh University David Monro, son of Monro *tertius*, emigrated to New Zealand where he took up sheep farming and entered politics, eventually becoming Speaker of the New Zealand House of Representatives. David Monro was intrumental in securing for the University of Otago the collection of Monro *tertius*' books now in the Medical School Library there. An item of particular interest in the collection is a manuscript of 46 pages with the binder's title inscribed on the spine 'Life of Monro by himself' and on the fly-leaf 'Life of A. R. Monro Sr. in his own handwriting'.[12]

Reverting to Australia our College was indebted to Dr J. O. Poynton of Melbourne for the gift in 1966 of a writing by Monro *secundus* dated 1755 and entitled 'Dissertatio medica inauguralis, de testibus et de semine in variis animalibus'.[6]

It has been said that to some extent *Singapore* and *Malaysia* are beginning to transfer their interest from the Edinburgh to the Australasian College. Certainly Australian surgeons have been credited with claiming Malaysia as coming within their rightful sphere of influence![13] Opinions may differ, however. Writing in 1972 an eminent physician in Singapore and Fellow of our College attributed the newly acquired influence of the College exerted in his country to the rapid expansion of medical services after World War II. At that time a considerable number of doctors were sent at Government expense to the United Kingdom. Edinburgh proved a particular attraction for these men partly because of the reputation of the postgraduate courses in medicine, and partly because 'there had always been a close association between Edinburgh and Singapore in medical matters' before the War. Many of those who were sent to Edinburgh acquired their Membership in the 1950s and, to quote again, 'many of these pioneers now in their late forties and early fifties, are leaders in medicine in Singapore. Government and University policies on medical care and education bear their imprint.' This being so there can be little doubt that the influence of Edinburgh medicine, and with it of our College, will continue in the foreseeable future—a probability which will surely perpetuate College co-operation. Had there been doubts about the unprejudiced nature of the information received, they would have been dispelled by the comments of a Fellow of the London College who summed up the situation after many years experience in the East by saying 'the Edinburgh College has played an influential part both in Singapore and Hong Kong and to a certain extent in Malaya'.[14] When visiting Hong Kong, the President of the College (Dr Halliday Croom) found to his gratification that, almost without exception, members of the Department of Medicine in the University were Fellows or Members of our College.

And what of the *Indian sub-continent* with a combined total of Fellows and Members of more than half the comparable total for Scotland, England, Wales, Northern Ireland and Eire? Vast although the continent is, to quote one frequent visitor to India, 'it is probably impossible to lecture in any centre without being overwhelmed by the hospitality of those one has examined in Queen Street'. Equally significant is the custom adopted by many heads of medical departments, themselves Fellows of our College, of making careful selections from their staff with a view to sending them to Edinburgh for postgraduate education. When the first University in Baroda (1963-4) entertained a member of the Edinburgh University Medical Faculty arrived from home, the seven members of the team 'alternated round the table with Members of the College'. Another occasion recalled by Dr James Farquhar was the opening at Poona in 1964 of the First Congress of the All India Academy of Paediatrics. Sir James Cameron took the Assembly by storm, as he avowed 'I am proud to be a Scot: I am proud that I come from Edinburgh: and I am proud to be President of the Royal College of Physicians of Edinburgh'. Words cannot describe the volume or intensity of the applause which greeted the declaration. A few days later, Sir James accompanied by Farquhar dined at the Poona Race Club as guests of General Bardhan, F.R.C.P.E. of the Indian Army College. The emotions of the occasion were heightened by the pipes and drums of the Punjabi soldiers, in a way reminiscent of festive occasions at the Palace of Holyroodhouse.

As the table (q.v.) indicates, there is a not inconsiderable number of Fellows and Members in *Pakistan*, with which country Sir James Cameron was associated after his premature retirement as senior physician of the Edinburgh Royal Infirmary. Among the most distinguished Fellows of the College in Pakistan is Dr Hamidali Khan who, while occupying the Chair of Paediatriacs in the University of Karachi, was simultaneously President of the Pakistan Medical Association and the British Medical Association. Another who never sought to disguise his pride in being a Fellow of our College and, casting his mind back to undergraduate and postgraduate days, his emotional attachment to Edinburgh, was Dr Ali Kassim. This was typified in his courteous request to be allowed to decline proferred hospitality in the home of a Fellow. And why?—because it would involve offending his old landlady. 'You do not know', he went on to elaborate, 'the treasures you have in those Edinburgh landladies who make it their duty to mother overseas students like us!'

Sri Lanka is another country where visiting Fellows can rely on meeting physicians with their Edinburgh College associations and where again they are assured of an overwhelming reception.

Passing from the sub-continent of India to the continent of *Africa*—the influence of Edinburgh medicine is very evident in both Johannesburg and Durban. The number of College Fellows and Members is considerable in both cities, and those who have been fortunate to visit them return greatly impressed by the high regard in which the College in general and its diplomas in particular are held. It is of interest that the examination for at least one diploma awarded by the South African College bears the imprint 'of the old Edinburgh Membership examinations'.[15]

In 1960 the President and Vice-President met Dr Rabinowitz, a Fellow of the College, who represented the desire of Fellows resident in South Africa to form a Regional Committee capable of co-operating with the College and of submitting recommendations for the promotion of Members to the Fellowship.[16] The suggestion was sympathetically received although importance was attached to any Committee which might be formed being of an informal nature, the recommendations of which would be subject to the scrutiny and approval of the Council and Fellowship Committee of the College.[17] The Council of the College was informed of the first meeting of the Regional Committee, and were constrained to inform the group that rejection of a nomination by secret ballot of all Fellows in South Africa did not preclude the nomination being submitted by any one Fellow should he so desire.[18] In the event the conception of a Regional Liaison Committee appears to have lapsed and the interests of Members are attended to by Fellows in the separate localities. It is probable that the deciding factor was the demands of long distance travel involved in attending meetings.[15]

As to developing African countries, there is no call for false modesty. Edinburgh College men have played a notable part in the development of medical services and the training of doctors in both *East and West Africa*. Mention has been made (Chap. XXVII) of the pioneer work of Dr Alexander Brown at Ibadan, and the advancement of medicine in Nigeria owes a great deal to Sir Samuel Manuwa, a Fellow of the College who was adviser to the Government at Lagos. An altogether impressive number of Fellows have held or hold professorial posts, a position which has been more than maintained with the return home to Britain of expatriates, and assumption of their duties by African and, to a decreasing extent, by Asian doctors. The influence of the College does not cease there. In some respects the influence has been cumulative and expansive. Thus at the time of writing a Tanzanian (Dr J. G. Ebrahim, F.R.C.P.E.) occupies a post of significant influence as senior lecturer at the London Institute of

Child Health. He plays a key rôle in a programme sponsored by UNICEF for senior paediatric teachers from developing countries. He thus has the opportunity to combine effectively his tropical and his Edinburgh professional experiences. Again, in Liverpool, a Fellow of our College and a former professor of paediatrics in Nigeria (Dr Ralph Hendrickse) is now responsible for the Diploma Course in Tropical Child Health at the University.

Without any semblance of bias, it can be claimed as a historical fact that the Edinburgh College of Physicians has played an altogether impressive part in the furtherance of the study of child life and health in the continents of Africa and India. This will be evident from what has already been said. There is further substantial evidence, allowing that it is neither desirable nor possible to consider separately the contribution of the College and the Edinburgh Post-Graduate School of Medicine. Professor Elaine Field, drawing on her experience in Malaya (1949–55), Singapore (1955–60) and Hong Kong (1962–71) wrote: 'It was the rule rather than the exception to send Paediatric trainees first, to the Institute of Child Health in London for three months, then to join the post-graduate Internal Medicine course in Edinburgh . . . The ultimate goal was the D.C.H. London and the M.R.C.P. Edinburgh. There were, of course variations to the above course.'[14] She gave as points in favour of Edinburgh that it offered an M.R.C.P. in which Paediatrics had special recognition without divorce from general medicine; and that being smaller than London, students were able to get more individual attention. Nevertheless it should in fairness be mentioned that the impression of the overseas students was that with increase in the size of classes there had been a lessening in the degree of this individual tuition.

In Africa there is a revealing situation in the developing countries. An Asiatic Fellow of the College assisted by two Edinburgh Members, occupies the Chair of Paediatrics in the University of Zambia, the staff having been recruited from College men practising paediatrics in Kenya. There are other Edinburgh men in Malawi, Uganda, Tanzania, Ethiopia, the Sudan and Mauritius. In West Africa, at Accra, the Professor of Paediatrics and his two most senior consultant colleagues are Ghanaian Fellows of our College; and at both Ibadan and Lagos the Professors of Paediatrics are Nigerian Fellows of the College, the former having among his colleagues at least four with the Edinburgh Membership. These are facts. They speak for themselves and are of undoubted historical significance.

Mention of all countries in which there are representatives of the College is not practicable. Information can be found in the Geographical List now a feature of the College Year Book and Calendar. Suffice it to say that links exist in both paediatrics and adult medicine with *Israel*, *Egypt*, the *Sudan* and the *Arab States* in the Middle

East. To claim a preponderating influence for our College in these countries would be wholly incorrect. In some of them American influence predominates and in others that of continental European medicine. Others again, with inclinations toward Britain look to London.

Reference to doctors from countries overseas would be incomplete were gracious mention not made to the contributions to the United Kingdom hospital services made by many of them during and after their postgraduate training. These contributions have been the subject of criticism in some places; in many more they have been highly valued by doctors (including the writer), nurses and patients with whom they have worked.

Withal may the College spare thoughts too for the Scottish expatriates among its numbers. Sentiment maybe—but the same sentiment which inspired Charles Murray to write:

> *Here on the Rand we freely grant*
> *We're blest wi' sunny weather;*
> *Fae cauld an' snaw we're weel awa'.*
> *But man, we miss the heather.'* [19]

REFERENCES

(1) FARQUHAR, J. W. (1972) Personal communication.

(2) College Minutes, 5.v.1959.

(3) Ibid., 3.v.1966.

(4) Ibid., 2.xi.1965.

(5) R.C.P.E. (1969) *Report by the President [Dr. C. Clayson] . . . 1967–68*. Edinburgh: Royal College of Physicians.

(6) R.C.P.E. (1968) *Report by the President [Dr. C. Clayson] . . . 1966–67*. Edinburgh: Royal College of Physicians.

(7) College Minutes, 7.ii.1967.

(8) Ibid., 5.xi.1963.

(9) R.C.P.E. (1963) *Report by the President [J. D. S. Cameron] . . . 1962–63*. Edinburgh: Royal College of Physicians.

(10) FARQUHAR, J. W. (1971) *Memorandum for the Overseas Committee of the University of Edinburgh.* (Typescript.)

(11) RUSSELL, K. F. & FORSTER, F. M. C. (1971) *A List of the Works of Sir James Young Simpson 1811–1870. A centenary tribute*, pp. 5–6. Melbourne: Dept. of Medical History, University of Melbourne.

(12) ERLAM, H. D. (1954) Alexander Monro, *primus. University of Edinburgh Journal*, **17**, 77.

(13) MONTGOMERY, H. M. (1972) Personal communication.
(14) FIELD, E. (1972) Personal communication.
(15) WALLACE, H. L. (1972) Personal communication.
(16) Council Minutes, 18.x.1960.
(17) Ibid., 22.xi.1960.
(18) Ibid., 8.iii.1961.
(19) MURRAY, C. (1909) *Hamewith*, p. vi. London: Constable.

Chapter XXXVI

ROYAL AND OTHER OCCASIONS

ROYAL OCCASIONS

Though God hath raised me high, yet this I count the glory of my crown: that I have reigned with your loves.

Queen Elizabeth, 1601

Early endeavours to found our College were pursued in an atmosphere of Royal, but unfortunately ineffective favour. An account has already been given of how James I of England issued an order to Parliament for the establishment of a College of Physicians in Edinburgh without result, and how Charles I's referral of the matter to his Privy Council rather more than a decade later was equally unproductive. Cromwell was more successful than his royal predecessors in so far as he was instrumental in having a Patent made out instituting a College of Physicians of Scotland. Together, delays arising from the protests of a seventeenth-century form of autocratic democracy and the death of the Protector served to nullify the intentions of the Patent (Chap. II). It remained for Charles II to succeed where others had failed, by granting our Charter of Erection, which duly had appended to it the Great Seal on St Andrew's Day 1681 (Chap. III).

Not until 1760 did another occasion occur meriting the description Royal. Seemingly with some hesitation the College resolved to present a loyal address to the new monarch, George III. Jolley ascribed the misgivings to prevailing political feelings in Edinburgh.[1] George IV visited Edinburgh in the summer of 1822. Poole's manuscripts cast an amusing if sensitive sidelight on the occasion as far as the College was concerned. An Address to His Majesty having been transmitted via the Home Office, the President (Dr Buchan) ' "attended by Dr. Hamilton Senr. and Dr. Spens, attended His Majestys levee, as a Deputation for the Royal College, the other members going in the capacity of Professors." They were—Dr. Hope, Duncan Senr., Home, Hamilton Junr. and Duncan Jnr.' Continuing Poole recorded: 'The proposal for a gown to be worn by the President was not carried into effect', and concluded with the rather incomprehensible comment that: 'Very evidently, the preponderance of Professors in the Council impaired the independence and dignity of the College on this occasion. Money, however, was got from it.'[2]

In 1863 the Social Science Congress met in Edinburgh and the College entertained the President and leading members of the Congress to Dinner. His Royal Highness Prince Alfred was present. Among many distinguished guests were the Chancellor of the Exchequer, the Right Honourable W. E. Gladstone and Sir Charles Hastings together with prominent representatives of the civic authority, the legal profession, surgeons and physicians.[3] Some two years previously the death of the Prince Consort was the subject of an Address of Condolence to the Queen.[4, 5] In 1863 Addresses of Congratulation were presented to the Queen and the Prince of Wales on the marriage of the Prince, and in 1864 appropriate Congratulatory Addresses were again sent to the Queen and Prince of Wales 'on the occasion of the birth of the Prince Royal'.[6] When the Prince of Wales attained his majority it was the Queen and not the Prince to whom an address was presented! Following the attempted assassination of His Royal Highness, the Duke of Edinburgh, the College submitted a suitable address to the Queen and sent congratulations to the Duke on his providential escape[7] and in due course loyal congratulations were sent to the Queen and Duke on the occasion of his marriage.[8] Two years previously loyal congratulations were sent to the Queen and Prince of Wales on the recovery of the Prince from a severe attack of enteric fever[9], and in 1885 another address was sent to the Queen on the occasion of the marriage of Princess Beatrice.[10]

Other royal occasions signalized by Loyal Addresses from the College were Queen Victoria's Jubilee in 1887[11] and her Diamond Jubilee in 1897[12]; and in 1901 Addresses of condolence on the death of Queen Victoria, and of congratulation on his Accession were presented to King Edward VII.[13] The new King visited Edinburgh in 1903 and the College marked the occasion by presenting a Loyal Address.[14] Within seven years it was the sad task of the College to convey loyal messages to His Majesty King George V and Her Majesty Queen Mary on the occasion of the death of King Edward VII.[15]

A touching occurrence in the College's history was the endowment in 1886 of a triennial prize, 'The Victoria Jubilee Cullen Prize' by His Excellency, Dr Gunning, in commemoration of the approaching Jubilee of Queen Victoria and in memory of Dr William Cullen.[16]

H.M. THE QUEEN MOTHER SIGNS THE ROLL OF HONORARY FELLOWS

The twentieth century opened auspiciously with the decision in 1911 by His Majesty King George V that the Royal College of Physicians should take precedence over the Royal College of Surgeons[17], and with the acceptance by His Royal Highness the Prince of Wales of, and his election to the Honorary Fellowship of our College in 1919 (Chap. XXX).[18] An occasion of no less if not greater significance was the acceptance by her beloved Majesty Queen Elizabeth, our Scots born Queen Mother, of the Honorary Fellowship of the College. On 5th May 1953 the Senior Fellow of the College present, Dr John Eason, at an Extraordinary Meeting moved:

'That Her Majesty Queen Elizabeth, the Queen Mother, having graciously signified her willingness to accept the Honorary Fellowship of the College, be elected an Honorary Fellow.' Most appropriately the privilege of seconding the motion was accorded to one of the first Lady Fellows of the College—Dr Agnes Macgregor. 'The motion . . . was carried by acclamation, the Fellows upstanding.'[19] To their undisguised immense gratification the College later heard the President's announcement that 'Her Majesty Queen Elizabeth the Queen Mother had graciously consented to visit the College to receive in person the Honorary Fellowship of the College'.[20]

Her Majesty's visit took place on 7th November 1959. She was received by the President, Dr Rae Gilchrist, and afterwards dined with the Fellows in the College Hall. A certain delay characterized the start of proceedings. Assuredly no one will take exception to the explanation given with all respect. Arrived at the College Her Majesty recognized in the College Servitor in attendance (Mr W. V. Pilcher) an old shipmate of her husband the late King George VI. Monarch—then Prince Albert—and Servitor both served on H.M.S. *Collingwood*, a ship of the line, at the Battle of Jutland. It was in keeping with the long admired human interests and kindness of Her Majesty, that she insisted on hearing the Servitor's reminiscences in informal fashion, before proceeding to the more formal part of the evening's programme. Formal may be the strictly correct word to use, but conveys no impression of the apparent enjoyment shown by the Queen Mother, an enjoyment sensed and loyally shared by all the Fellows present. Not surprisingly Fellows were drawn from all parts of the United Kingdom.

Replying to the Toast of Her Majesty's health, the Queen Mother referred to the pre-eminence of Scottish medicine to which the example and encouragement given by the Royal College of Physicians had contributed so much.

'The progress in medical science in the last few decades', Her Majesty said, 'has been prodigious. But we must not forget the pioneers of earlier years whose work did so much to advance the diagnosis and treatment of illness. It is a source of pride to reflect how many of these were Scotsmen practising in this city . . . Your services to hospitals and in the fields of discovery are often recorded—and rightly. But there is another place, less often quoted, where I think the doctor occupies a special niche and that is in the home. There can be few of us who cannot remember the sense of reassurance we have felt from childhood's days at the friendly spectacle, when we were ailing, of the family doctor—the friend of us all.'

In proposing the Toast of Queen Elizabeth the Queen Mother's health, Dr Rae Gilchrist expressed the College's profound gratitude for Her Majesty's presence. Referring to the particular pride which we in Scotland take in Queen Elizabeth the Queen Mother, he recalled Sir Winston Churchill's summation of her qualities— 'that valiant woman, with the famous blood of Scotland in her veins'. Continuing, Dr Gilchrist spoke of how honoured Fellows were to welcome to their Hall 'one who holds the admiration of the whole world—a noble and gentle Queen, the embodiment of personal courage, which stood this country well in the darkest days; the embodiment of personal charm and magnetism which enchants her admirers everywhere; and the embodiment of all that is best in family life'. Later Her Majesty accepted the gift of a silver rose-bowl as an enduring mark of gratitude for her visit and as a symbol of the lasting loyalty and affection of the Fellows of the College.

After dinner the Fellows reassembled in the New Library. There, Her Majesty the Queen Mother was formally presented as an Honorary Fellow by Dr Alister Alexander, a former President and a native of the County of Caithness in which Her Majesty resides when at her home, the Castle of Mey. 'It is not', said Dr Alexander, 'only because of what Her Majesty represents here that we are so happy to enrol Her Majesty as an Honorary Fellow. It is also because of what Her Majesty is . . . our revered Queen Mother is a source of inspiration and strength to this land, the value of which cannot be computed.' Thereafter Her Majesty signed the Promissory Obligation and was pleased to accept a copy of the History and Laws of the College, and a golden key; and having, in becoming an Honorary Fellow accepted the highest honour at the College's disposal, she received from the President the right hand of Fellowship.

Prior to dinner a number of Fellows and guests had the honour of being presented to Her Majesty. They included past Presidents, Members of Council, the Clerk, representatives of the Royal College of Surgeons of Edinburgh, the Royal Faculty of Physicians and Surgeons of Glasgow, and the Limner to Her Majesty the Queen in Scotland.

In truth, in the words of Dr Rae Gilchrist, 'Her Majesty's visit was a brilliant occasion, and an unforgettable experience'.[21]

Prior to the Queen Mother's visit to the College, her ready consent had been obtained to the proposal that Mr Stanley Cursiter, the Queen's Limner in Scotland, should paint Her Majesty's portrait for the College. Her graciousness in consenting was acknowledged on behalf of the College by the President.[22] Before coming into the final possession of the College the portrait was hung at the annual exhibition of the Royal Scottish Academy. Now it adorns the Adam Suite of the College where it was unveiled by Dr Rae Gilchrist on 15th March 1961, and where it is a constant reminder of the College's affectionate allegiance to the Crown and the Royal Family.

Generously, at a later date, Mr Cursiter donated to the College a painting of the rose-bowl which had been accepted by the Queen Mother.[23]

OUR ROYAL PATRON

In 1963 an event took place which as it were, set the seal on this chain of Royal Occasions. Her Majesty Queen Elizabeth graciously accepted an invitation to act as Patron of our College. This fact was intimated by the President at the Quarterly Meeting in May 1963.[24] Rather less than three years later the Fellows were greatly gratified to learn that Her Majesty the Queen had consented to pay a visit to the College in person.[25] This took place on 29th June 1966, the President at the time being (Sir) Ian G. Hill. The occasion took the form of a Reception graced by the presence of Her Majesty and His Royal Highness the Prince Philip, during which the Royal visitors mingled with Fellows and their wives assembled in the College Hall. At the express wish of Her Majesty the Queen those presented to her included the wives of Fellows. Altogether the occasion was an admirably happy blend of informality and profound respect. Especially appreciated was the fact that Her Majesty the Queen's visit was part of a crowded programme of engagements and that Her Majesty had not been deterred from coming to the College by an afternoon in exhausting heat at a Palace of Holyroodhouse Garden Party.

After the visit of Her Majesty to the College, a message was conveyed to Her Majesty's Private Secretary at the Palace of Holyroodhouse in the following terms:

> 'The President, Council and Fellows of the Royal College of Physicians of Edinburgh offer their humble duty to Her Majesty the Queen. They request that you convey to Her Majesty their deep appreciation of the honour done to the College by

the gracious presence of Her Majesty and His Royal Highness the Prince Philip, Duke of Edinburgh at the reception within the College on 29th June. The occasion was unique in the long history of the College, and the record of this momentous occasion will find a proud place in our annals.

Would you in conveying our thanks assure Her Majesty of our continuing loyalty and devotion?'

On the day after transmission of the message the President of the College received the following gracious message from the Palace of Holyroodhouse:

'The Queen has commanded me to thank you very much for the courteous telegram which I laid before her this morning. Her Majesty hopes that you will be able to convey an expression of her thanks and appreciation to the Council and Fellows of the Royal College of Physicians, Edinburgh, not only for their message of loyalty, but also for their kindness in entertaining her so agreeably yesterday evening.

Indeed when we returned last night to the Palace of Holyroodhouse and before your telegram arrived, Her Majesty instructed me to write to you this morning and to send you her warm thanks and those of the Duke of Edinburgh for the Reception. It gave Her Majesty and His Royal Highness the greatest pleasure to be able to meet so many Fellows of the Royal College in the splendid setting of the Queen Street Buildings and also to see some of the extremely interesting documents and possessions of the College.

The paper-weight which you gave to the Queen on her departure has given Her Majesty much pleasure and I can assure you that she will use it. The Golden Cock will always serve to remind her of a very pleasant evening at the Royal College of Physicians, Edinburgh.'[26]

OTHER OCCASIONS

Noscitur a sociis

Considering other occasions, more particularly but not entirely those occurring after World War II, two are of outstanding importance, although in markedly contrasting ways.

DEATH OF SIR WINSTON CHURCHILL

Of these the first was the death of Sir Winston Churchill. Surely there can be none regardless of race or creed, and regardless of what form or in what sphere they made their contribution to the war effort who were not conscious of an inexpressible loss on the passing of Sir Winston. Certainly that was the feeling shared by all Fellows present at the Quarterly Meeting in February 1965 when departing from precedent, the President Sir Ian Hill commenced the business of the meeting with a reference to the national loss. Sir Ian's words, delivered with impressive dignity, were admirably suited to his purpose and to the mood of the College.

'Fellows of the College', he began, 'it would seem fitting that, before I read the obituaries of those Fellows we have lost in recent weeks, we should stand for a moment in silent tribute to the man, whose death a few days ago marked the end of an epoch.

The Captains and the Kings have departed, and Sir Winston Churchill rests now from his labours in the peace of a rural churchyard, deep in the heart of England.

We stand not in mourning only, but in tribute to his many-sided genius, and above all to his lion-heart—the quality that personified the spirit of Britain in those darkest days a quarter of a century ago. Each and all of us owes an irredeemable debt to this one man, who literally saved our Western way of life.

In the words of another immortal of his race, we may say to him:

"Fear no more the heat o' the sun,
Nor the furious Winter's rages;
Thou thy earthly task hast done,
Home art gone—and ta'en thy wages"

Churchill's wages lie not in fame alone, but in the gratitude of free men the world over.'[27]

INAUGURAL CONFERENCE OF PRESIDENTS

The second occasion concerned a unique event which owed its conception and initiation to (Sir) James Cameron—the first meeting of Presidents of Colleges of Physicians of the Commonwealth and associated Republics. This was held on 4th and 5th October 1962. Rightly, considering the circumstances of its origin, it was held in Edinburgh, and the College knew proud satisfaction in acting as host. Presidents attending in addition to our own Dr (later Sir) J. D. S. Cameron, were Sir Charles Dodds of our sister Royal College in London; Drs R. E. Steen and K. B. Noad of the Royal Colleges of Physicians of Ireland and Australasia respectively; and Drs J. H. Wright and G. M. Brown of the Royal Faculty (now College) of Physicians and Surgeons of Glasgow and the Royal College of Physicians and Surgeons of Canada respectively. The College of Physicians, Surgeons and Obstetricians of South Africa was represented by their past President, Professor G. A. Elliot acting as deputy for the Surgeon President, Mr J. Douglas.

In all, the Conference consisted of four sessions. The first two were devoted to matters affecting the Colleges in general. Lord Cohen of Birkenhead opened the third with an address on 'The Common Market and Medicine' before an audience which included representatives from the Scottish Universities, the Royal College of Surgeons of Edinburgh, the Scottish Home and Health Department, the Ministry of Health, and the Ministry of Health and Local Government of Northern Ireland. At the fourth and final session the time was occupied in crystallizing the conclusions arrived at following the various discussions. The secretarial work was undertaken by Dr R. F. Robertson of our College. Important as the Conference consultations were, they were not alone in being of immense value. There was general agreement that a great advance had been achieved by enabling the various Colleges to understand each other's policies and difficulties.

The inaugural Conference was embellished by a dinner given to the Presidents by H.M. Government in Edinburgh Castle and by an invitation from the Scottish Society of Physicians to attend their annual meeting and dinner at Gleneagles.[28]

A far-reaching outcome of the Conference was agreement that similar meetings should follow. A second Conference took place in the Royal College of Physicians of London in 1964. The same medical bodies were represented as those at the inaugural meeting with, in addition, the President of the College of Physicians and Surgeons of Pakistan and a representative of the Academy of Medicine of India. Discussion was concerned in the main with the medical education of specialists and consultants, and reciprocity between Colleges.[29] Dublin was the venue of the third Conference in 1967, the Conference coinciding with the 300th Anniversary of the founding of the Royal College of Physicians of Ireland. Representatives from Australia, India and Pakistan were absent. Reciprocity between Colleges in the matter of examinations again came up for discussion as did the registration of specialists with particular reference to the possible implications of joining the European Economic Community.[30] A fourth Conference was held in London, but a fifth arranged for 1971 in Pakistan did not take place because of the international situation.

A COMMONWEALTH MEDICAL CONFERENCE

At this stage it is appropriate to mention another Conference with Commonwealth interests but not directly connected with the Conference of Presidents just described. The Commonwealth Medical Conference was a by-product of the 1963 Conference of Commonwealth Prime Ministers, and aimed at giving the Ministers of Health and

Chief Medical Officers of Commonwealth territories an opportunity to discuss problems of common interest. Edinburgh was chosen as a suitable centre and the College President (Sir Ian Hill) was a member of the British delegation. Subjects discussed included the available number of doctors, undergraduate and postgraduate education, the training of nurses and the deployment of skilled professional staff. Entertainment was provided by the two Edinburgh Colleges, and at a gathering in the Hall of the College of Physicians attended by seventy-five delegates and the same number of Fellows, the Minister for Overseas Development was present.[31]

Mainly social occasions

As to other occasions, they are in the main social in character and can be best considered according as they provide welcome to and appreciation of guests from abroad, or are related more to domestic activities within the College. Among those who have been entertained since 1955 have been members of the Danish Medical Association and their wives, Scandinavian physicians and visiting doctors from Russia. At one time or another Receptions have been given for such bodies as the World Health Organization, the European Association of Senior Hospital Physicians, the British Dietetic Association and the Association of Senior Administrative Officers of the Health Service. Others who have been our guests are the Faculty of Medicine of the University of Leyden and the American College of Physicians. There is a tradition extending back to 1858 that the College entertains the British Medical Association on the occasions when the Association holds its Annual Meeting in Edinburgh.

An aura of accepted tradition, conditioned only by unpredictable Treasury encroachments, has been or is being established in connection with many of the domestic social activities. Needless to say Honorary Fellows who have just signed the Roll do not depart without being guests of the Council at a small dinner party. A comparatively recent innovation is an annual reception for Final Year Medical Students and their wives. Of much longer standing is the dinner arranged for newly elected Fellows who have attended to sign the Promissory Obligation. The uninitiated should be wary on these occasions. He may be forewarned that he will be called upon to reply to a toast. He may make brief preparatory notes, but as he rises to speak the lights will slowly be completely dimmed. Only the candles set in beautiful ancient candelabra flicker bravely on, illuminating through the haze of cigar smoke the balding heads of Councillors sitting opposite: a magnificent traditional setting but potentially unnerving experience! But all in the spirit of a function admirably attuned to a memorable occasion.

Of other regular dinners some are essentially informal as in the case of the biennial occasions when Fellows and their wives meet, discuss and enjoy each other's company in complete relaxation. The same holds good when a necessarily small company dine and wine with a guest lecturer. Formality and traditional ceremony are more in evidence, at least in the earlier part of the proceedings, at the Biennial College dinners when leading representatives of the professions and civic authority adorn the head table and when after-dinner speeches of the highest order can be expected.

The 1960s and 1970s saw certain adjustments in the pattern of social occasions. These were intended to cater for the new situation arising from the policy of arranging for the contributions of guest lecturers to be grouped and integrated within a symposium programme. Another somewhat later purpose of adjustments was to promote greater participation by Collegiate Members in the social activities of the College. As a result receptions have come into increasing favour, and these have largely replaced the small dinners given to guest lecturers.

Whether formal or informal, whether attended by the many or the few, there is no gainsaying that in their own way each of these happy social occasions contributes to the spirit of Fellowship so fundamental for so many decades in the corporate life of the College.

The record would not be complete without circumspect reference to another annual event—the 'Greetin' dinner'. 'Circumspect' because doubt exists as to the extent to which Council continues to claim powers of censoring the written word or suspending a contumaciously orotund Fellow! Suffice it to say that at the end of their year of office, the Council indulges in an abundantly earned 'Greetin' dinner' at which the Treasurer is required to make a speech. Given the temperament and desire, it is his opportunity to cast diplomacy aside, subject always to the decorum imposed by the presence of wives!

REFERENCES

(1) JOLLEY, L. (1958) The records of the Royal College of Physicians of Edinburgh. *Bibliotheck*, **1**, 3, 22.
(2) POOLE, R. (1838) *Preparatory Notes for a History of the College. Memorandum.* (Ms.)
(3) College Minutes, 3.xi.1863.
(4) Ibid., 20.xii.1861.

(5) Ibid., 4.ii.1862.

(6) Ibid., 2.ii.1864.

(7) Ibid., 5.v.1868.

(8) Ibid., 3.ii.1874.

(9) Ibid., 7.v.1872.

(10) Ibid., 4.viii.1885.

(11) Ibid., 3.v.1887.

(12) Ibid., 27.vii.1897.

(13) Ibid., 5.ii.1901.

(14) Ibid., 5.v.1903.

(15) Ibid., 12.v.1910.

(16) Ibid., 2.xi.1886.

(17) Ibid., 27.vi.1911.

(18) Ibid., 8.viii.1919.

(19) Ibid., 5.v.1953.

(20) Ibid., 28.vii.1959.

(21) R.C.P.E. (1959) *Report by the President* [*A. R. Gilchrist*] ... *1958–59*. Edinburgh: Royal College of Physicians.

(22) College Minutes, 3.xi.1959.

(23) R.C.P.E. (1962) *Report by the President* [*J. D. S. Cameron*] ... *1960–61*. Edinburgh: Royal College of Physicians.

(24) College Minutes, 7.v.1963.

(25) Ibid., 1.ii.1966.

(26) Ibid., 26.vii.1966.

(27) Ibid., 2.ii.1965.

(28) R.C.P.E. (1963) *Report by the President* [*J. D. S. Cameron*] ... *1961–62*. Edinburgh: Royal College of Physicians.

(29) R.C.P.E. (1966) *Report by the President* [*I. G. W. Hill*] ... *1963–65*. Edinburgh: Royal College of Physicians.

(30) R.C.P.E. (1968) *Report by the President* [*C. W. Clayson*] ... *1966–67*. Edinburgh: Royal College of Physicians.

(31) College Minutes, 2.xi.1965.

Chapter XXXVII

FATA VIAM INVENIENT

If you consider the successive systems of philosophy; if you free yourself from the influence of persuasive rhetoric, intricate logic, and ancient authority; if you delve far down beneath the surface—what you will find more often than not, are but assumptions, which everyone is as free to deny as to accept; followed by speculation and assertion without proof.

Lord Samuel (Romanes lecture, 1947)

At the present time many questions concerning Medical Corporations are in the forefront of debate if not speculation. Among them are:

1. What circumstances gave rise to their foundation?
2. What have they accomplished during their several centuries of existence?
3. What functions do they perform at the present time? And
4. How are their policies being adjusted in the light of current and future changes in medical administration and medical practice?

FOUNDATION

The Royal College of Physicians in Edinburgh . . . the first small germ of Scotland's later reputation for great medical education.

T. C. Smout

As a generalization it can be said that all Medical Corporations had in common that they were established to curb the malpractices of those professing medicine despite a total lack of knowledge, and to enable the country to benefit from the experience of physicians who had trained in continental medical schools. The influence of the Colleges was aided by the powers conferred on them to license to practise.

In so far as the Royal College of Physicians of Edinburgh is concerned the writings of Sir Robert Sibbald best describe the events which took place before, during and immediately after the granting of a Royal Charter of Incorporation. Those with whom the idea of a College originated included Sir Robert's uncle Dr George Sibbald: they did not survive to see their hopes materialize. Sir Francis Darwin's words in another age are applicable: 'In science the credit goes to the man who convinces the world, not to the man to whom the idea first occurs.[1]

PAST ENDEAVOURS

Progress, man's distinctive mark alone.

Robert Browning

In broad terms the development and policies of the Medical Corporations over the years have been similar, although differently influenced by national and local aspirations. There are a number of publications which if studied collectively provide an historical, if somewhat disjointed, overall account of the achievements and setbacks of the Royal College of Physicians of Edinburgh during the first two and a half centuries of its existence. They include the *Autobiography*[2] and *Memoirs*,[3] both by Robert Sibbald; *Report on Examination of Medical Practitioners*[4] by a Committee of the College (1833); an *Address* by the President, Dr W. Beilby at the opening of the Queen Street College Hall in 1846[5]; *The Early Days of the Royall Colledge of Phisitians, Edinburgh*[6] by Dr R. Peel Ritchie (1899); *Historical Sketch and Laws of the Royal College of Physicians of Edinburgh*[7] from its institution—a College publication in 1925; and, noteworthy despite the restricted subject, *History of the Laboratory of the Royal College of Physicians of Edinburgh* by Dr John Ritchie (1953).[8] In addition to the above there are in the Library two valuable sets of manuscript notes: Dr George Paterson's *Abstract of the Minutes (1682–1731)*[9] and the other, *Notes for a History of the College* by Dr Richard Poole.[10] More recently Mr G. R. Pendrill, a former Librarian of the College, contributed a condensed account of the origins and functions of the College to the *Scottish Medical Journal*.[11]

As to College Minutes, records and correspondence: these relate virtually in their entirety to the activities and decisions of the College as a corporate body, contain virtually no information concerning the evolutionary progress of clinical medicine, and contribute little if anything to knowledge of the interests and work of Fellows who achieved professional or other eminence. This is fully in accordance with the Corporate Fellowship which has been a distinguishing feature of the College

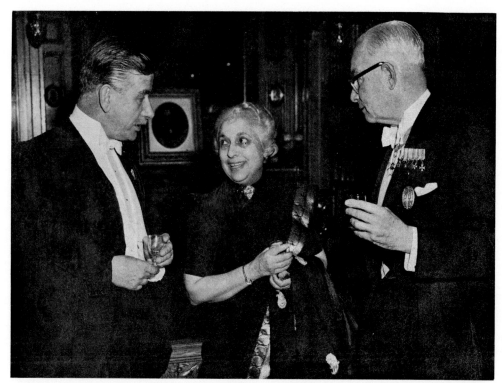

PLATE 53   A Distinguished Visitor: Her Excellency Mrs Pandit with (left to right) Dr J. Halliday
Croom and Sir Stanley Davidson (1960)
Photograph by the Scotsman Publications Ltd.

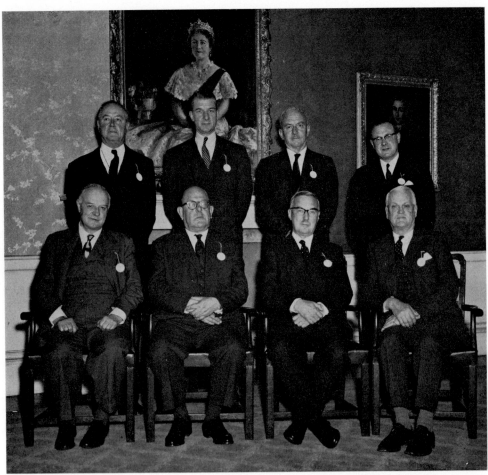

PLATE 54 Edinburgh: Inaugural Conference of the Presidents of the Colleges of Physicians of the Commonwealth and associated Republics (1962). Back row: Dr K. B. Noad (Australasia), Dr G. M. Brown (Canada), Professor G. A. Elliot (South Africa), Dr R. F. Robertson (Edinburgh, Secretary). Front row: Dr J. H. Wright (Glasgow), Sir Charles Dodd (London), Dr J. D. S. Cameron (Edinburgh), Professor R. E. Steen (Ireland)
Photograph by J. Campbell Harper, Edinburgh

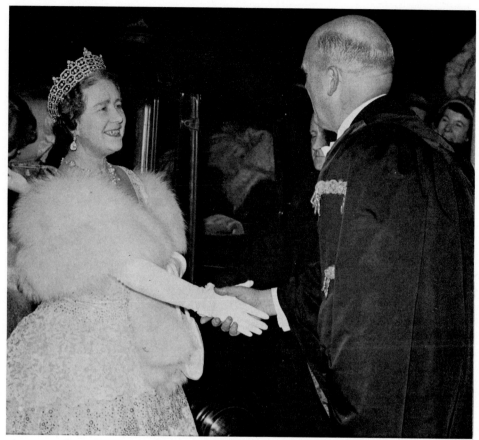

PLATE 55   Her Majesty Queen Elizabeth the Queen Mother, Honorary Fellow, being received by the
President, Dr A. Rae Gilchrist (1959)
Photograph by the Scotsman Publications Ltd.

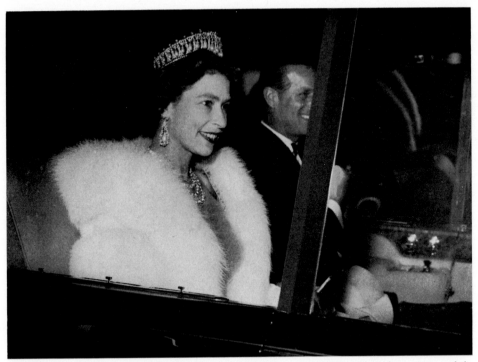

PLATE 56   Her Majesty Queen Elizabeth, Patron of the College, and His Royal Highness Prince Philip,
Duke of Edinburgh, leaving the College after a reception (1966)
Photograph by the Scotsman Publications Ltd.

throughout its existence, but gives little indication of *the spirit* of Fellowship known to and practised by Fellows throughout the ages.

AS PIONEERS

In what ways was this outlook applied to the ultimate enhancement of the prestige of the College? First and foremost it bred a pioneer spirit. It was revealed in the pertinacity of our predecessors in the second and subsequent decades of the seventeenth century. Receipt of the Charter was followed by the founding of a now world-famous library; the production of a classic *Pharmacopoeia* which for long stood the test of time; and the founding of a Dispensary for the Poor. Asked by the Town Council for epidemiological advice, the College did not miss the opportunity to enlarge upon matters of sanitation and public hygiene. With little delay the College was effective in encouraging the creation of a Medical Faculty in the University of Edinburgh, and played a leading part in the establishment of the Edinburgh Infirmary for the sick poor, and of an Asylum for the mentally afflicted. Considered in the context of their time these were great achievements manifesting a laudable visionary foresight embracing domiciliary and institutional care, physical and mental ill-health, poverty, malnutrition and environmental influences. This self-same breadth of outlook was to stand the College, and indeed the nation, in good stead in the nineteenth century with the problems which followed in the wake of industrialization, movements of population and immigration. The College was to the fore in its publicly declared concern for reliable statistical Bills of Mortality and Registers of Births, Deaths and Marriages.

The demands of patients, public health and administration did not deter the College from implementing the basic requirements of their Charter. A recognized place was secured for the physician in the practice of medicine, and certainly the College assisted in bringing order out of chaos among the many professing to practise the art of healing whether as physicians, surgeons, barber–surgeons, pharmacists or mountebanks. When in the nineteenth century an unquestioned need for comprehensive medical reform arose, the College's contribution was notable for its declared recognition of the inestimable value to the community of those who today would be referred to as general practitioners. It was Sir William Osler who urged '. . . the family doctor, the private in our great army, the essential factor in the battle, should be carefully nurtured by the schools and carefully guarded by the public'.[12] This truth was recognized by the College many years before it was expressed in words by Osler.

2K

There can be little doubt that the zeal displayed by the College in contributing to medical reform owed something to a resurgent nationalism. This can be explained by the sustained harrying of Scottish Licentiates practising south of Tweed. The reaction had sound basis. In 1890, in an address on medical education Sir William Turner submitted a powerful claim for educational freedom for the Scottish Universities. 'It is difficult to understand', he declared, 'why we in Scotland, with an educational history of which we have no cause to be ashamed, should be bound in swaddling clothes and impeded in our progress.' Turner's reaction was the more revealing in that he was a Lancastrian by birth.[13]

IN EDUCATION

Always concerned with medical education, the College combined with its sister Royal College of Surgeons in the supervision and management of the Edinburgh Extra-mural School of Medicine which in its heyday contributed great strength to Scottish medicine. The fact that it survived only fifty-three years was not the fault of the School or the Colleges but due to circumstances beyond their control. Sir Derrick Dunlop summed up the position succinctly: 'The empirical art of Medicine became more and more tinctured with a wholesome dose of science'[14] and medical teaching became almost completely dependent upon disbursements by the University Grants Committee. In its day the Laboratory was another pioneer project, which having proved itself in outstanding degree, did not acquire permanency. Again the determining factor was a wholly external one: expansion and reorganization of the National Health Service rendered an independent laboratory redundant.

In reality these two pioneer projects fell victims to the risks to which all such ventures have been exposed since time immemorial. Our national history abounds in examples of pioneer efforts being emulated, absorbed or replaced, in whole or part, by those possessed of greater resources.

AS COUNCILLOR

Study of the College history suggests that an element of complacency or more correctly, resignation entered the picture after the Report of the Royal Commission on the Scottish Universities. There was, however, evidence of purposeful rebound in the move towards an Extra-Mural School and the creation of a Research Laboratory —the first of its kind in the United Kingdom. Progress underwent deceleration as a result of two World Wars, and this was followed by the phenomenal influx of Membership candidates which resulted in a disproportionate amount of the College's time, energy and interest being devoted to examinations. Contrary to the view of one contributor to the *Chronicle*, preoccupation with examinations was *not* associated with a false sense of financial security.[15] Effective refutation is to be found in the Annual Reports of successive Treasurers for the years in question. Financial considerations apart, however, the College about this time seemed to withdraw into its ivory tower in a spirit of hauteur, assumed a somewhat parochial outlook and donned a mantle of benevolent historical superiority. Such an attitude sometimes masks inadequacy—and future historians may well refer to the period as one of inadequacy, not of the College but of its leadership. To the genuine distress of many Fellows this was obvious in the tactics adopted to impede closer association with the Glasgow Faculty (now Royal College). In 1971, Sir Stanley Davidson expressed the view of most Fellows and Members when he wrote 'the arguments which were mustered on behalf of a Scottish College in 1947 remain valid to-day'. Veiled contrition characterised Sir Stanley's rallying call.[16]

By way of contrast the late 1950s saw an enlivened awareness on the part of the College of existing links with overseas countries. For this the College was in large measure indebted to the presidential leadership of (Sir) James Cameron.

In its pioneering capacity the College early acquired the rôle of advisory body in relation to both national and civic affairs. Nor did it always wait to be approached as evidenced by the unsolicited advice given on more than one occasion to the Town Council on matters pertaining to community health, and the submission to the Government of a Petition for a Royal Commission on Venereal Diseases. Furthermore, initiative and catholicity were shown by the College in the constructively remonstrative memoranda and petitions submitted to central departments on such wide ranging subjects as the plight of the Highlands and Islands, the inadequacies of Poor Law Relief, and the circumstances of medical officers in the fighting services and Irish prison service. For a number of years, with justification, the College considered itself competent to advise on many aspects of medicine however widely interpreted. To an increasing extent its acknowledged expert advice was sought by public bodies and central and local authorities, and indeed the time was when in the view of many the College was the sole arbiter available on medical matters.

The present century has seen a change. The days of personal approach to Ministers are virtually things of the past. Perhaps comfortable tête-à-têtes in the Athenaeum or its Edinburgh equivalent are fast following suit! With the mushroom growth of many organizations with relatively narrow specialist interests, and of multiple departments directly or indirectly involved in matters concerning health and disease, the voice of the College has now often to compete as in a tower of Babel. To an increasing extent the submission of memoranda and petitions has largely given way to meeting requests from central Departments and Hospital Boards for comments and observations. Together with contributions to the work of local and national committees this now represents the bulk of the advisory activities of the College.

The beginnings of a change were evident at the time of the *National Insurance Act*, and the trend has not ceased to gain momentum with the progressive phase by phase expansion of the Welfare State concept. As a consequence the College has been involved in increased and not lessened administrative work. There is convincing evidence of this in the large number of Reports required of it during the planning, initial execution, and now reorganization of the National Health Service.

Inevitably the changes have necessitated considerable adjustment on the part of the College. Following the creation of Regional Hospital Boards (now Area Health Boards) many discussions have had to be conducted with a new type of official, best described as a curious cross between civil servant and local government officer. Evidences of incompatibility have not been lacking, but at least the Scottish Colleges have been spared the not always creditable confrontations elsewhere in the United Kingdom between Teaching and Regional Hospital Boards. One development which should put the College and other similar independent Corporations on the alert is the comparatively recent establishment of a Staff College for Hospital Lay Administrators. Certainly those concerned primarily with the clinical care of patients will require the carefully calculated support of the Medical Corporations in guarding against the insidious intrusion of excessive bureaucratic control. Warnings are not far to seek in other spheres. Scotland may well yet rue the day when hospitals dispensed with their altogether superb medical superintendents.

PRESENT ACTIVITIES

To travel hopefully is a better thing than to arrive, and the true success is to labour.
R. L. Stevenson

ADVISORY

Basic to all current activities is the maintenance and improvement of professional standards. The College continues to function in an advisory capacity by submitting its views to national bodies, Area Health Boards and District Executive Committees, either in the form of memoranda or through the agency of its appointed representatives on national and other committees. In this way the College is able, as in the past, to make representations concerning proposed legislation with a bearing on the health of the nation and of the local community. Representations may be in response to requests for advice, or spontaneous in origin. An admirable example of the latter is the Report published by the College on *The Care of the Elderly in Scotland*[17] which as a major contribution to community medicine may legitimately be regarded as having importance comparable to that of the London College's Report on *Smoking and Health Now*.[18]

The strength of our College as a Counselling Agent lies in its independence: its weakness in the fact that it cannot claim to be truly national.

EDUCATION

In the field of medical education College activities are confined to the needs of the postgraduate. Care has to be exercised that measures undertaken do not conflict with the work of the Edinburgh Post-Graduate Board for Medicine of which the College is a major constituent member with considerable influence on policy.

It is not without significance that the Croom Report on the Future of the College was produced by a College Committee appointed originally 'to consider the role of the College in the light of the Report of the Royal Commission on Medical Education'.[19] An early outcome was acceptance by the College of the Committee's Recommendation to establish a Standing College Committee to deal with Specialist Standards, Vocational Registration and Postgraduate Medical Education, and with powers to set up Specialty Committees. This was a timely prelude to discussions at a national level.

An early development was adoption of a policy to provide Instructional Courses at advanced level, these being organized by the appropriate Specialty Committees. *The courses are intended for the continuing education of Fellows and Members and not to provide preparation for Membership Examinations.* With the same object in mind the scientific symposia arranged by the College have been subject to modification. Not only have those held in the College Hall been expanded in number and scope but additional symposia have been organized in other centres in both Scotland and England. Of these additional symposia the Glasgow Royal College has to date been a co-sponsor in two, and local branches of the British Medical Association have co-operated in others. A further development has taken the form of separate joint symposia with the Royal College of Surgeons of Edinburgh, the Royal Society of Edinburgh and the Edinburgh Group of the Royal Statistical Society. The new symposia programme has met with an encouraging response as evidenced by greater participation in discussion and increased attendance. Plans are already in hand for several years ahead. Assuming these materialize, symposia in addition to those arranged to take place in Edinburgh will be held in several North of England centres. Certain symposia may from time to time be sponsored by the Pharmaceutical Industry.

Although not educational in the narrow sense, primarily social biennial meetings are now held by Fellows and Members in at least two centres in England. These have been attended by the President or other Members of Council as guests, and serve to consolidate the links between the College and 'distant exiles'.[20]

The examinations for the Membership, the Diploma in Psychological Medicine and those in connection with the Triple Qualification continue to exert a significant influence on medical education. Those in connection with the Membership have, without undue sacrifice of influence, undergone fundamental change with the introduction of the national multiple-choice screening examination and the Membership (U.K.). Nevertheless in agreeing to the abandonment of the long-established and well-proven characteristic Edinburgh examination the College made a sacrifice of considerable magnitude. Whether it was wholly justified in that by discouraging 'multiple diplomatosis' the concession enhanced the prestige of British medicine, remains an open question. There are many senior Fellows today with prolonged experience of examining, who think not—and their conviction is not attributable to parochialism or nationalism. Of particular importance was categorical rejection by the Croom Report of 'the inference which may be drawn from . . . the Royal Commission's Report that admission to the Membership of the College might be solely based on a series of training reports'. *Trainee physicians*, the Croom Report asserted, *will not be admitted to the Membership of the College without examination.*[21]

In so far as our College is concerned the Faculty of Community Medicine represents an entirely new development. Ostensibly a response to a recommendation of the Todd Report,[22] the Faculty aims at exercising a major rôle in the training of those in the field of Community Medicine. Rightly it has been said that doctors engaged in community medicine hold positions of relevance to key areas of College endeavour. Assuming that the Faculty attains its objective it may be accepted that both the College and Community Medicine stand to benefit from reasonably close association. Primarily the Faculty is to be evaluated as a contribution to furtherance of education within the overall field of social, preventive and administrative medicine.[23] In combining with the two sister Colleges, the Edinburgh College of Physicians has made its full contribution to trial of a new concept.

INTERNAL REFORM

Internal affairs have not escaped reform. Indeed they have been the subject of far-reaching developments opening up prospects of progress in an age of rapid changes in the medical scene. A careful review has been carried out of the procedure for elevation to the Fellowship with the object of dealing with anomalies and oversight. The institution of an order of Collegiate Members is a reform of outstanding historical and practical significance. With the privileges and rights accorded them, Collegiate Members are in a position to ensure that the moulding of policy is no longer the sole prerogative of seniors among Fellows, or for that matter of Fellows only.

The launching of the quarterly *Chronicle* is further evidence of a determination to progress. In the first few years of its existence this publication has provided a forum for healthy criticism and carefully considered constructive suggestions contributed by Fellows and Collegiate Members. If the infectious enthusiasm of the latter invades the College Hall, the silent acquiescent attitude characteristic of a goodly proportion of sederunts may soon be dispelled. An excellent feature, which should certainly become a routine, has been the inclusion of Council Committee Reports in recent issues of the *Chronicle*.[24]

THE FUTURE

Thou too, sail on, O Ship of State!
Sail on, O Union, strong and great!
Humanity with all its fears,
With all the hopes of future years,
Is hanging breathless on thy fate!

H. W. Longfellow

To those concerned for the prestige and welfare of our College nothing could be more heartening than the tenor and spirit of determination evident throughout the

Report of the Future of the College.[19] In an age dominated by administration and riddled with committees—an endemic disease more deeply rooted and more widely dispersed by far than 'multiple diplomatosis'—Reports are only too liable to speedy burial in the archives but not so in this instance. No time has been lost in implementing recommendations suited to prompt action. The institution of the order of Collegiate Membership with the avowed intention of 'securing the active participation of Members in College activities and affairs' is a case in point. Who knows how soon, to the ultimate benefit of the College, Fellows may find the pace being set for them by some twentieth-century Archibald Pitcairne, James Gregory, Alexander Wood or Robert Christison not yet emerged from chrysalis form? To say that is not to imply criticism of those, who as office bearers and committee members have so successfully and assiduously guided College affairs in recent years, but rather to suggest that those office bearers might in the past have had the encouragement of more active participation from 'the body of the Kirk'—with 'active' the operative word.

'NON-RESIDENT' FELLOWS AND MEMBERS

The advent of Collegiate Members, the revised policies with regard to postgraduate education activities, the manifest urge for intensified co-operation with other Royal Colleges, the Universities, selected specialist organizations and the British Medical Association, and the conception of the College becoming a prestigious focal meeting point for medical groups are all evidence of a raising of its sights by the College.

Widening outlook must not, however, be confined to internal administrative or to essentially local considerations—in the words of Sir Derrick Dunlop, 'the College . . . must . . . be more outward looking, remembering that it comprises a society which is not parochial, but is national and international'.[25] Whatever steps are taken in this direction, anything approaching complete success will not be achieved unless Diplomates, wherever they may be, are effectively encouraged to feel they are valued as *active* participants in the corporate life of the College. Should Regional Committees of Fellows be established along the lines proposed in the Croom Report, they would be ideally suited to fostering this feeling of mutual interest. Human nature being what it is, the initiative must be seen to come from the centre, and the *Chronicle* could give support by periodically including brief accounts of activities in—to borrow a term beloved by the Londoner!—'the provinces'. Regardless of their functions in the matter of recommendations for elevation to the Fellowship, the primary object of Regional Committees should be to foster and sustain affectionate allegiance to the parent body. The idea that the College has served its purpose in relation to the individual with the award of a Diploma must be ruthlessly discountenanced.

Sadly, of late, Graduate Associations of more than one Scottish University have found less favour among Scottish graduates domiciled in certain (but not all) parts of England. In one northern English city separate local associations, all with histories of over seventy years, representative of the Universities of Edinburgh, Aberdeen, Glasgow and St Andrews, have ceased their activities within the last few years. There are several explanations. One is that a growing tendency for functions to become dominantly medical, discouraged enrolment of graduates of other faculties. Far from inhibiting, this very finding should encourage the formation by the College of Regional Committees. Furthermore Regional Committees might well give valuable assistance to the College if, as would seem eminently desirable, it were in the words of one Fellow 'to keep information on its Fellows and Members as an ongoing project'. Certain American schools have established that interest in their alumni which, sustained in this way, serves to perpetuate strong and enduring loyalties.

OVERSEAS LINKS

Admittedly the varied situations in overseas countries present problems all their own, but there is no justification for regarding them as insoluble. Indebtedness is not all one-sided. The College is grateful for the opportunities it has had to help in the advancement of medicine overseas. It takes pride in the achievement of those of its Diplomates who are Fellows and Members of our corporate society in foreign lands, many of whom value their College associations—no matter how intangible links may have become with the passage of time. Surely it is not beyond the wit of multi-racial man to devise a means of extending further afield the spirit of warm genuine Fellowship which pervades the College at home. There are always in the United Kingdom a considerable number of Edinburgh Fellows and Members with first-hand knowledge of circumstances abroad. Is there not then, a good case for the establishment by the College of a Standing Committee, to keep under periodic review links with overseas countries? The suggestion merits consideration not as a defensive rearguard action nor as a move of imperialist expansion, but as the positive discharge of a responsibility inherited from our predecessors.

RESEARCH

In the present day and age the prosecution of Research is a hallmark of progress. The College has been fully alive to the deprivation experienced following closure of its Laboratory. Only the gratifying response to the Appeal, with Sir Derrick Dunlop as Chairman, has enabled the loss to be made good. Addressing an International Surgical Congress in 1949 Professor Grey Turner elaborated his views on Research. 'In greater medicine', he declared, 'all enquiry into the cause and natural history of disease, its response to environment and the reactions of the body to treatment . . . is real research and if such enquiries are made on careful lines which involve exactitude and measurement, then such enquiry has every right to be spoken about as scientific research. The common idea is that such work cannot be research, unless it is associated with laboratories, animal experiments, ultra-microscopic investigations, expensive apparatus, many assistants and so on.'[26]

Without question Grey Turner would have been in sympathy with the College's decision to promote research activities not dependent upon laboratory investigation, but directed towards solution of the epidemiological, statistical, social and genetic problems which figure so prominently in modern medicine. Proposals for the institution of two research Fellowships may be expected to result in necessary scientific information being readily available for Special College Committees and, of no less importance, for investigations upon which the College may decide to embark with a view to subsequent publication. Countless problems await investigation. Should a policy of promoting comprehensive research studies possessed of depth and breadth be adopted, the prestige of the College will be greatly enhanced.

The College must show, as it has done in the past, evidence of initiative and originality. Here again the need exists to avoid parochialism. The very nature of the fields of enquiry mentioned points to the desirability of co-operation with other centres. The other centres might consist of sister Corporations, Universities or groups of Fellows linked with the proposed College Regional Committees. To date medical research within the ambit of the National Health Service has failed to take full advantage of the possibilities of inter-regional co-operation and inter-regional controls. An example might be set by the College, which at the same time could endeavour to offset the element of professional isolationism hitherto inseparable from a primarily consultant body. Are all members of the College as well versed in domiciliary conditions as their predecessors were; are their views dominated disproportionately by urban as opposed to rural requirements; and to what extent are they becoming excessively conditioned by a wholly hospital outlook? In some parts of the country the priest and general practitioner are in process of losing their personal influence with the progressive decline in parish visiting. Broadly interpreted the College parish embraces town and country, hospital and home.

A ROYAL COLLEGE OF PHYSICIANS OF SCOTLAND?

A whole section of the Croom Report is devoted to the 'Relationship of the College to other Bodies'. This is fundamental to the future position of the College as an advisory and counselling body. Having regard to the trend towards centralization with concomitant acquisition of increasing directive powers by government departments, this facet of the College's function requires early priority consideration. None will question the desirability of closer relationship with the Universities and Boards responsible for the administration of hospitals when matters of mutual interest are under consideration. Of even greater importance is the need for greater collaboration with sister Royal Colleges. Past history serves as a reminder of the difficulties in the way of securing collaboration of the degree necessary if Medicine is to speak with one voice. Participants will require to show magnanimity and make concessions, and to consider proposals in a national and not a local context. Empire building and personal ambition must be eschewed.

These views are not hypothetical. Suffice it to say that *à propos* of some form of affiliation between the Edinburgh and Glasgow Colleges a senior Fellow of the latter recently expressed the opinion that 'the wounds are too deep to be healed'. None the less the Croom Report, despite our College's unhappy attitude in the past, has recommended that 'steps should be taken . . . to establish a closer association' between these two Colleges with, as ultimate aim, the creation of a Federation of Royal Colleges of Physicians of the United Kingdom.[27] Presumably consideration of a Scottish College of Physicians (or as some few would prefer, a Scottish Academy of Medicine) is not precluded. A Scottish College, it has been argued, would provide a united front in influencing 'medical and political affairs in Scotland and in England'.[28]

The argument is not attributable to irresponsible nationalistic fervour. Frankness demands admission to a wholesome respect for the influence and power of our elder sister College in London. Undoubtedly the London Royal College of Physicians speaks from strength in terms of the number and eminence of its Fellows, and of its history. It speaks for England and Wales. Transfer of its headquarters to a site with such enlightened associations as 'St Andrew's Place' is not assurance, however, that a Disraelian outlook no longer prevails! It is scarcely surprising that among those with allegiance to our College, some are apprehensive lest recent negotiations concerning the M.R.C.P. Diploma should prove to be the harbinger of a comprehensive 'take-over' by our London brethren. We live in equivocal times. If the methods adopted on the London Stock Exchange are any criteria the preliminaries to 'take-over bids' can be mysterious and multifarious.

On what other grounds then, can a case be made out for a Scottish College? It is not inappropriate to mention that the traditional perspicacity of the Scottish domiciled stockbroker has been ascribed to perspective derived from working at a distance from the southern metropolitan maelstrom. In a number of respects the Scottish approach to Medicine, and to medical education in particular, has differed from that in the south. The points of difference have varied from time to time over the centuries, and although essentially educational in character continue to be reflected in medical practice. In the circumstances the co-existence of a Scottish and London College would surely be to their mutual advantage. What better in the face of such a challenge then to ponder over the words of the seventeenth-century Scot, James Graham, Marquis of Montrose:

> *He either fears his fate too much,*
> *Or his deserts are small,*
> *That dares not put it to the touch,*
> *To gain or lose it all.*

ENLIGHTENING THE PUBLIC

Each year brings new challenges. To mention a few at random, there are the situations consequent upon entry into the European Common Market, prevalent concern over population control and pollution, euthanasia, and the consideration being given to future regulation of the Medical Profession. And what of genetic engineering with its ominous implications—moral, legal and scientific?

Obviously the future will witness no lessening in the total commitments undertaken by the College regardless of changes in emphases which may take place. Many if not most European colleagues are bewildered by the co-existence of Medical Corporations and Universities. Coming nearer home, to what extent are the activities of the College known outside medical circles in this country? The answer is, only to a limited extent, and then only very superficially. To know of its existence is not to know the College, and yet that is the sum total awareness of a large number of Edinburgh citizens. Perhaps understandably, confusion with the University is common.

Or—not infrequently the rhetorical question is heard—'something after the style of the Surgeons' Hall isn't it?', the 'after' clearly indicating a lesser degree of glamour! How many outside the profession know the full significance of the College's determination to maintain its professional and financial independence?

Not any one of these instances is vitally important, but cumulatively they point to the need for the place of the College in the civic life of Edinburgh to be more widely and accurately known. Historically we can claim that the City and not the College has reason to feel indebted. That which applies to Edinburgh, applies also in lesser degree to much of Scotland as a whole. The Croom Committee urged the College to be concerned with the projection of its own message to the medical profession, and the lay public. There is a crying need for this, a need which it should be the College's aim to convert to clamant demand. The time was when the Laws of the College deprecated if they did not actually forbid the reporting of such events as Receptions and Dinners. No such legal embargo obtains now although no one would question the need for continuing circumspection.

Whatever forms of publicity are employed, let there be no resort to the synthetic sensationalism and mischievous melodrama beloved of modern public media. However unfashionable let us have regard to the historical greatness of our College and the dignity of our profession. There is a rich abundance of proven facts dispensing with the necessity for prejudiced impressions and distorted comment. More especially where 'headlines' and their equivalent are concerned, Eastwood and Smith have drawn attention to the practical problems involved.[29]

A quarter of a century ago it was stated that the Scot 'likes to get his news unpredigested and unadorned, and to assess its implications independently'. Admittedly discernment of this nature is not now so much in evidence. None the less endeavours to reach the public should not underestimate 'the canny, critical and shrewd' temperament of those who have 'tended to idolize education'.

As it moves forward into the future let our College remain a bastion of some at least of the ancient graces. May G. K. Chesterton's warning be heeded:

> *'The modern innovation which has substituted journalism for history . . . has had at least one definite effect. It has insured that everybody should only hear the end of every story.'*[30]

Nor should it be forgotten that in the words of Trevelyan:

> *'The English language . . . had a pungency and a poetic power that it has . . . lost, in pursuit of scientific terms and journalistic phraseology.'*[31]

The trend is one our College should seek to arrest if not reverse.

In the interests of 'the Lieges', of Medicine and of our College let the lie be given to Bernard Shaw's assertion that: 'All professions are conspiracies against the laity'.[32] The truth is epitomized in the motto chosen by the Founders of the College of Physicians of Philadelphia:

Non sibi sed toti.

REFERENCES

FOUNDATION

(1) DARWIN, Sir F. (1914) Francis Galton. *Eugenics Review*, **6**, 1.

PAST ENDEAVOURS

(2) SIBBALD, Sir R. (1833) *The Autobiography of Sir Robert Sibbald, Knt., M.D.* Edinburgh: Thomas Stevenson.

(3) SIBBALD, Sir R. (1837) *Memoirs of the Royal College of Physicians at Edinburgh.* Edinburgh: Thomas Stevenson.

(4) R.C.P.E. (1833) *Report on Examination of Medical Practitioners.* Edinburgh: Neill.

(5) BEILBY, W. (1847) *Address Delivered at the Opening of the New Hall of the Royal College of Physicians, November 27, 1846.* Edinburgh: Constable.

(6) RITCHIE, R. P. (1899) *The Early Days of the Royall Colledge of Phisitians, Edinburgh.* Edinburgh: G. P. Johnston.

(7) R.C.P.E. (1925) *Historical Sketch and Laws of the Royal College of Physicians of Edinburgh from its Institution to 1925.* Edinburgh: Royal College of Physicians.

(8) RITCHIE, J. (1953) *History of the Laboratory of the Royal College of Physicians of Edinburgh.* Edinburgh: Royal College of Physicians.

(9) R.C.P.E. [c. 1850] *Abstracts of the Minutes, A.D. 1682–1731.* By George Paterson. (Ms.)

(10) POOLE, R. (1838) *Preparatory Notes for a History of the College.* (Ms.)

(11) PENDRILL, G. R. (1961) The Royal College of Physicians, its origins and functions. *Scottish Medical Journal*, **6**, 526–31.

(12) DOWLING, H. F. (1970). *Medicines for Man*, p. 285. New York: Knopf.

(13) TURNER, A. L. (1919) *Sir William Turner . . . Professor of anatomy and Principal and Vice-Chancellor of the University of Edinburgh. A chapter in medical history*, p. 336. Edinburgh: Blackwood.

(14) DUNLOP, Sir D. (1962) Medical education in Scotland. *Scottish Medical Journal*, **7**, 6, 247.

(15) WATSON, H. (1971) Conviction. *Chronicle*, **I**, 3, 32.

(16) DAVIDSON, Sir S. (1971) Letter. *Chronicle*, **I**, 3, 40.

PRESENT ACTIVITIES

(17) R.C.P.E. (1963) *The Care of the Elderly in Scotland.* Edinburgh: Royal College of Physicians. (Publication no. 22.)

(18) ROYAL COLLEGE OF PHYSICIANS OF LONDON (1971) *Smoking and Health now: a new report and summary on smoking and its effects on health.* London: Pitman Medical.

(19) R.C.P.E. (1969) *Report of College Committee to Consider the Future of the College.* (Convener: Dr. J. Halliday Croom.) Edinburgh: Royal College of Physicians.

(20) GRAY, J. A. (1972) Personal communication.

(21) R.C.P.E. (1969) *Report of the College Committee to Consider the Future of the College*, para. 43. Edinburgh: Royal College of Physicians.

(22) ROYAL COMMISSION ON MEDICAL EDUCATION 1965–68 (1968) *Report.* (Chairman: Lord Todd.) Para. 138. London: H.M.S.O.

(23) THE FACULTY OF COMMUNITY MEDICINE OF THE ROYAL COLLEGE OF PHYSICIANS OF EDINBURGH, ROYAL COLLEGE OF PHYSICIANS AND SURGEONS OF GLASGOW [and] ROYAL COLLEGE OF PHYSICIANS OF LONDON (1972) *Draft standing orders*, p. 1. [London: The Faculty.]

(24) Council Committee reports (1972) *Chronicle*, **2**, 4, 21–31.

THE FUTURE

(25) DUNLOP, Sir D. (1972). Personal impressions. *Chronicle*, **2**, 2, 5.

(26) TURNER, G. GREY (1950) Pillars of surgical wisdom. In *Congrès de la société internationale de chirurgie, 13th, New Orleans, 1949*, p. 219. Brussels: Imprimerie médicale et scientifique.

(27) R.C.P.E. (1969) *Report of College Committee to Consider the Future of the College*, para. 71. Edinburgh: Royal College of Physicians.

(28) OLIVER, M. F. (1971) Distinction or extinction? *Chronicle*, **1**, 2, 24.

(29) EASTWOOD, M. & SMITH, I. D. (1973) *Medicine and the Mass Media: answering Press questions*, p. 8. Edinburgh: Royal College of Physicians.

(30) CHESTERTON, G. K. (1946) *St. Francis of Assisi*, 25th Edition, p. 20. London: Hodder & Stoughton.

(31) TREVELYAN, G. M. (1954) *A Layman's Love of Letters*, p. 26. London: Longmans, Green & Co. (Clark lectures series—1953).

(32) SHAW, G. B. (1932) The doctor's dilemma, I. In *The Doctor's Dilemma* [and other plays]. Revised Edition, p. 106. London: Constable.

EPILOGUE

If to-day we have a broader vision of our science than the men of 25 years ago, it is not because our sight is better but because we stand on their shoulders.

Luther Emmett Holt

Appendix A

Chronological List of Events

Philosophy and science range farther than history. The mind must take its starting-point as far back as it can reach.

Lord Samuel

Year	College Events	Chap. Ref.	Related Historical and Contemporary Events	Year	Chap. Ref.
			Oxford University: foundation	1249	
			Balliol College, Oxford founded	1263	
			Cambridge University (foundation of first college)	1284	
			Bannockburn	1314	
			University of St Andrews founded by Bishop Wardlaw	1410	
			Edinburgh: arrival of Plague	1430	I
			Glasgow University: foundation	1451	
			Linacre: birth	c. 1460	
			London: Barber-Surgeons granted a Charter	1462	XXV
			Caxton's printing press introduced in England	1477	
			Aberdeen University: foundation	1494	
			Edinburgh Barbers and Surgeons: Seal of Cause	1505	I
			Vesalius: birth	1514	
			Royal College of Physicians, London: foundation	1518	VII
			Linacre Foundation of Medical Lectures at Oxford and Cambridge	1524	
			St Bartholomew's Hospital: refounded.	1544	
			St Mary of Bethlehem Asylum (Bedlam): conveyed to City of London by Henry VIII	1547	XX

Year	Event	Part
1561	Francis Bacon: birth	I
1561	*Book of Discipline* delivered	
1567–1625	King James VI	I
1575	University of Leyden: foundation	
1578	William Harvey: birth	
1582	University of Edinburgh: Charter for Town's College (James VI)	I
1588	Defeat of Spanish Armada	
c.1590	Edinburgh: hospital for lepers established	I
1593	Marischal College, Aberdeen: foundation	
1599	Glasgow Faculty of Physicians & Surgeons: foundation	I
1603	James VI of Scotland succeeded to English throne (James I)	I
1617	London: Worshipful Society of Apothecaries founded	
1617	First abortive attempt to found the College	II
1620	Pilgrims landed in America	
1621	Dr George Sibbald: Articles for consideration by Estates of Parliament	II
1625–1649	King Charles I	I
1629	(Sir) Archibald Stevensone: birth	III
1630	Second abortive attempt to found the College	II
1632	Edinburgh: House of Correction ('Bridewell') established	XX
1633	Edinburgh made a bishopric, acquired status of 'City' and recognition as 'Capital'	I
1636	Harvard College: foundation	
1641	(Sir) Robert Sibbald: birth	III
1642	(Sir) Issac Newton: birth	I
1643	Solemn League and Covenant	I

Year	College Events	Chap. Ref.	Related Historical and Contemporary Events	Year	Chap. Ref
			Edinburgh: Apothecaries admitted to Surgical Guild	1645	I
			Scotland free of the Plague after 200 years of recurrent epidemics	1649	I
1652	Archibald Pitcairne: birth	III			
			Cromwell's Protectorate	1653–1658	
1656	Third abortive attempt to found the College	II	Edinburgh: Surgeons laid out Physic Garden	1656	
1656	Desirability of a Scottish College of Physicians raised by Cromwell's Lords of Council	II			
1657	Physicians from Edinburgh and Aberdeen met in Dundee	II	Wm. Harvey: death	1657	
1657	Dr George Purves visited the London Royal College of Physicians	II	Edinburgh: Fraternity of Apothecaries founded	c. 1657	X
			King Charles II (of Scotland and England)	1660–1685	I
			Robert Sibbald at Leyden	1660–1661	XVII
			Royal Society: Charter granted	1662	
			Great Plague of London	1665	
			Great Fire of London	1666	
			Smallpox in Europe	1666–1675	I
			Ireland: Royal College of Physicians founded	1667	XXV
			Edinburgh: Sibbald and Balfour start Physick Garden	c. 1670	V
			Edinburgh: piped water supply introduced	1672	I
1680	'Discourses' arranged by Robert Sibbald	VIII			
1681	Great Seal appended to Charter of Erection on St Andrew's Day	III	Dispute between Surgeons and Apothecaries in Edinburgh. Four future original Fellows of College of Physicians gave evidence in Court of Session	1681	III
1681	First Meeting: December 7th	XXVI	Merchant Company of Edinburgh: Charter granted	1681	I

Year	Event	Ref.
1681	*Institutions of the Law of Scotland*: publication by Lord Stair	I
1681	Test Act imposed on Scotland	I
1681	Partially systematized emigration from Scotland: background of commercial enterprise and avoidance of religious persecution.	I
1682	Edinburgh: Surgeons and Apothecaries—'Decreit of Separation'	III & X
1682	Quaker Colony founded in America by William Penn	XXXV
1682	Edinburgh: Advocates' Library (National Library of Scotland) founded	I
1685	King James VII (II of England) succeeds Charles II	I

Ref.	Event	Year
XXVI	Election of first Office-Bearers	1681
XXVI	First Laws drafted	1681
VI	Gift of books from (Sir) Robert Sibbald	1682
VIII	FIRST SEDERUNTS (December 7th and 8th)	1682
V	Pharmacopoeia: referred to in first item of first Minutes	1682
XXVI	Promissory Obligation determined	1682
V	Two Fellows appointed to serve the poor of the City	1682
III	Doctors Sibbald, Stevensone and Balfour knighted	1682
VII	Admission of first Licentiate by examination	1682
VII	Formula for Licentiate's Diploma agreed	1683
VI	Dr William Stevensone appointed first Librarian	1683
VIII	First College Discourse given by Sir Archibald Stevensone	1684
V	College Minutes missing (Dec.) until March 21st, 1693	1684
III	Charter of Erection ratified by Scottish Parliament	1685
XVIII	Sibbald appointed Professor of Physick by Town Council: also Drs Halket and Pitcairne	1685
VII	Dr Irvin (Irving): absolution by Privy Council from adjudication by the College confirmed by Scottish Parliament	1685
X	Petition for reduction of proposed 'Patent for Chirurgions'	1686
III	Sibbald elected Fellow R.C.P. London. Embraced Roman Catholicism for brief period.	1686
I	'Anderson Pills'—Petition considered on instructions of the Lords of Session	1687

Year	College Events	Chap. Ref.	Related Historical and Contemporary Events ((F) = Fellow of R.C.P.Ed.)	Year	Chap. Ref.
1689	*Edinburgh Pharmacopoeia*: ready for publication	V	King William III	1689–1702	V
			Pitcairne appointed Professor of Medicine at University of Leyden: resigned following year	1692	XVII
			Massacre of Glencoe	1692	XXVII
1693	College Minutes again available	V	College of Surgeons of Edinburgh: Charter granted	1694	
1694	Publications by Fellows to have prior approval of College	VIII	Bank of Scotland founded	1695	I
1695	Withdrawal of opposition to reunion of Surgery and Pharmacy	X			
1695	'A ryot in the College': Pitcairne and Oliphant suspended	XIX			
1695	Suspension of a number of recalcitrant Fellows	XIX			
1696	Honorary Fellowship conferred for first time	VIII	Robert Sibbald (F) gave museum specimens to the Town's College Authorities	1697	V
1696–1707	Financial involvement in Darien Scheme	XXXIV	Edinburgh: Anatomical theatre established at Surgeon's Hall	1697	XVI & XXII
			Scottish Darien expedition	1698–1700	I
1699	Appeal for Relief of Poor by Sir Robert Sibbald	I			
1699	*Edinburgh Pharmacopoeia*: first published	V			
1700	Minutes missing from 5.xii.1700 to 16.v.1701	XXXIV			
1701	Minutes missing from 4.xii.1701 to 16.xi.1702	XXXIV			
1702	Jurisdiction of College rejected by (Dr) Drummond	VII	Queen Anne	1702–1714	I
1704	Fountain Close: first Physicians' 'Hall'	IV			
1704	Amnesty declared for suspended recalcitrant Fellows	XIX			

Year	Event	Ref
1705	Two Fellows examined the first candidate to receive degree of M.D. from Edinburgh Town's College	XVII
1706	Gift of 'curiosities' received from Sir Robert Sibbald	V
1707	Separation of Physicians and Surgeons: Act enacted by College, and signed Promissory Obligation required of Fellows	XXVI
1707	Beneficiary of Mary Erskine bequest	V
1708	Dispensary established in the Fountain Close Hall	V
1710	Status of 'Candidat' discarded	VII
1711	Garden and shrubbery established at Fountain Close Hall	V
1713	Archibald Pitcairne: death	XXXIV
1713	'Bath-House' ready for use	V
1714	Apothecary appointed to the Dispensary	V
1720–1	Approach by Town Council re 'Pestilentious Infection'	IX
1720–1	College Report on Sanitation of City sent to Town Council	IX
1722	The President (Dr Jas. Forrest) died in office	XXXIV
1722	Sir Robert Sibbald: death	XXXIV
1722	New 'Hall' erected in the garden of Fountain Close	IV
1725	Examination of candidates for M.D. of the Town's College ceased to be remitted to the College of Physicians	XVIII
1728	Dr Matthew Sinclaire (St Clair) died: last survivor of the original Fellows	III
1729	Hospital opened in Robertson's Close, staffed by Fellows: precursor of Infirmary	XX

Year	Event	Ref
1705	Edinburgh: Guild of Surgeons appoint Professor of Surgery (Robert Eliot)	XVI
1707	Treaty of Union	I
1708	Abolition of Scottish Privy Council	
1713	Dr James Crawford (F) elected Professor of Physic in University of Edinburgh	XVIII
1715	Jacobite Rising	XXVII
1720	Alexander Monro *primus* (F) appointed Professor of Anatomy by Edinburgh Town Council	XVII & XVIII
1724	Dr Porterfield (F) appointed Professor by the Town Council	XVIII
1726	Edinburgh: Mr Gibson appointed City Professor of Midwifery to instruct midwives	XVIII
1726	Four Fellows appointed Professors by the Town Council	XVIII
1726	Medical Faculty in the Town's College founded	XVIII
1727	Last Scottish 'witch' condemned to death	XVIII
1728	John Hunter: birth	I

Year	College Events	Chap. Ref.	Related Historical and Contemporary Events ((F) = Fellow of R.C.P.Ed.)	Year	Chap. Ref.
			Edinburgh: first Charity Workhouse opened	1731	XX
			Society for the Improvement of Medical Knowledge Founded by Monro *primus*	1731	VIII
			Edinburgh: Orphan Hospital founded (Dean Orphanage)	1733	XX
			Edinburgh Royal Infirmary: incorporated by Royal Charter	1736	XX
			Royal Medical Society: founded	1737	XXXIV
			University of Pennsylvania founded	1740	XVII
			Edinburgh: new Workhouse opened	1743	XX
			Sir John Pringle (F) urges immunity from military attack for hospitals	1743	XXVII
			Jacobite Rising	1745	XXVII
			Prestonpans	1745	XXVII
			Dr John Rutherford (F) delivered the first clinical lectures in the Edinburgh Royal Infirmary	1746	XX
			Falkirk	1746	XXVII
			Culloden	1746	XXVII
			Edinburgh–Glasgow stage coach inaugurated	1749	XXVII
1750	Fellows debarred from keeping shop, or being Members of the Corporation of Surgeons or Apothecaries	X & XIX			
			Philadelphia Hospital: foundation	1751	XVII
			Pringle's (F) *Observations on the Diseases of the Army*	1752	I
			Lind's (F) *Treatise of the Scurvy*	1753	XXI
1754	Conjoining of Medicine and Pharmacy prohibited	XIX & XXVI			
1756	Separation of Physicians and Surgeons: Fellows ceased to sign relevant Promissory Obligation (q.v.-1707)	XIX	Seven Years War (1756-1763)	1756	XXVII
1756	Monro *primus* and Wm. Cullen took seats as Fellows on same day	XVIII	Lind's (F) *Treatise on Naval Hygiene*	1757	XXI

Year	Event	Ref.
1758	'Bath House': last mention	V
1761	Separation of 'physick and pharmacy': College views advertised in local press	X & XIX
c. 1762	Wm. Shippen (F) organized extramural lectures in Philadelphia on Edinburgh pattern	XVII
1763	Licentiateship made a necessary stage before advancement to the Fellowship	VII
1763	Proposals for union of the College and University Libraries rejected	VI
1764	Indian Medical Service: foundation	XXVII
1764	Prohibition of membership of Corporations of Surgeons/Apothecaries reiterated	XIX
1765	Watt's Steam Engine	
1765	Fellows debarred from practising Surgery and Midwifery	X & XIX
1765	Medical Faculty of Pennsylvania University founded	XVII
1765	Election of first American (Dr John Morgan) to Fellowship	VII & XVII
1766	Meetings of the College and College Library transferred temporarily to Royal Infirmary	VI
1766	The President (Dr Robert Whytt) died while in office	XXXIV
1767	*Statuta Solennia* enacted	XVIII
1768	Forth and Clyde Canal: construction commenced	I
1769	Cullen's *Synopsis nosologiae*	
1771	'Mr' Eccles admitted Licentiate after losing Court Appeal	VII
1771	Asked by Town Council for advice on prevention of Smallpox	IX
1771	Admission of Fellows to be by Ballot	VIII
1771	Last Leyden candidate to become a Fellow in 1822 (David Campbell, M.D.)	XVII
1772	College Act prohibiting the practice of Surgery and Midwifery renewed after having been amended and rescinded in the interval since 1765	XIX
1773	President resigned office on leaving Edinburgh	XXXIV

Year	College Events	Chap. Ref.	Related Historical and Contemporary Events ((F = Fellow of R.C.P.Ed.))	Year	Chap. Ref.
1774	'Traffick of Degrees': Memorial by Wm. Cullen	VII & XIV	Edinburgh: (Royal) Public Dispensary founded	1776	XX
			American Declaration of Independence	1776	XVII
			Guild of Surgeons converted by Charter to Royal College of Surgeons of Edinburgh	1778	XVII
			'Brunonian Theory' source of contention between Wm. Cullen (F) and John Brown (F)	1778–1780	
1781	Removal to new Physicians' Hall in George Street	IV			
1781	Slaughter Houses: advice sought by Town Council and action taken	IX	Edinburgh: famine and destitution extreme	1782–1788	I
			Royal Society of Edinburgh founded	1783	XXXIV
1784	Committee appointed to prepare an Abstract of Laws enacted from 7.xii.1681 to 3.viii.1784	XIX			
			College of Physicians of Philadelphia founded	1787	XVII
1788	Right of Fellows to Practise Midwifery restored	XIX			
1789	First Code of Laws arranged and printed	VIII & XII	French Revolution: outbreak	1789	
1790	Committee appointed to consider institutional needs of Indigent Incurables	XX			
1791	Erection of Public Asylum recommended by College Committee	XX			
1792	Glass measures and laudanum vials introduced to apothecaries' shops at the instigation of the College	X			
1796	Stamp Duty imposed on Diplomas of Licentiates and Fellows	VIII & XIV			
1796	Proposal to permit Licentiates and Fellows to supply medicines to their own patients gave rise to violent and prolonged dissension culminating in expulsion of Dr James Gregory	XIX	Jenner introduced vaccination	1796	XIX
			Glasgow: Anderson's College of Medicine established	1799	

Year	Event	Ref.
1801	Library Committee appointed 'in terms of the Law'	VI
1805	Subject to Property and Income Tax	
1805	Old form of Promissory Engagement of 1682 lost: re-placement provided and signed by Fellows	XXVI
1809	Narrative of the conduct of Dr. James Gregory published by authority of the Royal College of Physicians	XIX
1809	Election of distinguished doctors and laymen as Honorary Fellows ceased temporarily	VIII
1817	Report to Attorney General on Regulation of Surgery Bill	X
1817	Police Bill (Edinburgh): draft considered	IX
1817	Request by Town Council for 'ascertainment' of Fever in city	IX
1822	Term 'Member' amended to 'Fellow' in Regulations	VIII
1823	Prohibition of Druggists Shops kept by Fellows, co-partners or servants	X
1823	Repeal of Acts relating to Surgery	X
1829	Issue of Licences granting right to practise in Edinburgh and environs discontinued: old order of Licentiates ceased to exist: Fellows now elected without passing through 'inferior' grade	VII

Year	Event	Ref.
1802	Edinburgh Review first published	I
1803–1815	Napoleonic Wars	XXVII
1805	Battle of Trafalgar	
1807	Royal Edinburgh Hospital (Morningside Asylum) received Charter	XX
1809	Treatise on Medical Police by Dr J. Roberton	XXI
1809	Quarterly Review first published	I
1812	S.S. 'Comet' launched	
1815	Battle of Waterloo	
1815	Apothecaries Act	XI & XII
1817	Scotsman founded	X
1820	Edinburgh: gas lighting introduced	I
1821	University of McGill founded	XVII
1823	Lancet founded by Thos. Wakley	X
1823	Edinburgh: first course of lectures in Britain on Mental Diseases delivered by Alexander Morison (F)	XX
1826	Edinburgh: 'New Town Epidemic'	I
1826	Royal Commission on Scottish Universities	XVIII
1828	Burke and Hare Trial	VIII

Year	College Events	Chap. Ref.	Related Historical and Contemporary Events ((F) = Fellow of R.C.P.Ed.)	Year	Chap. Ref.
			First Scottish Railway	1831	
			British Medical Association: foundation	1832	XI
			Anatomy Act	1832	VIII
1833	Petition to Parliament re monopolies enjoyed by Apothecaries' Company	IX & XII	University of Edinburgh: *Statuta Solemnia* adopted by Senate	1833	XXII
1833	Sibbald's *Autobiography* published	XXXVII			
1833	Protest to Home Secretary re new Regulations for medical degrees at St Andrew's University	XXII			
1834	Pauper Lunatics: historic letter from Dr Richard Poole (F)	IX & XX			
1834	Medical Education: principles agreed with University and Royal College of Surgeons of Edinburgh	X			
1835	Decision made to establish a Materia Medica Museum	V			
1835	Memorial to Home Secretary re proposed Metropolitan University	XXIII			
1836	Materia Medica Museum: Curator appointed	V	University of London: foundation	1836	XXIII
1838	Future of Profession: Joint Conference with University and Royal College of Surgeons of Edinburgh	X			
1838	Report on the Adulteration of Drugs	X			
			Postage stamps introduced by Rowland Hill	1839	
1840	Petition to Queen that Poor Law Commissioners extend enquiries to Scotland	IX	W. P. Alison's (F) *Observations on the Management of the Poor in Scotland*	1840	I
1841	Petition for more accurate Registration of Births, Deaths etc.	IX	Beginnings of Edinburgh Medical Missionary Society	1841–1858	XX
1841	*Edinburgh Pharmacopoeia*: issue of last (14th) edition	V			
1842	Homeopathy discussed in sederunt	VIII	Edinburgh and Glasgow Railway opened	1842–1850	
1843	Property of College to be invested in Trustees chosen by Council and approved by College	XXXIV	'The Disruption'	1843	I

Date	Event	Chapter
1843	Need for a Fever Hospital raised in sederunt	IX
1843	Temporary accommodation in 119 George Street	IV
1845	New Charter drafted and revised but no further action	XIV
1846	Transfer to new Physicians' Hall in Queen Street	IV
1847	Regulations re examination of Fellows proposing to Lecture agreed	XVI
1848	London Monopolies: Protest to Home Secretary	XII
1848	Cholera: General Board warned of need for action	XX
1848–9	Committee stressed need for a City M.O.H.	IX
1849	Failure of negotiations to consider unification with the Glasgow Faculty	XXIV
1849	Medical Reform: Scottish Colleges in acute disagreement	XII
1850	Failure to re-open negotiations with Glasgow Faculty	XII
1851	Coldstream's papers on Highlands and Islands	IX
1851	Proposals for Incorporation of General Practitioners opposed	XII
1852	Report of Deficiency of Practitioners in Highlands and Islands	IX
1854	Conditions for Insane: President approached by Miss Dorothea Dix	XXI
1854	English Nosology criticised	IX
1845	Edinburgh: last medical apprentice (Thos. Keith)	I
1846–1847	Potato famine in Ireland: extreme phase	I
1846	Scotland and England linked by railway	
1847	J. Y. Simpson (F) introduced chloroform for obstetric anaesthesia	I
1848–1854	Edinburgh: old Surgeons Hall used as Cholera Hospital	
1850	Apothecaries' Company agreed amendments to Apothecaries Act 1815	XII
1850	'Paraffin' Young pioneers shale mining in W. Lothian	XI
1850	Glasgow Faculty of Physicians & Surgeons relinquished jurisdiction over 'District'	XXV
1851	Royal College of Surgeons of Edinburgh ceased to be a City Trade Guild	IX
1854	Scotland: Compulsory Registration of Births, Deaths and Marriages	XXVII
1854–1856	Crimean War	XVI
1855	Edinburgh University recognised Extra-academical Teaching in Edinburgh	

Year	College Events	Chap. Ref.	Related Historical and Contemporary Events	Year	Chap. Ref.
			Edinburgh: Idiot Asylum for Feeble Minded opened in Gayfield Square	1855	
			Royal Commission on Lunatics and Asylums in Scotland	1855	XXI
			Indian Mutiny	1857–1858	
1857	Warburton Begbie commenced course on History of Medicine in Extra-Mural School	XVI	Medical Corporations and Universities discuss University Degrees	1857	XII
1858	Report of the position of the College under the new Medical Act etc.	XIII	Medical Reform Act	1858	XIV
			Edinburgh: Royal College of Surgeons relinquished exclusive 'District' rights	1858	XI
1858	Nomination of first Representative on G.M.C.	XIV	The Universities (Scotland) Act	1858	XXII
1859	'Year of Grace'	XIV & XIX			
1859	Double Qualification instituted	XIV	Florence Nightingale's *Notes on Nursing*	1859	
1859	Revival of Licentiateship in new form: candidates with no University degree required to sit examination	XIV			
1859	Candidates for the Licence and Fellowship no longer required to possess a medical degree but qualifications to be ascertained.	XIV			
1859	Stamp Duty removed from Diploma of Licentiate	XIV			
1859	Designations 'Resident' and 'Non-Resident' Fellow abandoned	XIV			
1860	College Licence recognised by English Poor Law Board	XIV	Edinburgh: Royal Hospital for Sick Children founded	1860	XX
1861	NEW CHARTER. Name of Royal College of Physicians of Edinburgh preferred to Royal College of Physicians of Scotland	XV	Edinburgh: collapse of High Street tenement with loss of 35 lives	1861	I
1861	Direct election of President: abolition of offices of Censor and Fiscal: power to institute an Order of Members	XV			

Year	Event	Ref.
1862	British Pharmacopoeia (G.M.C.) issued	V
1862	Henry Littlejohn appointed as Edinburgh's first M.O.H.	I
1864	Edinburgh: Chalmers Hospital—first physician appointed	XX
1865	Miss Garret obtained Licence of Apothecaries Hall	XXIII
1865	Henry Littlejohn's *Report on Sanitary Condition of Edinburgh*	XXI
1867	Lister introduced antiseptic surgery	I
1866–1867	Cholera: last epidemic to date in Scotland	
1867	Public Health (Scotland) Act	XXI
1870	Edinburgh: Craiglockhart Poor House opened	XX

Year	Event	Ref.
1862	The Order of Members instituted	XIV
1862	Lady's petition to sit preliminary examination rejected	XVI
1862	College recommended adoption of decimal system in Pharmacopoeia	V
1863	Vaccination: Representations to Government	XXI
1863	William Cullen: Memorial erected over grave	XXXIV
1864	Army Medical Organisation: Memorial to Lord Palmerston	XXVII
1865	Office of Registrar created to deal with Licence applications: capable of being conjoined with office of Secretary	XIV
1866	Request from Town Council for further advice on sanitary condition of Edinburgh	XXI
1866	Advice to Lord Provost on Sanitary Reform	XX
1866	Report on Lunacy Act (Scotland) Amendment Bill	XXI
1866	Petition that there should be not less than two Parliamentary representatives for Scottish Universities	XVIII
1868	Candidates for Licence required to produce a Certificate of having studied Vaccination	XXII
1868	Combination of Maternity Hospital with Royal Infirmary recommended	XIV
1870	State medicine: doubts re G.M.C. Report	XXI
1870	All candidates for Licence to be examined in Clinical Medicine	XIV

Year	College Events	Chap. Ref.	Related Historical and Contemporary Events ((F) = Fellow of R.C.P.Ed.)	Year	Chap. Ref.
1871	House of Commons Select Committee on Vaccination: Dr Alexander Wood (F) only Scottish medical witness	XXI	Edinburgh: City accepted responsibility for providing hospital care for infectious diseases patients	1871	XX
			Darwin's *Descent of Man*	1871	
1874	Candidates for the Licence required to pass an examination in Surgery	XIV			
1874	Resolution passed to establish a Certificate of Qualification in State Medicine	XXI			
1874	Declined to recognize London School of Medicine for Women	XXIII			
1874	Agreed that Infectious Diseases Returns be made to Local Authorities	XXI	Invention of modern telephone (A. G. Bell)	1874	
			Edinburgh: Cockburn Association founded	1874	
1875	First Report of G.M.C. Visitors	XIV	Edinburgh: Hospital for Incurables (Longmore) founded	1875	XX
1875	Regulations established for Certificate of Qualification in State Medicine	XXI			
			Visitations by Commissioners to Scottish Universities	1876	XIV & XXII
			Johns Hopkins University founded	1876	
			Edinburgh: Notification of Infectious Diseases made compulsory	1879	XXI
			Edinburgh: Royal Infirmary moved to Lauriston Place	1879	XX
			Edinburgh: (Royal) Maternity and Simpson Memorial Hospital opened	1879	XX
1881	New Laws relating to admission to Membership and Fellowship: Membership candidates required to sit an examination	XIV	Tubercle bacillus discovered by Koch	1881	
1881	BICENTENARY celebrated at Annual Dinner	XXXIV			
1883	Medical Amendment Bill: Joint letter to Prime Minister	XII			

Year	Event	Ref.
1883	Cholera bacillus isolated by Koch	XII
1884	Tercentenary of the University of Edinburgh	
1885	First official cremation in Britain	
1885	Post of Parliamentary Secretary of Scotland established	
1886	The Medical Act Amendment Act	XII
1887	Edinburgh: Victoria Dispensary opened by (Sir) R. W. Philip (F)	XVIII
1888	Edinburgh University applied unsuccessfully for M.D. degree to qualify for election to Royal Infirmary staff	XX
1889	Edinburgh University: degrees of M.B., Ch.B., M.D. and Ch.M. instituted	XXII
1891	University Commissioners issued 'Draft Ordinance—Edinburgh No. 1'	XXII

Year	Event	Ref.
1884	Medical Amendment Bill: Joint Petition to House of Lords	XII
1884	Medical Education: Report to G.M.C.	XXII
1884	Triple Qualification instituted	XIV
1884	Licence as Single Qualification issued only to those who had previously passed Surgery	XIV
1885	Preliminary Examination of Edinburgh Colleges discontinued	XXII
1886	Report on Lunacy Acts Amendment Bill	XXI
1886	Admission of Women to Conjoint Examinations	XVI & XXIII
1887	Decision to establish a Research Laboratory	V
1888	Joint petition by Scottish Corporations to Queen for powers to confer degrees	XXIII
1888	Dr Jex Blake accepted as qualified extra-mural lecturer	XVI
1888	Joint petition to Queen proposing Scottish Senate of Physicians and Surgeons	XXII
1888	Lunacy administration: Memorial to Parliament	XXI
1889	Decision to publish work of Laboratory annually	V
1889	Revision of Regulations for D.P.H.	XXI
1890	Statement submitted to Scottish University Commission	XXII
1890	Membership Examination: Medicine and Therapeutics included in addition to selected subjects	XIX
1890	Petition to Parliament re Habitual Drunkards	XXI
1891	Conjoint D.P.H. instituted	XXI
1891	Medical Officers of Health and Sanitary Inspectors: Whole-time appointments favoured	XXI

2L

Year	College Events	Chap. Ref.	Related Historical and Contemporary Events	Year	Chap. Ref.
1891	Albert University. Joint Petition to Privy Council	XXIII			
1892	Proposal for agreement with St Andrews University for conferment of M.B. degrees on Licentiates of Triple Qualification	XXII			
1894	New Fever Hospital: recommendations sent on request to Town Council	XX	Poor Relief: Parish Councils made responsible	1894	I & II
1895	Laboratory transferred to Forrest Road premises	V			
1895	Extra-Mural School of Medicine constituted with Royal College of Surgeons, Edinburgh as the School of Medicine of the Royal Colleges	XVI			
1896	Materia Medica Museum: decision to transfer to the Pharmaceutical Society of Great Britain	V	Wireless telegraphy introduced by Marconi	1896	
1896	Probationary period for Fellowship and Membership extended to three years	XIV & XIX			
1897	Recommendation to Royal Infirmary that connotation 'Gynaecologist' be adopted	X			
1898	G.M.C. proposals to prevent use of Diplomas by those removed from the Register: approved by College	XXVI	Royal Army Medical Corps established	1898	XXVII
			Edinburgh School of Tropical Medicine established	1898	
1899	Petition submitted to Parliament for Royal Commission on Venereal Disease	XXIX	Boer War	1899–1902	XXVII
1900	Matriculation of Arms	XXXIV			
1900	Agreement with Local Government Board to report cases of suspected Plague by the Laboratory	V			
			Edinburgh: beginnings of Antenatal Clinic at Simpson Memorial Hospital	1901	XXVII
1902	Electric lighting installed in the Hall	IV	Central Midwives Board created	1902	XXVIII
1902	Statement to Secretary for War re Advisory Board for R.A.M.C.	XXVII	Carnegie Trust for Universities of Scotland: founded	1902	

Year	Event	Ref.
1903	New Edinburgh City Fever Hospital (Colinton) opened	XX
1903	Royal Commission on Physical Training (in Scotland)	XXVIII
1904	Interdepartmental Committee on Physical Deterioration	XXVIII
1905	Royal Commission on the Poor Laws and Relief of Distress appointed	XXVIII
1906	Edinburgh: the beginnings of organized postgraduate teaching	XVI
1906	School Medical Services launched in Scotland	XXVIII
1906	Workmen's Compensation Act	XXVIII
1907	R.A.M.C.: Territorial Force created	XXVII
1908	Old Age Pensions instituted	XXVIII
1911	The National Insurance Act (Sickness: disablement: unemployment)	XXVIII
1913	Highlands and Islands Medical Service created	II
1913	College of Physicians and Surgeons of Bombay founded	XXXV

Year	Event	Ref.
1903	Consulted by Edinburgh Merchant Company re medical supervision in schools	XX
1904	Roll Call replaced by Card Records	XXXIV
1904	Royal Infirmary: agreed to age limit for staff	XX
1904	Report on Health of Scottish School Children	XXIX
1905	Education Bill for Scotland: Memorandum to Secretary of State	XXIX
1905	Joint Committee with the University on Postgraduate Education formed	XXIX
1908	Death of President (Dr Underhill) while in office	XXXIV
1909	Petition against draft Charter of B.M.A.	XXIII
1909	College represented by Dr James Ritchie at 350th anniversary of University of Geneva	XXVIII
1911	Report on National Insurance Scheme	XXVIII
1911	College precedence: Royal decision	XXV
1912	Joint Manifesto to Scottish Practitioners re National Insurance Act	XXVIII
1912	Suspension of Dr Axham	XXVI
1912	College Disciplinary Powers: correspondence with Privy Council and G.M.C.	XXVI
1913	Lister Memorial: draft agreement adopted	V
1913	Advice re Research Funds under National Insurance Act	XXVIII

Year	College Events	Chap. Ref.	Related Historical and Contemporary Events	Year	Chap. Ref.
1914	Committee appointed to consider City milk supply	XX			
1914	Prosecution of 'Dr Temple' and 'Dr Massey'	XXIX	First World War	1914–1918	XXVII
1914	Lister Memorial: agreement with University and Carnegie Trustees	V	Scottish Medical Service Emergency Committee established	1914	XXVII
1914	Midwives (Scotland) Bill: Petition to Parliament	XXIX			
1916	Graduates of any University in British Empire approved by Council, admissable as candidates for Fellowship and Membership	XIV	Midwives (Scotland) Act	1915	XXVIII
1916	Advisory Committee appointed to deal with medical problems of war	XVII			
1916	Membership without examination or fee, offered to four M.O.'s for eminent war services	XXVII			
1917	Statement favouring creation of Ministry of Health *but* after the War	XXVIII			
1917	Civic Welfare Scheme: co-ordinating action by College	XXIX			
1917	Honorary Membership instituted	XXXIV	Armistice	1918	XXVII
			Maternity and Child Welfare Act	1918	XXVIII
			Ministry of Health Act	1919	XXVIII
1919	Exemption from examination for Membership on score of age no longer permitted	XIV	Scottish Board of Health established (formed from Local Government Boards for Scotland; Scottish Insurance Commissioners; and Highlands and Islands (Medical Services) Board)	1919	XXVIII
1919	Council empowered to grant exemption from examination to Membership candidates of high scientific attainment	XIV	Nurses Registration (Scotland) Act	1919	XXVIII
			University Grants Commission: first grants to Universities	1919	
1919	His Royal Highness Prince of Wales accepted Honorary Fellowship	XXXVI	First transatlantic crossing by air (Alcock and Brown)	1919	

Year	Event	Ref.
1920	NEW CHARTER: making women eligible for Fellowship and Membership	XV & XXIII
1921	Presentation from 2nd Scottish General Hospital	XXVII
1921	Teaching on Tuberculosis: offer to mediate between the City and the University	XVIII
1921	Triple Qualification accepted for admission to examination for licence to practise in U.S.A.	XIV
1922	Members eligible for Staff appointments at Royal Infirmary	XX
1923	Library privileges extended to Fellows of Royal College of Surgeons of Edinburgh	VI
1925	Dr Ella Pringle: first Lady Member	XXIII
1926	Dr Axham: suspension removed	XXVI
1929	First Lady Fellow elected (Dr Pringle)	XXIII
1938	Statement to Royal Commission on Distribution of Industrial Population	XXIX
1938	Statement on Nursing Services	XXIX
1938	Statement on the Scottish Lunacy and Mental Deficiency Laws	XXIX
1920	Consultative Council on Medical and Allied Services: Interim (MacAlister) Report	XXVIII
1920	Medical Research Committee of Insurance Commission reconstituted as Medical Research Council	XXVIII
1928	Department of Health for Scotland established	XXVIII
1929	(Royal) College of Obstetricians and Gynaecologists: foundation	XXVIII
1929	Royal College of Physicians & Surgeons of Canada: foundation	XXXV
1929	Scottish Local Government Act	XXVIII
1932	Immigrant Refugee Doctors: London meeting of Licensing Authorities' representatives	XXVII
1936	Cathcart Report on Scottish Health Services	XXVIII
1937–1938	Emergency Medical Services: initial planning	XXVIII
1938	Royal Australasian College of Physicians: foundation	XXXV

Year	College Events	Chap. Ref.	Related Historical and Contemporary Events	Year	Chap. Ref.
1938	Members permitted to dispense medicines subject to specified conditions	XIV			
1939	Workmen's Compensation: Report to Royal Commission	XXIX	Second World War	1939–1946	XXVII
			Department of Health for Scotland: under Reorganisation of Offices (Scotland) Act 1939, independence of Department abolished and functions vested in the Secretary of State	1939	XXVIII
			Polish Faculty of Medicine at Edinburgh University established	1941	XXVII
1942	Post-war Hospital Problems: considered at the first of several Extraordinary Meetings	XXVIII	Medical Planning Commission: Draft Interim Report	1942	XXVIII
			Beveridge Committee: Report	1942	XXVIII
1943	Scottish Housing: views submitted to Scottish Housing Advisory Subcommittee	XXIX	Government acceptance of Beveridge's basic assumptions	1943	XXVIII
			Hetherington Committee: Report	1943	XXVIII
1944	B.M.A.: President invited to attend meetings of Scottish Committee	XXIII			
1944	N.H.S. Proposals: Memorandum sent to Secretary of State for Scotland	XXVIII	Goodenough Committee: Report	1944	XVI
1945	Conditions of Service of Medical Profession: views submitted to Department of Health	XXIX	Goodenough Report: Memorandum of Royal Scottish Medical Corporations	1945	XVI
			Hiroshima	1945	
			Spens Reports	1946 & 1948	XXXIII XXVIII
1946	Motion to explore the formation of a College of Physicians of Scotland keenly debated, won considerable support, but lost on technicality	XXIV	Cessation of hostilities	1946	
			Edinburgh: first full-time Director of Post-graduate Studies	1946	XXX
1948	School of Medicine of the Royal College of Edinburgh: ceased to function	XVI	National Health Service came into operation	1948	XXVIII

Year		Event	Ref.
1949	V	College Laboratory: research activities terminated	
1950	XXIV	Further efforts to promote a Scottish National College of Physicians failed	
1950	XV	SUPPLEMENTARY CHARTER: removal of Residential Qualification applicable to Members of Council	
1950	V	College Laboratory closed	
1952	VIII	Charitable Status granted for purposes of Inland Revenue	
1952	XXXIV	Pitcairne's tombstone renovated	
1953	XXXVI	Her Majesty Queen Elizabeth, the Queen Mother, elected an Honorary Fellow	
1953	XXXIV	Term 'Censor' revived temporarily but with new duties (q.v.–1861)	
1953	XXXI	Disabled Persons: evidence submitted to Committee of Enquiry	
1954	XXXI	National Health (Industrial Injuries) Act: evidence submitted to Departmental Committee	
1954	XXXIII	Cost of N.H.S.: Memo submitted to Committee of Enquiry	
1954	VIII & XXX	Decision to initiate R.C.P. Publication Series	
1955	XXXIII	Relationship between Hospital Doctors and Management: resolution	
1955	XXXVI	Physicians from U.S.S.R. entertained	
1955	XXXIV	Restoration of Adam Suite	
1957	XXXII	Report of College Committee on Clinical Teaching Facilities and Student Amenities in Scottish Hospitals	
1958	XXXIV	Roll of Attendance abolished	

Year	Event	Ref.
1948	World Health Organization: ratification by 26 countries	
1952	(Royal) College of General Practitioners: foundation	
1952	Standing Joint Committee of Scottish Royal Colleges: first meeting	
1953	Edinburgh Post-Graduate Board for Medicine came into operation	XXX
1954	First International Congress of World Federation of Occupational Therapists held in College Hall	XXXVI
1955	College of Medicine of South Africa (formerly College of Physicians, Surgeons and Gynaecologists of South Africa): foundation	XXXV
1957	Report of Committee of University Court on Post-Graduate Medical Education	XXXII

Year	College Events	Chap. Ref.	Related Historical and Contemporary Events	Year	Chap. Ref.
1958	B.M.A. Scottish Council: under constitution, one member to be nominated by College	XXIII			
1959	Revision of Pharmacopoeia: Report to Commission	XXXIII			
1959	Her Majesy Queen Elizabeth the Queen Mother dined with the Fellows in the College Hall, and signed the Roll of Honorary Fellows	XXXVI			
1959	SUPPLEMENTARY CHARTER: providing authority to grant Diplomas	XV			
1959	Drug Addiction: Report to the Inter-Departmental Committee	XXXI			
1959	Visit, by invitation, of President to the Royal Australasian College of Physicians on the occasion of their 21st Anniversary Celebrations	XXXV			
1959	Medical Staffing in Hospital Structure: Memo to Working Party	XXXIII			
1960	Her Excellency Mrs Pandit, High Commissioner of India visited College	XXXV			
1960	Registrar appointed after re-creation of office (q.v.–1865)	XXXIV			
1961	St Andrew's Day Festival initiated	XXX			
1962	Registration of Births, Deaths and Marriages: urgent modifications recommended	XXXI	Royal College of Physicians and Surgeons of Glasgow— new designation with Parliamentary approval	1962	XXXV
1962	Inaugural Conference in Edinburgh of the Presidents of the Colleges of Physicians of the Commonwealth and associated Republics: the Edinburgh College of Physicians acted as host	XXXVI	Scottish Home and Health Department: evolved in course of internal reorganisation of Secretary of State's departments	1962	
1962	The Structure of Edinburgh University: College Report	XXXII	College of Physicians and Surgeons of Pakistan: foundation	1962	
1962	Bequest of Dr Archibald Davidson of Australia	XXX			
1962	President attended as guest at the first area dinner of Yorkshire Fellows and Members—the first area meeting in England	XXXVII			

Year	Event	Ref
1963	Visit by Sir Robert Menzies, K.T., Prime Minister of Australia	XXXV
1963	Her Majesty The Queen graciously accepted invitation to act as Patron of the College	XXXVI
1963	Care of the Elderly in Scotland: Report of College Committee approved	XXXI
1963	Alcoholism: Evidence given to Standing Advisory Medical Committee	XXXI
1963	Visit by Medical Faculty of the University of Leyden	XXXV
1963	Scottish Post-graduate Medical Association founded	XXX
1964	SUPPLEMENTARY CHARTER: authorizing postal voting in certain circumstances	XV
1964	Visits by President to Pakistan, India, Burma, Ceylon, Hong Kong, Bahrain, Baghdad and Alexandria at invitation of Council under terms of the Verona Gow Bequest	XXXV
1965	Death of Sir Winston Churchill: the College represented at the services in St Giles' Cathedral, Edinburgh and St Paul's Cathedral, London	XXXVI
1965	Commonwealth Medical Conference: Delegates entertained	XXXVI
1965	Visit of President by invitation at the opening of the new Medical Faculty, University of Malaya	XXXV
1965	Report of Committee appointed to review the Membership Examination	XXX
1965	Pfizer Foundation Building opened by His Royal Highness the Prince Philip	XXX
1965	First Commonwealth Medical Conference	XXXVI
1966	Medical Education: Evidence given to Royal Commission	XXXII
1966	Her Majesty Queen Elizabeth and His Royal Highness the Prince Philip graced a Reception in the College	XXXVI
1966	Award of D.P.H. discontinued	XXI
1966	Visit by Students from University of Utrecht	XXXV
1967	College represented at 450th Anniversary of the Worshipful Society of Apothecaries	XXXV

Year	College Events	Chap.Ref.	Related Historical and Contemporary Events	Year	Chap. Ref.
1967	The President attended meetings of the Royal College of Physicians and Surgeons of Canada, and the Canadian College of Physicians	XXXV	Edinburgh: Lister Institute opened	1967	V & XXX
1967	Hospital Scientific and Technical Services: Memo to Ministry of Health	XXXIII	Joint Committee of the Three Royal Colleges of Physicians: first meeting	1967	
1967	A Fellow (Dr Girdwood) attended a meeting of the Pakistan Medical Association and a gathering of College Fellows and Members in Karachi		Ceylon (Sri Lanka) College of Physicians: foundation	1967	XXXV
1967	Postgraduate Medical Education: Report of Council Committee	XXX			
1967	Visit by Medical Faculty of Leyden University	XXXV			
1968	Decision to support in principle concept of single Library in Edinburgh of current medical literature	VI	Hospital Scientific and Technical Services: Zuckerman Report	1968	XXXIII
			Report of the Royal Commission on Medical Education (Todd)	1968	XXXII
1968	Introduction of Common Part I Examination and Multiple Choice Paper	XXX	Trainee Paediatricians: Evaluation of Scottish Royal Colleges	1968	XXXII
			R.C.P. London: 450th Anniversary	1968	XXXV
1968	College represented by the President at the Annual Meeting of the American College of Physicians	XXXV			
1969	M.R.C.P.: Advisory Committee on Examinations appointed	XXX			
1969	The Future of the College: unanimous approval given by College to Croom Report	XXX			
1969	College represented by the President at the Royal Australasian College of Physicians at Brisbane	XXXV	M.R.C.P. (U.K.): Award of first Diploma	1969	XXX
1970	M.R.C.P. Examination (Part II) in 'Medicine of Childhood'. New Regulations	XXXII	Scottish Council for Post-graduate Medical Education established	1970	XXX
1970	Hospital Pharmaceutical Service: Memorandum sent to Ministry of Health	XXXIII			

Year	College Events	Chap. Ref.	Related Historical and Contemporary Events ((F = Fellow of R.C.P.Ed.))	Year	Chap. Ref.
1971	Assessment of Children: Comments sent to Secretary of State	XXXI			
1971	Monopolies Commission Report: Comments sent to several Government Departments	XXXI			
1971	Reorganisation of N.H.S.: Observations on White Paper to Scottish Home and Health Department	XXXIII			
1971	Doctors in Integrated Health Service: Observations on Joint Working Party	XXXIII			
1971	Private Patients in N.H.S.: Written Evidence for House of Commons Subcommittee	XXXIII			
1972	Organisation of Government Research (Green Paper): Opinions conveyed to Joint Committee of Scottish Royal Colleges	XXXIII			
1972	Government Research: President communicated with Chief Scientific Officer	XXXIII			
1972	Common Part II Membership Examination introduced	XXX	Committee on Nursing: Briggs Report	1972	XXXIII
1972	Public Appeal launched by College for first time in its history	XXXVII			
1972	Joint Symposium with the Royal Society of Edinburgh	XXXVII			
1972	Scottish Licensing Laws: Report to Departmental Committee	XXXI			
1972	Blood Transfusion Service: Report to Scottish Home and Health Department	XXXIII			
1972	Future of Scientific Services in Scotland. Comments to Scottish Home & Health Department	XXXIII			
1972	Nurses in an Integrated Health Service: Comments to Scottish Home and Health Department on working Party Report	XXXIII			
1972	Rehabilitation: Criticism of Scottish Health Services Council Report	XXXI			

Appendix B

Royal College of Physicians of London
Extracts from Minutes of Comitia on
4th May 1657

'*Comitia majora extraordinaria*
4th May 1657

Present: the President Dr. Alston, Dr. Prujean, Mr. Maurice Williams, Dr. Hamey and Drs. Glisson, Ent, Bate, Staynes, Micklethwait, Paget, Goddard, Stanley, Whistler, Wharton, Merrett, Terne and Ringall.

Dr George Purves, a representative from the College of Physicians very recently founded at Edinburgh, presented a letter from certain members of that community addressed to our President and Fellows, and requested that he be given authority to examine our statutes, in order that they might frame their own more accurately on the model of ours. He received the reply that he had permission to run through our statutes forthwith; and the Registrar is instructed to give him assistance in that respect.'

Appendices B, C and D consist of Latin extracts translated by Professor I. M. Campbell and the Very Reverend A. C. Craig.

Appendix C

Royal College of Physicians of London
Extracts from Minutes of Comitia on
4th May 1657

'The Letter from Scotland.
To the Right Worshipful Dr. Alston President of the College
of Physicians and Fellows of the said College in London.
To the Very Renowned President and the other Very
Celebrated Fellows of the London College.

Your Excellencies,

We sincerely rejoice in the favour you show towards our endeavours on behalf of the Community of Medicine. Ever since this became known to us through our own distinguished and learned colleague, we have not ceased with one voice to proclaim your notable goodwill signalised by benefits conferred on him and us, and especially your having communicated to him the sacred laws of your Society, examination of which is your Society's own singular privilege. That this should be permitted by you is no small thing—by you who are revered by the Archiatri of all Britain, by luminaries the brightest of Europe in tracking down by their discoveries the most abstruse mysteries of Nature which were unknown to former generations— revered by the consenting vote of the whole world as an immortal glory of the Republic of Medicine.

What in truth we could not claim to have deserved at your hands and indeed scarcely dared to ask, that your indulgence and your ardent ambition to promote the cause of Medicine brought about of your own accord. Among posterity this will indeed stand out as a very worthy monument to your noble virtues. The fact is that by these good offices you have so closely bound us to you that we find it extremely difficult to know in what words to express our gratitude. For with you everything belongs to a plane too lofty to be reached by the weakness of our effort. Nevertheless, our longings remain, and if they do not match your kindness, we shall still, by our devotion to you, give the thanks we owe and you deserve, as far as we conceivably can.

Furthermore, by the good offices which you have already performed for the honour of Medicine, in consideration of your own dignity, and in the interest of the health of the human race in this kingdom, we most earnestly entreat and beseech you to take pity on the deviant course of Medicine among us, assailed as it is by empirics, quacks, barbers (*or* barber–surgeons), drug pedlars, and all kinds of false physicians.

And we humbly ask you to welcome with your accustomed kindness Purves, our representative, to help him with all good counsels bearing upon the common good of Medicine, and to deem him worthy of further examination of your records. You will thus be promoters of our Medical Republic; thus the splendour of your name will irradiate the darkness of Scotland* and it will not be extinguished either by any vicissitude of human affairs or the devouring force of time, but will be consecrated to eternity. Farewell.

Your Excellencies'
Most Humble Servants

ROBERT BURNETT, GEORGE RAY,
HEN. HENRYSON, RO. CUNNINGHAM,
JA. CALHOUN'

* *Scotiae* τὸ σκότος, a pun by using the Greek word for darkness.

Appendix D

Royal College of Physicians of London
Extracts from Minutes of Comitia on
7th May 1657

'Reply to the most distinguished and illustrious President and Fellows of the newly-founded College of Physicians of Edinburgh.

Most Distinguished and Illustrious Sirs,

While the recent storm of civil war was raging in our midst, the fear was that we should be dashed against that rock, ill-famed for a multitude of ship-wrecks, and be a plaything of those winds. The truth is that among the various disturbances that affected the Republic, our Art did also suffer no small loss of authority: once fear of the laws receded (neglect of which foments and feeds rascality) and while the atmosphere shone brightly upon hopes of immunity from punishment, impostors, quacks, pedlars of unguents, barbers, fortune-tellers, and other rank growths of that kind, seized upon our sacred rights. Doubtless a strong incentive to this kind of boundless audacity is avarice, especially on the part of those who have been reduced to extremities of hunger and stand in great fear of themselves paying the debt of Nature. [Literally, "of paying their own debts to Libitina", she being the goddess of corpses in whose temple at Rome a register of deaths was kept, and a piece of money deposited for every deceased person.]

But Apollo saved us: the reverence rightly due to so noble an Art and the inviolable authority long since granted to it by the supreme civil powers, has very largely repelled that lawless abuse of the healing art, and in a short time (as we hope) will restore in full the honour proper to a Profession so noble and so necessary.

In view of this, most learned sirs, we also congratulate you very much on having determined to found a College on the same pattern, and to deliver yourselves from the dregs of the people, and on having fortified your authority with ample privileges. By these laws you will of a surety keep within limits the unbridled audacity of those ignorant "Medicasters" who have the effrontery to undertake the cure of diseases they know nothing about; and the dignity of the Art, which has been so shamefully defiled, will be restored for posterity.

Another advantage will also accrue: by the activities and purposes of a society of this kind you will extend the bounds of Medicine with better promise, and men destined to be an ornament of the age and a glory of the Art of Apollo, whose breasts are imbued with honour and sagacity, will be all the more eager to extend the limits of our science and will establish its dignity by their own distinguished virtues.

Dr Purves, a man of remarkable humanity and erudition, has visited us and delivered your very welcome communication. We have given him facilities for examining our statutes, and if in any other way our work will appear to be of help to you, be sure that we shall not fall short of your requests. We take this opportunity of sincerely wishing you the best of health and success in every way. Farewell.

London 7th May
1657.

GEORGE ENT,
Doctor of Medicine,
Fellow and Registrar of the
London College.'

Appendix E

Translation of
Charter of Erection of the
Royal College of Physicians of Edinburgh,

Dated 29th November 1681.

CHARLES by the Grace of God of Great Britain, France and Ireland, King and Defender of the Faith to all his good men to whom these presents shall come, Health—KNOW YE in as much as we out of our natural goodness and paternal indulgence towards our People, seeing that we are the Father of our Country and the fostering Parent of all our Lieges and Subjects and also are most desirous and providently careful that not only the rights properties and possessions, and other enjoyments whatever of our subjects be secured provided for and confirmed, but also (what is of the greatest value to them and most nearly concerns them) their life and health of all other external benefits the foundation and subject, should be preserved by God's blessing accompanying the ordinary means, the diligence of honest faithful and approved physicians, and their faithful endeavours to cure and prevent the numerous dangerous diseases incident to human frailty: ALSO CONSIDERING that the practice of the legal and other professions and the exercise of the arts manufactures and mechanical trades have been so suitably regulated and adjusted by laws (enacted) through our own care and wisdom and those of our royal predecessors that allowance or permission is given to no one to practise in the law as a Counsel or Advocate, or in any duty or office having reference to the law or in any branch of knowledge profession or art, before being found of ability and fitness by a recognised examination and being admitted by men legally possessed of the requisite power and authority for this purpose; on account however of the excessive and too candid diffidence of the Physicians of this time (less they should seem to ascribe less to their own merit or to distrust it, or to direct and design a restriction upon others to their own interest and advantage) the practice of physic and medicine has been for a long time in the greatest disorder and confusion and without any warrant has used or rather abused an authority invaded usurped seized at will and exercised and that with great audacity and impunity without any hindrance or resistance by women and persons not only ignorant but vile and worthless without knowledge or liberal instruction or the least spark or tincture of literature or of the rudiments and principles of medicine; and not only gardeners and other rude and illiterate persons have dared to practise in diseases and to abuse, delude and impose upon our subjects, but also the rumour of this toleration of abuse being noised abroad foreign imposters charlatans and empirics looking to the absence of all prohibition have come and having remained long in the realm have professed and practised medicine and have sold their cures and drugs and without any use of the said College and to advance and promote the profession of Medicine and the practice and exercise of Physics, and for this purpose we deliver to the same persons the power and render them competent to acquire, procure, hold and possess lands, tenements, annual rents, possessions, tithes and other things and of possessing the same for the use of the said College and its Colleagues and successors, both within and without the Burgh and having a common seal to be designated the Common Seal of the Royal College of Physicians at Edinburgh, and of having, using and exercising all other liberties, powers and faculties competent to any other free College and Incorporation, or which they as incorporated bodies ought or can have, use or exercise.

And for the better government of the said College and for the administration of the funds and estate that may come to belong to the same we have given and by the tenor of these presents do give to the said Society and College the power and command the Fellows of the same to choose annually in all future time a Council consisting of seven of the Fellows of the said College the best informed, the most discerning, and the most conversant with the profession of medicine; which Council is to choose one of their number who shall be President for that year; with power also to the said President and Council to choose and appoint a Clerk, a Treasurer and other Officers requisite and necessary to the interest of the said Society, and we declare the said President, Council and Community under the name of the President of the Royal College of Physicians at Edinburgh shall be capable of conducting, prosecuting and maintaining causes before all Judges whatsoever and in whatsoever Courts and actions: And further to the said President and College and to their successors we deliver the power of making rules, precepts, acts and Statutes for promoting the science of medicine, and for duly ordering the practice of the same and for the good government, order, rule and correction of the said College and Community and of all practising the said profession within the said (jurisdiction of)

City of Edinburgh and its suburbs only namely, Leith, the Canongate, the West Port, St. Leonards and the Potter Row, when and as often as it shall be necessary. It being fully provided as by these presents it is provided and declared that notwithstanding these presents the Edinburgh Surgeon Apothecaries are to have the power of treating every kind of wounds, contusions, practises, dislocations, tumours, ulcers, and other evils of that kind which fall under surgical operations and the accidents thence arising; but that they shall by no means have the care of diseases originally internal, solely to be undertaken under the prescription and direction of the physicians of the said College.

And in like manner we have granted and by the tenor of these presents do grant to the said President and College and their successors that to no one shall it be allowed within the jurisdiction of the said City its suburbs and royalty to practise and exercise the forenamed profession before he shall have been admitted to the same by the said President and College and their successors for the time by a Warrant and Diploma to this purpose granted by the said President and College, and their successors for the time and signed with their Common Seal; and that under a penalty of Sixty Pounds of Scotch money for every month during which any one, not admitted and licensed in the forementioned manner, shall use and exercise the said profession and practice, of which fines one half we desire to be applied to the use of the Poor, the other to the use and benefit of the said College. If, however, any one after censure in the manner prescribed shall nevertheless persist in exercising the said profession without a license, we command the forementioned fine for every month during which they persist in practising to be doubled.

And in like manner we desire, grant and order that two of the said Society and College shall annually be chosen from the said Society and College by the said Council as Censors, who with the President for the time in the room and in the name of the said College shall have the power, authority and jurisdiction to call before them all persons practising and exercising within the jurisdiction of the said City, its liberties, and its said suburbs the said profession of Medicine without a license and to impose on them the fines above specified; yet the said College of Physicians or its President being about to hold a Court to punish delinquents duly informing the Provost of the said City or one of the Magistrates of the same, of the time and place of that Court, so that (if they shall think fit) they may appoint one of their Bailies to sit with them in a cumulative jurisdiction. It being duly provided, as by these presents it is provided and declared that it shall not yet be allowed to the College of Physicians to fine any Surgeon-Apothecary being a burgess of Edinburgh without the consent of the Provost or of some one of the Bailies of Edinburgh who shall act as Assessor and shall have been present at the judicial proceedings. And if they shall refuse to come and be present, this is to be made known to our Privy Council that they may proceed as is just and fit, without prejudice to the said College in the case of refusal and delay to proceed and in like manner watch, govern and call before them, and if it shall be necessary correct and punish all physicians and Doctors of Medicine, Associates or Licenciates exercising the said profession within the jurisdiction of the said City and the aforesaid limits on account of any crimes and offences committed by them in their practice against the Statutes and Acts of the said College; and that by exacting from them such amercements and fines as to the said President, Censors and Supervisors shall seem fit, and as the offence shall merit the said fines however not exceeding the sum of Forty Pounds; which amercements and fines indeed we desire and ordain to be applied to the uses already mentioned,—and for the same by distraining, using every other legal execution and imprisoning, and for the sentences and judgments to be from time set forth by these Supervisors by virtue of the power and authority committed to them by us we command and require by our authority through these presents, the Magistrates within the jurisdiction suburbs and liberties of the said City and our other Officers of the law to assist in the execution of the aforesaid sentences; and to direct the precepts of distraint and the other executions necessary for this end in the same manner in which they are wont to proceed on their own decrees and sentences; with power also to the said President, as often as it shall be necessary to search, examine and inspect the drugs and medicines, simple and compound, now or hereafter to be sold within the jurisdiction, suburbs and liberties of the said City, if these are fresh, good and real and such as may be trustfully used and applied in the treatment of the diseases and complaints of liege subjects: It being duly provided, as by these presents it is specially provided, that when such an inspection or search is to be made one of the Magistrates within the jurisdiction of the said City, with one Apothecary and one Surgeon Apothecary to be appointed visitors for the time who shall be required to be present in order to see, for the public advantage, that the same are well and according to rule compounded and prepared, and when drugs are found insufficient or spoiled, with the power to throw them into the public streets or to destroy them.

And further for ourselves and our successors that neither the President nor any other belonging to the said College of Physicians nor of their successors shall be cited or summoned in the Town or to proceed to the country upon any assize or inquest. And since their attention to the sick and ill is always so necessary that without the greatest injury and danger to the sick they ought not to be withdrawn from their attendance on any pretext or on any occasion; we therefore for ourselves and our successors for the future free and discharge all the Fellows and Associates of the said College from all watch and ward.

And by these presents we declare that every right power and jurisdiction belonging to the Magistrates of the City of Edinburgh and whatever rights and privileges belonging to the Surgeon Apothecaries are specially reserved to them and each of them respectively as is enjoined by law.

By these presents also it is specially provided that the concession of the above detailed rights and privileges to the said College of Physicians is in no respect to be extended to the erection of Schools to teach the said Art of Medicine or any part of the same, or to the conferring or granting of Degrees to any one in the same; this concession by these presents is specially declared to be without prejudice to the rights and privileges granted in favor of the University or College of St Andrews of Glasgow of Aberdeen and of Edinburgh; and notwithstanding these presents and certain clauses contained in them it shall be allowed and lawful to all who shall have obtained the Degree of Doctor from these Universities to have the liberty and power to practise in the said jurisdiction and in the other places above set down without being themselves liable to the foresaid fines and other penalties above described, unless within the said limits or any part of the same they shall have taken up their abode to practise; in which case they shall only be subjected to the precepts and rules of the said Incorporation and Society as others incorporated in the same, and the said College of Physicians to be established in the manner now detailed by these presents is obliged (to license any person or persons who shall have obtained the Degree of Doctor in these Universities) without any previous or antecedent examination, but only on the production to the President of the said College of their Diploma or Admission to a Degree.

In a special manner by these presents it is duly provided that the grant of the above detailed rights and privileges to the said College of Physicians shall in no way prejudice any one having obtained the Degree of Master of Arts in any University of the said Kingdom, and immediately exercising the practice of medicine or any one admitted to the Degree of Doctor of Medicine in any of the said Universities or in any celebrated foreign University to the extent that men provided with these qualities on the production of their letters patent from these Universities at home or abroad to the President of the said College may not be licensed to practise within the prescribed limits without examination.

It is also specially provided that the public Professors of Medicine of the respective Universities of this Kingdom on their application to the President of the College may be admitted as honorary Associates of the same Society.

And Lastly we faithfully promise upon the word of a Prince that this present Charter shall be confirmed in this present Parliament, and we require that the same shall be conformably ratified by the present States of Parliament. In testimony of which things we have commanded our great Seal to be appended to these presents at our Court of Whitehall on the Twenty ninth day of November in the year of our Lord 1681 and in the 33rd year of our reign.

(*Per signataram manu S. D. N. Regis suprascriptam.*)

Appendix F

Charter of Ratification
in Favour of the
Royal College of Physicians, Edinburgh,

Dated 16th June 1685.

ATT EDINBURGH *The Sixteenth day of June One thousand six hundred eighty and five years.*

OUR SOVERAIGNE LORD With advice and consent of the Estates of this present Parliament Ratifies and Approves and for His Majesty and His Successors Perpetually Confirms The Letters Patent granted by His Majestys dearest Brother King CHARLES the Second of ever blessed memory whereof the tenor follows.

[*Here the Letters Patent are engrossed* verbatim.]

Together with all Acts Decreets and sentances of His Majestys Privy Council or of the Lords of Session, or of any other Judicatory within this Kingdom conceived in favours of the Royal Colledge of Physicians for making the Patent above written and privileges therein contained effectuall And Specially but prejudice of the generality Ane act of His Majestys Privy Council of the date the tuentyfirst day of November one thousand six hundred eighty and four yeares Ordaining the said Royal College at least tuice a year to visit all Apothecarys Shops and Chambers within Edinburgh suburbs and libertys thereof calling to their assistance one or tuo of the eldest or ablest of the Brotherhood of the Apothecarys as also that they desire one of the Baillies of Edinburgh or respective Magistrats of the place where the shops to be visited doe lye to grant their concurrance in the said visitation and these Baillies or Magistrats are by the said Act ordained, upon any such desire to grant their effectual concurrance for ejecting and destroying all corrupt and insufficient drugs and also ordaining that the Apothecarys when required shall attend and assist the saids Physicians and that all Masters of Apothecarys Shops or Chambers, and their servants, receive the visitors of the Shops with all respect, and expose to their view all the drugs that shall be called for and that upon Oath to be administrat both to themselves and servants; and shall quietly and peaceably suffer the drugs that shall be found insufficient by the saids Physicians to be ejected and destroyed, as they will be ansuerable And Sicklike, ordaining that no person who have not already been examined and admitted by the Fraternity of Apothecarys, be suffered in any time coming, by the Magistrats aforsaid, to keep any Apothecarys shops or chambers, except such allennerly as shall be tryed and approven by the President and Censors of the said Royall College: And in like maner, ane Act of the Lords of Session, dated the tuentyfirst day of March last bypast, proceeding upon a suspension, at the instance of ane Chirurgeon Apothecary, of a sentence pronounced by the President and Censors of the said Royal Colledge, for unwarrantable practise of Medicine Whereby it was found by the saids Lords of Session, that where The Magistrats of Edinburgh refuse or delay to give concurrence to punish delinquents, that the Colledge, in that case, have both the Judicative and executive power, in all and sundry heads, points, articles, circumstances, and conditions, contained in the saids Letters Patents, and Acts above mentioned, and after the formes and tenors therof in all points And His Majesty with advice and consent foresaid, Wills and Grants, and for His Majesty and his Successors, Decerns and Ordains, That this present Ratification is, and shall be, as valid, sufficient and effectuall, to the said Royall Colledge, and their Successors, as if the Acts above mentioned were herein at lenth de verbo in verbum specially insert and ingrossed: Wheranent our said Soveraign Lord, with advice and consent forsaid, for His Majesty and his Successors, hath dispensed, and by thir presents dispenses forever Extracted forth of the Records of Parliament By George Viscount of Tarbat, Lord McLeod and Castlehaven, Clerk to His Majestys Parliament, Council Registers and Rolls, &c.

TARBAT,
Cler. Reg.

Appendix G

Royal Warrant for
Charter of Incorporation
in Favour of the
Royal College of Physicians of Edinburgh,
[*Translation*]

16th August 1861.

VICTORIA R.

VICTORIA, by the Grace of God, of the United Kingdom of Great Britain and Ireland, Queen; Defender of the Faith:

Whereas the Royal College of Physicians of Edinburgh have, by their Petition, humbly represented unto Us that our Royal Predecessor Charles the Second was pleased to erect and incorporate the said College by Charter or Letters Patent, bearing date at Whitehall, the twenty-ninth day of November, one thousand six hundred and eighty-one, in the thirty-third year of his reign, which Charter was afterwards ratified, approved, and confirmed by an Act of the Scottish Parliament, bearing date the sixteenth day of June, one thousand six hundred and eighty-five; and that the establishment of the said College has fulfilled the high purposes of consolidating the medical profession, elevating its character and dignity, and encouraging and advancing medical learning and science: And whereas the said College have also represented unto Us, that by an Act passed in the twenty-first and twenty-second year of our reign, intituled "An Act to regulate the Qualifications of Practitioners in Medicine and Surgery," it was enacted that it should be lawful for Us to grant to the Corporation of the Royal College of Physicians of Edinburgh a new Charter, and thereby to give to the said College of Physicians the name of 'The Royal College of Physicians of Scotland,' and that it should be lawful for the said Royal College of Physicians under their Common Seal, to accept such new Charter, and that such acceptance should operate as a surrender of all Charters heretofore granted to the said Corporation; and that by another Act, passed in the twenty-second year of our reign, intituled "An Act to amend the Medical Act (1858)," it was enacted that the term "Member" should be added to the Qualifications described in the schedule to the first-mentioned Act, in reference to the said College; and further, that by another Act, passed in the twenty-third and twenty-fourth year of our reign, intituled "An Act to amend the Medical Act (1858)," it was enacted that any new Charter to be granted to the said College may be granted either by and in its present name, or, as provided by the Medical Act, by and in the name of the Royal College of Physicians of Scotland: And whereas the said College have further represented to Us that the said Charter granted by our Royal Predecessor contains various provisions, which, by reason of the great changes that have taken place in the practice of medicine, have altogether gone into desuetude, and that it is expedient, and would be for the benefit of the said College, and of the medical profession, that a new Charter should be granted to the said College, by and in its present name, in pursuance of the provisions of the said Acts: Now know ye, that We, taking the premises into our Royal consideration of our especial grace, certain knowledge, and mere motion, have given, granted, and ordained, and by these presents, for Us, our heirs and successors, do give, grant, and ordain, as follows (that is to say):—

I. Alexander Wood, Doctor of Medicine, President; James Young Simpson, Doctor of Medicine, Vice-President; and Peter Fairbairn, William Seller, Charles Bell, William Henry Lowe, Alexander Keiller, and William Tennant Gairdner, Members of the Council of the said College, and their successors in office, and the other existing Fellows of the said College, and all other persons who shall hereafter be admitted or elected Fellows and Members of the said College, as hereinafter provided, shall be and are hereby united and incorporated into one body politic and corporate, by the name of "The Royal College of Physicians of Edinburgh," and shall by that name have perpetual succession, and a Common Seal, with power to break, alter, and renew the same from time to time, and may by that name sue and be sued; and the College shall at all times hereafter be capable in law to take, purchase, possess, hold, and enjoy, for the uses and purposes of the College, any lands, tenements or other heritages, and personal estate not exceeding in the whole the yearly value of Ten Thousand Pounds, and, if necessary, to sell, dispone, and convey the same, and to lend money on heritable or moveable, real or personal securities, and to hold goods and chattels for the uses and purposes of the College; and all charters, dispositions, securities, and other deeds or instruments affecting heritable or moveable, real or personal property, to be granted in favour of the College, may be taken in their corporate name, or to Trustees, on behalf of the College; and all charters, dispositions, or other deeds or instruments to be granted by the College, shall be under the

Common Seal, and shall be subscribed by three of the Trustees, and by the President, or Treasurer, or Secretary of the College, for the time being.

II. All property, heritable and moveable, real and personal, wheresoever situated, and all feu-charters, dispositions, bonds, instruments of sasine, leases, agreements, and other deeds and instruments, and vouchers of such property, or relating thereto, which have been already acquired by, or taken, granted, or executed in favour of the said Royal College of Physicians of Edinburgh, or any person or persons, as Trustee or Trustees, or otherwise, for the use or on behalf of the said College, whether the same be held absolutely or in security, and in general all estate and effects, and all debts, obligations, rights, interests, liberties, privileges, and immunities of and belonging to the said College, or vested in any person or persons for the benefit of the said College at the time of the granting of these presents, shall be, and the same are hereby transferred to and vested in the Royal College of Physicians of Edinburgh hereby incorporated, as fully as if the same had been acquired by, or taken, granted, or executed in favour of the College after the granting of these presents; and the same shall in future be held, managed, sold, conveyed, assigned, leased, discharged, or otherwise disposed of by the College, under their corporate name of "The Royal College of Physicians of Edinburgh," without the necessity of any connecting or continuing title, or separate investiture, or writing, or procedure, other than these presents.

III. The existing Fellows of the Royal College of Physicians of Edinburgh, at the time of the granting of these presents, shall be the first Fellows of the College hereby incorporated.

IV. The Fellows may, from time to time, elect and admit to be Fellows and Members of the College such persons as they shall think fit and qualified, in such manner, at such times, under such regulations, and on payment of such fees, as may, from time to time, be directed by the Bye-Laws.

V. The Fellows may, from time to time, admit to be Licentiates of the College, any persons who shall have gone through such course of studies, and passed such examinations, or submitted to such other regulations, and paid such fees, as may, from time to time, be directed by the Bye-Laws; and the existing Licentiates of the Royal College of Physicians of Edinburgh, at the time of the granting of these presents, shall be Licentiates of the College hereby incorporated.

VI. If it shall at any time hereafter appear that any Fellow, Member, or Licentiate of the College has obtained admission to or licence from the College, or the Royal College of Physicians of Edinburgh, by any fraud, false statement, or imposition, or that he has violated any bye-law, rule, or regulation of the College, then, and in every such case, and after such previous notice to, and such hearing of, such Fellow, Member, or Licentiate, as under the circumstances the Council shall think proper, it shall be lawful for the Fellows, with the concurrence of not less than three-fourths of their number, present at a Meeting, specially summoned for the purpose, to pass such censure or sentence of suspension against the Fellow, Member, or Licentiate so offending, as shall be determined at such Meeting, or to expel such Fellow, Member, or Licentiate from the College; and upon any such sentence of suspension or expulsion being passed, such Fellow, Member, or Licentiate shall cease to be a Fellow, Member, or Licentiate of the College, and to have any right or interest in or to the property or funds of the College, either absolutely, or for such time as shall be specified in the sentence of suspension; and all the rights and privileges granted to such Fellow, Member, or Licentiate, as the case may be, shall cease and determine upon such expulsion or during such suspension.

VII. Ordinary Meetings of the Fellows, for the transaction of the business of the College, shall be held at such times as shall, from time to time, be fixed by the Bye-Laws.

VIII. Extraordinary Meetings of the Fellows, for the consideration and disposal of any special business of the College, may be called by the President or the Council at any time when the same shall be deemed necessary; and it shall be incumbent on the President to call an Extraordinary Meeting of the Fellows on a requisition to that effect, specifying the purpose of such Meeting, and signed by any five of the Fellows, being delivered to him or to the Secretary of the College; and notice of all Extraordinary Meetings of the Fellows shall be given in such manner as shall be directed by the Bye-Laws.

IX. Ordinary Meetings of the Fellows and Members for the consideration of matters affecting the general interests of the medical profession and the public, shall be held at such times as shall from time to time be fixed by the Bye-Laws.

X. Extraordinary Meetings of the Fellows and Members may be called by the President or the Council at any time when the same shall be deemed necessary; and it shall be incumbent on the President to call an Extraordinary Meeting of the Fellows and Members on a requisition to that effect, specifying the purpose of such Meeting, and signed by any five of the Fellows or Members, being delivered to him or to the Secretary of the College; and notice of all Extraordinary Meetings of the Fellows and Members shall be given in such manner as shall be directed by the Bye-Laws; and any matters affecting the general interests of the medical profession and the public, which shall be specified in such requisition and notice, may be considered at any such Extraordinary Meeting of Fellows and Members.

XI. The Council of the College shall consist of the President and six of the Fellows resident in Edinburgh, or within seven miles of the General Post-Office in Edinburgh, by the nearest public highway.

XII. A meeting of the Fellows shall be held annually, on such day and at such hour as may, from time to time, be fixed by the Bye-Laws, for the election of the President and the Members of the Council.

XIII. The Council shall elect the Examiners of the College, and shall also elect a Treasurer, Secretary, Clerk, and such other officers as may be deemed necessary, annually, and as often as occasion may require, or vacancies occur, by death, resignation, or otherwise.

XIV. The Council shall, with the approval of the Fellows, nominate four Fellows, who, along with the Treasurer, shall be Trustees for the College; and as often as a vacancy shall arise by death, resignation, or otherwise, the Council shall fill up the same; and the existing Trustees of the said College at the time of the granting of these presents, shall be the first Trustees under these presents.

XV. The existing Members of the Council of the said College at the time of the granting of these presents shall continue in office, and be the first Council of the College under these presents; and the existing President shall continue in office, and be the first President of the College under these presents; and the existing Treasurer, Secretary, Clerk, and other officers of the said College shall continue to hold their several offices until the first Annual Meeting of the Fellows for the election of the Members of the Council and the President, to be held after the granting of these presents.

XVI. If it shall happen that any election of the President or of the Members of the Council, or any of them, shall not be made on the day appointed for that purpose, or if any Fellow elected to any such office shall not accept thereof, the person or persons then filling such office or offices shall continue to fill the same until another person or persons shall be appointed thereto; and the Fellows present at any Ordinary Meeting, or at an Extraordinary Meeting, to be called as herein provided, may elect out of the Fellows a person or persons to fill the said office or offices, or such of them as shall not have been filled up, or shall be vacant by reason of non-acceptance as aforesaid, for such part of the year of office as shall be then unexpired.

XVII. If the President or any Member of the Council shall die or resign before the expiration of the year, or other time for which he shall have been elected, the Fellows present at any Ordinary Meeting, or at an Extraordinary Meeting to be called as herein provided, may elect out of the Fellows a President or Member of the Council, as the case may be, in the place or stead of the President or Member of the

Council so dying or resigning; and the Fellow or Fellows so elected shall serve for the remainder of the year of office, or other time, for which the President or Member of the Council so dying or resigning was elected.

XVIII. The property and affairs of the College shall be managed and administered by the Fellows and the Council, in such manner, and under such regulations, as may from time to time be directed by the Bye-Laws.

XIX. All Acts done by the President, or by any Meeting of the Council, or by any person acting as President or Member of the Council, shall, notwithstanding it may be afterwards discovered that there was any defect or informality in the election or appointment of any such President or Member of the Council acting as aforesaid, or that they, or any of them, were or was disqualified, or that there was any vacancy in the office of President, or in the Council, be as valid as if every such person had been duly elected or appointed and was duly qualified, and as if no such vacancy had existed.

XX. It shall be lawful for the Fellows, and We do hereby grant full power and authority to them, from time to time, to make Bye-Laws, Rules, and Regulations, for promoting the Science of Medicine, for duly ordering the practice of the same, and for the good government, order, and direction of the College; for the admission and election of Fellows, Members, and Licentiates, and fixing and defining the qualifications of persons to be so admitted and elected; for the management of the property, funds and affairs of the College; for the regulation of all meetings, actings, and proceedings of the College, and of the Council and Fellows, and of the Fellows and Members, and of the several Office-Bearers and Officers of the College, and fixing the times for holding such meetings; and for the division of the persons composing the body corporate of the College into such orders of Resident and Non-resident Fellows or Members, or otherwise; and for giving and assigning to these orders such qualifications, powers, privileges, exemptions, and restrictions, as the Fellows may from time to time determine; and it shall be lawful for the Fellows, from time to time, to repeal, vary, or alter such Bye-Laws, Rules, and Regulations: Provided that every Bye-Law, Rule, and Regulation, to be hereafter made, and every repeal, variation, or alteration of any existing Bye-Law, Rule, or Regulation, shall be submitted to and approved by an Ordinary or Extraordinary Meeting of the Fellows, in such form and manner as they shall from time to time direct and appoint.

XXI. The Bye-Laws, Rules, and Regulations of the said Royal College of Physicians of Edinburgh existing and in force at the time of the granting of these presents, except in so far as the same may be inconsistent with these presents, shall be and continue to be the Bye-Laws, Rules, and Regulations of the College hereby incorporated, until the same are repealed, altered, or varied, in whole or in part.

XXII. The College hereby incorporated, and the Fellows, Members, and Licentiates thereof, shall and may have, exercise, and enjoy all such powers, functions, rights, and privileges, as the said Royal College of Physicians of Edinburgh, or the Fellows, Members, or Licentiates thereof respectively, before the granting of these presents, had or might have had, exercised or enjoyed under and by virtue of the several Acts of our reign hereinbefore recited.

XXIII. The following words and expressions in these presents shall have the several meanings hereby assigned to them; that is to say:—

> The expression "the College" shall mean "The Royal College of Physicians of Edinburgh," hereby incorporated; the words "Council," "Fellows," "Members," and "Licentiates," shall respectively mean the Council, Fellows, Members, and Licentiates of the College for the time being; and the word "Bye-Laws" shall mean and include the Bye-Laws, Rules, and Regulations of the College, made *or to be made, as herein* provided.

And with the consent of the College, testified by their acceptance of these presents, and by the authority of the Act of our reign first before recited, We do hereby accept the surrender made to Us by the Royal College of Physicians of Edinburgh of the said Charter or Letters Patent granted by our Royal Predecessor King Charles the Second, and do hereby revoke, annul, and make void the same: And We do hereby, for Us, our heirs and successors, further grant to the College, that this our Charter shall be in and by all things valid and effectual in law, according to the true intent and meaning of the same, and shall be held, construed, and adjudged in the most favourable and beneficial sense, and for the best advantage of the College, notwithstanding any misrecital, defect, uncertainty, or imperfections whatsoever: And We do hereby, for Us, our heirs and successors, covenant, grant, and agree to and with the College, that We, our heirs and successors, shall and will, from time to time, and at all times hereafter, upon their humble suit and request, give and grant to the College all such further and other powers, privileges, and authorities for rendering more effectual this our grant, according to the true intent and meaning of these presents, as We, our heirs and successors, can or may lawfully grant, and as shall be reasonably advised and devised by the Council learned in the law of the College for the time being.

And We further will and command that this our Charter do pass the Seal appointed by the Treaty of Union to be kept and used in Scotland in place of the

2M

Great Seal thereof *per saltum*, without passing any other Seal or Register: For which these presents shall be, as well to the Director of our Chancery for writing the same, as to the Keeper of the said Seal for causing the said Seal to be appended thereto, a sufficient warrant.

Given, at our Court at Saint James's the sixteenth day of August 1861, in the Twenty-fifth year of our reign.

By Her Majesty's Command,

G. GREY.

Appendix H

Supplementary Charter, 1919
in Favour of the
Royal College of Physicians of Edinburgh

GEORGE V., by the Grace of God of the United Kingdom of Great Britain and Ireland, and of the British Dominions beyond the Seas, King, Defender of the Faith, to all to whom these presents shall come—GREETING,—

WHEREAS

(i) Our Royal Predecessor, King Charles the Second, in the year 1681, by Royal Charter, dated the 29th of November 1681, and afterwards ratified by an Act of the Scottish Parliament, dated the 16th of June 1685, constituted the several persons therein named and their successors to be chosen as therein mentioned a body corporate and politic by the name of "THE ROYAL COLLEGE OF PHYSICIANS OF EDINBURGH," with perpetual succession and with the powers therein set forth.

(ii) Our Royal Predecessor, Queen Victoria, in the year 1861, accepted a surrender of the said original Charter, and by Royal Charter, dated the 16th of August 1861, constituted the several persons therein named who were then the Members of the Council of the Royal College of Physicians of Edinburgh, and their successors in office, and the then existing Fellows of the said College, and all other persons who should be admitted or elected Fellows and Members of the College as thereinafter provided one body politic and corporate by the name of "THE ROYAL COLLEGE OF PHYSICIANS OF EDINBURGH," with perpetual succession and with the powers therein set forth.

(iii) The said Charter, dated the 16th of August 1861, which is in the Latin language provides (among other things) as follows:—Clause 4, "Sociis licitum iri identidem eligere et in Societatem ejus Collegii Sociorum et Membrorum ascribere illos viros quos habiles idoneosque censeant eo modo iis temporibus sub iis regulis et eo soluto praemio sicut leges propriae Collegii alio atque alio tempore latae jusserint," and the provisions of the said Charter throughout contemplate that only persons of the male sex shall be capable of election and admission as Fellows and Members of the College.

(iv) It has been represented to us that a Motion in the following terms was unanimously passed at a Quarterly Meeting of the Royal College of Physicians of Edinburgh, duly held on the 5th of November 1918:—"The College authorises the Council to take steps to have the Constitution of the College altered or amended so as to permit of Women being admitted Members and Fellows of the College," and that it is expedient and will promote and facilitate the work of the said College, and will conduce to the encouragement and advancement of medical learning and science; that the said College shall be empowered to elect Women to be Fellows and Members thereof.

(v) Application has accordingly been made to Us to grant to the said College a Supplementary Charter making such alterations in its Constitution, and giving it such additional powers as are hereinafter set forth.

Now KNOW YE That We of Our Royal Will and pleasure, and moved thereto by Our goodwill to the said College, and Our desire to promote and facilitate the work carried on by it, and to encourage and advance Medical Learning and Science for Ourselves, Our Heirs, and Successors, in addition to and notwithstanding anything to the contrary contained in the said Charter, dated the 16th of August 1861, are graciously pleased to grant, ordain, and declare as follows:—

1. The Fellows for the time being of The Royal College of Physicians of Edinburgh may from time to time elect and admit to be Fellows or Members of the said College not only such persons of the male sex, but also such persons of the female sex as they shall think fit and qualified in such manner, at such times, under such regulations and on payment of such fees as may from time to time be directed by the Bye-Laws of the said College.

2. Each person of the female sex, so elected as aforesaid to be a Fellow or Member of the said College, shall, as such Fellow or Member of the said College, have, exercise, and enjoy the same powers, functions, rights and privileges, and be capable of election to the same offices (including the office of President, Vice-President, Member of the Council, or Representative of the College or any other Body), and shall be subject to the same duties, obligations, and incapacities, and to the like jurisdiction of the Fellows of the said College as if such person were of the male sex.

3. Unless, and until it shall be otherwise directed by any Bye-Law or Bye-Laws, the rules and regulations now directing and providing for the election of persons of the male sex to be Fellows or Members of the said College shall apply to and govern

the election of persons of the female sex to be Fellows or Members of the said College.

4. For the purposes and in the construction of the said Charter, dated the 16th of August 1861, and the Bye-Laws of the said College, words importing the masculine gender only shall be deemed to import also the feminine gender, where the context so admits:

IN WITNESS WHEREOF, We have ordered the Seal appointed by the Treaty of Union to be kept and used in Scotland in place of the Great Seal thereof to be appended to these presents: Given at our Court at St. James's the third day of December One thousand nine hundred and nineteen, in the Tenth year of our Reign.

Per Signaturam Manu S.D.N. Regis Supra Scriptam.

Sealed at Edinburgh the eighth day of January in the year One thousand nine hundred and twenty.

Written to the Seal and Registered the eighth day of January One thousand nine hundred and twenty.

WM. CROSBIE,
Substitute Keeper of the Seal.

J. C. STRETTELL MILLER,
Director of Chancery.

£80 *Scots.*

Appendix I

Supplementary Charter, 1950

GEORGE THE SIXTH by the Grace of God of Great Britain, Ireland and the British Dominions beyond the Seas King, Defender of the Faith To all to whom these presents may come Greeting!

WHEREAS

(i) Our Royal Predecessor, King Charles the Second, in the year 1681, by Royal Charter, dated the 29th day of November, 1681, and afterwards ratified by an Act of the Scottish Parliament dated the 16th day of June, 1685, constituted the several persons therein named and their successors to be chosen as therein mentioned a body corporate and politic by the name of "The Royal College of Physicians of Edinburgh," with perpetual succession and with the powers therein set forth.

(ii) Our Royal Predecessor, Queen Victoria, in the year 1861, accepted a surrender of the said original Charter, and by Royal Charter, dated the 16th day of August, 1861, consituted the several persons therein named who were then the Members of the Council of the Royal College of Physicians of Edinburgh, and their successors in office, and the then existing Fellows of the said College, and all other persons who should be admitted or elected Fellows and Members of the College as thereinafter provided one body politic and corporate by the name of "The Royal College of Physicians of Edinburgh" with perpetual succession and with the powers therein set forth.

(iii) Our Royal Predecessor, King George the Fifth, granted to the said College a Royal Charter dated the 3rd day of December, 1919, Supplementary to the said Royal Charter dated the 16th day of August, 1861, and making alterations in the constitution of the said College and giving it the additional powers therein set forth.

(iv) The said Charter dated the 16th day of August, 1861, which is in the Latin Language, provides (among other things) as follows:

Article XI. Concilium Collegii constituendum esse ex Praeside et sex Sociis Edinburgi habitantibus aut intra septem millia passuum a domo, vernaculo sermone, "the General Post Office of Edinburgh," appellata, per proximam viam publicam.

(v) It has been represented to Us that a Motion in the following terms was unanimously passed at a Quarterly Meeting of the Royal College of Physicians of Edinburgh, duly held on the 1st day of February, 1949:—"That the College authorises the Council to take steps to have Article XI of the Charter of the College altered or amended to read as follows:—"The Council of the College shall consist of the President and Six of the Fellows,' " and that it is expedient and will promote and facilitate the work of the said College, that the restriction on Membership of the Council of the College resulting from the residential qualification imposed by Article XI of the said Charter dated the 16th day of August, 1861, be removed.

(vi) Application has accordingly been made to Us to grant to the said College a further Supplementary Charter making such alteration in its Constitution as is hereinafter set forth.

Now KNOW YE THAT WE of Our Royal Will and pleasure, and moved thereto by Our goodwill to the said College, and Our desire to promote and facilitate the work carried on by it, for Ourselves, Our Heirs, and Successors in addition to the said Charter dated the 16th day of August, 1861, and the said Supplementary Charter dated the 3rd day of December, 1919, and notwithstanding anything to the contrary contained in the said Charter dated the 16th day of August, 1861, are graciously pleased to grant, ordain and declare as follows:—

The Council of the College shall consist of the President and six of the Fellows. IN WITNESS WHEREOF, We have ordered the Seal appointed by the Treaty of Union to be kept and used in Scotland in place of the Great Seal thereof to be appended to these Presents: GIVEN at Our Court at St. James's the Ninth day of March One thousand nine hundred and fifty in the Fourteenth year of Our Reign.

PER SIGNATURAM MANU S.D.N. REGIS SUPRA SCRIPTAM.

Written to the Seal and Registered and Sealed at Edinburgh the Fifteenth day of March in the year One thousand nine hundred and fifty.

JOHN McVIE
*Keeper of the Registers of Scotland and
Deputy Keeper of the Seal.*

Appendix J

Supplementary Charter, 1959

At the Court at Buckingham Palace
The 30th day of October, 1959.
Present,
The Queen's Most Excellent Majesty
in Council.

WHEREAS there was this day read at the Board a Report of a Committee of the Lords of Her Majesty's Most Honourable Privy Council, dated the 26th day of October, 1959, in the words following, viz.:—

"THE COUNSELLORS OF STATE, on Your Majesty's behalf, having by Order of the 28th day of July, 1959, referred unto this Committee the humble Petition of the Royal College of Physicians of Edinburgh praying for the grant of a Supplementary Charter:

"THE LORDS OF THE COMMITTEE, in obedience to the said Order of Reference, have taken the said Petition into consideration and do this day agree humbly to report, as their opinion, to Your Majesty, that a Supplementary Charter may be granted by Your Majesty in terms of the Draft hereunto annexed."

HER MAJESTY, having taken into consideration the said Report and the Draft Supplementary Charter accompanying it, was pleased, by and with the advice of Her Privy Council, to approve thereof, and to order, as it is hereby ordered, that the Right Honourable John Scott Maclay, one of Her Majesty's Principal Secretaries of State, do cause a Warrant to be prepared for Her Majesty's Royal Signature, for passing under the Seal appointed by the Act of Union to be used in Scotland in lieu of the Great Seal thereof, a Supplementary Charter in conformity with the said Draft, which is hereunto annexed.

W. G. AGNEW.

ELIZABETH THE SECOND by the Grace of God of the United Kingdom of Great Britain and Northern Ireland and of Our other Realms and Territories Queen, Head of the Commonwealth, Defender of the Faith. To all to whom these presents may come, Greeting!

WHEREAS

(i) Our Royal Predecessor, King Charles the Second, in the year 1681, by Royal Charter, dated the 29th day of November, 1681, and afterwards ratified by an Act of the Scottish Parliament, dated the 16th day of June, 1685, constituted the several persons therein named and their successors to be chosen as therein mentioned a body corporate and politic by the name of "The Royal College of Physicians of Edinburgh", with perpetual succession and with the powers therein set forth.

(ii) Our Royal Predecessor, Queen Victoria, in the year 1861, accepted a surrender of the said original Charter, and by Royal Charter, dated the 16th day of August, 1861, constituted the several persons therein named who were then the Members of the Council of the Royal College of Physicians of Edinburgh, and their successors in office, and the then existing Fellows of the said College, and all other persons who should be admitted or elected Fellows and Members of the College as thereinafter provided one body politic and corporate by the name of "The Royal College of Physicians of Edinburgh" with perpetual succession and with the powers therein set forth.

(iii) Our Royal Predecessor, King George the Fifth, granted to the said College a Royal Charter dated the 3rd day of December, 1919, Supplementary to the said Royal Charter dated the 16th day of August, 1861, and making alterations in the constitution of the said College and giving it the additional powers therein set forth.

(iv) Our Royal Predecessor, King George the Sixth, in the year 1950, granted to the said College a Royal Charter, dated the 9th day of March, 1950, in further supplement of the said Royal Charter dated the 16th day of August, 1861, and making alteration in the constitution of the Council of the said College.

(v) It has been represented to Us that a Motion in the following terms was unanimously passed at a Quarterly Meeting of the Royal College of Physicians of Edinburgh, duly held on the 5th day of May, 1959:—"That the College authorises the Council to take steps to have the Charter of the College altered or amended to read as follows:—

(1) By adding the following:—

GRANTING OF DIPLOMAS. It shall be lawful for the College, by themselves or in conjunction with any other Royal Scottish Medical Corporation having power to do so, to grant to persons who shall have passed such examinations as may be prescribed by the College, by themselves or in conjunction with any other Royal Scottish Medical Corporation, diplomas in special subjects in medicine.

(2) By amending Article I as follows:—

AMENDMENT OF ARTICLE I OF CHARTER DATED 16TH DAY OF AUGUST, 1861. Article I of the Royal Charter dated the 16th day of August, 1861, constituting the College shall have effect as if the words "fifty thousand pounds" were substituted therein for the words "Ten Thousand Pounds".

(3) By adding the following Section:—

INTERPRETATION. The following words and expressions in these Presents shall have the meanings hereby assigned to them, that is to say:—

The expression "the College" shall mean the Royal College of Physicians of Edinburgh;

the expression "special subjects in medicine" shall mean psychological medicine and such other subjects as the College may from time to time prescribe by byelaws, by themselves or in conjunction with any other Royal Scottish Medical Corporation having power to grant diplomas in special subjects in medicine."

(vi) Application has accordingly been made to Us to grant to the said College a further Supplementary Charter making such alteration in its Constitution as is hereinafter set forth.

Now KNOW YE THAT WE of Our Royal Will and pleasure, and moved thereto by Our goodwill to the said College, and Our desire to promote and facilitate the work carried on by it, for Ourselves, Our Heirs, and Successors, in addition to the said Charter dated the 16th day of August, 1861, the said Supplementary Charter dated the 3rd day of December, 1919, and the said further Supplementary Charter dated the 9th day of March, 1950, and notwithstanding anything to the contrary contained in the said Charter dated the 16th day of August, 1861, are graciously pleased to grant, ordain and declare as follows:—

1. Article I of the said Royal Charter dated the 16th day of August, 1861, constituting the College shall have effect as if the words "fifty thousand pounds" were substituted therein for the words "Ten Thousand Pounds".

2. It shall be lawful for the College by themselves or in conjunction with any other

Royal Scottish Medical Corporation having power to do so to grant to persons who shall have passed such examinations as may be prescribed by the College by themselves or in conjunction with any other Royal Scottish Medical Corporation having power to do so diplomas in special subjects in medicine.

3. The following words and expressions in these Presents shall have the meanings hereby assigned to them, that is to say:—

The expression "the College" shall mean the Royal College of Physicians of Edinburgh;

the expression "special subjects in medicine" shall mean psychological medicine and such other subjects as the College may from time to time prescribe by byelaws by themselves or in conjunction with any other Royal Scottish Medical Corporation having power to grant diplomas in special subjects in medicine.

IN WITNESS whereof We have ordered the Seal appointed by the Treaty of Union to be kept and used in Scotland in place of the Great Seal of Scotland to be appended to these Presents:

GIVEN at Our Court at Buckingham Palace, the Thirtieth day of October One thousand nine hundred and fifty-nine, in the eighth year of Our Reign.

Appendix K

Supplementary Charter, 1964

At the Court at Buckingham Palace
The 26th day of February, 1964.
Present,
The Queen's Most Excellent Majesty
in Council.

WHEREAS there was this day read at the Board a Report of a Committee of the Lords of Her Majesty's Most Honourable Privy Council, dated the 11th day of February, 1964, in the words following, viz.:—

"YOUR MAJESTY having been pleased, by Your Order of the 29th day of August, 1963, to refer unto this Committee the humble Petition of the Royal College of Physicians of Edinburgh, praying for the grant of a Supplementary Charter:

"THE LORDS OF THE COMMITTEE, in obedience to Your Majesty's said Order of Reference, have taken the said Petition into consideration, and do this day agree humbly to report, as their opinion, to Your Majesty, that a Supplementary Charter may be granted by Your Majesty in terms of the Draft hereunto annexed".

HER MAJESTY having taken into consideration the said Report, and the Draft Supplementary Charter accompanying it, was pleased, by and with the advice of Her Privy Council, to approve thereof, and to order, as it is hereby ordered, that the Right Honourable Michael Noble, one of Her Majesty's Secretaries of State, do cause a Warrant to be prepared for Her Majesty's Royal Signature, for passing under the Seal appointed by the Act of Union to be used in Scotland in lieu of the Great

Seal thereof, a Supplementary Charter in conformity with the said Draft, which is hereunto annexed.

W. G. AGNEW.

ELIZABETH THE SECOND by the Grace of God of the United Kingdom of Great Britain and Northern Ireland and of Our other Realms and Territories Queen, Head of the Commonwealth, Defender of the Faith: To all to whom these presents shall come, Greeting!

WHEREAS:

(i) Our Royal Predecessor King Charles the Second in the year 1681 by Royal Charter dated the 29th day of November, 1681, and afterwards ratified by an Act of the Scottish Parliament, dated the 16th day of June, 1685, constituted the several persons therein named and their successors to be chosen as therein mentioned a body corporate and politic by the name of "The Royal College of Physicians of Edinburgh", with perpetual succession and with the powers therein set forth.

(ii) Our Royal Predecessor Queen Victoria in the year 1861 accepted a surrender of the said original Charter, and by Royal Charter, dated the 16th day of August, 1861, (hereinafter referred to as "the Charter") constituted the several persons therein named who were then the Members of the Council of the Royal College of Physicians of Edinburgh, and their successors in office, and the then existing Fellows of the said College, and all other persons who should be admitted or elected Fellows and Members of the College as thereinafter provided one body politic and corporate by the name of "The Royal College of Physicians of Edinburgh" with perpetual succession and with the powers therein set forth.

(iii) Our Royal Predecessor King George the Fifth granted to the said College a Royal Charter dated the 3rd day of December, 1919, Supplementary to the Charter and making alterations in the constitution of the said College and giving it the additional powers therein set forth.

(iv) Our Royal Predecessor King George the Sixth granted to the said College a Royal Charter dated the 9th day of March, 1950, in further supplement of the Charter and making alteration in the constitution of the Council of the said College.

(v) We were pleased to grant to the said College a Royal Charter dated the 21st day of December, 1959, in further supplement of the Charter increasing the yearly value of lands, tenements or other heritages and personal estate which the said College are authorised to take, purchase, possess, hold and enjoy and empowering the said College to grant diplomas in special subjects in medicine.

(vi) Application has been made to Us to grant to the said College a further Supplementary Charter making such alterations in the Charter as are hereinafter set forth.

Now KNOW YE THAT WE of Our Royal Will and pleasure, and moved thereto by Our goodwill to the said College, and Our desire to promote and facilitate the work carried on by it, for Ourselves, Our Heirs, and Successors, in addition to the Charter, the said Supplementary Charter dated the 3rd day of December, 1919, the said further Supplementary Charter dated the 9th day of March, 1950, and the said further Supplementary Charter dated the 21st day of December, 1959, and notwithstanding anything to the contrary contained in the Charter are graciously pleased to grant, ordain and declare as follows:

1. Article V of the Charter, constituting the College, shall have effect as if the words "and Diplomates" were inserted after the word "Licentiates" where that word first appears in that Article.

Article VI of the Charter shall have effect as if

(i) the words "or diploma" were inserted after the word "licence" in that Article; and

(ii) the words "Licentiate or Diplomate" were substituted for the words "or Licentiate" wherever such last mentioned words appear in that Article.

Article XX of the Charter shall have effect as if the words "Licentiates and Diplomates" were substituted for the words "and Licentiates" in that Article.

Article XXIII of the Charter shall have effect as if the words "Licentiates and Diplomates" were substituted for the words "and Licentiates" in that Article.

2. Article XII of the Charter shall have effect as if

(i) the words "Vice-President" were inserted after the word "President" in that Article; and

(ii) the words "and for the election of Fellows to serve on the Fellowship Committee, the Library Committee and other Standing Committees of the College" were inserted after the word "Council" in that Article.

Article XVI of the Charter shall have effect as if the words "Vice-President" were inserted after the word "President" in that Article.

Article XVII of the Charter shall have effect as if the words "Vice-President" were inserted after the word "President" wherever such last-mentioned word appears in that Article.

Article XIX of the Charter shall have effect as if the words "Vice-President" were inserted after the word "President" wherever such last-mentioned word appears in that Article.

3. It shall be lawful for the Fellows (as defined in Article XXIII of the Charter), to provide by byelaws (as so defined) that a Fellow who has signed the Promissory Obligation referred to in byelaw 14 in Chapter II of the byelaws, and is unable to attend the Annual Meeting of the College, shall be entitled to vote by post for the election of Members of the Council of the College and the Charter shall be construed accordingly.

4. The following words and expressions in these Presents shall have the meanings hereby assigned to them, that is to say:

The expression "the College" shall mean The Royal College of Physicians of Edinburgh.

IN WITNESS whereof, We have ordered the Seal appointed by the Treaty of Union to be kept and used in Scotland in place of the Great Seal of Scotland to be appended to these Presents:

GIVEN at Our Court at Buckingham Palace the Twenty-sixth day of February One thousand nine hundred and sixty-four, in the thirteenth year of Our Reign.

Appendix L

Patron: Her Majesty The Queen

Honorary Fellows of the College

The Record is wanting from December 1682 to the year 1694.

	Elected		*Elected*
Patrick Hume, Bart., Baron Polwarth, *afterwards* 1st Earl of Marchmont	May 15, 1696	John Stuart, 3rd Earl of Bute	Nov. 3, 1761
James Scougal, Lord Whitehill★	May 15, 1696	James Mounsey, M.D.	Nov. 2, 1762
William Anstruther, Bart., Lord Anstruther★	Nov. 6, 1699	Giovanni Battista Carburi, Conte Carburi	Nov. 5, 1765
David Gregory, M.D. Oxon	Aug. 22, 1705	Carl von Linné, Kt., M.D. Harderwijk	Nov. 3, 1772
Robert Gray, M.D.	Oct. 4, 1705	Albrecht von Haller, M.D. Leiden	Nov. 3, 1772
Hans Sloane, Bart., M.D. Orange	Oct. 4, 1705	Henry Scott, 3rd Duke of Buccleuch	Dec. 2, 1773
David Wemyss, 3rd Earl of Wemyss	Dec. 13, 1705	Jerome David Gaubius, M.D. Leiden	Dec. 2, 1773
James Nasmyth, Bart., Laird of Posso	Nov. 14, 1706	James Flint, M.D. Glasg., *ex officio*	May 3, 1774
David Melville, 3rd Earl of Leven	April 22, 1707	Anton Stoerck, M.D. Vienna	Nov. 5, 1776
Charles Hay, 12th Earl of Erroll	June 3, 1707	Johann Georg Zimmermann, M.D. Göttingen	Dec. 5, 1782
John Boyle, 2nd Earl of Glasgow	June 3, 1707	Joseph Marie François de Lassone, M.D. Paris	Dec. 5, 1782
Roderick Mackenzie, Lord Prestonhall★	June 18, 1707	Joseph Banks, Bart.	Dec. 5, 1782
Gilbert Elliot, Bart., Baron Minto	June 18, 1707	John Rogerson, M.D.	Dec. 5, 1782
John Arbuthnot, M.D. St. And.	Dec. 12, 1707	George Brudenell, Duke of Montagu	Dec. 17, 1782
Alexander Russell, M.D. Aber.	Feb. 12, 1712	Pieter Camper, M.D. Leiden	Dec. 17, 1782
William Cockburn, M.D.	May 5, 1724	Felix Vicq-D'Azyr, M.D. Paris	Feb. 2, 1790
George Cheyne, M.D. Aber.	May 5, 1724	Johann Andreas Murray, M.D. Upsala	Feb. 2, 1790
James Campbell, M.D.	May 2, 1727	August Gottlieb Richter, M.D. Göttingen	Dec. 1, 1791
William Fullerton, M.D.	Nov. 5, 1728	Johann Gottlieb Walter, M.D. Königsberg	Dec. 1, 1791
George Martin, M.D.	Aug. 5, 1740	George Baker, Bart., M.D. Camb.	Mar. 27, 1792
David Balfour, M.D.	Feb. 7, 1744	Benjamin Thompson, Kt., Count von Rumford	Nov. 4, 1800
John Johnstoun, M.D. Utrecht	Feb. 7, 1744	Edward Jenner, M.D. St. And.	May 20, 1806
Thomas Simson, M.D. Glasg.	Feb. 7, 1744	Matthew Baillie, M.D. Oxon	Nov. 13, 1809
Richard Mead, M.D. Padua	May 7, 1745	Edward Albert, Prince of Wales	Aug. 8, 1919
James Mackenzie, M.D.	Oct. 2, 1755	David Beatty, 1st Earl Beatty	Nov. 4, 1919
John Huxham, M.D. Rheims	Oct. 2, 1755	Douglas Haig, 1st Earl Haig	Nov. 4, 1919
Gerard van Swieten, M.D. Leiden	Nov. 4, 1755		
Archibald Campbell, 3rd Duke of Argyll	Nov. 30, 1758		
Jean Baptiste Senac, M.D. Montpellier	Nov. 4, 1760		

★ Lords of Session.

	Elected		Elected
Edward Grey, 1st Viscount Grey of Fallodon	Nov. 4, 1919	Thorvald Johannes Marius Madsen, M.D., Denmark	June 14, 1927
Jan Christiaan Smuts, General, Rt. Hon.	Nov. 4, 1919	Arthur Logan Turner, F.R.C.S., Gt. Britain	June 14, 1927
Arthur Stanley, The Hon. Sir	Nov. 4, 1919	Donald Macalister of Tarbert, Bt., K.C.B., M.D., Gt. Britain	April 21, 1931
Henry Pomeroy Davidson	Nov. 4, 1919	Edward Albert Sharpey-Schafer, Kt., M.D., Gt. Britain	April 21, 1931
John Joseph Pershing, G.C.B., General, U.S.A.	Nov. 4, 1919	Archibald Edward Garrod, K.C.M.G., D.M., Gt. Britain	April 21, 1931
William Henry Welch, M.D. Columbia, N.Y.	Nov. 4, 1919	Robert Hutchison, M.D., Gt. Britain	April 21, 1931
Desire Joseph Mercier, Cardinal	Nov. 4, 1919	Thomas Lewis, C.B.E., M.D., Gt. Britain	April 21, 1931
Adolphe Max, Burgomaster of Brussels	Nov. 4, 1919	Charles Scott Sherrington, O.M., G.B.E., M.D., Gt. Britain	April 21, 1931
Ferdinand Foch, Marshal of France	Nov. 4, 1919	William Hale-White, K.B.E., M.D., Gt. Britain	April 21, 1931
Emile Roux, M.D.	Nov. 4, 1919	Frederick Grant Banting, M.C., M.B., Canada	April 21, 1931
Charles Louis Alphonse Laveran, M.D. Strassburg	Nov. 4, 1919	George Richards Minot, M.D., U.S.A.	April 21, 1931
Sidney Sonnino, Baron, LL.D., Pisa	Nov. 4, 1919	William Sydney Thayer, M.D., U.S.A.	April 21, 1931
Ettore Marchiafava, M.D.	Nov. 4, 1919	Julius Wagner-Jauregg, M.D., Austria	April 21, 1931
Hermann Michael Biggs, M.D. Bellevue, N.Y.	Dec. 4, 1919	Knud Faber, M.D., Denmark	April 21, 1931
Georges Eugene Benjamin Clemenceau, M.D. Paris	Dec. 4, 1919	Emile Charles Achard, M.D., France	April 21, 1931
Shibasaburo Kitasato, M.D.	Dec. 4, 1919	Friedrich von Müller, M.D., Germany	April 21, 1931
Eleutherios Venizelos, Prime Minister of Greece	Feb. 3, 1920	Albert Abraham Hijmans van den Bergh, Holland	April 21, 1931
Arthur William Currie, G.C.M.G., General	July 19, 1921	Hermann Sahli, M.D., Switzerland	April 21, 1931
Leon Charles Albert Calmette, M.D. Paris	May 2, 1922	Bertrand Edward Dawson, Baron Dawson of Penn, P.R.C.P.Lond., Gt. Britain	April 21, 1931
Jules Bordet, M.D. Brux.	Nov. 7, 1922	John Wheeler Dowden, P.R.C.S., Gt. Britain	Nov. 3, 1931
Theobald Smith, M.D.	Feb. 5, 1924	Karel Frederik Wenckebach, M.D., Austria	July 18, 1933
Arthur James Balfour, Earl of Balfour, Gt. Britain	June 14, 1927	Charles Bickerton Blackburn, Kt., O.B.E., M.D., Australia	Dec. 1, 1938
John Rose Bradford, K.C.M.G., M.D., Gt. Britain	June 14, 1927	Alexander Gordon Biggam, K.B.E., C.B., M.D. (Major-General), Gt. Britain	May 7, 1946
Hector Clare Cameron, Kt., M.D., Gt. Britain	June 14, 1927	Henry Hallet Dale, O.M., G.B.E., M.D., Gt. Britain	May 7, 1946
Arthur Neville Chamberlain (The Rt. Hon.), Gt. Britain	June 14, 1927		
William Watson Cheyne, Bt., F.R.C.S.Eng., Gt. Britain	June 14, 1927		
David Ferrier, Kt., M.D., Gt. Britain	June 14, 1927		
John Gilmour, Bt. (The Rt. Hon.), Gt. Britain	June 14, 1927		

	Elected		*Elected*

Neil Hamilton Fairley, C.B.E., M.D., Gt. Britain — May 7, 1946

Alexander Fleming, Kt., M.B., Gt. Britain — May 7, 1946

The Lord Moran of Manton, M.C., M.D., Gt. Britain — May 7, 1946

Percy Stanley Tomlinson, K.B.E., C.B., D.S.O. (Major-General), Gt. Britain — May 7, 1946

HER MAJESTY QUEEN ELIZABETH, THE QUEEN MOTHER — May 5, 1953

Charles Herbert Best, C.B.E., F.R.S., M.D., D.Sc., Canada — May 5, 1953

Walter Russell Brain, Bt., D.M., LL.D., Gt. Britain — May 5, 1953

Frank Macfarlane Burnet, Kt., F.R.S., M.D., Sc.D., Australia — May 5, 1953

Charles Ernest Hercus, Kt., D.S.O., O.B.E., M.D., New Zealand — May 5, 1953

Gordon Morgan Holmes, Kt., C.M.G., C.B.E., F.R.S., M.D., D.Sc., D.C.L., LL.D., Gt. Britain — May 5, 1953

Robert Muir, Kt., F.R.S., M.D., Sc.D., LL.D., D.C.L., Gt. Britain — May 5, 1953

John Parkinson, Kt., M.D., LL.D., Gt. Britain — May 5, 1953

William Boyd, M.D., D.Sc., LL.D., Canada — July 26, 1955

William Norman Pickles, M.D., D.Sc., Gt. Britain — July 26, 1955

The Rt. Hon. Lord Adrian, O.M., M.D., LL.D., F.R.S., Gt. Britain — May 3, 1960

John Smith Knox Boyd, Kt., O.B.E., M.D., LL.D., F.R.S. (Brigadier), Gt. Britain — May 3, 1960

John Crighton Bramwell, M.D., Gt. Britain — May 3, 1960

Wajid Ali Burki, C.B.E., M.D. (Lieut.-General), Pakistan — May 3, 1960

Howard Walter Florey, Kt., M.D., Ph.D., LL.D., P.R.S., Gt. Britain — May 3, 1960

Harold Himsworth, K.C.B., M.D., LL.D., F.R.S., Gt. Britain — May 3, 1960

Vasant Ramji Khanolkar, M.D., India — May 3, 1960

The Rt. Hon. The Viscount Malvern, C.H., K.C.M.G., D.C.L., LL.D., Rhodesia — May 3, 1960

The Rt. Hon. Robert Gordon Menzies, C.H., Q.C., LL.M., LL.D., Australia — May 3, 1960

Wilder Graves Penfield, O.M., C.M.G., D.Sc., M.D., LL.D., F.R.S., Canada — May 3, 1960

Edward George Sayers, C.M.G., M.D., New Zealand — May 3, 1960

The Rt. Hon. Lord Strathclyde, Gt. Britain — May 3, 1960

Robert Aitken, Kt., M.D., D.Phil., D.Sc., D.C.L., LL.D., Gt. Britain — Dec. 13, 1966

William B. Castle, M.D., D.Sc., LL.D., U.S.A. — Dec. 13, 1966

Ronald Victor Christie, M.D., D.Sc., Canada — Dec. 13, 1966

The Rt. Hon. Lord Cohen of Birkenhead, M.D., D.Sc., LL.D., Gt. Britain — Dec. 13, 1966

Percy Cyril Claude Garnham, C.M.G., M.D., D.Sc., F.R.S., Gt. Britain — Dec. 13, 1966

Peter Brian Medawar, Kt., C.B.E., M.A., D.Sc., F.R.S., Gt. Britain — Dec. 13, 1966

Arcot Mudaliar, Kt., B.A., M.D., D.Sc., D.C.L., LL.D., India — Dec. 13, 1966

Kenneth Beeson Noad, M.D., Aus. — Dec. 13, 1966

Claude Rimington, M.A., Ph.D., D.Sc., F.R.S., Gt. Britain — Dec. 13, 1966

George White Pickering, Kt., M.D., F.R.S., Gt. Britain — Dec. 13, 1966

Sir Charles Putnam Symonds, K.B.E., C.B., M.A., D.M., Gt. Britain — Dec. 13, 1966

The Rt. Hon. Lord Rosenheim, K.B.E., M.A., M.D.Camb., F.R.C.P.Lond., Gt. Britain — July 23, 1968

Edith Kate Dawson, M.B.E., M.A., M.D., F.R.C.S.Edin., Gt. Britain — July 15, 1969

Sir Robert Hay, K.C.I.E., M.B., Ch.B., D.P.H., Gt. Britain — July 15, 1969

Sir George Reid McRobert, Kt., C.I.E., M.D., F.R.C.P.Lond., Gt. Britain — July 15, 1969

	Elected		*Elected*
Sir Leybourne Stanley Patrick Davidson, Kt., LL.D., M.D., F.R.C.P.Edin. & Lond., Gt. Britain	Feb. 3, 1972	Professor M. Verstraete, Belgium	May 30, 1975
		Dr Christian Hamburger, Denmark	May 30, 1975
The Rt. Hon. Lord Erskine of Rerrick, D.L., J.P., LL.D., F.R.S.E., Gt. Britain	Feb. 3, 1972	Professor P. B. B. Gatenby, Eire	May 30, 1975
		Professor Jean Hamburger, France	May 30, 1975
		Professor Cesare Bartorelli, Italy	May 30, 1975
Professor Michael Swann, M.A., Ph.D., LL.D., D.Sc., D.Univ., F.R.S., F.R.S.E., F.R.C.S.E., Gt. Britain	Feb. 3, 1972	Dr Simon Hertz, Luxembourg	May 30, 1975
		Professor Dr D. Durrer, The Netherlands	May 30, 1975
Sir Derrick Melville Dunlop, Kt., B.A.Oxon., M.D., F.R.C.P.Edin. & Lond., Gt. Britain	July 19, 1973	Professor Dr G. A. Martini, West Germany	May 30, 1975

Honorary Members of the College

William Clarence Braisted, Admiral, U.S. Navy	Nov. 1, 1921	William Boog Leishman, Kt., Major-Gen.	May 1, 1923
Walter Lawrence Bierring, M.D.	Nov. 1, 1921	Robert Charles MacWatt, Kt., Major-Gen.	May 1, 1923
Temulji Bhicaji Nariman, Kt.	Nov. 7, 1922		

Appendix M

Presidents of the College

	Elected		*Elected*
Archibald Stevensone, Kt.	Dec. 8, 1681	William Wright	Dec. 3, 1801
Robert Sibbald, Kt.	Dec. 4, 1684	Thomas Spens	Dec. 1, 1803
Andrew Balfour, Bt.	Dec. 2, 1685	Charles Stuart	Dec. 4, 1806
Archibald Stevensone, Kt.	?	James Home	Nov. 30, 1809
Robert Trotter	Dec. 6, 1694	James Hamilton, jun.	Dec. 3, 1812
Thomas Burnet, Kt.	Dec. 3, 1696	Thomas Charles Hope	Nov. 30, 1815
Matthew Sinclare	Dec. 1, 1698	James Buchan	Dec. 2, 1819
Robert Trotter	Dec. 5, 1700	Andrew Duncan, jun.	Dec. 5, 1822
Alexander Dundas	Dec. 3, 1702	Andrew Duncan, sen.	Dec. 4, 1824
James Halket	Nov. 30, 1704	Alexander Monro *tertius*	Dec. 1, 1825
William Eccles	Dec. 5, 1706	Alexander Morison, Kt.	Dec. 6, 1827
Matthew Sinclare	Dec. 2, 1708	Joshua Henry Davidson	Dec. 3, 1829
William Stewart	Dec. 6, 1716	John Macwhirter	Dec. 1, 1831
James Forrest	Dec. 3, 1719	Joshua Henry Davidson	Dec. 5, 1833
John Drummond	Dec. 6, 1722	John Thomson	Dec. 4, 1834
Francis Pringle	Nov. 30, 1727	William Pulteney Alison	Dec. 1, 1836
John Riddell	Dec. 2, 1731	Robert Christison, Bt.	Dec. 6, 1838
Robert Lowis	Dec. 4, 1735	Robert Graham	Dec. 3, 1840
John Clerk	Dec. 4, 1740	Robert Renton	Dec. 1, 1842
William Cochrane	Dec. 6, 1744	William Beilby	Dec. 5, 1844
William Porterfield	Dec. 1, 1748	Robert Christison, Bt.	Dec. 3, 1846
John Rutherford	Nov. 30, 1752	William Seller	Nov. 30, 1848
Alexander Dick, Bt.	Dec. 2, 1756	James Young Simpson, Bt.	Dec. 5, 1850
Robert Whytt	Dec. 1, 1763	Thomas Stewart Traill	Dec. 2, 1852
Stuart Threipland, Bt.	Dec. 4, 1766	James Begbie	Nov. 30, 1854
John Boswell	Dec. 5, 1770	David Maclagan	Dec. 4, 1856
Colin Drummond	Dec. 3, 1772	Alexander Wood	Dec. 2, 1858
William Cullen	Aug. 3, 1773	David Craigie	Dec. 5, 1861
Francis Home	Nov. 30, 1775	John Graham Macdonald Burt	Dec. 3, 1863
Gregory Grant	Dec. 4, 1777	John Smith	Nov. 30, 1865
Alexander Monro *secundus*	Dec. 3, 1779	John Moir	Dec. 5, 1867
John Gardiner	Dec. 5, 1782	Andrew Halliday Douglas	Dec. 2, 1869
John Hope	Dec. 2, 1784	Robert Paterson	Nov. 30, 1871
James Hay, Bt.	Nov. 30, 1786	William Henry Lowe	Dec. 4, 1873
Joseph Black	Dec. 4, 1788	Alexander Keiller	Dec. 2, 1875
Andrew Duncan	Dec. 2, 1790	Alexander Peddie	Dec. 6, 1877
James Hamilton	Dec. 6, 1792	Daniel Rutherford Haldane	Dec. 4, 1879
Nathaniel Spens	Dec. 4, 1794	George William Balfour	Nov. 30, 1882
Daniel Rutherford	Dec. 1, 1796	Douglas Maclagan, Kt.	Dec. 4, 1884
James Gregory	Dec. 6, 1798	Robert Peel Ritchie	Dec. 1, 1887

	Elected		Elected
Thomas Grainger Stewart, Kt.	Dec. 5, 1889	Edwin Bramwell	Nov. 30, 1933
Alexander Russell Simpson, Kt.	Dec. 3, 1891	William Thomas Ritchie, O.B.E.	Dec. 5, 1935
William Tennant Gairdner, K.C.B.	Nov. 30, 1893	Alexander Goodall	Dec. 2, 1937
John Batty Tuke, Kt.	Dec. 5, 1895	Charles McNeil	Dec. 5, 1940
James Andrew	Dec. 1, 1898	Andrew Fergus Hewat	Dec. 2, 1943
Thomas Richard Fraser, Kt.	Dec. 6, 1900	David Murray Lyon	Dec. 6, 1945
Thomas Smith Clouston, Kt.	Dec. 4, 1902	William Douglas Denton Small,	
John Playfair	Dec. 1, 1904	C.B.E.	Dec. 4, 1947
Charles Edward Underhill	Dec. 6, 1906	David Kennedy Henderson, Kt.	Dec. 1, 1949
John Playfair	June 23, 1908	William Alister Alexander	Dec. 6, 1951
William Allan Jamieson	Dec. 3, 1908	Leybourne Stanley Patrick Davidson,	
Byrom Bramwell, Kt.	Dec. 1, 1910	Kt.	Dec. 3, 1953
John James Graham Brown	Dec. 5, 1912	Andrew Rae Gilchrist, C.B.E.	Dec. 5, 1957
Alexander Hugh Freeland Barbour	Dec. 3, 1914	James Davidson Stuart Cameron,	
William Russell	Nov. 30, 1916	C.B.E., T.D.	Dec. 1, 1960
Robert William Philip, Kt.	Dec. 5, 1918	Ian George Wilson Hill, Kt., C.B.E.,	
George Lovell Gulland, C.M.G.	Nov. 30, 1923	T.D.	Dec. 5, 1963
George Matthew Robertson	Dec. 3, 1925	Christopher William Clayson,	
Robert Alexander Fleming	Dec. 1, 1927	O.B.E.	Dec. 1, 1966
Norman Purvis Walker, Kt.	Dec. 5, 1929	John Halliday Croom, T.D.	Dec. 3, 1970
Robert Thin	Dec. 3, 1931	John Wenman Crofton	Dec. 6, 1973

Treasurers of the College

John Hutton	Dec. 9, 1681	Robert Lowis	Dec. 3, 1719
William Stevensone	May 1, 1682	John Lermont	Dec. 6, 1722
Alexander Cranstone	Aug. 20, 1683	David Kinneir, *alias* Bayne	Dec. 2, 1725
Robert Trotter	Dec. 7, 1684	James Eccles	Nov. 30, 1727
Thomas Spence	?	Andrew St. Clair	Dec. 4, 1729
William Eccles	?	Andrew Plummer	Dec. 2, 1731
Charles Oliphant	Nov. 30, 1693	James Dundas	Dec. 4, 1735
Adam Freer	Dec. 5, 1695	David Foulis	Dec. 4, 1740
Gilbert Rule	Dec. 3, 1696	James Baird	Dec. 6, 1744
James Forrest	Dec. 1, 1698	John Boswell	Dec. 1, 1748
William Gardyne	Dec. 5, 1700	James Lind	Dec. 2, 1756
John Hay	Dec. 3, 1702	John Boswell	Aug. 1, 1758
John Smelholme	Dec. 2, 1703	Colin Drummond	Dec. 1, 1763
John Riddell	Dec. 5, 1706	Adam Austin	Dec. 5, 1770
Francis Pringle	Dec. 2, 1708	James Hay	Dec. 2, 1773
William Leirmont	Nov. 30, 1710	Nathaniel Spens	Nov. 30, 1786
Nicholas Montgomery	Dec. 3, 1713	Thomas Spens	Dec. 4, 1794
Thomas Young	Dec. 1, 1715	Thomas Charles Hope	Dec. 1, 1803
William Cochrane	Dec. 6, 1716	Thomas Spens	Nov. 30, 1809

	Elected		Elected
Charles Ransford	Dec. 1, 1842	Norman Purvis Walker, Kt.	Jan. 31, 1908
John Taylor	May 1, 1848	George Freeland Barbour Simpson	Dec. 10, 1929
Andrew Halliday Douglas	Aug. 5, 1856	Douglas James Acworth Kerr	Dec. 9, 1941
Samuel Somerville	Mar. 31, 1863	John Alastair Bruce, T.D.	Dec. 5, 1950
John Alexander Smith	Nov. 3, 1874	Neil Macmichael, T.D.	Dec. 5, 1961
Robert Peel Ritchie	Nov. 6, 1883	William Macleod	Dec. 10, 1968
Peter Alexander Young	Dec. 1, 1887	James Cameron Gould	Dec. 10, 1974

Secretaries of the College

Robert Sibbald, Kt.	Nov. 30, 1682	Joshua Henry Davidson	Dec. 2, 1819
Archibald Pitcairne	Dec. 7, 1684	Alexander Morison, Kt.	Dec. 2, 1824
Alexander Dundas	Dec. 5, 1695	William Pulteney Alison	Dec. 1, 1825
David Mitchell	Dec. 1, 1698	Robert Renton	Dec. 2, 1830
William Gardyne	Dec. 7, 1699	William Gregory	Dec. 4, 1834
James Forrest	Dec. 5, 1700	David Craigie	Dec. 1, 1836
Adam Freer	Dec. 4, 1701	George Paterson	May 1, 1848
John Sinclair	Dec. 2, 1703	Alexander Wood	Feb. 5, 1850
Charles Preston	Dec. 6, 1705	William Seller	Nov. 4, 1856
John Drummond	Dec. 5, 1706	William Robertson	June 2, 1857
Robert Lowis	Dec. 2, 1708	Daniel Rutherford Haldane	May 18, 1858
James Crawford	Dec. 6, 1711	John Wyllie	Dec. 3, 1874
Nicholas Montgomery	April 14, 1713	George Alexander Gibson	Dec. 4, 1884
James Crawford	Dec. 3, 1713	Robert William Philip, Kt.	Dec. 11, 1894
William Arthur	Dec. 2, 1714	Harry Rainy	Dec. 6, 1904
James Crawford	Dec. 1, 1715	Alexander Dingwall-Fordyce	Dec. 8, 1914
Robert Thomsone	Dec. 6, 1716	James Stewart Fowler	Dec. 10, 1918
John Clerk	Dec. 5, 1717	Norman Purvis Walker, Kt.	Oct. 1, 1925
James Eccles	Dec. 3, 1719	George Herbert Rae Gibson, D.S.O.	Dec. 8, 1925
William Porterfield	Dec. 6, 1722	George Freeland Barbour Simpson	July 19, 1932
Charles Alston	Dec. 2, 1725	Andrew Fergus Hewat	Dec. 6, 1932
Robert Whytt	Dec. 4, 1746	Douglas James Acworth Kerr	Dec. 8, 1936
David Clerk	Nov. 30, 1752	James Kirkwood Slater, O.B.E.	Dec. 6, 1945
William Cullen	Dec. 2, 1756	Douglas James Acworth Kerr	April 29, 1946
Robert Ramsay	Dec. 6, 1764	John Halliday Croom, T.D.	Dec. 6, 1949
John Gregory	Sept. 14, 1765	Henry Johnston Scott Matthew	Dec. 7, 1954
Alexander Monro *secundus*	Dec. 3, 1772	Ronald Foote Robertson	Dec. 9, 1958
Daniel Rutherford	Dec. 3, 1779	John Bernard Stanton	Dec. 10, 1963
James Gregory	Dec. 2, 1790	Alexander John Keay	Dec. 5, 1967
Thomas Charles Hope	Dec. 6, 1798	James Syme	Dec. 2, 1971
James Home	Dec. 1, 1803	David Hugh Aird Boyd	Dec. 4, 1975
Alexander Monro *tertius*	Dec. 1, 1808		

Honorary Librarians of the College

	Elected		*Elected*
Archibald Stevenson ⎤		William Moncrieff	1824–1835
Archibald Pitcairne, *Depute* ⎦	1683–1685	Richard Poole	1835–1838
Charles Preston	1705–1706	William Thomson	1838–1841
John Smelholme	1706–1708	William Seller	1841–1848
Robert Lowis	1708–1711	John Brown	1848–1858
James Crawford	1711–1714	Charles Wilson	1858–1862
Robert Thomson	1715–1716	William Tennant Gairdner	1862
John Clerk	1717–1719	James Matthews Duncan	1862–1867
James Eccles	1719–1722	James Warburton Begbie	1867–1870
William Porterfield *Also Secretaries*	1722–1725	William Cumming	1871–1873
Charles Alston	1725–1746	George William Balfour	1873–1882
Robert Whytt	1746–1752	David James Brakenridge	1882–1886
David Clerk	1752–1756	James Ormiston Affleck	1886–1887
William Cullen	1756–1765	George William Balfour	1887–1902
John Gregory	1765–1772	David Berry Hart	1902–1920
John Gardiner	1772–1782	John William Ballantyne	1920–1923
James Hamilton	1782–1789	Robert Thin	1923–1931
Thomas Spens	1789–1794	Charles McNeil	1931–1947
Robert Freer	1794–1796	David Murray Lyon	1947–1954
James Home	1796–1801	John Ritchie	1954–1959
Andrew Duncan, jun.	1801–1806	William Alister Alexander	1959–1968
John Yule	1806–1807	James Douglas Stuart Cameron	1968–1969
John Barclay	1807–1810	Ian George Wilson Hill	1969–1970
Alexander Wylie	1810–1824	Chalmers Hunter Davidson	1970–

Registrars of the College

William Macleod	Dec. 6, 1960	Hugh M. MacLeod	Dec. 10, 1968

Librarians of the College

John Small, sen.	1823–1847	T. H. Graham, O.B.E.	1909–1950
John Small, jun.	1847–1886	L. Jolley, M.A., F.L.A.	1950–1956
Thomas G. Law	1887–1888	G. R. Pendrill, M.A., A.L.A.	1957–1965
John Matheson Shaw	1888–1903	Miss J. P. S. Ferguson, M.A., A.L.A.	1966–
F. C. Nicholson, M.A.	1903–1909		

Clerks to the College

	Elected		Elected
Hugh Stevensone	1681–1695	James D. Haig	1854–1856
Robert Trotter, W.S.	1695–?1697	Christopher Douglas, W.S.	1856–1891
William Riddell	?1697–1727	Christopher Douglas, W.S.	
Henry Balcanquall, W.S.	1727–1771	Alexander Sholto Douglas, W.S. } Jointly	1891–1894
Robert Boswell, W.S.	1771–1800	Alexander Sholto Douglas, W.S.	1894–1908
Alexander Boswell, W.S.	1800–1836	Andrew Gray Muir, W.S.	1908–1938
William Spens, Accountant	1836–1839	K. M. Oliphant, M.C., W.S.	1938–1947
Kenneth Mackenzie, Accountant	1839–1854	Alexander Macfie, W.S.	1947–

INDEX I: NAMES

See also Appendix C

Compiled by D. Dainty

Note: An italicized name indicates an additional entry in Index II

2N

INDEX II: GENERAL SUBJECT

Compiled by D. Dainty

Note: RCPE and College indicate throughout the Royal College of Physicians of Edinburgh

R. Sibbald

Wortesfield P. C. R. M. E.

Ja. Rutherford C. R. M. E. P.

Alexander Dick C. R. m. & p.

Robert Whytt C. R.

Stuart Threipland P. C. R. M. E.

B. Boswell.

William Cullen C. R. M. E. P.

Andrew Duncan. P.

Alex. Morison

David Maclagan

J. Y. Simpson M. D.

Some signatures of Presidents of the College

J. Wood

Thomas R. Fraser.

Dr Allan Jamieson

Byrom Bramwell.

Alexander Hugh Barbour.

Sir Robert Philip

W.A. Alexander.

Elij Davies

a. Rae Gilchrist

James D.S. Cameron.

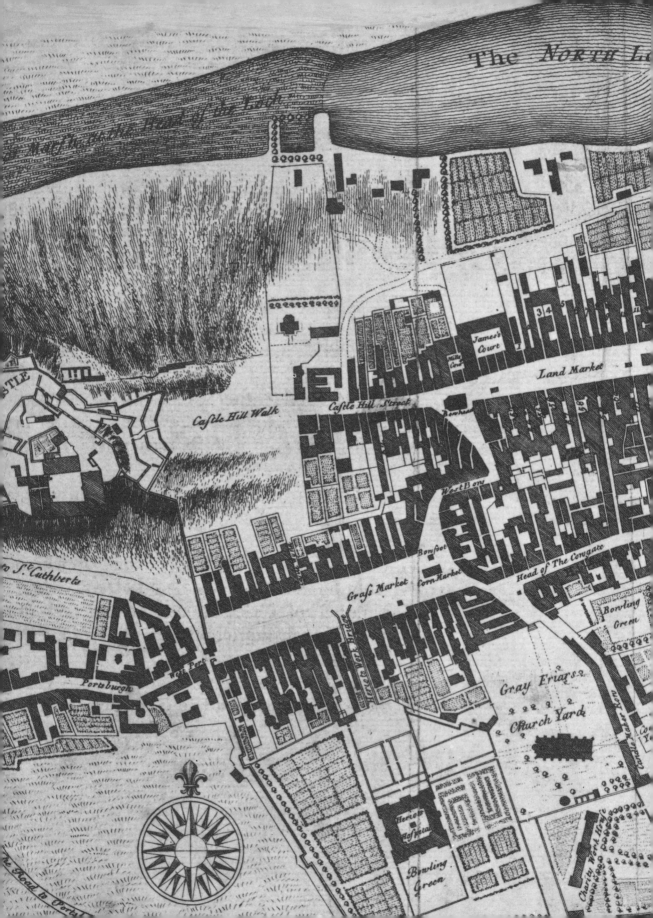